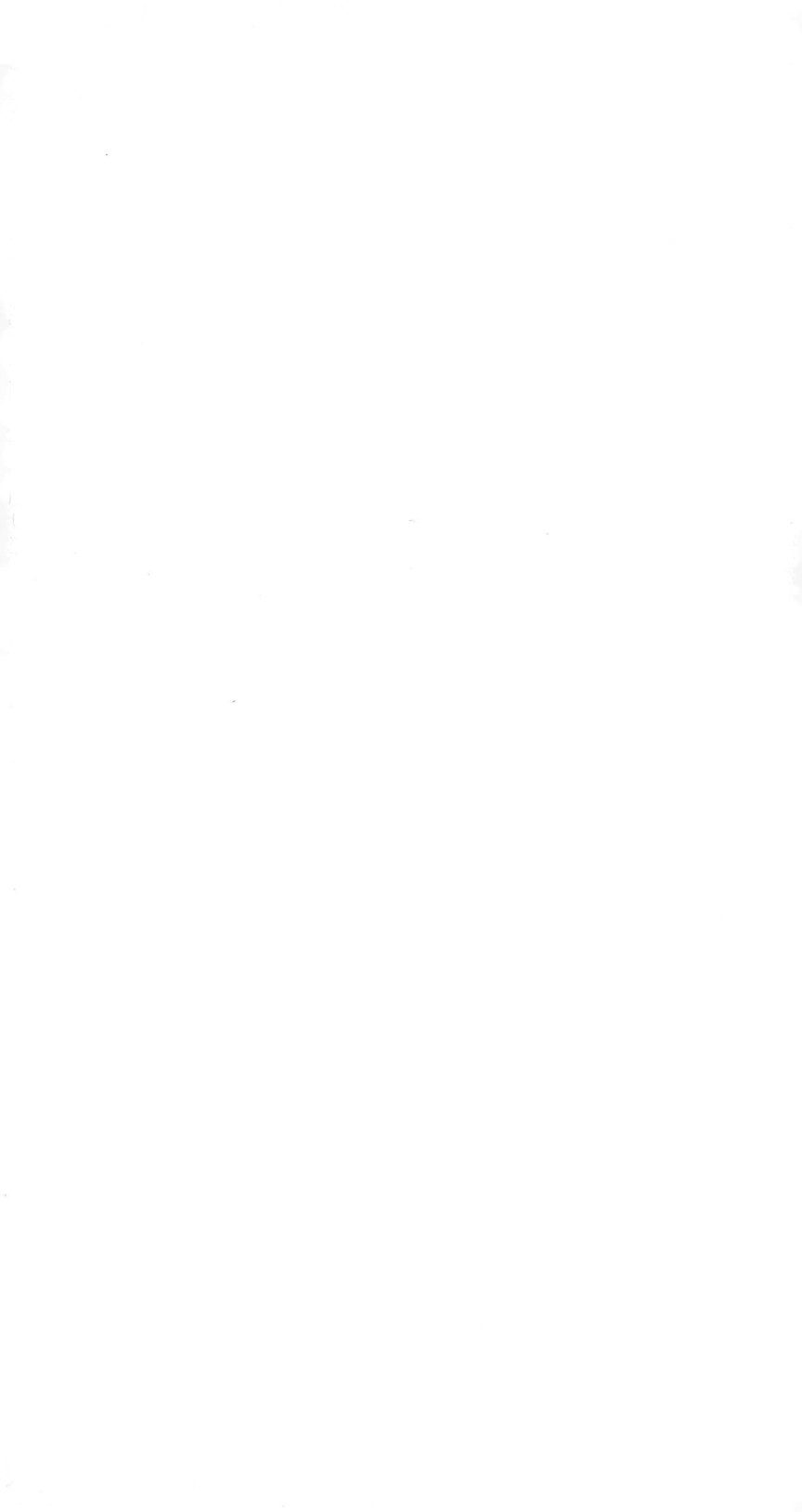

The Manual of Emergency Medicine Therapeutics

Editor-in-Chief
Gideon Bosker, MD, FACEP
Associate Clinical Professor of Emergency Medicine
Oregon Health Sciences University
Director, Continuing Education Programs,
Department of Emergency Medicine,
Good Samaritan Medical Center,
Portland, Oregon

Editors
David A. Talan, MD, FACEP
Associate Professor of Medicine
University of California Los Angeles School of Medicine
Chairman, Department of Emergency Medicine,
Olive View Medical Center,
Sylmar, California

H. Brian Goldman, MD, ABEM, MCFP (EM)
Assistant Professor of Family and Community Medicine
University of Toronto Faculty of Medicine
Staff Emergency Physician,
Mount Sinai Hospital,
Toronto, Ontario, Canada

J. Michael Albrich, MD, FACP, FACEP
Assistant Clinical Professor of Emergency Medicine
Oregon Health Sciences University
Attending Staff Physician,
Good Samaritan Hospital,
Portland, Oregon

Mosby

St. Louis   Baltimore   Boston
Carlsbad   Chicago   Naples   New York   Philadelphia   Portland
London   Madrid   Mexico City   Singapore   Sydney   Tokyo   Toronto   Wiesbaden

Mosby
Dedicated to Publishing Excellence

A Times Mirror
Company

Editor: Laurel Craven
Associate Developmental Editor: Wendy Buckwalter
Project Manager: Carol Sullivan Weis
Production Editor: Darrick Dudley
Cover Design: Frank Loose Design
Manufacturing Supervisor: Theresa Fuchs

A note to the reader:
The authors have made every attempt to ensure that dosages are in accordance with current recommendations. We suggest referring to the Physician's Desk Reference before using a drug for the first time. It is the reader's responsibility to stay informed of changes in emergency medicine therapeutics.

Copyright © 1995 by Mosby–Year Book, Inc.

All rights reserved. No part of this publication may be reproduced, stored in a retrieval system, or transmitted, in any form or by any means, electronic, mechanical, photocopying, recording, or otherwise, without prior written permission from the publisher.

Permission to photocopy or reproduce solely for internal or personal use is permitted for libraries or other users registered with the Copyright Clearance Center, provided that the base fee of $4.00 per chapter plus $.10 per page is paid directly to the Copyright Clearance Center, 27 Congress Street, Salem, MA 01970. This consent does not extend to other kinds of copying, such as copying for general distribution, for advertising or promotional purposes, for creating new collected works, or for resale.

Printed in the United States of America
Composition by Top Graphics, Inc.
Printing/binding by Phoenix

Mosby–Year Book, Inc.
11830 Westline Industrial Drive
St. Louis, Missouri 63146

International Standard Book Number ISBN 0-8016-0445-1

94 95 96 97 98 / 9 8 7 6 5 4 3 2 1

Contributors

J. MICHAEL ALBRICH, M.D., F.A.C.P., F.A.C.E.P.
Assistant Professor of Emergency Medicine,
Oregon Health Sciences University;
Staff Physician, Emergency Department,
Good Samaritan Hospital and Legacy Portland Hospitals,
Portland, Oregon

JEFFREY ARNOLD, M.D.
Clinical Instructor,
Harbor-UCLA Medical Center;
Attending Physician,
Department of Emergency Medicine,
Cedars-Sinai Medical Center,
Los Angeles, California

MARC J. BAYER, M.D., F.A.C.E.P.
Professor of Surgery and Medicine,
University of Connecticut School of Medicine;
Chief, Medical Toxicology
Medical Director,
Connecticut Poison Control Center,
Farmington, Connecticut

GIDEON BOSKER, M.D., F.A.C.E.P.
Associate Clinical Professor of Emergency Medicine,
Oregon Health Sciences University,
Portland, Oregon

STEPHAN A. BILLSTEIN, M.D., M.P.H.
Staff Dermatologist,
St. Michael's Medical Center, Newark,
Director of Medical Services,
Roche Laboratories,
Nutley, New Jersey

NORMAN CHRISTOPHER, M.D., F.A.A.P., F.A.C.E.P.
Assistant Professor of Pediatrics,
Case Western Reserve University School of Medicine;
Coordinator, Pediatric Emergency Medicine,
MetroHealth Medical Center,
Cleveland, Ohio

MOHAMUD DAYA, M.D., F.A.C.E.P.
Assistant Professor of Emergency Medicine,
Oregon Health Sciences University,
Portland, Oregon

JAMES DOUGHERTY, M.D., F.A.C.E.P.
Associate Professor of Emergency Medicine,
Northeastern Ohio University College of Medicine;
Research Director and Emergency Medicine Residency Program,
Akron General Medical Center,
Akron, Ohio

MATTHEW G. FAHEY, M.D., F.A.C.E.P.
Staff, Good Samaritan Hospital,
Portland, Oregon
Mercy Medical Center,
Redding, California

ROBERT FERM, M.D., F.A.A.P., A.B.E.M., A.B.M.T.
Assistant Professor of Medicine and Director of Toxicology Fellowship,
University of Massachusetts Medical Center,
Worcester, Massachusetts

JOEL M. GEIDERMAN, M.D., F.A.C.E.P.
Assistant Clinical Professor of Medicine,
Division of Emergency Medicine,
University of California, Los Angeles,
UCLA School of Medicine;
Director and Co-Chair,
Department of Emergency Medicine,
Cedars-Sinai Medical Center,
Los Angeles, California

H. BRIAN GOLDMAN, M.D., A.B.E.M., M.C.F.P. (EM)
Assistant Professor of Family and
Community Medicine, University of
Toronto Faculty of Medicine;
Staff Emergency Physician,
Mount Sinai Hospital,
Toronto, Ontario, Canada

DAN A. HENRY, M.D., F.A.C.E.P.
Associate Professor of Clinical Medicine,
University of Connecticut School of
Medicine;
Chief of Medicine,
Mount Sinai Hospital,
Hartford, Connecticut

PATRICIA L. JOHNSON, B.Sc., M.D., C.C.F.P. (EM)
Vancouver, British Columbia, Canada

JONATHAN JUI, M.D., M.P.H., F.A.C.E.P.
Associate Professor of Emergency
Medicine,
Oregon Health Sciences University,
Portland, Oregon

MARC KAMIN, M.D.
Director of Clinical Research, CNS
Drugs,
Wallace Laboratories,
Princeton, New Jersey

CHARLES A. KENNEDY, M.D., F.A.C.P.
Clinical Assistant Professor of Medicine,
University of Kentucky School of
Medicine;
Attending Physician,
Infectious Disease Section,
Lexington Clinic,
Lexington, Kentucky

ERNEST A. KOPECKY, B.Sc., PH.D. (CANDIDATE)
Faculty of Pharmacy, University of
Toronto Faculty of Medicine;
Clinical Researcher,
Department of Clinical Pharmacology
and Toxicology,
Hospital for Sick Children,
Toronto, Ontario, Canada

LAWRENCE LEVINE, M.D.
Chairman, Department of Emergency
Medicine,
Bristol Hospital,
Bristol, Connecticut

JUDITH R. LOGAN, M.D., F.A.C.E.P.
Clinical Instructor of Emergency
Medicine,
Oregon Health Sciences University,
Emergency Physician,
Good Samaritan Hospital and Medical
Center,
Portland, Oregon

RICARDO MARTINEZ, M.D., F.A.C.E.P.
Associate Professor of Emergency
Medicine,
Department of Surgery,
Emory University School of Medicine;
Associate Director,
Center for Injury Control,
Emory University School of Public
Health,
Atlanta, Georgia

LOUIS J. PERRETTA, M.D., F.A.C.E.P.
Assistant Professor of Emergency Medicine,
Oregon Health Sciences University;
Attending Physician,
Legacy Portland Hospitals,
Portland, Oregon

THOMAS D. SABIN, M.D.
Professor of Neurology and Psychiatry,
Boston University School of Medicine;
Lecturer, Harvard and Tufts Medical Schools;
Director, Neurological Unit,
Boston City Hospital,
Boston, Massachusetts

GEORGE R. SCHWARTZ, M.D., F.A.C.E.P.
Staff, Emergency Medicine,
Los Alamos Medical Center,
Los Alamos, New Mexico
Visiting Associate Professor of Emergency Medicine,
Medical College of Pennsylvania,
Philadelphia, Pennsylvania

VAL SELIVANOV, M.D.
Working Surgeon,
Santa Theresa Hospital,
San Jose, California

MARC SMITH, M.D., F.A.C.E.P.
Staff Physician,
Good Samaritan Hospital,
Portland, Oregon

DAVID A. TALAN, M.D., F.A.C.E.P.
Associate Professor of Medicine,
University of California Los Angeles School of Medicine;
Chairman, Department of Emergency Medicine
Faculty, Division of Infectious Diseases,
Olive View-University of California Los Angeles Medical Center,
Sylmar, California

RICHARD Y. WANG, D.O., F.A.C.E.P., A.B.M.T.
Assistant Professor of Medicine,
Brown University School of Medicine;
Director, Medical Toxicology Service,
Department of Emergency Medicine,
Rhode Island Hospital,
Providence, Rhode Island

CRAIG A. WOOD, M.D.
Assistant Professor of Medicine,
Division of Infectious Diseases,
Hahnemann University School of Medicine,
Philadelphia, Pennsylvania

To Lena Lencek, who taught me
the meaning of scholarship
G.B.

To my wife and parents, who give
me so much love and support
D.A.T.

To my wife, Debra Jeremias, and my
parents, Shirley and Samuel Goldman
H.B.G.

To Alice, Kelsey, and Peter
J.M.A.

Preface

The First Edition of *The Manual of Emergency Medicine Therapeutics* comes at a very critical junction in the relatively short but distinguished history of the specialty of emergency medicine. Although many of the fundamentals remain unchanged, the practice of emergency medicine, especially as it relates to such areas as drug therapy, detection of medication-related adverse patient events, and pharmacotherapeutic management of serious and life-threatening disorders, has become increasingly complex and sophisticated.

Until recently, most emergency physicians were able to deliver acceptable standards of clinical care simply by gaining familiarity with the indications, contraindications, and common adverse reactions associated with a relatively limited number of medications and drug classes—among them, antibiotics, non-steroidal antiinflammatory drugs (NSAIDs), narcotic analgesics, and antiarrhythmic agents. Unfortunately, this rudimentary approach to drug therapy for emergency disorders is no longer sufficient for achieving optimal therapeutic outcomes and minimizing the risk of drug-related adverse patient events.

For one thing, the emergency medicine pharmacopea has swelled dramatically over the past decade, and as a result the practitioner has had to become familiar with the indications and potential side effects for hundreds of new agents. There are now 12,000 drugs approved for human use, a new chemical entity is approved for clinical practice every 2-3 weeks, and physicians now write more than 1.3 billion prescriptions per year. Approximately 25% of all nonelective hospital admissions through emergency department patients over the age of 65 are precipitated or associated with a drug-related adverse patient event.

Cost-consciousness in the area of drug therapy has also reared its head in our day-to-day practice. In this regard, it has become increasingly important to examine new drugs in a much more critical light, and determine when these agents—among them sumatriptin, azithromycin, and adenosine—represent bona fide therapeutic advances, and when less expensive, established drugs will produce equivalent clinical results. In addition, many widely used drug *classes,* from the cephalosporins, macrolides, and quinolones to calcium channel blockers, thrombolytics, and antiepileptics, now consist of *several* different agents, some of which may offer unique therapeutic advantages in one patient subgroup but present potential liabilities in others.

Not surprisingly, this dramatic explosion in therapeutic options has required emergency physicians to become "splitters" rather than "lumpers" when selecting medications. In other words, the practitioner is now faced with the challenge of carefully evaluating the specific properties of *individual* drugs for a wide range of diseases and then selecting the most appropriate agent for a particular patient. This means taking into account *all* the factors that influence therapeutic outcomes, from medication compliance and cost issues to drug-drug and drug-disease incompatibilities. Moreover, the difficulty of keeping abreast of and identifying "the best drugs" for a particular condition has been complicated by the emergence of treatment recommendations and guidelines issuing from a large number of consensus panels, professional colleges, and societies, many of which are outside the mainstream of emergency medicine practice. Evaluating and incorporating expert opinion and recommendations from these sources continues to be an important mechanism for ensuring that pharmacotherapeutic guidelines in emergency medicine are synchronized with developments in the subspecialty areas encompassed by our practice.

Finally, the demographic and pharmacologic infrastructure of our practice has changed. New clinical disorders (AIDS, opportunistic infections), emerging patient subgroups (the elderly), and the rapid introduction of new medications have justified production of an authoritative resource devoted exclusively to emergency medicine therapeutics. In this regard, emergency physicians are increasingly treating older patients who present with the life-threatening complications of polypharmacy, individuals with HIV-related complications who are at risk for many drug-related complications and side effects, as well as patients with complex cardiovascular disorders (i.e., myocardial infarction) that require many simultaneous drug interventions. These evolutionary changes in the scope of our practice demand a special sensitivity to a patient's *preexisting* pharmacologic and pathophysiological landscape before medications are introduced into the treatment plan.

With these clinical issues in mind, the primary purpose of *The Manual of Emergency Medicine Therapeutics* is to provide an easily accessed, authoritative source for *pharmacotherapeutic* management (i.e., drug therapy) of acute medical and surgical disorders. It should be stressed that this manual is not designed to be a primer for diagnostic evaluations, procedural interventions, or surgical management. Rather, it is written and organized to provide practicing emergency physicians—as well as emergency nurses, physician assistants, and paramedics—with a definitive, easy-to-use, one-stop, hands-on, "in-the-heat-of-battle" resource that will guide practitioners toward start-of-the-art choices, strategies, and treatment plans for drug-based intervention emergency medicine. If we have succeeded in our mission, this book will permit emergency physicians to generate cost-effective, compliance-promoting, and therapeutically effective treatment plans for patients with a wide range of emergency conditions.

Gideon Bosker, M.D., F.A.C.E.P.
Editor-in-Chief
First Edition

Introduction

Rational and intelligent use of pharmacotherapeutic agents represents a special challenge for emergency department physicians. Because of the broad spectrum and ever-increasing number of potent drugs that are available to treat acute clinical disorders, emergency physicians must be aware of the precise indications and contraindications for a wide range of medications. What makes drug therapy in the emergency setting especially treacherous is the fact that many of the agents employed for medical and surgical emergencies—among them, antiarrhythmics, thrombolytic agents, and sedatives—can have serious adverse side effects, especially in pharmacologically or pathophysiologically vulnerable patients (i.e., the elderly, patients on polypharmacy, individuals with cardiovascular or renal compromise). Consequently, the selection, dose, and route of administration of many commonly used medications must be tailored to specific patient subgroups.

Strategies for recognizing and preventing the perilous pitfalls of polypharmacy are stressed throughout the *Manual*. For example, some drugs—among them, nonsteroidal antiinflammatory (NSAIDs) medications, beta-blockers, and certain calcium channel blockers—are more likely to cause adverse side effects in the elderly than in younger individuals, and therefore specialized approaches to drug selection, prevention of drug-drug interactions, and dose modification are mandatory in this age group. The fact is, medications within a given drug class are not all created equally, and in this regard one of the primary objectives of *The Manual of Emergency Medicine Therapeutics* is to highlight specific pharmacologic features that make some drugs preferable in one clinical situation and other agents more desirable in another.

The pitfalls of drug prescribing and pharmacologic assessment in the emergency department are legion. First, emergency physicians are frequently faced with the challenge of detecting drug-related adverse patient events (DRAPEs) associated with a patient's existing medication regimen. Identifying medications that might explain a patient's symptoms or deterioration requires an awareness of a broad range of side effect profiles—ranging in severity from mild to life-threatening—for a large number of drugs. In addition, both when prescribing oral medications for discharged patients as well as when using parenteral drugs in the department, emergency physicians must engage in prudent prescribing practices that attempt to minimize the risk of introducing potential drug-drug interactions. A chapter on "General Principles of Drug Prescribing and Systematic Detection of Adverse Drug Reactions" has been included to clarify these issues. It has been designed to provide an overview of side effects associated with commonly used medications and to establish a practical foundation for prudent, effective, and patient-specific drug selection, especially in vulnerable populations.

The purpose of this *Manual* is to guide the practicing emergency physician toward drug-oriented therapies that have been proven both effective and safe. With these issues in clear focus, each chapter is written with attention to both prevention and intervention issues as they relate to drug therapy. To accomplish these objectives, the risks of introducing *drug-drug* interactions are highlighted in nearly all the chapters, while the potential complications associated with *drug-host* interactions are summarized in sections devoted to drug therapy in pregnancy, medication use in breast-feeding mothers, and drug-induced side effects in the elderly.

Drug administration can be a treacherous exercise, especially in the emergency medicine setting. In fact, studies have shown that emergency physicians are at high risk for introducing potential drug interactions, especially in patients who are already taking three or more drugs as part of their therapeutic regimen. Many of these pitfalls are discussed in detail. For example, cardiovascular drugs are well-known for their potential to cause drug-related adverse patient events (DRAPEs). In the world of calcium channel blockers, drugs such as verapamil and diltiazem, when used concurrently with beta-blockers, can cause symptomatic bradyarrhythmias or congestive heart failure, whereas other calcium blockers are less likely to produce these complications. Among the H2-antagonists, cimetidine inhibits the P450 cytochrome oxidase system and, therefore, it has the potential to affect the blood levels of many different drugs including theophylline, tegretol, and many antiarrhythmic agents.

Not surprisingly, the contributors to this *Manual* have had to make many difficult choices regarding their therapeutic recommendations. The fact is, there are better drugs and worse drugs. Choices must be made. No two drugs are created equally. Moreoever, because more than one acceptable pharmacotherapeutic option usually exists for managing a particular clinical disorder, it is frequently necessary for emergency physicians to carefully weigh the advantages and disadvantages of different drugs within the same or related classes, and select those agents which are best-suited for specific situations.

Whenever possible, drug therapy options in this *Manual* have been analyzed with a number of considerations in mind: (1) Cost of the drug; (2) compliance profile; (3) side effects; (4) drug-drug interactions; (5) drug-disease incompatibility; and (6) the "smartness" of a drug, i.e., the capacity of a single prescription ingredient to simultaneously service more than one target organ, or in the case of infection, more than one etiologic organism using only one agent. Finally, when well-designed, published trials can help shed light on why one medication might be preferable in one clinical situation or patient subgroup versus another, the contributors have been encouraged to support their therapeutic recommendations with sound analyses based on these evidentiary studies.

Finally, this book is not intended to replace comprehensive, multi-volume textbooks in the field of emergency medicine. Rather, it should be considered a therapeutic adjunct/companion volume to these expansive works. Accordingly, diagnosis- and assessment-oriented information is included in this *Manual* only if it might affect drug therapy. In this vein, one of the principal objectives of this book is to build upon the pharmacotherapeutic information contained in comprehensive textbooks of emergency medicine. To achieve this goal, the material in this *Manual* has been organized to provide a "last stop"—and for that matter, a "one-stop"—resource that facilitates *rapid access* to detailed, authoritative, application-oriented drug therapy and treatment guidelines. Moreover, comprehensive chapters on management of HIV-infected individuals, detection of drug-seeking patients, mortality-reducing measures in myocardial infarction, and acute stroke management have been included to reflect current pharmacotherapeutic interventions in these conditions. Using detailed and comprehensive tables, charts, figures, algorithms, and treatment plans, the information in this book is designed to maximize clinical outcomes for a large number of conditions, ranging from urgent, potentially serious medical and surgical disorders to life-threatening, catastrophic emergencies. In the final analysis, if this *Manual* is able to guide emergency physicians toward optimal therapeutic outcomes that are based on safe, cost-effective drug therapy, it will have served its purpose.

Gideon Bosker, M.D., F.A.C.E.P.
Editor-in-Chief

Acknowledgments

As is the case for every book, the process of conceiving, writing, editing, and finally publishing *The Manual of Emergency Medicine Therapeutics* has had a beginning, middle, and end. With these evolutionary stages in clear focus, the authors and editors wish to express their thanks to a number of talented, highly professional, and committed individuals at Mosby–Year Book. First, we wish to express our gratitude to George Stamathis who, at the inception of this project, had the vision to recognize that the discipline of emergency medicine could benefit greatly from a book devoted to drug therapy.

Stephanie Manning and Jim Shanahan are gratefully acknowledged for their diligent editorial efforts during the early stages of this project. They succeeded admirably at transferring editorial responsibility from one editor to another during a very delicate stage of the project. In addition, the editors are especially indebted to Anne Patterson, Editor-in-Chief, who provided outstanding editorial suggestions, insightful design guidance, and publication-saving diplomacy during all stages of the project. Kind appreciation is also due to Laurel Craven, Medical Editor, who, during critical stages of the publishing process, demonstrated the willingness and flexibility to discuss and eventually implement editorial, design, and logistical options that helped the *Manual* stay on course.

Sheilah Barrett deserves high praise for her patience, talent, and follow-through during the final design process. Our special thanks also go to Rick Dudley, who took a special interest in this project and who facilitated a number of important design modifications that enhanced the user-friendliness of this book.

Finally, this *Manual*, like every book project that must bring together an eclectic mix of scholars, writers, and clinicians, requires an editorial beacon. Wendy Buckwalter has been that giant behind-the-scenes, i.e., a persevering and quietly, but enormously, talented individual skilled in the fine points of both editorial execution and diplomacy, and whose sheer force of will and determination provided the octane necessary to bring a project of this scope to completion. In this regard, the editors are deeply indebted to Ms. Buckwalter, who, at various phases in this project's evolution, has worn a number of different hats and assumed a number of linchpin roles, from backstage manager and book design consultant to editorial impressario and labor arbitrator. In every sense of the word, she must be given the lion's share of credit for delivering this book into the hands of the emergency medicine community.

The editors of the *Manual* take enormous pleasure in recognizing Ms. Buckwalter's talent as an editorial manager. In particular, we have admired her stamina—galvanized, in this case, by a rare brand of visceral courage and patience—that permitted her to keep slugging at this project, even after a number of bruising blows and ten-counts threatened to end the fight. Stated simply, the completion of this book is testimonial that in *any* editorial league, she is a heavyweight and, one day, will certainly be a contender.

Contents

1 **General Principles of Drug Prescribing and Systematic Detection of Adverse Drug Reactions: An Overview, 1**
Gideon Bosker, J. Michael Albrich

2 **Oral Pain Management, 72**
H. Brian Goldman

3 **Parenteral Pain Management, 97**
H. Brian Goldman

4 **Detecting the Drug Seeker, 131**
H. Brian Goldman

5 **Acute Myocardial Infarction: Initial Stabilization, Mortality Reduction, and Treatment of Complications, 144**
J. Michael Albrich

6 **Rational Use of Poison Antidotes, 179**
Robert Ferm, Lawrence Levine, Marc J. Bayer, Richard Y. Wang

7 **Cardiac Arrhythmias and Antiarrhythmic Drugs, 205**
Ernest A. Kopecky

8 **Emergency Neurologic Therapeutics, 252**
Marc Kamin, Thomas D. Sabin

9 **Noninfectious Pulmonary Diseases, 275**
Louis J. Perretta

10 **Drug Therapy for Gastrointestinal Emergencies, 293**
Marc Smith

11 **Acute Food-Related and Toxic Plant Emergencies, 312**
George R. Schwartz

12 **Metabolic Emergencies, 349**
Dan A. Henry, Gideon Bosker

13 **Antimicrobial Agents: Uses, Indications, and Interactions, 400**
David A. Talan

14 Treatment of Common Infections, 432
Craig A. Wood

15 Management of Common Infectious Diseases: Rapid Access Guidelines, 453
Jon Jui

16 Antimicrobial Therapy for Sexually Transmitted Diseases, 467
Charles A. Kennedy, Gideon Bosker

17 Human Immunodeficiency Virus (HIV) Infection, 479
Jon Jui, Mohamud Daya

18 Empiric Antibiotic Selection for Infectious Disease Emergencies in the Pediatric Age Group, 509
Norman Christopher

19 Empiric Antibiotic Selection for Infectious Disease Emergencies in the Elderly Patient, 524
Gideon Bosker

20 Immunization, 529
Jeffrey L. Arnold, Joel M. Geiderman

21 Trauma, 547
Ricardo Martinez, Val Selivanov

22 Ear, Nose, and Throat Emergencies, 563
H. Brian Goldman, Patricia L. Johnson

23. Ophthalmologic Disorders, 580
James Dougherty

24 Dermatologic Disorders, 606
Stephan A. Billstein

25 Rheumatoid Emergencies, 632
Ernest A. Kopecky

26 Psychiatric Emergencies, 646
H. Brian Goldman

27 Drugs in Pregnancy, 661
Matthew G. Fahey

28 Drugs in Lactation, 669
Judith R. Logan

29 Thermoregulatory Disorders, 682
Louis J. Perretta

Index, 692

1

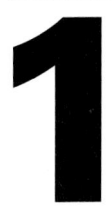

General Principles of Drug Prescribing and Systematic Detection of Adverse Drug Reactions: An Overview for the Emergency Physician

Gideon Bosker, M.D., F.A.C.E.P.
J. Michael Albrich, M.D., F.A.C.P., F.A.C.E.P

As the United States enters the twenty-first century, a large fraction of its population will approach old age. Mean survival has increased over 60% since the turn of the last century so that elderly Americans 65 years and older will constitute 20% of the population by the year 2010. Moreover, by the year 2000, there will be 15 million Americans over the age of 85 which, at present, is the fastest growing segment of the geriatric population.

With advancing age, individuals become susceptible to a number of clinical disorders. Current approaches to most geriatric disorders use drug therapy. Thus, the elderly find themselves burdened not only by diseases of old age, but with the consumption—for therapeutic purposes—of an ever-increasing number of potent drugs, many of which can precipitate adverse side effects and compromise quality of life.

Adverse Drug Reactions

Treatment with medications is associated with a wide variety of adverse drug reactions (ADRs) including adverse drug interactions (ADIs). While there is fierce debate regarding the risks and benefits of drug therapy in many disorders endemic to the elderly population, one thing remains clear: Adverse drug reactions and interactions are directly related to the *number of drugs* taken concurrently, and medication compliance patterns.

I. **Polypharmacy.** Regardless of whether drug therapy is provided in the acute hospital setting, the ambulatory environment, or the chronic care institution, no other risk factor or group of risk factors compares with polypharmacy as a cause of adverse drug reactions and interactions in the geriatric population. A number of British and American studies have corroborated that person over 65 years of age living independently take an average of 2.8 drugs per day. In nursing homes the number increases to an average of 3.4, while about 9 drugs per day are prescribed for the hospitalized elderly **(Table 1-1)**.

   A. **One recent study** conducted by Larsen at the University of Washington has demonstrated that there is a ninefold increased risk of having an adverse drug reaction when four or more drugs are taken simultaneously. Not surprisingly, 3 to 5% of all hospital admissions are related to adverse drug reactions, and of all hospital admissions for the elderly, 15 to 25% are complicated by an adverse drug reaction. Some of these reactions are life threatening, and it is estimated that adverse drug reactions in the United States may account for up to 30,000 deaths each year.

Table 1-1. Medications for Hospitalized Elderly

Country	Average drugs per hospitalized patient
United States	9.1
Canada	7.1
Israel	6.3
New Zealand	5.8
Scotland	4.6

- **B. Availability.** The potential toxicity of drugs in the elderly is exacerbated by the burgeoning pharmaceutical landscape. At present, 8,000 prescription drugs are available in the United States, including 14 beta-blockers, 15 cephalosporins, 16 nonsteroidal anti-inflammatory drugs (NSAIDs), 10 oral sulfonylureas, 13 diuretic preparations, 7 ACE inhibitors, 15 penicillins, and 8 calcium channel blockers. A new entity is approved for human use every 2 to 3 weeks and two thirds of all physician visits culminate in a prescription for a drug. In 1993, American physicians wrote 2.3 billion prescriptions, an average of 8.1 prescriptions for every woman, man, and child in the country. Over the past 8 years, it is estimated that the total number of prescriptions and pills have increased by 27% and 35%, respectively.
- **C. As the number of geriatric patients** receiving pharmacologic treatment continues to rise, physicians are increasingly challenged with the diagnosis, identification, and management of adverse drug reactions among the elderly.

II. Inaccurate diagnoses of adverse drug reactions in elderly patients are common. Patients often experience multiple, nonspecific symptoms—a problem further complicated because many elderly patients on potent drug regimens suffer from dementia, depression, or other psychiatric disturbances. In addition, because in this age group drug toxicity usually affects the central nervous system, its symptoms are frequently attributed to other underlying causes, such as sepsis, neurologic disease, and metabolic derangements. Finally, because medical illnesses in the elderly may be difficult to recognize, drugs may be prescribed for the incorrect diagnosis, thereby confusing the clinical picture even more. This exposes the patient to the risk of taking unnecessary medications, while neglecting the underlying condition.

III. Noncompliance. Complicating assessment of drug-related toxicity is poor drug compliance, which is frequent among the elderly **(Table 1-2).** In addition to not taking their medications, some elderly patients make unauthorized changes in their dosing intervals. Up to 70% of the geriatric population take over-the-counter (OTC) drugs that may interfere with, inhibit, or potentiate prescribed medications. Complex regimens can confuse the geriatric patient, particularly if the patient has cognitive impairments. Physical limitations may also hinder drug compliance.

IV. Awareness. Pharmacologic therapy of the elderly, therefore, requires knowledge not only of appropriate drug dosages, potential side effects, and altered pharmacokinetics of drugs, but an increased awareness of potential interactions between chronic and acute medications.
- **A. Other factors.** Although it is generally assumed that the elderly are more susceptible to adverse drug reactions, some investigators argue that no good evidence exists in the medical literature to support this contention. Rather,

Table 1-2. Causes of Unintentional Drug Toxicity Among the Elderly

- Duplications
- Self-selection of drugs
- Taking p.r.n. drugs too frequently
- Automatic refills
- Omissions
- Pharmacy error
- Drug-induced confusion
- Recreational misuse
- Multiple MDs

Table 1-3. Risk Factors for Adverse Drug Reactions

- Multiple drug regimens
- Incorrect diagnosis
- Lack of compliance
- Poor OTC drug history
- Changes in drug metabolism
- Changes in drug effect
- Multiple physicians
- Generic versus trade names

these experts suggest that drug treatment of the elderly is complicated by the presence of coexisting diseases, multiple medications, self-selection of drugs, inappropriate dosing, multiple doctors, difficulty with compliance, and other factors inherent to the geriatric age group **(Table 1-3).**

B. Categories. Based on numerous reports and clinical reviews, it is clear that in order to reduce the risks of drug therapy in the elderly, it is useful to categorize precipitating factors into physician-, patient-, and drug-related groups.

Physician-Related Risk Factors for Adverse Drug Reactions (Table 1-4)

I. Detection. The majority of adverse drug reactions in the elderly are difficult to detect because symptoms are vague and nonspecific and, not infrequently, mimic symptoms of illnesses common to the geriatric age group. As a result, manifestations of many drug reactions and side effects are often overlooked or ignored by the physician. Difficulty in obtaining a history in this age group, the lack of specific physical findings, and the inability to alter the progression of disease can lull the clinician into unsafe prescribing habits and poor case detection patterns.

A. For example, physicians who prescribe drugs primarily in response to symptoms may fail to detect adverse drug reactions and interactions which, in many cases, obscure the underlying medical condition that prompted initial drug therapy. In these cases, the clinician is at risk for prescribing a compensatory drug which, unwittingly, has been added to treat an adverse reaction caused by another drug rather than the primary illness against which the physician thinks the treatment is being directed.

II. Patterns. Two common—and potentially harmful—patterns that have emerged include prescribing a cyclic antidepressant (CA) to treat the clinical depression induced by a lipophilic (e.g., propranolol) beta-blocker and the addition of a major tranquilizer to the drug regimen of patients with Alzheimer's disease to treat unrecognized benzodiazepine agitation. Another well-described pitfall is

Table 1-4. Causes of Adverse Drug Reactions in the Elderly

Physician factors

- Physician prescribes a high-risk drug to vulnerable host (i.e., ASA for patient with peptic ulcer disease)
- Physician prescribes highly interactive drug to "pharmacologically vulnerable" patient (i.e., captopril to patient on potassium-sparing agent, diphenhydramine to patient on anticholinergics, etc.)
- Physician prescribes inappropriate compensatory drug for unrecognized drug effect (i.e., tricyclic antidepressant to treat beta-blocker depression, major tranquilizer to treat benzodiazepine agitation, etc.)
- Automatic drug prescribing (i.e., standard orders for ICU, CCU, or chronic care facilities)
- Lack of follow-up on drug effects or poor longitudinal monitoring of drug interactions
- Failure to adjust dosage

---

the propensity of the subspecialist to focus on a single organ system and institute treatment that neglects drug effects on other organ systems as well as the patient's global pharmacologic landscape.

III. **Noncompliance** with prescription medications contributes significantly to the incidence of adverse drug reactions and interactions in the geriatric age group. Rates of noncompliance with prescribed medications have been shown to be substantially higher if the patient is unaware of the purpose for which the drug is prescribed. Interestingly, studies show that elderly patients are more likely to understand the use of OTC drugs when the medication is given to them by a friend or family member than when it is prescribed by a physician. In this regard, *physician instructions for drug use,* complemented by written information, have been shown to be integral to a patient's understanding of the purpose of prescribed medication; this approach is associated with increased compliance rates.

IV. **Prescribing new drugs** that are touted to be effective in the elderly but whose clinical safety and efficacy has been proven primarily in only younger, otherwise well patients is a particularly insidious problem. Most large pharmaceutical studies tend to exclude the very old and extremely ill patient because of the difficulty in evaluating drug efficacy and side effects. And, almost without exception, pharmaceutical trials are short term, and rarely exceed four months in duration. Consequently, in all but the most unusual and urgent circumstances, the clinician is on safer ground waiting until careful trials with older patients appear in the literature so that the risk of adverse reactions, drug interaction, and the long-term effects of newer drugs can be fully assessed in this vulnerable patient population.

V. **Compulsion to prescribe.** Perhaps the first—and simplest—step toward eliminating the most important risk factor (i.e., the total number of drugs consumed) burdening the elderly is to recognize and combat the physician's *compulsion to prescribe* drugs for this age group **(Table 1-5).** It is estimated that 75% of all geriatric patient-physician contacts result in the addition of a prescription drug to the patient's therapeutic regimen. Part of the problem appears to be a discrepancy between physician and patient expectations regarding the necessity for drug administration. One large study has shown that up to 80 to 90% of physi-

Table 1-5. Physician Prescribing Behavior: Patterns and Pitfalls

- Two thirds of all physician visits lead to prescription for drug.
- American patients receive about four times more medication for a specific complaint than patients in Scotland.
- In one study, 60% of physicians prescribed antibiotics for common cold.
- Duke University study suggested 64% of antibiotic usage in hospitalized patients was either unnecessary or inappropriately dosed.

cians are under the impression that their patients expect a prescription drug as part of their outpatient therapy.

A. Patient proclivity. However, when patients are interviewed regarding their desires for drug intake, they indicate the need primarily for a thorough examination, consultation, and reassurance and for a prescription in only 30 to 50% of physician contacts. This proclivity for drug use has been instilled into the general population by the pharmaceutical industry and, perhaps more importantly, by their own experiences with physicians who prescribe with such great avidity. Thus, it appears that the unfounded expectations of both physicians and patients contribute to excessive prescribing of medications.

B. The pharmaceutical industry has long recognized the pivotal role of the physician in sales of their products. To this end, the medical community is the target of a multibillion dollar annual drug promotion and continuing education campaign. Some studies suggest that these efforts are the most important external influence on physician prescribing habits. For example, 85% of all prescriptions written by practitioners graduating in 1960 are for medications introduced after graduation about which they have no formal education. It is not surprising, then, that the date of graduation from medical school has been shown to be a critical factor affecting physician choice of therapeutic agents.

C. Physician prescribing knowledge. Until recently, physician prescribing knowledge in geriatric therapeutics had not been examined in a systematic way. Early studies documented significant misuse of psychotropic drugs in nursing homes and suggested that the physician's knowledge base in geriatric clinical therapeutics may be inadequate. Ferry and his associates devised a questionnaire to test the prescribing knowledge of primary care physicians in Pennsylvania. They concluded that less than 30% of responding doctors "exhibited adequate knowledge of prescribing for the elderly." They also identified physician variables positively and negatively associated with an adequate knowledge of geriatric pharmacotherapy. Positive associations included the importance of professional meetings, perception of the need for continuing medical education, board eligibility or certification, group (rather than sole) practice, and a practice which had at least 25 to 50% geriatric patients. Negative associations were the number of years since licensure and the belief that drug advertisements are an important source of drug information. These associations speak eloquently for themselves. It is generally assumed by the lay public that physicians continually update their prescribing knowledge. Most doctors do attend conferences, read literature, and discuss topics in therapeutics with colleagues and pharmaceutical representatives. But this and other studies question the adequacy of these methods for staying current with geriatric drug prescribing.

D. Physician supervision of medications for the elderly, particularly in the nursing home environment, has been judged inadequate by several authors in England who reviewed repeat prescriptions for psychotropic drugs without a physician visit. These studies demonstrated a strong association between the number of times a prescription was refilled without seeing a physician and the age of the patient. In a large general practice in England, 70% of patients taking psychotropic and/or cardiovascular drugs had not contacted their physician in more than a month, and, of these, half had not been in contact with their physicians for a 6-month period. Inasmuch as psychotropics are capable of producing a variety of adverse reactions, their use demands constant vigilance. Ironically, those patients least able to monitor their own medications (i.e., the oldest and most frail elderly) were most likely to be taking these drugs without supervision. Attitude surveys of these older patients found them very receptive to physician intervention aimed at withdrawing drugs judged detrimental or no longer useful.

E. Medication surveillance is one of several areas in geriatric medicine well suited to the use of computer technology. This area has been pioneered by pharmacists maintaining records for nursing homes in California. Currently, it is feasible to modify computer software designed for medical offices to facilitate drug surveillance. *The Medical Letter* publishes IBM-based software and a handbook that allows the physician to anticipate and avoid adverse drug interactions.

Patient-Related Risk Factors for Adverse Drug Reactions

The two major patient-related risk factors associated with adverse drug reactions are compliance and age-associated changes in drug distribution and metabolism.

I. If compliance is defined as taking prescribed medications in a specified manner, then the elderly as a group are noncompliant at least 50% of the time in the community setting. The complexity of a three-drug regimen, for example, is sufficiently great so that even patients under age 45 demonstrate noncompliance rates equal to those of the elderly. Patient noncompliance is a diverse category that includes errors of omission and commission. In a group of elderly diabetics with heart failure, analysis of noncompliance rates found a number of factors that, interestingly enough, were not associated with altered or inappropriate drug intake. These include age, number of associated diseases, functional impairment of the patient, and frequency of hospitalization. Only one factor clearly correlated with both errors of omission and commission: *the number of drugs* in the patients' regimen. Level of confusion and dementia were not assessed in this study, but other investigations have suggested that compliance suffers even with the limited forgetfulness so common in this age group.

A. Compliance errors of *commission* include mixing of *alcohol* or *over-the-counter drugs* with prescribed drugs. It is estimated that alcoholism is present in up to 10% of the elderly population. Alcohol interacts adversely with all sedative drugs (e.g. benzodiazepines, antipsychotics, and some antihypertensives) while such OTC drugs as the antihistamines may add to the anticholinergic effects of prescribed antipsychotics, antidepressants, and anti-parkinsonian medica-

tions. *Laxative abuse* is thought to increase with age, and this may result in fluid and electrolyte disorders. Self-overmedication by *repeat dosing* or overuse also represents errors of commission, although their prevalence is unknown.
   B. **Environmental limitations** are a major obstacle to compliance and play a major role in inappropriate drug intake in the elderly. For example, the elderly patient with arthritis may be unable to open childproof bottles or split pills to obtain a fractional dose, whereas the patient with limited mobility may have difficulty getting to the bathroom and, therefore, discontinue or disrupt regular use of diuretics. Retinopathy and peripheral neuropathy may make use of insulin impossible for the older patient who lives alone.
II. **Changes in drug effect and metabolism with aging** vary widely among individuals in old age. The greater the age the greater the divergence between chronologic and biologic aging; said another way, not everyone's biologic functions decline at the same rate. Thus, the "appropriate dose" will usually follow the maxim, "Start low, go slow" in order to accommodate wide patient variability in the elderly.

Pathophysiology and Pharmacokinetics

A number of age-related changes in pharmacokinetics affect drugs commonly prescribed for the elderly. Alterations in absorption, distribution, metabolism, and elimination can precipitate adverse reactions or potentiate drug toxicity.

I. **Absorption.** Because drugs are taken up passively and are not transported in active forms, absorption generally does not change with increasing age. However, distribution may be altered because the fat-muscle ratio increases with age and because of achlorhydria. The fat portion of body weight increases from midlife averages of about 18% for men and 33% for women to 36% and 48% respectively for individuals aged 65 or over. As a result, the volume of distribution for water-soluble drugs decreases with age, whereas that for fat-soluble drugs increases with age.

II. **Metabolism**
   A. **Relatively water-soluble drugs** include acetaminophen (Tylenol) and alcohol. Diazepam (Valium) and lidocaine are examples of fat-soluble drugs. In the elderly, acetaminophen and other water-soluble drugs will attain higher plasma levels. On the other hand, diazepam and lidocaine will be distributed across a greater volume of fat, causing markedly delayed metabolism and a prolonged half-life elimination.
   B. **Serum albumin** also decreases with age, which means a lower dose may be required. This alteration is important for highly protein-bound drugs, such as sulfonylureas, for which effective concentrations depend upon the amount of unbound drug. Thus, drug interactions that decrease protein binding for such drugs as chlorpropamide (Diabinese) and tolbutamide (Orinase) may lead to toxicity in the elderly patient.

III. **Elimination**
   A. **Renal and hepatic clearance** of drugs may also be affected by the aging process. Liver blood flow is decreased 40 to 50% in the elderly. But hepatic drug metabolism varies widely with individuals, and there are no predictable age-related alterations.
   B. **The glomerular filtration rate** (GFR), however, is reduced by approximately 35% in the geriatric age group. Unlike hepatic clearance, the GFR reduction

leads to predictable, directly proportional decreases in the clearance of drugs dependent on the kidney for excretion. Serum creatinine is less useful. Examples of such drugs include lithium, digoxin, cimetidine (Tagamet), procainamide (Pronestyl), most commonly used antimicrobials, and chlorpropamide (Diabinese).

IV. Age-related changes in pharmacodynamics affect the use of a number of drugs. For example, the number of beta-adrenergic receptors is markedly reduced on lymphocytes of elderly patients. Therefore, plasma levels of propranolol (Inderal) and metoprolol (Lopressor) are higher and can cause marked hypotension, bradycardia, or central nervous system depression in the susceptible elderly patient.

Types of Adverse Drug Reactions

When evaluating and identifying potential drug reactions in the ambulatory setting, classifying adverse geriatric pharmacologic events into four groups is helpful **(Tables 1-6 and 1-7)**:

1. Primary drug reactions
2. Secondary drug reactions
3. Drug withdrawal syndromes
4. Tertiary extrapharmacologic drug effects

I. Primary drug reactions. These occur when a single medication, usually one with a narrow toxic-to-therapeutic ratio, is responsible for the patient's symptoms. Common examples include cimetidine psychosis, theophylline-induced seizures, propranolol depression, and digitalis toxicity. Other primary reactions are narcotic-induced respiratory depression, chronic salicylism, and lidocaine psychosis.

II. Secondary drug interactions. These toxic reactions result from the interaction between two medications, one causing an increased plasma level of the other drug. Common examples include the interaction between first-generation sulfonylurea agents (chlorpropamide, tolbutamide) and sulfonamide antibiotics. The sulfonamides impair hepatic metabolism of sulfonylureas, thus causing elevated plasma levels, which may lead to increased insulin release and symptomatic hypoglycemia. Salicylates, phenylbutazone, and nonsteroidal anti-inflammatory

---

Table 1-6. Assessment of Adverse Drug Reactions

Primary Drug Reaction
Single drug causing single target organ side effect
Secondary Drug Reaction
Two drugs interact: one potentiates or negates the effect of the other through competition at metabolic breakdown sites, displacement from protein-binding sites, or some other mechanism
Drug Withdrawal
Narcotics, benzodiazepines, beta-blockers
Tertiary Drug Reaction
"Falling drugs," psychometric changes, etc.

Table 1-7. Evaluation of Drug Toxicity in the Elderly

Toxic/therapeutic ratio: A time-honored concept that is valuable primarily when measuring dose-related adverse effects of a single drug in a patient with uncomplicated disease pattern

Interdrug toxicity: Much more applicable concept in the elderly, where there is a ninefold increase in adverse drug toxicity with consumption of four or more drugs

Extrapharmacologic toxicity: Tertiary clinical pathology (falls, hip fractures) not included in classic categories of drug toxicity and measurable only through large-scale epidemiologic surveys; not included as "adverse" drug reaction in package insert (i.e., propensity to cause falling)

drugs (NSAIDs) can also displace sulfonylurea from its serum protein binding sites, causing hyperinsulinemia and hypoglycemia.

A. Cimetidine. Because it is a potent inhibitor of the P-450 cytochrome oxidase system in the liver, cimetidine (Tagamet) has the potential for increasing the effective plasma concentration of a number of important drugs that undergo hepatic metabolism. These drugs include lidocaine, phenytoin (Dilantin), aminophylline, benzodiazepines (Valium, Dalmane), propranolol (Inderal), and warfarin (Coumadin). Thus, any elderly patient who is taking cimetidine in addition to one of these medications is at high risk for developing a secondary drug interaction.

B. Erythromycin and ciprofloxacin inhibit hepatic breakdown of aminophylline and theophylline compounds—as well as carbamazepine—and can induce elevations of these agents into the toxic range. Other examples of secondary drug interactions include blunted beta-receptor site sensitivity to propranolol caused by indomethacin (Indocin) and the mutual inhibition of cyclic antidepressants and centrally acting alpha-sympatholytic antihypertensives such as alpha-methyldopa (Aldomet) and clonidine (Catapres).

III. Drug withdrawal syndromes

A. Additional risks. In the elderly, traditional drug withdrawal syndromes caused by addicting medications such as phenobarbital, benzodiazepine, and alcohol usually do not differ in their clinical presentations from those seen in younger patients. However, older patients carry an additional risk of drug withdrawal syndromes from nonaddicting medications such as beta-blockers or other antihypertensives.

B. Sudden cessation of beta-blockers or calcium channel blockers, for example, can produce angina and rebound hypertension in susceptible elderly patients. The two classes of agents are not cross-protective with respect to their antianginal properties. In fact, myocardial infarction is precipitated in 2 to 3% of patients when propranolol is abruptly withdrawn, usually in elderly patients at high cardiovascular risk. The proposed mechanism for rebound symptoms is an extended period of beta-receptor supersensitivity to endogenous catecholamine stimulation.

IV. Extrapharmacologic effects.
Finally, tertiary extrapharmacologic effects are a consideration for elderly patients taking a large number of medications. Recent studies have reported that the elderly have a 50% to 150% increased risk of falling and sustaining a hip fracture when taking cyclics, long-acting anxiolytics, or antipsychotic medications **(Table 1-8).**

Table 1-8. Types of Adverse Drug Reactions in the Elderly

Primary Drug Reactions
(One drug—one side effect)
- Cimetidine psychosis
- Narcotic-induced respiratory depression
- Lidocaine psychosis
- Theophylline seizures
- Insulin reaction
- Chronic salicylism

Secondary Drug Interactions
(Requires at least two drugs to cause interaction)
- Sulfonylurea/sulfonamide
- Cimetidine/lidocaine
- Erythromycin/theophylline
- Indomethacin/propranolol
- Tricyclic antidepressant/alpha-sympatholytic

Drug Withdrawal Syndromes
(Addictive and nonaddictive withdrawal)
- Beta-blocker withdrawal (angina)
- Calcium channel-blocker withdrawal (angina, hypertension)
- "Addictive drug" withdrawal syndromes (benzodiazepines, narcotics, etc.)

Tertiary "Extrapharmacologic" Effects
(Measurable only by epidemiologic studies)
- Falls caused by tricyclics, anxiolytics, and antipsychotics (short half-life versus long half-life agents)
- Traumatic injuries caused by drug-induced orthostatic hypotension

General Principles and Patient Evaluation

Although clinical manifestations of drug toxicity are legion, they may be particularly subtle in the elderly **(Table 1-9)**. In the case of digoxin or insulin toxicity, the nature of the drug reaction can frequently be diagnosed from the history, physical examination, and laboratory data base alone. However, when a drug reaction is expressed as a minimal alteration in mental status or mood, fatigue, focal neurologic lesion, coma, seizure disorder, cardiac arrest, myopathy, or nonspecific symptoms complex, the diagnosis may be much more elusive. In such cases, if the clinician does not use a systematic approach to drug evaluation, the disease may go undiagnosed in the ambulatory setting and, hence, may go untreated.

To ensure rapid recognition of adverse drug reactions and the institution of appropriate therapy, familiarity with common medications and the ability to assess drug toxicity with little quickly available historical, physical, and laboratory data are essential.

I. **History.** To evaluate the possibility of drug toxicity, the physician should obtain a complete drug history, noting recent medication changes, including deletions, additions, and adjustments in dosages. Inquiry should be made about OTC drug use, especially formulations containing salicylates, antihistamines, and sympathomimetics. Aspirin-containing compounds can lead to gastritis in addition to chronic salicylism. Moreover, antihistamines such as diphenhydramine (Benadryl) can produce anticholinergic symptoms that may be potentiated by other commonly prescribed medications, such as cyclic antidepressants and antipsychotics. Finally, sympathomimetics such as pseudoephedrine (Sudafed) and

Table 1-9. Some Presenting Symptoms of Drug Toxicity and Adverse Drug Reactions in the Elderly

- Acute delirium
- Akathisia
- Altered vision
- Bradycardia
- Cardiac arrhythmias
- Chorea
- Coma
- Confusion
- Constipation
- Fatigue
- Glaucoma
- Hypokalemia
- Orthostatic hypotension
- Paresthesias
- Psychic disturbance
- Pulmonary edema
- Severe bleeding
- Tardive dyskinesia
- Urinary hesitancy

phenylpropanolamine-containing compounds can precipitate hypertension, angina, or even myocardial infarction.

II. Physical examination. A thorough physical exam and vital signs can help detect abnormalities frequently associated with adverse drug reactions and toxicity. Such alterations in body temperature as hypothermia are associated with drug-induced hypoglycemia, whereas temperature elevations may be caused by anticholinergic drugs. Elevated blood pressure may reflect abrupt withdrawal from beta-blockers or clonidine. Increases in resting heart rate may indicate not only beta-blocker withdrawal, but occult toxicity due to cyclic antidepressants or aminophylline. Profound, symptomatic bradycardia may be the first manifestation of beta-blocker toxicity, which is potentiated by concomitant use of calcium channel blockers such as diltiazem.

  A. Hyperventilation, especially when associated with respiratory alkalosis, is a nonspecific finding but may be the first manifestation of chronic salicylism in the elderly patient. An irregular or rapid pulse may reflect digoxin, aminophylline, or cyclic antidepressant toxicity. Neurologic findings, such as nystagmus, may suggest sedative (phenobarbital, benzodiazepine) intoxication, while constricted pupils may reflect opiate intoxication. Wheezing may be the first sign of beta-blocker or salicylate toxicity.

  B. The physical exam should assess abnormalities in the skin, mucous membranes, and pupillary size. Dry mouth, hypertension, and mydriasis suggest anticholinergic toxicity. A recent history of mental fatigue, depression, or altered thought processes may indicate beta-blocker toxicity or exaggerated effects from anxiolytic drugs of the benzodiazepine group.

III. Laboratory evaluation

  A. Indication. The laboratory exam is invaluable and may reveal metabolic and electrolyte abnormalities associated with drug toxicity. Thiazide and loop diuretics may cause hyponatremia and hypokalemia, the former sometimes severe enough to induce coma and seizures. A decreased serum bicarbonate level may indicate chronic salicylism or an anion gap acidosis. Azotemia may reflect not only excessive diuretic use but also renal failure precipitated by NSAIDs.

  B. Mental status alterations that cannot be explained by sepsis, myocardial infarction, hypotension, or metabolic abnormalities should be evaluated for the possibility of drug toxicity. Blood levels of phenytoin, digoxin, phenobarbitol, aminophylline, and salicylates are frequently helpful to detect adverse drug reactions caused by these agents. Ultimately, accurate assessment and diagnosis of drug toxicity depends on the association of recent changes in the drug dosage or frequency with the recent onset of central nervous system (CNS), gastrointestinal, cardiac, or metabolic derangements.

Important Adverse Reactions Encountered in the Emergency Department

A British study of nearly 2,000 geriatric patients admitted to the hospital examined the drugs most often associated with adverse reactions **(Table 1-10)**. Diuretics were responsible for the greatest absolute number of side effects, but they were also the most frequently used medications. Drug groups with the highest risk of adverse reactions were antihypertensives and antiparkinsonian drugs (13%), diuretics (11%), psychotropic drugs (12%), and digitalis (11.5%). Smaller studies in both the extended care and home setting have confirmed these findings.

I. Cardiovascular medications—beta-blocking agents. Toxicity from beta-blockers primarily involves the cardiovascular and central nervous systems. The most common cardiovascular side effects include hypotension, congestive heart failure, bradycardia, and high-degree heart block. The most common respiratory manifestation is bronchoconstriction. Central nervous system alterations—associated primarily with beta-blockers of the lipophilic class (e.g., propranolol)—include depression, altered mental status, and decreased libido. Some of the newer hydrophilic agents, such as atenolol, are associated with less CNS toxicity.

  A. **A number of medications,** including cimetidine, furosemide, and hydralazine, increase beta-blocker effects and may produce clinical symptoms. Concomitant use of intravenous verapamil and beta-blockers is contraindicated, because the combination may produce irreversible hypotension and profound bradycardia.

  B. **Diabetes.** Beta-blockers may also abolish symptoms of hypoglycemia and should be avoided in patients with diabetes mellitus. Diabetics who are taking a concomitant beta-blocker should be treated with $D_{50}W$ intravenously if they present with focal deficits or any mental status changes.

  C. **Glucagon.** In addition to supportive treatment, glucagon is recommended for severe beta-blocker overdose. Glucagon directly activates adenyl cyclase and mimics beta-agonist activity. Treatment with an IV bolus (50 µg/kg), an IV infusion (1 to 5 µg/hr), or a combination of the two has been successful in several cases. Severe overdoses unresponsive to glucagon may require administration of epinephrine or a pacemaker.

  D. **Heart disease.** For a variety of reasons, outpatients with heart disease frequently require adjustments—as well as additions and subtractions—in their antianginal regimen. Dramatic cardiac events, however, including unstable angina, rebound hypertension, and myocardial infarction have been described following abrupt cessation of beta-adrenoceptor blocking agents, such as propranolol. While such observable—and relatively uncommon—clinical events are sufficient to argue persuasively against the abrupt withdrawal of antianginal agents in patients with chronic stable angina, the association and frequency of silent myocardial ischemia from beta-blockade withdrawal has been less well studied. Furthermore, given the steadily increasing number of outpatients taking calcium antagonists alone and in combination with beta-blockers for treat-

Important Adverse Reactions Encountered in the Ambulatory/Emergency Setting

Table 1-10. Indicators of Possible Toxicity

Selected drugs	Reactions
Chlorpropamide (Diabinese)	Hepatic changes, signs of congestive heart failure, bone marrow depression, seizures. STADH.
Digitalis	Anorexia, nausea, vomiting, arrhythmias, blurred vision, other visual disturbances (colored halos around objects)
Furosemide (Lasix)	Severe electrolyte imbalance, impaired hearing and/or balance (ototoxicity), hepatic changes, pancreatitis, leukopenia, thrombocytopenia
Ibuprofen (Advil, Motrin, Nuprin)	Nephrotic syndrome, fluid retention, ototoxicity, blood dyscrasias
Lithium	Diarrhea, drowsiness, anorexia, vomiting, slurred speech, tremors, blurred vision, unsteadiness, polyuria, seizures
Methyldopa (Aldomet)	Hepatic changes, mental depression, nightmares, dyspnea, fever, tachycardia, tremors
Phenothiazine tranquilizers	Tachycardia, arrhythmias, dyspnea, hyperthermia, excessive anticholinergic effects
Procainamide (Pronestyl, Procan, others)	Arrhythmias, mental depression, leukopenia, agranulocytosis, thrombocytopenia, joint pain, fever, dyspnea, skin rash
Theophylline (Bronkodyl, Elixophyllin, others)	Anorexia, nausea, vomiting, GI bleeding, tachycardia, arrhythmias, irritability, insomnia, muscle twitching, seizures
Tricyclic antidepressants	Arrhythmias, congestive heart failure, seizures, hallucinations, jaundice, hyperthermia, excessive anticholinergic effects

ment of chronic angina, two important questions regarding pharmacologic manipulation of these patients have surfaced: (1) does the presence of calcium blockers in individuals also taking beta-blockers protect against the beta-blockade withdrawal syndrome, and (2) what is the frequency of transient myocardial ischemia from abrupt cessation of calcium antagonist monotherapy?

1. In an attempt to answer these questions, a study from Denmark investigated the occurrence of transient myocardial ischemia as detected by ambulatory electrocardiographic monitoring. In 47 patients with chronic stable angina and proven coronary artery disease, abrupt withdrawal of beta-blockers, either as monotherapy or in combination with calcium antagonists (group 1, n = 25), was compared with abrupt cessation of calcium antagonist monotherapy (group 2, n = 22) as regards the occurrence of symptomatic cardiac events and total ischemic activity as measured by ambulatory monitoring. The first two monitorings were performed in the hospital (at entry into study and at 48 hours after withdrawal of drugs) and the third monitoring, 5 days after withdrawal, was performed out of the hospital and during daily activity (monitoring occasions 1, 2, and 3).

2. **The investigators found** that in group 1, the frequency of total ischemia increased by 64% and 148% from monitoring occasions 1 and 2 and 1 to 3, respectively, and silent ischemia increased by 100% and 129%, respectively. However, no significant change in transient myocardial ischemia following cessation of drug was noted in group 2 (calcium monotherapy). The heart rate at onset of ischemia increased significantly in group 1 in contrast to group 2, which had significant increases only during out-of-hospital monitoring periods. Based on these results, the researchers concluded that a rebound in ischemic activity—predominantly silent—occurs after abrupt withdrawal of beta-blockers and that angina does not, in itself, seem to be a reliable parameter for assessing ischemic activity. Furthermore, it seems that combined therapy with calcium antagonists neither protects against the effects of beta-blocker withdrawal nor increases ischemic activity.

3. The results of this investigation make it clear that **abrupt withdrawal from beta-blockade** may result in transient myocardial ischemia whether or not patients manifest clinical symptoms (e.g., angina). In fact, the finding of predominantly silent ischemia with beta-blocker cessation suggests that all patients should be considered at risk for potential morbid cardiac events when such therapy is abruptly discontinued. Put another way, this study suggests that relying exclusively on clinical symptomatology to indicate adverse effects of antianginal drug withdrawal may lead to a serious underestimation of ischemic phenomena as measured by ST-segment depression on ambulatory electrocardiogram (ECG). Unfortunately, this study did not address the question as to whether gradual withdrawal of beta-receptor blockade is preferable to sudden cessation.

4. **The role of calcium antagonists** has also been clarified. Based on this study, it appears as if abrupt withdrawal of this class of antianginal agents is not associated with significant transient myocardial ischemia. And, finally, the presence of calcium antagonists does not protect against ischemic events produced by beta-blocker withdrawal.

II. **Calcium channel blockers.** Patients with calcium channel blocker toxicity usually present with an accentuation of the drug's desired clinical effects, i.e., high degree of atrioventricular (AV) block, hypotension, and, on occasion, CNS changes or congestive heart failure.

   A. **Hypotension** results from the drug's direct effect on ventricular and vascular smooth muscle and has been reported in 3.4 to 6% of patients taking nifedipine and in 5 to 10% of patients treated with verapamil for supraventricular tachycardia. Although most cases of hypotension are mild, some patients will require aggressive treatment. Infusion of IV calcium appears to be the best available treatment for such overdoses. The initial dose of 10 to 20 ml of a 10% calcium gluconate solution may be repeated every 8 hours. For cases refractory to IV calcium, fluids and vasopressors may be necessary.

   B. **Bradycardia and a high degree of AV block** may also occur. They are most often associated with verapamil or diltiazem use because of their potent, negative effect on the sinus and AV nodes. In such cases, temporary pacing may be required. Because of its potent, negative inotropic effect on the ventricle, verapamil or diltiazem can precipitate congestive heart failure in patients with depressed myocardial contractility. Headache is a common side effect and is most commonly seen in patients taking nifedipine. Other CNS side effects include dizziness, sleep disturbance, and mood changes.

C. **The variability of action** among calcium antagonists is so pronounced that interchanging one calcium channel blocker for another sometimes proves impossible. In contrast to the case of beta-blockers or theophylline derivatives, in which differences among agents basically involve such minor factors as duration of action, appearance of CNS side effects, or receptor subselectivity, the various calcium channel blockers often cannot treat the same disease process.

D. **Amlodipine.** Such differences in clinical effect do offer distinct advances in terms of individualizing therapy, however. A patient with angina, AV node conduction disturbance, and mild congestive heart failure, for instance, would benefit most from amlodipine. In this patient, amlodipine (1) relaxes coronary artery tone, which helps the angina, (2) does not change directly SA or AV node conduction, which leaves the conduction disturbance unaffected, and (3) dilates peripheral vessels (decreasing afterload and, thereby, myocardial oxygen demand), which aids the congestive heart failure. Using either diltiazem or verapamil in the same patient would primarily treat the anginal symptoms, may possibly exacerbate the conduction disturbance, would probably not affect the congestive heart failure significantly, and may even make it worse.

   1. **Electrical conduction.** In contrast to verapamil and diltiazem, which should not be prescribed to patients with sinoatrial disease, atrioventricular block, congestive heart failure, or severe ventricular dysfunction (and only cautiously to those on a beta-blocker), amlodipine does not affect electrical conduction anywhere in the heart and can be used safely in patients with the aforementioned conditions. The net physiologic effects of amlodipine's actions are (1) increased coronary blood flow, (2) decreased afterload, (3) reduced myocardial oxygen consumption, and (4) increased cardiac output.

   2. **Combined therapy.** Because amlodipine is a potent peripheral and coronary vasodilator, and because it decreases systemic vascular resistance—thus decreasing afterload and improving cardiac output—it is more suitable for combined therapy with a beta-blocker or digitalis. Its pharmacologic advantages make amlodipine the initial drug of choice in elderly patients who have marginal cardiac output, are prone to episodes of congestive heart failure, are taking beta-blockers or digitalis, or have a history of conduction disturbances. Amlodipine has also been used as monotherapy in elderly patients and seems to be very effective.

   3. **Several studies have concluded** that combined treatment with beta-blockers and calcium blockers increases antianginal efficacy compared with monotherapies, without increasing adverse effects. Moreover, amlodipine does not precipitate congestive heart failure or profound bradycardia, two adverse consequences that have been observed with the other calcium channel blockers.

   4. **In one large study** designed to measure the safety of combined intravenous diltiazem and propranolol therapy for angina, cardiac output was lowered in all patients, and because of the additive negative dromotropic activities of these two drugs, the researchers concluded that ECG monitoring was warranted. Frequent episodes of profound asymptomatic bradycardia (rates less than 50) have also been observed with combined oral therapy of diltiazem and beta-blockers.

E. **Coronary artery disease.** There has been considerable controversy regarding the appropriate use of the different calcium channel blockers (nifedipine, verapamil, and diltiazem) in patients with coronary artery disease. Some experts have argued that because of its depressive effect on sinoatrial node automaticity, increase in AV node conduction time, and decrease in cardiac muscle contractility, diltiazem (Cardizem) should not be used in patients with left ventricular dysfunction. The calcium blocker, nifedipine (Procardia), on the other hand, does not suppress sinus node rate, decreases afterload, and increases cardiac output, which has prompted some cardiologists to recommend its use as an angina agent in the subpopulation of cardiac patients with left ventricular dysfunction.

F. Diltiazem. The potential wisdom of these approaches is now somewhat clearer. According to a 5-year multicenter trial, there is now strong evidence to suggest that postinfarction patients with left ventricular dysfunction (i.e., ejection fraction less than 40%) should not be given the calcium antagonist diltiazem. The 23-center study with 2,466 patients who had isoenzyme-proven Q-wave or non-Q-wave myocardial infarction were randomized to 60 mg of diltiazem 4 times a day or placebo and then followed for 12 to 52 months. Although total cardiac mortality appeared to be equal for placebo and diltiazem-treated groups, when investigators began to look at results in specific patient subgroups, they found marked differences between diltiazem and placebo.

   1. When ejection fraction fell below 40%, diltiazem was associated with significantly increased risk represented by a 1.31 hazard ratio as compared to the control group (hazard ratio = 1.0). Moreover, the risk of adverse cardiac consequences increased as the ejection fraction fell. Although a deleterious effect of diltiazem (1.41 hazard ratio) was also observed in those patients who had x-ray manifestations of pulmonary congestion upon admission, the drug seemed to benefit those patients without congestion and ejection fractions greater than 40%.

   2. Investigators cited left ventricular dysfunction as the principal factor determining the potential benefits versus drawbacks of diltiazem therapy. Based on this multicenter trial, it seems prudent to withhold therapy with the calcium antagonist diltiazem in those postinfarction patients with either 1) an ejection fraction less than 40%, 2) x-ray proven pulmonary congestion upon admission, or 3) chronic congestive heart failure. Although, at present, no comparative data are available for the calcium antagonist nifedipine, it may be that its potent vasodilatory effects and capacity for increasing cardiac output will make it the calcium channel blocker of choice in this prespecified patient population.

III. Angiotensin-converting enzyme (ACE) inhibitors

A. Preventing complications of congestive heart failure (CHF). Many older patients suffer from cardiovascular disease and, consequently, use drugs that reflect long-term therapy directed at preventing recurrence and/or deterioration of heart-related conditions. In this vein, the rationale for including aspirin, estrogen, and/or beta-blockers as part of the permanent foundation for selected geriatric patients has been discussed in detail above. Now, it appears that ACE inhibitors also should be considered for their preventative properties in patients with heart disease. Initially, ACE inhibitors were introduced for management of hypertension. In recent years, however, studies have confirmed their usefulness in prolonging longevity and decreasing morbidity (including the need for hospitalization) in patients who have symptomatic CHF and for improving their exercise tolerance and functional status. Accordingly, this drug class has become the mainstay of patients with early, symptomatic CHF.

1. **Asymptomatic patients.** The role of these agents in asymptomatic patients has been less clear. But recent trials now confirm that such ACE inhibitors as enalapril and captopril may play an equally important therapeutic and prevention-oriented role in patients with *asymptomatic* left ventricular (LV) dysfunction after myocardial infarction. In particular, the evidence confirms that long-term administration of captopril (25 to 50 mg PO TID) is associated with a reduction in morbidity and mortality from major cardiovascular events and prolonged survival. The effects on survival in the *absence* of LV dysfunction are minimal, at best.

2. **Based on these studies,** *it is reasonable to include ACE inhibitors in the blueprint for older patients who have ejection fractions less than 0.40 and who are recovering from myocardial infarction.* Benefits are possible when ACE inhibition is instituted within 3 to 16 days after myocardial infarction and are independent of the advantages conferred by use of beta-blockers and aspirin, as discussed above. To summarize, these agents should not be used routinely after myocardial infarction but, at present, are reserved for patients with LV dysfunction, even if it is asymptomatic, who are recovering from a myocardial infarction. When ACE inhibitors are indicated for inclusion in a prevention-oriented regimen, a dosage of 25 to 50 mg of captopril taken orally three times a day, or 20 mg daily of enalapril is usually required.

B. **Prevention of diabetic renal disease.** The ability of ACE inhibitors to prevent morbidity and mortality associated with CHF is well documented; therefore the inclusion of this drug for preventive maintenance in selected patients is justified. There is now increasing evidence that ACE inhibitors should also be considered as essential pharmacologic building blocks in the drug houses of type II *normotensive* diabetics with microalbuminuria and normal renal function. Although the exact mechanism of the beneficial effects of ACE inhibitors on preservation of renal function is unclear, it most likely relates in part to the ability of these drugs to dilate the efferent arteriole of the glomerulus and thereby decrease intraglomerular capillary pressure and reduce capillary membrane permeability. Studies with such calcium channel blockers as nifedipine GITS have suggested these agents also reduce protein excretion and improve renal function in diabetic patients, but these results have been less uniform than those with ACE inhibitors.

1. **Preserving renal function.** Most of the evidence regarding the benefits of ACE inhibitors on preserving renal function in diabetics has accrued from relatively short-term studies primarily involving patients with type I diabetes. Although approximately 40% of type I diabetics eventually develop nephropathy compared with 20% of type II patients, there are 10 times as many patients with type II disease as compared with type I, so the number of patients with end-stage renal disease with type II diabetes far exceeds those with type I.

2. **Slowing nephropathy.** That ACE inhibitors help slow the progression of nephropathy in type II diabetes has been confirmed by a very carefully conducted Israeli study that demonstrates amelioration of proteinuria and preservation of renal function in normotensive patients with type II diabetes. This relatively long trial consisted of type II diabetics whose blood pressure was normal at entry and was controlled as necessary during the

study. Normotensive patients were given enalapril, 10 mg/day, and were seen every 3 to 4 months over a period of 5 years at which time values of blood glucose, creatinine, electrolytes, glycosylated hemoglobin, and 24-hour urine protein excretion were determined. During the study, if elevated blood pressure (SBP >145 mm Hg or DBP >95 mm Hg) was detected on two separate occasions, treatment with long-acting nifedipine (Procardia XL) was instituted. During the study period, albuminuria essentially remained stable in the enalapril group, while increasing significantly in patients on placebo. Renal function declined by only 1% in the enalapril group, whereas in the placebo group renal function steadily deteriorated by 13% overall between the initial evaluation and 5-year end point.

3. **Evidence.** This study provides compelling evidence for inclusion of ACE inhibitors for prevention of renal disease in patients who have had type II diabetes for less than 10 years and who demonstrate microalbuminuria. Although similar findings have been noted in the past, they were generally of shorter duration and/or included type I diabetics.

4. **Tight blood pressure control** is clearly the most effective means of slowing the progression of nephropathy in diabetic patients with hypertension and renal insufficiency. ACE inhibitors have become important agents in these patients because they have demonstrated the most consistent effects on reducing proteinuria and preserving renal function in this population. Because of the cost and potential toxicities of ACE inhibitors, it is still premature to prescribe these drugs uniformly to all patients with type II diabetes, at least until even longer-term trials with more precise measurements of renal function are available. Nevertheless, ACE inhibitors are probably justified routinely in type I diabetics in whom microalbuminuria and a positive family history for cardiovascular disease, hypertension, or both are known to be risk factors for nephropathy.

   In patients with type II diabetes, only microalbuminuria has been shown to predict nephropathy and increased morbidity associated with renal deterioration. Based on recent studies, it seems justified to consider the routine, prophylactic use of low-dose ACE inhibitors (e.g., enalapril 10 mg daily) in patients with type II diabetes *and* microalbuminuria, even in the absence of hypertension. When hypertension is present with microalbuminuria, compared with other blood pressure–lowering agents, ACE inhibitors can be considered smart drugs because they service two target organs (peripheral vasculature and kidneys) within the framework of a single prescription ingredient. This prevention-oriented approach to drug house construction is likely to reduce the long-term costs associated with treating renal deterioration and related complications associated with this common clinical disorder.

IV. **Antiarrhythmics.** Appropriate therapy for ventricular arrhythmias remains a dilemma for the practicing clinician. While a host of potent antiarrhythmic agents are now available that can ameliorate or eradicate most serious rhythm disturbances, the long-term survival benefit of such therapy is unproven. Furthermore, these agents have numerous adverse effects well known to primary care practitioners, ranging from benign problems, such as rash or gastrointestinal intolerance, to serious hematologic or immunologic derangements.

   A. **Proarrhythmias.** In recent years, the paradoxical tendency for these drugs to induce rather than control arrhythmias has become more widely recognized and a cause for great concern. Drug-associated arrhythmias, or proarrhythmias, have ranged from an increase in premature ventricular contractions in life-threatening phenomena, such as refractory ventricular tachycardia, torsades de pointes ventricular tachycardia associated with marked prolongation of the QT interval, and ventricular fibrillation.

1. The **purpose of one retrospective study** was to evaluate the clinical and electrocardiographic features of drug-associated ventricular fibrillation in a large group of patients seen at a referral center over a 5-year period. In particular, the investigators sought to define the time between the initiation of therapy and the onset of fibrillation, and to identify clinical or laboratory parameters that predicted this occurrence.

2. The **study group consisted of 28 patients,** from among 603 referred for evaluation, who had 38 episodes of drug-associated ventricular fibrillation. Data on each patient were obtained from review of available medical records, including age, sex, type of heart disease, functional class, and left ventricular ejection fraction when available. For each episode of fibrillation, dosage of antiarrhythmic and duration of therapy prior to the event, serum drug and potassium levels on the day fibrillation occurred, and electrocardiograms after fibrillation, as well as in the control of drug-free state, were obtained. In addition, a subgroup of 26 patients receiving quinidine, procainamide, or disopyramide as a single antiarrhythmic agent who developed fibrillation was compared to a control group of 62 patients who received these same agents but did not develop fibrillation.

3. **Short interval**. The most striking finding from this review was that the interval between the initiation of antiarrhythmic therapy and onset of ventricular fibrillation was usually very short. For the whole study group, the median duration of therapy before fibrillation onset was 4 days, while, for the group receiving quinidine, procainamide, or disopyramide, the median duration was only 3 days. Over 70% of drug-induced fibrillation occurred within 10 days of the onset of therapy.

4. **In comparing the study group** that developed fibrillation versus the control group that did not, the left ventricular ejection fraction was significantly lower in the study group (0.28 versus 0.43). These individuals were also more likely to have received concomitant therapy with digitalis, diuretics, and potassium supplements, although there was no clinical or laboratory evidence of digitalis toxicity in any of these cases and the serum potassium level was less than 3.5 mEq/L in only eight of the fibrillation episodes. The QT interval before drug therapy was slightly longer in the study group, but there was no significant difference between the groups in the degree of QT prolongation while receiving antiarrhythmics.

B. **Antiarrhythmics.** Given the number of patients who manifest simple or complex premature ventricular contractions (PVCs) after acute myocardial infarction (MI) and the documented adverse effects of potent antiarrhythmic agents, it is important to establish guidelines regarding the safety and efficacy of empiric antiarrhythmic therapy in this patient population. Because sudden death after MI remains a significant public health concern, primary care practitioners sometimes feel compelled to initiate antiarrhythmic therapy in patients who have PVCs during the period after their MI. The presence of PVCs has been shown to be a risk factor for increased mortality and sudden death after MI, although whether such arrhythmias represent a primary myocardial derangement or are a more general marker of underlying coronary artery disease has not yet been established. Nevertheless, there have been a number of randomized clinical trials (RCTs) designed to test whether secondary prevention of sudden death after MI with Type I antiarrhythmics is associated with improved survival. In general, these investigations have yielded mixed results, with one recent and highly publicized trial, the Cardiac Arrhythmia Pilot Study (CAST), demonstrating a significant disadvantage for those treated with Type I antiarrhythmics.

1. **Harvard investigators** conducted an English-language literature search of published RCTs that evaluated the use of prophylactic Type I antiarrhythmics in patients with documented MI. Patients had to be enrolled within 60 days after MI, continued on therapy for at least 3 months, and only those trials about which a complete report was published in the medical literature were included. Ten such studies were examined by using a metaanalysis approach. Not surprisingly, individual study designs differed with respect to follow-up (range 3 to 24 months), Type I antiarrhythmic employed, and underlying arrhythmia profile satisfying inclusion criteria, which ranged from the presence of simple PVCs to ventricular tachycardia. Investigators successfully isolated a total of 4122 patients randomly selected to receive either antiarrhythmic therapy or placebo. The 10 studies tested 9 antiarrhythmic agents including mexiletine hydrochloride, phenytoin sodium, tocainide hydrochloride, flecainide acetate, encainide hydrochloride, procainamide hydrochloride, aprindrine hydrochloride, amiodarone, imipramine hydrochloride, and moricizine.

2. **Precise risk profiles** of enrolled patients were characterized. Four studies specifically selected patients at relatively high risk (i.e., those with mechanical complications, those with sustained ventricular tachycardia) for late mortality and sudden death after MI. Based on previously reported classifications of risk stratification after MI, 2 of the 10 studies examined patients that would be considered "low risk" (i.e., no mechanical complications and infrequent PVCs), while the remaining 8 studies enrolled patients that would be considered at moderate to high risk after MI (i.e., patients with high-grade arrhythmias, complex PVCs, or mechanical complications).

3. **Results.** Although six of the seven studies that specifically assessed arrhythmias found significantly reduced numbers of PVCs sometime during the trial period, the overall effects on mortality were discouraging. Overall, three studies showed small beneficial effects of treatment, two showed no difference, four showed small adverse effects of treatment, and one study (CAST) showed a statistically significant deleterious effect on mortality. Although this metaanalysis meets recently proposed study standards, it is weakened somewhat because the included studies evaluated nine separate antiarrhythmic agents. Despite these limitations, these investigators conclude that empiric therapy of unselected patients with Type I antiarrhythmic agents is currently unwarranted, even in those patients deemed to be at "moderate" risk for late mortality after MI.

4. **The recently published CAST report** has done much to make physicians aware of the potentially lethal consequences of treating unselected post-MI patients with such potent Type I antiarrhythmics as encainide and flecainide. In that study, which eventually prompted warnings about the use of these agents from their manufacturers, investigators reported 48 to 56

deaths in the treated group and 22 deaths in the placebo groups, resulting in a relative mortality rate of about of 7.5% and 3.0%, respectively. These early mortality data ultimately precipitated discontinuation of the trial.
5. **The current metaanalysis study** is also important, however, because it extends the CAST-induced cautionary note to other Type I antiarrhythmics. Given the inclusion criteria for enrolling patients in the 10 studies reviewed, it appears that even patients at moderate risk (i.e., complex PVCs, mechanical complications, short runs of nonsustained ventricular tachycardia) for late mortality after MI do not demonstrate any advantage over placebo when treated with Type I antiarrhythmic agents. Given the potent and sometimes adverse consequences associated with these drugs, emergency physicians are best advised not to begin empiric prophylactic therapy with these agents, even when faced with post-MI patients whose ambulatory electrocardiograms demonstrate complex PVCs. It is conceivable that a small subset of patients who are at an unusually high risk for sudden death after MI (i.e., mechanical complications, recurrent ventricular tachycardia, cardiac arrest, etc.) may benefit from such therapy. At present, however, only invasive electrophysiologic studies can identify such patients and, even in this subgroup, the benefits of therapy have not been conclusively proven. In any event, initiation of long-term, empiric antiarrhythmic therapy in these patients is probably better left to the cardiac specialist who has considerable experience in arrhythmia management.
6. **Potential hazards.** Primary care practitioners need to recognize the significant potential hazards of antiarrhythmic drug therapy. In particular, the proarrhythmic potential of these agents can be life threatening. Left ventricular dysfunction and concomitant treatment with digitalis and diuretics predispose patients to be development of ventricular fibrillation during antiarrhythmic therapy. Drug-induced ventricular fibrillation seems to be a very early event, frequently occurring within 3 days of initiating treatment and most often by 10 days.

C. **Setting.** Based on these findings, it seems prudent to initiate antiarrhythmic therapy in a monitored inpatient setting whenever possible, especially in those at increased risk for ventricular fibrillation (i.e., those on digitalis therapy or the presence of low left ventricular ejection fraction). Furthermore, until more data are available regarding the long-term survival benefit of antiarrhythmic therapy, these agents should be used very judiciously and reserved for those with malignant and symptomatic ventricular arrhythmias. Finally, with respect to assessment and triage of patients on antiarrhythmic therapy, physicians should maintain a high index of suspicion in those patients complaining of syncopal symptoms, palpitations, or other manifestations of cerebral hypoperfusion within a few days of initiation of such therapy.

D. **Lidocaine.** It most often affects the central nervous system and usually occurs during rapid IV infusion. CNS effects include light-headedness, somnolence, coma, and seizures. Supportive care and discontinuation of lidocaine infusion are generally sufficient treatment in the emergency setting. Fluid repletion or pharmacologic cardiac acceleration may be necessary for hypotension due to heart block or negative inotropic actions. Treat seizures with benzodiazepines (Valium, 5 to 10 mg IV) rather than phenytoin.

E. **Quinidine.** Quinidine toxicity may be either acute or chronic. Many of the gastrointestinal, CNS, ECG, and other findings (headache, flushed skin, blurred vision with mydriasis) are similar to findings seen in anticholinergic stimulation. This correspondence suggests that quinidine and other anticholinergic drugs, such as cyclic antidepressants and antipsychotics, may produce an additive effect.

    1. **The ECG changes,** which consist primarily of conduction delays including PR, QRS, and QT prolongation, correlate closely with the severity of the clinical course. Quinidine toxicity may also cause severe hypotension and severe systemic acidosis.

    2. **In addition to supportive treatment,** studies suggest that alkalinization may be appropriate for quinidine toxicity since alkaline serum decreases the free levels of the highly protein-bound drug.

F. The newer antiarrhythmic oral agents, tocainide, mexiletine, and flecainide, produce a number of CNS and gastrointestinal side effects, some of which may necessitate discontinuing the drug in an elderly patient. Approximately 20% of all elderly patients taking tocainide stop the drug because of dizziness, confusion, nightmares, coma, or seizures. Gastrointestinal side effects that precipitate discontinuance include nausea, vomiting, and constipation. Mexiletine produces the same CNS and GI symptomatology as tocainide, and discontinuance rates as high as 40% have been reported.

V. Digitalis. Geriatric patients are at high risk for developing toxicity from digitalis glycosides. Several factors lead to increased risk, including concurrent administration of other drugs such as quinidine or disopyramide and metabolic abnormalities such as hypokalemia, hypomagnesemia, and renal failure. Toxicity should be suspected in any patient taking digoxin who develops new gastrointestinal, ocular, or central nervous system complaints, or in whom sinus bradycardia, AV conduction defects, junctional tachycardia, or premature ventricular contractions (PVCs) develop without an underlying cause.

A. Symptoms. Anorexia, confusion, and depression are the most common symptoms of digoxin intoxication, while nausea, vomiting, and visual changes, so common in young patients, are frequently absent in the elderly. However, elderly patients may develop CNS symptoms of digoxin toxicity even with normal plasma digoxin levels. Geriatric patients' complaints are nonspecific and include anorexia, abdominal pain, fatigue, malaise, headache, and visual disturbances. Cardiac toxicity may be present, with increased vagal tone or enhanced automaticity producing sinus bradycardia, variable degrees of AV conduction block, or ventricular ectopy. Ventricular arrhythmias are the most common dysrhythmic derangements, but atrial and junctional tachycardias with variable nodal conduction blocks also occur in 2 to 6% of patients.

B. Serum digoxin levels should be obtained whenever you suspect underdigitalization or overdigitalization, or when progressive cardiac or renal failure occurs. Levels above 2 ng/ml are associated with increased risk of toxic effects.

C. Delayed absorption. The clinical pharmacology of digoxin depends on various parameters, including absorption, distribution, metabolism, and elimination. Increasing age seems to be associated with delayed absorption of digoxin. Other medications, including kaolin pectate, cholestyramine, neomycin, and metoclopramide may also delay absorption when given concurrently.

D. Drug interactions further complicate digoxin therapy. Disopyramide and quinidine reduce digoxin clearance by nearly 50%. Spironolactone amiodarone and verapamil may also increase the serum digoxin level. Therefore, levels should be obtained to anticipate toxicity when these drugs are part of the patient's regimen. Hypokalemia associated with concurrent diuretic therapy augments digitalis cardiotoxicity.

E. Management consists of stopping digoxin therapy, cardiac monitoring, maintaining normal to high-normal serum potassium levels, and, when toxicity is life threatening, initiating appropriate antiarrhythmic therapy (phenytoin 50 mg/min until a loading dose of 1,000 mg is achieved) in combination with antidigoxin antibodies.

1. **Controversy.** Although digitalis has been the cornerstone of therapy for congestive heart failure for more than two centuries, the use of digoxin in such patients remains controversial. Some studies have shown that digoxin may be discontinued without adverse consequences in up to 75% of patients with stable heart failure and sinus rhythm, while other experts consider atrial fibrillation with a rapid ventricular response to be the only absolute indication for digoxin therapy. Additional debate over the potential CNS depressive effects of the drug (especially in the postmyocardial infarction [MI] period), its potential proarrhythmic properties, and controversy regarding the effect of digoxin on the long-term survival of patients with ischemic heart disease have induced the Captopril-Digoxin Multicenter Research Group to examine the comparative efficacy and safety of digoxin versus captopril therapy in patients with mild to moderate heart failure.

2. **Trial.** The principal objective of their randomized, double-blind multicenter trial was: (1) to determine whether treatment with captopril or digoxin, in addition to diuretic maintenance therapy, was associated with improved exercise tolerance during a period of 6 months and (2) to assess the relative proportions of patients on each drug requiring hospitalization or emergency department visits for exacerbations of congestive heart failure.

   a. **Entry criteria** included patients younger than age 75 years who had a left ventricular ejection fraction less than 40%, a treadmill exercise time (greater than 4 minutes, but less than the age- and sex-predicted average maximum) limited by dyspnea or fatigue, and sinus rhythm and heart failure secondary to ischemic heart disease or primary myocardial disease. The investigators concluded that compared with placebo, captopril therapy resulted in significantly improved treadmill exercise time (mean increase 82 s versus 35 s) and improved New York Heart Association class (41% versus 22%), but digoxin therapy did not. Although digoxin treatment increased ejection fraction (4.4% increase) compared with captopril (1.8% increase) and placebo (0.9% increase), the number of ventricular premature beats (VPBs) decreased 45% in the captopril group and increased 4% in the digoxin group in those patients whose baseline ambulatory electrocardiogram revealed more than 10 premature beats per hour.

   b. With respect to treatment failures, the requirements for stepped-up diuretic therapy, hospitalization, and emergency visits were significantly more in the patients receiving placebo compared with those receiving either active drug. A greater number of possible adverse side effects such as transitory hypotension, dizziness, or light-headedness, were attributable to captopril (44.2% of patients) during the blinded portion of the study than to either digoxin (30.2%) or placebo, even though the rate of discontinuation was lower in the captopril (2.9%) versus digoxin group (4.2%). Based on this study, the authors conclude that captopril treatment is significantly more effective than placebo and is an alternative to digoxin therapy in patients with mild to moderate heart failure who are receiving diuretic maintenance therapy.

3. **Diuretics and digoxin.** A recent study of outpatient prescribing practices in the elderly suggests that most physicians prescribe diuretics alone or in combination with digoxin for the initial pharmacologic maintenance of patients with mild to moderate heart failure and sinus rhythm. Based on the results of this first placebo-controlled trial comparing the effects of digoxin and captopril treatment, in which exercise time and functional class improved significantly in the captopril but not digoxin group, it now appears reasonable for physicians to prescribe captopril (25 mg t.i.d. for the first week, and then increase to 50 mg t.i.d., if tolerated) as a first-line adjunct to diuretic therapy in the patient with mild to moderate heart failure. Although this group of patients can be expected to have both a diminished mean VPB and lower treatment failure rate, the physician should still observe for potential side effects attributable to captopril therapy.

VI. Cardiovascular drugs in the elderly: cost-effective maintenance.
Drugs with cardiovascular effects must be used with special care, especially in the older age group in which one half of all drug-related adverse patient events are associated with drugs used to treat coronary artery disease, high blood pressure, and CHF. The pitfalls associated with cardiovascular drugs come in many different forms. For example, digoxin half-life may increase by 40% in normal elderly patients, and even levels of digoxin in the therapeutic range may produce nonspecific symptoms (such as anorexia or changes in mental status) normally attributed to chronic illness. Elderly hypertensive patients have impaired homeostatic mechanisms and are prone to postural hypotension. Diuretics can produce hypokalemia, hypovolemia, fatigue, and hypotension, especially in combination with potent vasodilators and anticholinergic antidepressants. The cost savings associated with using diuretics as *initial* therapy in hypertension must be weighed against the resulting quality-of-life disturbances which, although usually not life threatening, can be irksome and irritating over the long term. Other antihypertensive agents, such as ACE inhibitors, can cause cough, especially in elderly women. Among the calcium channel blockers, verapamil should be noted for its propensity to cause bradycardia, conduction disturbances, and myocardial suppression, especially when used in combination with cardioprotective beta-blockers. In general, vigilance is required when selecting drugs used to treat cardiovascular disorders. Special design considerations, with respect to prescribing for cardiovascular conditions, apply to the following therapeutic agents and drug classes:

A. **Digoxin: cost-effective maintenance.** Perhaps for no single drug is the application of total pharmacotherapeutic quality management more important than it is for the time-honored cardiac glycoside, digoxin (Lanoxin). Digoxin is the third most commonly prescribed drug in the United States. It has a long and distinguished history that dates to antiquity, and yet, debate still rages concerning its appropriate use for long-term therapy of cardiovascular conditions. Because of its widespread use and narrow toxic/therapeutic ratio, many pharmacists and physicians have become sympathetic with the growing sentiment to curtail indiscriminate digoxin use in the outpatient setting and identify more precisely those subsets of patients most likely to benefit from its long-term use. Although a number of studies have gone so far as to question the appropriateness of digoxin therapy for patients with CHF—as well as its relative efficacy compared with ACE inhibitors—most experts still agree that at least one of the following indications must be met to justify inclusion of digoxin in the drug house of patients with cardiovascular disease: (1) digoxin is indicated for the control of rapid ventricular rate in patients with chronic atrial fibrillation; and (2) digoxin is indicated for improvement of myocardial performance in patients with CHF associated with left ventricular systolic dysfunction.

B. Prescribing digoxin. As a rule, prescribing digoxin to patients with rapid ventricular rates precipitated by atrial fibrillation is usually straightforward and rarely poses a clinical dilemma. Stated simply, when chronic atrial fibrillation is present and attempts at cardioversion have been unsuccessful, digoxin is indicated for rate control. Lower dosages (digoxin 0.125 mg daily) should be tried first to achieve rate control, and only if unsuccessful, should the dosage be increased. Digoxin, then, should be included in the pharmacologic environment of patients with atrial fibrillation and rapid ventricular rate. The drug regimen should also include either Coumadin or aspirin to prevent thromboembolic stroke associated with this cardiac arrhythmia.

C. Selecting patients. If the use of digoxin in atrial fibrillation is rather straightforward, selecting patients with ventricular systolic dysfunction (i.e., those patients with CHF who are considered appropriate candidates for digoxin therapy) is much more problematic. Digoxin is still an *overused* drug to treat CHF. Interestingly, digoxin is overused in this patient population not because it isn't useful for the management of CHF—it is extremely effective for the treatment of systolic dysfunction—but because CHF is *overdiagnosed* in the outpatient setting. Hence, digoxin is overprescribed for patients who do not require the drug. In fact, there are studies that suggest that up to 42% of patients presently receiving digoxin are taking the drug for questionable reasons and that digoxin can be discontinued in these patients without compromising their clinical status.

D. Adverse events. Because digoxin is a widely prescribed agent known to cause drug-related adverse patient events, both the pharmacoeconomic and clinical consequences of inappropriate prescribing are significant. To determine what clinical criteria must be satisfied to justify cost-effective use of digoxin in patients in *normal sinus rhythm,* a Veterans Administration Hospital Study in San Francisco evaluated 242 patients in order to identify potential pitfalls associated with digoxin use. Specifically, to reduce the risk of unnecessary prescribing for this drug, they attempted to determine whether noninvasive testing (i.e., echocardiography) is indicated in outpatients to establish the diagnosis of CHF. In this investigation, patients with documented atrial fibrillation and confirmed left ventricular systolic dysfunction (ejection fraction less than 45%) were classified as appropriate candidates for digoxin therapy. With respect to establishing guidelines for digoxin use, the two most important observations were as follows: (1) the finding that 18% of patients receiving digoxin for CHF and normal sinus rhythm had preserved systolic function; and (2) the finding that detection of an S_3 gallop on physical examination was neither specific nor sensitive for confirming a decreased ejection fraction.

E. Assessing left ventricular systolic dysfunction. Based on these findings, it was concluded that the major problem associated with excessive use of digoxin in this population is the difficulty of assessing left ventricular systolic dysfunction. Based on the finding that a substantial percentage of patients with normal sinus rhythm are at risk for being *inaccurately* diagnosed as having systolic dysfunction—and, consequently, being started on digoxin therapy—the investigators recommended that all patients in whom digoxin therapy is contemplated undergo noninvasive left ventricular assessment to ensure that appropriate criteria are met for institution of digoxin therapy.

F. Risk factors. This well-designed study is helpful because it illuminates the risk factors associated with overprescribing digoxin in outpatients who have normal sinus rhythm (those with atrial fibrillation are almost always appropriate candidates for the drug). The proarrhythmogenic potential, narrow therapeutic/toxic ratio, and central nervous system (CNS) side effects of digoxin therapy are widely appreciated. This investigation is important from a pharmacoeconomic and drug maintenance standpoint because it identifies a specific subset of patients (i.e., those with normal sinus rhythm) who, in the absence of noninvasive echocardiographic studies, are at especially high risk for being inaccurately diagnosed as having systolic ventricular dysfunction. Because of the potential hazards associated with long-term digoxin use, it is prudent to recommend that all outpatients in whom the drug is being considered undergo noninvasive assessment of myocardial function.

G. Cost. Although the cost of this diagnostic evaluation is approximately $330, a 1-year supply of digoxin costs only $85. But when the costs of monitoring drug levels ($70 per digoxin level) and additional office visits are considered over time, noninvasive confirmation that digoxin is indicated can prove cost-effective. Even more important, perhaps, is that echocardiographic assessment can provide valuable information that enhances patient management, suggests clinical conditions not appreciated on physical examination, and spares a large number of patients the unnecessary risks and subtle toxic effects of long-term digoxin therapy.

H. Discontinuation. At present, patients who are in normal sinus rhythm and living in drug houses that include digoxin as a basic building block should be evaluated for the possibility of digoxin discontinuation. Noninvasive assessment of cardiac function is the best method for evaluating a patient's suitability for digoxin cessation. In this regard, if echocardiographic assessment demonstrates normal left ventricular systolic function and the patient is not taking an ACE inhibitor, the dosage of digoxin can be gradually decreased over a 12-week period. The patient's progress should be monitored every 4 weeks to ensure that clinical deterioration has not resulted from the drug's discontinuation.

  1. Patients on ACE inhibitors. Whether digoxin can or should be discontinued *in patients already on an ACE inhibitor is another matter altogether.* Although digoxin has been the traditional choice for treatment of CHF, in recent years ACE inhibitors have been shown to improve clinical status and survival in patients with CHF. Not surprisingly, they have become increasingly popular for management of this common condition. With more and more patients being treated with ACE inhibitors, one of the important issues that has surfaced is whether the use of ACE inhibitors obviates the need for digoxin therapy. In other words, can digoxin be eliminated from a drug house that contains an ACE inhibitor as one of its structural elements? This is an important issue because it suggests an opportunity to streamline drug therapy in patients with cardiovascular conditions.

2. **Patients with chronic CHF.** To answer this question, a multicenter group conducted a study on the effect of withdrawing digoxin from patients with chronic CHF. The patients had New York Heart Association class II or III heart failure, with a left ventricular ejection fraction of less than 35%, and were clinically stable on a regimen of digoxin, diuretics, and ACE inhibitors. Heart failure was found to worsen severely enough in 23 of the 93 patients randomized to withdrawal of digoxin to warrant their dropping out of the study, compared with 4 of the 85 patients who continued to receive the cardiac glycoside. The risk of increasing the severity of heart failure was six times greater in the group in whom digoxin was discontinued. Similar deteriorations in quality of life, ejection fraction, heart rate, and body weight were also noted. Interestingly many of the changes did not occur until several weeks after discontinuing digoxin therapy.
3. **Adverse effects from discontinuation.** This study demonstrates that discontinuing digoxin in patients who have CHF, even if they are on an ACE inhibitor, is a treacherous plan of action. For chronic CHF patients in sinus rhythm with systolic dysfunction and an ejection fraction less than 35%, digoxin can be an important component of the medical regimen. Patients responding favorably to a regimen of digoxin, diuretics, and ACE inhibitors should not have their digoxin withdrawn because there is a significant risk of functional deterioration. Unfortunately, there are insufficient data at present comparing the relative benefits and adverse effects of digoxin and ACE inhibitors in chronic CHF to determine which drug should be used first—an important clinical decision. Given the proven efficacy of ACE inhibitors in diastolic ventricular dysfunction, its relatively well-tolerated side effect profile, and its improvement in survival in patients with CHF, many pharmacists and physicians have advocated that initial therapy for CHF include this drug class. Whether it is the drug of choice is still to be determined, although what is clear is that patients with documented CHF who live in drug houses that already contain digoxin, diuretics, and ACE inhibitors are not ideal candidates for elimination of agents directed at improvement of cardiac function.

VII. **Antihypertensive drug toxicity.** **Optimal therapy** for high blood pressure remains an extremely controversial issue. Put another way, the noise level emanating from the antihypertensive drug landscapes is virtually deafening. As recently as 15 years ago, state-of-the-art management of patients who had mild to moderate elevations in blood pressure and who required drug therapy for their disease was relatively simple and consisted of merely selecting an agent that would lower diastolic blood pressure to a range between 80 and 90 mm Hg. Because the primary emphasis at that time was on normalizing *numbers* of blood pressure, with minimal concern for other comorbid metabolic, renal, cardiovascular, and quality-of-life parameters associated with hypertension, it is not surprising pharmacists and physicians felt comfortable choosing among a smorgasbord of what, in retrospect, are relatively primitive—some would call them barbaric—medications for hypertension. They included, among others, reserpine, guanethidine, hydralazine, alpha-methyldopa, hydrochlorothiazide, and propranolol.

   A. **Lowering the numbers.** Times have changed, and we now recognize that lowering the numbers of high blood pressure is a necessary but not sufficient condition for patients with hypertension. After a decade of clinical, interventional, and epidemiologic trials, it has become clear that hypertension is a multietiologic entity that is either associated with or capable of producing a cluster of comorbid cardiovascular, metabolic, psychobehavioral, and renovascular abnormalities, some of them associated with therapeutic intervention.

B. Complexity. The plethora of clinical studies—and the multiplicity of possible interpretations—evaluating the efficacy of various drugs for hypertension has created a therapeutic schizophrenia surrounding the treatment of high blood pressure that no amount of thorazine seems able to put to sleep. It is as if drug house construction for the hypertensive patient has been submitted to a design competition, with two different stylistic approaches, that of the Joint National Committee and that of pharmatecture competing for the building contract. Published in 1993, the Fifth report of the Joint National Committee on Detection, Evaluation, and Treatment of High Blood Pressure (JNC V) attempts to set standards based on a consensus analysis of leaders in the field and contribute to progress in the primary prevention and control of high blood pressure. Despite a number of recommendations and an overwhelming amount of information, pharmacotherapeutic choices for management of hypertension have become increasingly complex and controversial.

C. The JNC V Report introduces a number of new recommendations and some *Back to the Future* wrinkles in time, many of which appear motivated primarily by drug acquisition cost issues, rather than by the expanded range of concerns—quality of life, compliance, comprehensive pharmacologic servicing, smart drug therapy, and reduction in total outcome costs accruing from preventive pharmacologic maintenance—that characterize pharmatectural approaches to long-term drug therapy. Although JNC V appropriately expanded the list of agents suitable for initial monotherapy from diuretics, beta-blockers, calcium antagonists, and ACE inhibitors to include the alpha-1-receptor blockers (i.e., doxazosin, Cardura) and the alpha-beta-blocker (labetolol), the Report also made recommendations that signal a return to stylistic approaches to drug house design that are associated with many potential pitfalls. With respect to initial monotherapy for high blood pressure, JNC V argues that because beta-blockers and diuretics reduce cardiovascular morbidity and mortality in controlled clinical trials, these two classes of drugs are preferred for initial drug therapy. The alternative drugs—calcium antagonists, ACE inhibitors, alpha-1 receptor blockers, and alpha-beta blockers—are equally effective in reducing blood pressure. Although these alternative drugs have potentially important benefits, argues the Report, they have not been used in long-term controlled clinical trials to demonstrate their efficacy in reducing morbidity and mortality and, therefore, should be reserved for "special indications" or when diuretics or beta-blockers have proved unacceptable or ineffective.

D. Comprehensive pharmacologic servicing. This strategy represents a very rigid position that ignores comprehensive pharmacologic servicing of the patient with hypertension. Specifically, JNC V fails to account sufficiently either for the well-documented pitfalls associated with diuretic and beta-blocker therapy, or for the technological advances and clinical outcome studies that document multifactorial improvements—delayed progression of diabetic renal disease, improved survival in CHF, enhanced exercise tolerance in angina, lipid-lowering effects, 24-hour blood pressure maintenance with once-daily dosing, and quality-of-life improvements—associated with more recent, post-Framingham additions (calcium antagonists, ACE inhibitors, and alpha-blockers) to the antihypertensive pharmacopea. Given the present fiscal belt-tightening in health care, the reality is that large-scale, long-term investigations such as the Framingham Study can probably never be implemented again. Therefore the incentives for using agents other than beta-blockers and diuretics must be based on other real world factors, on clinical trials of shorter duration, and on innovative—yet scientifically rigorous—strategies that shape pharmacotherapeutic practices.

E. Symptoms. Seventy percent of the elderly individuals treated with antihypertensive medications show symptoms of sadness, fatigue, apathy, agitation, or insomnia. Reserpine, propranolol, and methyldopa are the worse offenders, but clonidine, guanethidine, and hydralazine are also capable of producing symptoms of mental depression. Other nonantihypertensive agents with similar effects include neuroleptics, tranquilizers, hypnotics, digoxin, antiparkinsonian drugs, anticancer agents, corticosteroids, and nonsteroidal antiinflammatory agents (NSAIDs). **(See Table 1-11.)**

F. Diuretics. Used both in the management of congestive heart failure and hypertension, diuretics are associated with more adverse reactions than any other drug. They are also among the most commonly prescribed drugs for the elderly. Hypovolemia and postural hypotension, electrolyte imbalances (hyponatremia, hypercalcemia, and hypokalemia), glucose intolerance, and hyperuricemia are the most common adverse reactions **(Table 1-12)**.

1. **Hypokalemia** may induce or augment digoxin toxicity, while severe hyponatremia may produce stupor, seizures, and coma. Mild hyperuricemia is common but rarely induces an acute gouty attack. Serum uric acid levels, however, can be helpful when the patient presents with a monoarticular arthritis.
2. **Finally, loop diuretics** can induce painful urinary retention and symptoms of prostatism in elderly men with gland enlargement. Spironolactone and triamterene and amiloride may induce hyperkalemia in patients with reduced renal failure or those taking ACE inhibitors.

Table 1-11. Evolution of Antihypertensive Drug Therapy

Step	1970	1980	Current
I	Diuretic	Beta-blocker/diuretic	Vasodilator, alpha-blocker, angiotensin converting enzyme (ACE) inhibitor, calcium antagonist
II	Sympatholytic, methyldopa, beta-blocker, reserpine, etc.	Diuretic/beta-blocker	Diuretic/beta-blocker
III	Vasodilator hydralazine, minoxidil	Vasodilator hydralazine, minoxidil, alpha-blocker, ACE inhibitor, calcium antagonist	Beta-blocker/diuretic
IV	Others	Others	Others

Table 1-12. Side Effects of Commonly Used Diuretics

Diuretic	Hypo-kalemia	Hyper-kalemia	Acidosis	Alkalosis	Hyper-uricemia	Hyper-calcemia	Hyper-glycemia	Hypertri-glyceridemia	Hypo-natremia	Hypo-magnessemia
Thiazide	+	−	−	+	+	+	+	+	+	+
Loop diuretics	+	−	−	+	+	−	+	+	+	+
Potassium-sparing	−	+	+	−	−	−	−	−	−	+

Important Adverse Reactions Encountered in the Ambulatory/Emergency Setting

Table 1-13. Adverse Side Effects of Antihypertensive Drugs

	Impotence	Ejaculation difficulties	Decreased libido	Gynecomastia
Thiazides	?	−	+	−
Spironolactone	+	−	+	+
Methyldopa	+	+	+	+
Clonidine	+	+	−	+
Propranolol	+	−	+	−
Hydralazine	?	−	−	−
Prazosin	+	−	−	−
Doxazosin	−	−	−	−

- **G.** The centrally acting sympatholytic drugs, clonidine and methyldopa, can cause postural hypotension, CNS depression, and sexual dysfunction **(Table 1-13)**. The CNS depression associated with clonidine decreases mental acuity so that patients can appear "senile" or demented in addition to feeling tired or drowsy. Moreover, sudden discontinuation of clonidine can cause a withdrawal syndrome of headache, sweating, and rebound hypertension. If a patient on clonidine therapy presents with symptoms of rebound hypertension, insomnia, headache, or arrhythmias, suspect that the patient may have discontinued the drug abruptly.
- **H. Sexual dysfunction.** All antihypertensives, including thiazide diuretics and spironolactone, may cause sexual dysfunction. Patients may complain of depression and fatigue in an attempt to mask underlying sexual dysfunction. Methyldopa and clonidine can also cause gynecomastia.
- **I. Peripheral vasodilators** used to treat hypertension may produce symptoms that induce the elderly to seek emergency care. Hydralazine (Apresoline) and alpha blockers (Minipress) are useful for either hypertension alone or in association with congestive heart failure. Enalapril, lisinopril, captopril, and other ACEIs are also vasodilators that block the formation of angiotensin II **(Table 1-14)**.
  - **1. Sudden syncope.** Elderly patients may experience sudden syncope after taking the first dose of prazosin or report some combination of dizziness, headache, or lethargy. Usually, these symptoms will clear after 2 or 3 days of therapy. The concomitant intake of beta-blockers or diuretics may enhance this first-dose side effect **(Table 1-15)**.
  - **2. Hydralazine** can produce CNS manifestations, such as headache or depression. Reflex tachycardia, angina, lupus syndrome, and fluid retention have also been reported.
- **J. ACE inhibitors.** Although they are associated with fewer side effects and are increasingly popular in treating hypertension, ACE inhibitors can produce a number of symptoms and side effects including hyperkalemia. ACE inhibitors may produce proteinuria, reversible neutropenia, dermatitis, and angioedema. Enalapril (Vasotec) produces syncope in 1% of elderly patients who use the drug, as well as headache and dizziness. ACE inhibitors may cause hypotension in patients who are hypovolemic or on diuretic therapy. Consequently, stopping diuretic therapy one week before beginning therapy with ACE inhibitors is generally recommended. The hypotensive effect of

Table 1-14. Antihypertensive Drug and Disease Interaction Profiles

	Alpha-blockers	ACE inhibitors	Beta-blockers	Calcium antagonists	Diuretics
Effects of antihypertensive agents on coexisting disease					
Angina	No effect	Beneficial (?)	Beneficial	Beneficial	No effect
CHF	± Beneficial	Beneficial	Worsen	± Beneficial	Beneficial
Arrhythmias	No effect	No effect	± Beneficial	Beneficial	May worsen
COPD	No effect	No effect	Worsen	Beneficial (?)	No effect
Effects of antihypertensive agents on concomitant metabolic disorders					
Hyperlipidemia	Improve	No effect	Worsen	No effect	Worsen
Diabetes	No effect	No effect	May worsen	May worsen (?)	Worsen
Hypokalemia	No effect	May correct	No effect	No effect	Worsen
Hyperuricemia	No effect	No effect	No effect	No effect	Worsen

Table 1-15. Drugs Causing Orthostatic Hypotension

Benzothiadiazides	Methotrimeprazine
Bretylium	Methyldopa
Captopril	Methysergide
Chlorisondamine	Minoxidil
Clonidine	Nifedipine
Cyclic antidepressants	Nitroglycerin
Furosemide	Pentolinium
Guanethidine	Phenothiazines
Guanidine	Phenoxybenzamine
Hexamethonium	Prazosin
Hydralazine	Procarbazine
Iopanoic acid	Reserpine
Levodopa	Thiothixene
Lidocaine	

these drugs is also enhanced by the calcium channel blocker nifedipine—or significantly diminished by NSAIDs.

K. New pharmaceuticals. Over the past decade, the pharmacotherapeutic landscape for the treatment of hypertension has witnessed major tectonic shifts. Recently, physicians have been deluged by an avalanche of newly approved pharmaceuticals—from ACE inhibitors to long-acting, cardioselective beta-antagonists and combinations thereof—aimed at the primary treatment of hypertension.

1. **Selecting a regimen.** Given the wide variety and proven efficacy of so many available agents, optimal antihypertensive therapy has become less a matter of selecting a drug that adequately controls diastolic and systolic blood pressure than of selecting an agent or regimen that is predictably associated with high patient compliance, a low incidence of adverse drug reactions, minimal interdrug toxicity, and preservation of quality of life, including cognitive and sexual function. As better-tolerated agents become available and long-term, large-scale studies on hypertension begin to yield statistically significant morbidity and mortality data, the focus has now shifted on the comparative ability of different antihypertensives to reduce total, cardiac, and stroke morbidity and mortality.

L. Captopril. Left ventricular enlargement is a well-recognized marker of cardiac dysfunction of various causes and, in coronary artery disease, left ventricular volume is the best predictor of long-term survival. Dilatation of the left ventricle begins soon after an acute myocardial infarction and, in animal models, continues well after healing of the infarcted area has been documented histologically. This sustained enlargement of the left ventricle in animal models has been moderated by the long-term use of the ACE inhibitor captopril, with resultant improved survival.

1. **Trial.** One prospective, randomized, double-blind, placebo-controlled trial had three objectives: to determine whether left ventricular dilatation continues beyond the acute phase of myocardial infarction in humans; whether persistent ACE inhibition changes the long-term process; and whether captopril treatment improves exercise performance in patients

with diminished left ventricular function without overt congestive heart failure.

    a. Fifty-nine patients who had sustained a first myocardial infarction involving the anterior wall and with a radionuclide ejection fraction of 45% or less were randomized. Thirty patients received captopril in a blinded fashion beginning an average of 20 days after infarction and titrated to a target dose of 50 mg three times per day, and 29 patients received placebo. The two groups were comparable in terms of coronary risk factors, peak creatine kinase concentration, pretreatment hemodynamics and functional status, and prior use of thrombolytic or angioplasty therapy. The study medication was added to optimal conventional therapy, including diuretics, digitalis, antiarrhythmics, and beta-blockade as deemed appropriate by the treating physician. Baseline catheterization was performed in all patients and repeated 1 year later, and exercise stress testing was performed quarterly.

    b. At 1-year follow-up, left ventricular size as measured by end-diastolic volume increased significantly and left ventricular filling pressure remained elevated in the placebo group. In those treated with captopril, the increase in end-diastolic volume was not significant and filling pressure decreased. In a subset of patients with persistent occlusion of the left anterior descending artery and, therefore, at high risk for ventricular enlargement, captopril prevented further dilatation. The exercise duration in the captopril group consistently exceeded that in the placebo group at 3, 9, and 12 months.

    c. The authors conclude that left ventricular enlargement following anterior myocardial infarction is a progressive process that may be moderated by treatment with captopril resulting in reduced filling pressures and improved exercise tolerance.

    d. Salvage of ischemic myocardium in an effort to preserve left ventricular function in the setting of acute myocardial infarction has been a major focus of cardiologists in recent years. Primary care physicians, often entrusted with the long-term management of patients post-MI, have concentrated on risk factor modification and the use of antiplatelet or beta-blocker therapy to reduce the chances of recurrent infarction. This study provides preliminary evidence to suggest that it may become common to add ACE inhibitor therapy to the long-term outpatient treatment regimen of patients who have sustained a myocardial infarction.

    e. Although the size of the study was small and restricted to those with anterior infarction and reduced ventricular function and the follow-up was only for 1 year, the salutary benefits of captopril therapy were significant. Coupled with results of other studies that have shown survival benefits in patients with congestive heart failure treated with ACE inhibition, it suggests that these agents interrupt a pathophysiologic sequence that promotes ventricular enlargement and dysfunction post-MI and in other situations causing heart failure.

2. Larger studies. It is interesting to speculate on the results of larger studies (currently ongoing) of longer term captopril therapy and whether any beneficial effects will be demonstrated with other ACE inhibitors. Most likely, evidence will continue to mount to support the use of ACE inhibitors as cornerstone therapy for heart failure precipitated by myocardial infarction and other causes.

a. Metoprolol. Using data collected as part of the European MAPHY (Metoprolol Atherosclerosis Prevention in Hypertensives) Trial, a randomized, prospective study was designed to investigate whether metoprolol, a relatively beta-1-selective beta-blocker, given as initial antihypertensive treatment to white men aged 40 to 64 years, lowers cardiovascular complications of high blood pressure to a greater extent than thiazide diuretics. The investigators randomized 1,609 (8,110 patient years) patients to metoprolol and 1,625 (8,070 patient years) to a thiazide diuretic, with a mean follow-up time of 4.2 years. the mean dose of metoprolol was 174 mg/d and, of thiazide diuretics, 46 mg/d of hydrochlorothiazide. Both study groups achieved identical control of blood pressure using a fixed therapeutic schedule. The investigators randomized both previously treated patients and those with newly detected and untreated hypertension. The patients' diastolic blood pressure in the sitting position was 100 mm Hg or greater and less than 130 mm Hg at randomization. Since this was a study of primary prevention, previous myocardial infarction, angina pectoris, and stroke were exclusive criteria. Also excluded were patients with secondary hypertension, second- and third-degree atrioventricular block, cardiac failure, obstructive lung disease not well-controlled by beta-2 stimulants, and diabetes mellitus.

b. The investigators concluded that starting antihypertensive therapy in men with mild to moderate hypertension with the beta-1-selective beta-blocker—metoprolol—instead of a thiazide diuretic leads to a total mortality reduction of -68% to -17% (95% confidence limits). The lower total mortality can be ascribed to fewer deaths from coronary heart disease and stroke, a benefit that also extends to hypertensive smokers. Whether the improved mortality data are in any way specific to metoprolol or can be extended to other beta-blockers or nondiuretic antihypertensive drugs could not be answered by the present trial.

c. Several widely cited studies reported during the late 1970s and early 1980s proved conclusively that first-line treatment of hypertension with diuretics prevented or delayed several well-known complications of hypertension, including renal failure, heart failure, accelerated hypertension, and stroke. Despite these well-documented advantages, the effect of diuretics on reduction of deaths from coronary heart disease was not encouraging. This large, randomized study is significant, then, because it attempts to provide scientific proof that beta-blocker therapy used as initial therapy in mild to moderate hypertensives can lower total mortality from coronary heart disease better than thiazide diuretics.

d. Based on the findings from the MAPHY Trial, it is reasonable for physicians to use metoprolol as initial therapy for mild to moderate hypertension in white middle-aged men who have no previous history of heart disease, stroke, or diabetes. Compared to thiazide diuretics, this agent can be expected to lower total mortality in both smokers and nonsmokers. The value of other beta-1-selective beta-blockers for primary prevention of death from coronary heart disease and stroke cannot be assessed from this study. **(See Table 1-16.)**

M. Antihypertensives and quality of life. Until the late 1980s, little or no attention was directed at the effects of antihypertensive therapy on quality of life. Fortunately, recent studies have attempted to qualitate and quantitate quality-of-life issues as they relate to antihypertensive drug therapy. Previous studies have attempted to compare a number of different drug classes but were limited by the absence of placebo control groups, thus making it difficult to determine the true effects of monotherapeutic agents. Also

Table 1-16. Drug Interactions in Antihypertensive Therapy

Diuretics

Diuretics can raise lithium blood levels by enhancing proximal tubular reabsorption of lithium

NSAIDs, including aspirin, may antagonize antihypertensive and natriuretic effectiveness of diuretics

ACE inhibitors magnify potassium-sparing effects of triamterene, amiloride, or spironolactone

ACE inhibitors blunt hypokalemia induced by thiazide diuretics

Sympatholytic Agents

Guanethidine monosulfate and guanadrel sulfate. Ephedrine and amphetamine displace guanethidine and guanadrel from storage vesicles. Tricyclic antidepressants inhibit uptake of guanethidine and guanadrel into these vesicles. Cocaine may inhibit neuronal pump that actively transports guanethidine and guanadrel into nerve endings. These actions may reduce antihypertensive effects of guanethidine and guanadrel

Hypertension can occur with concomitant therapy with phenothiazines or sympathomimetic amines

Monoamine oxidase inhibitors may prevent degradation and metabolism of released norepinephrine produced by tyramine-containing foods and may thereby cause hypertension

Tricyclic antidepressant drugs may reduce effects of clonidine and guanabenz

Beta-blockers

Cimetidine may reduce bioavailability of beta-blockers metabolized primarily by the liver by inducing hepatic oxidative enzymes. Hydralazine, by reducing hepatic blood flow, may increase plasma concentration of beta-blockers

Cholesterol-binding resins, i.e., cholestyramine and colestipol, may reduce plasma levels of propranolol hydrochloride

Beta-blockers may reduce plasma clearance of drugs metabolized by the liver (e.g., lidocaine, chlorpromazine, coumarin)

Combinations of calcium channel blockers and beta-blockers may promote negative inotropic effects on the failing myocardium

Combinations of beta-blockers and reserpine may cause marked bradycardia and syncope

ACE inhibitors. Nonsteroidal anti-inflammatory drugs, including aspirin, may magnify potassium-retaining effects of ACE inhibitors

Calcium Antagonists

Combinations of calcium antagonists with quinidine may induce hypotension, particularly in patients with idiopathic hypertrophic subaortic stenosis

Calcium antagonists may induce increase in plasma digoxin levels

Cimetidine may increase blood levels of nifedipine

absent in earlier studies was a comprehensive assessment of the potential effects that dietary modifications (i.e., weight loss, sodium restriction, etc.) might have in conjunction with pharmacotherapeutic interventions. This is of special importance because drug therapy is often used in conjunction with a program of dietary restriction or modification. Finally, of all quality-of-life parameters that are potentially affected by antihypertensive drug therapy, sexual function is, perhaps, one of the most important. Because beta-blockers and diuretics are still widely used in the management of hypertension, a randomized, placebo-controlled clinical trial evaluating the effects of these agents on sexual function is especially timely.

1. **Study.** Investigators from three university-based tertiary care centers enrolled 696 mildly hypertensive (diastolic blood pressure between 90 and 100 mm Hg) and mildly to moderately obese (weight between 110% and 160% of ideal weight) patients, ranging in age from 21 to 65 years, into a randomized, placebo-controlled trial (called the Trial of Antihypertensive Interventions and Management [TAIM] Study) to evaluate the effects of chlorthalidone and atenolol on quality of life and sexual function. The patients were stratified by clinical center and race and then assigned to one of three diets (usual, low sodium and high potassium, weight loss) and one of three agents (placebo, chlorthalidone 25 mg/day, and atenolol 50 mg/day). Patients were evaluated at baseline and at 6 months with respect to blood pressure parameters and satisfaction with various aspects of life as measured by the following instruments: (1) Life Satisfaction Scale, (2) Physical Complaints Inventory, and (3) Symptom Check List. Drug dosages remained unchanged for the first 6 months of the study. With respect to dietary counseling, patients who were randomly assigned to the usual diet group received no further nutritional counseling, whereas those randomly assigned to the weight reduction or low-sodium and high-potassium diet groups participated in 10 weekly group sessions and, thereafter, in monthly individual sessions with nutritionists.

2. **Between baseline and 6 months** for all drugs and all diets, improvement was significant on all subscales measuring distress except that on the Sexual Physical Complaint Scale. Low-dose chlorthalidone and atenolol produced few side effects, except in men, which tended to be primarily sexual in nature. Erection-related problems worsened in 28% (95% confidence interval, 15% to 41%) of men receiving chlorthalidone and the usual diet, in 11% (confidence interval, 2% to 20% of men receiving atenolol and the usual diet, compared with 3% (confidence interval, <0% to 9%) of men receiving placebo in combination with the usual diet. Of female patients receiving chlorthalidone therapy, 24% had worsening sexual problems when following their usual diet. Patients taking chlorthalidone or atenolol had their sexual problems ameliorated if they followed a weight loss diet (average weight loss of 10.4 pounds in the atenolol group and 15.1 pounds in the chlorthalidone group).

3. **Other parameters.** With respect to other quality-of-life parameters, the low-sodium diet with placebo was associated with greater fatigue (34%; confidence interval, 23% to 45%) than was either the usual diet or weight reduction diet. The low-sodium diet with chlorthalidone increased problems with sleep (32%; confidence interval, 22% to 42%) compared with chlorthalidone and the usual diet.

4. **Atenolol and chlorthalidone.** This is a useful study because it compares quality-of-life parameters associated with two commonly used antihypertensive agents, atenolol and chlorthalidone, with placebo therapy under varying dietary regimens. It is, perhaps, the only study to evaluate these parameters according to dietary variations, a feature that may explain findings that conflict with previous trials. Overall, the study design is clean and straightforward, although because two thirds of the patients enrolled were previously treated for hypertension may affect the validity of the data. Moreover, the 6-month follow-up period is relatively short and therefore may not reflect long-term trends observed at this point in the trial.

5. **Given these limitations,** it is important to note that within the parameters of this study design, both male and female patients who are placed on either low-dose chlorthalidone or atenolol therapy and who are maintained on their normal diets can be expected to have a statistically significant impairment in sexual function. These effects are considerably attenuated when a successful weight loss regimen has been followed. Moreover, patients placed on a combination of chlorthalidone and sodium restriction are more likely to have sleep problems. Based on these results, the investigators conclude that when either chlorthalidone or atenolol are used for antihypertensive therapy, weight reduction should be used in addition to drug regimens to minimize impairment of sexual function.

6. **Sexual function.** Although we have suspected that diuretics and beta-blockers adversely affect sexual function in hypertensive patients, this good study suggests that we are now on solid ground when we avoid these drugs as first-line agents in patient populations where maintenance of sexual function is a high priority. What is of special interest from this trial is that sexual impairment of low-dose chlorthalidone therapy can be detected in both men and women. The real mystery of this investigation, however, emerges from the observation that sexual dysfunction induced by either chlorthalidone or atenolol is affected greatly by the choice of dietary regimen (i.e., those patients following their usual diet have dramatic deterioration in sexual function, whereas patients following a successful weight loss program have a significantly reduced deterioration in sexual function). Just why this happens the investigators cannot fully explain, although the study suggests that all quality-of-life parameters improve when weight loss is achieved, and that blood pressure reduction with weight loss alone is as good as low-dose chlorthalidone with a usual diet. Therefore patients who are unable to follow a long-term weight reduction program may have sexual dysfunction when placed on diuretic or beta-blocker therapy. If a weight loss dietary regimen cannot be followed and sexual dysfunction occurs, then these agents are best avoided. Instead, patients should be placed on one of the agents (i.e., ACE inhibitors, calcium blockers, doxazosin) that do not produce significant impairments in sexual function compared with placebo therapy. In all cases, however, weight loss counseling should be considered a high priority modification that affects remediable coronary heart disease risk, as well as quality-of-life parameters.

Antihypertensive Agents: Management Overview

Since publication in 1984 of the last report of the Joint National Committee (JNC) on Detection, Evaluation, and Treatment of High Blood Pressure, there has been a significant decline in both national age-adjusted stroke mortality and in mortality associated with coronary artery disease. These impressive improvements have been accompanied by dramatic alterations in the pharmacologic and nonpharmacologic treatment of hypertension, the majority of which were addressed in the 1988 JNC report. Based on the latest scientific research, this comprehensive federal blueprint, produced under the auspices of a multimember committee chaired by Boston University's Aram V. Chobanian, represents state-of-the-art thinking regarding evaluation and management of high blood pressure.

I. **Initial pharmacologic therapy.** Updating findings contained in previous reports, the 1988 JNC report is intended to serve as a guide for practicing physicians in their care of hypertensive patients and to guide health professionals participating in community-based high blood pressure programs. Directing its recommendations toward the treatment of 58 million Americans with high blood pressure, the 1988 white paper broadens the time-honored step-care approach to provide more flexibility for clinicians. Perhaps the most important change introduced by the JNC is the expansion of initial pharmacologic monotherapy to include both ACE inhibitors and calcium channel antagonists *in addition* to thiazide-type diuretics and beta-blockers recommended by the 1984 JNC report. Addressing special populations with management problems, the authors of the current report observe that, with respect to drug therapy, black patients usually do not respond as well to beta-blockers or ACE inhibitors as do whites and that diuretics are generally more effective monotherapy than either beta-blockers or ACE inhibitors. With respect to elderly hypertensives, the report notes the efficacy of calcium antagonists as monotherapy and recommends centrally and peripherally acting adrenergic inhibitors as step 2 drugs.

II. **Step-care approach.** In addition to making specific pharmacologic recommendations, the step-care approach to antihypertensive therapy has been refined considerably. Its equation now includes implementation of one among three options in the event that, after a 1- to 3-month interval, the patient's response to the initial agent has been *inadequate* and is not experiencing significant side effects from the initial agent. In such cases, it is recommended that the physician 1) increase the dose of the initial drug if it was prescribed below the recommended maximum dose, 2) add an agent from another class, or 3) discontinue the initial choice and substitute a drug from another class. A step-down (i.e., drug withdrawal) option is also suggested for those patients with mild hypertension who have satisfactorily controlled their blood pressure through treatment for at least 1 year.

   A. **Ongoing monitoring.** Comprehensive in its scope and presentation of adverse drug reactions and interactions, the 1988 JNC report makes a plea not only for a systematic, judicious approach to pharmacologic therapy of high blood pressure but for ongoing physician monitoring of the impact of such therapy on quality of life.

   B. **Upgrade.** Although much of the 1988 JNC report confirms and highlights the significant improvements in stroke and cardiac morbidity that can be achieved with treatment of high blood pressure, there are some new wrinkles worthy of note in the pharmacologic treatment sphere, especially the addition—or, put another way, upgrading—of calcium blockers and ACE inhibitors to the revered step 1 class of monotherapy agents. For example, the inclusion of ACE inhibitors now provides a unique therapeutic option for those hypertensive patients who may also require treatment for chronic congestive heart failure, whereas hypertensive patients suffering from chronic stable angina are uniquely positioned to benefit from both the antianginal and blood pressure–lowering effects of a single agent (e.g., calcium blocker). Moreover, the elderly patient who requires treatment with a NSAID can, by using a calcium antagonist, be spared the potential potassium-retaining complications of combined NSAID-ACE inhibitor therapy. The addition of these two classes also provides salutary options for a number of patients—diabetics, asthmatics, and individuals with left ventricular dysfunction—who, under the 1984 JNC regimens, might have been adversely affected by the negative inotropic properties of beta-blockers or the alterations in plasma lipids and blood glucose associated with thiazide diuretics.

III. Compliance. Recently, large clinical trials and metaanalytical studies have repeatedly demonstrated that antihypertensive therapy will reduce stroke morbidity and may reduce incidence and mortality of cardiovascular disease caused by hypertension. The elderly have been shown to be among the most compliant patients (HDFP trial) of any hypertensive age group. In spite of their fragility, careful antihypertensive therapy can be expected to prolong their useful lives.

A. Quality of life. Studies show that physicians are notably poor at judging the effect of hypertensive therapy on quality of life. Interestingly, patients were found to be only marginally better at assessing their general well-being in a British study of the effects of antihypertensive therapy. The spouse or house mate was the most sensitive indicator of adverse effect on well-being and, thus, is the individual to be queried by the physician to give the best assessment in this regard.

B. Failure of an antihypertensive regimen to lower blood pressure must not necessarily be assumed to be failure of the drug. Compliance must be verified before additional drugs are added to prevent hypotension.

C. Nonpharmacologic therapy must be tried first, but the clinician must be realistic about expectations for a change of long-established behaviors. Salt restriction, weight reduction, and avoidance of alcohol are all admirable goals if the patient can be persuaded.

IV. Response. In general, the elderly respond to all available antihypertensive agents. Some trials suggest they may respond to a calcium channel blocker better than to a beta-blocker or an ACE inhibitor, although any one of these classes may be used as monotherapy in the elderly. Since concomitant diseases are prevalent in the elderly, tailoring therapy to these disorders and vigilant anticipation of side effects is the most important part of antihypertensive management. Hypertensives with angina may improve with a beta-blocker or a calcium channel blocker. Congestive heart failure is frequently accompanied by, and even caused by, hypertension. These patients benefit from diuretics and vasodilators of all types, especially ACE inhibitors.

Nitrate Therapy

The sublingual (nitroglycerin) and oral (isosorbide dinitrate) nitrate preparations are the principal antianginal agents, and promote vasodilation of both venous and, to a lesser extent, arterial vascular beds. In the coronary beds, nitrates redistribute blood flow among collateral routes to the underperfused myocardium.

I. **Adverse drug reactions.** Orthostatic hypotension occurs commonly in the elderly. Tolerance and cross-tolerance between nitrates develops with repeated usage. Headache occurs early in the use and with excessive doses. Angina may develop or worsen with sudden withdrawal of nitrates.

II. **Adverse drug interactions.** Orthostatic hypotension occurs with the antihypertensives, especially the calcium channel blockers, phenothiazines, and alcohol.

III. **Management.** Patients inexperienced with nitrates should lie down for the first few doses in case of hypotension. This is usually associated with dehydration.
   A. **The onset of action** of nitroglycerin topical ointment is 20 to 60 minutes and transdermal patch is 40 to 60 minutes. These are adequate for prophylaxis but too slow to respond to the immediate need during angina. Only sublingual nitroglycerin or sublingual/chewable isosorbide with an onset of action of 1 to 3 minutes should be used for the acute anginal attack.
   B. **To avoid nitrate tolerance,** a low-nitrate or nitrate-free period each 24 hours should be provided. Transdermal patch or ointment should be left on only for 14 to 16 hours and then removed. Oral nitrate such as isosorbide should be used three times per day with the last dose near the evening meal. Oral nitrate schedules that provide the last dose at bedtime are associated with tolerance. If angina persists, a beta-blocker or a calcium channel blocker should be added.

Nonsteroidal Anti-Inflammatory Drugs (NSAIDs)

Current NSAIDs
Aspirin
Ibuprofen
Indomethacin (Indocin)
Diflunisal (Dolobid)
Fenoprofen (Nalfon)
Ketoprofen (Orudis)
Meclofenamic acid (Ponstel)
Naproxen (Naproxyn)
Piroxicam (Feldene)
Sulindac (Clinoril)
Tolmetin (Tolectin)
Ketorolac
Diclofenac

Ch 1. Drug Prescribing and Systematic Detection of Adverse Drug Reactions

I. Adverse drug reactions. After the psychotropic and cardiovascular drugs, the NSAIDs, including aspirin, are the most frequent causes of drug-related morbidity and mortality in the elderly. Important forms of toxicity include gastritis, peptic ulceration and blood loss, and renal insufficiency. All NSAIDs are associated with these adverse drug reactions although some studies have identified piroxicam (Feldene) and sulindac (Clinoril) as clinically safer with respect to renal toxicity. All NSAIDs, except aspirin, cause readily reversible inhibition of platelet function. Aspirin has an irreversible effect on platelet function that lasts for the life of the platelet, 4 to 7 days. All of the NSAIDs can cause allergic reactions ranging from rash to anaphylaxis in patients allergic to aspirin. Aspirin taken chronically even in recommended amounts by the elderly may lead to chronic salicylism, which is characterized by deafness, marked fatigue, confused and withdrawn behavior, metabolic acidosis, and noncardiogenic pulmonary edema. CNS effects include dizziness, anxiety, tinnitus, and confusion and may occur in up to 10 to 20% of the elderly on chronic salicylate therapy. Hepatic reactions are usually mild when they occur, but severe hepatitis has been reported. Aplastic anemia has also been reported with all of the available NSAIDs.

   A. Women older than 65 seem to be at greatest risk of gastrointestinal bleeding and gastric perforation associated with NSAIDs. A history of gastrointestinal (GI) bleeding and concomitant diuretic therapy are the two risk factors identified in this group of patients that predict poor outcome. These patients are also frequently dehydrated. In one retrospective study, sulindac was a statistically significant more common cause of GI bleeding than ibuprofen. It is not clear whether this drug is more ulcerogenic than ibuprofen because of inadequate controls.

   B. A review of Medicaid administrations for elderly patients from two states with diagnoses of nephritis, nephropathy, and hyperkalemia showed a strong correlation with NSAID use. Three distinct renal syndromes are now associated with NSAIDs:
      1. Patients with **dehydration, congestive heart failure, nephrosis, or pre-existing renal insufficiency** develop acute renal failure within days of initiating NSAID therapy. The urine sediment is normal.
      2. Acute interstitial nephritis may occur at any time but usually occurs after months of NSAID exposure. There is no eosinophilia or eosinophiluria or rash. Patients present with the nephrotic syndrome (usually edematous).
      3. Chronic interstitial nephritis has been associated with high-dose NSAIDs and other analgesics for years. Papillary necrosis is frequently present.

II. Adverse drug interactions. NSAIDs increased the bleeding tendency of patients on *Coumadin anticoagulants*. Mixing NSAIDs has no theoretical advantage and may delay excretion of one of the drugs. *Probenecid* reduces excretion of most NSAIDs. All NSAIDs blunt the antihypertensive effects of thiazides, beta-blockers, and ACE inhibitors. Diuretics, in general, have been associated with renal failure in some patients using NSAIDs. Specifically, triamterene and indomethacin, and HCTZ and ketoprofen, are interacting pairs reported to cause renal failure. *Lithium* levels may rise or fall and need to be monitored with concomitant NSAID therapy.

III. Management. Elderly patients at risk of renal failure or GI bleeding need to be advised of these risks when taking OTC ibuprofen. If at all possible, NSAIDs should be reserved for acute inflammation associated with rheumatoid arthritis or osteoarthritis. GI blood loss is usually minimal even in predisposed patients during the first 7 to 10 days unless an active ulcer is present. After the acute flare, NSAIDs should be withdrawn in favor of acetaminophen for chronic pain control. Hypertensives should be warned that OTC ibuprofen and all NSAIDs may elevate blood pressure. Patients should be warned to stop NSAIDs if they become weak or dizzy or develop diarrhea, vomiting, or loss of appetite. The NSAIDs piroxicam (Feldene) and sulindac (Clinoril) appear to have renal-sparing effects in the elderly population.

Oral Hypoglycemic Agents

I. **Management** of non-insulin-dependent, type II diabetes mellitus usually relies on diet, weight control, exercise, and oral sulfonylurea agents **(Table 1-17)**. Although newer oral sulfonylureas, such as glipizide (Glucotrol), appear to offer significant advantages in reducing adverse side effects, be aware of unusual manifestations of hypoglycemic syndromes in the geriatric population. Hypoglycemia, which can be precipitated by oral agents, is a frequently encountered metabolic derangement—especially in the frail elderly—and can present a broad range of neuropsychiatric syndromes and dysfunctions. Typically, CNS findings in the acutely hypoglycemic geriatric patient consist of confusion, mental impairment, delirium, focal deficits, or frank coma.

A. **Renal impairment.** Physicians should maintain a high index of suspicion for hypoglycemic reactions in elderly patients with mild or progressive renal impairment (reflected in a decreased glomerular filtration rate) who are concomitantly taking an oral hypoglycemic agent. Because approximately two thirds of circulating insulin is metabolized in the renal parenchyma, patients with reduced renal mass who are taking insulin-releasing agents are especially prone to elevated circulating insulin levels and secondary hypoglycemia. Thus, in this clinical situation, oral sulfonylurea agents may precipitate hypoglycemia, even though the drug is being taken as prescribed and with adequate, food intake. Initial treatment consists of IV glucose administration with $D_{50}W$ followed by patient education and readjustment of the sulfonylurea dose.

B. Large studies usually point to the **first-generation sulfonylureas** such as chlorpropamide (Diabinese) and tolbutamide (Orinase) as the agents most likely to cause hypoglycemia in the elderly population. Chlorpropamide has a long duration of effect (24 to 60 hours) and elimination half-life (35 hours) and should be used with caution in the elderly. Moreover, secondary drug interactions with phenylbutazone, sulfonamides, salicylates, and NSAIDs can precipitate an increased hypoglycemic effect among the first-generation oral agents.

C. **Glipizide.** A newer, more potent second-generation oral sulfonylurea agent, glipizide (Glucotrol), has a shorter half-life and more rapid onset of action, making it the current oral sulfonylurea of choice in the elderly population. Glyburide (Micronase, Diabeta) is another second-generation agent, but one study of its effects reported 57 cases of severe hypoglycemia, including 24 protracted cases and 10 fatalities. In contrast, glipizide caused neither long-lasting cases of hypoglycemia nor hypoglycemia-induced fatalities in a 7-year study conducted by the Swedish Board of Health and Welfare's Adverse Drug Reaction Advisory Committee.

D. **Glyburide** is also subject to erratic absorption and produces two active metabolites with 1/40 and 1/400 the potencies of the parent compound. The

Table 1-17. Pharmacologic and Pharmacokinetic Activity of Sulfonylurea Agents

Generic name	Brand	Daily dose range (mg)	Duration of effect (hr)	Elimination of half-life (hr)
Tolbutamide	Orinase	500-3,000	6-12	4-5
Tolazamide	Tolinase	100-750	10-16	7
Acetohexamide	Dymelor	500-1,500	12-24	5
Chlorpropamide	Diabinese	100-500	24-60	35
Glyburide	Micronase	2.5-20	24	10
Glipizide	Glucotrol	2.4-50	24	2-4

former metabolite is still five times more potent than the typical first-generation sulfonylurea and, therefore, can produce severe hypoglycemic reactions. In contrast, glipizide does not produce significantly active metabolic breakdown products.

   E. **Insulin-release pattern.** Perhaps most importantly, among all oral sulfonylurea agents, glipizide has the unique capacity to induce a selective glucose (nutrient)-mediated insulin release that closely mimics in vivo insulin release patterns in response to postprandial nutrient loading. This selective release, which appears to be maintained as long as 48 months after glipizide therapy, offers special advantages and reduces adverse side effects in the elderly patient with type II diabetes. Finally, because glipizide, unlike the first-generation agents, is bound nonionically to serum proteins, it is less prone to producing hypoglycemia due to secondary drug interactions. Glipizide has a milligram-for-milligram potency equivalence with glyburide, and has been shown to reduce insulin requirements when used in type I diabetics.

II. **Insulin versus oral agents for adult-onset diabetes.** A major unresolved issue in management of non-insulin-dependent diabetes mellitus (NIDDM) is whether insulin or an oral agent is the treatment of choice for patients who fail dietary therapy. An intense debate among diabetologists has raged ever since the University Group Diabetes Program (UGDP) study cast some doubt on the safety of oral agent therapy. A small but statistically significant increase in cardiac deaths was found in patients treated with oral agents as compared to those treated with insulin. Proponents of oral agent therapy criticized the UGDP study design and argued that oral agents are ideally suited for NIDDM, since they act to lessen peripheral resistance to endogenous insulin, a major cause of NIDDM.

   A. **Oral agents.** The issue of cardiovascular morbidity remains unresolved, although new data may be forthcoming. In the meantime, the advent of a more potent generation of oral agents raises the issue of how well these new preparations compare with insulin regarding control of hyperglycemia, risk of hypoglycemia, correction of hyperlipidemia, and other important risk/benefit parameters. A randomized, double-blind, placebo-controlled study of glyburide versus insulin for long-term metabolic control of NIDDM has just been reported, providing a prospective, controlled comparison of these two modes of therapy.

   1. **The study population** consisted of 31 patients with NIDDM who failed to achieve normal glucose control on a program of diet alone. They were randomized to once-per-day insulin and glyburide placebo, or to glyburide and once-per-day placebo insulin injection. Active agent and placebo were adjusted according to fasting plasma glucose level to achieve a level of less than 115 mg/dL without hypoglycemia. Parameters monitored included weight, fasting serum glucose, hemoglobin A_{1c}, triglyceride, cholesterol, high-density lipoprotein (HDL), and the ratio of HDL to cholesterol. Patients were observed for 9 months.

   2. **Both agents produced similar improvements** in fasting blood sugar and hemoglobin A_{1c} levels, similar degrees of weight gain, similar frequencies of mild symptomatic hypoglycemia, and significant reductions in serum lipid levels. Nearly normal degrees of blood glucose control were achieved. Patients in both treatment groups showed significant improvements in HDL levels and HDL: cholesterol, but those treated with insulin had a signifi-

cantly greater improvements in these parameters than did those treated with glyburide.
3. **The authors concluded** that glyburide and once-per-day insulin therapy provide similar and very adequate degrees of glucose control in NIDDM patients who have failed on diet alone. Insulin appears to have the advantage of producing a more favorable lipid profile, although the long-term benefits of this effect are not known.

Cholesterol-Reducing Agents

I. **Diabetic patients.** According to the Framingham Heart Study, the prevalence of coronary artery disease in the diabetic patient is about twice that in the general population. Although the increased susceptibility to heart disease is almost certainly related in part to impaired glucose homeostasis, the patient with NIDDM is also susceptible to abnormalities in the lipoprotein metabolism that include increases in plasma VLDL triglycerides and VLDL and LDL cholesterol and decreases in HDL cholesterol. Based on epidemiologic studies in the general population, there is evidence to suggest that pharmacologic and/or dietary interventions that achieve beneficial effects on plasma lipid levels (i.e., reduction in serum LDL and VLDL cholesterol and elevation of HDL cholesterol) may decrease the risk of coronary heart disease in patients with NIDDM.

II. **Lovastatin.** The investigators of this double-blind, randomized, placebo-controlled study employed lovastatin, a potent inhibitor of 3-hydroxy-3-methylglutaryl-coenzyme-A reductase, to determine whether significant reductions in plasma cholesterol levels could be achieved in 16 NIDDM patients on glyburide therapy with mild to moderate elevations of plasma lipids. Patients ranged in age from 41 to 70 years, with a mean age of 61 years. Based on plasma lipid levels determined at the beginning of the study and 28 days after therapy, the authors concluded that, when compared to placebo, lovastatin reduced total cholesterol by 26%, LDL by 28%, and LDL apolipoprotein B by 26%. In addition, lovastatin therapy reduced plasma triglycerides and VLDL cholesterol by 31% and 42%, respectively. Although there was no change in the plasma level of HDL cholesterol, the ratio of total cholesterol to HDL cholesterol fell by 29%. No side effects or abnormalities in the serum values of hepatic enzymes or creatine kinase were noted during short-term lovastatin therapy.

A. **Risk reduction.** These investigators point out that, according to available data, an average reduction in total cholesterol levels of 26%, as observed with lovastatin therapy, should reduce the risk of coronary heart disease by about 50%. This reduction in risk, they conclude, should put patients with NIDDM at about the same baseline risk for heart disease as the general population.

B. **Effectiveness.** The relative importance of multiple factors that place patients with NIDDM at increased risk for heart disease is not precisely known. Nevertheless, reduction of elevated plasma cholesterol and triglyceride levels with dietary or pharmacologic intervention is advisable in diabetic patients with risk factors for coronary artery disease. Although this study was conducted on a limited number of patients for a short period of time, it demonstrates the efficacy of lovastatin therapy in significantly reducing total cholesterol levels. Based on these data, lovastatin can be expected to improve the plasma lipid

Anxiolytic and Sedative-Hypnotic Drugs
(Table 1-18)

I. **Benzodiazepines.** These agents are frequently used to relieve short-term anxiety in geriatric patients. Diazepam (Valium) has a longer half-life than most other benzodiazepines. Other such agents with long half-lives include chlordiazepoxide (Librium), flurazepam (Dalmane), clorazepate (Tranxene), and prazepam (Centrax). In general, these drugs should be avoided in the elderly population. Somnolence, confusion, and depression are the most common presenting symptoms of anxiolytic toxicity associated with long-acting benzodiazepines. Drugs with shorter half-lives, such as triazolam (Halcion), oxazepam (Serax), alprazolam (Xanax), and lorazepam (Ativan) are preferable anxiolytics for the elderly. Benzodiazepines are also effective sedative hypnotics. Flurazepam is the most common, but, like diazepam, it has a long half-life. Thirty-nine percent of elderly patients receiving the usual 30 mg dose of flurazepam have significant CNS depression due to accumulation of the drug. A shorter-acting benzodiazepine, such as temazepam (Restoril) or alprazolam, may be an improvement, requiring only a dosage reduction.

II. **Minimizing symptoms of benzodiazepine withdrawal syndrome: guidelines and strategies for drug cessation in benzodiazepine-addicted patients.** Although some patients are appropriate candidates for long-term benzodiazepine use, studies show that approximately 25% to 55% of patients presently on chronic anxiolytic therapy do not demonstrate sufficient indications for long-term use and should be discontinued from the drug. Unfortunately, managing benzodiazepine withdrawal can be a frustrating and challenging clinical problem in addicted patients who have agitation, nervousness, anxiety, lethargy, and perceptual disturbances as the drug is discontinued. Although the difficulties associated with physician-limited benzodiazepine cessation are bandied about through the oral tradition, few good studies are available that provide a workable clinical strategy for facilitating discontinuation of this overused medication.

   A. **Two thorough investigations** from the psychopharmacology research units at the University of Pennsylvania and Tufts University School of Medicine compared the effects of abrupt (57 patients) versus gradual taper (63 patients) of therapeutic doses of short half-life (SHL) and long half-life (LHL) benzodiazepines in benzodiazepine-addicted patients (daily use >1 year). For evaluation of the withdrawal syndrome associated with abrupt cessation, benzodiazepine intake was stabilized for 3 weeks before double-blind assignment to placebo (n = 47), or continued benzodiazepine use (n = 20). Depending on outcome criteria used, investigators found that 58% to 100% of patients had a withdrawal reaction, with peak severity of such symptoms observed at 2 days for SHL and 4 to 7 days for LHL benzodiazepines. Many of the withdrawal reactions were judged to be moderate to severe. Relapse back to benzodiazepine use occurred in 27% of patients receiving LHL benzodiazepines and in 57% of patients receiving SHL preparations. The presence of non-

Table 1-18. Sedative-Hypnotic and Anxiolytic Drugs in the Elderly

Drug	FDA approved	Half-life (hr)	Usual initial dose for the elderly	Drug name
Flurazepam	Hypnotic	50-100 (major metabolite)	15 mg at bedtime	Dalmane
Temazepam	Hypnotic	5-15	15 mg at bedtime	Restoril
Oxazepam	Anxiolytic	5-20	10 mg three times a day	Serax
Diazepam	Anxiolytic	20-100 (major metabolite)	2 mg per day or twice a day	Valium
Lorazepam	Anxiolytic	10-20	0.5-2 mg/day	Ativan
Triazolam	Hypnotic	2.3	0.125 mg	Halcion
Alprazolam	Anxiolytic	12-15	0.25 mg-1.0 mg three times a day	Xanax

panic diagnosis, higher benzodiazepine dose, and high scores on tests for neuroticism predicted relapse. For the abrupt discontinuation arm of the study, only 46% of LHL and 48% of SHL benzodiazepine-treated patients were free of the drug at 5 weeks.

B. **For the gradual taper arm** of the study, patients were permitted an incremental reduction of benzodiazepines, at a dose reduction rate of 25% per week, whether they were taking SHL or LHL compounds. Patients who were unable to tolerate the taper at the aforementioned rate were permitted to slow the taper rate as needed. Among those permitted the gradual taper option, 90% had a withdrawal syndrome, but it was rarely more than mild to moderate as judged by the absence of precipitated seizures, psychosis, or other serious withdrawal symptoms, or the need for inpatient management. Overall, 32% of LHL and 42% of SHL benzodiazepine-treated patients were unable to tolerate taper and either continued or resumed their daily use of benzodiazepines. At 5 weeks, 56% of LHL and 53% of SHL benzodiazepine-treated patients were drug-free according to inquiry and drug-level evaluations.

C. **Minimizing withdrawal severity.** This study is helpful because it tries to support anecdotal clinical experience, which endorses gradual rather than abrupt taper for benzodiazepine-addicted patients. Using well-matched groups and performing double-blind assessments of the withdrawal syndrome, this study confirms that use of a gradual taper schedule minimizes the contribution of benzodiazepine daily dose and half-life to withdrawal severity that is observed with abrupt benzodiazepine withdrawal.

D. **Discontinuation.** This study suggests a rational approach to discontinuation of benzodiazepines in patients who have used the drug daily for at least 1 year. The results confirm that in long-term benzodiazepine users, a withdrawal syndrome can be expected, even when low-to-moderate therapeutic doses of benzodiazepines are gradually tapered at the rate of 25% per week or less. More importantly, however, gradual taper significantly minimizes withdrawal symptoms to the point that no statistically significant differences in 5-week drug-free outcome or in withdrawal severity were observed in SHL and LHL benzodiazepines. It should be emphasized that more than one half of patients who undergo gradual taper will require an extended taper requiring dose reductions of less than 25% per week. Because of the severity of the withdrawal symptoms observed in the abrupt discontinuation group, we support the investigators' conclusion that gradual benzodiazepine taper offers distinct advantages over precipitous cessation, especially for those taking SHL benzodiazepines.

III. **Midazolam** (Versed) is a new ultra-short-acting parenteral benzodiazepine with excellent amnestic properties. It is particularly advantageous for inducing conscious sedation in elderly patients. An average dose not exceeding 1.0 or 1.5 mg of midazolam by slow IV infusion (0.018 mg/kg) is recommended. Versed has an average elimination half-life of about 2 1/2 hours, and sedation usually occurs within 2 to 4 minutes. Because respiratory depression can occur, the use of midazolam should be restricted to settings where emergency intubation can be performed.

IV. **Cimetidine** (Tagamet) and disulfiram (Antabuse) both inhibit metabolism of the long-acting benzodiazepines, diazepam and chlordiazepoxide. Oxazepam (Serax), bracepam, temazepam, and alprazolcem are unaffected by these drugs. Alcohol potentiates the CNS depression of all benzodiazepines.

V. Triazolam. Triazolam is the most widely prescribed hypnotic in the United States. Its relatively short serum half-life (approximately 6 hours) reduces the risks of daytime sedation and cumulative sedation compared with longer-acting hypnotics such as flurazepam (Dalmane). However, behavioral disturbances and impairment of memory have been reported, with particular concern for the elderly who seem to be more "sensitive" to the medication. The mechanism(s) and severity of the susceptibility to the adverse effects of triazolam remain incompletely defined and the subject of considerable research.

  A. Investigators at the New England Medical Center in Boston conducted a four-way crossover study of the effects of triazolam, comparing psychomotor performance, memory, and degree of sedation in 26 young volunteers (mean age, 30 years) and 21 healthy elderly persons (mean age, 69 years). The study began with a single-blind adaptation trial with placebo, followed by random, double-blind single doses of placebo, 0.125 mg of triazolam, and 0.25 mg of triazolam. In addition to the parameters noted above, plasma drug levels were monitored and clearances determined. Given the same doses, elderly subjects manifested higher serum levels than did the younger participants, resulting from a 50% reduction in drug clearance. Degree of sedation and psychomotor retardation were greater in the elderly, paralleling their increases in serum triazolam levels. Recall of information presented 1½ hours after a dose and requested at 24 hours was equally impaired in both young and old subjects.

  B. Single-dose therapy. This study examines only a very discrete situation, namely single-dose therapy in healthy patients. Although such usage is common, the data presented here do not address the effects of repeated doses or the impact of such use on patients who are ill or taking other drugs that may add to the sedative effect. Moreover, there is no attempt to study the important issue of behavioral disturbances resulting from the drug's use. The study's strength is in defining an important mechanism of the drug's heightened effects in the elderly, namely reduced clearance. Therefore, a given single dose of triazolam causes greater sedation and impairment of psychomotor function in the elderly than in the young. This appears to be due to a 50% reduction in drug clearance in the elderly. No intrinsic sensitivity to the drug was demonstrated.

  C. The approximately 50% reduction in drug clearance and the absence of evidence for a specific drug sensitivity suggests that reduced single doses of triazolam can be used in the elderly for sleep. Dosage should be cut by 50% from that which would be appropriate for a young patient. A reasonable single dose might be 0.125 mg. One might even consider prescribing just half of a 0.125 mg tablet, as this is likely to have the same sedative effect of 0.125 mg would have in a young person. It is essential that the cause of insomnia be determined before it is deemed safe to use any sedative. Nocturnal heart failure, sleep apnea, and depression are among the very important conditions that may cause insomnia but not be appropriate for sedative use. Even when it is appropriate to use triazolam, only a small number of pills should be dispensed at any one time, and the patient and family should be carefully instructed against the routine or daily use of the medication. The issue of an idiosyncratic behavioral disturbance triggered by triazolam remains a concern, and the literature should be followed carefully for more details about its occurrence and identifying patients at risk.

Antidepressants

The necessity for distinguishing between better and worse pharmacologic options is especially important in geriatric patients, where side effects, drug interactions, half-life of medications, and functional considerations play a critical role in pharmacologic management. In the treatment of major depression in the elderly, for example, selective serotonin reuptake inhibitors (SSRIs) have clear advantages over other classes of antidepressants. Although all SSRIs are free of the myocardial and CNS effects characteristic of tricyclic antidepressants (TCAs), there are still significant differences among the three marketed drugs in this class that indicate sertraline (Zoloft) may represent a better choice for the management of depression in the elderly. Unlike fluoxetine (Prozac) and paroxetine (Paxil), sertraline has linear pharmacokinetics in both young and elderly patients. Thus, special dosing is not required in older patients. Moreover, unlike fluoxetine, neither sertraline nor paroxetine has metabolites with clinically significant activity with regard to serotonin reuptake inhibition. A final advantage is that sertraline does not produce clinically meaningful inhibition of the P-450 IID6 isoenzyme at its effective, minimum dose, unlike paroxetine and fluoxetine. The reduced potential for pharmacokinetic drug-drug interactions with sertraline is especially important in elderly patients who are likely to be taking a variety of medications concomitantly. The elderly are particularly sensitive to the adverse effects of cyclic antidepressants (CAs). The most common presenting symptoms of CA toxicity include sedation, anticholinergic effects, adrenergic hyperactivity (tremulousness, sweating), and cardiovascular toxicity. Anticholinergic effects include dry mouth, constipation, blurred vision, urinary retention, decreased sweating, and hyperthermic reactions **(Table 1-19)**.

I. **Anticholinergic CNS effects**—which may cause delirium, agitation, visual hallucinations, decreased thirst—precipitated by CAs are frequently underdiagnosed. Lack of sweating and decreased thirst can produce dehydration and electrolyte imbalances that can be fatal in the elderly population. Orthostatic hypotension due to anticholinergic toxicity can cause falls, myocardial infarction, and cerebrovascular events. Cardiovascular effects due to antidepressant toxicity in the elderly include an anticholinergic effect which can increase the heart rate and a quinidine-like effect which may increase PR, QRS, and QTc intervals.

II. **CA overdose has serious cardiotoxic effects** that are not usually present at the therapeutic doses. Because of the cardiovascular effects associated with overdose, researchers anticipated an increased incidence of sudden death and arrhythmia among elderly patients using cyclic antidepressants. The Boston Collaborative Drug Surveillance Program, however, has demonstrated that neither occurs, even in the presence of organic heart disease, which is so common in the elderly.

III. **Monoamine oxidase inhibitors.** Although pharmacologic treatment of depression is effective in the elderly, monoamine oxidase inhibitors should be avoided because of the risks of serious drug interactions and the frequency of orthostatic hypotension. Common practice dictates that agitated or anxious depressions should be treated with sedating drugs (amitriptyline or doxepin) and retarded depressions should be treated with less sedating agents (nortriptyline or desipramine). Orthostatic hypotension, which can cause falls, is probably the most dangerous side effect. Doxepin and nortriptyline cause fewer incidents of postural hypotension. Their major cardiac toxicity is interference with cardiac

Table 1-19. Adverse Effects and Toxicity of Tricyclic and Tetracyclic Antidepressants

Structural class	Trade name	Young adult	Elderly	Sedative properties	Anticholinergic properties
Tricyclic					
Tertiary amine					
Amitriptyline	Elavil	100-300 mg	25-150 mg	+++	+++
Imipramine	Tofranil	100-300 mg	25-150 mg	++	+++
Doxepin	Sinequan	100-300 mg	25-150 mg	+++	+++
Trimipramine	Surmontil	100-300 mg	25-150 mg	+++	+++
Secondary amine					
Nortriptyline	Pamelor	50-100 mg	10-60 mg	+	+++
Desipramine	Norpramin	100-300 mg	25-150 mg	0	++
Protriptyline	Vivactil	20-60 mg	5-30 mg	0	+++
Dibenzoxazepine (amoxapine)	Asendin	150-300 mg	25-150 mg	++	+++
Triazolopyridine (trazodone)	Desyrel	150-400 mg	50-300 mg	+++	+
Tetracyclic maprotiline	Ludiomil	100-300 mg	25-150 mg	++	+++
Selective serotonin reuptake inhibitor (SSRI):					
Sertraline	Zoloft	50-200 mg	50-100 mg	0	0
Fluoxetine	Prozac	20-40 mg	10-20 mg	0	0
Paroxetine	Paxil	20-50 mg	10-40 mg	0	0

conduction. At high risk are patients with pre-existing bundle branch block or sinus node dysfunction.
IV. **Doxepin** has the fewest adverse effects on the heart. However, anticholinergic effects, such as dry mouth, urinary hesitance or retention, and constipation, are common. The most serious anticholinergic effect is confusion or delirium, for which the underlying cause frequently goes unrecognized in the emergency department setting. Amitriptyline and doxepin are the most potent anticholinergics, and desipramine is the least. Other miscellaneous side effects include increased appetite and weight gain, decreased seizure threshold, and increased anxiety.

Treatment of Diabetic Neuropathy: The Role of Antidepressants

Diabetic peripheral neuropathy can be very painful and difficult to manage. Although there is some suspicion that improved glycemic control may help prevent severe neuropathy, treatment of established disease remains a challenge. Tricyclic antidepressants have been used for more than a decade to control pain in patients with diabetic peripheral neuropathy, and controlled studies demonstrate some efficacy. The mechanism of pain control is a subject of research interest, with practical implications for drug selection. Amitriptyline, the prototype tricyclic used for diabetic peripheral neuropathy, inhibits reuptake of norepinephrine and serotonin in the central nervous system. Desipramine, another tricyclic, is more selective than amitriptyline for inhibition of norepinephrine reuptake. Often, the anticholinergic side effects of many tricyclics are difficult to tolerate, leading to a search for an alternative antidepressant. The nontricyclic antidepressant fluoxetine (Prozac) has been suggested as an alternative. It selectively inhibits reuptake of serotonin.

I. **Painful diabetic peripheral neuropathy.** Researchers at the National Institutes of Health conducted a series of randomized, double-blind, crossover studies of patients with painful diabetic peripheral neuropathy, comparing amitriptyline, desipramine, and fluoxetine. The study objectives were to assess relative efficacy and to better understand the mechanism(s) of their effect on diabetic neuropathic pain. Recruitment was done by advertisement; 57 patients qualified and entered one or both of the studies. Two separate studies were conducted: one compared desipramine with amitriptyline, and the other compared fluoxetine with placebo. The outcome measures examined were daily pain score and end-of-study global pain rating. Appropriate periods of washout before and during each phase were included. Each treatment phase lasted 7 weeks, followed by a washout period and crossover for another 7 weeks of treatment. Doses were titrated to the maximum tolerated.

   A. **Mean daily dose** was 105 mg for amitriptyline, 111 mg for desipramine, and 40 mg for fluoxetine. Seventy-four percent of patients reported moderate or greater pain relief during the "blinded" use of amitriptyline; 61% during the use of desipramine; and 41% during the use of placebo. The differences between amitriptyline and desipramine were not significant, nor were those between fluoxetine and placebo. Amitriptyline and desipramine were effective even in patients who were not depressed, whereas fluoxetine worked only when there was an underlying depression.

   B. **Protocol.** This set of studies is well designed in that there was randomization and a double-blinded, placebo-controlled crossover protocol. Patient selection

was probably biased because it depended on responses to advertisements, but careful patient evaluation and diagnosis ensured full confirmation and characterization of each patient's condition, including the presence of concurrent depression. The sample sizes were sufficient to give the studies a power of 0.8, the usually accepted standard for detecting a meaningful difference between treatments. The presence of depression was also taken into account as a potentially important factor in determining response to therapy. The study indicates that amitriptyline and desipramine are equally effective for treatment of pain caused by diabetic peripheral neuropathy, regardless of the presence of depression. Fluoxetine appears to work only in the context of depression, suggesting it has no direct effect on the mechanism of pain in diabetic peripheral neuropathy.

II. Tricyclic therapy. Painful diabetic peripheral neuropathy unresponsive to mild analgesics such as aspirin or acetaminophen should be considered a reasonable indication for a trial of tricyclic therapy. However, many patients find it difficult to tolerate the marked anticholinergic side effects of amitriptyline, especially when the drug is used in dosages approaching 100 mg/day. This study indicates that desipramine and other tricyclics with lesser anticholinergic activity (e.g., nortriptyline) may be reasonable alternatives to amitriptyline. The study suggests that the reason for the beneficial effect of these agents is related to their blockade of norepinephrine reuptake, distinguishing them from fluoxetine, which does not block norepinephrine reuptake and which did not provide significant pain relief. We recommend that patients with neuropathic pain caused by diabetic neuropathy be given a 6-week trial of tricyclic therapy, building up to a dosage of approximately 100 mg/day. Fluoxetine appears to have no direct effect on neuropathic pain.

Antipsychotic Drugs

Several major psychiatric disorders in the elderly are treated with antipsychotic and neurologic agents. Complications of this treatment include tardive dyskinesia (five times more common in the elderly), akathisias, dystonias, pseudoparkinsonism, and anticholinergic side effects similar to those discussed above **(Table 1-20)**.

I. NMS. A major adverse reaction to neuroleptics is neuroleptic malignant syndrome (NMS), which is frequently unrecognized in the elderly. NMS consists of fever, rigidity, autonomic instability, and mental status changes.

II. Symptoms. With the widespread use of both cyclic antidepressants and antipsychotics, 12% of all elderly ambulatory patients and 25% of those hospitalized in nursing homes now receive two or more drugs with anticholinergic effects. In general, studies show that clinicians do not choose drugs within a given class to minimize anticholinergic effects. Consequently, suspect an anticholinergic reaction in elderly patients with symptoms of urinary retention, acute glaucoma, delirium, hallucinations, seizures, dysarthria, hyperthermia, tachycardia, and even heart block—especially if the patient has taken drugs in one or more of the anticholinergic classes.

Anticoagulants

Heparin and warfarin (Coumadin) causes complications in the elderly population. Oral anticoagulants are also associated with a high incidence of skin necrosis in obese, elderly women, especially in areas rich in fat (breast, buttock, and thighs). Drugs can

Table 1-20. Adverse Effects of Antipsychotic Medications in the Elderly

Drug and dose for elderly	Relative potency	Sedation	Extra-pyramidal	Anticholinergic	Orthostatic hypotension
Chlorpromazine (Thorazine) 10-25 mg b.i.d. t.i.d.	100	+++	++	+++	++
Thioridazine (Mellaril) 10-25 mg b.i.d. t.i.d.	95-100	+++	+	+++	++
Thiothixene (Navane) 2-3 mg	5	+	+++	+	+
Haloperidol (Haldol) 0.5-2 mg	2	+	+++	+	+
Fluphenazine (Prolixin) 0.5-2 mg	2	+	+++	+	+

Table 1-21. Possible Drug Interactions with Anticoagulants

Decrease vitamin K	Displace anticoagulant	Inhibit metabolism	Other
Antibiotics	Phenylbutazone	Chloramphenicol	Thyroid drugs
Cholestyramine	Salicylates	Allopurinol	Anabolic steroids
Mineral oil	Sulfonamides	Nortriptyline	Quinidine
	Sulfonylureas	Disulfiram	Glucagon
	Ethacrynic acid	Metronidazole	
	Mefenamic acid	Alcohol (acute ingestion)	
	Nalidixic acid	Phenylbutazone	
	Diazoxide	Cimetidine	
		Fluconazole	

Table 1-22. Drugs That Diminish Anticoagulant Drug Activity

Induction of enzymes	Increased procoagulant factors
Barbiturates	Estrogens
Glutethimide	Oral contraceptives
Ethchlorvynol	Vitamin K
Griseofulvin	
Phenytoin	
Carbamazepine	
Rifampin	
Chlorinated insecticides	

Table 1-23. Drugs Potentiating Anticoagulant Drug Effects

Inhibition of platelet aggregation	Inhibition of procoagulant factors	Ulcerogenic drugs
Salicylates	Quinidine	Sulfinpyrazone
Sulfinpyrazone	Antimetabolites	Salicylates
Dipyridamole	Alkylating agents	Adrenal corticosteroids
NSAIDs	Salicylates	

increase the anticoagulant effect in the elderly by the following mechanisms: displacement of anticoagulant from binding sites, inhibition of hepatic microsomal enzymes, or other mechanisms not understood (Tables 1-21 through 1-23).

I. **Thromboembolic prophylaxis: Coumadin.** Overall, the stroke rate for patients with chronic atrial fibrillation is about 5% per year. However, this arrhythmia is a heterogenous disorder, and in certain subgroups (i.e., the elderly, those with recent MI, and those with a history of hypertension), the stroke rate is greater than 5% per year. At one time, rheumatic heart disease was the disorder most commonly associated with atrial fibrillation, but currently nonvalvular heart disease accounts for more than 70% of the cases of atrial fibrillation. Despite the clear association between atrial fibrillation and stroke, the role of long-term anticoagulant therapy or long-term antiplatelet therapy for prevention of thromboembolic cerebral infarction remains unclear. Fortunately, in the last few years there have been four, large prospective randomized trials that have examined the risks and benefits of antithrombotic therapy for patients with nonvalvular atrial fibrillation. The results were presented during a recent symposium at Stanford University Medical Center, and the highlights of this conference were published in the *Annals of Internal Medicine*. Collectively, these studies represent more than 4300 patient years of follow-up observation in subjects who were randomly assigned to warfarin (Coumadin; DuPont, Wilmington, Del.), aspirin, or control groups. The purpose of this symposium was to review the evaluation and management of patients with atrial fibrillation, with a special emphasis on assessing the risks and benefits associated with low-dose anticoagulant therapy and antiplatelet stroke prevention.

II. **Criteria.** Not surprisingly, the treatment in each study focused on elderly patients, with the average age in most trials about 70 years. In general, patients who were not good candidates for anticoagulant therapy were excluded from prospective trials (except in the Stroke Prevention in Atrial Fibrillation Trial, where such patients were assigned to receive either aspirin or placebo). Generally, exclusionary criteria were based on the anticipated risk for bleeding with oral anticoagulants and included a history of bleeding disorders, previous hemorrhage, active peptic ulcer disease, alcoholism, uncontrolled hypertension, gait disorders predisposing to falls, and severe renal or hepatic disease. Because recommendations for optimal intensity of anticoagulant therapy have been substantially modified during the past 2 years, the target range for optimal intensity of therapy varied between prothrombin time (PT) ratios of 1.5 to 2.0 (the highest) in The Copenhagen Atrial Fibrillation, Aspirin, and Anticoagulant Study (AFASAK) to PT ratios of 1.2 to 1.5 in the Boston Area Anticoagulation Trial for Atrial Fibrillation (BAATAF).

III. **The Copenhagen Atrial Fibrillation, Aspirin, and Anticoagulant Study.** The AFASAK trial provided the first prospective, randomized evaluation of treatment options for patients with atrial fibrillation. The study included 1,007 patients with nonrheumatic atrial fibrillation who were randomly assigned to treatment with aspirin, 75 mg/day, warfarin (PT ratio, 1.5 to 2.0), or placebo. The investigators planned a 2-year treatment duration. Perhaps the most important drawback of AFASAK was the large dropout rate in the warfarin group; overall, 38% of the patients assigned to warfarin ceased therapy before completion of the study, compared with only 13% to 15% in the aspirin and placebo groups, respectively. The most common reason cited for withdrawal from the warfarin group was the inconvenience of frequent blood sampling required for monitoring of bleeding times. Bleeding-related side effects occurred in 6% of patients assigned to receive warfarin (two considered serious, including one fatality) and in 1% of patients assigned to receive aspirin.

- **A. Premature end.** The AFASAK trial was stopped prematurely by the data-monitoring statistician because a substantial reduction in thromboembolic complications (stroke, transient ischemic attack, systemic embolization, or intracranial hemorrhage) was observed in the warfarin group. Overall, only 4 cerebral infarctions and 1 fatal intracerebral hemorrhage occurred in the warfarin group, whereas 20 and 21 thromboembolic complications occurred in the aspirin and placebo groups, respectively. It is interesting and perhaps clinically important to note that of the four patients in the warfarin group who had cerebral infarctions, only one was receiving adequate anticoagulant therapy at the time of the event.
- **B. Despite the large dropout rate** in the warfarin group, the intention-to-treat analysis showed a significant reduction in total thromboembolic events (risk reduction, 56%) in the warfarin group, but no such reduction in thromboembolic events among those receiving aspirin, 75 mg/day.

IV. The Stroke Prevention in Atrial Fibrillation Study (SPAF). The SPAF was a multicenter trial comparing warfarin and aspirin therapy with placebo in patients with nonrheumatic atrial fibrillation. The design called for the enrollment of 1,644 patients during a 3-year period, with an additional year of follow-up observation before termination. Like AFASAK, SPAF was terminated by the safety monitoring committee because significant benefit was found with active aspirin or warfarin therapy. When the study was interrupted, 627 patients were enrolled in the anticoagulation group and 703 in the nonanticoagulation group. Analysis of the data at the time of study cessation demonstrated an acceptably low bleeding risk and a thromboembolic event rate of 2.3% per year in the warfarin group, 3.6% in the aspirin group, and 7.4% in the placebo group, for an overall warfarin-associated risk reduction of 67%. Interestingly, once again, only two of the six patients with strokes on warfarin were receiving adequate anticoagulant therapy. The advantage of aspirin in this study was limited to younger patients, with no stroke reduction observed in patients older than 75 years.

V. Boston Area Anticoagulation Trial for Atrial Fibrillation (BAATAF). The BAATAF was an unblinded, randomized, controlled study performed to test the safety and efficacy of low-dose warfarin therapy for preventing stroke in patients with nonrheumatic atrial fibrillation. Overall, 212 patients received anticoagulant therapy for an average of 2.3 patient years, and the control group consisted of 208 subjects. Only 10% of those started on warfarin discontinued the drug. The mean PT ratio of those with active therapy was 1.33. Thirteen strokes occurred in the control group, whereas only two occurred in the warfarin group, yielding a stroke rate of 0.4% per patient year for the warfarin group and 3.0% in the control group. Minor bleeding occurred in 7.8% of those patients in the warfarin group, with only 4 of 38 patients requiring hospitalization. Of special note is that patients with "lone atrial fibrillation" (no overt evidence of clinical heart disease) had one third of the incidence of stroke. The Boston study demonstrated that low-intensity anticoagulation in patients with nonrheumatic atrial fibrillation was safe and effective, and could yield a stroke reduction rate as high as 86% per patient year.

VI. The Canadian Atrial Fibrillation Anticoagulation Study (CAFA). The CAFA was a randomized, double-blind, multicentered, placebo-controlled trial of warfarin in patients with nonrheumatic atrial fibrillation. Consisting of

187 patients in the warfarin group and 191 in the placebo group, the study yielded an annual combined event rate for nonlacunar stroke and non-CNS embolism of 2.5% in the warfarin group and 5.2% in the placebo control group. Although the reduction in the risk for systemic embolization that was attributable to warfarin therapy was not statistically significant, the study lacked statistical power. Nevertheless, the discussant emphasized that the trend in warfarin therapy seen in this study is consistent with and supportive of the positive results with warfarin found in the other three aforementioned randomized studies of atrial fibrillation.

VII. **Follow-up.** Although each of the trials discussed was different with respect to entry criteria, patient profile, level of intensity of anticoagulation, and end points measured, the large number of patient follow-up years evaluated (4,300) in a subgroup of patients with nonvalvular atrial fibrillation provides statistically significant data for directing clinical management of patients with this condition. All studies show a substantially reduced incidence of stroke and a low incidence of significant bleeding in patients treated with warfarin. Overall, the benefits in stroke reduction appear to outweigh the risks for serious bleeding in patients with atrial fibrillation. Clearly, further studies will be required to identify the precise role of aspirin in such patients, and the relative risks and benefits of using warfarin for prevention of stroke in patients with lone atrial fibrillation.

VIII. **Atrial fibrillation.** With its propensity for causing thromboembolic cerebrovascular infarction; atrial fibrillation is a common disease that has the potential for killing and disabling thousands of elderly Americans each year. It should be emphasized that atrial fibrillation has a prevalence of about 2% in the general population but is more common in the elderly, affecting about 5% of persons older than 60 years. With an association between 6% and 24% in ischemic strokes and 50% in cardioembolic strokes, clinicians now recognize that chronic atrial fibrillation in older patients with coronary artery disease is a quietly festering but deadly condition that, before the aforementioned studies were published and discussed, many physicians chose not to treat because of the perception that the hemorrhagic risks of anticoagulant therapy would outweigh the benefits.

   A. **Nonvalvular atrial fibrillation.** It is clear from these four major trials that this perception has been irrevocably altered, for it now appears that most patients with nonvalvular atrial fibrillation, especially those at high risk for stroke and who are candidates for anticoagulation, will benefit from long-term warfarin therapy. Despite overall trial results showing a statistical benefit of low-intensity (PT ratio 1.3 to 1.5) warfarin therapy, it is critical to identify the precise subgroup of patients who would benefit the most from this intervention and to identify those patients in whom the risk/benefit equation with anticoagulation therapy is not yet entirely proven.

   B. **"State-of-the-stroke"** clinical strategies for prevention of thromboembolic cerebral infarction can be summarized as follows:

      1. **Chronic atrial fibrillation with coronary artery disease.** The elderly patient with chronic nonvalvular atrial fibrillation and underlying coronary heart disease is perhaps the most likely to benefit from long-term, low-intensity warfarin therapy. If attempts at restoration of normal sinus rhythm have failed or are contraindicated, patients with chronic atrial fibrillation who are good candidates for warfarin therapy (i.e., low risk of bleeding, well-controlled hypertension, no history of falling, etc.) should

be started on long-term warfarin therapy; however, it should be stressed that because studies looking at clinical end points have been conducted for less than 2 years, the precise benefits and risks of long-term anticoagulation are simply not known.

2. **Chronic atrial fibrillation without coronary artery disease.** The stroke rate in younger patients without underlying cardiovascular disease appears to be less than 0.5% per year. At present, the degree of stroke reduction that could be anticipated from anticoagulant therapy favors treatment.

3. **Paroxysmal atrial fibrillation (PAF).** Because patients with PAF are not well represented in these studies, few specific conclusions can be drawn regarding warfarin use in this subgroup. In general, anticoagulation is not recommended in this group, with the following exception: the small minority of patients with PAF who have had thromboembolic events (transient ischemic attacks, etc.). These patients have demonstrated that they are at high risk for such events and should be considered for long-term warfarin therapy.

4. **Aspirin versus warfarin.** The value of aspirin in stroke prevention is less clear. One study (AFASAK) demonstrated no benefit with 75 mg/day of aspirin, whereas another (SPAF) using 325 mg/day showed a statistically significant improvement in stroke reduction. A recent study, however, evaluating low-dose aspirin (30 mg/day) in prevention of transient ischemic attacks tends to cast a generally favorable cast on aspirin as a useful pharmacotherapeutic adjunct in cerebrovascular disease. The role of aspirin-mediated antiplatelet action, although undefined, is best characterized as a low-risk, potentially beneficial maneuver in (1) patients with lone atrial fibrillation and (2) in patients with chronic nonvalvular atrial fibrillation who are tenuous candidates for anticoagulation but would probably tolerate long-term aspirin therapy.

5. **Intensity of therapy.** Although intensity of anticoagulation varied in the studies cited, it appears as if PT ratios between 1.4 and 1.5 are as effective as ratios of 1.5 to 2.0. Consequently, the lower range is recommended with the qualification that subsequent studies may demonstrate that stroke prevention can be accomplished with still lower PT ratios.

6. **Monitoring anticoagulation therapy.** An important empirical observation to emerge from two of these studies is that a significant minority of patients who sustained a thromboembolus while on warfarin had a subtherapeutic PT ratio. This observation stresses the importance of vigilant monitoring of warfarin therapy to prevent morbidity associated with overcoagulation and undercoagulation.

H_2 Antagonists

I. **Cimetidine.** A commonly prescribed drug among the elderly population, cimetidine (Tagamet) can cause sedation and confusion, especially in doses above 1,000 mg/day. Aside from this direct adverse reaction, side effects are very few **(Table 1-24).**

　A. **Dangers.** However, because cimetidine is a potent inhibitor of the P-450 hepatic microsomal oxidation enzymes, it blocks metabolism of many other drugs that may be taken concurrently, increasing their effect on plasma levels. This leads to a number of potentially dangerous drug interactions. In patients

Table 1-24. Adverse Drug Interactions in Combination with Cimetidine (Tagamet)

- With warfarin, prothrombin time rises 20 to 200%.
- With benzodiazepines, increases sedation.
- With theophylline, increases in theophylline from therapeutic to toxic range (narrow therapeutic range).
- With beta-blockers, toxic effects may appear, such as bradycardia, hypotension, arrhythmias.
- With carbamazepine (Tegretol) and phenytoin (Dilantin), elevated levels of anticonvulsants, especially in the elderly, over several days.
- With lidocaine, 60 to 90% increase in serum levels occurred with maintenance infusion; study conducted in the elderly. Cimetidine therapy was new in these patients.

taking warfarin (Coumadin), the prothrombin time can rise 20 to 200%. Both diazepam (Valium) and chlordiazepoxide (Librium) can cause increased sedation. Theophylline levels can increase from the therapeutic to the toxic range in patients who are on cimetidine therapy. Toxic effects, such as bradycardia, hypotension, and arrhythmias, may appear with beta-blockers. Elevated levels of anticonvulsants, especially in the elderly, can be seen over a period of several days in patients taking carbamazepine (Tegretol) and phenytoin (Dilantin). With lidocaine, an increase in serum levels of 60 to 90% can occur with maintenance infusions in patients on cimetidine therapy.

II. **Ranitidine.** The newer, selective H_2 antagonists, ranitidine (Zantac) and famotidine (Pepcid), produce very mild CNS depression. As a result, neither produces adverse secondary drug interactions such as those described with cimetidine.

Bronchodilators

I. **Aminophylline and theophylline** represent the cornerstone of oral bronchodilator therapy for the elderly asthmatic, bronchitic, or cardiac patient. They are metabolized by the liver, and clearance is remarkably sensitive to hepatic dysfunction caused by disease (primary and hypoxia induced) or low-flow states (congestive heart failure and propranolol induced).

 A. **Complications** of aminophylline include seizures, which may even occur at therapeutic levels, increased angina, palpitations, and arrhythmias. Nervousness and lack of sleep are also encountered in the geriatric population. Aminophylline toxicity in the elderly may also mimic chronic organic brain syndrome, multi-infarct dementia, and psychosis. Draw blood levels on patients who have this constellation of symptoms and who are taking an aminophylline preparation.

 B. **Certain drug interactions may precipitate aminophylline toxicity.** Cimetidine and other liver-metabolized antibiotics (erythromycin, clindamycin) decrease excretion of aminophylline. Ephedrine and other sympathomimetic agents in combination with aminophylline may cause excessive CNS stimulation, precipitating bizarre behavior and sleeplessness.

II. **Epinephrine.** Asthma is a reversible but serious respiratory condition that still claims more than 2,000 lives annually in the United States. For the past 80 years, the rapid reversal of acute bronchospasm and hypoxemia associated with asthma using subcutaneous epinephrine has been confirmed by numerous investigators.

Despite its efficacy, many physicians are reluctant to administer subcutaneous epinephrine to acute asthmatics 40 years of age or older, especially those with concomitant heart disease or a history of hypertension, because of the potent cardiovascular effects of the drug. Cydulka and associates conducted a study to determine whether the administration of subcutaneous epinephrine (0.3 mL, 1:1,000) is associated with an increased risk of cardiovascular side effects—adverse hemodynamic consequences and arrhythmias—in patients more than 40 years of age as compared with patients younger than 40.

A. Investigation. Conducting their prospective investigation in a large urban teaching hospital, these researchers administered three subcutaneous doses of 0.3 mL 1:1,000 epinephrine 20 minutes apart to 95 adult asthmatics 15 to 96 years of age during 108 asthma exacerbations. Thirty-nine of the 108 episodes occurred in patients over the age of 40, 48.7% of which were men. Patients were diagnosed as having an acute asthmatic attack if they had had an established history of reversible bronchospasm, dyspnea, or wheezing on presentation, and diminished peak expiratory flow rates. Individuals with a previous history of chronic obstructive lung disease, chronic bronchitis, or an acute myocardial infarction, as well as patients presenting with angina or those who had received epinephrine prior to admission, were considered ineligible. In addition, the use of aerosolized adrenergic agents was prohibited during the study period.

   1. Systolic blood pressure. Heart rhythm and rate, blood pressure, respiratory rate, and clinical response were prospectively evaluated before, during, and after administration of epinephrine doses. The investigators found that initial systolic blood pressures were higher in the older than younger age group (146 ± 4.2 versus 130.6 ± 3.2 mm Hg), while the incidence of sinus tachycardia was not significantly different (49.3% older versus 59% younger) between the two groups. The only significant difference ($p < .0033$) between asthmatics in the two age groups occurred after the first dose of epinephrine when mean systolic blood pressure was observed to decrease by 9.5 ± 3.3 mm Hg in patients older than 40 years, while it increased 1.3 ± 1.9 mm Hg in the younger age group.

   2. Ventricular arrhythmias. The authors noted there was no significant difference in the occurrence of ventricular arrhythmias between patients less than and older than 40 years of age, although isolated VPBs <10/hr were observed after treatment in 11.6% of the younger patients and in 21.6% of those over 40 ($p > .05$). There were no adverse consequences from these ventricular irregularities. While atrial premature beats occurred significantly more often in the older than younger age group (32.4% versus 10.1%, $p < .05$), all atrial tachycardias resolved spontaneously without symptomatology or adverse cardiac consequences. Of special interest is the fact that mean systolic and diastolic blood pressures, heart rate, and respiratory rate decreased as bronchoconstriction was relieved and respiratory flow rates improved with epinephrine therapy in the older age group.

   3. Clinical improvement was similar in each of the populations studied, with an average increase in peak flow rates of 47.1%, 24.5%, and 25.1% after the first, second, and third doses of subcutaneous epinephrine, respectively.

   4. Initial treatment. This study has important implications for the initial pharmacologic treatment of the adult asthmatic. A nonselective alpha- and beta-adrenergic agonist, epinephrine has long been considered standard therapy for acute asthma. It relaxes bronchial smooth muscle and constricts bronchial arterioles, reaching detectable serum levels within 5 to 10 minutes after subcutaneous injection, and attaining peak blood levels between 20 to 40 minutes. Because of its chronotropic effect on the sinoatrial node and positive inotropic effect on the myocardium, however, epinephrine can increase myocardial irritability and oxygen consumption, thereby precipitating cardiac arrhythmias in susceptible individuals.

B. Controversy. While many practitioners routinely use epinephrine to relieve asthma in the young adult and pediatric patient, the proarrhythmogenic potential of epinephrine has deterred its use in older adults, especially those with preexisting cardiac disease or hypertension. This is unfortunate, since subcutaneous epinephrine is a relatively inexpensive, easily administered, and efficacious bronchodilator. In the older age group, many experts advocate aerosolized, inhaled selective sympathomimetic agents which, although just as efficacious as parenteral epinephrine, have been associated with fewer cardiovascular side effects. It should be noted, however, that the cost difference between injection and inhalation treatment is substantial. In most institutions, subcutaneous epinephrine 1:1,000 is approximately one third of the cost of sympathomimetic inhalation therapy.

   1. Age. The results of this limited study suggest that use of subcutaneous epinephrine can probably be safely expanded to include selected asthmatic patients over 40 years of age, providing these individuals have not had a recent myocardial infarction and do not report anginal symptoms on presentation. The use of epinephrine in older patients with recent, silent myocardial infarction or severe coronary ischemia as determined by ECG findings was not specifically evaluated in this study and, therefore, the safety of its use in this population remains questionable.

   2. Older age group. Although the investigators report findings for 39 patients over the age of 40 years, they fail to indicate the mean age and specific breakdown of ages within the older population studied. Lacking such age-adjusted, fractionated data for the 40 years and older group, it is difficult to draw conclusions about the drug's overall safety in the "elderly" population, per se. In this regard, the authors conclude that a larger population must be studied before this modality can be recommended without reservation for all age groups. Moreover, in an age when selective, aerosolized bronchodilating agents are readily available—and have proven efficacy—the rationale for an expanded role for subcutaneous epinephrine therapy is debatable.

III. Optimal corticosteroid tapering schedule following exacerbation of asthma. Although corticosteroids have been known to be effective in the treatment of severe asthma for more than 30 years, no adequate data exist to help the physician determine how rapidly steroids can safely be withdrawn in patients who have experienced an acute exacerbation of their illness. Published recommendations run the gamut, from a few days to several months, but controversy persists, with some experts claiming that rapid tapering (i.e., 4 to 10 days) of corticosteroid therapy is associated with a higher exacerbation and hospital readmission rate, while other experts claim that long tapering schedules (2 to 3 weeks) place patients at risk for complications of long-term corticosteroid therapy.

  A. Investigation. Given the clinical importance, economic implication, and widespread use of this outpatient prescribing practice, the investigators conducted a randomized, double-blind, placebo-controlled trial to determine whether a long corticosteroid tapering following an exacerbation of asthma reduced the likelihood of re-exacerbation and/or readmission to the hospital.

1. **Non-steroid-dependent adult men** (n = 43) hospitalized for asthma exacerbations and treated with steroids acutely during a 1-year period were randomly assigned to corticosteroid tapering regimens of 1 or 7 weeks, following an 8-day course of high-dose corticosteroid therapy. Specifically, the short taper consisted of 7 days using daily prednisone doses of 45, 30, 25, 20, 15, 10, and 5 mg; the long tapering consisted of each of the above doses for 7 days each for a total of 7 weeks.
2. With respect to clinical deterioration for each dosage schedule, **this study found no significant difference** between the long-taper and short-taper groups in the rate of re-exacerbation (41% versus 52%) or readmission (22% versus 21%) during the 12-week study period. Failure was defined as a re-exacerbation of asthma requiring additional high-dose corticosteroid therapy during the 12-week study period. Patients who did not have a re-exacerbation during the 12 weeks were evaluated with spirometry, with no significant differences occurring between the two groups. Those patients who required mechanical ventilation for their initial hospitalization (n = 7) or who reported more than 2 days of worse than usual dyspnea during the 12-week period (n = 20) had high rates of re-exacerbation (86% and 80%, respectively). And confirming the clinical impressions of some experts, the results of this trial also indicate that more patients in the long-term taper group reported corticosteroid side effects (41% versus 14%), including weight gain, edema, easy bruising, and acne. Based on rigorous statistical analysis (Cox's F test), the authors contend that their results provide reasonable certainty (90%) that a long taper does not result in a large reduction (50% or more) in re-exacerbations compared with a short taper. Moreover, they conclude that the relapse rate is high in this population regardless of the corticosteroid tapering regimen employed and that a long taper does not justify its routine use.

B. **Corticosteroid therapy is pivotal** to the management of exacerbations of asthma that fail to respond to conventional bronchodilator therapy. Curiously, despite the universal use of high-dose, short-course steroid therapy to treat this disorder, no previous studies have addressed the important question of how rapidly corticosteroid therapy should be withdrawn following an exacerbation. The value of conducting such a study is clear. If not associated with an increased readmission of treatment failure rates, the use of a short-term tapering schedule, because of its reduced likelihood of steroid-induced side effects, would have a significant clinical advantage over a long-term tapering regimen.

1. **Short-term therapy.** Based on this clinical trial, physicians can expect a short-term (7 days) tapering of prednisone therapy in adult men to be just as effective as a long-term (7 weeks) tapering regimen and to be associated with a significantly lower incidence of side effects. Although this recommendation will apply to large numbers of patients, three aspects of this study deserve comment.
2. **Comments on study.** First, the patients receiving systemic corticosteroids at the time of initial exacerbation were excluded from the study. Second, most of the patients in this study were older men (mean age, 63 years) with histories of heavy smoking and abnormal spirometry, whose clinical picture would be considered consistent with chronic obstructive pul-

Salicylates

More than 200 OTC preparations contain aspirin, which can adversely affect the elderly. Presenting symptoms can include gastritis with gastrointestinal blood loss leading to iron deficiency anemia and peptic ulcer with or without serious hemorrhagic manifestations. The elderly are particularly prone to chronic salicylate intoxication, which presents as tinnitus, confusion, respiratory alkalosis, and noncardiogenic pulmonary edema. Even patients taking therapeutic doses of salicylates are prone to chronic salicylism. Consequently, any elderly patient who presents with confusion, respiratory alkalosis, and pulmonary edema of unknown etiology should have a salicylate level drawn, even if the patient has taken salicylates as prescribed by a physician. The diagnosis depends on a thorough drug history and elevated blood salicylate level.

Antihistamines

I. **The early stages of diphenhydramine intoxication** are characterized by acute psychosis, hallucinations, autism, loosened associations, cardiotoxicity affective blunting, and inappropriateness. As time passes, the symptom complex may become more similar to an acute brain syndrome with confusion, disorientation, inability to concentrate, and loss of short-term memory. These symptoms present an interesting differential diagnosis. However, based on the physical exam, drug overdose should always be suspected. Initial lab analysis should include serum electrolytes, prothrombin time, calcium, blood urea nitrogen (BUN), glucose, arterial gases, blood alcohol, and urine toxicologic screening. In addition, an ECG, chest and skull x-rays, and lumbar puncture may be necessary, depending on the clinical presentation.

II. **A history of drug ingestion** is frequently unreliable or unobtainable from the patient. Friends or relatives may be questioned concerning the availability of medications, prior history of drug use, and ingestion of hallucinogenic plants or seeds (jimsonweed, mushrooms). However, autonomic signs or symptoms may be the key to diagnosis. Anticholinergic poisoning is associated with tachycardia, mydriasis, flushing, hyperpyrexia, urinary retention, decreased intestinal motility, hypertension, dry skin, and decreased salivation. This clinical picture may be obscured by the frequency of hypertension, tachycardia, and mydriasis with many of the hallucinogens, including sympathetic stimulants (LSD, amphetamines) **(Table 1-25).**

III. **A vast array of antihistamines, hypnotics, antidepressants, and tranquilizing agents** pose significant anticholinergic activity. An increasing number of these drugs are now available in OTC preparation and may, in acute poisoning, produce a picture typical of central anticholinergic toxicity. This syndrome refers to an acute psychosis of delirium resulting from a primary blockade of cerebral cholinergic inhibitory pathways accompanied by signs of peripheral muscarinic blockage.

Table 1-25. Anticholinergic Agents

Antihistamines
Antiparkinsonian drugs
Antipsychotics (phenothiazines and butyrophenones)
Antispasmodics
Belladonna alkaloids
Ophthalmic products (myriatics)
Plants (jimsonweed)
Thioxanthenes
Tricyclic antidepressants

Table 1-26. Central Effects of Anticholinergic Toxicity

Anxiety	Hallucinations (visual/auditory)
Ataxia	Hyperactivity
Choreoathetoid movements	Lethargy
Coma	Loss of short-term memory
Delirium	Myoclonus
Disorientation	Paranoid ideation
Dizziness	Respiratory failure
Dysarthria	Seizures
Expressive aphasia	Tinnitus
Frank psychosis	Tremor

IV. The presentation may vary from confusion, hallucinations, and convulsions to deepening coma and respiratory arrest. Toxic psychosis is a recognized complication of antihistamine poisoning. Ethanolamine derivatives, such as diphenhydramine, are distinct because of their proven safety and are noted for their sedative and anticholinergic properties **(Table 1-26).**

   A. Clinical presentation of the diphenhydramine overdose patient depends on age. Adults commonly present with central nervous system depression, such as drowsiness, dizziness, and ataxia. Occasionally, there can be coma and cardiovascular collapse. Fever and flushing are not usually seen. Temporary ECG changes, such as prolonged QT interval, nonspecific ST-T changes, wandering pacemaker, and left bundle branch block, may be seen. A fatal dose in adults is approximately 20 to 40 mg/kg. In children, as little as 500 mg of diphenhydramine may be fatal. Children and young adults are remarkably susceptible to the anticholinergic action of this drug and commonly present with excitement, tremors, hyperactivity, hyperpyrexia, and tonic-clonic seizures.

   B. The central effects of antihistamines constitute their greatest danger in acute poisoning. The first report of toxic psychosis resulting from diphenhydramine was reported by Borman in 1947. Since then, there have been few reported cases. All the cases were characterized by amnesia for the entire toxic episode and returned to a normal mental state within 48 hours. Possible predisposing factors in diphenhydramine-induced psychosis include parenteral administration, underlying psychosis, organic brain disease, combined use

with other anticholinergic drugs, and reduced clearance of drug secondary to altered renal or hepatic function.
V. **The treatment** of a diphenhydramine overdose is generally supportive, particularly in regard to airway management and the maintenance of vital signs. The patient in a psychotic episode may require constant supervision for up to several days to guard against potentially serious complications, such as aspiration, accidental injury, hyperthermia, and seizures. Diphenhydramine is well absorbed following ingestion and is widely distributed throughout the body, including the CNS. The drug appears in plasma within 15 minutes and may reach peak concentrations within 1 hour. Gastric lavage or emesis should be initiated immediately on the patient's arrival at the emergency department. After emesis, administration of activated charcoal and a cathartic may help to minimize absorption. Forced diuresis, hemodialysis, and hemoperfusion are generally ineffective since little free drug remains in the plasma.
  A. **For a mild case** of intoxication or in elderly, confused patients with uncertain cardiac status, one can manage the patient with conservative treatment and reassurance. Central nervous system depressants, which themselves have anticholinergic properties (phenothiazine), should be avoided. Convulsions may be treated with phenytoin at 10 to 15 mg/kg intravenously. *Severe intoxications* should be admitted to intensive care and monitored closely for cardiac arrhythmias, hypotension, and cardiovascular collapse.
VI. **The major controversy** surrounding the treatment of any anticholinergic syndrome concerns the use of physostigmine (Antilirium). This drug is a reversible cholinesterase inhibitor capable of crossing the blood-brain barrier. Physostigmine (2 mg IV) has been shown to rapidly reverse coma, delirium, seizures, and other signs of the central anticholinergic syndrome. A patient may have dramatic symptomatic relief from low doses of intravenous physostigmine. However, the benefits of this therapy must be weighed against the major side effects, including seizures, cholinergic crises, bradyarrhythmias, and asystole. We feel that physostigmine should be reversed for use in patients with refractory tachyarrhythmias or convulsions. In summary, any patient with an acute onset of bizarre mental and neurologic symptoms should be suspected of poisoning by an anticholinergic drug, including antihistamines. A careful history, with specific attention to OTC drugs, is vital for confirming the diagnosis.

Summary

Although the elderly constitute only 11% of the U.S. population, they consume approximately 20 to 30% of all drugs **(Table 1-27).** Moreover, many of the elderly are simultaneously taking more than one prescription drug for more than one chronic condition, over variable periods of time; and they may supplement their prescription drugs with OTC medications and alcohol. Medication storage is often inadequate. For these reasons, this age group is at high risk for sustaining drug toxicity and adverse drug interactions. Many ineffective medications can be discontinued.
  I. **Behavior.** One large study of hospitalized elderly patients with a mean age of 71 years found that each patient consumed an average of 3.1 prescription drugs and one OTC preparation. Initially, one sixth of the persons surveyed denied using OTC medications, but further questioning revealed that these patients did, in fact, take OTC drugs. Moreover, 50% of these elderly patients needed prompting to remember to take their medications, so noncompliance was a serious problem.

Table 1-27. Twenty Suggestions for Preventing Drug Toxicity in the Elderly

- Strive for a diagnosis prior to treating
- Take a careful drug history
- Know the pharmacokinetics of the drug(s)
- Adjust the dose
- Use smaller doses in the elderly
- Work to simplify the regimen
- Regularly review the regimen
- Avoid polypharmacy at all costs
- Use medication cards
- Keep a record of the Rx on the problem list
- Use medication diary (or containers, such as egg cartons, for daily doses)
- Have patient bring in all medicine bottles
- Check the labels
- Instruct family
- Destroy old medicines
- Use the services of visiting nurses
- Check serum drug levels when appropriate
- Support community education
- Consider overdose risk in elderly patients with clinically evident psychiatric conditions
- Be sure patients are aware that medicines can cause, as well as cure, illness

Among the implications of that study for the diagnosis and identification of adverse drug reactions in the emergency setting is the importance of focused assessment and interview techniques to examine drug behavior and compliance in the elderly, particularly for OTC drugs.

II. **Adverse drug reactions as a cause.** Finally, any elderly patient who presents to the emergency physician with nonspecific CNS, cardiac, or gastrointestinal signs and symptoms must have a careful drug history, including OTC medications, antiulcer agents, cardiac medications, and antihypertensives. Always consider adverse drug reactions, especially the anticholinergic syndrome, and secondary drug interactions, as a cause of illness.

Suggested Readings

Albrich JM: Geriatric pharmacology. In Schwartz GR, Bosker G, Grigsby JW, editors: *Geriatric emergencies,* Bowie, Md, 1984, Robert J Brady.

Alegro S, Fenster PE, Marcus FI: Digitalis therapy in the elderly, *Geriatrics* 38:93, 1983.

American College of Physicians: Improving medical education in therapeutics, *Ann Intern Med* 108:145-147, 1988.

American Society of Hospital Pharmacists: Antidiabetic agents-sulfonylureas, *Drug Information TM* '86 68:1579, 1986.

Amery A et al: Mortality and morbidity results from the European working part on high blood pressure in the elderly, *Lancet* 1:1349-1354, 1985.

Asplund K, Wilholm BE, Lithner F: Glibenclamide-associated hypoglycemia: a report on 57 cases, *Diabetologia* 26:412, 1984.

Bauman JH, Kimelblatt BJ: Cimetidines as an inhibitor of drug metabolism: therapeutic implications and review of the literature, *Drug Intell Clin Pharm* 16:380, 1982.

Ben-Ishay D, Leibel B, Stessman J: Calcium channel blockers in the management of hypertension in the elderly, *Am J Med* 81(suppl 6a): 1:30-34, 1986.

Blazer DG et al: The risk of anticholinergic toxicity in the elderly: a study of prescribing practices in two populations, *J Gerontol* 38(1):31, 1983.

Bliss MR: Prescribing for the elderly, *Br Med J* 282:203-206, 1981.

Borland C et al: Biochemical and clinical correlates of diuretics therapy in the elderly, *Age Ageing* 15:357-363, 1986.

Cassel CK, Walsh JR, editors: Medical, psychiatric, and pharmacological topics, *Geriatr Med* 1:554, 1984.

Christopher CD: The role of the pharmacist in a geriatric nursing home: a literature review, *Drug Intell Clin Pharm* 18:428-433, 1984.

Coope J, Warrender TS: Randomized trial of treatment of hypertension in elderly patients in primary care, *Br Med J* 293:1145, 1148, 1986.

Cydulka R et al: The use of epinephrine in the treatment of older asthmatics, *Ann Emerg Med* 17:322-326, 1988.

Dall JLC: Maintenance digoxin in elderly patients, *Br Med J* 2:702, 1970.

Darnell JC et al: Medication used by ambulatory elderly: an inhome survey, *J Am Geriatr Soc* 34:1, 1986.

Douglas WW: Histamine and 5-hydroxytryptamine (serotonin) and their antagonists. In Goodman LS, Gilman A, editors: *The pharmacological basis of therapeutics,* ed 6, New York, 1979, Macmillan.

Downs GE, Linkewich JA, DiPalma JR: Drug interactions in elderly diabetics, *Geriatrics* 36(7):45, 1986.

Duvoisin RC, Kat R: Reversal of central anticholinergic syndrome in man by physostigmine, *JAMA* 206(9):1963, 1968.

Egstrup K: Transient myocardial ischemia after abrupt withdrawal of antianginal therapy in chronic stable angina, *Am J Cardiol* 61:1219, 1988.

Emanueli A et al: Glipizede—new sulfonylurea in the treatment of diabetes mellitus: summary of clinical experiences in 1,064 cases, *Arzneimittelforschung* 22:1881, 1971.

Goldfrank LR, Melinek M: Locoweed and other anticholinergics (the telltale heart). In Goldfrank LR, editor: *Toxicologic emergencies,* New York, 1982, Prentice-Hall.

Granacher RP, Baldessarini RJ: Physostigmine: its use in acute anticholinergic syndrome with antidepressant and antiparkinson drugs, *Arch Gen Psychiatry* 32:375, 1975.

Granek E et al: Medications and diagnosis in relation to falls in a long-term care facility, *J Am Geriatr Soc* 35:505, 1987.

Greenblatt DJ, Shader RI: Anticholinergics, *N Engl J Med* 288(23):1215-1218, 1984.

Greenblatt DJ, Sellers EM, Shader RI: Drug therapy: drug disposition in old age, *N Engl J Med* 306(18):1081, 1982.

Gryfe CI, Gryfe BM: Drug therapy for the aged: the problems of compliance and the roles of physicians and pharmacists, *J Am Geriatr Soc* 32(4):301, 1984.

Hall RCW et al: Anticholinergic delirium: etiology, presentation, diagnosis, and management, *J Psychedel Drugs* 10:237, 1978.

Hansten PD: *Drug interactions,* ed 5, Philadelphia, 1985, Lea & Febiger.

Heifetz S, Day D: Inadvertent chlorpropamide hypoglycemia—no longer once in a blue moon? *N Engl J Med* 316(4):223, 1987 (letter).

Hestand HE, Teske DW: Diphenhydramine hydrochloride intoxication, *J Pediatr* 90(6):1017, 1977.

Hoffman JR: Overdose with cardiotherapeutic agents, *Geriatrics* 38:51, 1983.

Hollifield JW, Slaton PE: Thiazide diuretics, hypokalemia, and cardiac arrhythmias, *Acta Med Scand* 647(suppl):67, 1981.

Hutchinson TA et al: Frequency, severity, and risk factors for adverse drug reactions in adult out-patients: prospective study, *J Chronic Dis* 39(7):533, 1986.

Iserson KV, Hackney KU: Antihistamines. In Haddad LM, Winchester JF: *Clinical management of poisoning and drug overdose,* Philadelphia, 1983, WB Saunders.

Jenike MA: Cimetidine in elderly patients: review of uses and risks, *J Am Geriatr Soc* 30(3):170, 1987.

Keller MB et al: Treatment received by depressed patients, *JAMA* 248(15):1848, 1982.

Knapp DA et al: Drug prescribing for ambulatory patients 85 years of age and older, *J Am Geriatr Soc* 32(2):138, 1984.

Kramer MS et al: An algorithm for the operational assessment of adverse drug reactions. I. Background, description, and instructions for use. II. Demonstration of reproducibility and validity, *JAMA* 242(7):623-633, 1979.

Kranzelok EP, Anderson GM, Mirik M: Massive diphenhydramine overdose resulting in death, *Ann Emerg Med* 11(4):212, 1982.

Kulig K, Rumack BH: Anticholinergic poisoning. In Haddad LM and Winchester JF, editors: *Clinical management of poisoning and drug overdose,* Philadelphia, 1983, WB Saunders.

Lamy PP: Geriatric pharmacology, *Geriatrics* 36(12):41-49, 1986.

Lamy PP: A "risk" approach to adverse drug reactions, *J Am Geriatr Soc* 36:79, 1988.

Larson EB et al: Adverse drug reactions associated with global cognitive impairment in elderly persons, *Ann Intern Med* 107:169-173, 1987.

Leach S, Roy SS: Adverse drug reactions: an investigation on an acute geriatric ward, *Age Ageing* 15:241, 1986.

Lee JH, Turndorf H, Poppers PJ: Physostigmine reversal of antihistamine-induced excitement and depression, *Anesthesiology* 43(6):683, 1975.

Leichter S: A prospective double-blind clinical trial of glipizide and glyburide in type II diabetes mellitus, *Communication,* 1986.

Leventhal JM et al: An algorithm for the operational assessment of adverse drug reactions. III. Results of tests among clinicians, *JAMA* 242(18):1991, 1979.

Levy DW, Lye M: Diuretics and potassium in the elderly, *J R Coll Physicians Lond* 21(2):148, 1987.

Litovitz T: Hallucinogens. In Hadden LM, Winchester JF, editors: *Clinical management of poisoning and drug overdose,* Philadelphia, 1983, WB Saunders.

Loew ER, MacMillan R, Katser ME: The antihistamine properties of benadryl, β-dimethylaminoethyl ether hydrochloride, *J Pharmacol Exp Ther* 86:229, 1946.

May FE, Stewart B, Cluff LE: Drug Interactions and multiple drug administrations, *Clin Pharmacol Ther* 2:705, 1970.

McEvoy G, editor: *American Hospital formulary service drug information 85,* Bethesda, 1985, American Society of Hospital Pharmacists.

Melander A: Clinical pharmacology of sulfonylureas, *Metabolism* 36(2)(suppl 1):1987.

Minardo JD et al: Clinical characteristics of patients with ventricular fibrillation during antiarrhythmic drug therapy, *N Engl J Med* 319:257, 1988.

Monroe R, Jacobson G, Ervin F: Activation of psychosis by combination of scopolamine and alpha-chloralose, *Arch Neurol* 76:536, 1957.

National Poison Center Network: Annual statistical report, Pittsburgh, 1979.

Nigro SA: Toxic psychosis due to diphenhydramine hydrochloride, *JAMA* 203(4):139, 1968.

Nilsson E: Physostigmine treatment in various drug-induced intoxications, *Ann Clin Res* 14:165, 1982.

Nolan L, O'Malley K: Prescribing for the elderly. I. Sensitivity of the elderly to adverse drug reactions, *J Am Geriatr Soc* 36:142-149, 1988.

Ouslander JG: Drug therapy in the elderly, *Ann Intern Med* 95:711-722, 1981.

Pickles H, Fuller S: Prescriptions, adverse reactions, and the elderly, *Lancet* 2(8497):40, 1986.

Plum F, Posner JB, editors: *The diagnosis of stupor and coma,* Philadelphia, 1982, FA Davis.

Podolsky S: Diabetes and aging: the type II patient. 1986 (abstract).

Ray WA et al: Psychotropic drug use and the risk of hip fracture, *N Engl J Med* 316:363, 1987.

Report of the Royal College of General Physicians: Medication for the elderly, *J R Coll Physicians Lond* 18:7, 1984.

Rizack MA, Hillman CDM: *The Medical Letter handbook of adverse drug interactions,* New Rochelle, NY, 1987, The Medical Letter.

Rumack BH: Anticholinergic poisoning: treatment with physostigmine, *Pediatrics* 52:449, 1973.

Sachs BA: The toxicity of benadryl: report of a case and review of the literature, *Ann Intern Med* 29:135, 1948.

Shrimp LA et al: Potential medication-related problems in noninstitutionalized elderly, *Drug Intell Clin Pharm* 19:766, 1985.

Spector R, editor: *The scientific basis of clinical pharmacology: principles and examples,* Boston, 1986, Little, Brown.

Sternberg L: Unusual side reactions of hysteria from benadryl, *J Allergy* 18:417, 1947.

Stults BM: Digoxin use in the elderly, *J Am Geriatr Soc* 30(3):158, 1985.

Symposium: managing medication in an aging population: physician, pharmacist, and patient perspectives, *J Am Geriatr Soc* (suppl 30):11, 1985.

Thompson JF et al: Clinical pharmacists prescribing drug therapy in a geriatric setting: outcome of a trial, *J Am Geriatr Soc* 32(2):154, 1984.

Thompson TT, Moran MG, Nies AS: Psychotropic drug use in the elderly, *N Engl J Med* 308(3):134, 1983.

Tilson HH: Social policy and drug safety, *Clin Geriatr Med* 2(1):165, 1987.

Tintinalli JE: Emergency psychiatric evaluation: medical history and physical exam. In Tintinalli JE, Rothstein RJ, Krome RL, editors: *Emergency medicine: a comprehensive study guide,* New York, 1985, McGraw-Hill.

Todd B: Drugs and the elderly: identifying drug toxicity, *Geriatr Nurs* 12:231, 1985.

Vestal RE: Drug use in the elderly: a review of problems and special considerations, *Drugs* 16:358, 1978.

Williamson J, Chopin JM: Adverse reactions to prescribed drugs in the elderly: a multicenter investigation, *Age Ageing* 9:73, 1980.

World Health Organization: Health care in the elderly: report of the technical group on the use of medications in the elderly, *Drugs* 22:279, 1981.

Wyngaarden JB, Severs MH: The toxic effects of antihistamine drugs, *JAMA* 145:277, 1951.

This chapter is modified from Albrich JM, Bosker G. Drug Prescribing and Systematic Detection of Adverse Drug Reactions. In Bosker et al: Geriatric Emergency Medicine. St. Louis: Mosby, 1990, 33–61.

Oral Pain Management

H. Brian Goldman, M.D., A.B.E.M., M.C.F.P. (EM)

Oral analgesics have an important role to play in emergency medicine. Parenteral analgesics and sedatives are generally indicated for the management of severe pain. However, many patients who are seen in the emergency department have mild to moderate pain; in such cases, oral analgesics may be appropriate and necessary. Moreover, patients who receive parenteral analgesics in the emergency department usually require a prescription for an oral analgesic.

Analgesics Available

There is an enormous choice of analgesics available to emergency physicians. There are numerous oral narcotics. Despite this, relatively weak opioids such as oxycodone and acetaminophen with codeine are the most widely prescribed analgesics in the emergency department. Patients with severe pain who receive analgesics suitable for moderate pain are often inadequately treated and thus require increasing doses of the prescribed analgesic. Such dosage escalations increase the risk of adverse effects, as well as invite physicians to conclude that the patient is addicted to their analgesics. By taking a detailed history and using simple techniques for evaluating the patient's level of pain, it is usually possible to choose the most appropriate opioid drug with the fewest adverse effects.

I. **Nonsteroidal antiinflammatory drugs (NSAIDs).** A growing number of NSAIDs are also available. These are indicated for the management of mild to moderate pain and are similar in potency to acetaminophen with 30 to 60 mg of codeine. However, NSAIDs carry a greater potential for toxicity than do narcotics, particularly in the elderly. Knowledge of the adverse effects of NSAIDs and the contraindications to their use is essential.

II. **Nonnarcotic analgesics.** A new category of oral analgesic has recently emerged; these drugs are referred to as nonnarcotic analgesics. They offer similar potency to NSAIDs but with less toxicity. Acetaminophen belongs in this category.

III. **Skeletal muscle relaxants.** There is a widely held misconception that skeletal muscle relaxants are not effective in relieving pain due to muscle spasms. Despite this, numerous placebo-controlled studies have demonstrated they are extremely effective when used on a short-term basis.

IV. **Other agents** have specific indications. For example, the antidepressants amitriptyline and fluoxetine are effective in the management of pain due to fibromyalgia. Carbamazepine is effective in the relief of pain due to trigeminal neuralgia.

V. **Transelectrical nerve stimulation (TNS).** Transelectrical nerve stimulation is an increasingly useful modality of analgesia. Like oral analgesics, TNS can be self-administered by the patient at home.

Narcotic Analgesics

I. **General considerations**
   A. **Comparison to parenteral potency.** In general, orally administered opioids have a slower onset of action, a delayed peak efficacy, and a longer duration of action than parenterally administered opioids. As shown in **Table 2-1**, a number of opioid analgesics are available for oral administration; however, oral administration robs opioids of much of their potency. Before reaching the systemic circulation, some of the drug is either inactivated during absorption or metabolized by the liver. The ratio of oral parenteral potency varies according to the drug. Morphine and hydromorphone have ratios of 1:6 and 1:5, respectively. Levorphanol has a much narrower ratio, on the order of 1:2. Meperidine has a ratio of 1:4, while pentazocine has a ratio of 1:3. These ratios remain constant and can be used to compare equipotent doses of opioid analgesics as shown in **Table 2-1**.
   B. **Relative potencies.** In theory, different opioids can be matched for potency by giving equipotent doses. In practice, however, this is not always possible; for example, adverse effects prevent the use of oral codeine and pentazocine in doses equipotent to morphine. Thus oral opioid drugs are effectively ranked according to their ability to relieve mild, moderate, and severe pain.
   C. **Response to opioids as a function of age.** In patients older than 50 years, the clearance of opioid drugs is reduced. In addition, opioid binding sites in the central nervous system (CNS) are more sensitive to opioids in the elderly than they are in younger adults. Thus elderly patients tend to be more sensitive to a given dose of narcotics than are young adults. They also tend to have more adverse effects from opioid drugs. Therefore it is prudent to minimize the risk of adverse effects by using starting doses that are 50% to 75% of those recommended in healthy young adults. It is also prudent to lengthen the recommended dosage interval by 50%.
   D. **Adverse effects**
      1. **Constipation.** Codeine causes the greatest degree of constipation, but all oral opioid drugs cause some degree of constipation when used for at least 4 to 7 days. It is a particular problem in elderly patients. Constipation should be prevented by encouraging the patient to exercise regularly if possible, and to increase consumption of bran-containing foods. In addition, most patients should be instructed to start a bulk-forming laxative such as psyllium (Metamucil). Patients with a previous history of constipation should be started on a stool softener such as docusate sodium, 100 mg orally twice a day. The goal of treatment is at least one bowel movement every 2 to 3 days.
      2. **Nausea.** All narcotics cause nausea and vomiting after repeated dosing. Nausea is produced by direct stimulation of the chemotrigger receptor zone in the brain stem. It is worse when the patient is ambulatory and is improved when the patient is recumbent. It usually responds to antiemetics such as prochlorperazine, 10 mg suppositories; metoclopramide, 5 to 10 mg orally every 6 to 8 hours as needed; or prochlorperazine, 5 to 10 mg orally or rectally every 6 to 8 hours as needed.
      3. **Respiratory depression.** This adverse effect occurs primarily in patients who ingest a large dose of narcotics for the first time. The peak incidence

Table 2-1. The Narcotic Equivalency Index

	Equianalgesic dose (mg)	Relative potency (compared with parenteral morphine)	Duration of action (hr)	Relative duration of action (compared with parenteral morphine)	Narcotic equivalency index conversion factor
Morphine					
Parenteral	10.0	1.00	4.0	1.000	1.00
Oral	60.0	0.17	4.0	1.000	0.17
Hydromorphone					
Parenteral	1.5	6.67	4.0	1.000	6.67
Oral	7.5	1.33	4.0	1.000	1.33
Codeine					
Parenteral	130.0	0.08	4.0	1.000	0.08
Oral	200.0*	0.05	4.0	1.000	0.05
Oxycodone					
Oral	30.0*	0.33	4.0	1.000	0.33
Levorphanol					
Parenteral	2.0	5.00	5.0	1.250	6.25
Oral	4.0	2.50	5.0	1.250	3.13
Meperidine					
Parenteral	75.0	0.13	3.0	0.750	0.10
Oral	300.0	0.03	4.0	1.000	0.03
Fentanyl					
Parenteral	0.01	100.0	1.0	0.250	25.00
Nalbuphine					
Parenteral	12.5	0.80	4.0	1.000	0.80
Pentazocine					
Parenteral	60	0.17	4.0	1.000	0.17
Oral	180*	0.056	4.0	1.000	0.056

*Exceeds recommended dose.

Table 2-2. Plasma Half-lives of Various Opioid Drugs

Opioids with Short Plasma Half-lives	Plasma Half-life (hr)
Codeine	3
Hydromorphone	2-3
Meperidine	3-4
Morphine	4
Nalbuphine	5
Pentazocine	3
Opioids with Long Plasma Half-lives	
Levorphanol	15
Methadone	24-48
Normeperidine (metabolite of meperidine)	18

of respiratory depression occurs 60 to 90 minutes after oral administration of narcotics, as compared with 7 minutes after intravenous administration. Tolerance rapidly develops for narcotic-induced respiratory depression.

4. **Sedation.** This is a common adverse effect that is associated with drowsiness, poor concentration, and memory deficits. It sometimes occurs after ingestion of a large dose of oral narcotic. More frequently, sedation occurs because of accumulation of a long-acting narcotic or its metabolite. The sedative and analgesic effects of narcotics have different durations of action. The duration of analgesia for most opioid drugs, as shown in **Table 2-1**, is fairly similar. However, the sedative effect of narcotics varies with the plasma half-life. As shown in **Table 2-2**, oral narcotics can be subdivided into opioids with short plasma half-lives and those with long half-lives. Sedation is rapidly reversed by administering naloxone, a narcotic antagonist. It is gradually reversed by substituting lower doses of a shorter-acting opioid. Ironically, meperidine, which has a short duration of analgesia, has a long duration of sedation, and is not recommended for long-term use.

5. **Urinary retention.** Opioid analgesics cause urinary retention by increasing sphincter tone. The effect is usually transient but can be a problem in elderly men with prostatic hypertrophy.

6. **Addiction.** This is a behavioral syndrome manifested by drug craving, unsanctioned dosage escalations by the patient, and an overwhelming preoccupation with acquiring a drug. There is a widely held misconception that the routine prescribing of opioid drugs frequently leads to addiction. In prospective studies, the true incidence of iatrogenic addiction to oral narcotics is approximately 1 per 1000. **Emergency physicians who prescribe oral narcotics should screen patients for a history of narcotic abuse.** In addition, they should learn to recognize the ruses used by entrepreneurial drug seekers as described in the chapter "Detecting the Drug Seeker." However, bear in mind that the vast majority of patients who receive oral narcotics for pain do not become addicted to them.

7. **Withdrawal symptoms.** This phenomenon is often confused with addiction. Withdrawal is a physiologic phenomenon with a characteristic set of symptoms that include anxiety, irritability, insomnia, diaphoresis, rhinorrhea, lacrimation, nausea, vomiting, cramps, diarrhea, and myoclonus. It occurs because the body increases production of substances that counteract some of the effects of narcotics. Withdrawal occurs in virtually every

patient when chronically administered narcotics are precipitously withdrawn. Withdrawal per se is not a marker for addictive behavior, and its symptoms do not cause addictive behavior. The easiest way to avoid withdrawal symptoms is to slowly taper the dose of narcotics over several days. One protocol is to reduce the total daily dose of narcotics by 15% per day. Clonidine is also used to manage withdrawal symptoms. The usual dosage of clonidine is 17 µg/kg/day in divided doses, once it is determined that the drug does not cause an unacceptable degree of hypotension in the patient. Clonidine is administered for 10 days, after which it is rapidly tapered. Clonidine is best administered in a hospital where the blood pressure can be readily monitored.

II. Opioid drugs for mild pain

A. Codeine. This is the most commonly prescribed oral narcotic, despite that its utility is limited by weak potency and by bothersome adverse effects. To increase its potency, codeine is usually combined with a mild analgesic such as acetylsalicylic acid (ASA) or acetaminophen. The main advantages of codeine are its minimal euphoric effects and low abuse potential. A growing selection of nonnarcotic analgesics are equipotent to acetaminophen with 30 to 60 mg of codeine.

  1. **Dosage and recommended use.** The dosage of codeine is 30 to 60 mg orally every 4 hours as needed, up to a maximum of 3 mg/kg/day. It is recommended for the short-term relief of mild to moderate pain due to fractures, burns, abscesses, headaches, as well as strains and sprains. The recommended pediatric dose is 0.5 mg/kg. Codeine elixir is frequently prescribed in children as an analgesic after tonsillectomy.
  2. **Precautions and contraindications.** Codeine causes significant nausea and vomiting, and is particularly constipating. If prescribing codeine to elderly patients, prescribe bulk-forming laxatives, stool softeners, or both at the same time.

B. Pentazocine. This narcotic agonist–antagonist is classified as a weak opioid, since its equipotent oral dose far exceeds recommended guidelines.

  1. **Dosage and recommended use.** The dosage of pentazocine is 50 to 100 mg orally every 3 to 4 hours as needed. It is recommended for mild to moderate pain.
  2. **Precautions and contraindications.** The most significant adverse effects are psychotomimetic effects such as auditory hallucinations, disorientation, episodes of panic, and feelings of depersonalization. Sedation can be severe in the elderly. Pentazocine should not be used in patients who are habituated to pure narcotic agonists because it can precipitate narcotic withdrawal. It should not be used in the elderly because of the aforementioned sedative effects, and should not be administered to patients with obstructive uropathy.

C. Propoxyphene. This narcotic agonist is equipotent with most NSAIDs but carries a more severe toxicity profile than do other pure agonists. Overdoses of propoxyphene can cause refractory seizures and respiratory depression that often relapse after successful treatment with naloxone. Accordingly, propoxyphene is not recommended for routine use in emergency medicine.

III. Opioid drugs for moderate pain

A. Hydrocodone. A derivative of codeine, hydrocodone is more effective than codeine and is less constipating. Like codeine, hydrocodone produces little euphoria. It is also formulated as an antitussive elixir.

1. **Dosage and recommended use.** The recommended dosage of hydrocodone is 5 to 10 mg orally every 4 to 6 hours as needed for moderate to moderately severe pain. Vicodin-Es is a combination analgesic; each tablet contains 7.5 mg of hydrocodone and 750 mg of acetaminophen. The recommended dosage of Vicodin-Es is one tablet every 4 to 6 hours as needed, up to a maximum of five tablets per day (See Acetaminophen, **III B 1**). Elixirs containing hydrocodone (e.g., Hycodan) are indicated for children with moderately severe pain who are unable to swallow tablets. The dosage in children is 1.25 to 2.5 mg orally every 4 hours as needed.
2. **Precautions and contraindications.** The most frequent adverse effects are sedation, dizziness, nausea, and vomiting. Patients using hydrocodone should be cautioned not to operate a motor vehicle or heavy equipment.

B. Oxycodone. Most preparations of this analgesic combine either 2.5 or 5 mg of oxycodone with a weak nonnarcotic analgesic such as ASA or acetaminophen. Various proprietary preparations contain oxycodone including Percodan, Percocet, Tylox, Roxicet, Roxiprin, Oxycocet, and Oxycodan.

1. **Dosage and recommended use.** The usual dosage is 5 mg orally every 6 hours as needed for moderate to moderately severe pain, and 2.5 mg orally every 6 hours as needed for moderate pain. Conditions for which oxycodone is useful include fractures, burns, after incision and drainage of abscesses, severe low back pain, moderate cancer pain, and severe dental pain. Occasionally, oxycodone is indicated for the temporary relief of headaches of vascular, tension, or mixed cause. If necessary, the dosage may be slowly titrated for optimal effect. Oxycodone, 2.5 mg, may be administered to children as young as 6 years.
2. **Precautions and contraindications.** See the section on hydrocodone. Oxycodone has a higher dependence liability than does codeine. Patients with headaches should not be given oxycodone if increased intracranial pressure has not been ruled out. Oxycodone is contraindicated in patients with severe asthma or chronic obstructive pulmonary disease (COPD), or hypersensitivity to the drug. Patients with peptic ulcer disease should not use preparations that contain ASA.

IV. Opioid drugs for severe pain

A. Hydromorphone. This short-acting narcotic is exquisitely potent when given orally or by rectal suppository.

1. **Dosage and recommended use.** The recommended dosage for hydromorphone is 2 to 4 mg orally every 4 to 6 hours as needed for moderately severe to severe pain due to severe trauma, biliary and renal colic, metastatic cancer, gangrene, and as a postoperative analgesic. Hydromorphone is among the few narcotic analgesics to be formulated in a rectal suppository (containing 3 mg), making it ideal for patients who cannot tolerate oral narcotics because of nausea. Its euphoric effects make hydromorphone extremely useful in patients with severe cancer pain.
2. **Precautions and contraindications.** Hydromorphone is not recommended for widespread use because the drug causes extreme euphoria and is highly prized by narcotic abusers as a substitute for heroin. Contraindications include increased intracranial pressure, pulmonary edema, and severe asthma. It is also not recommended for use in children.

B. Levorphanol. This is a strong opioid that is similar to morphine, although it has a much longer plasma half-life.

1. **Dosage and recommended use.** The recommended dosage is 1 to 3 mg orally as needed for severe pain due to myocardial infarction, biliary or renal colic, severe trauma, gangrene, and advanced cancer. Because the elimination half-life is 15 hours, levorphanol should not be routinely used for the ongoing management of severe pain.
2. **Precautions and contraindications.** Levorphanol may accumulate to toxic levels if given more frequently than once or twice a day, causing excessive sedation. The drug should not be used in patients who are elderly, have renal or liver disease, or raised intracranial pressure.

C. **Meperidine.** Although extremely popular as a parenteral agent, meperidine is not particularly useful in emergency medicine as an oral analgesic. Its duration of action is only 2 to 3 hours, requiring frequent doses. Taking meperidine as frequently as required for optimal analgesic effect over several days increases the risk of CNS toxicity resulting from the accumulation of toxic metabolites.
  1. **Dosage and recommended use.** Although meperidine is classified as a strong narcotic analgesic, its oral form cannot be used as such in severe pain. The average recommended dosage of meperidine is 100 to 150 mg orally every 3 to 4 hours as needed, which is well below the 300 mg that is required to reach the potency of parenterally administered morphine.
  2. **Precautions and contraindications.** Meperidine causes adverse effects in the CNS including tremors, hallucinations, anxiety, myoclonus, and seizures. Meperidine is contraindicated in patients with severe renal or hepatic disease, those with hypersensitivity to meperidine, and those who have taken a monoamine oxidase (MAO) inhibitor within the previous 14 days. Meperidine should be used with extreme caution in patients with severe asthma and COPD.

D. **Morphine.** This is the standard narcotic against which all others are measured. There are numerous oral preparations of morphine available. Orally administered morphine is available in tablets and elixirs of various strengths; morphine is also formulated in rectal suppositories. The peak analgesic effect occurs 1 to 2 hours after ingestion, and the duration of action is 3 to 5 hours. Newer sustained-release preparations reach a peak concentration 4 to 5 hours after ingestion and last up to 12 hours.
  1. **Dosage and recommended use.** Oral morphine is indicated for the management of severe acute pain due to burns, severe trauma, gangrene, and advanced cancer. Morphine may also be indicated for severe chronic pain of various causes, including trigeminal neuralgia and other forms of neuropathic pain, radiculopathies, myelopathies, and severe forms of headaches such as cluster headaches. The use of morphine for chronic pain is controversial. Recent data suggest that a subgroup of patients with chronic pain can be maintained on stable dosages of morphine and its equivalents without becoming addicted. Until the controversy is settled, it is prudent to reserve morphine for cases of chronic pain in which other treatment approaches have been exhausted. It is prudent to begin therapy with a short-acting form of morphine. There is no fixed dose of the drug **(Table 2-3).** The usual starting dosage of morphine is 15 to 30 mg orally every 4 hours; titrate upwards in increments of 25% to 50% every 8 to 12 hours until adequate analgesia is reached. If the pain is expected to persist, then switch to a long-acting form of morphine once adequate analgesia has been reached.

Table 2-3. Oral and Rectal Preparations of Morphine

Short-acting Preparations

Tablets	Dose (mg)
Morphine sulfate	15 or 30
M.O.S.-10	10
M.O.S.-20	20
M.O.S.-40	40
M.O.S.-60	60

Syrups	Dose (mg/ml)
Morphitec-1	1
Morphitec-5	5
Morphitec-10	10
Morphitec-20	20
M.O.S.-1	1
M.O.S.-5	5
M.O.S.-10	10
M.O.S.-20 (concentrate)	20
M.O.S.-50 (concentrate)	50

Suppositories	Dose (mg)
M.O.S.-10	10
M.O.S.-20	20
M.O.S.-30	30

Sustained-release Preparations

Tablets	Dose (mg)
M.O.S.-SR	30 or 60
MS CONTIN	15, 30, 60, 100

2. **Precautions and contraindications.** Morphine should be used with caution in patients with obstructive uropathy, Addison's disease, hypothyroidism, and renal failure. The drug can potentiate the anticholinergic effects of drugs such as antihistamines, tricyclic antidepressants, and phenothiazines. Contraindications to the use of morphine include hypersensitivity to the drug, concomitant or recent use of MAO inhibitors, severe asthma or COPD, increased intracranial pressure, convulsive disorders, cardiac arrhythmias, and severe liver disease.

E. **Methadone.** Methadone is not recommended for the routine oral management of pain. The duration of analgesic action of the drug is 4 to 6 hours. However, the drug has a plasma half-life of 24 to 48 hours, making rapid adjustments in the drug's dosage nearly impossible. In Canada, methadone is routinely prescribed for addicts undergoing withdrawal from narcotics and is occasionally prescribed for patients with cancer pain or chronic pain. However, emergency physicians practicing in the United States may only prescribe methadone on an emergent basis as an analgesic. Because such patients occasionally require admission to acute care hospitals, emergency physicians should be aware of the potency of methadone relative to morphine. Methadone, 20 mg orally, is equivalent to 60 mg of oral morphine or 10 mg of parenteral morphine.

NSAIDs

I. General considerations. The NSAIDs are a heterogenous group of pharmaceuticals with antiinflammatory and antipyretic properties. The NSAIDs were originally classified as analgesics for mild pain. However, it is increasingly becoming evident that some NSAIDs possess an analgesic potency similar to oral opioid drugs.

  A. Mechanism of action. The NSAIDs prevent or reduce the production of prostaglandins by inhibiting the enzyme cyclooxygenase. A subgroup of NSAIDs also prevents the production of leukotrienes by inhibiting the enzyme lipoxygenase.

  1. Prostaglandin synthesis is associated with acute pain for several reasons. First, prostaglandins E_1 and E_2, as well as leukotriene B_4, produce hyperalgesia by lowering the threshold of nociceptors to painful stimuli. This usually occurs at peripheral sites where acute tissue damage has occurred. Second, NSAIDs probably exert a hyperalgesic effect within the CNS. Third, prostaglandin F_2 appears to mediate the uterine smooth muscle contraction associated with dysmenorrhea. Fourth, prostaglandins may cause the increase in pressure within the renal pelvis of patients with renal colic.

  2. NSAIDs undoubtedly possess analgesic effects through unknown mechanisms. For instance, although the nonacetylated salicylates diflusinal and magnesium trisalicylate do not block cyclooxygenase, they do inhibit prostaglandin activity.

  3. The NSAIDs tend to have a delayed onset of effect. This is because they inhibit the production of fresh prostaglandin but have no effect on the prostaglandin already produced because of acute tissue damage and inflammation. Therefore, NSAIDs should be started as soon as possible after an injury. Also, some patients may require a narcotic in addition to the NSAID to meet their needs until the NSAID begins to work.

  B. Classification of NSAIDs. The NSAIDs are divided into five broad categories: salicylate derivatives, fenamates, propionic acid derivatives, oxicams, and acetic acid derivatives. Commonly-prescribed NSAIDs belonging to each of these categories are shown in **Table 2-4.**

  C. Relative potency of NSAIDs. There is little precise data on the relative potencies of various NSAIDs. Most studies have tended to compare the NSAID under investigation with acetaminophen, ASA, or a narcotic analgesic such as pentazocine or codeine. All NSAIDs relieve mild to moderate pain. However, parenterally administered NSAIDs such as ketorolac and indomethacin are effective in relieving severe pain due to fractures, renal colic, and postsurgical pain.

  The following generalizations may be made regarding the relative potencies of nonnarcotic analgesics based on evidence from the literature.

  1. Salicylate derivatives. Acetylsalicylic acid is a relatively weak analgesic when compared with other NSAIDs in analgesic dosages. It is equipotent with acetaminophen. It may potentiate the effects of narcotic analgesics. Diflusinal is as potent as ASA, ibuprofen, and acetaminophen with codeine. Choline magnesium trisalicylate is as effective as ASA, but it is longer acting.

  2. Propionic acid derivatives. Ibuprofen has been shown to be superior to ASA and acetaminophen with or without codeine in analgesic dosages of 1200 mg/day. It is the therapeutic benchmark against which all other propionic acid derivatives are compared. Ibuprofen is also considered the safest drug in this category. Although there is some evidence that naproxen is the

Table 2-4. Categories of NSAIDs and Their Analgesic Dosages

Category	Drug	Analgesic dose
Acetic acid derivatives	Diclofenac*	25 mg TID or 75-100 mg/day
	Indomethacin*	25 mg q8-12h for moderate pain and up to 100 mg BID for severe pain
	Ketorolac	10 mg q4-6h
	Sulindac	200 mg BID
	Tolmetin†	Adults: 400 mg q84 Children: 20 mg/kg/day divided q8h
Fenamates	Meclofenamate	Not available
	Mefenamic acid	500 mg followed by 250 mg q6h
Oxicams	Piroxicam	10 mg OD or BID
Propionic acid derivatives	Fenoprofen	200 mg q4-6h
	Flurbiprofen	50 mg q8-12h
	Ibuprofen	200-400 mg q4-6h
	Ketoprofen*	50 mg q6-8h (reduce dosage by 50% if elderly or renal failure)
	Naproxen*	500 mg followed by 250 mg q6-8h (reduce dosage by 50% in patients with cirrhosis)
	Suprofen	200 mg q6h
Salicylate derivatives	ASA†‡	325-650 mg q4h
	Choline magnesium trisalicylate‡	1000-1500 mg BID
	Diflusinal‡	1 gm followed by 500 mg q8-12h

*Available in sustained release preparation.
†Approved for use in children.
‡Considered safe for use in the elderly.

most potent propionic acid derivative, each member of the group has comparable analgesic potency. Ketoprofen possesses analgesic potency roughly equivalent to indomethacin. Flurbiprofen is as effective an analgesic as morphine, 10 mg given intramuscularly after gynecologic surgery.
3. **Acetic acid derivatives.** Indomethacin is the reference drug against which acetic acid derivatives are compared. Intravenous indomethacin, as well as indomethacin suppositories, are effective in relieving pain due to renal colic, biliary colic, and postoperative pain. Sulindac has a potency comparable to ASA and ibuprofen. Tolmetin has analgesic potency that is comparable to ASA, indomethacin, and ibuprofen.
4. **Oxicams.** Piroxicam is equivalent in potency to ASA, indomethacin, sulindac, naproxen, and ibuprofen.
5. **Fenamates.** Meclofenamate is as effective as most other NSAIDs.
6. **Ketorolac tromethamine (Toradol)**
    a. **Mechanism of action.** Ketorolac is an acetic acid derivative with predominantly analgesic activity.
    b. **Indications and relative potency.** Ketorolac is indicated for the management of mild to moderately severe acute pain. Parenterally administered ketorolac is as effective as meperidine, 75 mg, or morphine, 10 to 12 mg, in the management of postoperative pain. However, there is little data comparing oral ketorolac with other analgesics.
    c. **Contraindications and precautions.** Ketorolac is contraindicated in patients with hypersensitivity to ASA or NSAIDs, as well as patients with peptic ulcer disease.
    d. **Dosage.** The dosage of ketorolac is 10 mg orally every 4 to 6 hours, with a maximum daily dose of 40 mg.
    e. **Caution:** Ketorolac was originally marketed as a nonnarcotic analgesic. It is critical for the ED physician to realize that Ketorolac is an NSAID with all its attendant risks. Use with extreme caution in patients with known contraindications.
D. **Adverse effects.** The NSAIDs have a number of significant adverse effects.
    1. **Gastrointestinal.** Most NSAIDs cause nausea, vomiting, and epigastric pain, especially if taken on an empty stomach; instruct patients to take NSAIDs with a small amount of food and 8 to 10 ounces of water. In small but significant numbers, NSAIDs have been shown to cause gastric erosions or frank ulceration (with or without perforation), gastrointestinal (GI) hemorrhage, and severe abdominal pain. The inhibition of platelet aggregation contributes to GI hemorrhages. These effects tend to be worse in the elderly, making it mandatory that the decision to start an NSAID in this age group be a well-considered decision. The NSAIDs producing the most severe adverse GI effects are indomethacin, piroxicam, ASA, and meclofenamate. Administration of sucralfate or H_2-receptor blocker drugs such as ranitidine do not prevent NSAID-induced GI ulcers. However, misoprostil, a synthetic analogue of prostaglandin E_1, lowers the incidence of gastric ulceration caused by NSAIDs. It is not known whether the drug prevents serious GI bleeding. The dosage of misoprostil is 200 μg orally with each meal and at bedtime.
    2. **Renal.** NSAIDs are well-known causes of renal disease. They cause acute renal failure and exacerbate chronic renal disease. Fortunately, the renal impairment is generally reversible on discontinuation of the drug. Indomethacin and fenoprofen are two commonly prescribed NSAIDs that are

most likely to cause renal impairment. Suprofen causes a syndrome in young adults of flank pain, hematuria, and decreased renal function. The syndrome is usually reversible on discontinuation of the drug. The drugs least likely to cause renal impairment are ASA and sulindac.
3. **Hypersensitivity.** This is a syndrome characterized by urticaria, bronchospasm, and angioedema. Occasionally a full-blown anaphylactic reaction occurs. Hypersensitivity reactions are commonest with ASA but have been reported with every NSAID. Patients who have a history of allergy to ASA should avoid taking NSAIDs of any kind. Also, NSAIDs should be used with caution in patients who give a history of chronic urticaria, asthma, as well as nasal congestion or polyps.
4. **Other adverse effects.** Indomethacin is associated with CNS toxicity manifesting as dizziness, confusion, depression, feelings of depersonalization, and headaches. Other less common adverse effects include hematologic abnormalities such as agranulocytosis or aplastic anemia, thrombocytopenia, and pancytopenia, as well as hepatic adverse effects such as hepatitis, jaundice, hepatomegaly, as well as transient elevations in hepatic transaminases.
5. **Drug interactions.** NSAIDs are associated with a number of potentially serious drug interactions. Since NSAIDs are highly bound to plasma proteins, they will compete with other drugs for protein binding sites. The result is either an increase in the free concentration of NSAIDs or the drugs with which they compete.
    a. Drugs that are displaced from protein binding sites include oral hypoglycemic agents, phenytoin, and Coumadin. Patients who take an NSAID in addition to an oral hypoglycemic agent should have their blood glucose level checked often. In patients who are on Coumadin, NSAIDs should be used with extreme caution. In this situation, prothrombin times should be checked regularly, and patients should be asked to report abnormal bleeding at once.
    b. Other drug interactions work by different mechanisms. Both corticosteroids and cimetidine increase the metabolism of NSAIDs. In addition, NSAIDs appear to blunt the action of a variety of antihypertensive agents including thiazide diuretics, β-adrenergic blockers, and angiotensin converting enzyme inhibitors such as captopril.
E. Contraindications and precautions. The NSAIDs are contraindicated in patients with active peptic ulcer disease or active GI bleeding, a history of allergic conditions such as nasal polyps or rhinitis, as well as a history of renal or hepatic disease. Because of the risk of Reye's syndrome, children with an influenza-like illness or varicella zoster should not be given ASA. If patients are taking NSAIDs for persistently painful conditions such as lumbar strain and osteoarthritis, obtain a complete blood cell count and serum levels of liver enzymes, blood urea nitrogen (BUN), and creatinine before starting therapy. Advise the patient's attending physician to repeat these tests at 1- to 3-month intervals. In patients on oral anticoagulants, NSAIDs should be prescribed sparingly.
F. Which NSAID to choose? There is a variety of NSAIDs licensed for use by the Food and Drug Administration (FDA). With more agents becoming available, the choice is getting more difficult. Two factors make things even more difficult for emergency physicians. First, there is insufficient data comparing the potency of the various agents. Second, patients respond to NSAIDs in different

ways. For instance, a patient may respond well to a propionic acid derivative, yet not respond to an acetic acid derivative. The choice should be based on a combination of factors including efficacy (patient response), adverse effects and safety, cost, and convenience.

1. **Efficacy.** No individual NSAID is clearly superior to the others. However, for unknown reasons, some patients respond well to NSAIDs from some categories but not from others. Therefore it is prudent to become familiar with at least one NSAID from each category. The following are NSAIDs from every category that are efficacious, relatively free of serious adverse effects, and inexpensive.
   a. Propionic acid derivatives
      Safe and inexpensive—ibuprofen, naproxen
      Safe but relatively expensive—fenoprofen
   b. Acetic acid derivatives
      Safe and inexpensive—indomethacin
      Safe and relatively expensive—diclofenac, tolmetin
   c. Salicylate derivatives
      Safe and inexpensive—ASA
      Safe and relatively expensive—diflusinal
2. **Children.** The NSAIDs of choice in children are ASA and tolmetin. The dose of tolmetin is 20 mg/kg/day in divided doses every 8 hours. Children with an influenza-like illness or with suspected varicella zoster should not receive ASA.
3. **Safety.** Because of debilitating or potentially serious adverse effects, the following NSAIDs approved for clinical use should not be prescribed as frontline analgesics: meclofenamate, phenylbutazone, piroxicam, and suprofen.

Other Nonnarcotic Analgesics

I. **General considerations.** There are a number of nonnarcotic analgesics that do not belong in the NSAID category. These agents are analgesics; they possess little, if any, antiinflammatory properties.
II. **Agents for mild pain: acetaminophen.** Acetaminophen is a centrally acting cyclooxygenase inhibitor. In analgesic dosages, acetaminophen is equal in analgesic and antipyretic potency to ASA. The drug is not highly bound to plasma proteins. Its only significant drug interaction is a mild tendency to potentiate the action of oral anticoagulants; check prothrombin times regularly in this case.
   A. **Acetaminophen is well tolerated.** There are extremely rare reports of acetaminophen causing leukopenia and pancytopenia. In overdoses of 140 to 250 mg/kg, acetaminophen causes severe and frequently fatal hepatotoxicity. The management of acetaminophen poisoning is discussed elsewhere. Concerns have been raised regarding the adverse consequences of taking acetaminophen on a long-term basis for chronic pain.
   B. **The dosage** of acetaminophen in adults is 325 to 650 mg orally every 4 to 6 hours as needed. The dosage in children is 10 to 15 mg/kg every 4 to 6 hours up to a maximum of 60 mg/kg/day. The maximum recommended dose in adults is 4 grams per day.
III. **Agents for moderate pain**
   A. Floctafenine (Idarac)

1. **Mechanism of action.** Floctafenine is an anthranillic acid derivative. Like NSAIDs, the drug is an inhibitor of prostaglandin synthesis. However, the drug does not have potent antiinflammatory effects.
2. **Indications and relative potency.** Floctafenine is indicated for the management of mild to moderate pain due to soft tissue injuries, fractures, acute low back pain, headache, dental pain, and mild to moderate cancer pain. Floctafenine may be moderately effective in managing the pain due to trigeminal neuralgia and other causes of neuritis. In clinical studies, floctafenine is superior to acetaminophen with 15 mg of codeine, ASA, pentazocine, and propoxyphene; it is as effective as acetaminophen with 30 mg of codeine, ibuprofen, and dihydrocodeine.
3. **Contraindications and precautions.** Floctafenine has few adverse effects. It causes GI upset that is comparable to that produced by ibuprofen. It has also reportedly exacerbated GI symptoms in patients with active peptic ulcer disease. There are no significant drug interactions except for several case reports of severe bleeding in patients who concomitantly take oral anticoagulants. **Floctafenine** is contraindicated in patients with renal disease, known hypersensitivity to ASA or NSAIDs, as well as those with active GI inflammation or peptic ulcer disease. It should be used with extreme caution in patients who take oral Coumadin; check prothrombin times frequently.
4. **Dosage.** The dosage of floctafenine is 200 to 400 mg orally every 4 to 6 hours as needed for moderate pain. The maximum daily dose is 1200 mg.

Skeletal Muscle Relaxants

I. **General considerations.** The pathophysiology of skeletal muscle spasm is not yet well understood. It appears as if muscle spasm occurs in response to either blunt trauma or stretching of muscle fibers. Pain and muscle spasm go hand in hand in a vicious cycle. Motor neurons and spinal interneurons likely play a pivotal role in causing and perpetuating muscle spasm. Higher centers in the CNS also play a significant, if unclear role.

II. **Mechanism of action.** Skeletal muscle relaxants likely work by a variety of mechanisms. First, most muscle relaxants depress spinal polysynaptic reflexes. Second, many of the agents depress motor tracts within the extrapyramidal system. Finally, skeletal muscle relaxants may promote muscle relaxation by acting on higher centers in the CNS.

III. **Specific agents.** There are numerous skeletal muscle relaxants that are currently licensed for use to treat muscle spasm. A detailed discussion of each preparation is beyond the scope of this book. However, the following points should make it easier to navigate through a bewildering array of products.

   A. **Treating acute muscle spasm.** In numerous controlled clinical trials, the following skeletal muscle relaxants have been shown to be superior to placebo in treating acute muscle spasm: chlorphenesin, carisprodol, chlorzoxazone, diazepam, metaxalone, orphenadrine, and methocarbamol.

   B. **The maximum benefit** of skeletal muscle relaxants occurs in the first 7 days of treatment. Generally, there is little point in continuing therapy with the above agents beyond the first 2 to 3 weeks after the onset of acute muscle spasm.

   C. **Cyclobenzaprine.** The only agent with proven benefit in the relief of chronic muscle spasm is cyclobenzaprine. As shown below, cyclobenzaprine has also

been shown to provide symptomatic improvement in patients with fibromyalgia.
- **D. Combinations products** containing a muscle relaxant with one or two analgesics appear to work better than skeletal muscle relaxants alone.
- **E. Adverse effects.** These tend to be common to all muscle relaxants. Up to one third of all patients taking muscle relaxants complain of drowsiness. Some patients complain of anticholinergic symptoms such as dry mouth, blurred vision, as well dizziness, nausea, and epigastric distress.
    1. **Carisprodol** occasionally causes extreme weakness and transient quadriplegia shortly after starting the drug. Fortunately, these effects subside several hours after discontinuing the drug. Both metaxalone and chlorzoxazone can reportedly cause liver abnormalities.
    2. **Orphenadrine** has the strongest anticholinergic effects. It is the only muscle relaxant in which an overdose has been associated with death.
- **F. Contraindications.** The following skeletal muscle relaxants have specific contraindications:
    1. **Chlorzoxazone**—hepatic disease
    2. **Cyclobenzaprine**—urinary retention, narrow-angle glaucoma, hyperthyroidism, congestive heart failure, arrhythmias, and myocardial conduction disturbances
    3. **Metaxalone**—hepatic disease
    4. **Orphenadrine**—urinary retention, prostatic hypertrophy, acute glaucoma, and recent onset of depression and suicidal ideation
- **G. Dosage recommendations.** These are listed in **Table 2-5.**
- **H. Abuse potential:** Carisprodol is reportedly ingested with hydrocodone as a recreational drug.

Miscellaneous Oral Agents

- **I. General considerations.** A number of oral agents are not analgesics. Nevertheless, they are of value in relieving specific conditions that cause pain.
- **II. Antidepressants**
    - **A. Amitriptyline.** This antidepressant has proven itself an invaluable addition to the arsenal of oral agents against a disparate group of painful conditions.
        1. **Mechanism of action.** When used for painful conditions, it is unlikely that amitriptyline acts primarily as an antidepressant, since the dosage of amitriptyline falls far below that recommended for depression. The neurotransmitter serotonin appears to be very important in the inhibition of pain transmission. Fibromyalgia (previously referred to as fibrositis) is a condition in which chronic pain is associated with a deficiency of serotonin. Amitriptyline prevents the reuptake of serotonin in selected neuronal pathways that inhibit the transmission of painful stimuli. Thus it helps restore the depletion of serotonin associated with fibromyalgia. Likewise, migraine headache appears to be caused by vasodilation of extracranial blood vessels; the vasodilation is caused by a lack of serotonin.
        2. **Indications.** Amitriptyline is indicated for the relief of pain due to fibromyalgia, postherpetic neuralgia, and neuropathic pain associated with cancer. Amitriptyline is also indicated for the prophylaxis of migraine headaches, although it is unlikely that emergency physicians will use amitriptyline for this purpose.

Table 2-5. Skeletal Muscle Relaxants

Agent	Dosage	Contraindications
Carisoprodol	350 mg q8h; 25 mg/kg/day in children	History of drug abuse
Chlorzoxazone	250-500 mg q6-8h; 20 mg/kg/day in children	Hepatic disease
Cyclobenzaprine	20-40 mg/day	Hyperthyroidism, congestive heart failure, arrhythmias and blocks, urinary retention, prostatic hypertrophy, acute glaucoma
Diazepam	5 mg q6h	
Metaxalone	800 mg q6-8h	Hepatic disease
Methocarbamol	1-1.5 gm q6h	
Orphenadrine	10 mg q12h	Acute glaucoma, urinary retention, prostatic hypertrophy, depression with suicidal ideation

3. **Dosage.** Since the serum half-life of amitriptyline is approximately 24 hours, the drug may be taken once daily. In fibromyalgia, the usual starting dose of amitriptyline is 10 to 20 mg at bedtime; the dose may be increased in 10 mg increments to a maximum of 50 mg. In symptomatic postherpetic neuralgia, the usual dosage is 25 to 75 mg orally at bedtime along with fluphenazine, 1.0 gm at bedtime. The dosage of amitriptyline for migraine prophylaxis is 25 to 50 mg orally at bedtime.
4. **Precautions and contraindications.** Amitriptyline causes anticholinergic effects such as dry mouth, constipation, increased intraocular pressure, urinary hesitancy, hyperthermia, and toxic delirium. The drug is contraindicated in patients with acute glaucoma, prostatic enlargement, and urinary retention. It should be used with caution in the elderly and in patients suffering from depression associated with acute suicidal ideation.

B. **Fluoxetine**
  1. **Mechanism of action.** Like amitriptyline, fluoxetine is a serotonin reuptake inhibitor. However, it lacks the anticholinergic action of tricyclic antidepressants. Recently, fluoxetine has been used in the treatment of fibromyalgia.
  2. **Pharmacology.** Fluoxetine has a serum half-life of 4 days, and its active metabolite has a half-life of 8 days.
  3. **Indications.** Fluoxetine is indicated for the treatment of depression, as well as panic disorder. It has been used experimentally in the management of fibromyalgia. The usual starting dosage for fibromyalgia is 10 mg orally every day. The starting dosage should be maintained for 3 to 4 weeks as response to therapy is measured. The dosage may be increased to 20 to 30 mg/day; increasing the dosage above 30 mg daily does not appear to result in further improvement. Since elderly patients are particularly vulnerable to the anticholinergic side effects of tricyclic antidepressants, fluoxetine may well be the drug of choice for fibromyalgia in that age group.

4. **Precautions and contraindications.** Fluoxetine can cause nausea, orthostatic hypotension, insomnia, and anxiety. It lacks the anticholinergic adverse effects associated with tricyclic antidepressants and does not cause weight gain. There have been concerns raised about fluoxetine possibly increasing violent behavior or suicidal ideation; however, such concerns have yet to be validated by scientific evidence.

C. Cyclobenziprene (see **Table 2-5**)
1. **Mechanism.** Like amitriptyline, cyclobenzamine prevents reuptake of serotonin.
2. **Indications.** Cyclobenzamine is indicated for acute muscle spasm, as well as fibromyalgia.
3. **Dosage.** The starting dosage for fibromyalgia is 10 to 20 mg at bedtime. The maximum recommended dosage for this disorder is 40 mg at bedtime.
4. **Precautions and contraindications.** Cyclobenzamine causes anticholinergic side effects. Both amitriptyline and cyclobenzamine share the same contraindications.

III. **Anticonvulsants**
A. Carbamazepine. This anticonvulsant is extremely effective in relieving the lancinating pain associated with trigeminal neuralgia. The mechanism by which carbamazepine works is uncertain.
1. **Indications.** Carbamazepine is indicated for the treatment of trigeminal neuralgia, complex partial seizures, bipolar affective disorder, and in borderline personality, as well as schizoaffective disorder.
2. **Dosage.** For patients with trigeminal neuralgia, the starting dosage of carbamazepine is 50 mg twice a day. The dosage is gradually increased until the patient is either free of pain or has significant adverse effects. The response to therapy is often rapid and quite dramatic. Therefore if a patient is seen with a convincing history of neuralgia, it is worthwhile to initiate therapy in the emergency department.
3. **Precautions and contraindications.** Most patients complain of sedation, ataxia, and dizziness. Leukopenia is the most serious adverse effect associated with the use of carbamazepine. Patients on the anticonvulsant should have a complete blood cell count checked every 2 to 3 weeks for the first 2 to 3 months, and 2 to 3 times yearly thereafter. Discontinue therapy immediately if the total leukocyte count falls below 3000 cells/µl or if the total neutrophil count is less than 1500 cells/µl.
B. Phenytoin. The anticonvulsant phenytoin is considered a second-line drug in the treatment of trigeminal neuralgia. It is indicated for neuralgia that does not respond to carbamazepine.
C. Valproic acid. This anticonvulsant is considered a second-line drug.

IV. **Baclofen.** This is a potent muscle relaxant used primarily to relieve muscle spasms associated with spinal cord injuries. It also appears to be effective in treating trigeminal neuralgia. The mechanism of action with respect to trigeminal neuralgia is unknown.
A. **Indications.** Baclofen is indicated for the treatment of trigeminal neuralgia that has not responded to carbamazepine. It is also indicated for the treatment of postherpetic neuralgia not responding to a combination of amitriptyline and fluphenazine.

B. Dosage. The dosage of baclofen used to treat trigeminal neuralgia is 10 mg orally three times a day. The daily dose is increased by 10 mg every other day until either the pain is relieved or sedation develops.

V. Fluphenazine. This phenothiazine is combined with amitriptyline in the management of postherpetic neuralgia. The dosage of fluphenazine is 1 to 3 mg given orally at bedtime. Like amitriptyline, fluphenazine causes anticholinergic adverse effects; the two drugs have similar contraindications.

VI. Oral therapy for vascular headaches
  A. Ergotamine tartrate.
  1. **Mechanism of action.** Ergotamine tartrate is a potent vasoconstrictor that reverses the extracranial vasodilation associated with acute migraine headache. The drug also has seritonergic effects that may play a role in attenuating an acute attack.
  2. **Indications.** Ergotamine tartrate is indicated for the abortion of an acute migraine headache. It is also somewhat useful in reversing established headaches. Ergotamine is sometimes helpful in the treatment of cluster headaches. Its use is limited in cluster headaches because the headache is usually well established by the time the drug is given.
  3. **Dosage.** The initial dosage of ergotamine is 2 mg, followed by 1 mg every 30 to 60 minutes to a maximum of 5 to 6 mg/day and 10 mg/week. The drug may be administered orally, sublingually, by inhalation, and by rectal suppository. Preparations containing caffeine seem to potentiate the action of ergotamine.
  4. **Precautions and contraindications.** Ergotamine causes nausea and vomiting. In patients who are prone to nausea, it is prudent to administer metoclopramide, 10 to 20 mg orally, before administering ergotamine. Ergotamine can cause vascular occlusion and gangrene when used in dosages above the limits mentioned (see Section **VI. A. 3.**). The effects of ergotamine are potentiated by concurrent use of β-adrenergic blockers and erythromycin. Rebound headaches occasionally occur on discontinuation of the drug. Frequent use of ergotamine should be discouraged because dependence has reportedly occurred after taking regular doses of as little as 0.5 to 1.0 mg. **Contraindications** to the use of ergotamine include pregnancy, uncontrolled hypertension, angina, peripheral vascular disease, and vasospastic disorders.
  B. Isometheptene mucate. This is a sympathetic vasoconstrictor that is formulated in combination with acetaminophen and the sedative dichloralphenazone. The drug is not as effective as ergotamine in severe migraine but is better tolerated and has fewer side effects. Isometheptene is indicated for the treatment of acute migraine headache of mild to moderate severity. The dosage is two capsules orally at the first sign of a headache followed by one capsule every hour as required, up to a maximum of five capsules.
  C. Metoclopramide. This drug is a useful adjunct in the treatment of acute migraine headaches. During an acute headache, gastric motility appears to be depressed and oral analgesics are poorly absorbed. Metoclopramide promotes gastric motility and thereby increases absorption of oral analgesics. The dosage is 10 to 20 mg taken orally.
  D. Nasal oxygen. Nasally administered oxygen abolishes acute cluster headaches by causing cerebral vasoconstriction. Administer the highest con-

centration of oxygen by nasal cannula until the headache is over or until 30 minutes have elapsed. Nasally administered oxygen is effective in 50% of cases.
- **E. Cocaine.** Nasally administered cocaine can be very effective in abolishing cluster headaches. A total of 1 to 2 ml of a 5% solution of cocaine is administered by gauze nasal packing to the sphenopalatine region.
- **F. Prednisone.** Oral corticosteroids are indicated for the management of acute cluster headaches that are refractory to other agents. Therapy with prednisone is occasionally initiated in the emergency department. The initial dosage of 50 to 60 mg orally every day is maintained for 1 week, and then the dosage is slowly tapered.
- **G. Sumatriptan.** Oral sumatriptan is a selective 5-hydroxytryptamine-like receptor agonist. It has been shown to be effective in relieving migraine headaches. It is not a prophylactic agent. The recommended oral dosage is a single 100 mg. If ineffective, the dose should not be repeated. Sumatriptan is contraindicated in patients with ischemic and vasospastic coronary artery disease, complex migraine (e.g. hemiplegic migraine), previous myocardial infarction, and uncontrolled hypertension. In addition, sumatriptan should not be ingested by patients who are taking any of the following: ergotamine preparations, monoamine oxidase inhibitors, selective 5-hydroxytryptamine re-uptake inhibitors, and lithium.

VII. Quinine sulfate. Quinine has been used for years in the management of night cramps.
- **A. Mechanism.** Quinine sulfate is both an analgesic and a muscle relaxant. It increases the refractory period of skeletal muscle and reduces the excitability of the motor end-plate. Although there is considerable anecdotal evidence that quinine reduces the pain associated with night cramps, this has not yet been confirmed by controlled clinical trials.
- **B. Indications.** Quinine sulfate is indicated for the symptomatic relief of nocturnal muscle cramps that have not responded to mild analgesics, as well as physical measures such as elevating the foot of the bed. It is also important to search for metabolic abnormalities associated with muscle cramps such as disorders of sodium and calcium metabolism.
- **C. Dosage.** The dosage of quinine sulfate is 130 to 260 mg orally at bedtime.
- **D. Precautions and contraindications.** Quinine can cause thrombocytopenia. Thus patients should be advised to observe for abnormal bleeding and petechiae. The physician should check the platelet count at regular intervals. Regular use of quinine occasionally causes cinchonism, a syndrome characterized by tinnitus, nausea, headache, and distorted vision. If therapy is not discontinued at this point, patients may develop severe symptoms such as delirium, renal failure, and cardiac arrhythmias. Quinine sulfate is contraindicated in pregnancy.

VIII. Acyclovir. Oral acyclovir helps prevent the onset of postherpetic neuralgia. The drug is useful even when started after the first vesicles of herpes zoster have appeared. The dosage of oral acyclovir is 800 mg five times per day for 10 days.

Other Modalities

I. **Topical anesthetics.** *Lidocaine* base, 5% or 10% in gel (Lido-derm gel). In uncontrolled studies, topical lidocaine gel is effective in reducing the pain associated with postherpetic neuralgia. The dose for use in areas involving the trigeminal nerve is 140 to 300 mg. For the thoracic region, the dose is 250 to 500 mg. The lidocaine gel is administered under an occlusive dressing.

II. **Trigger point therapy.** Trigger points are tender areas of muscle in which the muscle fibers are shortening; thus, range of motion is decreased. They can exist in any skeletal muscle. Trigger points develop spontaneously or after an injury. They tend to be present in patients which chronic myofascial pain syndromes of the neck, back, and shoulders. On examination, trigger points can be palpated inside skeletal muscles. The trigger point feels like a nodule and is tender to palpation. The skin overlying the trigger point is cool and has an edematous "peau d'orange" appearance. There are **two techniques** that can reduce the tenderness of trigger points, thereby decreasing pain and improving range of motion.

   A. **Stretch and spray technique.** A fine stream of a vapocoolant such as Fluori-Methane is sprayed toward the skin overlying the trigger point. The spray is administered in even sweeps across the skin at an acute angle from 30 to 50 cm away. At the same time, the underlying muscle is progressively and passively stretched. The sequence of spraying and passive stretching of the underlying muscle is repeated until the range of motion is improved and the trigger point is no longer tender.

   B. **Trigger point injections.** This is an invasive form of trigger point therapy that can easily be performed in the emergency department for the relief of myofascial pain in any location of the body. The technique is a two-phased process. First, the trigger point is identified and probed with a sterile needle. Second, the trigger point is injected with local anesthetic. Immediately after the injection, the muscle just needled is passively stretched for 1 to 2 minutes to restore the muscle's full resting length to normal. If the technique is done correctly, immediate improvement is noted in 89% of patients and long-term improvement is noted in 30%.

   1. **Technique.** Trigger points are located by palpation of specific muscle groups; the skin overlying the trigger point is marked. Aseptic technique is used when injecting trigger points. A 30-gauge needle is mounted on a syringe containing a local anesthetic. Either chlorpromazine 3% or procaine 5% are recommended. A long-acting corticosteroid such as depomethylprednisolone (Depomedrol) may be added to the syringe, although it is not essential to do so. After cleansing the skin, the needle is quickly brought through the skin and then slowly advanced into the muscle. The trigger point is reached when the needle causes the local band of muscle fibers to twitch. In addition, the presence of the needle inside the trigger point elicits a dull ache inside the muscle. As soon as either of these findings are elicited, inject 0.5 ml of local anesthetic into the trigger point. After the injection, remove the needle and begin stretching the injected muscle passively for 1 to 2 minutes. Other muscles may be needled in the same manner.

2. **Contraindications.** Trigger point therapy is contraindicated in patients with severe acute muscle trauma or pain, allergies to local anesthetics, bleeding disorders, or cellulitis overlying the trigger point.

III. Transcutaneous nerve stimulation (TNS). The TNS technique is widely used for the relief of acute and chronic pain of many causes. The technique is easy to master and easy to teach to patients.

  A. **Mechanism.** The mechanism by which TNS relieves pain remains controversial. Pain impulses are carried along peripheral nerves inside small diameter fibers called C fibers. Touch, proprioception, and kinesthesia impulses are conveyed from the periphery along large myelinated fibers called A fibers. Preferentially, TNS stimulates A fibers, possibly making it difficult for pain impulses to be transmitted. It may also stimulate the release of endorphins.

  B. **Equipment.** The TNS machines require a pulse generator, an amplifier, and electrodes. The most practical pulse generator produces a rectangular pulse that is balanced to avoid a net positive or negative current that would damage the skin. The amplitude determines the strength of the pulse that is delivered to the peripheral nerve. Electrodes attached to the skin deliver the current to the peripheral nerve.

  C. **Technique.** The electrodes are empirically placed on the skin overlying trigger points and other tender areas of skin. One electrode is placed at the proximal end of a tender area, while the other is placed at the distal end. The TNS machine is then turned on. Optimal parameters for TNS have not been established.

  D. **Indications.** Treatment with TNS is indicated for the relief of acute pain due to musculoskeletal injuries and strains, such as low back pain, cervical strain, and torticollis. It is also indicated for the relief of acute orofacial pain due to periodontitis, facial abscess, and dry socket. Transcutaneous nerve stimulation is useful in reducing the pain due to rib fractures, thus permitting the patient to inspire deeply and obviating the need for large doses of oral narcotics. Treatment with TNS relieves pain due to dysmenorrhea. Finally, since studies have shown that TNS reduces postoperative pain, the technique may also be a useful adjunct in relieving pain due to painful procedures.

  E. Transcutaneous nerve stimulation is also effective in relieving **chronic pain** of many causes. Unfortunately, the effect of TNS appears to decline over time in a majority of patients. Nevertheless, TNS continues to help 25% of patients with chronic pain on a long-term basis.

  F. **Adverse effects and contraindications.** The side effects caused by TNS are minimal and include mild erythemas and allergic skin rashes of the skin. The technique is contraindicated in patients who have implanted electrical devices such as cardiac pacemakers. The TNS electrodes should not be applied near the carotid sinus in patients with cardiac arrhythmias, and should not be applied to the head and neck of patients with a history of seizure disorder or cerebrovascular disease.

Modalities of Choice in Various Painful Conditions

General considerations. The general principles of pain management are covered in the chapter on parenteral pain management (see Chapter 3, **I.A.-J.**). **Table 2-6** presents a list of oral analgesics that are currently indicated for mild, moderate, and severe pain. **Table 2-7** lists the specific agents of choice, as well as alternative agents and adjuncts, in a variety of painful conditions.

Suggested Readings

Basmajian JV: Acute back pain and spasm. A controlled multicenter trial of combined analgesic and antispasm agents, *Spine* 14:438-439, 1989.

Bentley K, et al: Floctafenine, acetaminophen/codeine combinations, and placebo in dental pain, *Current Therapeutic Research* 49:147-154, 1991.

Cole RS, et al: Indomethacin as prophylaxis against ureteral colic following extracorporeal shock wave lithotripsy, *J Urol* 141:9-12 1989.

Drugs for migraine, *Med Lett Drugs Ther* 29:27-28, 1987.

Fricton JR: Management of myofascial pain syndrome, *Advances in Pain Research and Therapy* 17:325-346, 1990.

Goldman B, editor, Stewart RD, consulting editor: Providing effective analgesia and sedation in the emergency department, *Emergency Medicine Reports* 10:73-82, 1989.

Ketorolac tromethamine, *Med Lett Drugs Ther* 32:79-81, 1990.

Lee VC: Non-narcotic modalities for the management of acute pain, *Anesthesiology Clinics of North America* 7:101-123, 1989.

McClain GA: Management of the fibromyalgia syndrome, *Advances in Pain Research and Therapy* 17:289-303, 1990.

Minotti V, et al: Double-blind evaluation of analgesic efficacy of orally administered diclofenac, nefopam, and acetylsalicylic acid (ASA) plus codeine in chronic cancer pain, *Pain* 36:177-183, 1989.

O'Hara DA, et al: Ketorolac tromethamine as compared with morphine sulfate for treatment of postoperative pain, *Clin Pharmacol Ther* 41:556-561, 1987.

Paris PM, Stewart RD: *Pain management in emergency medicine,* East Norwalk, 1988, Appleton & Lange.

Rowbotham MC, Fields HL: Topical lidocaine reduces pain in postherpetic neuralgia, *Pain* 38:297-301, 1989.

Ventafridda F, et al: Non-steroidal anti-inflammatory drugs as the first step in cancer pain therapy: double-blind, within-patient study comparing nine drugs, *J Int Med Res* 18:21-29, 1990.

Weissman DE, et al: *Handbook of cancer pain management,* ed 1, Madison, 1988, Wisconsin Cancer Pain Initiative.

Yrjola H, et al: Intravenous indomethacin for postoperative pain. A double-blind study of ankle surgery, *Acta Orthop Scand* 59:43-45, 1988.

Table 2-6. Oral Analgesics for Mild, Moderate, and Severe Pain

Analgesic	Indications (pain intensity)	Contraindications	Dosage
Acetaminophen with oxycodone 2.5 mg	Mild to moderate	Asthma/COPD, seizures	1-2 tabs q6h
ASA with oxycodone 2.5 mg	Mild to moderate	Asthma/COPD plus GI ulcer, hypersensitivity to ASA	1-2 tabs q6h
Acetaminophen with codeine 15-30 mg	Mild to moderate	Asthma/COPD, seizures	1-2 tabs q4-6h
ASA with codeine 15-30 mg	Mild to moderate	Asthma/COPD plus GI ulcer, hypersensitivity to ASA	1-2 tabs q4-6h
Floctafenine	Mild to moderate	GI ulcer, GI inflammation, Coumadin therapy	200-400 mg q6-8h
Ketorolac	Mild to moderately severe	ASA hypersensitivity	10 mg q4-6h
Acetaminophen with codeine 60 mg	Moderate to moderately severe	Allergy to acetaminophen or codeine	1 tab q4-6h
Acetaminophen with oxycodone 5 mg	Moderate to moderately severe	Asthma/COPD, seizures	1-2 tabs q6h
ASA with oxycodone 5 mg	Moderate to moderately severe	Asthma/COPD plus GI ulcer, hypersensitivity to ASA	1-2 tabs q6h
Hydrocodone 7.5 mg (with or without acetaminophen)	Moderate to moderately severe	Hypersensitivity to hydrocodone or acetaminophen	Maximum 5 tabs/24h
Pentazocine	Moderate to severe	Hypersensitivity, habituated to narcotics	50 mg q3-4h
Hydromorphone	Moderate to severe	Increased intracranial pressure, asthma/pulmonary edema	Titrated q4-6h
Morphine sulfate	Moderate to severe	Asthma/COPD, pulmonary edema, seizures, MAO inhibitors	Titrated q4-12h*

*Given every 12 hours for sustained-release preparations.

Table 2-7. Analgesic Modalities of Choice for Specific Conditions

Condition	Agent(s) of choice	Alternative(s)	Adjuncts
Cancer*			
Somatic pain†			
Mild	Acetaminophen, ASA, ibuprofen, naproxen	None	Anticonvulsants
Moderate	Acetaminophen or ASA with codeine 30-60 mg, **or** with oxycodone 5 mg, hydrocodone‡	None	Moderate stimulants (Ritalin), glucocorticoids Prochlorperazine, metoclopramide, anxiolytics
Severe	Morphine, hydromorphone		
Neuropathic§	Amitriptyline		Tricylic agents
Chest wall injuries	Floctafenine, ketorolac, naproxen	Carbamazepine, phenytoin	Nerve blocks
Dental pain	Ketorolac, floctafenine, ibuprofen	Hydrocodone, oxycodone	Nerve blocks, TNS
		Acetaminophen with codeine, oxycodone with acetaminophen	TNS
Dysmenorrhea	Naproxen, ibuprofen	Floctafenine, ketorolac, acetaminophen with codeine	TNS
Fibromyalgia or fibrositis	Amitriptyline, fluoxetine‖	Cyclobenzamine	TNS, trigger point therapy
Fractures			
Moderate pain	Floctafenine, ketorolac, naproxen, acetaminophen with codeine 30 mg	None	Rest, elevate injured area
Moderate to severe pain	Hydrocodone, oxycodone‡	Floctafenine, naproxen	None
Gout—acute	Naproxen, indomethacin	Colchicine	None
Headaches			
Migraine	Ergotamine tartrate, isometheptene mucate, naproxen, ibuprofen	Acetaminophen with codeine, oxycodone with acetaminophen Oxycodone with acetaminophen, prednisone¶	Metoclopramide
Cluster	Ergotamine tartrate, nasal oxygen		Cocaine 5% intranasal

Continued on next page

Table 2-7. Analgesic Modalities of Choice for Specific Conditions—cont'd

Condition	Agent(s) of choice	Alternative(s)	Adjuncts
Muscle spasms			
Acute	See Table 2-5	Naproxen, ibuprofen, acetaminophen with codeine, oxycodone with acetaminophen	TNS
Chronic	Cyclobenzaprine	See acute muscle spasm	TNS
Neuralgias			
Postherpetic	Acyclovir, amitriptyline with fluphenazine	Baclofen, narcotic analgesics, floctafenine	Nerve blocks
Trigeminal	Carbamazepine	Baclofen, phenytoin, floctafenine, nonnarcotic analgesics	Nerve blocks, ablative surgery
Night cramps	Correct underlying abnormality, elevate legs	Quinine sulfate	None
Pericarditis	NSAIDs	Narcotic analgesics, corticosteroids	None
After painful procedures	Hydrocodone, oxycodone	Floctafenine, ketorolac, ibuprofen/naproxen	Rest
Renal colic (prophylaxis against colic after lithotripsy)	Indomethacin suppositories, other NSAIDs	Narcotic analgesics, ketorolac	None
Sickle crisis	Nonnarcotic analgesics, pentazocine	Narcotic analgesics	None
Strains and sprains	Floctafenine, ketorolac, naproxen	Hydrocodone, oxycodone, codeine‡	Ice, rest, elevate‡

*Antineoplastic therapy is assumed.
†Due to direct tumor involvement.
‡With or without acetaminophen.
§Due to tumor compressing or invading nerves.
‖Preferred drug in elderly.
¶Refractory cluster headaches.

Parenteral Pain Management

H. Brian Goldman, M.D., A.B.E.M., M.C.F.P. (EM)

Physicians regard pain as a symptom, a key that unlocks the door to a diagnosis and treatment. The strategy was first developed several hundred years ago, and it's seductively simple. Doctors use a chief complaint of pain as a clue to a diseased or broken body part. Once found, the diseased or broken body part can be treated or removed, and the pain goes away. Without such a strategy, many patients would suffer great harm before seeking medical attention.

Pain and Diagnosis

- **A. There are many examples** that prove the strategy works. For example, both a detailed history on the quality of chest pain, and appropriate laboratory tests help distinguish the pain of myocardial ischemia from that caused by a pulmonary embolus. Moreover, it would be foolhardy to treat the pain in either case without interrupting the process that caused the pain in the first place.
- **B. Extremes.** Unfortunately, the strategy is all too frequently carried to extremes. Many emergency physicians make no attempt to treat the pain until they make a definitive diagnosis. This is borne out in some alarming statistics. More than half of all patients who are seen in emergency departments because of pain do not receive an analgesic during the visit. Emergency physicians cite two reasons for not treating acute pain. The first is a concern that analgesics mask symptoms and compromise attempts to make a diagnosis. The second is a pervasive fear that the liberal prescribing of narcotic analgesics leads to widespread abuse. Recent evidence suggests that both concerns are far more trivial than widely believed.
- **C. Pain relievers.** There is a vast arsenal of potent analgesics that relieve pain effectively and without worrisome side effects or abuse liability. Thus, the emergency physician's approach to painful conditions is two-pronged. As always, the physician must search for the cause of the pain. This approach is the focus of many other chapters in this book.
- **D. Understanding acute pain.** In addition, every effort should be made to relieve pain as completely and as expeditiously as possible. This requires an understanding that acute pain causes a nociceptive sensation, as well as an emotional impact, usually anxiety. Either of the two may predominate; depending on the situation, both may have to be treated. Analgesia and sedation often go hand in hand.
- **E. Parenteral agents.** There is a large selection of analgesics and sedatives suitable for use in the emergency department. Parenteral agents are the focus of this chapter. (Oral agents were discussed in the preceding chapter.) Narcotic agonists such as morphine and meperidine are used by most emergency physicians. The short-acting narcotic fentanyl is emerging as the analgesic of choice for painful procedures. Narcotic agonist–antagonists are useful because they cause

less respiratory depression than pure agonists and have a longer duration of action. Nalbuphine is the drug of choice among this group. Ketamine is a dissociative agent with potent analgesic action. Parenterally administered nonsteroidal antiinflammatory drugs (NSAIDs) provide an efficacious alternative to narcotics, with fewer side effects. Ketorolac tromethamine is the only drug of this class approved for use in the United States. In addition, a variety of nonnarcotic analgesics have proven effective in the treatment of acute migraine headaches. These include prochlorperazine, chlorpromazine, and ergotamine tartrate. Sumatriptan, a selective 5-hydroxytryptamine receptor agonist, has also been shown to be highly effective in the treatment of acute migraine.

F. Parenteral anxiolytics such as diazepam and midazolam are useful for sedating patients who undergo painful procedures such as reduction of fractures and dislocations. Inhaled nitrous oxide plays a similar adjunctive role.

Mechanisms of Acute Pain

Despite extensive research, the definitive mechanism for acute pain perception has not been established. However, it is clear that pain has both a physiologic and psychologic dimension.

I. Physiologic aspects. The pathways of acute pain transmission are better understood. An impulse of the acute pain pathway begins in the periphery, where specialized pain receptors are activated by mechanical, thermal, and chemical stimuli. This stimulation is mediated by some of the mediators of inflammation, namely histamine, leukotrienes, kinins, and slow-reacting substance of anaphylaxis (SRS-A). There are two fiber pathways for pain transmission. Large myelinated fibers known as A fibers carry acute pain impulses. These are responsible for the acute pain experienced at the instant an acute injury (e.g., a laceration or a fracture) occurs. Small unmyelinated fibers known as C fibers also carry acute pain impulses but at a much slower rate. The C fibers are responsible for the diffuse ache that sets in several minutes after an acute injury. The diffuse ache is associated with release of prostaglandins. Not surprisingly, NSAIDs are effective in relieving this kind of pain.

A. Pain impulses. Once generated, pain impulses travel to the dorsal root ganglion of the same spinal level, then cross the midline where they synapse with ascending pathways. These pathways carry pain impulses to the thalamus and other centers of the limbic system, where acute pain messages are modified by the patient's own memories of and experiences with pain.

B. Endorphins play a crucial role in modifying both the perception and the experience of pain. Endorphins are a heterogeneous group of neuropeptides that exert analgesic and other effects by binding to opiate receptors in the central nervous system. As shown in **Table 3-1,** there are six opiate receptors. Two receptors—mu and kappa—are responsible for the analgesic effects of opiates. This has clinical significance. Opiates that bind to the mu receptor—such as morphine—produce analgesia, as well as euphoria, physical dependence, and withdrawal symptoms. Kappa opiate agonists, such as nalbuphine, produce analgesia without euphoria or dependence.

C. Mu receptor. In addition, mu receptor was recently reclassified into two receptors: mu^1 and mu^2. Activation of the mu^1 receptor causes spinal analgesia, while activation of the mu^2 receptor causes respiratory depression. This subdivision means that it may be possible to synthesize potent opioid analgesics that do not cause respiratory depression.

Table 3-1. Opiate Receptors

Receptor	Action	Agonist(s)	Antagonist(s)
mu[1]	Supraspinal analgesia, euphoria, physical dependence, suppression of withdrawal	Morphine, meperidine, fentanyl, hydromorphone	Naloxone, naltrexone, butorphanol, pentazocine, nalbuphine
mu[2]	Respiratory depression	See mu[1]	See mu[1]
kappa	Spinal analgesia, miosis, sedation	Morphine, pentazocine, butorphanol, nalbuphine	Naloxone, naltrexone
sigma	Dysphoria, hallucinations, vasomotor stimulation	Pentazocine, nalbuphine,* butorphanol*	Naloxone, naltrexone
delta	No actions discovered	None	None
epsilon	No actions discovered	None	None

*Weak agonist.

II. **Psychologic aspects.** Pain perception is as individual as are fingerprints. No two patients have identical thresholds for pain. For this reason, pain management must be individualized. There is no standard dose of opioid analgesics. Therefore it is counterproductive to compare one patient's response to a given dose of opiate with that of another.

A. Scales for measuring. Unfortunately, there are no established ways of objectively measuring the patient's level of discomfort. Most scales for measuring pain are based on the patient's subjective level of discomfort. The easiest way to determine this is to ask the patient to score his or her pain as a number between 0 and 10, where 10 is the highest possible level of pain. As various analgesic modalities are administered, the level of pain can be easily compared to baseline.

B. Psychology plays an important role in determining how well patients respond to analgesics. In addition to the pain, many patients suffer from associated anxiety. Anxiety magnifies the experience of pain. Thus effective management of anxiety can improve a patient's response to analgesics. The easiest way to manage anxiety associated with pain is to give the patient confidence that his or her pain will be promptly relieved (see Pain Management, General Principles).

Analgesic Agents

Table 3-2 lists the properties of the ideal analgesic. At present, no single agent has all of those properties. With each analgesic, there are trade-offs. Opiate agonists are both potent and titratable, but they cause respiratory depression and are associated with physical dependence and abuse. Ketorolac is as potent as morphine or meperidine, but it cannot be titrated as opiates can, since it is approved for intramuscular administration only.

Fortunately there are more than enough agents to cover almost every contingency in emergency medicine. Selecting the most appropriate agent means knowing the pharmacologic profile of each agent, as well as its side effects and contraindications.

I. **Narcotics or opioids (Table 3-3).** This group of agents consists of morphine as well as its synthetic derivatives. Some of the agents described below produce analgesia by binding to both mu receptors and kappa receptors, while others produce analgesia by binding to kappa receptors alone. Narcotic agents are classified according to their receptor activity. Thus, there are opioid agonists, partial agonists, agonist-antagonists, and pure antagonists.

Table 3-2. Properties of the Ideal Analgesic

General procedures
- Potent
- Rapid onset
- Titratable
- Easily administered
- Painless administration
- No serious side effects
- Safe for use in the elderly
- Effects easily reversible
- No physical dependence
- No abuse potential

Painful procedures
- Short duration of action
- Sedative or anxiolytic effects
- Amnesic effect
- No serious side effects
- Easily reversible

Analgesic Agents 101

Table 3-3. The Narcotic Equivalency Index

	Equianalgesic dose (mg)	Relative potency (compared with parenteral morphine)	Duration of action (hr)	Relative duration of action (compared with parenteral morphine)	Narcotic equivalency index conversion factor
Morphine					
Parenteral	10.0	1.00	4.0	1.000	1.00
Oral	60.0	0.17	4.0	1.000	0.17
Hydromorphone					
Parenteral	1.5	6.67	4.0	1.000	6.67
Oral	7.5	1.33	4.0	1.000	1.33
Codeine					
Parenteral	130.0	0.08	4.0	1.000	0.08
Oral	200.0	0.05	4.0	1.000	0.05
Oxycodone					
Oral	30.0	0.33	4.0	1.000	0.33
Levorphanol					
Parenteral	2.0	5.00	5.0	1.250	6.25
Oral	4.0	2.50	5.0	1.250	3.13
Meperidine					
Parenteral	75.0	0.13	3.0	0.750	0.10
Oral	300.0	0.03	4.0	1.000	0.03
Fentanyl					
Parenteral	0.1	100.00	1.0	0.250	25.00
Nalbuphine					
Parenteral	12.5	0.80	4.0	1.000	0.80

A. Narcotic agonists. These agents are the most useful drugs available for the relief of acute pain of most causes. If given in equipotent doses **(Table 3-3)**, all of the narcotic agonists are interchangeable. They are differentiated by their duration of action and their side effects.

1. **Agonists useful in emergency medicine.** Of those agonists listed in **Table 3-3,** the ones most useful in emergency medicine are morphine, meperidine, hydrocodone, levorphanol, and fentanyl. Parenteral hydromorphone is highly efficacious, but its tendency to cause euphoria increases its dependence liability. The only indication for parenteral hydromorphone in the emergency department should be for the management of terminal cancer pain. Parenteral codeine is not particularly useful, since at equipotent doses, it produces an unacceptable degree of nausea and constipation. Methadone is not licensed for use by physicians other than addiction specialists who practice in recognized drug treatment centers. Opiate agonists that are only available in oral form were discussed in the previous chapter.

2. **General principles.** The agents discussed in this section may each be administered intravenously or intramuscularly. Although the intramuscular route is more convenient to the emergency department staff than is the intravenous route, the latter route is more efficacious. Narcotics given intravenously have a rapid onset of analgesia, reach a consistent plasma level, and are easily titrated to the patient's response. By contrast, narcotics given intramuscularly have a slower onset of efficacy, reach variable plasma levels, and are not easily titrated to the patient's response (titration is possible but much slower than with intravenous administration). Where possible, parenteral narcotics should be given intravenously.

   a. **There is no correct dosage of narcotics.** In general, it is best to administer small boluses of narcotic intravenously over 1 to 2 minutes at intervals of 5 minutes, observing the patient between doses for signs of efficacy. These include decreased sweating, reduced anxiety, return of normal skin color, and normalization of vital signs.

   b. **Level of pain.** Patients should be asked to report frequently on their level of pain, so that it can be relieved at the first indication of recurrence. When pain is treated before reaching maximum severity, the total dose of analgesic required is lower than it is when pain is allowed to progress to maximum severity.

   c. **Addiction.** Despite a good deal of evidence to the contrary, it is widely held that patients receiving parenteral narcotics are at high risk of becoming addicted to them. The actual incidence of iatrogenic addiction to parenteral narcotics for the treatment of acute pain is roughly 4 per 10,000. The vast majority of patients who take narcotics for the relief of acute pain stop taking them when the cause of the pain is removed.

3. **Morphine**

   a. **Pharmacokinetics.** Intravenous morphine has a serum half-life of 2 to 3 hours. The drug is metabolized by hepatic glucuronidation and is excreted by the liver. Hepatic disease does not lead to altered metabolism unless there is overwhelming liver failure. The usual duration of action is 4 hours. The half-life is 50% longer in **elderly patients.** Elderly patients have effective analgesia, as well as side effects, at smaller doses than do young adults.

   b. **Dosage and routes of administration**

Analgesic Agents 103

Table 3-4. Parenteral Analgesics and Sedatives

Agent	Dose/Route	Indications	Contraindications	Precautions
Narcotic Agonists				
Morphine sulfate	2-5 mg IV q5 min till pain relieved; Children, 0.1-0.2 mg/kg/dose	1) Acute pain relief 2) Analgesic for procedures	1) Severe COPD 2) Asthma 3) Hepatic failure	1) Respiratory depression (have naloxone 2-5 mg IV at bedside) 2) O_2 saturation monitor 3) Vomiting: give promethazine 5-10 mg IV or 25 mg IM 4) Histamine release
Meperidine	40-50 mg IV titrated to pain relief, max dose range 100-125 mg; Children, 0.5-1.0 mg/kg/dose	See morphine	1) Same as morphine 2) MAO inhibitors	1) Reduce dosage if renal or hepatic dysfunction 2) Not ideal for pain >3 hours 3) Vomiting: see morphine
Fentanyl	25-50 µg q5 min IV to max of 150-300 µg; Children, 2-3 µg/kg	1) See Morphine 2) Drug of choice for brief procedures 3) Drug of choice if history of asthma	Severe COPD	Truncal rigidity in anesthetic dose (responds to naloxone)
Narcotic Agonist–Antagonists				
Nalbuphine*	10-20 mg IV in 2-5 mg boluses q5-6h	1) Drug of choice for new onset sickle cell crisis 2) ? Drug of choice for biliary colic	Physical dependence on narcotics	Precipitates withdrawal in narcotic dependency

Continued on next page

Table 3-4. Parenteral Analgesics and Sedatives—cont'd

Agent	Dose/Route	Indications	Contraindications	Precautions
Parenteral NSAIDs				
Ketorolac*	Indomethacin—not approved as a parenteral analgesic 30-60 mg IM followed by 15-30 mg q6h	1) Moderate to severe pain of various causes 2) Drug of choice when risk of narcotic abuse is high 3) May be drug of choice for renal colic	1) Peptic ulcer disease 2) Inflammatory bowel disease 3) Allergy to NSAIDs 4) Labor	1) Decrease dose by 50% in renal failure
Benzodiazepines				
Diazepam*	5-15 mg slow IV push; Children, 0.1-0.3 mg/kg	1) Sedation for procedures 2) Prevents ketamine-induced nightmares	Altered mental status of unknown cause	1) Respiratory depression if given with IV narcotic 2) Reduce dose in hepatic failure
Midazolam	1-2 mg slow IV push in boluses of 0.5 mg; Children, 0.04-0.10 mg/kg	1) See diazepam 2) Ideal for brief procedures	See diazepam	See diazepam
Dissociative Agents				
Ketamine	Loading dose, 0.5-1.0 mg/kg IM or slow IV push; Maintenance infusion, 0.01-0.02 mg/kg/min for procedures >20 min	1) Painful procedures 2) Useful analgesic if narcotics contraindicated 3) Useful in children	1) History of psychosis 2) Hallucinogen abuse 3) Severe hypertension	1) Exacerbates hypertension 2) Emergence nightmares prevented by pretreatment with IV midazolam or diazepam

Table 3-4. Parenteral Analgesics and Sedatives—cont'd

Agent	Dose/Route	Indications	Contraindications	Precautions
Muscle Relaxants				
Methocarbamol	1 gm IV or IM q8h prn	Acute muscle spasm	1) Hypersensitivity 2) Renal failure	Causes drowsiness and syncope
Orphenadrine	60 mg IV or IM q12h × 2 doses	Acute muscle spasm	1) Glaucoma 2) Prostatic hypertrophy 3) History of bowel obstruction 4) Stenosing peptic ulcer 5) Hypersensitivity	1) May cause anticholinergic syndrome in elderly 2) Dry mouth 3) Drowsiness
Nitrous oxide	Self-administered via mask with O_2 in 50:50 mixture	Adjunctive analgesic	1) Altered LOC 2) Pneumothorax 3) Abdominal pain with distension 4) Bowel obstruction 5) COPD	1) Self-administration only 2) Discontinue if patient too drowsy to operate mask 3) Use scavenging device to protect staff
Antimigraine Therapy				
Dihydroergotamine	0.5-1.0 mg IV over 2-3 min; may repeat × 1 in 1 hour	1) Acute migraine 2) Cluster headaches	1) Thrombophlebitis 2) Hypertension 3) Sepsis 4) Peptic ulcer 5) Coronary artery disease 6) Collagen vascular diseases 7) Renal or liver disease	1) Causes nausea; give antiemetic 2) Numbness of extremities 3) Precordial chest pain

Continued on next page

Table 3-4. Parenteral Analgesics and Sedatives—cont'd

Agent	Dose/Route	Indications	Contraindications	Precautions
Antimigraine Therapy, cont'd				
Chlorpromazine	5-10 mg IV	Acute migraine	Patients at risk of anticholinergic syndrome (see orphenadrine)	Prolonged orthostatic hypotension; may require IV bolus of saline solution
Prochlorperazine	5-10 mg IV	1) Acute migraine 2) Adjunct when administering narcotics	See chlorpromazine	Doses not cause orthostatic hypotension
Metoclopramide	5-10 mg IV; 10-20 mg IM	Same as prochlorperazine	1) Hypersensitivity 2) Mechanical bowel obstruction 3) Gastrointestinal bleeding	Extrapyramidal side effects

COPD, Chronic obstructive pulmonary disease; *MAO*, monoamine oxidase; *LOC*, level of consciousness.
*Not recommended in children

(1) Intravenous administration. The intravenous route is the preferred route of administration. The dosage should be individualized. Begin with a 2 to 3 mg bolus (given over 1 minute), and titrate in increments of 2 to 3 mg given intravenously every 5 minutes until the patient is comfortable. Reduce the dosage by 25% to 50% for elderly patients and those concomitantly receiving intravenous sedation. There is no maximum dose of morphine. Some patients require as much as 30 to 50 mg intravenously. Once analgesia is obtained, the total titrated dose may be given intravenously every 4 hours.

(2) Intramuscular and subcutaneous administration. Either route produces the same plasma levels. The subcutaneous route is preferable because it is less painful than an intramuscular injection. Intramuscular absorption varies with the individual and also varies with the injection site. Patients with sickle trait and a past history of frequent painful crises have very poor and unpredictable absorption of narcotic administered intramuscularly. As with intravenous administration, there is no specific starting dose and precise titration is not possible; an average starting dose is 5 to 10 mg given intramuscularly or subcutaneously. Peak levels are reached 10 to 20 minutes after administration.

c. Clinical use. Morphine is effective in relieving pain of almost any cause. It is a tried and tested analgesic used during painful procedures. Since it has a longer duration of action than meperidine, morphine is preferable to meperidine in relieving painful conditions expected to last more than 3 hours, such as sickle crisis and renal colic.

d. Adverse effects and contraindications. The most significant adverse effect is respiratory depression. The peak incidence of respiratory depression occurs 4 to 6 minutes after an intravenous injection, 30 minutes after an intramuscular injection, and up to 90 minutes after a subcutaneous injection.

(1) Morphine. Like many narcotics, morphine causes nausea and vomiting by direct stimulation of the chemotrigger zone located in the brain stem. The nausea is exacerbated when the patient is either sitting up or ambulatory. Patients placed in the supine or recumbent position have less nausea. The nausea may also be relieved by administering dramamine, 50 mg IM q4h; promethazine, 25 mg IM (starting dose) and 10 to 25 mg IM q4h thereafter; or haloperidol, 1 mg SC.

(2) Constipation. Morphine also increases constipation; in cases of ulcerative colitis it can precipitate a toxic megacolon. Morphine has long been believed to worsen the pain associated with biliary colic by causing spasm of the sphincter of Oddi. Biliary pressure rises after a bolus of either morphine or meperidine. Narcotic agonist–antagonists do not have the same effect.

(3) Asthma. Morphine can exacerbate asthma by releasing histamine. It should be used with caution in patients with mild to moderate asthma.

(4) Contraindications. The contraindications to the use of morphine include hypersensitivity to opiates, severe asthma, chronic obstructive lung disease, liver failure, increased intracranial pressure, as well as the concomitant use of monoamine oxidase (MAO) inhibitors.

4. **Meperidine**
   a. **Pharmacokinetics.** The serum half-life of meperidine is 2½ hours. The drug is metabolized by hepatic demethylation; thus metabolism will be affected by mild to moderate liver disease. The metabolite normeperidine, which is responsible for central nervous system (CNS) side effects such as tremors and hyperreflexia, is excreted by the kidney. As with morphine, elderly patients have increased sensitivity to meperidine. In patients with renal disease, normeperidine accumulates. The maximum duration of action of meperidine is 3 hours.
   b. **Dosage and routes of administration**
      (1) **Intravenous administration.** This is the preferred route of administration (see **b) 2)**). Begin with an intravenous bolus of 15 to 25 mg (over 1 minute) and titrate in increments of 15 to 25 mg given intravenously every 5 minutes until the patient is comfortable. Careful titration is critical to the administration of meperidine because the drug has a steep dose-response curve. Near the dosage required for optimal analgesia, an incremental intravenous dose of 10 to 15 mg may mean the difference between adequate and inadequate analgesia. Once a baseline analgesic dose is determined, the same dose should be given every 2 to 3 hours. If the drug is given every 4 hours, the pain will almost certainly recur.
      (2) **Intramuscular or subcutaneous administration.** The same considerations apply as in the case of morphine. An average intramuscular or subcutaneous dosage of meperidine is 75 to 100 mg given every 3 hours.
   c. **Adverse effects and contraindications.** Meperidine shares many of the same adverse effects as morphine. Meperidine causes nausea and vomiting. Like morphine, meperidine exacerbates asthma because is causes histamine release. Despite teaching to the contrary, both morphine and meperidine increase biliary pressure by causing spasm of the sphincter of Oddi.
      (1) **Meperidine** causes CNS adverse effects such as tremors, hyperreflexia, anxiety, disorientation, hallucinations, psychosis, and seizures.
      (2) **The absolute contraindications** to the use of meperidine include hepatic disease, severe asthma, and the concomitant or recent (within 10 days of starting meperidine) use of MAO inhibitors. The combination of meperidine with an MAO inhibitor can cause the malignant neuroleptic syndrome.
   d. **Clinical use.** Like morphine, meperidine has a long track record in the treatment of pain of various causes. It is useful in the treatment of pain during painful procedures such as incision and drainage of abscesses, as well as reduction of fractures. However, there is no apparent justification for establishing meperidine as a drug of choice over morphine. The main limitation of meperidine is its brief duration of action. Painful conditions likely to last longer than 3 hours, such as renal colic, sickle crisis, cancer pain, and postoperative pain, should not be treated with this drug.

5. **Fentanyl**
   a. **Pharmacokinetics.** Fentanyl is a potent narcotic analgesic. It is highly lipophilic and penetrates the CNS quickly. Fentanyl has a duration of action of only 20 to 40 minutes because of a rapid redistribution of the drug. The drug also produces potent sedation. These two properties make fentanyl an ideal analgesic for brief procedures. The drug is metabolized by the liver and excreted by the kidneys.
   b. **Dosage and routes of administration**
      (1) **Intravenous administration.** As with other narcotics, fentanyl is titrated to optimal analgesia and sedation. The average adult requires 100 to 200 µg, or 2 to 3 µg/kg. Adults should receive an initial dose of 50 to 100 µg by slow intravenous push; thereafter, they should receive 25 to 50 µg intravenously every 5 minutes until the patient has adequate analgesia or is sedated. Use one half the recommended starting and incremental dosages in elderly patients, as well as those patients concomitantly receiving a benzodiazepine sedative such as diazepam or midazolam.
      (2) **Oral administration.** Because of its extensive first pass effect, there is no oral form of fentanyl. However, research is under way on the development of a fentanyl lollipop that can be administered to children. Absorption of the drug occurs transmucosally in the oral cavity. In studies, fentanyl lollipops have been used successfully to premedicate children about to undergo a variety of surgical procedures.
   c. **Adverse effects and contraindications.** This drug is known to cause very few serious side effects. There are no significant effects on vital signs, aside from respiratory depression. The most serious side effect of fentanyl is muscular rigidity. This occurs at anesthetic doses used during surgery (>10 µg/kg) and responds to narcotic antagonists such as naloxone, as well as to muscle relaxants. In studies involving the use of fentanyl at doses of 2 to 3 µg/kg, no cases of muscular rigidity have been documented. Fentanyl does not cause histamine release and thus may be used as an analgesic in **severe asthmatics**. The main contraindications to the use of the drug are documented hypersensitivity, as well as a history of truncal rigidity on previous exposure to fentanyl. Since there is little clinical experience, fentanyl should not be given to pregnant women.
   d. **Clinical use.** Fentanyl has emerged as the analgesic of choice for brief, painful procedures such as reduction of fractures and dislocations, incision and drainage of abscesses and external thrombosed hemorrhoids, changing of burn dressings, and insertion of a chest tube. Because of its sedating effects, fentanyl is also useful in the premedication of patients undergoing elective cardioversion.
6. **Alfentanil and sufentanil.** These two drugs are derivatives of fentanyl. Alfentanil is of similar potency to fentanyl but has a shorter duration of action. The drug may be useful for pain control in brief outpatient procedures, but there is little experience using this drug in the emergency department. Sufentanil is 10 times as potent as fentanyl and is not considered safe enough for use in emergency medicine.

B. **Partial agonists.** Opioids is this category owe their analgesic properties to partial agonist activity at the mu opioid receptor. Unlike the agonist-antagonists, partial agonists are not mu receptor antagonists. Both partial agonists and agonist-antagonists have a much lower abuse potential than do pure agonists. Buprenorphine is the only partial agonist currently licensed for use in the United States.

1. **Buprenorphine**
   a. **Pharmacokinetics.** Buprenorphine is well absorbed when administered orally or intramuscularly. It is also well absorbed when administered sublingually, and is the only opioid drug widely available in that form. The drug is excreted in both urine and feces. The serum half-life is 3 hours. However, buprenorphine binds tightly to opioid receptors, and its duration of action is 6 to 8 hours, much longer than that of morphine or meperidine. This makes buprenorphine very useful in the management of painful conditions lasting longer than 4 hours.
   b. **Dosage and routes of administration.** The dosage of buprenorphine is 0.3 to 0.6 mg administered intravenously or intramuscularly every 6 to 8 hours as needed. The intravenous route is the preferred route.
   c. **Adverse effects and contraindications.** Buprenorphine can precipitate withdrawal in patients who are physically dependent on narcotics. The drug can reverse the respiratory depression caused by narcotic administration. However, buprenorphine can itself cause respiratory depression that is difficult to reverse. Drowsiness is also a feature of the drug. Buprenorphine is contraindicated in patients who are habituated to narcotics, patients with severe COPD, and those with a history of hypersensitivity to the drug.
   d. **Clinical use.** With its long duration of action and low abuse potential, buprenorphine is ideal for the treatment of painful conditions lasting more than 4 hours, such as low back pain and renal colic. Since the drug does not increase biliary pressure, it is also useful in patients with biliary colic. Buprenorphine should be strongly considered in patients with newly diagnosed sickle cell disease. It is less likely to be useful in patients with well-established sickle disease because the majority of such patients are habituated to narcotics.

C. Narcotic agonist–antagonists. The opioid analgesics in this category are mu antagonists and kappa agonists; they owe their analgesic properties to the latter. Drugs in this group have a much lower dependence liability then do pure agonists. They produce little euphoria, and tolerance to these drugs occurs more slowly than with morphine. Withdrawal symptoms tend to be mild, although the drugs can cause severe withdrawal symptoms when administered to patients habituated to pure agonists.

1. **Nalbuphine.** This agonist-antagonist has a potency roughly equivalent to that of morphine and three times that of pentazocine.
   a. **Pharmacokinetics.** Nalbuphine is well absorbed, is metabolized by the liver, and is excreted by the kidneys. The serum half-life is 5 hours, and the duration of action is 3 to 6 hours.
   b. **Dosage and routes of administration**
      (1) **Intravenous administration.** This is the preferred route of administration. The onset of action after an intravenous bolus is 2 to 3 minutes, compared with 15 minutes after subcutaneous or intramuscular administration. The dosage of nalbuphine is similar to that of morphine, except that nalbuphine has a maximum single

dose of 20 mg, and maximum daily dose of 160 mg. Begin with an intravenous bolus of 2 to 3 mg (over 1 minute), and titrate in 2 to 3 mg aliquots every 5 minutes up to a maximum dose of 0.15 to 0.30 mg/kg or 20 mg, whichever is less. The optimal analgesic dosage can be repeated every 3 to 6 hours, up to a maximum of 160 mg/day.

   (2) Intramuscular and subcutaneous administration. See intravenous administration guidelines.

   c. **Adverse effects and contraindications.** Nalbuphine is remarkably free of worrisome side effects. The drug is almost as potent as morphine but causes much less euphoria and potential for abuse. The incidence of psychotomimetic effects is far less than that of pentazocine. The most common side effect is sedation. A 10 mg dose of nalbuphine causes the same degree of respiratory depression as does a 10 mg dose of morphine. However, at doses of 30 mg or higher, nalbuphine has a respiratory depressant effect comparable to only 20 mg of morphine. The only **absolute contraindication** is a history of hypersensitivity to the drug. Relative contraindications include advanced liver or renal disease, severe COPD, and a history of narcotic abuse.

   d. **Clinical use.** Nalbuphine is useful as an alternative to morphine in the management of moderate to severe pain in patients at high risk of narcotic addiction or abuse. For example, nalbuphine may be the opioid of choice in patients with sickle disease not yet habituated to narcotics. Note that the administration of nalbuphine to patients habituated to narcotics may precipitate withdrawal symptoms. Nalbuphine does not increase biliary pressure and thus may be the *drug of choice for biliary colic*. Nalbuphine is also indicated for the management of respiratory depression in patients receiving narcotics for pain control (e.g., cancer pain). In this situation, nalbuphine reverses respiratory depression without reversing analgesia.

2. **Pentazocine.** This narcotic agonist–antagonist has been largely superseded by nalbuphine, which is three times more potent than pentazocine and has fewer side effects.

   a. **Pharmacokinetics.** Pentazocine is well absorbed orally. The drug is conjugated in the liver and excreted by the kidneys. The serum half-life is 2 to 3 hours, and the duration of action is 3 to 4 hours.

   b. **Dosages and routes of administration.** The onset of analgesia occurs 2 to 3 minutes after an intravenous bolus of pentazocine, and 15 to 30 minutes after an intramuscular or subcutaneous injection.

   (1) Intravenous administration. The maximum intravenous dosage is 30 mg every 3 to 4 hours.

   (2) Intramuscular or subcutaneous administration. The dosage is 30 to 60 mg subcutaneously every 3 to 4 hours up to a maximum dose of 360 mg/day. Intramuscular administration of pentazocine is not recommended because repeated injections may cause fibrous myopathy.

   c. **Adverse effects and contraindications.** The most serious side effects seen with pentazocine are psychotomimetic effects such as hallucinations, delusions, dysphoria, and psychosis. These occur in up to 10% of patients receiving pentazocine, and less so with nalbuphine. As with nalbuphine, administration of pentazocine may induce withdrawal in patients habituated to narcotics. The only *absolute contraindication* is hypersensitivity to pentazocine.

- **d. Clinical use.** Pentazocine is recommended for patients with moderate pain due to biliary colic. It is also recommended as an analgesic in patients who are at risk of becoming addicted to narcotics and where no other alternative such as nalbuphine is available.

D. Narcotic antagonists. Naloxone is the only pure narcotic antagonist available for clinical use. Nalmefene, another pure antagonist that is not yet available for use in the United States, has shown promise in clinical research. Its main advantage is that its duration of action is 3 to 5 hours.

1. **Naloxone**
   a. **Pharmacokinetics.** Naloxone has an onset of action 30 to 60 seconds after an intravenous bolus injection. The duration of action depends on the dose of naloxone, as well as the narcotic being antagonized.
   b. **Dosage and routes of administration**
      (1) **Intravenous administration.** Administer an intravenous bolus of naloxone, 1 to 2 mg, for respiratory depression caused by the administration of narcotic analgesics. Repeat as required. An infusion of naloxone is only indicated for known or suspected overdoses of methadone and propoxyphene.
      (2) **Intramuscular or subcutaneous administration.** Not recommended.
   c. **Adverse effects and contraindications.** Administration of naloxone reverses respiratory depression and analgesic actions of narcotics. Patients who are habituated to narcotics may manifest symptoms of withdrawal. The **only contraindication** to the use of naloxone is known hypersensitivity.
   d. **Clinical use.** Naloxone is the current narcotic antagonist of choice for respiratory depression and excessive sedation caused by overdoses of narcotics.
2. **Nalbuphine.** This drug may be the treatment of choice for respiratory depression due to narcotic overdose in patients receiving narcotics for pain control.

II. Parenteral NSAIDs.
Oral NSAIDs have been part of the analgesic arsenal of emergency physicians for years. Oral NSAIDs are effective in relieving acute pain of mild to moderate severity. Until recently, it was a matter of speculation whether parenteral NSAIDs might be effective in the relief of severe acute pain.

A. Ketorolac tromethamine (Toradol). Ketorolac is the first parenteral NSAID approved by the United States Food and Drug Administration for the relief of moderate to severe pain. At present, it is only licensed for intramuscular administration.

1. **Mechanism of action.** Ketorolac decreases prostaglandin synthesis by inhibiting arachidonic acid metabolism. The drug appears to be more potent as an analgesic than as an antipyretic or antiinflammatory agent.
2. **Pharmacokinetics.** Ketorolac is well absorbed after intramuscular injection. It has a serum half-life of 4 to 6 hours in young adults, and up to 9 hours in elderly patients. Ketorolac has a duration of action of 6 hours. The drug and its metabolites are excreted primarily by the kidney. The clearance of ketorolac is reduced in the elderly, as well as in those patients

with moderately impaired renal function. Salicylates, which displace ketorolac from its protein binding sites, can increase the serum's free concentration of the drug.
3. **Dosage and administration.** *Intramuscular administration.* The recommended initial intramuscular dosage is 30 to 60 mg, followed by 15 to 30 mg every 6 hours. Patients older than 65 years or with impaired renal function should receive the lower dose. The recommended maximum daily dose is 150 mg on the first day and 120 mg/day thereafter.
4. **Adverse effects and contraindications.** Ketorolac has fewer side effects than morphine or meperidine. Unlike narcotics, it has no dependence liability and does not cause respiratory depression. It does not cause constipation.
    a. Ketorolac causes dyspepsia, nausea, and drowsiness. Although it causes reversible platelet dysfunction, ketorolac has not been associated with postoperative bleeding when prescribed as a postsurgical analgesic.
    b. **The contraindications** to the use of ketorolac include known hypersensitivity to NSAIDs, previous history of peptic ulcer disease, or conditions causing active inflammation of the gastrointestinal tract such as diverticulitis and ulcerative colitis. Ketorolac should not be used as an obstetric analgesic because of its effects on uterine contractility and fetal circulation.
5. **Clinical use.** Ketorolac given intramuscularly is indicated for the short-term management of moderate to severe pain after abdominal, orthopedic, and gynecologic procedures. The drug is as effective and longer lasting than morphine, 12 mg, or meperidine, 100 mg, administered intramuscularly.
    a. **The main limitation of ketorolac** is that it is not titratable. It cannot be administered intravenously. Besides, incremental doses above the maximum dose do not increase the analgesic effect of the drug.
    b. In theory, ketorolac should be efficacious in the relief of pain due to **renal colic**. Prostaglandins have been shown to mediate the increase in pressure inside the renal pelvis that is associated with a ureteral calculus. Intravenous indomethacin has been used in Europe for years for the relief of pain due to renal calculi. However, there have been no studies testing ketorolac in the management of pain due to renal colic.
    c. **Acute pain.** Likewise, there is little data on the efficacy of ketorolac in the relief of acute pain for conditions seen by emergency physicians. Ketorolac could potentially be of use in the management of acute pains such as low back pain, pelvic pain, dental pain, sickle crisis, and headaches. However, no studies have been published evaluating ketorolac in the above conditions.
    d. **In summary,** ketorolac may be the drug of choice in situations in which narcotic analgesics are contraindicated, such as advanced COPD, a history of narcotic abuse, and patients who are concomitantly taking MAO inhibitors. Ketorolac should also be considered in situations in which excessive sedation is undesirable. The list includes patients with head injuries, the elderly, patients whose initial presentation is complicated by ethanol or other sedating drugs, and those patients who require intravenous sedation as part of their management.

III. **Ketamine.** Ketamine is a dissociative sedative that has been used for years as a general anesthetic. Recently the drug has been used in emergency medicine as a highly potent analgesic agent.
  1. **Mechanism of action.** Ketamine produces a state of dissociation between the thalamus and the cortex. At a dose of 0.4 mg/kg, ketamine depresses the medial thalamic nuclei and blocks afferent pain signals, producing a profound state of analgesia such that even a local anesthetic is seldom required. Patients receiving this dose remain conscious and cooperative, albeit in a trance-like state. Ketamine does not cause respiratory depression or loss of airway reflexes; cardiovascular function remains normal. Ketamine also has an amnesic effect.
  2. **Pharmacokinetics.** Ketamine can be given intravenously or intramuscularly. It is rapidly taken up by the CNS, accounting for its rapid onset of action. The drug is metabolized by the liver and cleared by the kidney. The serum half-life is 3 to 4 hours, longer if diazepam is administered concomitantly.
  3. **Dosage and administration**
      a. **Intravenous administration.** Ketamine is administered as a bolus of 0.4 mg/kg over 1 minute. Sedation begins within seconds and lasts for 20 minutes. Alternatively, ketamine may be administered as a constant infusion of 0.01 to 0.02 mg/kg/min. If oral secretions become bothersome, administer atropine, 0.4 mg in adults, and 0.1 mg in children.
      b. Up to 5% of patients given ketamine have unpleasant dreams as they emerge from dissociative sedation. These may be attenuated by administering diazepam, 0.08 mg/kg, before giving ketamine.
      c. **Intramuscular administration.** Administer an intramuscular bolus of ketamine, 0.4 mg. Sedation reaches its peak in 5 minutes and lasts for 20 minutes. Repeated boluses of 0.4 mg/kg every 20 minutes may be given as required. Administer atropine and diazepam as per intravenous technique.
  4. **Adverse effects and contraindications.** Ketamine causes a centrally mediated increase in heart rate and blood pressure. It also increases cerebrospinal fluid pressure. Ketamine potentiates the effects of both depolarizing and nondepolarizing neuromuscular blocking agents. The drug does not precipitate malignant hyperthermia.
      a. The most significant **side effects** are increased oral and tracheal secretions, and emergence nightmares. Both are attenuated as described above.
      b. **Contraindications** to the use of ketamine include severe hypertension, a history of psychosis, and a history of abuse of hallucinogens such as lysergic acid diethylamide (LSD).
  5. **Clinical use.** When narcotics such as fentanyl are contraindicated, ketamine should be considered as the analgesic of choice for brief painful procedures such as reduction of fractures, incision and drainage of abscesses, dental procedures, and cardioversion. It is particularly useful in children undergoing painful procedures.
IV. **Muscle relaxants.** Most soft tissue injuries have associated muscle spasm. Frequently the spasm becomes part of a vicious cycle; the spasm causes increased pain, which in turn causes increased spasm. Skeletal muscle relaxants act centrally to minimize spasm. The precise mechanism is unknown.

While there is a plethora of skeletal muscle relaxants on the market, only three may be administered parenterally. They are orphenadrine, methocarbamol, and the benzodiazepines. The latter are discussed elsewhere.

A. Orphenadrine.
  1. Pharmacokinetics. Orphenadrine is a skeletal muscle relaxant with both antihistaminic and anticholinergic properties. It is metabolized by the liver and excreted by the kidney.
  2. Dosage and routes of administration.
    a. Intravenous administration. The intravenous dose is 60 mg by bolus injection. If necessary, a second bolus injection may be repeated 12 hours later.
    b. Intramuscular administration. As per intravenous administration.
  3. Adverse effects and contraindications. Orphenadrine causes typical anticholinergic effects such as dry mouth and difficulty voiding. Drowsiness is a common side effect. If taken in overdose or combined with other anticholinergic agents, orphenadrine can produce an anticholinergic syndrome that is potentially fatal.

  Orphenadrine is contraindicated in patients with stenosing peptic ulcers, prostatic hypertrophy, glaucoma, a history of bowel obstruction, and hypersensitivity.
  4. Clinical use. Orphenadrine is indicated for the treatment of acute muscle spasm when vomiting prevents oral administration. Treatment does not obviate the need to determine the cause of the muscle spasm.

B. Methocarbamol
  1. Pharmacokinetics. See orphenadrine. The plasma half-life of methocarbamol is 2 hours.
  2. Dosage and administration
    a. Intravenous administration. Administer intravenously 1 gm in 10 ml saline over 3 minutes every 8 hours up to three times daily.
    b. Intramuscular administration. Administer 0.5 gm in 5 ml saline every 8 hours as required to each gluteal region. The maximum dosage is 3 gm/day.
  3. Adverse effects and contraindications. Methocarbamol causes drowsiness, syncope, gastrointestinal upset, and allergic phenomena such as urticaria and rhinitis. Contraindications include renal disease and a history of hypersensitivity reactions.
  4. Clinical use. Methocarbamol is indicated for the treatment of acute muscle spasm.

V. Nitrous oxide. Nitrous oxide is a colorless gas that is used as a general anesthetic and as an analgesic. It is administered in a gaseous mixture of nitrous oxide and oxygen. At a concentration of 70% nitrous oxide and 30% oxygen, the gas acts as a general anesthetic. In a 50:50 mixture, nitrous oxide acts as a weak analgesic. The peak analgesic effect occurs in 1 to 2 minutes and disappears several minutes after the patient stops inhaling the drug.
  1. Administration. Nitrous oxide (contained in a 50:50 mixture with oxygen) is self-administered by using an aviator-style mask. The patient holds the mask, which falls harmlessly away if the patient becomes excessively sedated.
  2. Adverse effects and contraindications. Aside from drowsiness, no serious adverse effects have been found. Nitrous oxide may be teratogenic in

the first trimester of pregnancy. Health care workers may be protected from the effects of nitrous oxide if the delivery device is equipped with a scavenging device. Contraindications to the use of nitrous oxide include severe COPD, suspected bowel obstruction, decompression sickness, suspected pneumothorax, and impaired consciousness from any cause.

3. **Clinical use.** Because of its relatively weak analgesic properties, nitrous oxide is not considered an agent of choice for moderate to severe pain. However, it is indicated as an adjunct in acute pain of virtually any cause. Nitrous oxide is an extremely useful adjunct **in children**. The gas mixture is the same for children as it is for adults. Other analgesics and sedatives require that an intravenous drip be established, a procedure which is both painful and frightening for children. Nitrous oxide has the advantage of obviating the need for an intravenous drip. In addition, children given nitrous oxide become highly suggestible and can be encouraged to recall images of cartoon characters and other fond memories.

VI. Miscellaneous analgesics. A number of parenteral agents have demonstrated efficacy in the management of acute migraine, cluster headaches, and tension headaches.

  A. Dihydroergotamine (DHE). Dihydroergotamine is an α-adrenergic blocking agent with serotonin receptor activity.

  1. **Mechanism of action.** Acute migraine headaches are associated with dilation of extracranial blood vessels. The vasodilation is thought to be due to a fall in platelet levels of 5-hydroxytryptamine (5-HT, also known as serotonin). Administered intravenously, serotonin acts as a vasoconstricting agent. The precise mechanism by which DHE works is unknown. However, it has been shown to be 70% effective in aborting acute migraine attacks.

  2. **Pharmacokinetics.** The onset of action of DHE is 15 to 30 minutes after an intramuscular injection. The duration of action is 3 to 4 hours. Dihydroergotamine is metabolized by the liver; it has a distribution half-life of 90 minutes and an elimination half-life of 18 hours.

  3. **Dosage and administration**

     a. **Intravenous administration.** Administer DHE, 0.5 to 1.0 mg, by slow intravenous push over 2 to 3 minutes. Because of nausea caused by the drug, administer prochlorperazine, 5 mg intravenously, before giving the DHE. The dose may be repeated 1 hour after the first dose of DHE. The same protocol may be used in acute cluster headache.

     b. **Intramuscular and subcutaneous administration.** See intravenous administration.

  4. **Adverse effects and contraindications.** Dihydroergotamine causes nausea, numbness of the fingers and toes, tachycardia, weakness, and precordial chest pain. The contraindications to DHE include sepsis, collagen vascular diseases, severe atherosclerosis, coronary artery disease, thrombophlebitis, hypertension, peptic ulcer, renal or liver impairment, severe pruritus, pregnancy, lactation, and a history of hypersensitivity.

  5. **Clinical use.** The indications for DHE include the abortion of acute vascular headaches such as migraine and cluster headaches, as well as the management of established vascular headaches.

  B. Sumatriptan. This new antimigraine agent is a selective 5-HT_1 receptor agonist. Sumatriptan is believed to relieve migraine headaches by causing vasoconstriction of arteriovenous anastomoses within the carotid circulation.

Studies have shown that sumatriptan, 2 mg intravenously or subcutaneously, is at least as effective as DHE in relieving acute migraine headaches but without the side effects and contraindications of DHE.

C. Chlorpromazine
 1. **Mechanism of action.** Chlorpromazine is a phenothiazine that is highly effective in the rapid relief of established migraine headaches. The mechanism of action is unclear. Chlorpromazine has antiserotonergic and antiemetic activity. Both may play a role in the drug's effectiveness against migraine.
 2. **Dosage and administration.** Chlorpromazine is most effective when given intravenously; the dose is 5 to 10 mg. Because the drug causes pronounced orthostatic hypotension, many emergency physicians consider it advisable to administer 500 to 1000 ml of normal saline solution before administration of chlorpromazine.
 3. **Adverse effects.** Chlorpromazine causes orthostatic hypotension when given intravenously. The drug also causes drowsiness and anticholinergic effects.
 4. **Clinical use.** Chlorpromazine is indicated for the rapid relief of acute migraine headache.

D. **Prochlorperazine (Compazine).** Prochlorperazine is a phenothiazine that works in the same fashion as chlorpromazine. The main advantage of prochlorperazine is that it appears to cause far less orthostatic hypotension when given intravenously. The intravenous dose of prochlorperazine is 5 mg. Like chlorpromazine, it is indicated for the relief of acute migraine headaches.

E. **Metoclopramide.** Metoclopramide is a benzamide derivative with antiemetic and antidopaminergic activity. Although the mechanism of action is unclear, metoclopramide can be extremely efficacious in the treatment of acute migraine headache. The dosage is 10 to 20 mg given intramuscularly.

Sedative Agents

Parenteral agents are extremely useful adjuncts in the management of acute pain in the emergency department. They serve several important functions. First, by reducing anxiety, they blunt the emotional experience of pain. Second, their calming effects enhance the cooperation of the patient during outpatient procedures. Third, such agents induce muscle relaxation, making it much easier to successfully complete orthopedic procedures.

Benzodiazepines are the sedatives of choice in emergency medicine. However, haloperidol (administered intravenously) and nitrous oxide are also useful agents.

I. **Benzodiazepines.** These agents are the adjuncts of choice for painful or unpleasant emergency procedures. As anxiolytics, they reduce the anxiety associated with most procedures. By acting in the CNS, as well as at spinal interneurons, they induce skeletal muscle relaxation. This makes it easier to reduce fractures and dislocations. Benzodiazepines also induce anterograde amnesia; patients thus forget the pain associated with procedures. The parenteral agents of choice in emergency medicine are *diazepam* and *midazolam*. Diazepam is the benzodiazepine with which emergency physicians are most familiar. However, midazolam, with its shorter half-life, is emerging as the benzodiazepine of choice.

A. Diazepam
 1. **Pharmacokinetics.** Diazepam initially binds with high affinity to the CNS (particularly the limbic system and the cerebral cortex). Redistribu-

tion throughout the body occurs within 30 to 60 minutes, after which the CNS effects usually (but not always) wear off. The elimination half-life is 24 to 48 hours. The half-life is prolonged in infants and the elderly, and is also prolonged in patients with liver disease. The combined sedative effects of benzodiazepines and parenteral narcotics are additive, not synergistic.

2. **Dosage and routes of administration.** The intravenous route is the preferred route of parenteral administration because intramuscular absorption is erratic and unpredictable.

   a. **Intravenous administration.** Diazepam is titrated to optimal sedation. This is evidenced by slurred speech, loss of the blink reflex when the eyelids are touched, and positioning of the eyelids below the midpoint of the pupils. The usual adult dose is 5 to 15 mg by slow intravenous push, administered in 2 to 4 mg aliquots. The dose in children is 0.15 to 0.25 mg/kg. Use half of the recommended dose in patients who are elderly, have liver disease, or who are receiving concomitant narcotics.

   b. Because of the risk of severe **respiratory depression,** equipment for endotracheal intubation and bag ventilation must be kept near the patient's bedside. Continuous monitoring of oxygen saturation is recommended. Since circulatory impairment has been observed after an intravenous bolus injection, it is advisable to use a cardiac monitor and to maintain a secure intravenous drip during and after the procedure.

3. **Adverse effects and contraindications.** The most common adverse effects are drowsiness and ataxia. Less frequent adverse effects include headache, vertigo, tremors, euphoria, dysarthria, hypotension, and paradoxical excitement. Contraindications to the use of intravenous diazepam include myasthenia gravis, acute angle closure glaucoma, coma of unknown cause, shock, severe COPD, advanced liver disease, and hypersensitivity reactions.

4. **Clinical use.** Intravenous diazepam is indicated as an adjunct for emergency procedures requiring muscle relaxation, including closed reduction of fractures and dislocations. It is also recommended as an adjunct for procedures associated with anxiety, such as incision and drainage of abscesses, proctosigmoidoscopy, disimpaction, bronchoscopy, and the changing of burn dressings.

   a. Diazepam is useful of procedures in which *amnesia is desirable,* such as cardioversion. The drug also is indicated for patients who require sedation to complete urgent procedures such as computed tomography. In addition, diazepam is also indicated for the prevention of emergence nightmares when ketamine is used as the primary analgesic agent.

   b. Diazepam is the sedative of choice in *children* because of the lack of experience using midazolam in such patients.

B. Midazolam

1. **Pharmacokinetics.** Peak sedation occurs 3 to 6 minutes after an intravenous bolus injection, and 30 to 60 minutes after an intramuscular injection. The elimination half-life in normal subjects is 1 to 3 hours. However, the half-life is 4 hours in patients with severe alcoholic liver disease, and 6.5 hours in patients with congestive heart failure. In critical care settings, the half-life has been as high as 10 hours.

2. **Dosage and administration.** Unlike diazepam, midazolam may be given intravenously or intramuscularly. However, since titration must be precise, the intramuscular route is not recommended for emergency department use.
   a. **Intravenous administration.** Like diazepam, midazolam is titrated to optimal sedation (see **I.A.2.a**). Administer midazolam in 0.5 mg aliquots (iv push over 2-3 minutes) until the patient is adequately sedated or until an initial dose of 2 to 2.5 mg has been given. Wait at least 6 minutes before giving further increments. If the patient is still not sedated after receiving 2.5 mg, cautiously administer boluses of 0.5 mg every 2 to 3 minutes up to a maximum dose of 4 mg.
   b. Use half the recommended dosages in debilitated or elderly patients, as well as those who have mild liver disease, COPD, or who have been concomitantly given parenteral narcotics.
   c. Because of the risk of cardiorespiratory depression, take the same precautionary measures as described under diazepam (see **I. A.2.b**). The use of midazolam in children has not been well studied. A dose of 0.04 to 0.1 mg/kg appears safe.
3. **Adverse effects and contraindications.** The most common adverse effects are sedation and hypotension. Less common adverse effects include hypertension, cardiac arrhythmias, restlessness, agitation, dysphoria, excessive salivation, skin rashes, and muscle stiffness. Transient elevations in liver enzymes have also been observed. Contraindications to the use of midazolam include known hypersensitivity to benzodiazepines, myasthenia gravis, severe COPD and other causes of severe respiratory insufficiency, shock, coma, acute alcoholic intoxication, and severe renal impairment.
4. **Clinical indications.** The indications for midazolam are the same as for diazepam. Because of its shorter duration of action, midazolam is now regarded as the benzodiazepine of choice. Because of a lack of published experience, diazepam is preferred over midazolam for use in children.

II. Nitrous oxide (see **Analgesic Agents, V. I.-3.**). Nitrous oxide has sedative and analgesic properties. As such, it is indicated as the sedative of choice when benzodiazepines are contraindicated.

III. **Haloperidol**
   A. High-dose intravenous administration. Physicians are familiar with the therapeutic profile of haloperidol when administered in small intramuscular boluses. The drug has been used for decades in the management of acute schizophrenia and other psychoses. Concern over hemodynamic and extrapyramidal adverse effects has resulted in a reluctance to use larger dosages. However, recent studies have shown that haloperidol may be administered intravenously in much larger doses than previously believed. In light of these recent developments, intravenous haloperidol has emerged as a **first line drug in the treatment** of agitation of virtually any cause. In particular, it has been used to sedate agitated patients requiring diagnostic procedures such as magnetic resonance imaging and computed tomography.
   B. **Research.** The use of intravenous haloperidol as described below is currently the focus of intensive research. The results of preliminary studies are extremely encouraging. However, until definitive studies are completed, the use of intravenous haloperidol as recommended below must be considered experimental.

1. **Pharmacokinetics.** Haloperidol produces peak sedation effects 5 to 10 minutes after an intravenous bolus, compared with 20 minutes after an intramuscular injection. The elimination half-life is 20 hours.
2. **Dosage and route of administration.** As is the case with intravenous benzodiazepines, haloperidol is titrated for optimal effect. The starting dose is 5 to 10 mg administered by slow intravenous push. If the patient tolerates this dose, increments of 5 to 10 mg may be given every 10 minutes until the patient is calm. In elderly patients, administer 1 to 2 mg intravenously every 5 to 10 minutes for three doses, and increase the increments to 5 mg every 10 minutes if tolerated. There is **no maximum dose** of intravenous haloperidol. Severely agitated patients in critical care settings have required boluses as large as 50 to 75 mg every 30 to 60 minutes.
3. **Adverse effects and contraindications.** Intravenously given haloperidol does not cause adverse hemodynamic, respiratory, or neurological effects. Extrapyramidal effects are rarely observed and tend to be milder than those occurring after intramuscular administration; they respond well to diphenhydramine.
4. **Clinical indications.** Intravenous haloperidol is indicated for the rapid relief of agitation from any cause such as psychosis, organic brain disease, CNS pathology, metabolic or endocrine abnormalities, major organ failure, and drug-induced delirium. Haloperidol is also indicated for the sedation of patients requiring diagnostic imaging or painful procedures when benzodiazepines are contraindicated.

Principles of Parenteral Pain Management

I. **General considerations.** Emergency physicians are called on to manage pain from a wide variety of conditions in patients with an equally wide variety of tolerances to pain. The priorities and approaches to pain management vary with the condition, as explained below. Despite this variation, the general principles of pain management remain the same.
   A. Keep the goals of diagnosis and pain management separate. Arriving at a correct diagnosis and treatment often leads to relief of pain, but this is not always the case. Besides, there is often a significant time lag between the patient's arrival in the emergency department and diagnosis. Keeping diagnosis and pain management separate allows the emergency physician to tackle both at the same time, instead of handling them sequentially. Sometimes it is important to treat pain immediately, even before a thorough history and physical examination can be completed. The concern that parenteral analgesics compromise the diagnosis has been greatly exaggerated. Treating pain promptly often improves the patient's cooperation in history taking.
   B. **Pain management should be individualized.** Current knowledge of pain perception suggests that patients have distinct and individual responses to painful stimuli of all kinds. Moreover, the response to analgesics is likewise distinct. Thus it is pointless to compare one patient with another.
   C. The only practical way to measure acute pain is to elicit the patient's subjective measurement of pain. This is done by asking the patient to rate his level of pain on a scale from 0 to 10, with 10 being the worst pain the patient has ever had. Once a baseline is established, subsequent ratings can be elicited to gauge response to therapy.

D. Determine the patient's level of anxiety. Manage pain and anxiety separately. If appropriate, as is the case with painful or uncomfortable procedures, administer a short-acting anxiolytic, as well as an analgesic.

E. Choose the most appropriate analgesic available. The choice depends on the clinical situation, the duration of action required, as well as the side effects and contraindications.

F. When possible, administer analgesics and sedatives by intravenous drip. This permits rapid and closely titrated management of pain.

G. Therapy should be individualized. With many of the agents described in this chapter, there are no standard dosages. For example, there is a wide variation in patient response to intravenous narcotics. Frequently, physicians and nurses tend to suspect a patient of malingering when he or she fails to respond to a specific dose of narcotics. This advice does not apply when using medications such as ketorolac, which has a maximum recommended dosage.

H. Treat anticipatory pain. It is best to treat pain promptly (i.e., before it has a chance to reach its maximum level). When this strategy is used, the patient's anxiety decreases, as does his or her perception of pain.

I. Provide psychologic support. Let the patient know that providing pain relief is as important to the medical staff as is making a diagnosis. The following specific measures can assist the physician.

1. **Permit parents to remain in the treatment room** while their children are having painful procedures. This is less disruptive than generally thought. The presence of the parent reduces the child's anxiety, thus reducing the experience of pain. Parents who are reluctant to watch the procedure may be seated off to the side of the procedure, within calling distance of the child.
2. **Use music to create a relaxed atmosphere.** A radio or personal stereo tape player with headphones can be used to play the patient's favorite music. This strategy reduces the patient's anxiety and improves cooperation.
3. **Patient choice.** When possible, give the patient a measure of control regarding the choice of analgesic, as well as the dosage interval. This strategy reduces anxiety. Studies have shown that patients receiving narcotics via patient controlled analgesia (PCA) devices require lower doses of narcotic than those receiving doses as needed. The PCA devices are seldom used in the emergency department. Nevertheless, patients can be given a partial sense of control over their analgesics.

J. Anticipate the cardiorespiratory complications of parenteral narcotics and benzodiazepines. Physicians using either or both medications should have resuscitative equipment nearby. An oxygen saturation monitor and cardiac monitor are also recommended. In addition, a vial or syringe containing naloxone should be immediately available.

II. Disease-specific pain management (Tables 3-4 and 3-5)

A. Abdominal pain of unknown etiology

1. **Approach.** In treating the patient with acute abdominal pain of unknown cause, emergency physicians have two priorities.
    a. **Find the cause of the pain.** A detailed approach to the diagnosis of acute abdominal pain is beyond the scope of this chapter, but some points bear emphasis. A thorough history should help determine whether the pain is abdominal, pelvic, or urinary in origin. Crucial points on physical examination include a search for signs suggestive of peritonitis; a pelvic examination should be considered in any female of

Table 3-5. Disease-Specific Pain Management

Condition	Analgesic(s) of choice	Alternatives	Adjuncts
Abdominal pain	Fentanyl, 50-100 µg IV	Nalbuphine, 10-20 mg IV	Nitrous oxide
Acute musculoskeletal injury	Ketorolac, 30-60 mg IM	Nalbuphine, morphine, methocarbamol, 500-1000 mg IV	TNS*
Biliary colic	Nalbuphine, 10-20 mg IV	Ketorolac, meperidine	Nitrous oxide
Chest Pain			
Angina	Nitrates IV, SL, transdermal	—	Oxygen
Myocardial infarction	Morphine IV, nitroglycerin IV	Nalbuphine	Oxygen, nitrous oxide
Pericarditis	Morphine	Ketorolac	Methylprednisolone IV
Thoracic aortic aneurysm	Morphine IV, antihypertensives IV	Nalbuphine	—
Diffuse esophageal	Nitroglycerine SL	Nifedipine, 10 mg SL	—
Costochondritis spasm	Local infiltration bupivacaine 0.25%, ± methylprednisolone	Ketorolac, NSAIDs PO, narcotics PO	—
Rib fractures	Intercostal nerve block bupivacaine 0.25%; ketorolac, 30-60 mg IM	Nalbuphine, morphine	TNS, nitrous oxide (rule out pneumothorax)
Diagnostic imaging: sedation	Midazolam IV	Diazepam IV, Haloperidol IV	—
Cardioversion	Midazolam IV, sodium pentobarbital	Diazepam, ketamine IM/IV	Nitrous oxide, fentanyl IV

Principles of Parenteral Pain Management 123

Table 3-5. Disease-Specific Pain Management—cont'd

Condition	Analgesic(s) of choice	Alternatives	Adjuncts
Headaches			
Cluster	DHE, 0.5-1.0 mg IV, liquid cocaine 5-10% intranasally	Nalbuphine, Morphine	Oxygen by nasal prongs
Migraine	DHE, 0.5-1.0 mg IV; prochlorperazine, 5-10 mg IV	Chlorpromazine IV, ketorolac, nalbuphine, morphine	Normal saline IV, antiemetic
Tension	Ketorolac	Methocarbamol, nalbuphine	
Painful Procedures			
Incision and drainage of abscess, reduction of fracture, multiple lacerations, burn management	Fentanyl IV, midazolam IV	Morphine IV, diazepam IV, ketamine IM/IV, nalbuphine IV for patients with COPD	Nitrous oxide
Colles fracture	Fentanyl IV, midazolam IV	Add hematoma block	—
Renal colic	Morphine IV; Ketorolac IM or IV	Nalbuphine IV; indomethacin, 100 mg suppository q8-12h; diclofenac, 50-100 µg suppository	Nitrous oxide
Sickle crisis			
Habituated to narcotics	Morphine IV	—	Nitrous oxide
Not habituated to narcotics	Ketorolac IM	Nalbuphine	Nitrous oxide

TNS, Transelectrical nerve stimulation.

childbearing age. Relevant laboratory evaluation includes a complete blood cell count, urinalysis, and determination of serum levels of amylase, lipase, lactate, electrolytes, creatinine, and liver enzymes. In women of childbearing age, consider obtaining a serum human chorionic gonadotropin level. **Relevant diagnostic imaging studies** include abdominal and chest radiographs, as well as an ultrasound of the abdomen, pelvis, or both.

    b. **Treat the pain.** If the patient is comfortable, the emergency physician may defer pain management until the diagnosis has been made. However, in many cases, the patient is forced to remain in pain for several hours while diagnostic tests and consultations are completed. Also, some patients in extreme pain are unable to cooperate through a history and physical examination. Because there is no compelling evidence that the administration of an analgesic compromises the diagnosis of abdominal pain, there is no need to withhold analgesics in such cases. In particular, parenteral narcotics have not been shown to mask the signs of peritonitis.

    c. **Manage the patient's anxiety.** Patients with abdominal pain of unknown cause are anxious; the anxiety magnifies the intensity of pain. While an anxiolytic is not indicated in this case, the emergency staff should reassure the patient that the cause of the pain will be found. In addition, the patient should be encouraged to inform the staff of any increase in pain; he should also be reassured that the pain will be treated promptly.

2. **Drugs of choice.** The ideal drug in this case is fentanyl, 50 to 100 µg given intravenously. Unlike other narcotics, fentanyl is extremely short-acting. Thus the patient remains alert, cooperative, and competent to sign a consent form should the need arise. A good second choice is a narcotic agonist–antagonist such as nalbuphine, 10 mg given intravenously or subcutaneously.

3. **Adjuncts.** Nitrous oxide may be administered as described above. Although the gas is sedating, its effects wear off within minutes of discontinuation. Nitrous oxide is contraindicated in cases of suspected bowel obstruction.

B. **Acute musculoskeletal pain** such as lumbar strain, disk herniation, cervical strain, and ligamentous injuries.

1. **Approach.** The primary goals of acute therapy are pain relief and muscle relaxation lasting at least several hours. Once the acute episode is relieved, the patient can be switched to oral therapy.

2. **Drugs of choice.** For analgesia with a rapid onset, the narcotic agonist of choice is morphine, while the narcotic agonist–antagonist of choice is nalbuphine. Alternatively, if muscle spasm is present, administer a muscle relaxant such as methocarbamol or orphenadrine instead of a narcotic. **If rapid onset is not considered necessary**, the drug of choice is ketorolac, 30 to 60 mg given intramuscularly. If therapy is successful, the patient can be discharged with a prescription for oral ketorolac.

3. **Adjuncts.** Nitrous oxide can be used in the initial management of pain due to acute musculoskeletal strains. Transelectrical nerve stimulation (TNS) can also provide significant relief and can be used both in the emergency department and at home.

C. **Biliary colic.** Since the diagnosis is known, the main goal is to treat the pain pending definitive management.

1. **Drugs of choice.** Initiate therapy with a potent intravenously administered narcotic. Because narcotic agonists such as morphine and meperidine cause an increase in biliary pressure, it may be prudent to use a potent narcotic agonist–antagonist such as nalbuphine. Administer intravenous boluses of 2 to 5 mg every 5 to 10 minutes up to a maximum dose of 20 mg or until the patient is comfortable. Once reached, the optimal dose may be repeated every 3 to 6 hours as necessary.
2. **Alternatives.** Despite the theoretical risk of exacerbating the pain of biliary colic, many patients have substantial relief with morphine and meperidine. Administer either drug intravenously as described above, along with an antinauseant such as promethazine or dimenhydrinate.
   a. **Ketorolac** is an acceptable alternative to narcotics. The main disadvantage of the drug is its relatively slow onset of action. However, once adequate analgesia is obtained with narcotics, it may be prudent to switch to ketorolac. To expedite the switch, administer ketorolac intramuscularly (as described above) as soon as possible after the patient arrives. Likewise, indomethacin suppositories (100 mg every 8 to 12 hours as needed) may be administered as a substitute for narcotics. Its onset of action is similar to that of intramuscular ketorolac.
   b. **Nitrous oxide** is another alternative to intravenous narcotics. It provides a weak analgesic effect of rapid onset.
D. **Chest pain.** Chest pain can arise from disorders of the myocardium, pericardium, great vessels, lungs, pleura, esophagus, and chest wall. Frequently, the cause remains unknown. The specific management of the following conditions is discussed elsewhere. The discussion that follows is confined to the management of pain.
   1. **Angina.** The goal of therapy is to treat the pain by terminating the episode of angina. The drug of choice for relieving angina is nitroglycerine, administered sublingually or by nasal spray.
   2. **Myocardial infarction.** The main goals of therapy are to limit the size of the infarction and to prevent or manage the usual complications. Relief of pain and anxiety are the other key goals in the management of acute myocardial infarction. Pain and anxiety both increase sympathetic tone, which increases afterload and can increase the size of the infarct.
      a. **Morphine sulfate.** The drug of choice for the relief of both pain and anxiety is morphine sulfate. The dosage is 2 to 5 mg given intravenously in incremental doses until the pain is relieved. To prevent nausea and vomiting, administer promethazine or dimenhydrinate. The use of intravenous agents such as thrombolytic therapy and nitroglycerine does not obviate the need for morphine.
      b. **Intravenous nitroglycerine** is indicated for ongoing chest pain that does not resolve with morphine and for recurrent chest pain after successful treatment with morphine.
      c. **Nitrous oxide** is partially effective in treating **ischemic chest pain.** However, it should not be combined with narcotics because the combination causes significant hypotension.
   3. **Pericarditis.** The objectives of therapy are to treat the underlying cause of the disease and to reduce pain by reducing pericardial inflammation. Potent analgesics such as intravenous narcotics may be used for the initial management of pain. Because of its antiinflammatory action, ketorolac, 30 to 60 mg, may be as effective as intravenous narcotics. Intravenous steroids

such as solucortef, 500 mg given intravenously, cause relief of pain within several hours.

4. **Thoracic dissection of the aorta.** The main goal of therapy is to reduce blood pressure and sympathetic tone. Intravenous antihypertensive therapy often relieves pain. However, pain should be managed separately by using long-acting intravenous narcotics such as morphine. Alternatively, administer a narcotic agonist–antagonist such as nalbuphine.
5. **Pleuritis.** This is a disparate group of disorders including pleurodynia, pneumonia, and pulmonary embolus. The definitive therapy varies with the condition. If necessary, administer an intravenous narcotic such as morphine for the relief of pain pending investigations. With elderly patients, as well as those with advanced COPD, a narcotic agonist–antagonist such as nalbuphine (10 mg intravenously) may be substituted for morphine.
6. **Diffuse esophageal spasm.** The drug of choice for acute relief of this condition is sublingual nitroglycerine. Pain relief usually begins 5 to 6 minutes after administration and lasts up to an hour. Sublingual nifedipine, 10 mg, is also effective. Neither drug prevents recurrences of esophageal spasm. Long-term oral therapy is described in the chapter on oral analgesia.
7. **Costochondritis (Tietze syndrome).** Oral antiinflammatory agents relieve pain by relieving inflammation; however, these work on a delayed basis. For acute relief, inject 1 to 1.5 ml of 1% lidocaine (or 1 to 2 ml of bupivacaine 0.25%) into the affected costochondral junction. This area may be identified by palpating the skin; the area where palpation reproduces the patient's chest pain is the site of the inflamed costochondral junction. Concomitant administration of a steroid such as methylprednisolone (20 to 40 mg) may provide longer lasting relief than local anesthetic alone.
8. **Rib fractures.** The priorities in this case are pain control and prevention of atelectasis through the promotion of deep breathing. The ideal agent is a long-acting local anesthetic such as bupivacaine. There are two ways of administering the bupivacaine.
   a. **Local infiltration at the site of the rib fracture.** Locate the site of the fracture by direct palpation and by chest radiographs. After cleansing the skin, inject 2 to 3 ml of bupivacaine 0.5% at the fracture line and into the surrounding intercostal tissue. This injection will last up to 12 hours, and may be repeated on a daily basis.
   b. **Intercostal nerve block.** Bupivacaine 0.25% is the preferred agent because it is longer acting than lidocaine. The maximum dose of bupivacaine 0.25% is 2 mg/kg; the maximum for lidocaine 1% is 5 mg/kg (7 mg/kg if the mixture contains epinephrine).
   c. **The location** for the intercostal nerve block depends on the location of the fracture. With posterior rib fractures, the nerve is best blocked just lateral to the paraspinal muscles. Fractures anterior to this location are best infiltrated in the midaxillary line. After preparing the skin with an antiseptic solution, the skin is infiltrated with local anesthetic and the needle is advanced until it reaches the periosteum of the rib. The needle is then walked inferiorly until it is 2 to 3 mm below the inferior surface of the rib. Inject 2 to 3 ml of local anesthetic at this location. It is advisable to block the intercostal nerves immediately above and immediately below the segment containing the fractured rib.
   d. **Oral narcotic analgesics.** Although local anesthetics often provide excellent pain relief, a potent oral narcotic analgesic such as oxycodone, 5

to 10 mg every 4 to 6 hours as needed, should also be prescribed. Oral NSAIDs have a potency roughly equivalent to that of acetaminophen with 30 mg of codeine. Relative contraindications to the use of potent oral narcotics include elderly patients with severe COPD.
  - e. **Transelectrical nerve stimulation.** A useful adjunct is a portable TNS unit. The advantages of TNS are its ease of use at home and a lack of adverse effects. The only absolute contraindication to TNS is a demand cardiac pacemaker.
- E. Direct current (DC) cardioversion
  1. **Approach.** The main goal is to relax and sedate the patient. Pain management, while important, is less of a priority than it is in painful procedures such as reduction of fractures. The technique that follows does not require the assistance of an anesthesiologist.
  2. **Drugs of choice.** The combination of midazolam and fentanyl should be used. Both are short-acting drugs. Midazolam provides sedation, muscle relaxation, and amnesia. It is also short acting. **Administer midazolam** first in boluses of 0.5 mg over 2 to 3 minutes per bolus until a maximum dose of 2 mg is reached. Then, administer fentanyl in 25 to 50 µg aliquots up to a maximum dose of 100 to150 µg. The combination of drugs is safe as long as the midazolam is administered over 2 to 5 minutes. Observe closely for respiratory depression and monitor oxygen saturation at all times. In children, intravenous diazepam should be substituted for midazolam.
  3. **Alternatives and adjuncts.** Nitrous oxide is a useful adjunct to midazolam and fentanyl because it does not act synergistically with either agent. Ketamine is a useful alternative in patients who cannot tolerate either midazolam or fentanyl.
- F. Headaches
  1. **Cluster headache.** The drug of choice for the initial management of cluster headache of recent onset is DHE, 0.5 to 1.0 mg given intravenously over 2 to 3 minutes. Administer oxygen by nasal prongs; oxygen promotes cerebral vasoconstriction and relieves cluster headaches in a significant percentage of patients. Administration of 5% liquid cocaine, 1-2 ml by nasal gauze packing, sometimes relieves the pain within 2 to 3 minutes. If the above measures fail, a **parenterally administered opioid drug** should be given. If the patient has not been given a narcotic agonist recently, then give the narcotic agonist–antagonist nalbuphine. The narcotic agonist morphine (with an antiemetic) should be reserved for patients who are habituated to narcotic agonists. Alternatively, administer **sumatriptan**, 2 to 4 mg subcutaneously.
  2. **Migraine headache.** During the first 1 to 2 hours of a typical migraine headache, the drug of choice is DHE, 0.5 to 1.0 mg given intravenously. To prevent nausea, administer promethazine, 15 to 25 mg intramuscularly or intravenously.
     - a. If the headache is well established, then the current drugs of choice are **prochlorperazine**, 5 to 10 mg given intravenously, or **chlorpromazine**, 5 to 10 mg given intravenously. An alternative drug is metoclopramide, 10 mg intravenously, or 10 to 20 mg intramuscularly. If the headache is still present 20 minutes after administration of any of the above three drugs, administer an oral or parenteral nonnarcotic analgesic such as ketorolac or naproxen. Because of the risk of orthostatic hypotension associated with chlorpromazine, it is recommended that patients receiving

the drug also receive a bolus of 500 to 1000 ml of normal saline solution intravenously.
   - **b.** If all of the above agents fail, then a **potent narcotic** should be administered. The choice depends on the patient's history of using narcotics (see section on cluster headaches). The long-term use of narcotics is associated with an increased frequency, duration, and severity of headaches. It is not certain whether this is a cause and effect relationship.
3. **Tension headache.** The use of narcotics should be restricted to severe cases. The drug of choice is ketorolac, 30 to 60 mg intramuscularly, followed by 15 to 30 mg intramuscularly every 6 hours as needed. Because migraine and tension headache are often overlapping syndromes, a trial of antimigraine therapy as described above is quite appropriate. A muscle relaxant such as methocarbamol or orphenadrine may also be tried.

   Patients who do not respond to any of the above agents should be treated with either a potent narcotic such as morphine (with an antiemetic) or a narcotic agonist–antagonist such as nalbuphine.
4. **Headache of unknown etiology.** The diagnostic investigation of the patient with headache of potentially serious cause is described elsewhere. However, a favorable response to empiric antimigraine therapy is not diagnostic of migraine and does not eliminate more serious causes of headaches.

G. Painful procedures including reduction of fractures and dislocations, incision and drainage of abscesses, suturing of multiple lacerations, changing of burn dressings, and insertion of chest tubes should be addressed as follows.
1. **Approach.** In this case, there are three priorities. The first is to relieve the pain of the procedure. The second is to sedate the patient to relieve anxiety and improve cooperation. With fractures and dislocations, the third priority is to obtain muscle relaxation sufficient to permit a successful reduction.
2. **Drugs of choice.** To achieve all three goals, a narcotic and a benzodiazepine should be administered intravenously. In order to expedite a rapid recovery, the most appropriate agents are short acting, such as fentanyl and midazolam. In most cases, completion of the procedure will substantially reduce the patient's level of pain.
   - **a. Children** should receive diazepam instead of midazolam. Elderly patients (the majority of those patients with Colles fractures) should receive half the recommended dose of midazolam and fentanyl.
   - **b. After the procedure,** the patient may be continued on an oral narcotic such as hydrocodone or oxycodone (as described in the previous chapter) or switched to a nonnarcotic analgesic such as ketorolac or floctafenine.
3. **Alternatives and adjuncts.** Intravenous morphine or meperidine may be substituted for fentanyl. Likewise, intravenous diazepam may be substituted for midazolam. Patients with COPD, as well as elderly patients requiring insertion of a chest tube, should receive a narcotic agonist–antagonist such as nalbuphine.
   - **a. Ketamine** is a useful alternative sedative-analgesic in patients for whom the above therapy is contraindicated. It is particularly useful in children.
   - **b. Nitrous oxide** is a useful adjunct in most of the situations listed above except for insertion of a chest tube. Patients receiving morphine or meperidine should also receive an antiemetic such as promethazine or dimenhydrinate.

c. In the case of **Colles fractures,** a hematoma block with lidocaine 1% (3 to 5 ml) can provide additional pain relief but is not necessary, since fentanyl alone usually provides adequate analgesia.

H. Renal colic
  1. **Approach.** In managing the pain caused by renal calculi, the priority is to manage pain and nausea as rapidly and completely as possible with the fewest side effects. The pain can be expected to last from 4 to 6 hours to several days.
  2. **Drugs of choice.** The drug of choice for initial pain relief is intravenous morphine because it is potent, works quickly, and can be titrated. Once determined, the optimum dose of morphine can be administered every 4 hours. Alternatively, once pain relief is obtained, administer **ketorolac**, 15 to 30 mg intramuscularly, or **indomethacin**, 100 mg by rectal suppository (as described in the section on biliary colic), or **diclofenac**, 50 to 100 μg by rectal suppository.
  3. **Alternatives and adjuncts.** An antiemetic such as promethazine or dimenhydrinate should be administered along with morphine. Barring contraindications, nitrous oxide may be administered as described elsewhere.

I. Sedation for diagnostic imaging
  1. **Approach.** The goals are to reduce anxiety and improve cooperation.
  2. **Drugs of choice.** The drugs of choice are midazolam, followed by diazepam.
  3. **Alternatives.** Intravenously administered haloperidol is indicated for agitated patients requiring sedation for diagnostic imaging procedures. Another useful alternative medication is ketamine administered intramuscularly or intravenously.

J. Sickle crisis and other recurrently painful conditions.
  1. **Approach.** The management of painful sickle crisis includes the administration of oxygen, intravenous fluids, and a parenterally administered analgesic. Because most painful crises tend to last for several days, choose an analgesic with a relatively long duration of action. Patients with sickle crisis can be expected to require analgesics on an intermittent basis for the rest of their lives. Such patients have an increased risk of becoming addicted to narcotics. The same considerations apply for other recurrently painful conditions such as recurrent pancreatitis.
  2. **Drugs of choice**
     a. **Patients who have never used narcotics.** When possible, treat patients with newly diagnosed recurrent pain with analgesics that carry a low risk of psychologic dependence. Thus the initial drug of choice should be a nonnarcotic such as ketorolac. This drug is both long acting and nonaddictive; moreover, ketorolac is available in oral form. If ketorolac is ineffective, the next best choice is a potent narcotic agonist–antagonist such as **nalbuphine.** Nalbuphine last for 5 to 6 hours. Drugs in this category have a lower potential for abuse than do narcotic agonists.
     b. **Patients who are habituated to narcotic agonists.** The drug of choice is morphine because it is the parenteral narcotic with the longest duration of action. Narcotic agonist–antagonists such as nalbuphine are contraindicated because they can precipitate withdrawal in patients habituated to narcotics. Narcotics should not be administered intramuscu-

larly because absorption by this route is highly variable in patients with sickle cell disease.

3. **Alternatives and adjuncts**. Nitrous oxide may be substituted for opioid drugs. If a narcotic is given, an antiemetic such as promethazine should also be administered.

Suggested Readings

Attard AR, et al: Safety of early pain relief for acute abdominal pain. *Br Med J* 305:554, 1992.

Chudnofsky CR, et al: The safety of fentanyl use in the emergency department, *Ann Emerg Med* 18:635-9, 1989.

Goldman B, editor, Stewart RD, consulting editor: Providing effective analgesia and sedation in the emergency department, *Emergency Medicine Reports* 10:73-82, 1989.

Heller MB: Emergency management of acute pain. New options and strategies. *Postgrad Med Spec* No:39-46, 1992.

Ketorolac tromethamine, *Med Lett Drugs Ther* 32:79-81, 1990.

Klapper J: The pharmacologic treatment of acute migraine headaches. *J Pain Symptom Manage* 8:140-7, 1993.

Labrecque M, et al: Efficacy of nonsteroidal antiinflammatory drugs in the treatment of acute renal colic. A metaanalysis. *Arch Intern Med* 154:1381-7, 1994.

Lewis IM, et al: Are emergency physicians too stingy with analgesics? *South Med J* 87:7-9, 1994.

Miller DL, Wall RT: Fentanyl and diazepam for analgesia and sedation during radiologic special procedures, *Radiology* 162:195-8, 1987.

Paris PM, Stewart RD: *Pain management in emergency medicine,* East Norwalk, 1988, Appleton & Lange.

Perlmutter A, et al: Toradol, an NSAID used for renal colic, decreases renal perfusion and ureteral pressure in a canine model of unilateral renal obstruction. *J Urol* 149:926-930, 1993.

Shapiro BS, et al: Patient-controlled analgesia for sickle-cell-related pain. *J Pain Symptom Manage* 8:22-28, 1993.

Silverstein S, et al: Parenteral haloperidol in combative patients: a prospective study, *Ann Emerg Med* 15:636, 1986.

Tesar GE, et al: Use of high-dose intravenous haloperidol in the treatment of agitated cardiac patients, *J Clin Psychopharmacol* 5:344-7, 1985.

Tverskoy M, et al: Midazolam-morphine sedative interaction in patients, *Anesth Analg* 68:282-5, 1989.

Weissman DE, et al: *Handbook of cancer pain management,* ed 2, Madison, 1988, Wisconsin Cancer Pain Initiative.

Yrjola H, et al: Intravenous indomethacin for postoperative pain. A double-blind study of ankle surgery, *Acta Orthop Scand* 59:43-45, 1988.

4

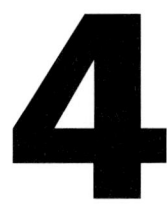

Detecting the Drug Seeker

H. Brian Goldman, M.D., A.B.E.M., M.C.F.P. (EM)

The vast majority of patients come to an emergency department to find out the cause of their symptoms and to obtain relief from them. In most cases, the doctor–patient relationship is founded on mutual trust and good faith.

Definition

I. **Prescription drug seekers** are people who exploit that trust to obtain pharmaceuticals that they consume themselves or sell to drug dealers and other users to make a profit. In a sense, the doctor–drug seeker relationship is a mirror image of the usual doctor-patient relationship. Ordinarily, the doctor is the experienced professional, while the patient is naive and trusting. In the doctor–drug seeker relationship, the drug seeker is the experienced professional, while the doctor is often naive and trusting.
   A. **Feigning illness.** Drug seekers do this by feigning illnesses and by convincing the physician that there is no choice but to write a prescription for the desired drug. In many cases, the drug seeker alters the prescription to increase the quantity of medication dispensed. Since drug seekers tend to travel from city to city, they frequently target emergency departments and urgent care centers.
   B. **Diverting drugs.** Drug seekers are highly successful in diverting drugs for their own purposes. The Federal Drug Enforcement Administration estimates that prescription drug diversion is a $25 billion year business. There are no scientific studies to verify that claim.
   C. **Robberies.** Although pharmacy break-ins and robberies account for a significant percentage of drug diversion, the largest percentage of prescription drugs are diverted as a result of the doctor-patient encounter.
II. **Systematic approach.** In general, emergency doctors fall for the schemes of drug seekers when they fail to use a systematic approach to detection and disposition. Fortunately it is possible to frustrate a large number of prescription drug seekers by learning the stereotypic ways in which they come to emergency departments and by learning how to confront and frustrate them.

Preferred Drugs

I. **Why drug seekers prefer prescription drugs.** Drug seekers often come from the ranks of those addicted to heroin and other illicit drugs. However, a growing number of drug abusers prefer prescription drugs for the following reasons:

- **A. Safety and strength are guaranteed.** Illicit drugs have variable potency and may be laced with dangerous adjuvants. By contrast, pharmaceuticals are made under stringent quality control.
- **B. Legitimacy of possession.** Simple possession of illicit drugs is a crime; possession of prescription drugs is not a crime, as long as the pharmaceuticals are stored in a legitimate prescription bottle with an appropriate label.
- **C. Dealing with reputable sources.** Illicit drug abusers constantly run the risks of dealing with unsavory drug dealers or undercover police officers. Prescription drug seekers deal mainly with physicians and pharmacists.
- **D. No risk of human immunodeficiency virus (HIV) transmission.** With the risk of HIV transmission from contaminated intravenous needles, many heroin addicts have now switched to potent oral pharmaceutical narcotics.

II. **Controlled substances preferred by prescription drug seekers.** Prescription drug seekers mainly visit emergency departments in search of the following drugs that are classified as controlled substances.
- **A. Narcotics.** Narcotics are the drugs most sought after by drug seekers. They prefer narcotic analgesics in tablet form because they can be easily carried in lots of 100 tablets or more. Because of its potent euphoric effects, drug seekers prefer hydromorphone (4 mg) tablets. They also seek less potent narcotics, such as oxycodone, propoxyphene, codeine, pentazocine, and meperidine. In addition, analgesic cough syrups that contain dihydrocodone are also in high demand. The effects of consuming 1 to 2 ounces of such cough syrups are similar to those achieved by injecting an intravenous bolus of heroin.
- **B. Benzodiazepines.** Benzodiazepines are also highly sought after by prescription drug seekers. The drugs preferred in this category include diazepam, alprazolam, clorazepate dipotassium, and oxazepam. Benzodiazepines have traditionally been desirable because of their mild euphoric effects. Today, a growing number of cocaine users consume the anxiolytic to alleviate the symptoms of cocaine withdrawal. In addition, heroin addicts use benzodiazepines to augment the psychotropic effects of methadone.
- **C. Barbiturates.** Barbiturates are less in demand than they were years ago, when secobarbital was the drug of choice for insomnia. A notable exception is Fiorinal, a combination drug that contains the barbiturate butalbital, with acetylsalicylic acid (ASA) and caffeine. This drug, used commonly for migraine headaches, is in rapidly increasing demand by drug seekers.
- **D. Amphetamine-like drugs.** This heterogeneous group of pharmaceuticals includes appetite suppressants such as phenmetrazine, as well as methylphenidate (Ritalin), which is used in the treatment of attention deficit disorder and narcolepsy.

III. **Street value of prescription drugs.** Prescription pharmaceuticals are sold to drug abusers at prices much higher than the cost inside pharmacies. For example, a tablet of acetaminophen with 30 mg of codeine sells in pharmacies for between $.75 and $1; the same pill can be sold on the street for up to $8. A 4 mg tablet of hydromorphone has a street value of between $50 and $100, depending on the supply of heroin. The street prices of these and other pharmaceuticals are shown in **Table 4-1.**

IV. **Noncontrolled prescription drugs preferred by drug seekers.**
- **A. β-Blockers.** These are taken to alleviate the tremor and tachycardia associated with cocaine use or benzodiazepine withdrawal.

Table 4-1. The Street Prices of Prescription Pharmaceuticals

Drug	Price on street ($ per tablet)
Acetaminophen with codeine 30 mg	5-8
Diazepam 5-10 mg	2-3
Fiorinal with codeine 30 mg (ASA/caffeine/butalbital)	8
Hydromorphone 4 mg	50-100
Methylphenidate 20 mg	15
Oxycodone 5 mg	6
Hydromorphone compound–containing cough syrups	$16 per ounce

  B. **Clonidine.** This drug is used to blunt the effects of narcotic withdrawal. An increase in the number of bogus patients complaining of hypertension is a sure sign that the supply of heroin available to addicts has dried up.
  C. **Nonsteroidal antiinflammatory drugs** (NSAIDs). They are popular in some urban centers in North America.

Prescription Drug Seekers

I. **General considerations.** Drug seekers have a stereotypic appearance, but it is not the one society would have physicians believe. Although some of them have tattoos on their arms and a skid-row appearance, they are in the minority and are not very good at fooling doctors. There are three categories of drug seekers **(Table 4-2)**.
   A. **Drug addicts.** This is a heterogeneous group of men and women of all ages. They range from the middle-aged executive who consumes 10 to 12 oxycodone tablets per week to the unemployed or disabled person who has been labeled by society as an addict and who has attended drug rehabilitation programs. As a group, they tend to cluster around middle age and hold middle-class values. They see themselves as bona fide patients, not con artists. Most of them take the pills they receive for medicinal, not recreational purposes. The physician is their only source of medication; they would never contemplate buying pills from a drug dealer or selling off their excess supply to make a profit. They tend to seek out emergency physicians when their attending physician is either unavailable or unwilling to write more prescriptions for them. In other words, they come to emergency departments when they are desperate for a prescription.
   B. **Entrepreneurial drug seekers.** Unlike the drug addicts described above, entrepreneurial drug seekers are a homogeneous group of men and women who are in the business of buying and selling prescription drugs. Very few are middle-aged; most are in their 20s and 30s. They tend to consume prescription drugs for recreational, not medicinal purposes. Unlike middle-class drug addicts, they buy pharmaceuticals from drug dealers when unable to obtain them from doctors.
      1. **Obtaining prescriptions.** These self-styled entrepreneurs obtain prescriptions from doctors by feigning illnesses or by purchasing prescriptions from unsavory physicians. Often they alter the doctor's prescription to increase

Table 4-2. Types of Prescription Drug Seekers

	Drug addicts	Entrepreneurial drug seekers	Professional patients
Ages	All	20s and 30s	All
Sees self as bona fide patient	Yes	No	No
Purpose of drug use	Medicinal	Recreational	Recreational (infrequent)
Purchases supply from drug dealers	No	Yes	N/A
Sells drugs for profit	No	Yes	N/A

N/A, Not applicable.

the number of tablets dispensed. Thus it is important for emergency physicians to realize that entrepreneurial drug seekers primarily want prescriptions from doctors, not the pills themselves.

2. **Appearance.** They usually appear well-to-do and frequently dress conservatively. They are invariably articulate and affable. The most successful drug seekers are inconspicuous in manner. They blend in with the crowd so as to avoid suspicions, and seldom get into arguments with physicians who refuse their requests for drugs.

C. Professional patients. These are men and women who possess an obvious physical deformity; they use the deformity as part of their pitch to obtain prescriptions. The three most common types of professional patients are amputees, paraplegics, and obese women. Amputees and paraplegics use their deformities to obtain narcotics analgesics; they often claim that they were injured during a tour of duty in the armed services to elicit sympathy. Professional patients seldom consume or sell drugs. They are hired by a drug dealer to portray a patient and are paid a set fee for every prescription obtained.

Techniques Used by Drug Seekers to Obtain Prescriptions from Emergency Physicians

I. **General considerations.** To obtain prescriptions from emergency physicians, entrepreneurial drug seekers use several strategies. First, they feign illnesses for which doctors are accustomed to prescribing drugs such as narcotics and benzodiazepines. Since they do not wish to arouse suspicion, drug seekers learn about the diseases they intend to feign by reading about them in medical textbooks, as well as the *Physicians' Desk Reference*. That way, they know the symptoms and signs to mimic, as well as the contraindications to drugs they do not want.

A. Feigning disease. For example, a drug seeker who pretends to have low back pain may claim a past history of peptic ulcer disease to discourage the emergency physician from prescribing an NSAID. Alternatively, a drug seeker pretending to have renal colic may claim to be allergic to radioopaque dyes to avoid getting an intravenous pyelogram.

B. Psychological pressure. Besides feigning a disease, drug seekers use psychologic pressure to lead the doctor to the conclusion that a prescription is both necessary and urgent. They tend to visit crowded emergency departments at busy times, such as evenings and weekends. They know that physicians are under increased pressure at these times to see patients quickly and discharge them. Often they employ elaborate scams to increase the likelihood of getting a drug.

II. Conditions feigned by drug seekers.
These are summarized in **Table 4-3,** along with the drugs sought.

A. Conditions with subjective symptoms only. This category is made up of disorders for which there is no way of objectively verifying the drug seeker's complaints. This group includes migraine and cluster headaches, tic douloureux, psychiatric disorders, attention deficit syndrome, and low back pain.

B. Conditions that are difficult to verify in the emergency department. These include narcolepsy, inflammatory bowel disease, and metastatic cancer. Although all three disorders can be verified objectively, none can be verified quickly by using tests easily available to most emergency physicians. In many such cases, the bogus patient has photocopies of hospital records that apparently confirm the diagnosis. The confirmatory hospital records have been pilfered from a legitimate patient's chart. For example, drug seekers feigning narcolepsy have gone to the emergency department with copies of abnormal sleep electroencephalograms.

Table 4-3. Conditions Feigned By Drug Seekers

Condition	Drugs sought
Acute or chronic pain	Narcotics such as oxycodone and hydromorphone
Attention deficit syndrome	Methylphenidate
Bronchitis	Cough syrups containing dihydrocodone compound
Colitis	Narcotics, antidiarrheals such as loperamide
Metastatic cancer	Narcotics such as dihydromorphone and morphine
Migraine	Fiorinal with codeine, oxycodone, acetaminophen with codeine
Narcolepsy	Methylphenidate
Obesity	Phenmetrazine
Old orthopedic injuries (e.g., nonunion of scaphoid, compression fracture of vertebrae, acromioclavicular separation)	Narcotic analgesics
Psychiatric disorders	Benzodiazepines
Renal colic	Narcotics such as dihydromorphone and oxycodone
Sickle crisis	Narcotic analgesics
Tic douloureux	Narcotic analgesics
Toothache	Narcotic analgesics

Table 4-4. Conditions With Flawed Objective Tests

Condition	Flawed objective test	Reason why test is flawed
Renal colic	Blood in urine	Alternative ways of introducing blood into urine
Sickle cell crisis	Sickle preparation	Does not correlate with severity of pain
Bronchitis	Sputum sample	Easy to simulate
Some orthopedic injuries	Abnormal radiograph	Radiographic abnormalities may be old
Dental caries	Inspection, dental radiographs	Abnormalities may be old

- **C. Conditions for which standard objective tests are flawed.** This group includes disorders such as renal colic, sickle cell crisis, bronchitis, old orthopedic injuries, and dental caries **(Table 4-4).**
  1. **Renal colic.** Drug seekers feigning renal colic have several means of introducing blood into a urine sample. They may do so by puncturing their fingers or toes, or biting their lips or tongue. such sites can be detected by a careful physical examination. Some drug seekers cause genuine hematuria by injuring their urethra.
  2. **Bronchitis** is mimicked in two ways. First, the drug seeker inhales black pepper to make the mucous membranes hyperemic. Second, sputum can be simulated by ingesting a viscous substance just before seeing the physician, then coughing it up in the presence of the doctor.
- **D. Using genuine conditions to obtain drugs.** Some drug seekers exploit genuine, acute conditions to obtain drugs from numerous sources. For example, drug seekers who sustain acute fractures reportedly go from hospital to hospital, receiving a cast and a prescription for narcotics at each stop. They remove the cast as soon as they leave one hospital and go to the next hospital with an "untreated fracture". Other drug seekers use the same strategy with dental abscesses.

III. **Psychologic tactics.** Experienced con artists employ a number of psychologic techniques that are designed to throw the emergency physician off balance. Faced with such tactics, many physicians find themselves reacting to the demands of such patients, often abandoning their critical judgment. Simply recognizing that these techniques exist can often help to neutralize their effect.
- **A. Creating a false sense of urgency.** This strategy is an adjunct to virtually every bogus presentation. In almost every scenario, the drug seeker tries to persuade the emergency physician that a prescription is the only sensible or compassionate option available. This is done in one of two ways.
  1. **Unbearable symptoms that must be treated at once.** Some patients go to the emergency department complaining of such severe pain that they insist it be treated without delay. Any attempt to take a history and perform a physical examination is met with resistance or accusations that the physician lacks compassion. This tactic often works best when the drug seeker has a companion who verifies the drug seeker's assertion that he is not receiving compassionate care. In many cases, it may be appropriate

and compassionate to give analgesics before a diagnosis is reached. However, the persistent attempt to prevent the physician from making a diagnosis once the initial pain is relieved should be viewed with suspicion.
    2. **Substitute doctor.** With this technique, the drug seeker tries to convince the emergency doctor that he either has run out of his medication or has lost it, and needs a fresh supply. There are several possible tip-offs to this scam.
        a. The patient states he has lost his prescription.
        b. The patient states he is a visitor from another town and did not bring his usual medication with him.
        c. The patient goes to the emergency department on a weekend, needs a refill of his prescription, and cannot reach his regular physician.
        d. The patient states he is about to fly to a foreign country for several months and cannot reach his regular physician for a prescription.
    B. **Manipulation.** Some drug seekers use flattery or even outright seduction to influence physicians. Others are overly friendly to nearby patients and staff in an effort to gain their sympathy. Should the emergency physician refuse to give them a prescription, the drug seeker tries to enlist the help of bystanders to change the physician's mind.
    C. **Implied or overt threats.** This is a risky strategy for drug seekers because it makes them very conspicuous. Once frustrated, some con artists threaten to sue the doctor or to complain to the state licensing authorities. Death threats are sometimes uttered in anger, but prescription drug seekers rarely resort to violence. The most successful drug entrepreneurs seldom raise the specter of retaliation.
    D. **Desperation.** This is the dominant affect of the true prescription drug addict. In this case, it is not an act. Anxiety or overt desperation is part of the psychologic profile of an addict. Other features of addictive behavior include excessive preoccupation with the drug of choice, concern or anxiety that builds as the supply of the drug runs out, and unsupervised escalations of the dosage of drug. Faced with an emotional onslaught from such patients, it is treacherously easy for emergency physicians to fall into the trap of writing a prescription.
IV. **Prescription drug scams.** In addition to the above techniques of manipulation, professional drug seekers try a variety of stereotypic scams on emergency physicians. These change from time to time, but some key elements seldom vary.
    A. **Parent and child scams.** In this case, an adult goes to the emergency department seeking medication for themselves or their children. The child may or may not be present for the scam. In every case, the parent uses the child to add plausibility or sympathy to their "pitch for pills."
        1. **Parent seeking medication for self.** Parents using this scam claim that they have arrived in town to take their child to the local pediatric hospital for tests or for surgery. Then the parents make a pitch for medication, stating that they suffer from a condition such as headaches, and have run out of their usual analgesic.
        2. **Parent seeking medication for their child.** To obtain prescription narcotics, parents of children who suffer from sickle cell anemia have coached their children to pretend as if they are having a painful crisis. To obtain a supply of methylphenidate, parents have coached their children to mimic the behavior associated with attention deficit syndrome (hyperkinesis).

B. Confessing to Drug Addiction. Some drug seekers freely admit to being addicts as part of a scam to obtain prescription drugs. In this scam, the drug seeker expresses a desire to stop taking drugs. They may even claim that they are on a waiting list to enter a drug rehabilitation program. The drug seeker invariably asks for an interim supply of drugs to ward off the symptoms of drug withdrawal. The only certain way to verify this is to contact the addiction specialist the drug seeker claims to be seeing.

V. Prescription forgery. As mentioned before, entrepreneurial drug seekers are in the business of acquiring prescription drugs and then selling them to make a profit. To maximize their supply, drug seekers often alter the prescriptions provided by emergency physicians. Prescriptions written in Arabic or Roman numerals, or longhand can be altered by skilled forgers. Techniques for discouraging forgeries are described below.

Diagnosis of Drug-seeking Behavior

I. General considerations. As with any other condition, the diagnosis of drug-seeking behavior requires a thorough history and physical examination. Laboratory testing helps to confirm the diagnosis and rule out other conditions. In the majority of cases, the drug seeker is seen is the emergency department with a chief complaint that points to a specific diagnosis. The history, physical examination, and laboratory tests should always focus on that complaint. This should be well documented in the patient's emergency department chart. There are two reasons for this. First, drug seekers, like other patients, have genuine illnesses. Second, it is often difficult to confirm that a patient is a drug seeker during a single visit to the emergency department. If in doubt, it is best to give the patient the benefit of the doubt.

II. History (Table 4-5). The diagnosis of drug-seeking behavior can sometimes be made when the patient registers for treatment. Establish a departmental policy of asking all new patients for two or three pieces of identification such as a driver's license and Social Security card. Many drug seekers use aliases; few carry two or three forged documents.

A. Precautions. Several features should arouse suspicion during history taking. Be wary of patients who are evasive during the interview. In addition, be suspicious of patients who request commonly abused prescription drugs by name, particularly if the request seems overly urgent. Drug seekers also tend to control the flow and pace of the interview.

Table 4-5. History of Suspicious Features

Lack of confirmatory identification
Diagnosis commonly feigned by drug seekers
Evasive or controlling historian
Overly flattering or seductive behavior
Request commonly abused medications by name
Out-of-towner
Past history of alcohol or drug abuse
Allergic to codeine, NSAIDs, pentazocine, local anesthetics, and radioopaque dyes

B. False claims. Drug seekers often claim to have allergies to medications that ordinarily serve as alternatives to abused pain relievers. These include codeine, local anesthetics, and NSAIDs. Narcotic seekers may claim an allergy to pentazocine because they are aware that the drug precipitates withdrawal in narcotic addicts. Drug seekers pretending to have renal colic will often claim to be allergic to radioopaque dyes to avoid having an intravenous pyelogram performed.

C. Behavior. One of the most useful tip-offs to suspicious behavior is the drug seeker who maintains continuous eye contact with the emergency physician. For genuine patients, a visit to the doctor is both embarrassing and worrisome; most patients look away from the doctor from time to time. Drug seekers stare constantly at the doctor to gauge the reaction of the physician.

D. Substance abuse history. Ask all unfamiliar patients whether they have a past history of drug or alcohol abuse. For reasons unknown, many drug seekers admit previous substance abuse.

III. Physical examination. If the patient complains of acute pain, look for sympathetic manifestations such as sweating, tachycardia, peripheral vasoconstriction, and dilated pupils. Remember that such manifestations should not be expected in patients with chronic pain.

A. Orthopedic injuries. Examine patients who complain of orthopedic injuries for signs of acute trauma such as bruising, erythema, induration, and point tenderness. Many drug seekers have difficulty mimicking the latter sign. Drug seekers complaining of low back pain may be aware of the significance of the straight leg raising test. Perform a surreptitious straight leg raise by asking to examine the patient's foot while the patient is seated in a chair.

B. Dental complaints. Look carefully for evidence of dental abscesses in patients who complain of toothache. These include gingival erythema and fluctuation. The most important sign is tenderness of the infected tooth when percussed by a tongue depressor.

C. Hematuria. Check suspicious patients who complain of hematuria for bite marks inside the mouth, puncture wounds of the fingers and toes, and signs of local trauma to the urethra.

D. Intoxication. Examine all suspicious patients for signs of acute intoxication caused by alcohol or drugs. These include slurred speech, altered mental status, facial flushing, and abnormal vital signs. In addition, look for the cutaneous manifestations of long-standing drug or alcohol abuse, such as needle tracks, cutaneous abscesses, spider nevi, gynecomastia, hyperpigmented marks or tattoos over venipuncture sites, tourniquet pigmentation, and ulceration or perforation of the nasal septum.

IV. Laboratory tests

A. Blood tests. When an unfamiliar patient claims to have an established diagnosis, serum and urine tests can sometimes be used to confirm the diagnosis. For example, patients who complain of recurrent pancreatitis or cancer with liver metastases may have elevated levels of liver enzymes, as well as elevated levels of amylase or lipase. Suspicious patients who claim they are having a sickle crisis should have a sickle test. Obtain serum ethanol levels and drug screens on patients with suspected acute intoxication. In patients with alcoholic lever disease, obtain serum levels of liver enzymes, magnesium, total proteins, and ketones, as well as a prothrombin time and complete blood cell count.

B. Radiographs. Suspicious patients who complain of acute trauma to the back or extremities should have radiographs done. If an abnormality is found, try to determine whether the injury is new or old. Drug seekers frequently recycle old orthopedic injuries, such as compression fractures of the vertebrae, nonunion of fractures, and chronic separation of the acromioclavicular joint, to obtain narcotic analgesics. If in doubt, obtain additional confirmatory tests such as bone scans, or consult with an orthopedic surgeon.

C. Intravenous pyelogram. Confirm the diagnosis of renal colic by ordering an intravenous pyelogram. Consult the attending physician of patients who claim to be allergic to radioopaque dyes.

Other Diagnostic Strategies

I. Confirm the patient's stated history. The key to detecting drug seekers is to expose their fictitious and fraudulent history. The easiest way to do that is to contact the patient's attending physician. Most drug seekers who give a fictitious history are hoping that the emergency physician will not do this. More often than not, the drug seeker leaves the emergency department while such contacts are being made.

  A. Even on weekends and evenings, try to contact the patient's personal physician. Most physicians have an on-call system. If the attending physician is not available, speak with the physician on call and ask him to inform the attending physician of the patient's attempt to obtain drugs.

  B. Out-of-town patients. Use the same strategy with out-of-town patients. If the patient's personal physician cannot be reached, telephone the main emergency department in the patient's hometown. If the patient is a drug seeker, the chances are high that the emergency staff has heard of him or her.

  C. Local emergency departments. In addition, it sometimes helps to contact other nearby emergency departments and urgent care centers. Drug seekers may well have visited other local emergency departments before the current visit.

II. Golden rule: make at least one phone call

  A. Other sources of information about suspicious patients. Pharmacists are often in the best position to spot drug-seeking behavior early on. For instance, they are often aware of patients who are receiving drugs of abuse from more than one physician at the same time. Listen to warnings from pharmacists who raise concerns about prescriptions written by emergency physicians.

  B. In addition, it is sometimes helpful to contact the **state medical board** or the nearest office of the Drug Enforcement Administration. Either office has information on known drug seekers.

III. Other methods

  A. Consultations. If unable to contact another physician who knows the patient, consult with local specialists. Try to arrive at a consensus regarding the genuineness of the patient's history.

  B. Behavior. Be aware of other tip-offs to drug-seeking behavior. Genuine patients tend to be more reasonable than drug seekers; conversely, drug seekers tend to be more manipulative than legitimate patients. For instance, drug seekers tend to get angry when asked for several pieces of identification or for evidence confirming their past history; legitimate patients almost always react to such questioning with equanimity.

C. **Refusal.** Sometimes it is possible to make a diagnosis of drug-seeking behavior by refusing the patient's request for medication. Legitimate patients tend to accept this, while drug seekers frequently become angry and abusive.

D. **Narcotic agonist–antagonist.** Also, if a patient asks for an analgesic and denies taking narcotics, it is possible to test the patient by administering a narcotic agonist–antagonist such as pentazocine. Legitimate patients have relief from their pain; narcotic abusers have withdrawal symptoms. Use this strategy only with the patient's knowledge and consent.

Frustrating Entrepreneurial Drug Seekers

I. **General considerations.** The primary goal is to prevent the entrepreneurial drug seeker from obtaining a prescription for pharmaceuticals that are ultimately sold to drug dealers. If a drug seeker does not obtain a prescription, the visit is regarded as unsuccessful. Fortunately, there are strategies that permit the physician to frustrate entrepreneurial drug seekers while giving all other patients the benefit of the doubt.

II. **Administrative policies.** Develop a consistent policy to be used by all emergency physicians for dealing with suspected drug seekers. For example, the emergency physicians may decide not to prescribe narcotics for acute migraine headaches. Likewise, emergency physicians should meet regularly to discuss problem patients. By developing such a policy and sticking to it, drug seekers will not be able to play one emergency physician against the other.

  A. **Suspicious patients** should be noted in some sort of departmental record. Besides recording the patient's name, write down identifying features such as height, weight, approximate age, and any distinguishing features such as tattoos. That way, a drug seeker who uses an alias will still be recognizable. In addition, flag the charts of suspicious patients so that the patient's hospital records are retrieved whenever they arrive.

  B. **Do not label patients** in writing as drug addicts or drug seekers under any circumstances. Such references needlessly call the compassion of health care workers into question.

III. **Alternatives to abusable prescriptions.** A variety of potent **nonnarcotic analgesics** provide pain relief without the risk of dependence or diversion **(Table 4-6).**

  A. **Local nerve block.** For patients with a toothache or herpes zoster, a local nerve block with a long-acting local anesthetic such as bupivacaine hydrochloride (maximum dose 1.5 mg/kg) may be given instead of an analgesic. Note that bupivacaine is not recommended for pudendal blocks or for regional intravenous anesthesia.

  B. **Nonsteroidal antiinflammatory drugs** may be prescribed instead of narcotics for the relief of painful conditions such as acute low back pain, fractures, sprains, and headaches.

  C. **Floctafenine and ketorolac tromethamine.** One analgesic has analgesic effects without the toxicity associated with NSAIDs. Floctafenine, 400 mg, is as effective as acetaminophen with 30 mg of codeine in patients with toothaches. The dosage of floctafenine (Idarac) is 200 to 400 mg every 6 to 8 hours. The maximum recommended daily dose is 1200 mg. Alternatively, ketorolac tromethamine (Toradol) is effective for acute pain. The dosage is

Table 4-6. Alternatives to Prescriptions for Abused Pharmaceuticals

Condition	Alternative
Acute sprains and fractures	Ketorolac 10 mg PO QID as needed, floctafenine 400 mg PO TID as needed
Low back pain	Ketorolac 15-30 mg IM (10 mg PO QID as needed), floctafenine 400 mg PO TID as needed
Migraine headache	Prochlorperazine 5 mg IV or IM, chlorpromazine 5-10 mg IV, ketorolac 15-30 mg IM
Renal colic	Ketorolac 15-30 mg IM, indomethacin 50-75 mg IV, indomethacin rectal suppository 100 mg as needed
Tic douloureux	Carbamazepine 50-100 mg PO BID (start at 25 mg BID and increase slowly)
Toothache	Local anesthetic (bupivacaine), floctafenine 400 mg PO TID, ketorolac 10 mg PO QID

10 mg every 4 to 6 hours, up to a maximum dose of 40 mg/day. **Caution:** Remember that ketorolac is an NSAID, with all its attendant risks.

D. A number of nonnarcotic analgesics may be used instead of narcotics for the relief of acute migraine headaches. These include prochlorperazine (Compazine), 5 mg by intravenous or intramuscular injection, as well as chlorpromazine, 5 mg given intravenously.

E. If a narcotic must be given, it is best to administer one parenterally or to provide several tablets of oral narcotics. This strategy often helps in identifying drug seekers. Legitimate patients will be satisfied with a few tablets or an injection, but many drug seekers become angry at not receiving a prescription.

IV. Confronting the drug seeker. It is unwise to accuse a patient of being a drug addict or a prescription drug seeker on the evidence obtained from a single visit to the emergency department.

  A. Chief complaint. In general, it is best to keep referring to the patient's chief complaint. The advice given should be specific to the chief complaint. The emergency physician has a duty to examine all patients and to render aid and assistance. That does not include a duty to provide drugs on demand. It is acceptable to tell a patient who has a headache that narcotics will not be prescribed, as long as a viable alternative is made available.

  B. Advise the patient in a respectful, nonjudgmental manner. Drug seekers often become overtly hostile when not given medication. At times this is part of the drug seeker's con—an attempt to intimidate the emergency physician into acceding to the drug seeker's demands. Call security or the police in response to abusive or threatening behavior.

V. Dealing with drug addicts. Sometimes it is possible to gather sufficient evidence to directly confront the patient about suspected addiction. Often such patients have been returning to the emergency department so many times that the diagnosis is obvious. Confront such patients gently but firmly. Note the addictive properties of the drug they are taking and express concern for the patient's well-being. Ask whether the patient is concerned about becoming addicted to

prescription drugs. If confronted in this way, some patients will admit to being drug addicts. Refer such patients to the nearest drug rehabilitation center.
VI. **Withdrawal symptoms. Withdrawal from benzodiazepines** and barbiturates can be fatal. Patients addicted to such medications should either be admitted to the hospital for controlled withdrawal or referred immediately for close follow-up. **Withdrawal from narcotics** is not considered fatal. There is no pressing reason to admit such patients to a hospital or to provide them with a small supply of narcotics.
VII. **Drug laws and regulations**
   A. **Under the Controlled Substances Act,** physicians may not prescribe narcotics for detoxification or as part of a drug rehabilitation program unless given expressed permission by federal authorities. Emergency physicians may prescribe narcotics to so-called drug addicts for a maximum of 3 days. At the same time, arrangements should be made to enroll the patient in a recognized drug treatment program.
   B. **State laws vary** from jurisdiction to jurisdiction, but they tend to be more stringent than federal laws. In general, such laws compel the physician to prescribe controlled substances for pain relief; it is a crime in some states to prescribe narcotics for the maintenance of an addiction. For further information, consult the state licensing board.

Suggested Readings

Coleman N: Check…checkmate. Countering the con games of drug abusers, *Postgrad Med* 77:68, 1985.

Goldman B: The prescription drug sting: be careful out there, *Can Med Assoc J* 136:629, 1987.

Goldman B: Part II. The difficult patient: detecting drug seekers in primary care, *Canadian Family Physician* 35:2047-2173, 1989.

Goldman B, editor, Carlisle JR, Wilford BB, consulting editors: Frustrating prescription drug seekers, *Emergency Medicine Reports* 9:203-210, 1988.

PADS: A look at prescription drug abuse, *Ohio Med* 82:33, 1986.

The Missouri Task Force on Misuse, Abuse and Diversion of Prescription Drugs: *The scam of the month,* ed 2, Jefferson City, 1986.

Weiss KJ, Greenfield DP: Prescription drug abuse, *Psychiatr Clin North Am* 9:475, 1986.

Wilford BB: *Drug abuse: a guide for the primary care physician,* Chicago, 1981, American Medical Association.

5

Acute Myocardial Infarction: Initial Stabilization, Mortality Reduction, and Treatment of Complications

J. Michael Albrich, M.D., F.A.C.P., F.A.C.E.P.

Acute myocardial infarction (AMI) is a life-threatening emergency most often caused by thrombotic occlusion of an atherosclerotic coronary artery and subsequent myocardial necrosis. In the United States, 1.3 million people suffer myocardial infarction annually, and approximately 40% die before reaching the hospital. Those who reach the hospital are at risk of the complications of AMI (death, cardiogenic shock, congestive heart failure (CHF), and arrhythmias), particularly in the first 24 hours. In this early period, the greatest mortality reductions are possible when the complications of AMI are treated with advanced cardiac life support (ACLS), and the mortality-reducing drugs—aspirin, thrombolytic agents, beta-blockers, and angiotensin-converting enzyme (ACE) inhibitors—are employed as soon as possible after onset of symptoms. Emergent direct percutaneous transluminal coronary angioplasty (PTCA) may reduce mortality as effectively as thrombolysis when thrombolysis is contraindicated. *Delay* in instituting treatment of all types is recognized as a significant cause of avoidable mortality in AMI (GISSI: *Lancet* i:397–402, 1986).

The **diagnosis of** myocardial infarction is based on (1) history and physical examination; (2) electrocardiographic (ECG) changes compatible with myocardial infarction; and (3) the characteristic rise and fall of cardiac isoenzyme, creatine kinase, MB fraction (CK-MB), and rarely, lactic dehydrogenase, isoenzyme 1 (LDH_1) is useful in late presentations (Herr CH: *J Emerg Med* 10:455–461, 1992). Symptoms may be vague, signs are infrequently useful, the initial ECG is nondiagnostic in 50% to 60% of proven AMIs, and cardiac enzymes are elevated in only a small minority of AMI patients at presentation in the emergency department. Of all AMIs, 25% to 30% occur in patients who do not seek medical care either because the AMI is truly silent or because the symptoms are atypical. The emergency physician must maintain a high index of suspicion in all clinical presentations that are suggestive of AMI. Even in the best institutions, up to 1% to 2% of patients with AMIs are sent home and up to 26% of these patients die. These deaths result in the single largest source of malpractice awards in emergency medicine. Unstable angina (angina that is new or increasing in frequency, intensity, or duration) is often indistinguishable from myocardial infarction in the emergency department. Both require admission. Because the diagnosis of AMI is initially uncertain in many patients who ultimately develop AMI, it is important to begin pharmacologic mortality reduction in selected patients by administering aspirin, beta-blockers, and in some cases, thrombolytic agents in the emergency department *before* the diagnosis of AMI is confirmed.

This chapter depends heavily on large, double-blind, randomized, controlled multicenter trials in AMI for the recommendations it contains. Recently, two therapeutic agents for AMI, intravenous nitroglycerin and magnesium, which produced significant mortality reduction in multiple, small randomized trials, have not proven substantially effective in large multicenter trials (GISSI-3 and ISIS-4, respectively, preliminary communication; see IV Nitroglycerin and Agents Ineffective or Harmful in AMI). In the case of magnesium, over 3600 patients were randomly selected in eight controlled trials of magnesium versus placebo in AMI. One of these, the LIMIT-2 trial, randomly selected over 2300 patients (Woods KL et al: *Lancet* 339:1553–1558, 1992). Metaanalysis of multiple small trials of both of these agents (Lau J et al: *N Engl J Med* 327:248–254, 1992) predicted substantial mortality reduction, greater even than the thrombolytic agents, aspirin, and beta-blockers. The failure of metaanalysis requires investigation and, for the present, casts some doubt on the method (in particular, when total patients number under 3000 to 4000). The failure of the LIMIT-2 trial, a well-designed, moderate-sized trial of 2300 patients to predict intravenous magnesium's behavior in a large trial (ISIS-4; 54,000 patients) further encourages dependence on large, double-blind, randomized, controlled multicenter trials.

History and Physical Examination

I. **History**
   A. **Chest pain.** Classic chest pain of AMI is crushing pain or pressure in the substernal area and/or left side of the chest. Chest pain is present in 80% to 85% of patients with AMIs and usually occurs suddenly. The pain may resemble previous angina or AMI but is poorly responsive to nitroglycerin and oxygen. Prodromal angina may preceed the current episode by days or weeks. More often, the presenting episode of chest pain is the first. Radiation of chest pain to the jaw, neck, back, shoulders, arms, or epigastrium (indigestion) increases the probability that the pain is ischemic. Most commonly the pain radiates to the left arm. Radiation to the right arm is uncommon but more specific for AMI than other patterns of radiated pain. Radiation to the back is common with inferior AMIs. Chest pain of AMI may be pleuritic or worsen with movement in 5% to 8% of AMI patients. Increased severity of pain is associated with a poorer prognosis.
   B. **Absence of chest pain.** AMI may occur without chest pain, especially in patients with CHF or arrhythmias (premature ventricular contractions [PVCs], ventricular tachycardia, and atrial flutter or fibrillation with ventricular rates of 120 or more). The mortality of these patients is substantially higher than those with chest pain.
   C. **The elderly.** Chest pain is increasingly less specific with age. Classic symptoms are less specific with advancing age. Patients 85 years and older have no pain in over 60% of myocardial infarctions. As age increases, symptoms such as syncope, acute confusion, and stroke become more common and chest pain and diaphoresis, less common. In the very old, AMI must be considered in all acutely ill patients.
   D. **Associated symptoms.** Diaphoresis, nausea, vomiting, dyspnea, palpitations, and dizziness or lightheadedness are frequent but nonspecific complaints in AMI. They do, however, add weight to the more diagnostic complaints.
   E. **Cardiac risk factors.** Smoking, hypertension, diabetes mellitus, hypercholesterolemia (and low high-density lipoprotein [HDL] cholesterol), previous angina or MI, peripheral vascular disease, and an immediate family history of MI are all risk factors for AMI, but *none* of these independently discriminates between patients with chest pain of AMI and other causes. Only a history of

angina or MI discriminates as an independent variable among AMI and other causes of chest pain. Use of cocaine by all routes (intranasal, intravenous, and inhaled) is associated with AMI.

F. Medication history. Various medications (antianginals, antiarrhythmics, antihypertensives, anticoagulants, and digitalis) increase suspicion of ischemic origin of the presenting complaint. The use of gastrointestinal medications such as antacids, sucralfate, and H_2-blockers (cimetidine, ranitidine) for presumed dyspepsia or non-steroidal antiinflammatory drugs for presumed musculoskeletal chest pain should alert the physician to the possibility that myocardial ischemia is the cause of the patient's symptoms.

II. Physical examination. Most patients suffering AMI appear acutely ill.

A. Vital signs. Tachycardia, bradycardia, irregular pulse, tachypnea, and marked hypertension or hypotension are all consistent with AMI.

B. Skin. Diaphoresis is common. Cyanosis (peripheral or central), mottling, or pallor suggests shock.

C. Cardiopulmonary. Rales and an S_3 gallop are associated with left ventricular failure; jugular venous distension, hepatojugular reflux, and peripheral edema suggest right ventricular failure. Pure right-sided heart failure suggests right ventricular infarction. An S_4 gallop is of dubious value.

1. **The Killip classification** of heart failure in AMI is based on bedside clinical findings of left ventricular dysfunction and is useful prognostically and in selection of patients for thrombolysis **(Table 5-1).**
2. **A new systolic murmur** is associated with ischemic mitral regurgitation or ventricular septal defect (VSD), particularly in the presence of heart failure or cardiogenic shock. A pericardial rub implies pericarditis and may be present briefly in 5% of AMIs. It is an important clinical finding because pericarditis is difficult to diagnose by ECG in AMI and its presence contraindicates thrombolysis.

Electrocardiography

Most ECGs will demonstrate some abnormality in patients ultimately proven to have AMI. An ECG should be obtained immediately in patients with chest pain, pressure, or symptoms suggestive of AMI (dyspnea without obvious cause, syncope, acute confusion, or stroke). The ECG should be repeated with recurrence of chest pain or sudden improvement or decline in the patient's clinical condition. Several subsequent ECGs in the emergency department may discover diagnostic criteria not present on initial ECG.

Table 5-1. The Killip Classification of Heart Failure in AMI

Class I	No clinical heart failure
Class II	Rales heard bilaterally up to 50% of the lung fields
Class III	Pulmonary edema: rales heard in all lung fields
Class IV	Cardiogenic shock: stuporous; BP <90; cold, clammy skin; pulmonary edema; decreased urine output

I. **Criteria.** Numerous ECG findings have been used as criteria for the diagnosis of AMI. Large thrombolytic trials have used the GISSI ECG criteria to establish the presence of AMI; these criteria have a specificity of 94% (GISSI: *Lancet* i:397–402, 1986). The criteria are (1) ≥1 mm ST segment elevation or depression in any limb lead, or (2) ≥2 mm ST segment elevation in any precordial lead. The sensitivity of these criteria on the initial ECG even with a strong clinical history is only about 40% for patients ultimately shown to have AMI (see Rationale for the Guideline: ECG criteria).

II. **Sensitivity.** Early studies of the sensitivity of the ECG to detect AMI in the emergency department by using a variety of criteria indicate a sensitivity from 43% to 65% (Herr CH: *J Emerg Med* 10:455–461, 1992). The Multicenter Chest Pain Study of 7115 patients with chest pain seen in the emergency departments of seven hospitals used three liberal ECG criteria that, taken together, achieved 79% sensitivity but only 44% specificity. These criteria assume that changes are new or that no old ECG is available. The criteria are as follows:
   A. **Probable new transmural AMI:** sensitivity, 45%; positive predictive value, 76%.
      1. ≥1 mm ST segment elevation in two or more leads, or
      2. abnormal Q waves in two or more leads.
   B. **New strain or ischemia:** sensitivity, 20%; positive predictive value, 38%.
      1. ≥1 mm ST segment depression in two or more leads.
   C. **New ST or T wave changes of ischemia or strain:** sensitivity, 14%; positive predictive value, 21%.
      1. ST segment depression <1 mm and T wave inversions thought to represent ischemia or strain.

III. **All inferior and/or lateral AMIs** should have lead V_4R included in the ECG to detect a right ventricular infarction. The prognosis is much worse than inferior AMI only **(Table 5-2)**.

Table 5-2. Occurrence of AMI in Patients With Other ECG Findings

Normal ECG	3%
Old infarct, ischemia or strain	5%
Nonspecific ST-T changes	7%

IV. **The false-positive rate** for ≥1 mm ST segment elevation in the diagnosis of AMI on the initial ECG is 12% to 15%. Non-AMI causes of a newly or persistently abnormal ECG suggestive of AMI include the following:

Diagnosis	ECG abnormality	Evaluation
Myocarditis	ST segment and T wave changes	Coronary angiography, echocardiography, endocardial biopsy
Pericarditis	ST segment elevation	Echocardiography
Hemorrhagic stroke	T wave inversion	CT of the head
Ventricular aneurysm	ST segment elevation	Echocardiography, LV angiography

Cardiac Enzymes

I. **CK and CK-MB.** The "gold standard" for the diagnosis of AMI is the characteristic rise and fall of both total creatine kinase (CK) and its cardiac isoenzyme, the MB fraction (CK-MB), which is specific for cardiac muscle. These enzymes are released from necrotic myocardial cells and appear in the serum within 4 to 8 hours and peak in 12 to 20 hours of onset of AMI. Total CK may be elevated because of contributions from muscle (MM fraction) and brain (BB fraction) unrelated to AMI. Initial determinations of both CK and CK-MB have low sensitivity (30% to 40%) to detect AMI in patients in the emergency department, but a markedly positive CK-MB greatly increases the probability of AMI. CK-MB is considered positive in most studies when it exceeds 3% to 6% of total CK. Initial determinations of CK-MB or CK can neither reliably diagnose AMI or exclude it so that the patient can be safely sent home. Serial measurement of total CK and CK-MB initially, and 12 and 24 hours later, has a sensitivity approaching 100% for the detection of AMI and is currently recommended. CK and CK-MB should also be measured at these intervals for recurrent ischemia.

  A. **Serial immunochemical measurement** of CK-MB performed in the emergency department when the patient is first seen and 3 hours later increases the sensitivity to detect AMI to about 80, with a specificity of 94% of all patients tested. Decisions regarding in-hospital disposition (intensive care unit or monitored bed on a medical floor) may be improved with initial and 3-hour serial CK-MB determinations, but use of these criteria to determine thrombolysis candidacy in patients with ECG findings other than diagnostic GISSI criteria would lead to exposure of one in four patients without AMI to thrombolytic agents. (This may be acceptable; see Rationale for the Guideline; ECG criteria.)

  B. **CK-MB false-positive elevations** occur in certain clinical situations that are readily apparent such as muscular dystrophy, renal failure, rhabdomyolysis, prostate surgery or Cesarean section (specific tissue sources), and athletic activity. If true CK-MB elevation is found but the typical rise and fall of total CK and CK-MB are not observed, these other causes of elevated CK-MB should be considered. False-negative CK and CK-MB results in AMI are invariably due to inadequate sampling.

II. **LDH isoenzymes.** Lactate dehydrogenase occurs in five isomeric forms. LDH_1 and to a lesser extent, LDH_2 isoenzymes predominate in the heart. Total LDH levels rise 8 to 12 hours after AMI and peak at 72 to 144 hours. An LDH_1/LDH_2 ratio >0.76 has both a sensitivity and specificity greater than 90% for the detection of AMI. Erythrocytes and myocardial muscle have similar isoenzyme distributions; therefore hemolysis, either endogenous or mechanical, invalidates the test. Other interfering conditions are pregnancy and myopathy. Current recommendations for LDH determination to confirm AMI are as follows:

  A. **>24 hours of symptoms of AMI.**
  B. **CK and CK-MB are nondiagnostic.**
  C. **Elevated total LDH.**
  D. **If LDH_1/LDH_2 ratio is between 0.76 and 1.0,** a second determination should be considered.

Other Serum Markers of AMI

I. **Myoglobin.** Myoglobin is a small protein involved in muscle oxygen transport. It is released earlier than CK-MB from injured cardiac muscle after onset of AMI (1 to 2 hours). A new immunoturbidimetric method allows myoglobin determination in less than 10 minutes. Sensitivity to AMI approaches 90% from 4 to 6 hours after onset of symptoms. Unfortunately, myoglobin is not specific for cardiac muscle, but consideration of the principal interfering clinical situations (acute or chronic muscle injury and impaired renal function) allows the assay to maintain a high specificity. Large prospective trials of myoglobin in the early diagnosis of AMI are not yet available.

II. **Troponin T and I.** Troponin T and I are regulatory proteins specific for myocardial cells. Immunoassay of these proteins provides specific and sensitive detection of myocardial injury. Troponin I, in particular, appears to have a low false-positive rate. Clinical experience with these assays in prospective identification of AMI is limited, and they are not currently available in the United States.

III. **Chest x-ray.** Cardiomegaly and pulmonary congestion on chest X-ray are more sensitive than auscultation for the diagnosis of CHF. Other causes of chest pain such as pneumonia, pneumothorax, malignancy, or trauma may be identified. Chest X-ray is also required to confirm endotracheal tube and central venous line placement and complications.

Echocardiography

I. **Transthoracic.** Wall motion abnormalities are a hallmark of AMI and are present even when the ECG is nondiagnostic. Unfortunately, these abnormalities may be old, so the diagnosis of AMI is not possible unless recent, prior echocardiography establishes that they are new. Absence of wall motion abnormality implies a very low probability of ischemia and is unknown in AMI. Echocardiography detects the large mural thrombi associated with up to 40% of transmural myocardial infarctions. Echocardiography in AMI also examines the abnormalities of the valves (mitral regurgitation), septum (ventricular septal defect), ventricular wall (ventricular aneurysm), and pericardium (effusion), which are associated with CHF and cardiogenic shock in AMI. Most patients with new AMI, especially those with CHF, anterior and large AMIs, and those who develop complications, should receive echocardiographic evaluation (see Complications, p. 164).

II. **Transesophageal.** This method of echocardiography is potentially a bedside diagnostic technique with superior imaging of the great vessels (to exclude aortic dissection), and atrial and ventricles (to exclude AMI-associated thrombi).

III. **Nuclear scanning.** Technetium-99 pyrophosphate is bound to the infarct site, but many factors determine binding. Sensitivity and specificity depend on type of abnormality considered to be diagnostic. Highly focal uptake is insensitive but highly specific for AMI (>99%). Alternatively, diffuse uptake is 94% sensitive for transmural AMI but only 70% specific. This test is not available in many institutions. It is recommended for those cases where ECG and cardiac enzymes are not diagnostic and suspicion is still high for AMI.

Clinical Management of Acute Myocardial Infarction

The principal components of AMI management are initial stabilization, pharmacologic mortality reduction, and vigilant anticipation and treatment of the complications of AMI.

INITIAL STABILIZATION

In patients with chest pain or clinical presentation suggestive of AMI (new CHF in the elderly), the history, physical examination, laboratory data (ECG, chest X-ray, complete blood cell count [CBC], and serum levels of electrolytes, creatinine, glucose, and cardiac enzymes), and the treatments described below are obtained and performed simultaneously. Physicians and nurses evaluate and deliver care to the patient together as part of a cardiac team. Only a team approach provides the rapid assessment and treatment needed in AMI. Delay in providing the therapies for AMI is becoming a significant cause of unnecessary mortality and morbidity. Patients with suspected AMI should receive the following initial treatment:

Intervention I: Sitting Position

Patients often wish to sit up; this increases tidal volume and decreases the work of breathing.

Intervention II: Oxygen (O_2)

All patients should be placed on supplemental oxygen. Monitor oxygen saturation (SaO_2) by pulse oximetry, continuously if available, and maintain at ≥95%. The stable patient is given oxygen by nasal prongs at flow rates of 2 to 4 L/min. Unstable patients are given oxygen at 5 to 6 L/min by mask, or at 12 to 15 L/min by nonrebreather mask as needed to maintain SaO_2 at ≥95%. Continuous positive airway pressure (CPAP) applied with a tight fitting mask may improve oxygenation. If these efforts fail to maintain SaO_2 at ≥95%, arterial blood gases should be drawn. If arterial oxygen pressure (PaO_2) is less than 60 mm Hg or acidosis is present, the patient should have an endotracheal tube placed and mechanical ventilation begun.

Intervention III: Intravenous Access

Two large-bore (16 to 18 gauge) lines should be secured. Antecubital sites are preferred if there are no large forearm veins.

Intervention IV: Cardiac Monitor

Should be applied on all patients.

Intervention V: Blood Pressure

Automatic blood pressure monitoring is available with some cardiac monitors and provides blood pressure measurements at frequent intervals. Initial values should be confirmed manually by mercury sphygmomanometer. Blood pressure should be measured in both arms if pain radiates to the back or legs or is associated with asymmetrically weak or absent upper extremity pulses.

Intervention VI: Initial Relief of Pain and Pulmonary Congestion

Mortality reduction in AMI has not been demonstrated for either sublingual nitroglycerin or intravenous morphine sulfate. Despite this, these agents are administered first as standard practice because of the clinical benefits of preload reduction and pain relief.

DRUG THERAPY OPTIONS

Step 1: Sublingual Nitroglycerin

Sublingual nitroglycerin, 0.3 or 0.4 mg tablet (Nitrostat) or 0.4 mg spray (Nitrolingual), should be administered every 5 minutes if the systolic BP remains above 110 mm Hg. In these dosages nitroglycerin causes preload reduction by venodilation. If symptoms are not relieved with three doses, particularly if there is no change with the first two, intravenous nitroglycerin should be prepared and intravenous morphine sulfate should be given. Between 2% and 3% of patients given sublingual nitroglycerin will have hypotension secondary to hypovolemia and/or right ventricular infarction. After intravenous normal saline solution is given to correct the hypotension, an ECG with leads V_3R and V_4R should be obtained to rule out right ventricular infarction. Rarely, symptomatic sinus bradycardia may occur and may be treated with atropine (see Bradycardia).

Step 2: Intravenous Morphine

Intravenous morphine, 2 to 4 mg, should be given every 5 to 10 minutes as needed for pain if the systolic BP remains above 110 mm Hg. Complications of morphine include hypotension, treated with normal saline solution infusion; nausea and vomiting, treated by discontinuing the drug; and itching at the site, treated by discontinuing the drug. If the itching becomes generalized—an uncommon event—diphenhydramine (Benadryl), 25 to 50 mg intravenously, is effective. Symptomatic sinus bradycardia is treated with atropine if persistent. Respiratory depression rarely occurs, but the effects of morphine can be reversed by naloxone (Narcan) in small doses of 0.1 to 0.2 mg intravenously to avoid sudden analgesic withdrawal. Pulse oximetry and blood pressure should be monitored carefully during such episodes.

Step 3: Intravenous Nitroglycerin

For persistent chest pain, hypertension, or pulmonary rales, if systolic BP >110 mm Hg, intravenous nitroglycerin is indicated in the AMI patient. Begin titration at 10 to 20 µg/min, and advance to 50 to 180 µg/min in increments of 5 to 10 µg/min every 5 minutes. Blood pressure response and hemodynamic improvement depend more on the volume status of the patient than the absolute dose of nitroglycerin. Hypovolemia, which is common in AMI, must be corrected before intravenous nitroglycerin is fully effective. Intravenous nitroglycerin has been studied versus placebo in a small number of patients. Metaanalysis of the six available randomized controlled trials (951 patients total) indicated a mortality reduction of 49% compared with the control group in the treatment of AMI, but results (preliminary) of GISSI-3, a randomized, controlled 232 design trial (like ISIS-2) of approximately 19,000 patients, suggest that the mortality reduction at 42 days in patients treated with intravenous nitroglycerin followed by topical nitroglycerin is much less than previously believed **(Table 5-3)**.

Currently, intravenous nitroglycerin offers benefit in the treatment of hypertension, chest pain, and CHF in AMI. Dosage is given in the "Guideline". Topical and oral nitroglycerin are of benefit when combined with ACE inhibitors after the first 24 hours. The dosage from GISSI-3 is one 10 mg patch per day or 50 mg of oral isosorbide per day. In patients with persistent headache, hypotension, or tachycardia, the dosage is one 5 mg patch daily or 20 mg of isosorbide twice per day. Hypotension is the principal complication of intravenous nitroglycerin and responds to reduction or termination of infusion, and fluid resuscitation of hypovolemia or right ventricular myocardial infarction. Careful blood pressure monitoring is essential. Other medications commonly used in the treatment of AMI such as diuretics (furosemide), beta-blockers, and the thrombolytic agents, streptokinase and anisoylated plasminogen streptokinase activator complex (APSAC), can cause hypotension. If hypotension develops while intravenous nitroglycerin and either of these thrombolytic agents or the beta-blockers are employed, intravenous nitroglycerin should be withdrawn first in order to continue therapy with agents known to reduce mortality (see Thrombolytic Therapy and Beta-blockade on pp. 152 and 153).

Step 4: Intravenous Furosemide

In patients with adequate blood pressure who have pulmonary rales, the loop diuretic furosemide may reduce pulmonary congestion. The initial dose is 40 to 80 mg given intravenously, although higher doses may be required for patients with chronic CHF who routinely use furosemide. Urine output should be carefully monitored, and in many patients this may require Foley catheter insertion.

Table 5-3. Preliminary Results of the GISSI-3 Trial

Treatment group	Mortality at 42 days
Double placebo	7.2%
Nitroglycerin only	7.0%
Lisinopril only	6.6%
Nitroglycerin and lisinopril	6.0%

Guidelines for Mortality Reduction in Acute Myocardial Infarction

Once the patient is stabilized, pharmacologic therapy aimed at morbidity and mortality reduction should be initiated as soon as possible. The emergency department management of the AMI patient begins before the patient ever arrives at the department. All impediments to delivery of these lifesaving agents should be anticipated and removed to the extent that the emergency department has authority to establish policies regarding their expedited use. The "Guideline" below reflects the results of the most recent therapeutic trials (including ISIS-4 and GISSI-3; both preliminary conference reports of results) and is presented to facilitate rapid delivery of these drugs. Note that because aspirin is of very high benefit with very low risk, it should be used in patients *even remotely* suspected of having AMI. Each of the subsequent three sections of the "Guideline" should be considered for *all* patients with suspected AMI. The rationale for the "Guideline" is discussed below.

CHEST PAIN AND/OR CLINICAL PRESENTATION SUGGESTIVE OF AMI

Consider interventions below.

Phase I

325 mg; four baby aspirin or one adult aspirin, chew and swallow; if vomiting, 325 mg suppository per rectum.
ECG *not* required; *No* age limit; symptoms up to 24 hours or more.

Exclusion Criteria

Allergy to ASA.

Phase II: Thrombolysis

1. Entry Criteria

a. No age limit.
b. Killip class I and II only.
c. **Time.** Up to 12 hours from onset of symptoms; up to 24 hours of symptoms in patients with stuttering pattern of symptoms.
d. **ECG.** Obtain leads V_3R and V_4R with inferior or lateral changes
  (1) ST-elevation. >1 mm in two contiguous leads (GISSI-2).
  (2) Any of the following with strong clinical history: left bundle branch block (LBBB), pathologic Q waves >2 mm, T wave inversion, second- or third-degree atrioventricular (AV) block, any arrhythmia (ISIS-2).

2. Limitation Criteria

Prior exposure to APSAC or streptokinase, or recent streptococcal infection; **only** tissue-type plasminogen activator (t-PA) is appropriate.

3. Exclusion Criteria

a. **Aortic dissection,** suspected; *immediate* thoracic CT with contrast or transesophageal echocardiography.
  For patients excluded below: **Consider Immediate PTCA.**
b. **History of stroke** or transient ischemic attack (TIA) in past 6 months.
c. **Recent head trauma** or known intracranial mass.

d. **Surgery,** PTCA, or severe trauma in last 2 weeks.
   e. **Recent GI bleed** or ulcer.
   f. **BP >110 diastolic,** >200 systolic, persistent despite intravenous nitroglycerin.
   g. **Noncompressible venous** *or arterial puncture.*
   h. **History of bleeding** disorder or anticoagulation.
   i. **Cardiopulmonary resuscitation** >10 minutes (relative contraindication).
   j. **Pulmonary edema** and/or cardiogenic shock (Killip class III or IV).
   k. **Pericarditis.**
   l. **Pregnancy.**
   m. **ECG.** ST-T segment depression alone.

CHOICE OF THROMBOLYTIC AGENTS

1. Preferred
Streptokinase, 1.5 million U IV over 1 hour.

2. Optional. Accelerated t-PA with Intravenous Heparin
For patients <75, anterior AMI and symptoms:
   a. **Accelerated t-PA**
      (1) **t-PA**
         (a) 15 mg bolus.
         (b) 0.75 mg/kg up to 50 mg over 30 minutes.
         (c) 0.5 mg/kg up to 35 mg over 60 minutes.
      (2) **Heparin:** 5000 U IV bolus and 1000 U/hr (1200 U/hr if >80 kg); keep PTT between 60 and 85 seconds.
   b. **Standard t-PA,** 100 mg IV over 3 hours (GISSI-2/International Study Group).
   c. **Standard APSAC,** 30 U IV over 3 minutes (ISIS-3).

Phase III: Beta-blockade

Elderly patients (>65) benefit most (ISIS-1); useful with recurrent symptoms of ischemia, hypertension, sinus tachycardia.

1. Entry Criteria
   a. **Clinically stable** after thrombolytic agent (BP >110, no wheezes).
   b. **Killip class I** only.

2. Exclusion Criteria
   a. **Asthma** (as an adult) or chronic obstructive pulmonary disease (COPD).
   b. **AV block.**
   c. **Hypotension** (BP <100).

3. Available Beta-Blockers
   a. **Atenolol,** 5 mg IV every 10 minutes to a total of 10 mg, followed in 15 minutes by 50 mg PO as tolerated.
   b. **Metoprolol,** 5 mg IV every 5 to 10 minutes to a total of 15 mg, followed in 15 minutes by 100 mg PO as tolerated.

Phase IV: ACE Inhibitors (ACEIs)

When clinically stable, first 24 hours.

1. Entry Criteria
Killip class I and II.

2. Exclusion Criteria
   a. **Allergy** to ACEIs.
   b. **Killip class III and IV.**
   c. **History of renal failure or** bilateral renal artery stenosis.

3. Available ACEIs
   a. **Lisinopril.** BP >120, 5 mg orally q24h; (GISSI-3) BP ≤120, >100, 2.5 mg orally q24h.
   b. **Captopril.** BP ≥120, 6.25 mg initially, then 1.25 mg TID (ISIS-4).

Mortality-Reducing Intervention in AMI

I. Rationale for the guideline

A. Aspirin. The use of aspirin (ASA) in AMI is based on the data from one large randomized controlled trial, ISIS-2 (*Lancet* 2:349–360, 1988). This 2×2 factorial design trial randomly assigned the entire study population of 17,187 patients to either receive ASA or placebo, and also randomly assigned all patients to receive streptokinase (SK) or placebo. This design created three treatment groups and a placebo group: (1) ASA only, (2) SK only, (3) ASA and SK, and (4) double placebo. Aspirin, 162.5 mg, was given immediately and every day for 1 month. Streptokinase, 1.5 million U over 1 hour, was infused as soon as possible. Mortality reduction and stroke reduction for the first three treatment groups as compared with the placebo group, and rates of reinfarction of all groups at 35 days appear in **Table 5-4.**

B. These results demonstrate that aspirin is as effective as streptokinase in the reduction of AMI mortality (each drug, $p < 10^{-5}$) and that the effect of ASA is additive to, and independent of, SK. Aspirin is much more effective than SK for reduction of all strokes (hemorrhagic and thrombotic). Further, ASA reduced the rate of reinfarction of the placebo group and eliminated all excess reinfarction due to SK alone (note that it is greater than placebo). This excess reinfarction rate associated with SK was also noted in the GISSI-1 trial, which compared SK with placebo in 11,806 patients (GISSI: *Lancet* i:397–402, 1986). Aspirin reduces mortality by over 25% in the first 4 hours after onset of symptoms, and reduces mortality by 21% from 5 to 24 hours after onset of symptoms. The mechanism of action appears to be aspirin inhibition of cyclooxygenase-dependent platelet aggregation, which is thought to be important in acute coronary thrombosis associated with both infarction and reinfarction. The survival benefits of aspirin therapy persisted and remained highly significant after a median survival of 15 months.

C. Complications of aspirin therapy are limited to allergic reactions and gastrointestinal symptoms.

D. The utility of aspirin in AMI as demonstrated by ISIS-2 is so significant that it is unlikely that future trials will ever again compare aspirin with placebo in AMI. Indeed, all subsequent large direct comparison trials of various thrombolytic agents and dosing regimens in AMI included ASA as standard-of-care treatment.

Table 5-4. Results of the ISIS-2 Trial

Treatment group	Mortality reduction	Total stroke reduction	Reinfarction rate
ASA only	23%	42%	1.9%
SK only	25%	9%	3/8%
ASA and SK	42%	44%	1.8%
Double placebo	—	—	2.9%

Thrombolytic Therapy: Overview

Acute myocardial infarction is most often caused by acute thrombotic occlusion of a fissured or ruptured atherosclerotic coronary artery plaque. A natural fibrinolytic system is activated when this occurs, converting plasminogen to plasmin, to lyse the coronary thrombus. Three drugs that promote plasminogen activation to plasmin, thereby increasing thrombolysis, have been evaluated in many large therapeutic trials: SK, APSAC, and t-PA. Urokinase has been used for this indication but has not been as extensively studied. A list of the trials establishing the efficacy and risks of SK, APSAC, and t-PA are given in **Table 5-5**.

I. **Thrombolytic vs. usual care trials.** Mortality reduction for all trials of thrombolytic agents versus usual care is approximately 27% when the drug is infused within 6 hours of onset of symptoms. The results of GISSI-1, the SK only and double-placebo arms of ISIS-2, and ASSET (ASSET Study Group: *Lancet* 2:525–530, 1988) are similar. The AIMS trial mortality reduction was greater (50%), but the results of this small trial were not confirmed in the much larger direct comparison trials (AIMS Trial Study Group: *Lancet* 1:545–549, 1988) **(Table 5-6).**

II. **Direct comparison of thrombolytic trials.** Much larger trials were needed to detect mortality differences among the various thrombolytic agents. In spite of the size of GISSI-2 and the International Study Group Trial (International Study Group: *Lancet* 336:71–75, 1990) and the ISIS-3 trial (ISIS-3: *Lancet* 339:753–770, 1992), no difference in hospital mortality between SK and t-PA was found. Subcutaneous heparin added nothing to mortality reduction. Indeed, when combined with SK, heparin caused significantly more major bleeds. Heparin did not reduce either reinfarction or stroke. In addition, t-PA was associated with higher rates of total stroke (thrombotic and hemorrhagic) and hemorrhagic stroke than SK. The results of these two trials and ISIS-2 lead to the conclusion that the ISIS-2 drugs, ASA and SK, are the preferred combination in the treatment of AMI. The GUSTO trial was designed to determine whether intravenous or subcutaneous heparin added to SK was superior to two regimens of t-PA plus intravenous heparin. The first utilized an accelerated t-PA (two-thirds of the dose in the first 30 minutes; see the "Guideline: Choice of Thrombolytic Agents") and the second, a t-PA infusion (half in the first 30 minutes) plus a reduced dose of SK (1 million U). Both t-PA regimens included intravenous heparin (GUSTO:

Table 5-5. Major Trials of Thrombolytic Therapy versus Usual Care (Mortality as Endpoint)

Trial	Study drug	Year	Patients randomized
GISSI-1	SK vs open placebo	1986	11,712
ISIS-2	SK vs placebo	1988	8,600*
AIMS	APSAC vs placebo	1988	1,004
ASSET	t-PA vs placebo	1988	5,011

*The sum of those in the SK only and double-placebo arms of the trial.

Table 5-6. Direct Comparisons of Thrombolytic Agents (All Patients Receive Aspirin)

Trial	Drugs compared	Year	Patients randomized
GISSI-2/International Study Group (2 × 2 design)	SK vs t-PA; subcutaneous (SC) heparin vs no heparin	1990	20,891
ISIS-3 (3 × 2 design)	SK vs APSAC vs t-PA; SC vs no heparin	1992	41,299
GUSTO	1) SK + SC heparin 2) SK + IV heparin 3) Accelerated t-PA + IV heparin 4) SK + t-PA + IV heparin	1993	41,021

N Engl J Med 329:673–682, 1993). The accelerated t-PA arm of the trial had an overall 14% mortality reduction advantage. Subgroup analysis identified younger (<75 years) patients, with anterior or large (inferior and lateral) AMIs as the population that benefited from this regimen. However, for the majority of AMI patients who have smaller infarcts (inferior or lateral), and who are elderly (>75 years), there was no t-PA advantage over SK. Since the ISIS-3 trial could not identify any benefit from adding heparin to SK, these patients are best treated with SK and ASA. Criticisms of the GUSTO trial include the following: (1) The trial was open label, and all participants were aware of the agents used during the trial. (2) The 14% advantage of the accelerated t-PA arm was derived from a comparison of it with *both* the SK plus high-dose subcutaneous heparin and the SK plus intravenous heparin arms of the trial, combined. The ISIS-3 trial (41,000 patients) was unable to identify any benefit from the addition of high-dose subcutaneous heparin to SK and ASA. In addition, the outcome of SK plus intravenous heparin arm in the GUSTO trial was worse than the SK plus high-dose subcutaneous heparin. Thus, the benefit of accelerated t-PA was derived by comparing it with two inferior SK regimens. (3) The rate of potentially life-saving coronary artery bypass grafting (CABG) was 9.5% for the accelerated t-PA arm versus 8.5% for the SK regimens. This 12% additional CABG rate may have contributed significantly to the 14% mortality reduction of accelerated t-PA and represents one of the perils of an open-label trial. (4) Finally, the accelerated t-PA arm of the GUSTO trial enjoyed significant advantage over the SK regimens *only* in the United States where the rates of CABG and PTCA were up to three times those of all other participating countries. In those countries, which contributed 44% of all GUSTO patients, the outcome of the accelerated t-PA arm was not significantly different from the SK regimens. For these reasons and the significant cost advantage of SK over t-PA (about $2000), SK and ASA is the preferred regimen in the "Guideline".

III. **Choice of agent.** Despite the large size of the three direct comparison trials (total, over 100,000 patients), very little mortality reduction gains were realized over the ISIS-2 regimen of ASA and SK. These trials emphasize that the mortality reduction differences among the thrombolytic agents are insignificant so that *the choice of agent is of much less importance than the decision to employ some thrombolytic agent and aspirin early in the treatment of AMI.*

Thrombolytic Therapy: Patient Selection

I. **Age.** Age alone is no longer a reason for withholding thrombolytic therapy. In GISSI-1 (GISSI: *Lancet* i:397–402, 1986), there was no significant benefit of SK over placebo in elderly patients. When ASA was added to SK in ISIS-2 (ISIS-2: Lancet 2:349–360, 1988), mortality for patients older than 70 years declined from 23.8% in the placebo arm to 15.8%, a highly significant reduction. The incidence and mortality rate of AMI increases dramatically with age, and thus the absolute number of deaths prevented by thrombolysis and aspirin is greater than in younger patients. The increased risk of stroke with advancing age did not limit the cost-effective benefits of treatment.

II. **Killip Classification.** In GISSI-1, only Killip class I and II benefited from thrombolysis. Killip class III (pulmonary edema) had a mortality rate of 33% when treated with SK and 39% when treated with placebo (not significant). Killip IV (cardiogenic shock) treated with either SK or placebo had a mortality rate of 70%. This mortality rate may be reduced dramatically with PTCA (see **PTCA**).

III. **Time of symptoms.** Only the trials of thrombolytic agents versus placebo could determine the effect of delay. The mortality reduction in GISSI-1 (SK vs placebo) are given in **Table 5-7**. After 6 hours there was no further significant reduction in mortality with SK treatment in this trial. In ISIS-2, treatment with SK and ASA resulted in a 53% mortality reduction for patients treated in the first 4 hours. Unlike GISSI-1, the SK and ASA treatment produced 33% mortality reduction in the 5- to 24-hour interval after symptom onset. Aspirin alone appeared to continue to reduce mortality well after the first 4 hours.

IV. **Shortening the time to treat: prehospital thrombolysis.** The logical extrapolation of these results is the careful use of thrombolysis in the prehospital setting. The European Myocardial Infarction Project (EMIP) Group studied prehospital thrombolysis in 5469 patients randomly assigned to receive prehospital or emergency department administration of APSAC. They were unable to demonstrate a decrease in the overall mortality rate, although death from cardiac causes was reduced (The European Myocardial Infarction Group: *N Engl J Med* 329:383–389, 1993). Use of the EMIP protocol led to a 15 minute "door-to-needle" time during the study, demonstrating the effectiveness of prehospital triage and coordination with the emergency department. The Myocardial Infarction Triage and Intervention (MITI) trial randomly assigned 360 patients to prehospital or emergency department thrombolysis with t-PA. In this trial there was no demonstrated benefit to prehospital thrombolysis; if thrombolysis occurred before 70 minutes, whether prehospital or in the emergency department, patient outcome was superior to later treatment. Similar reductions in door-to-needle time were noted in the MITI trial.

V. **Extending the time to treat: "LATE" and "EMERAS" trials.** GISSI-1 did not demonstrate significant mortality reduction after the first 6 hours. Subsequently, GISSI-2/International Study Group and GUSTO trials limited patients to 6 hours of symptoms. But ISIS-2 found benefit in the 5- to 24-hour interval after onset of symptoms, and ISIS-3 randomly assigned patients with symptoms up to 24 hours. The LATE trial randomly assigned 5711 patients with 6 to 24 hours of symptoms to receive t-PA (100 mg over 3 hours) or placebo to test efficacy in this time interval (LATE Study Group: *Lancet* 342:759–766, 1993). Both groups received ASA. Benefit was demonstrated only for patients with 6 to 12 hours of symptoms. The authors conclude that t-PA should be offered at least up to 12 hours after onset of symptoms and that patients with a "stuttering pattern" of pain may benefit beyond that time.

The EMERAS (Estudio Multcentrico Estreptoquinasa Republicas de America del Sur) trial of SK (1.5 million U over 1 hour) versus placebo randomly as-

Table 5-7. Mortality By Hours From Onset of Symptoms in GISSI-1

Hours of symptoms	Mortality reduction	p
Less than 1	51%	0.0001
Less than 3	26%	0.0005
3 to 6	20%	0.03

signed 4534 patients with 7 to 24 hours of symptoms but was unable to show significant benefit even in the 7- to 12-hour interval (EMERAS Collaborative Group: *Lancet* 342:767–772, 1993). Since all patients after the first 300 received ASA, this study actually compared SK plus ASA versus ASA for the vast majority of the study population. From ISIS-2, ASA alone provides such significant mortality reduction in the 5- to 24-hour interval after symptom onset (21%) that the *difference* in mortality reduction between SK plus ASA and ASA may have been too small to detect by a trial of this size. Because ISIS-2, a larger study, demonstrated significant mortality reduction 5 to 24 hours after onset of symptoms, it seems reasonable to offer SK and ASA to patients with up to 12 hours of symptoms and to those with a stuttering pattern of pain up to 24 hours after onset of symptoms.

VI. ECG criteria. Most large trials of thrombolytic agents (GISSI, GISSI-2/International Group Study, and GUSTO trials) required ST-segment changes for entry to the study and reported a high rate of confirmed AMI by typical CK-MB rise and fall (all >92%; GUSTO >97%). The ISIS-2 and ISIS-3 trials required only that the physician believe that the patient was within 24 hours of the onset of a suspected AMI. These later two trials did not require consideration of the ECG for entry into the study nor did they report their incidence of confirmed AMI. In the GISSI trial, over 95% of patients had ≥1 mm ST-segment elevation in one or more leads, and the remainder had ST depression in one or more leads. The trial had a confirmed AMI rate of 95%. However, only 56% of patients in the ISIS-2 trial had ST elevation, and thus this study may have had only a 60% to 70% AMI rate (LIMIT-2, a trial of magnesium vs placebo in AMI with entry criteria similar to ISIS-2, reported a 65% incidence of AMI with similar distribution of ECG findings [Woods KL et al: *Lancet* 339:1553–1558, 1992]). In spite of these differences, the ISIS-2 and GISSI trials (thrombolytic vs usual care trials) both found highly significant benefit for their study populations. The implication is that a range of patients with ECG findings including, but not limited to, ST-segment elevation appear to derive benefit from thrombolysis and aspirin.

   A. In ISIS-2, the only large trial of thrombolytic drug therapy versus placebo that did not require an ECG—yet retrospective subset analysis was performed on the ECGs obtained on enrollees—found that patients with the following ECG abnormalities had significant mortality reduction: LBBB, pathologic Q waves ≥2 mm, T-wave inversion, any conduction abnormality, and any arrhythmia. Patients with ST-T segment depression were the only ECG subgroup that did not benefit from thrombolysis in ISIS-2.

   B. Gibler et al. studied 616 patients who presented to eight emergency departments with chest pain. Only 39 (36%) of the 108 patients ultimately shown to have an AMI had ST-segment elevation >1 mm in any two or more contiguous leads. This observation was corroborated by a Swedish study of 7157 patients with chest pain seen in the emergency department. A total of 921 patients were ultimately shown to have an AMI; only 368 (40%) had ST-segment elevation at the time of presentation. Thus, if the GISSI trial criteria (above) or the GUSTO trial criteria (ST-segment elevation ≥1 mm in two contiguous limb leads or ≥2 mm in two contiguous precordial leads) are used exclusively, nearly two patients in three who ultimately develop AMIs will be excluded from thrombolytic therapy. For this reason the "Guideline" also contains the more liberal criteria of ISIS-2.

VII. Coronary angioplasty (PTCA). Angioplasty is as effective as thrombolysis and aspirin for reduction of mortality in AMI. There are no large comparison trials that suggest that PTCA is superior to thrombolysis and aspirin. Less than 18% of all hospitals have the facilities to perform PTCA, and far fewer can do it emergently. However, when available, *PTCA should be considered when thrombolysis is contraindicated.* Routine use of PTCA after thrombolytic therapy has not been found to be of benefit; it is best reserved for patients who have persistent ischemia.

Complications of Thrombolytic Therapy

I. Bleeding. The majority of bleeding episodes (70%) associated with thrombolysis occur at vascular access sites and rarely require transfusion. Other common sites of bleeding are the gastrointestinal and genitourinary tracts, central lines, and the central nervous system (see "Stroke"). The exclusion criteria in the "Guideline" are those imposed by many large thrombolytic trials mainly to avoid bleeding of all types. If significant bleeding occurs during thrombolysis, the following management steps have been recommended:

A. Conservative measures
1. **Manual compression of site** if accessible; if not accessible, such as a central line, surgical intervention may be required.
2. **Replace volume** as needed; secure two large-bore (18 gauge or larger) intravenous lines.
3. **Reduce heparin dose.**
4. **Transfusion therapy.**

B. In patients who do not respond to the above, the following measures may be used for life-threatening bleeding. It should be remembered that these measures defeat the purpose of thrombolysis and may actually promote thrombosis at the coronary site of obstruction.
1. **Discontinue any remaining thrombolytic** or heparin infusion. Aspirin effects will persist for at least several days.
2. **Protamine** should be considered if heparin infusion has been terminated within 4 hours (see "Heparin").
3. **Measure hematocrit** every 4 to 6 hours.
4. **Draw baseline aPTT.**
5. **Give 10 units cryoprecipitate.**
6. **Check fibrinogen level;** if less than 1.0 gm/L and the patient is still bleeding, give another 10 units of cryoprecipitate.
7. **If still bleeding, give 2 units** of fresh frozen plasma (FFP).
8. **If still bleeding, check Ivy bleeding time;** if >9 minutes, give 10 units of platelets.
9. **If still bleeding, consult a hematologist.**

II. Stroke: Stroke is a complication of AMI as demonstrated by the double-placebo arm of the ISIS-2 trial (see "Aspirin"). In that study the incidence of total stroke was reduced by SK alone and by SK plus ASA, but SK was associated with an increase in hemorrhagic stroke over placebo (less than 1 per 1000 treated). The GISSI-2/International Group Study and ISIS-3 trials found that SK was associated with a lower incidence of hemorrhagic (p <0.0001) and total stroke (p <0.01) than t-PA. These trials also showed that high-dose subcutaneous heparin (12,500 U twice per day) added to a thrombolytic agent (SK or t-PA) had no effect on total stroke or mortality. In the GUSTO trial, t-PA was associated with more hemorrhagic stroke than SK. In all three large thrombolytic comparison trials (over 100,000 patients), t-PA was consistently associated with an increase in cerebral hemorrhage compared with SK.

III. **Allergy.** Allergic reactions to APSAC (5.1%), SK (3.6%), and t-PA (0.8%) were usually minor in ISIS-3 (ISIS-3: *Lancet* 339:753–770, 1992). Approximately 1 of 10 reactions were persistent in each group.

IV. **Hypotension.** APSAC (12.5%), SK (11.8%), and t-PA (7.1%) frequently cause transient hypotension, which is treated with intravenous fluids (ISIS-3: *Lancet* 339:753–770, 1992). Approximately half of these episodes required some drug therapy. If hypotension is persistent, other drugs used concurrently to treat AMI should be reviewed. When multiple agents capable of causing hypotension are used simultaneously, the order of withdrawal should be commensurate with the drug's increasing ability to reduce AMI mortality: first, morphine and intravenous nitroglycerin, then beta-blockers or ACE inhibitors, and lastly, thrombolytic agents.

Other Agents Used in Thrombolysis

I. **Heparin.** Heparin is included in the "Guideline" because it was used intravenously with accelerated t-PA in the GUSTO trial (see "Thrombolysis: Overview"). This combination had a marginal but statistically significant advantage over the other treatment arms of the trial, which all included SK. The superiority of accelerated t-PA and intravenous heparin cannot be attributed to heparin because accelerated t-PA has not been studied without it. The widespread use of intravenous heparin for the treatment of AMI in the United States is based on the belief that it promotes coronary artery patency after thrombolysis with t-PA and that improved patency reduces mortality. However, no large controlled trials have evaluated the efficacy of intravenous heparin to reduce mortality in AMI.

A. **Adverse reactions.** The principle adverse reaction to heparin in the emergency department is bleeding. If severe bleeding occurs during heparin therapy, it should be stopped and protamine should be considered. If heparin infusion has been terminated more than 4 hours, it is unlikely that protamine will be useful because the half-life of heparin is 1 to 2 hours. If the infusion was very recently terminated, 1 mg of protamine is used for each 100 U of heparin given in the last 4 hours of infusion. If a recent bolus of heparin was given, 1 mg of protamine is given for each 100 U of heparin in the bolus. If the heparin infusion was stopped or the heparin bolus given 30 minutes before, half of the protamine dose is given. Protamine should be infused at 5 mg/min to avoid hypotension. Other adverse reactions to protamine include allergy, particularly in patients previously exposed to protamine during previous neutralization of heparin, in diabetics who receive insulin (NPH, neutral protamine Hagedorn; PZI, protamine zinc insulin), and in patients with fish allergy.

B. **Other uses.** Heparin alone has been found to be effective treatment of unstable angina in a trial of heparin vs. ASA vs. heparin and ASA. Since it is often impossible to distinguish unstable angina from AMI early in their clinical courses, this use commonly overlaps the recognition of AMI. In this small study, heparin was found to be superior to ASA alone but not to the combination of heparin and ASA for the treatment of unstable angina. Withdrawal of heparin alone was associated with a significant rate of reactivation of angina in 5 to 15 hours, which appears to be avoidable with the addition of ASA.

II. **Evidence of reperfusion.** Reperfusion is often but not invariably accompanied by resolution of chest pain and ST-T segment changes. Transient accelerated idioventricular rhythm, which usually requires no treatment, is seen in up to 50% of patients who reperfuse.

Beta-Blockade

I. **Mortality reduction.** Beta-blocking agents have been shown to provide some mortality reduction when used early in AMI by two large trials: ISIS-1 (ISIS-1: *Lancet* 2:57–66, 1986) and the MIAMI (Metoprolol in Acute Myocardial Infarction) trial (MIAMI Trial Research Group: *Eur Heart J* 6:199–226, 1985). The MIAMI trial randomly assigned patients who were less than 75 years of age and within 24 hours of onset of symptoms to metoprolol (three 5 mg doses IV, followed by 100 mg twice daily) or placebo. This trial of 5778 patients was unable to demonstrate a significant overall mortality reduction at 15 days or 1 year, but a subgroup of high-risk patients had a significant 15-day mortality reduction from 8.5% to 6%. These patients were found retrospectively to have three or more of the following risk factors: age over 60 years, history of AMI, diabetes, CHF, ECG diagnostic of AMI, a history of angina, or use of diuretics or digoxin. The ISIS-1 trial of 16,027 patients randomly assigned patients to atenolol (two 5 mg IV doses 10 minutes apart, followed 10 minutes later by 50 mg orally if IV doses tolerated) or placebo. This trial was able to demonstrate a significant 15% mortality reduction that occurred entirely on the first day of treatment and was due solely to the prevention of cardiac rupture. Although not conventionally significant, virtually all the mortality reduction occurred in patients ≥65 years. Recently, the GISSI-2 investigators reviewed the 9720 patients who suffered their first AMI in the GISSI-2 trial and found that the incidence of cardiac rupture as a terminal event increased from 19% in patients younger than 60 years to 86% in patients older than 70 years in those autopsied. The dramatic rise in the incidence of cardiac rupture as the terminal event with advancing age and the demonstrated ability of early beta-blocker therapy to reduce the incidence of this complication suggests that *the elderly may be the principal beneficiaries of beta-blockage in AMI.*

II. **Beta-blocker therapy is limited** to approximately one-fourth to one-half of the AMI population by preexisting medical conditions and Killip classification (GISSI-2: *Lancet* 336:65–71, 1990). Contraindications and dosages are given in the "Guideline."

Angiotensin-Converting Enzyme Inhibitors (ACEIs)

These antihypertensive agents have been shown to prolong life and reduce the development of CHF and recurrent MI when long-term therapy is given after AMI. In the SAVE Trial (Survival and Ventricular Enlargement Trial), oral captopril or placebo was begun 3 to 16 days after AMI and was continued for 2 years in patients who initially had ejection fractions ≤0.40 and were asymptomatic. The mortality reduction was 19% in the captopril group, the development of severe CHF was reduced by 37%, and

Table 5-8. ACEI Trial Mortality Summary

ACEI trial	Mortality/treated, (%)	Mortality/control, (%)
ISIS-4 (captopril)	1,886/27,442 (6.87)	2,008/27,382 (7.33)
GISSI-3 (lisinopril)	597/9,435 (6.3)	673/9,460 (7.1)

reinfarction was reduced by 25%. The CONSENSUS II Trial studied enalapril given as the intravenous form, enalaprilat, for the first 24 hours, then orally for 6 months versus placebo. Treatment was initiated within 24 hours of onset of chest pain in patients with BP ≥100/60 mm Hg. The study found no benefit in survival at 6 months. Significantly more hypotension was observed in the treatment group (12% vs 3%). Recently, results of the GISSI-3 trial (see "IV nitroglycerin") of nearly 19,000 patients has become available. Oral lisinopril, started within 24 hours of symptoms of AMI was compared with placebo in patients with AMI who were Killip class I or II (see "Guideline" for dosage). In this trial and in an even larger trial, ISIS-4 (nearly 55,000 patients), that studied the oral ACEI, captopril versus placebo, *ACEIs were found to significantly reduce mortality* (at 35 days in the ISIS-4 trial and 42 days in the GISSI-3 trial). These trials allowed aspirin, thrombolytic agents, beta-blockers, and other medications deemed appropriate by the treating physician **(Table 5-8).** These agents appear to be effective in the first 24 hours of AMI symptoms after the patient's clinical condition stabilizes. The subgroups that benefit most are not known at this time. This class of medications may be particularly useful when the use of beta-blockers is contraindicated. The ACEIs are not currently FDA approved for this indication.

Agents Thought To Be Ineffective or Harmful in AMI

I. **Magnesium.** Though eight, small, randomized clinical trials demonstrated benefit with use of magnesium in AMI, the preliminary results of the ISIS-4 trial indicate no benefit. Since this trial is over 20 times larger than the largest of the small trials (LIMIT-2 trial [Woods KL et al: *Lancet* 339:1553–1558, 1992]) and well designed, it must be concluded that magnesium should no longer be used in AMI. The 35-day mortality rates for the magnesium arm of the trial were 7.28% (1997 deaths in 27,413 patients) and 6.92% (1897 deaths in 27,411 patients) for the nontreatment arm (open-label study for magnesium only). The difference was not significant.

II. **Calcium channel blockers: routine use.** A review and metaanalysis of 16 randomized controlled trials (6400 patients) of the calcium channel blockers, diltiazem, verapamil, or nifedipine versus placebo concluded that there was no mortality benefit or reduction in reinfarction. These observations do not preclude the use of calcium channel blockers in the treatment of tachyarrhythmias.

III. **Prophylactic lidocaine.** An analysis similar to that of the calcium channel blockers was performed on 15 trials of prophylactic lidocaine (8745 patients), and no benefit was found. Indeed, mortality was greater in the treated group (Lau J et al: *N Eng J Med* 327:248–254, 1992).

Complications of Acute Myocardial Infarction: Overview

The complications of AMI increase with age, size of infarction, and coexisting conditions at the time of infarction such as previous AMI, angina, CHF, and diabetes. The incidence of these complications in the thrombolytic era can be obtained from recent large thrombolytic trials (GISSI-2: *Lancet* 336:65–71, 1990; GUSTO: *N Engl J Med* 329:673–682, 1993).

The complications reported by these two trials are different as indicated by the absent data in **Table 5-9**. The large differences between these trials in the categories of sustained ventricular tachycardia, asystole, and cardiogenic shock are not explained.

Congestive Heart Failure and Cardiogenic Shock

Emergency department management of CHF and cardiogenic shock requires pharmacologic treatment and initiation of aggressive diagnostic evaluation, especially for Killip class III (pulmonary edema) and IV (cardiogenic shock). Advanced cardiac life support (ACLS) guidelines from the 1992 National Conference of the Emergency Cardiac Care Committee of the American Heart Association provide the framework for management of CHF and cardiogenic shock in AMI. Detailed discussion of the rationale for the guidelines appears in that reference. The approach to hypotension and shock utilizes a conceptual model that divides the causes of shock into three "problem" categories: problems with rate, volume, and the pump.

I. Rate. Significant symptomatic bradycardia (<60 beats/min, or <70 beats/min with BP <100 mm Hg) or tachyarrhythmias (>140 to 150 beats/min) that are not sinus require immediate treatment (see "Arrhythmias"). Volume and pump problems are addressed when the abnormal rhythms are corrected.

II. Volume. Adequate filling pressure is required to produce sufficient cardiac output to avoid hypotension. Inotropic agents and vasopressors may be detrimental if volume is not first repleted. Many patients, particularly the elderly, are dehydrated, and hypotension in the absence of pulmonary edema will improve with 250 to 500 ml of 0.9% normal saline solution or lactated Ringer's solution.

Table 5-9. Incidence of Complications from the GISSI-2 and GUSTO Trials

Complication	GISSI-2 (%)	GUSTO (%)
Killip class II	18	16.7
Killip class III (pulmonary edema)	2.8	—
Killip class IV (cardiogenic shock)	1.2	6.1
Acute mitral regurgitation	—	1.7
Acute ventricular septal defect	—	0.5
Ventricular fibrillation	6.6	6.8
Sustained ventricular tachycardia	3.7	6.4
Asystole	2.4	6.0
Second- and third-degree AV block	—	8.3
Third-degree AV block	5.3	—
Atrial fibrillation/flutter	—	9.4
Pericarditis	6.0	—

III. **Pump.** Primary myocardial failure is the most common cause of pump failure in AMI and can be temporized with inotropic agents, vasodilators, and diuretics as discussed below. Secondary myocardial failure occurs when critical myocardial substrates are depleted (oxygen, glucose, adenosine triphosphate [ATP]) in protracted shock. Thus, it is important to define the cause of pump failure and correct it before tissue depletion occurs.

IV. **Intravenous inotropic and vasopressor support** for hypotensive, normovolemic patients follows "Initial Stabilization" and is dependent on the systolic blood pressure.
   A. **Systolic BP >100.** Dobutamine, 2 to 20 µg/kg/min (do not use if BP falls below 100).
   B. **Systolic BP 70 to 100.** Dopamine, 2.5 to 20 µg/kg/min; add Norepinephrine if dopamine >20 µg/kg/min.
   C. **Systolic BP <70.** Norepinephrine, 0.5 to 30 µg/min, or Dopamine, 5 to 20 µg/kg/min.

V. **If pulmonary edema is present** and systolic BP >100, consider vasodilators (hemodynamic monitoring necessary) and intraaortic balloon counterpulsation support as a bridge to revascularization (see below).

VI. **For marked hypertension,** diastolic BP >110, and/or pulmonary edema (in obese patients, use a large blood pressure cuff):
   A. **Vasodilator therapy.** Nitroglycerin (the preferred agent in ischemic states; see "Guideline" and "Rationale: IV Nitroglycerin") and/or Nitroprusside, 0.1 to 5.0 µg/kg/min.
   B. **Hemodynamic monitoring** allows optimal management of these agents but is usually not available in the emergency department. The important characteristics of these agents above are described below.
      1. **Dobutamine.** A potent synthetic beta-adrenergic inotrope that usually produces peripheral vasodilation, which limits use to patients with systolic BPs >100 mm Hg. It may cause tachycardia, particularly as the dosage approaches 20 µg/kg/min. This may exacerbate myocardial ischemia.
      2. **Dopamine.** Dopamine is a naturally occurring precursor of norepinephrine with potent alpha- and beta-adrenergic actions. At lower doses (1 to 2 µg/kg/min), renal and mesenteric vasodilation occur with little change in heart rate or blood pressure. From 2 to 10 µg/kg/min, dopamine increases cardiac output (beta-adrenergic effect) without widespread vasoconstriction. Above 10 µg/kg/min, alpha-adrenergic effects appear, causing vasoconstriction peripherally and centrally. Monoamine oxidase inhibitors potentiate dopamine's effect.
      3. **Norepinephrine.** Norepinephrine is a very potent vasoconstrictor and inotropic agent. It is useful in low peripheral resistance states associated with shock. It usually reduces renal and mesenteric flow, which limits the duration of its use. Low dosages are recommended (0.5 to 1.0 µg/min) initially, but dosages from 8 to 30 µg/min may be required. Norepinephrine is contraindicated in hypovolemic patients. Infiltration of a norepinephrine infusion is often associated with necrosis of superficial tissues, and infiltration of the area with 10 mg of phentolamine in 10 to 15 ml of normal saline solution is recommended as soon as possible.
      4. **Nitroprusside.** Nitroprusside is a potent arterial vasodilator that acts rapidly and has a short half-life. Nitroprusside is more likely to lower

coronary perfusion than nitroglycerin. Thus, nitroglycerin is preferred in AMI. Nitroprusside is metabolized to cyanide and thiocyanate. The cyanide is further metabolized to thiocyanate. Toxicity to cyanide and thiocyanate usually does not occur before 72 hours of infusion at 3 µg/kg/min.

VII. PTCA. The available series, although retrospective, suggest that mortality in cardiogenic shock caused by primary myocardial failure in AMI can be substantially reduced by successful emergent PTCA. In the series by Bengtson, the principal determinant of survival was a patent infarct-related artery (IRA); the mortality rate of patients with a patent IRA was 33% versus 75% with an occluded IRA. Other smaller series corroborate this observation. The successful angioplasty rates vary from 62% to 85% in the three studies, with an overall success rate of 79% in the 314 patients studied. Coronary artery bypass graft may be successful in patients not suitable for PTCA, but very few patients treated with this procedure have been reported. Others have demonstrated benefit of CABG in cardiogenic shock. These studies also suffer from small numbers and retrospective design, but until more reliable data are available, reperfusion, either by PTCA or CABG, appears to offer the only alternative to the dismal prognosis of cardiogenic shock. Inotropic and vasopressor agents alone are associated with high in-hospital mortality. Thrombolytic therapy is minimally helpful for Killip III and virtually useless for Killip IV (GISSI: *Lancet* i:397–402, 1986).

VIII. Other causes. In addition to primary myocardial failure, other causes of cardiogenic shock to be considered are the mechanical consequences of ischemia. Acute ischemic mitral regurgitation, ischemic ventricular septal defect (VSD), and ventricular aneurysm are surgically correctable causes of congestive failure and shock. Incomplete rupture of the myocardial wall with hemopericardium may also present as cardiogenic shock. Acute mitral regurgitation may be both severe and silent (absent systolic murmur of mitral regurgitation) in up to 50% of patients. Severe mitral regurgitation carries a poor prognosis (50% mortality rate at 1 year). Ischemic VSD is usually associated with a loud holosystolic murmur and also carries a poor prognosis. Doppler transthoracic echocardiography or, where available, transesophageal echocardiography will provide the diagnosis for all surgically managed conditions and should be employed early in congestive failure and shock in AMI if cardiac catheterization is not readily available.

Arrhythmias

The drugs recommended in the "Guideline" will reduce but not eliminate arrhythmias that are inherent to ischemic myocardium. Other metabolic conditions that predispose to arrhythmia include hypoxemia, metabolic acidosis, and abnormal serum potassium, calcium, and magnesium levels. The highest incidence of arrhythmia occurs during the first 24 hours of symptoms. Most rhythm disturbances require immediate treatment to prevent further ischemic injury or death. The 1992 Guidelines from the American Heart Association provide algorithms for specific arrhythmia management, which are briefly summarized (American Heart Association: *JAMA* 268:2171–2302, 1992).

I. Ventricular fibrillation/pulseless ventricular tachycardia (VF/VT). These rhythms are immediately fatal because cardiac output is negligible. Cardiopulmonary resuscitation (CPR) is performed until a defibrillator is attached. Rapid defibrillation is the principal determinant of survival. Three shocks of increasing energy are delivered: 200 joules (J), 200 to 300 J, and 360 J. Pulse should not be checked between shocks if the cardiac monitor is properly functioning. If this is unsuccessful, CPR should be continued, the patient should have an endotracheal tube placed, and intravenous access should be established. Epinephrine is the most effective drug to improve clinical outcome. As soon as intravenous access is secured, 1 mg of epinephrine is given by intravenous push and this dose is repeated every 3 to 5 minutes. Within 30 to 60 seconds after epinephrine is given, defibrillate at 360 J, and check the monitor and the pulse. Then begin a repeating pattern of intravenous medication followed in 30 to 60 seconds by defibrillation at 360 J, as the drugs below are given up to their maximums.

  A. Lidocaine, 1.5 mg/kg by intravenous push; repeat in 3 to 5 minutes to a total dose of 3 mg/kg.

  B. Bretylium, 5 mg/kg by intravenous push; repeat in 5 minutes at 10 mg/kg by intravenous push.

  C. For refractory VF/VT

  1. **Magnesium,** 1 to 2 gm over 1 to 2 minutes intravenously.
  2. **Procainamide,** 30 mg/min to a maximum of 17 mg/kg.
  3. **If defibrillation is achieved,** an intravenous drip of the antiarrhythmic agent used last is started.

  D. High-dose epinephrine (0.1 mg/kg) has been recommended, but no evidence of significantly improved survival or neurologic outcome could be demonstrated in a small trial of 650 patients randomly assigned to receive standard and high-dose epinephrine. This trial was too small to exclude a small benefit.

II. **Pulseless electrical activity (PEA).** This is defined as any pulseless rhythm except VF/VT. The nonspecific interventions for this group of rhythms are as follows: begin CPR; perform endotracheal intubation; establish intravenous access; 1 mg of epinephrine by intravenous push every 3 to 5 minutes; and if heart rate <60, give atropine, 1 mg intravenous push every 3 to 5 minutes up to a total dose of 0.04 mg/kg.

  A. Causes. Hypovolemia is the most common; Doppler ultrasound may detect blood flow.

  B. Other causes. Hyperkalemia, metabolic acidosis, hypoxia, drug overdose (tricyclic antidepressants, beta-blockers, calcium channel blockers, digitalis), pericardial tamponade, tension pneumothorax, massive pulmonary embolism, and hypothermia.

III. **Asystole.** Confirm asystole in more than one lead. Begin CPR, perform endotracheal intubation, and obtain intravenous access. Consider immediate transcutaneous pacing (TCP). Give epinephrine, 1 mg by intravenous push every 3 to 5 minutes, and atropine, 1 mg by intravenous push every 3 to 5 minutes up to a total dose of 0.04 mg/kg. If the rhythm remains asystolic after intubation and initial medications, and reversible causes are not identified, consider termination of resuscitation.

IV. **Bradycardias.** Bradycardia is defined as a heart rate <60, or inappropriately low for blood pressure. If serious symptoms (chest pain, shortness of breath, or decreased level of consciousness) and/or signs (hypotension or shock, CHF, premature ventricular contractions [PVCs]) are present, therapeutic options are as follows:

- **A. Atropine,** 0.5 to 1.0 mg by intravenous push every 3 to 5 minutes to a total dose of 0.04 mg/kg; avoid atropine in patients with wide QRS complex second- and third-degree AV block and cardiac transplants.
- **B. Transcutaneous pacing** is appropriate for all symptomatic bradycardias; some sedation and analgesia may be required.
- **C. Dopamine,** 5 to 20 µg/kg/min (advance rapidly to 20 µg/kg/min), or if symptoms are severe:
- **D. Epinephrine,** 2 to 10 µg/min.
- **E. Consider right ventricular AMI** in patients with bradycardia and hypotension (obtain ECG leads V_3R and V_4R); fluid challenge with saline solution may be lifesaving.

V. Tachycardias. If serious symptoms (chest pain, shortness of breath, or decreased level of consciousness) and/or signs (hypotension or shock, CHF, PVCs) are present and the rhythm is not sinus tachycardia and the ventricular rate is ≥150 beats/min, prepare for immediate cardioversion (below).

- **A. Atrial fibrillation.** While spontaneous conversion occurs, in the setting of AMI the ventricular response must be controlled. Beta-blockers (see "Guideline: Beta-blockade") or the calcium channel blockers are recommended. The calcium channel blocker diltiazem given intravenously is preferred for this purpose over intravenous verapamil because of the lower incidence of hypotension. The dose of diltiazem is 0.25 mg/kg given intravenously over 2 minutes (20 mg is a reasonable dose for the average patient). If the ventricular response is inadequate, give 0.35 mg/kg of diltiazem intravenously over 2 minutes (25 mg is a reasonable dose). A continuous infusion will control the rate (up to 24 hours). After the bolus(es) above, an initial infusion rate of 10 mg/hr should be started, followed by dosage adjustments for ventricular rate. The range of infusion dosage is 5 to 15 mg/hr. After the ventricular rate is controlled, beta-blockade or digoxin therapy may be used to maintain control of the ventricular rate and avoid prolonged use of a calcium channel blocker (diltiazem). Pharmacologic conversion of stable atrial fibrillation is usually achieved with procainamide or quinidine (see "Arrhythmias" chapter). If atrial fibrillation is thought to be present for several days or more, conversion should not be attempted before anticoagulation because of the high incidence of atrial thrombi.
- **B. Atrial flutter.** Atrial flutter is an unstable rhythm because ventricular response can be quite rapid (≥150 beats/min). Carotid sinus massage (contraindicated if carotid bruit is present; avoid in the elderly) or adenosine administration (see "PSVT") may unmask the flutter waves if the diagnosis is uncertain. This rhythm responds well to cardioversion. If pharmacologic control of ventricular rate is preferred, see "Atrial Fibrillation" above.
- **C. Paroxysmal supraventricular tachycardia (PSVT).** Adenosine given intravenously is preferred over intravenous verapamil because it produces less hypotension, is equally effective in converting PSVT, and is rapidly cleared from the circulation (1 to 2 minutes). The dose of adenosine is 6 mg given by intravenous push over 1 to 3 seconds. If that is unsuccessful, 12 mg of adenosine is given by intravenous push over 1 to 3 seconds. Drugs that interact with adenosine are carbamazepine (increases AV block produced by adenosine), dipyridamole (potentiates adenosine's effect, use half the dose), and theophylline (blocks adenosine's cellular entry, use higher doses). If two doses of adenosine have not lowered the BP and the QRS complexes are nar-

row (<0.10 seconds on 12-lead ECG), intravenous verapamil, 2.5 to 5.0 mg over 3 to 4 minutes may be given (*never* after intravenous or long-term oral beta-blocker therapy). A second dose of verapamil, 5 to 10 mg over 3 to 4 minutes may be given in 15 to 30 minutes if PSVT persists or recurs. Verapamil is contraindicated in any wide complex tachycardia not known from electrophysiologic testing to be supraventricular. If both adenosine and verapamil are unsuccessful, consider cardioversion, intravenous diltiazem, and other antiarrhythmic agents.

D. **Wide complex tachycardia (WCT), uncertain type.** No attempt should be made to determine ventricular versus supraventricular origin from the ECG in the AMI setting. Lidocaine, 1 to 1.5 mg/kg given by intravenous push, followed in 5 to 10 minutes by doses of 0.5 to 0.75 mg/kg to a total dose of 3 mg/kg is recommended. If that is unsuccessful, adenosine, as for PSVT, may be tried. Some physicians might try adenosine first in stable WCT because it can be done safely and quickly. If these medications are unsuccessful and the patient remains stable, administer procainamide, 20 mg/min to a total dose of 17 mg/kg, unless hypotension or QRS widening by 50% of the original width occurs.

E. **Ventricular tachycardia.** If serious symptoms (chest pain, shortness of breath, or decreased level of consciousness) and/or signs (hypotension or shock, or CHF) are present, cardiovert immediately. In stable VT, lidocaine followed by procainamide as for WCT above are recommended. After conversion of VT, an intravenous drip of the drug in use at the time of conversion is recommended (lidocaine: 2 to 4 mg/min; procainamide: 1 to 4 mg/min). Bretylium is the third agent for VT. Bretylium, in a dose of 5 mg/kg, is given slowly over 8 to 10 minutes to avoid nausea (which may occur even at this rate) in the conscious patient. If bretylium converts VT, an infusion of 1 to 2 mg/min should be given to a maximum of 30 mg/kg over a 24-hour period.

F. **Torsades de pointes.** This VT variant is treated with electrical overdrive pacing (TCP at rates up to 180 beats/min) or magnesium infusion of 1 to 2 gm over 1 to 2 minutes. Procainamide, quinidine, and disopyramide are contraindicated. Defibrillation as for VF/pulseless VT is indicated for sustained episodes.

VI. **Cardioversion of the tachycardias.** In patients with serious symptoms and/or signs, and in particular, if the ventricular rate is over 150 beats/min, immediate cardioversion is indicated. Intravenous access, supplemental oxygen, and all equipment for intubation are requirements for cardioversion. A respiratory therapist or nurse should be available to assist ventilation if necessary. The patient should be given diazepam, 5 to 10 mg intravenously or midazolam, 1 to 3 mg intravenously with or without morphine and another analgesic. *Synchronized* cardioversion should be attempted for patients who are relatively stable and the ventricular rate is 150 to 160 beats/min. *Unsynchronized* cardioversion is indicated for unstable patients with rapid tachycardias or whenever synchronization is delayed for any reason. Energy requirements for conversion depend on the rhythm; the sequence for VT and atrial fibrillation (AF) is 100 J, 200 J, and 300 J. Paroxysmal supraventricular tachycardia and atrial flutter can be converted at lower energies: begin their sequence at 50 J, then proceed as with VT/AF. Polymorphic VT (irregular form and rate) is treated as VF/pulseless VT, with the same defibrillation sequence.

Ch 5. Acute Myocardial Infarction

Emergency Guideline Algorithms

The algorithms in this section are derived from *JAMA's* Adult Advanced Cardiac Life Support Guidelines (*JAMA* 268:2199, 1992). These guidelines focus on early treatment for cardiopulmonary arrest, as well as stabilization of the resuscitated patient and proper management of situations leading to cardiac arrest **(Figures 5-1** to **5-6).**

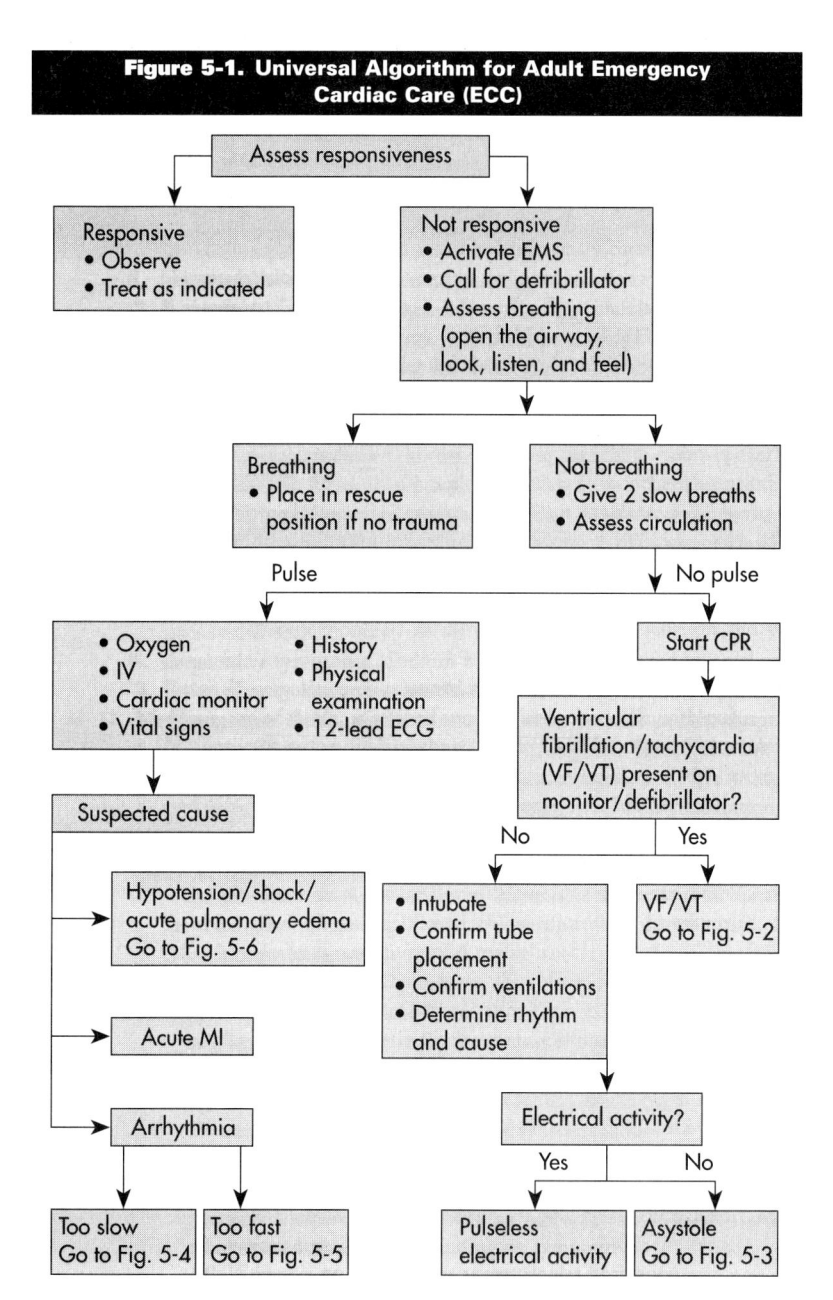

Figure 5-1. Universal Algorithm for Adult Emergency Cardiac Care (ECC)

Assess responsiveness

Responsive
- Observe
- Treat as indicated

Not responsive
- Activate EMS
- Call for defibrillator
- Assess breathing (open the airway, look, listen, and feel)

Breathing
- Place in rescue position if no trauma

Not breathing
- Give 2 slow breaths
- Assess circulation

Pulse
- Oxygen
- IV
- Cardiac monitor
- Vital signs
- History
- Physical examination
- 12-lead ECG

Suspected cause
- Hypotension/shock/acute pulmonary edema — Go to Fig. 5-6
- Acute MI
- Arrhythmia
  - Too slow — Go to Fig. 5-4
  - Too fast — Go to Fig. 5-5

No pulse
- Start CPR

Ventricular fibrillation/tachycardia (VF/VT) present on monitor/defibrillator?
- Yes → VF/VT Go to Fig. 5-2
- No →
  - Intubate
  - Confirm tube placement
  - Confirm ventilations
  - Determine rhythm and cause

Electrical activity?
- Yes → Pulseless electrical activity
- No → Asystole Go to Fig. 5-3

Figure 5-2. Algorithm for Ventricular Fibrillation and Pulseless Ventricular Tachycardia (VF/VT)

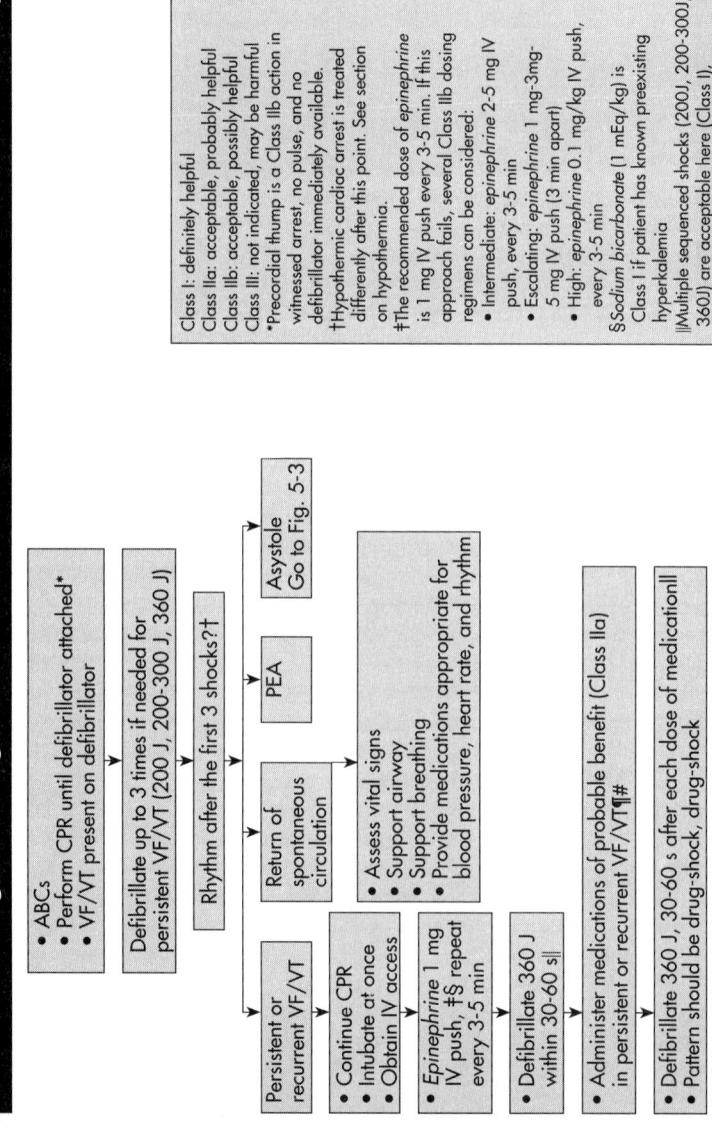

- ABCs
- Perform CPR until defibrillator attached*
- VF/VT present on defibrillator

↓

Defibrillate up to 3 times if needed for persistent VF/VT (200 J, 200-300 J, 360 J)

↓

Rhythm after the first 3 shocks?†

- Asystole → Go to Fig. 5-3
- PEA
- Return of spontaneous circulation
  - Assess vital signs
  - Support airway
  - Support breathing
  - Provide medications appropriate for blood pressure, heart rate, and rhythm
- Persistent or recurrent VF/VT
  - Continue CPR
  - Intubate at once
  - Obtain IV access

↓

- *Epinephrine* 1 mg IV push, ‡§ repeat every 3-5 min

↓

- Defibrillate 360 J within 30-60 s‖

↓

- Administer medications of probable benefit (Class IIa) in persistent or recurrent VF/VT¶#

↓

- Defibrillate 360 J, 30-60 s after each dose of medication‖
- Pattern should be drug-shock, drug-shock

Class I: definitely helpful
Class IIa: acceptable, probably helpful
Class IIb: acceptable, possibly helpful
Class III: not indicated, may be harmful

*Precordial thump is a Class IIb action in witnessed arrest, no pulse, and no defibrillator immediately available.
†Hypothermic cardiac arrest is treated differently after this point. See section on hypothermia.
‡The recommended dose of epinephrine is 1 mg IV push every 3-5 min. If this approach fails, several Class IIb dosing regimens can be considered:
- Intermediate: epinephrine 2-5 mg IV push, every 3-5 min
- Escalating: epinephrine 1 mg-3 mg-5 mg IV push (3 min apart)
- High: epinephrine 0.1 mg/kg IV push, every 3-5 min

§Sodium bicarbonate (1 mEq/kg) is Class I if patient has known preexisting hyperkalemia
‖Multiple sequenced shocks (200J, 200-300J, 360J) are acceptable here (Class I), especially when medications are delayed

¶ • *Lidocaine* 1.5 mg/kg IV push. Repeat in 3-5 min to total loading dose of 3 mg/kg; then use
- *Bretylium* 5 mg/kg IV push. Repeat in 5 min at 10 mg/kg
- *Magnesium sulfate* 1-2 g IV in torsades de pointes or suspected hypomagnesemic state or severe refractory VF
- *Procainamide* 30 mg/min in refractory VF (maximum total 17 mg/kg)
- *Sodium bicarbonate* (1 mEq/kg IV):

Class IIa
- if known preexisting bicarbonate-responsive acidosis
- if overdose with tricyclic antidepressants
- to alkalinize the urine in drug overdoses

Class IIb
- if intubated and continued long arrest interval
- upon return of spontaneous circulation after long arrest interval

Class III
- hypoxic lactic acidosis

Ch 5. Acute Myocardial Infarction

Figure 5-3. Asystole Treatment Algorithm

- Continue CPR
- Intubate at once
- Obtain IV access
- Confirm asystole in more than one lead

↓

Consider possible causes
- Hypoxia
- Hyperkalemia
- Hypokalemia
- Preexisting acidosis
- Drug overdose
- Hypothermia

↓

Consider immediate transcutaneous pacing (TCP)*

↓

- *Epinephrine* 1 mg IV push, †‡
  repeat every 3-5 min

↓

- *Atropine* 1 mg IV, repeat every
  3-5 min up to a total of 0.04 mg/kg§||

↓

Consider
- Termination of efforts¶

Class I: definitely helpful
Class IIa: acceptable, probably helpful
Class IIb: acceptable, possibly helpful
Class III: not indicated, may be harmful

*TCP is a Class IIb intervention. Lack of success may be due to delays in pacing. To be effective TCP must be performed early, simultaneously with drugs. Evidence does not support routine use of TCP for asystole.

†The recommended dose of *epinephrine* is 1 mg IV push every 3-5 min. If this approach fails, several Class IIb dosing regimens can be considered:
- Intermediate: *epinephrine* 2-5 mg IV push, every 3-5 min
- Escalating: *epinephrine* 1 mg-3mg-5 mg IV push (3 min apart)
- High: *epinephrine* 0.1 mg/kg IV push, every 3-5 min

‡*Sodium bicarbonate* 1 mEq/kg is Class I if patient has known preexisting hyperkalemia.

§Shorter *atropine* dosing intervals are Class IIb in asystolic arrest.

||*Sodium bicarbonate* 1 mEq/kg:
Class IIa
- if known preexisting bicarbonate-responsive acidosis
- if overdose with tricyclic antidepressants
- to alkalinize the urine in drug overdoses

Class IIb
- if intubated and continued long arrest interval
- upon return of spontaneous circulation after long arrest interval

Class III
- hypoxic lactic acidosis

¶If patient remains in asystole or other agonal rhythms after successful intubation and initial medications and no reversible causes are identified, consider termination of resuscitative efforts by a physician. Consider interval since arrest.

Figure 5-4. Bradycardia Algorithm (with the Patient Not in Cardiac Arrest)

- Assess ABCs
- Secure airway
- Administer oxygen
- Start IV
- Attach monitor, pulse oximeter, and automatic sphygmomanometer
- Assess vital signs
- Review history
- Perform physical examination
- Order 12-lead ECG
- Order portable chest roentgenogram

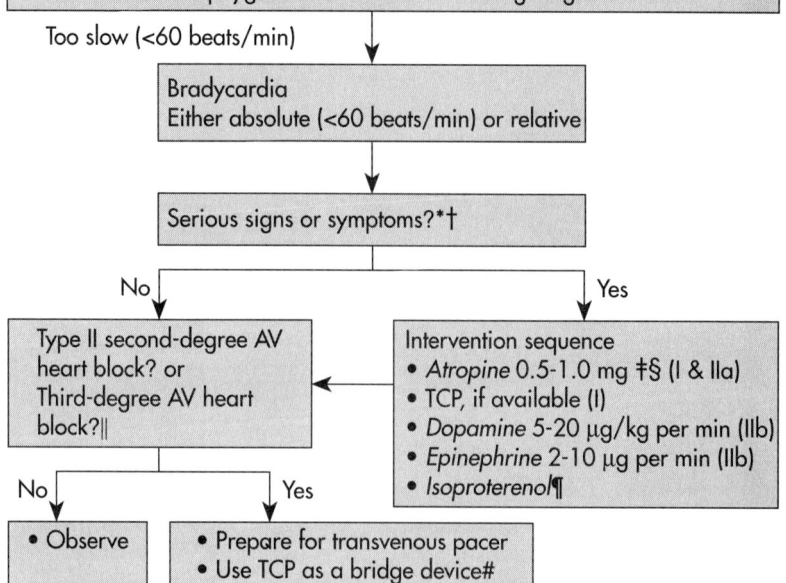

↓ Too slow (<60 beats/min)

Bradycardia
Either absolute (<60 beats/min) or relative

↓

Serious signs or symptoms?*†

No →

Type II second-degree AV heart block? or Third-degree AV heart block?‖

- **No** → Observe
- **Yes** → Prepare for transvenous pacer; Use TCP as a bridge device#

Yes →

Intervention sequence
- *Atropine* 0.5-1.0 mg ‡§ (I & IIa)
- TCP, if available (I)
- *Dopamine* 5-20 µg/kg per min (IIb)
- *Epinephrine* 2-10 µg per min (IIb)
- *Isoproterenol*¶

---

*Serious signs or symptoms must be related to the slow rate. Clinical manifestations include:
symptoms (chest pain, shortness of breath, decreased level of consciousness) and
signs (low BP, shock, pulmonary congestion, CHF, acute MI).

†Do not delay TCP while awaiting IV access or for *atropine* to take effect if patient is symptomatic.

‡Denervated transplanted hearts will not respond to *atropine*. Go at once to pacing, *catecholamine* infusion, or both.

§*Atropine* should be given in repeat doses in 3-5 min up to total of 0.04 mg/kg. Consider shorter dosing intervals in severe clinical conditions. It has been suggested that atropine should be used with caution in atrioventricular (AV) block at the His-Purkinje level (type II AV block and new third-degree block with wide QRS complexes) (Class IIb).

‖Never treat third-degree heart block plus ventricular escape beats with *lidocaine*.

¶*Isoproterenol* should be used, if at all, with extreme caution. At low doses it is Class IIb (possibly helpful); at higher doses it is Class III (harmful).

#Verify patient tolerance and mechanical capture. Use analgesia and sedation as needed.

Figure 5-5. Tachycardia Algorithm

- Assess ABCs
- Secure airway
- Administer oxygen
- Start IV
- Attach monitor, pulse oximeter, and automatic sphygmomanometer
- Assess vital signs
- Review history
- Perform physical examination
- Order 12-lead ECG
- Order portable chest roentgenogram

Unstable, with serious signs or symptoms*

No or borderline →

Atrial fibrillation / Atrial flutter†

Consider
- *Dilliazem*
- *β-Blockers*
- *Verapamil*
- *Digoxin*
- *Procainamide*
- *Quinidine*
- *Anticoagulants*

Paroxysmal supraventricular tachycardia (PSVT)

Vagal maneuvers†

- *Adenosine* 6 mg, rapid IV push over 1-3 s

1-2 min

- *Adenosine* 12 mg, rapid IV push over 1-3 s (may repeat once in 1-2 min)

Yes →

If ventricular rate >150 beats/min
- Prepare for immediate cardioversion
- May give brief trial of medications based on arrhythmia
- Immediate cardioversion is seldom needed for heart rates <150 beats/min

Wide-complex tachycardia of uncertain type

- *Lidocaine* 1-1.5 mg/kg IV push

Every 5-10 min

- *Lidocaine* 0.5-0.75 mg/kg IV push, maximum total 3 mg/kg

- *Adenosine* 6 mg, rapid IV push over 1-3 s

Ventricular tachycardia (VT)

- *Lidocaine* 1-1.5 mg/kg IV push

Every 5-10 min

- *Lidocaine* 0.5-0.75 mg/kg IV push, maximum total 3 mg/kg

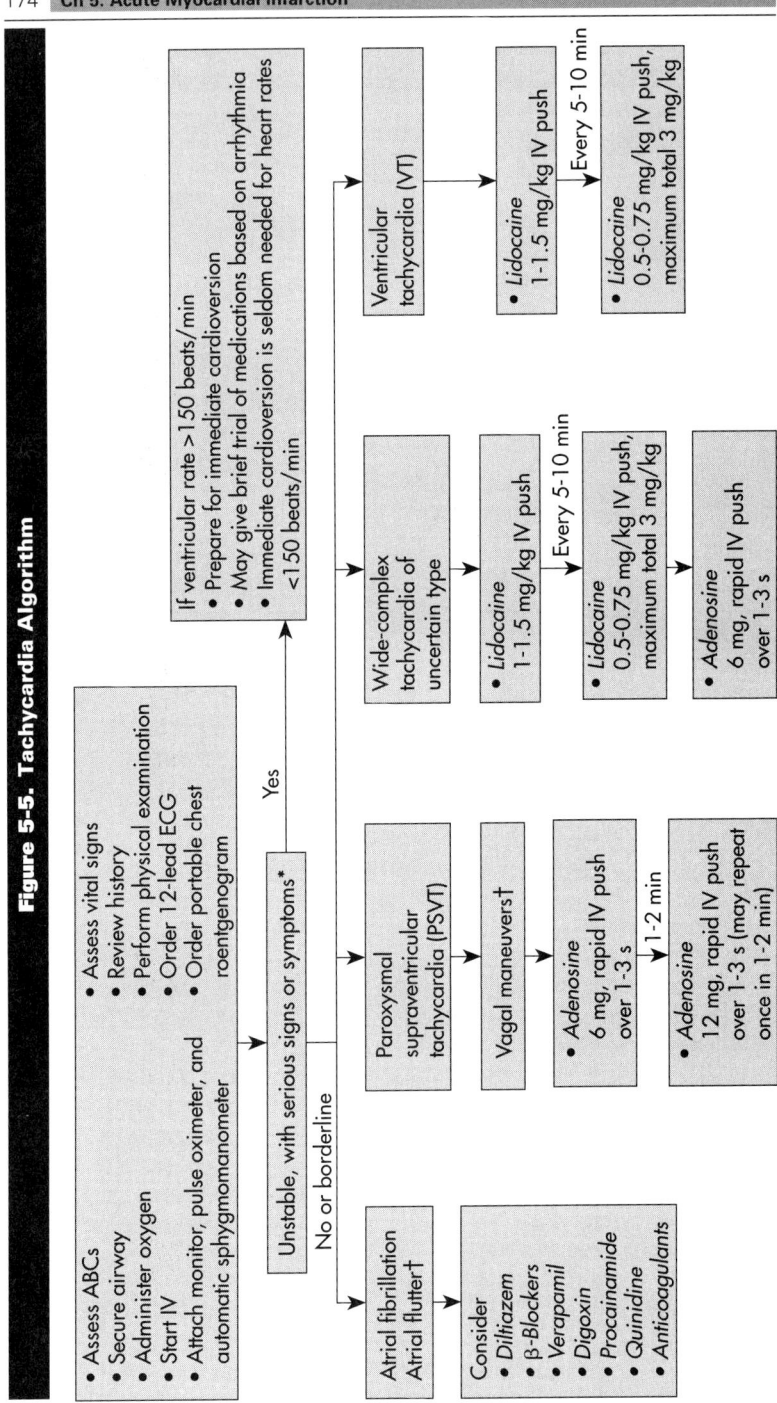

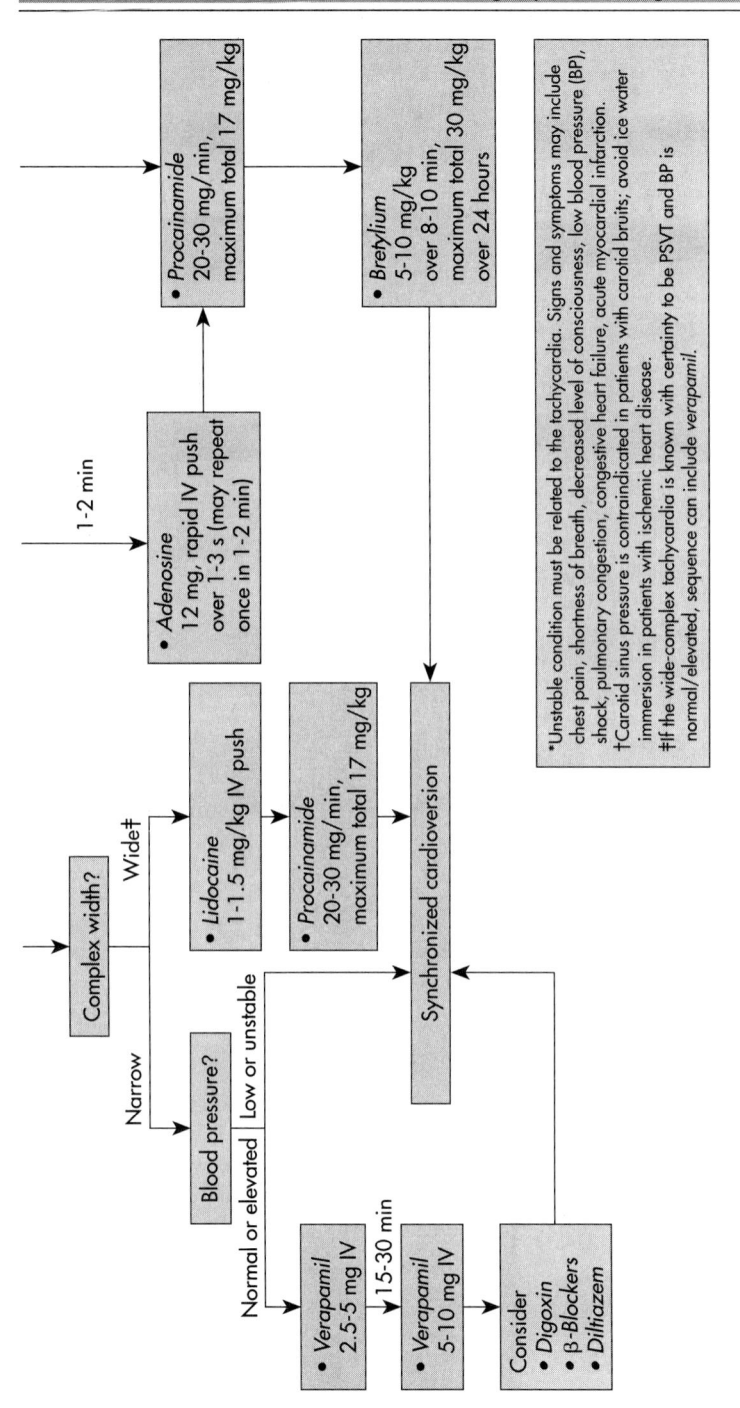

Emergency Guideline Algorithms

- *Adenosine* 12 mg, rapid IV push over 1-3 s (may repeat once in 1-2 min)

- *Procainamide* 20-30 mg/min, maximum total 17 mg/kg

- *Bretylium* 5-10 mg/kg over 8-10 min, maximum total 30 mg/kg over 24 hours

Complex width?

Wide‡:
- *Lidocaine* 1-1.5 mg/kg IV push
- *Procainamide* 20-30 mg/min, maximum total 17 mg/kg

Narrow → **Blood pressure?**

Low or unstable → Synchronized cardioversion

Normal or elevated:
- *Verapamil* 2.5-5 mg IV
- 15-30 min
- *Verapamil* 5-10 mg IV

Consider:
- *Digoxin*
- *β-Blockers*
- *Diltiazem*

---

*Unstable condition must be related to the tachycardia. Signs and symptoms may include chest pain, shortness of breath, decreased level of consciousness, low blood pressure (BP), shock, pulmonary congestion, congestive heart failure, acute myocardial infarction.

†Carotid sinus pressure is contraindicated in patients with carotid bruits; avoid ice water immersion in patients with ischemic heart disease.

‡If the wide-complex tachycardia is known with certainty to be PSVT and BP is normal/elevated, sequence can include *verapamil*.

Figure 5-6. Algorithm for Hypotension, Shock, and Acute Pulmonary Edema

Clinical signs of hypoperfusion, congestive heart failure, acute pulmonary edema
- Assess ABCs
- Secure airway
- Administer oxygen
- Start IV
- Attach monitor, pulse oximeter, automatic sphygmomanometer
- Assess vital signs
- Review history
- Perform physical examination
- Order 12-lead ECG
- Order portable chest roentgenogram

What is the nature of the problem?

Volume problem
Administer
- Fluids
- Blood transfusions
- Cause-specific interventions
- Consider vasopressors, if indicated

Pump problem
What is the blood pressure (BP)?*

- Systolic BP <70 mm Hg†
- Systolic BP 70-100 mm Hg†
- Systolic BP >100 mm Hg and diastolic BP normal
- Diastolic BP >110 mm Hg

Rate problem
- Too slow — Go to Fig. 5-4
- Too fast — Go to Fig. 5-5

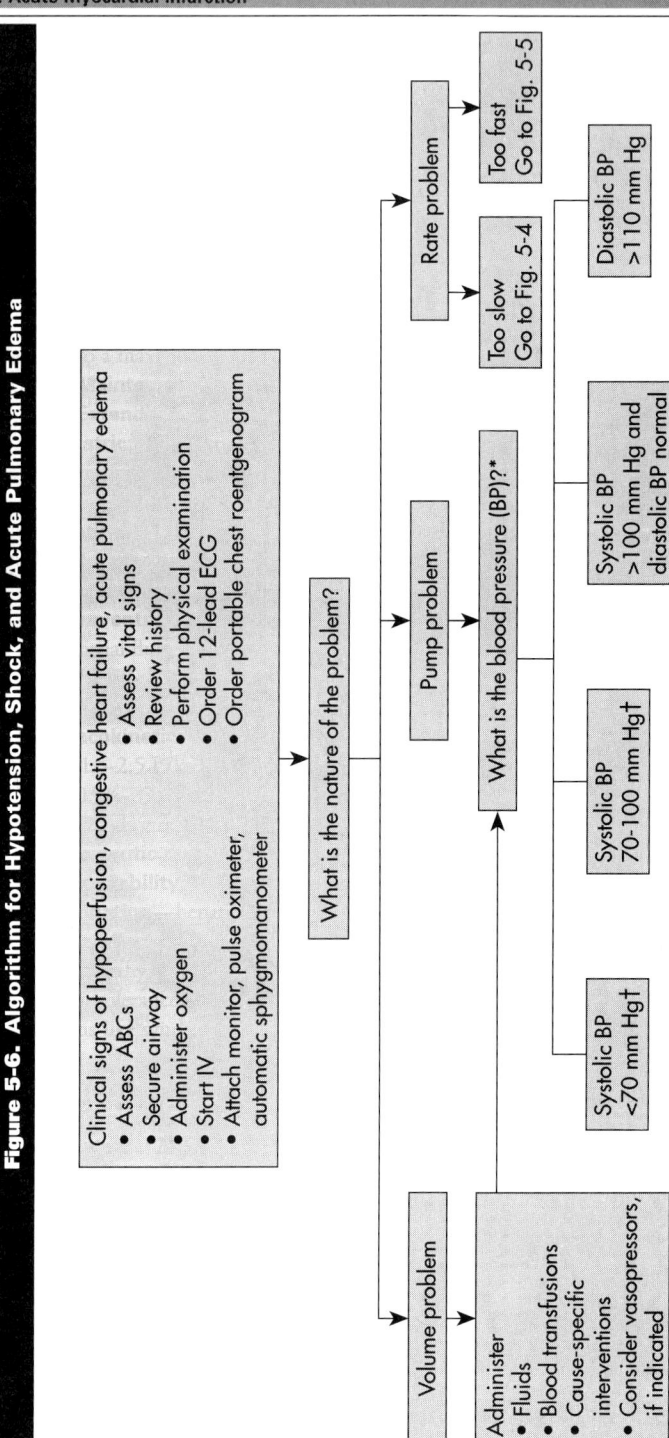

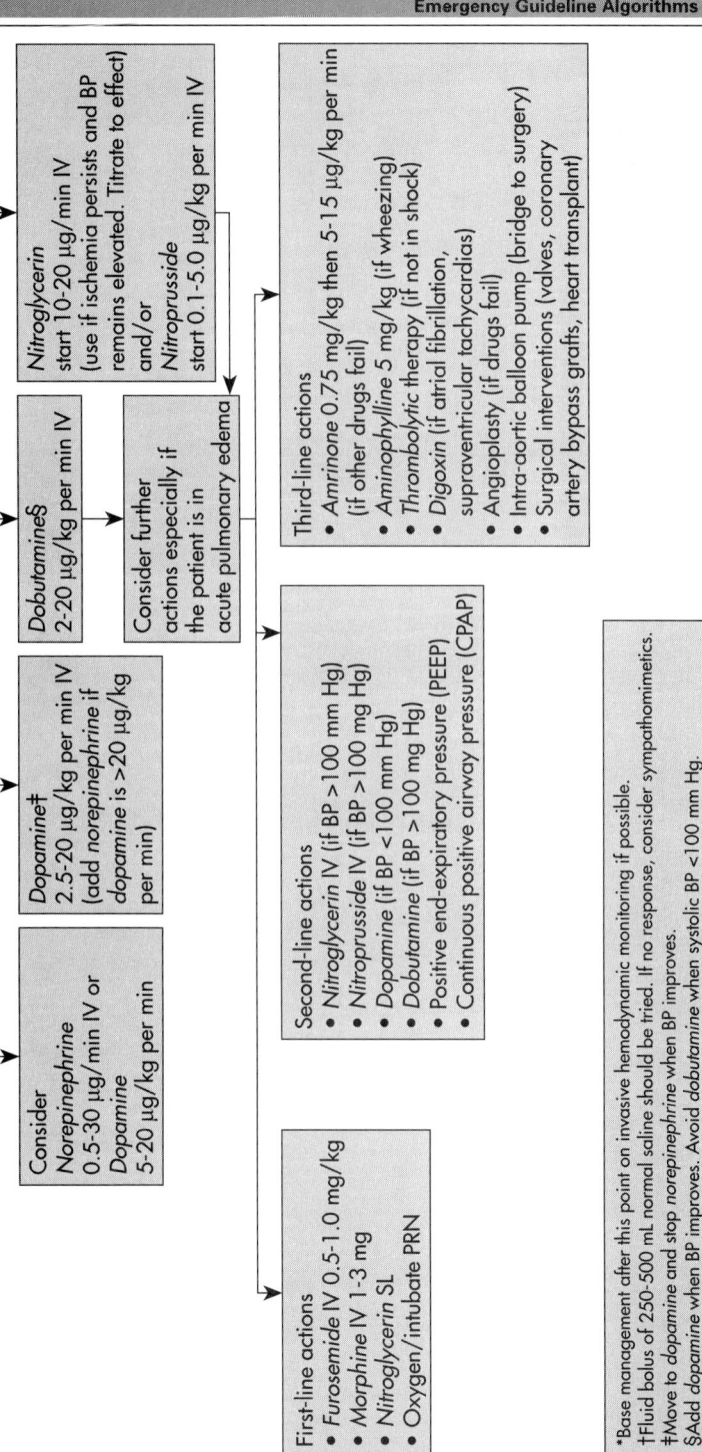

Emergency Guideline Algorithms

Nitroglycerin
start 10-20 µg/min IV
(use if ischemia persists and BP remains elevated. Titrate to effect)
and/or
Nitroprusside
start 0.1-5.0 µg/kg per min IV

Dobutamine§
2-20 µg/kg per min IV

Consider further actions especially if the patient is in acute pulmonary edema

Dopamine‡
2.5-20 µg/kg per min IV
(add *norepinephrine* if dopamine is >20 µg/kg per min)

Consider
Norepinephrine
0.5-30 µg/min IV or
Dopamine
5-20 µg/kg per min

Third-line actions
- *Amrinone* 0.75 mg/kg then 5-15 µg/kg per min (if other drugs fail)
- *Aminophylline* 5 mg/kg (if wheezing)
- *Thrombolytic therapy* (if not in shock)
- *Digoxin* (if atrial fibrillation, supraventricular tachycardias)
- *Angioplasty* (if drugs fail)
- *Intra-aortic balloon pump* (bridge to surgery)
- *Surgical interventions* (valves, coronary artery bypass grafts, heart transplant)

Second-line actions
- *Nitroglycerin* IV (if BP >100 mm Hg)
- *Nitroprusside* IV (if BP >100 mm Hg)
- *Dopamine* (if BP <100 mm Hg)
- *Dobutamine* (if BP >100 mm Hg)
- Positive end-expiratory pressure (PEEP)
- Continuous positive airway pressure (CPAP)

First-line actions
- *Furosemide* IV 0.5-1.0 mg/kg
- *Morphine* IV 1-3 mg
- *Nitroglycerin* SL
- Oxygen/intubate PRN

*Base management after this point on invasive hemodynamic monitoring if possible.
†Fluid bolus of 250-500 mL normal saline should be tried. If no response, consider sympathomimetics.
‡Move to *dopamine* and stop *norepinephrine* when BP improves.
§Add *dopamine* when BP improves. Avoid *dobutamine* when systolic BP <100 mm Hg.

Suggested Readings

AIMS Trial Study Group: Effect of intravenous APSAC on mortality after acute myocardial infarction: preliminary report of a placebo-controlled clinical trial, *Lancet* 1:545-49, 1988.

American Heart Association: Emergency Cardiac Care Committee and Subcommittees: Guidelines for cardiopulmonary resuscitation and emergency cardiac care, *JAMA* 268(16):2171-302, 1992.

ASSET Study Group: Trial of tissue plasminogen activator for mortality reduction in acute myocardial infarction, *Lancet* 2:525-30, 1988.

EMERAS Collaborative Group: Randomized trial of late thrombolysis in patients with suspected acute myocardial infarction, *Lancet* 342:767-72, 1993.

The European Myocardial Infarction Project Group: Prehospital thrombolytic therapy in patients with suspected acute myocardial infarction, *N Engl J Med* 329(6):383-9, 1993.

GISSI-2: A factorial randomized trial of alteplase versus streptokinase and heparin versus no heparin among 12,490 patients with acute myocardial infarction, *Lancet* 336:65-71, 1990.

Gruppo Italiano per lo Studio della Streptokinasi nell'Infarto Miocardico (GISSI): Effectiveness of intravenous thrombolytic treatment in acute myocardial infarction, *Lancet* i:397-402, 1986.

GUSTO: An international randomized trial comparing four thrombolytic strategies for acute myocardial infarction. The GUSTO investigators, *N Engl J Med* 329(10):673-82, 1993.

Herr CH: The diagnosis of acute myocardial infarction in the emergency department; Part 1 and 2, *J Emerg Med* 10(4,5):455-61, 591-9, 1992.

ISIS-1. First International Study of Infarct Survival Collaborative Group: Randomised trial of intravenous atenolol among 16,027 cases of suspected acute myocardial infarction: ISIS-1, *Lancet* 2(8498):57-66, 1986.

ISIS-2. Second International Study of Infarct Survival Collaborative Group: Randomised trial of intravenous streptokinase, oral aspirin, both, or neither among 17,187 cases of suspected acute myocardial infarction: ISIS-2, *Lancet* 2(8607):349-60, 1988.

ISIS-3. Third International Study of Infarct Survival Collaborative Group: A randomised comparison of streptokinase vs tissue plasminogen activator vs anistreplase and of aspirin plus heparin vs aspirin alone among 41,299 cases of suspected acute myocardial infarction, *Lancet* 339(8796):753-70, 1993.

International Study Group: In-hospital mortality and clinical course of 20,891 patients with suspected acute myocardial infarction randomized between alteplase and streptokinase with or without heparin, *Lancet* 336:71-5, 1990.

LATE Study Group: Late assessment of thrombolytic efficacy (LATE) study with alteplase 6-24 hours after onset of acute myocardial infarction, *Lancet* 342(8874):759-66, 1993.

Lau J et al: Cumulative meta-analysis of therapeutic trials for myocardial infarction, *N Engl J Med* 327(4):248-54, 1992.

MIAMI Trial Research Group: Metoprolol in acute myocardial infarction (MIAMI): a randomized placebo-controlled international trial, *Eur Heart J* 6:199-226, 1985.

Woods KL et al: Intravenous magnesium sulfate in suspected acute myocardial infarction: results of the second Leicester Intravenous Magnesium Intervention Trial (LIMIT-2), *Lancet* 339(8809):1553-8, 1992.

6

Rational Use of Poison Antidotes

Robert Ferm, M.D., F.A.A.P., A.B.E.M., A.B.M.T.
Lawrence Levine, M.D.
Marc J. Bayer, M.D.
Revised by Richard Y. Wang, D.O., F.A.C.E.P., A.B.M.T.

General Principles of Supportive Care

Specific antidotal therapy exists for relatively few poisonings. Appropriate stabilization, resuscitation, and supportive measures are the most important factors to a successful outcome for these patients. The general guidelines and principles are the same as those for any other critically ill patients presenting to an emergency department. Of primary importance is attention to the "ABCDs" of patient management.

I. **Airway: establish a patent airway.** In the mildly obtunded patient, this may require simple maneuvers such as the jaw thrust or the chin lift. However, intubation may be required, especially in the more deeply obtunded patient who may have lost protective reflexes.

II. **Breathing: provide adequate oxygen.** Supply sufficient supplemental oxygen to achieve adequate oxygenation of the blood. Oxygen therapy may enhance the toxicity of certain poisons. These include adriamycin, bleomycin, and daunorubicin. In paraquat poisoning, supplemental O_2 should be avoided unless necessary to maintain the arterial pO_2 over 50 mm Hg. Ensure adequate gas exchange by assisting ventilation as needed.

III. **Circulation.** Hypotension should be corrected to ensure adequate tissue perfusion. Initial measures should include positioning (Trendelenburg) and intravenous fluid challenges. Vasopressors should be used only if these initial measures are inadequate.

IV. **Drugs**
   A. **ACLS.** The ACLS protocols are appropriate in most instances, with certain modifications (e.g., bicarbonate for hypotension or dysrhythmias encountered in tricyclic antidepressant toxicity). All patients presenting with a depressed level of consciousness should receive glucose (1 to 2 mL/kg D50W and naloxone (2 to 10 mg). If there is suspicion that the patient might be thiamine deficient (e.g., chronic alcoholism, AIDS), 100 mg of this vitamin should be administered with glucose to avoid precipitation of a Wernicke's encephalopathy.
   B. **Effective antidotes.** The remainder of this chapter will limit its scope to the specific drug therapies for poisons. The field of medical toxicology is ever evolving as new information is presented on a continuous basis. To provide patients with the most appropriate care, medical management will need to change accordingly. The information presented within this chapter is deemed appropriate at the time of its writing; although, this may not be the situation at the time of its publication. It is recommended that clinicians who are not familiar with the following antidotes and their most current indications should call their regional poison control center for fur-

ther assistance. Otherwise, the local poison center should be notified of the patient case, so the information may be used to further our understanding of this disease.

Principles of Antidotal Action

Antidotes may counteract the toxic effects of poisons by a variety of mechanisms. Some of these are as follows.

I. **Direct detoxification of poison.** This is one of the several potential antidotal mechanisms of *N*-acetylcysteine (NAC) for acetaminophen (APAP) poisoning. NAC may serve as a scavenger for the toxic free radical intermediate that is responsible for APAP-induced hepatotoxicity. Also, NAC may be converted to glutathione, which serves as an endogenous reducing agent for the free radical. Another example is the role of pralidoxime in the treatment of poisoning by organophosphate insecticides. Pralidoxime (2PAM) regenerates cholinesterase activity by binding to the phosphate group of the insecticide.

II. **Prevention of formation of poisonous product.** This is a relatively common and important mechanism of antidotal action. Examples include ethanol for poisoning by methanol or ethylene glycol, and the use of N-acetyl-L-cysteine (NAC) for acetaminophen (APAP) toxicity. In the former case, ethanol is a competitive substrate for alcohol dehydrogenase and can effectively inhibit the formation of the toxic metabolites of the parent alcohols (formic acid from methanol and oxalic acid from ethylene glycol). In addition to detoxifying the free radical intermediate, NAC may also limit its production by shunting the metabolism of APAP to nontoxic byproducts.

III. **Removal of poison.** This may occur by chemical sequestration of the toxin as in chelation of heavy metals (e.g., by calcium disodium ethylenediaminetetraacetate [CaNa$_2$EDTA], deferoxamine, dimercaprol [BAL], and D-penicillamine), antibody-antigen binding with snake antivenin and digoxin Fab, or simple ionic complexing. The latter process is the mechanism by which calcium and magnesium salts limit tissue damage in hydrofluoric acid burns. In many of these cases, the binding of the toxin also enhances its elimination.

IV. **Antagonism of toxic effects.** This may occur through competitive inhibition by the antidote at the toxin's binding site. This is observed in atropine therapy for organophosphate toxicity, naloxone treatment for opioid induced coma, and sodium bicarbonate therapy for tricyclic antidepressant cardiac toxicity. In a similar manner, flumazenil is effective in reversing central nervous system (CNS) depression due to benzodiazepines. Glucagon's beneficial cardiac effects in beta-adrenergic and calcium channel blocker toxicity is through its binding at a different receptor site on the myocardial cell membrane.

V. **Reversal of toxic effect.** Examples of this mechanism include methylene blue treatment for nitrite-induced methemoglobinemia, and folinic acid (leucovorin) therapy for methotrexate toxicity. Methylene blue facilitates the reduction of the physiologically inactive methemoglobin (Fe+3) back to the oxygen transporting hemoglobin (Fe+2). Folinic acid limits bone marrow suppression by providing the necessary enzyme dependent cofactors that are blocked by methotrexate.

Specific Antidotes
(Table 6-1)

I. **Antivenins.** Commercially available antivenins are lyophilized antibodies derived from the serum of animals inoculated with venoms. They act by binding to the components of the venom and inhibit the activity of the various toxins (enzymes and polypeptides). Three FDA approved antivenins are commercially available in the United States: *Crotalidae polyvalent* (rattlesnake), Coral snake, and *Latrodectus mactans* (black widow spider).

   A. *Crotalidae* polyvalent antivenin (Wyeth)
   1. **Uses and indications.** This preparation is active against the water moccasin (cotton mouth), copper-head, North American rattlesnakes, some Asian snakes, and South American pit vipers. Clinical factors determine the use of these agents on a case by case basis. An exception would be an envenomation by the Mojave rattlesnake *(Crotalus scutulatus)* where local tissue response may not be a good estimate of the extent of toxicity, and immediate antivenin therapy should be initiated. More specific guidelines are provided in **Table 6-2**.
   2. **Dosage.** Once the decision to use antivenin therapy has been made, an intradermal testing to determine sensitivity to horse serum should be performed. Mild envenomations may often be treated supportively and symptomatically without use of antivenin. Moderate envenomations require an initial treatment with 4-5 vials IV over 1-2 hours. Serious envenomations with signs of systemic toxicity may require 30-40 vials. Children may require relatively more antivenin per body weight than adult victims. When indicated, antivenin treatment should be begun as soon as possible; therapy is most effective when administered within 4-5 hours of envenomation, and of uncertain efficacy when administered more than 12-24 hours post-envenomation. **Reconstituted antivenin** should be infused slowly as a 1:10-1:100 dilution with saline. The first dose is given over an hour and the remaining dose over 3-4 hours. Therapy for anaphylaxis should be immediately available.
   3. **Adverse effects and toxicity.** The major risk with antivenin therapy is hypersensitivity reactions (e.g., anaphylaxis). Treatment should always be preceded by skin testing for sensitivity to horse serum. In serious life-threatening envenomations, concurrent use of epinephrine infusions and antihistamines may blunt the allergic response and allow use of antivenin even in hypersensitive patients. Since the skin testing can yield false negative results, the clinician should always be ready to treat for anaphylaxis. Delayed onset of serum sickness can be anticipated in days to weeks, especially if more than 4-5 vials are employed. Symptoms include urticaria, fever, malaise, arthralgias, myalgias, lymphadenopathy, nausea, and vomiting. Mild cases may be managed with antihistamines and close outpatient follow-up. More severe cases may require the use of systemic corticosteroids.

   B. Coral snake antivenin
   1. **Uses and indications.** This antivenin is effective against the Eastern or Texas coral snake *(Micrurus fulvius)*, but is not for the Sonoran or Arizona coral snake *(Micrurus euryxanthus)*.

Table 6-1. Specific Antidotes

Poisons	Antidotes
Acetaminophen	N-acetylcysteine (NAC, Mucomyst)
Anticholinergics	Physostigmine
Arsenic	Dimercaprol (BAL), D-penicillamine
Beta adrenergic antagonists	Glucagon
Benzodiazepine	Flumazenil
Botulism	Botulinum Antitoxin (ABE Trivalent)
Cadmium	CaNa2EDTA, D-penicillamine
Calcium channel blocker	Calcium Chloride
Cardiac glycosides	Digoxin immune FAB (Digibind)
Carbamates	Atropine, Pralidoxime (2PAM)
Chlorine gas	Sodium Bicarbonate
Cobalt	CaNa2EDTA
Copper	Dimercaprol (BAL), D-penicillamine, CaNa2EDTA
Coumarin Derivatives	Vitamin K1 (Phytonadione)
Cyanide	Amyl Nitrite, Sodium Nitrite, Sodium Thiosulfate, Oxygen, Hydroxocobalamin
Cyclic antidepressant	Sodium Bicarbonate
Ethylene glycol	Ethanol, Pyridoxine, Thiamine
Hydrazines	Pyridoxine (Vitamin B6)
Hydrogen Sulfide	Amyl Nitrite, Sodium Nitrite, Oxygen
Hydrofluoric acid	Calcium gluconate, magnesium sulfate
Hypoglycemics	Dextrose, glucagon, hydrocortisone, diazoxide
Iron	Deferoxamine
Inorganic Mercury	Dimercaprol (BAL), Dimercaptosuccinic acid (DMSA), D-penicillamine
Lead	Dimercaprol (BAL), CaNa2EDTA, Dimercaptosuccinic acid (DMSA), D-penicillamine
Magnesium	Calcium Gluconate
Methanol	Ethanol, Folinic acid (Leucovorin)
Methemoglobinemia	Methylene Blue
Methotrexate	Folinic acid (Leucovorin)
Mushrooms	
Clitocybe/Inocybe	Atropine
Amanita Phalloides	Penicillin G, Silibinin, Silimaryn
Gyromitra Esculenta	Pyridoxine
Neuroleptics (Extrapyramidal symptoms)	Diphenhydramine Benztropine
Phenothiazines	
Butyrophenones	
Thioxanthenes	
Metoclopramide	
Opioids	Naloxone
Zinc	CaNa2EDTA, Dimercaprol (BAL)

From Roberts JR, Otten EJ: Snakes and other reptiles. In Goldfrank L. *Goldfrank's toxicological emergencies.* Norwalk: Appleton and Lange, 1994.

Table 6-2. Evaluation and Treatment of Crotalid Envenomation

Extent of envenomation	Clinical observations	Antivenin recommendation	Other treatment	Disposition
None	Fang marks may be seen, but there are no local or systemic manifestations after 6-8 h observation.	None	Local wounds care Tetanus prohylaxis Value of prophylactic antibiotic unknown	Discharge with follow-up after 6 h observation
Minimal	Minor local swelling and discomfort. No systemic symptoms, normal laboratory findings. No blisters, ecchymosis, or necrosis. No progression after 6 h of observation.	None	Same as above	Same as above
Moderate	Progression of swelling beyond area of bite. Moderate to severe pain. Petechiae and ecchymosis of bite area. Minor systemic symptoms such as anxiety, nausea, tingling, may be seen. May note minor laboratory value abnormalities.	4-10 vials depending on severity.	Tetanus prophylaxis Broad spectrum antibiotics Cardiac and vital sign monitoring IV fluids Pain medication Assess for compartment syndrome, debridement as necessary Follow-up laboratory abnormalities	Admit for observation

Table 6-2. Evaluation and Treatment of Crotalid Envenomation—cont'd

Extent of envenomation	Clinical observations	Antivenin recommendation	Other treatment	Disposition
Severe	Marked progressive swelling and pain, early blisters, ecchymosis, and necrosis. Systemic symptoms such as vomiting, fasciculations, weakness, tachycardia, hypotension, incontinence, epistaxis, hematuria, or cardiopulmonary arrest. Coagulopathy, hemolysis, renal failure.	10-40 vials	Tetanus prophylaxis, prophylactic antibiotics, cardiac and vital sign monitoring, IV fluids, vasopressors, oxygen, monitor coagulopathy, assess for compartment syndrome, debridement as necessary	Admit to intensive care unit

From Goldfrank L, Flomenbaum NE, Lewin NA, eds, et al: Goldfrank's toxicologic emergencies, ed 4, New York, 1987, Appleton and Lange.

2. **Dosage.** Intradermal testing for horse sensitivity serum should be performed only after the decision to use antivenin therapy has been made. Therapy should be initiated for any case of coral snake bite, even in the absence of specific clinical manifestations. This is because systemic toxicity may develop even without any apparent evidence of local injury. Initial dosage is 3-5 vials, with further treatment as determined by the clinical status. If neurological symptoms develop, an additional 3-5 vials should be administered.
3. **Adverse effects and toxicity.** As for crotalid antivenin, the major risk is anaphylaxis. The subsequent development of serum sickness should be anticipated in the majority of cases receiving 5 or more vials. Management of these complications is as discussed for Crotalidae antivenin.

C. *Latrodectus mactans* antivenin
   1. **Uses and indications.** This antivenin is effective against all North American widow species *(Latrodectus sp)*. Antivenin administration is not necessary for most *Latrodectus* envenomations, which can be managed supportively and symptomatically. However, this agent may be of use in infants, the elderly, and those with serious underlying cardiovascular disease due to their propensity for worse outcome.
   2. **Dosage.** In patients requiring antivenin therapy, the average dose is 1-2 vials IV, infused over an hour. This antivenin is also a horse serum product, and requires the same cautions and skin testing procedure as described for crotalidae antivenin.
   3. **Adverse effects and toxicity.** As with any horse serum product, hypersensitivity reactions and serum sickness are the most significant adverse effects.

D. **Other antivenins.** These preparations are not approved for use by the FDA; therefore, they cannot be legally transported across state lines.
   1. **Exotic snake species.** These antivenins may be available in zoos (where such envenomations are most likely to occur).
   2. **Sea snake.** The Commonwealth Serum Laboratory in Melbourne, Australia produces a polyvalent horse serum antivenin. Following skin testing, the initial dosage is one vial, with further doses as determined by the patient's clinical status.
   3. **Stonefish.** A horse serum antivenin is produced by Commonwealth Serum Laboratories in Melbourne Australia, and is recommended for most stonefish stings.
   4. **Scorpion.** This product is derived from goat serum and is stocked by the Arizona State University Antivenom Product Laboratory in Tempe. Based on cases reported in the literature, 1 to 2 vials have appeared to be effective in severe envenomations.
   5. **Sea wasp.** Commonwealth Serum Laboratories in Melbourne Australia produces a sheep serum derived antivenin to the toxins of this extremely poisonous Southern Pacific jelly fish. After intradermal skin testing, one vial is administered intravenously in all cases with significant envenomation.

II. **Atropine**
   A. **Uses and indications.** Atropine is effective in reversing the muscarinic signs of cholinergic poisoning as seen with organophosphate/carbamate insecticides; Clitocybe or Inocybe mushrooms; synthetic cholinergic agonists (bethanechol, carbachol), and physostigmine.

B. Dosage. Initial dosages are 1-4 mg for adults, 0.015-0.05 mg/kg in children (minimum 0.15 mg), and the dose repeated every 15-30 minutes as necessary to control symptoms of cholinergic excess. The end point is drying of pulmonary secretions, rather than pupillary dilatation, which may be seen at lower (and inadequate) doses. Extremely high cumulative daily doses (in grams) may be required for days in severe organophosphate intoxications.

C. Adverse effects and toxicity. Adverse effects are those of anticholinergic excess, including tachycardia, fever, ileus, delirium, urinary retention and excessive drying of secretions. Supplemental O_2 should be administered prior to giving atropine as ventricular fibrillation may occur in the setting of hypoxia. Atropine should be used with caution in patients with hypertension, fever, or hyperthyroidism and is relatively contraindicated in narrow angle glaucoma.

III. Botulinum antitoxin

A. Uses and indications. There are a total of eight botulinum strains (A-G), of which horse derived antitoxins are available for the more common varieties. The botulinum toxin causes muscle paralysis by binding irreversibly to presynaptic neuromuscular receptors and prevent the release of acetylcholine. The antitoxin binds to circulating toxin and prevents their receptor binding. Thus, the benefit of the antitoxin is in preventing and halting paralysis, but not in reversing already paralyzed muscle groups. Lower fatality rates, and shorter durations of illness are reported with antitoxin use. It is important to provide both symptomatic and asymptomatic victims of exposure the antitoxin when it is recognized. However, the benefit of antitoxin therapy late in the course of disease remains in question. Whenever an exposure is of suspect, the local Department of Health and the Center for Disease Control (CDC) (404-639-3753/days, 404-639-2888/off hours) should be contacted for reporting and further assistance. **The botulinum antitoxin is not effective in infant botulism** because most cases do not have circulating toxin.

B. Dosages. Botulinum antitoxin is available as Type A, Type B, Type AB, Type E, and Type ABE (trivalent), and is administered intravenously. The trivalent antitoxin should be used when the specific type of toxin has not yet been identified. For availability of antitoxin and dosages, contact the local Department of Health and the CDC.

C. Adverse effects and toxicity. Since the antitoxin is horse derived, anaphylaxis and serum sickness needs to be observed for.

IV. Calcium salts.
Calcium salts are effective for a variety of poisonings. These include *Latrodectus* envenomation, hydrofluoric acid burn, calcium channel blocker toxicity, and magnesium toxicity. It is also indicated as replacement therapy in ethylene glycol toxicity. Two types of calcium salts are available, calcium gluconate and calcium chloride. It is important to note that they do not contain the same amount of ionized calcium per percent volume. Three times more volume of 10% calcium gluconate is needed to deliver the same amount of ionized calcium of an equal volume of 10% calcium chloride. Thus, depending on the nature and severity of the poisoning, one calcium salt would be indicated over another.

A. Calcium gluconate 10% solution

  1. Uses and Indications. Intravenous calcium gluconate may ameliorate muscle spasms from *Latrodectus* envenomation, and reverse the neuro-

muscular paralysis in hypermagnesemia. It is also effective for hydrofluoric acid burns, in limiting tissue destruction and controlling pain.
   2. **Dosage.** Intravenous calcium must be given slowly through a well-established vascular access and with constant monitoring of blood pressure and heart rate. The recommended dose is 0.2 mL/kg of 10% solution. For mild hydrofluoric acid burns, a calcium gluconate gel may be adequate therapy. The gel is prepared by mixing 3.5 gms of calcium gluconate powder and 150 mL of a water soluble lubricant. If pain persists for more than 45 minutes after the application of the gel, or the degree of the injury is more significant, then parenteral calcium therapy is warranted. Intradermal calcium gluconate is administered through a narrow gauge needle in the burn site, and around it for a distance of about 0.5 cm at a dose of not more than 0.5 mL/cm2. For digital burns, intradermal injections and nail plate removal is not longer recommended. Intraarterial administration of calcium salts is the preferred method of managing significant digital injuries. A 2% calcium gluconate solution is infused through a standard radial intraarterial catheter, whose placement has been ensured to be good. A volume of 50 mL is administered by an infusion pump over a period of 4 hours. The infusion can be repeated if pain recurs.
 B. Calcium chloride 10% solution
   1. **Uses and indications.** Calcium chloride is indicated for the treatment of hypotension and bradycardia due to calcium channel blocker toxicity, and significant hypocalcemia.
   2. **Dosage.** For calcium channel blocker toxicity, adults should be initially treated with 10-20 mL 10% calcium chloride IV (pediatrics 0.2-0.25 mL/kg) before moving onto another agent. If found to be effective, the dose can be repeated, as necessary, but the serum calcium should be monitored of severe hypercalcemia.
   3. **Adverse effects and toxicity.** Calcium salts are themselves irritating to tissues and may cause sloughing upon extravasation. Use with great caution in patients on digitalis or with renal failure. If mixed with bicarbonate, calcium carbonate salts will precipitate out of solution. Serum calcium levels needs to be monitored for hypercalcemia during therapy.
V. **Chelators.** These antidotes are used for heavy metal toxicities, both chronic and acute. They contain either oxygen, sulfur or nitrogen ligands, that form coordinate bonds with the metal to produce a complex of less toxicity than the free metal. Chelators currently in use include the following.
 A. Calcium disodium ethylenediaminetetraacetate (CaNa$_2$EDTA)
   1. **Uses and indications.** CaNa$_2$EDTA is indicated for lead, cadmium, copper, cobalt, and zinc toxicities.
   2. **Dosage.** A daily dosage of 50-75 mg/kg per day is given IV or IM in two to four divided doses for 5 days. A 2-day rest period should include assessment of efficacy of treatment and need for further treatment.
   3. **Adverse effects and toxicity.** CaNa$_2$EDTA must be given slowly IV, over 15-20 mins. Adequate fluids must be provided and urine output and renal functions monitored, as acute tubular necrosis can occur with CaNa$_2$EDTA use. In addition, prolonged use has been associated with zinc and pyridoxine (B$_6$) deficiency. Patients with significant lead toxicity should receive dimercaprol (BAL) before CaNa$_2$EDTA.

B. Deferoxamine

1. **Uses and indications.** Deferoxamine is a specific chelator of iron and enhances the renal elimination of excess body iron. The intravenous route should be used in patients with significant toxicity or hypotension. Otherwise, the intramuscular route is adequate. If the diagnosis of iron toxicity is in doubt, then a single intramuscular dose may be administered and the urine observed for color changes consistent with toxicity.
2. **Dosage.** The intravenous dose is 15 mg/kg/hour up to a total of 90 mg/kg over 8 hours (maximum recommended dose is 6 grams over 24 hours). The infusion should be started at a rate of 5 mg/kg/hr and titrated to 15 mg/kg/hr as quickly as possible. The intramuscular dose is 90 mg/kg every 8 hours; a maximum of 1.0 gm in children and 2.0 gms in adults per dose. Chelation therapy is continued until the resolution of toxic manifestations, and the urine is no longer of a "vin rose" or dark orange color.
3. **Adverse effects and toxicity.** Hypotension may occur with the rapid intravenous administration of deferoxamine. Protracted treatment (e.g. in treatment of chronic iron overload in patients requiring chronic transfusion therapy) is associated with cataract formation, sensory deficits, visual loss, night blindness, retinal pigmentary degeneration, sensorineural hearing loss, and yersinia enterocolitica septicemia.

C. Dimercaprol (British anti-Lewisite/BAL)

1. **Uses and indications.** Used in poisoning of several metals, including arsenic (not from arsine gas), cobalt, gold, lead, and mercury. It is possibly useful in poisonings by antimony, bismuth, chromium, nickel, copper, zinc, and tungsten.
2. **Dosage.** Start with 3-5 mg/kg administered as deep intramuscular injections every 4 hours for the first two days. Continual therapy is dependent on patient's response, and severity of illness.
3. **Adverse effects and toxicity.** Pain and sterile abscesses may occur at the injection site. Hypertension and tachycardia occur frequently, as does fever in children. Urticaria has also been reported and is responsive to therapy with diphenhydramine. Dimercaprol is contraindicated in patients with peanut allergy due to the oil in which BAL is suspended, alkyl mercury toxicity, hepatic insufficiency, and G6PD deficiency.

D. D-penicillamine

1. **Uses and indications.** This agent is an orally administered drug for the chelation of lead, mercury, and copper. It is investigational for cadmium, arsenic, and bismuth toxicity. D-penicillamine should not be administered if there are still lead contaminants in the patient's gut, as this agent may enhance the metal's absorption. This may also be so for the other heavy metals.
2. **Dosage.** 15-40 mg/kg/day (up to 1-2 gms) in four divided doses for five days. The drug should be given on an empty stomach, as the drug's absorption is poor in the presence of food, antacids, or iron salts. The urine should be monitored for heavy metal content to determine the efficacy of treatment.
3. **Adverse effects and toxicity**
   a. **Side effects** include fever, rash, bone marrow suppression, gastrointestinal distress, kidney and liver dysfunction, and auto-immune disorders.

b. **Pyridoxine 10-25 mg/day** should be given concurrently, as D-penicillamine inhibits pyridoxal-dependent enzymes.
   c. **Penicillin allergy** is a contraindication to use.
E. DMSA and DMPS
   1. **Uses and indications.** DMSA (Dimercaptosuccinic acid, CHEMET®) and DMPS (2,3 dimercapto 1-propane sulfonic acid) are two new derivatives of BAL that are effective as heavy metal chelators. DMPS is not approved for use in the United States. These agents are water soluble, relatively safe and effective orally.
      a. **DMSA** was used in the Iraqi methylmercury mass poisoning where it was shown to decrease the half-life of methylmercury from 65 to 10 days. DMSA is approved in the United States for the treatment of childhood lead poisoning with blood lead levels greater than 45 mcg/dL. DMSA is not recommended for the treatment of either lead encephalopathy, or extremely elevated blood lead levels. In these instances, parenteral chelation therapy would be indicated.
      b. **Animal data** suggest that DMSA may be most beneficial in treating arsenic, lead and mercury poisonings, while DMPS may be best suited for chromium, inorganic mercury, lead and copper exposures.
   2. **Dosage for DMSA.** The recommended dose for children is 10 mg/kg p.o. three times a day for five days. The same dose is then administered two times a day for 14 more days. Continual use of DMSA is dependent on patient toxicity, and courses of therapy should be separated by two weeks.
   3. **Adverse effects and toxicity.** The more common side effects from DMSA therapy include: nausea, vomiting, diarrhea, urticaria, transaminitis, and eosinophilia. These are transient and resolve upon the discontinuance of therapy.
VI. **Cyanide antidote kit.** The Eli Lilly Cyanide antidote kit consists of three components: amyl nitrite, sodium nitrite, and sodium thiosulfate. The nitrites form methemoglobin (Fe+3), which removes CN from cellular cytochrome oxidases and allows for the resumption of aerobic metabolism. Sodium thiosulfate converts CN to the less toxic thiocyanate (SCN) derivative, which is excreted renally.
   A. **Uses and indications.** Use of all three components of the antidote kit is indicated in symptomatic acute cyanide poisonings. The nitrite components of the kit are also indicated for symptomatic hydrogen sulfide and sodium azide exposures. In victims of smoke inhalation where both carbon monoxide and cyanide toxicities are of suspect, administer only the sodium thiosulfate.
   B. Dosage
      1. **For adults:** one **amyl nitrite** ampule (0.2 mL) is crushed and held under the nose or at the intake of the ventilator bag for 30 seconds of every minute. When an intravenous line is established, 10 mL of the **sodium nitrite** is given slowly IV over 4 minutes. This therapy should result in a methemoglobin level of approximately 20-30%. Nitrite treatment is followed by the administration of **sodium thiosulfate:** 50 mL of a 25% solution as a slow IV infusion over 10-15 minutes.
      2. **Dosage in children:** 3% sodium nitrite 0.15-0.33 mL/kg (maximum 10 mL) at a rate of 2.5 mL/min; sodium thiosulfate dosage is 1.65 mL/kg (maximum 50 mL). These doses are based on a hemoglobin concentration of 12 g/dL, and should be reduced in patients with anemia.

C. Adverse effects and toxicity. Nitrites are potent vasodilators and may cause hypotension, nausea, vomiting, headache, and syncope. If hypotension occurs during sodium nitrite therapy, the rate of administration should be decreased and a saline fluid bolus given. Methemoglobin levels should be measured 30 minutes upon completion of sodium nitrite therapy, to monitor response. Methemoglobin may produce symptoms of toxicity at levels greater than 30%, and death may occur at levels of approximately 70%. In patients with borderline cardiorespiratory function or anemia, significant symptoms may occur at lower levels. Dosage must be accurately determined in children and in the setting of anemia. Thiocyanate can cause psychosis, nausea, vomiting, muscle cramps, and arthralgias at levels greater than 10 mg/mL. Thiocyanate is excreted by the kidney and may accumulate in renal failure.

VII. Dextrose

A. Uses and Indications. The primary use of dextrose therapy is for symptomatic hypoglycemia induced by hypoglycemic agents. Dextrose is also used in the management of hyperkalemia along with sodium bicarbonate, insulin, and calcium. Initial therapy for drug induced hypoglycemia or hyperkalemia can begin with bolus therapy. However, a maintenance dextrose infusion is often required for overdoses involving hypoglycemic agents.

B. Dosage. Bolus: 50-100 mL D50W IV for adults (2-4 mL/kg D25W IV in pediatrics). Maintenance: D10W IV titrated to effect.

C. Adverse effects and toxicity: The consequences associated with the administration of dextrose are few and minor in comparison to those related to prolonged unrecognized hypoglycemia. Delayed dextrose therapy for symptomatic hypoglycemia is associated with permanent neurologic deficit, and slow clinical response to treatment. There is theoretical concern regarding the precipitation of Wernicke's encephalopathy by giving dextrose to a nutritionally deficient patient. Thus, it is recommended to administer thiamine along with dextrose in patients that are malnourished. **High concentrations of dextrose** can be irritating to blood vessels, and concentrations greater than 10% dextrose are to be delivered by the central venous route.

VIII. Digoxin-specific antibody fragments.

These are the Fab fragments derived from papain cleavage of antibodies produced by immunization of sheep with a digoxin-albumin conjugate.

A. Uses and indications. Digoxin-specific antibody fragments are effective for both chronic and acute intoxication by either digoxin or digitoxin. These antibody fragments can also be used for plant cardiac glycoside toxicity (i.e., oleander, foxglove, and dogbane).

B. Dosage. Digoxin antibodies are derived from goat serum and patients that are to be treated with this agent should be considered for skin testing prior to drug administration. If sensitivity is demonstrated, the decision to proceed with treatment must be based on the relative risks and benefits of that individual case. The effective dose of Fab is approximately equimolar to that of the ingested digitalis compound. This is 50-100 mg of Fab per mg of digoxin or approximately 65 mg of Fab per mg of digitoxin. If the amount ingested is unknown, then empiric therapy is as follows: Acute toxicity—400-800 mg (10-20 vials), Chronic toxicity—80-200 mg (2-5 vials). In the clinically stable patient, the agent is reconstituted and administered through a 0.22 micron filter over 30 minutes. If the patient is clinically unstable, the rate of administration should be quicker.

C. **Adverse effects and toxicity.** Minimal hypersensitivity reactions have been reported with digoxin Fab use. Signs of hypersensitivity must be observed for and immediate therapy available. Monitor the serum potassium level as hypokalemia may occur when the sodium-potassium pump is disinhibited. Patients who are dependent on the inotropic support of their digitalis may require alternative treatment as the digitalis effect is withdrawn.

IX. **Diphenhydramine and benztropine.** These compounds act by the blockade of dopamine uptake and the competitive inhibition of muscarinic receptors.

   A. **Uses and indications.** These drugs are useful for the reversal of extrapyramidal symptoms induced by butyrophenones, phenothiazines, thioxanthenes, or metoclopramide.

   B. **Dosage.** For acute dystonic reactions, the parenteral dose of diphenhydramine is 1-2 mg/kg (IM or slow IV, 50 mg maximum). This should be followed by 25 mg (1 mg/kg in children) po tid for 3 days to prevent recurrences. For benztropine the adult dosage is 1-2 mg IV or IM then 1-2 mg po bid for 3 days.

   C. **Adverse effects and toxicity.** The side effects of these agents are related to their anticholinergic effects. These clinical manifestations include mydriasis, urinary retention, paralytic ileus, flushed skin, dry mucous membranes, sedation, and psychomotor agitation.

X. **Ethanol**

   A. **Uses and indications.** Ethanol prevents the metabolism of methanol and ethylene glycol to their toxic byproducts by acting as a competitive substrate for the enzyme alcohol dehydrogenase. Therapy is indicated either in the presence of manifestations of toxicity or when peak plasma levels are greater than 20 mg/dL. Treatment should be instituted prior to confirmatory laboratory results if the patient is symptomatic or there is a suspicion of significant methanol or ethylene glycol ingestion (>0.4 mL/kg).

   B. **Dosage.** The desired serum concentration of ethanol in the management of methanol or ethylene glycol toxicity is 100 mg/dL, or at least 25% of the toxic alcohol concentration, whichever is greater. To achieve 100 mg/dL:

   1. **Loading ethanol dose:** 0.6-0.8 g/kg (this is equal to 0.75-1.0 mL/kg of 100% ethanol, or 7.5-10 mL/kg of 10% ethanol for intravenous use, or 1.5-2.0 mL/kg of oral 100-proof ethanol). This load need not be adjusted in the chronic alcoholic, but should be adjusted downward if the patient already has a significant serum ethanol level.

   2. **Maintenance ethanol infusion:** Upon completion of the loading dose, a constant infusion is required to maintain the serum concentration. The recommended infusion rate is 0.07 g/kg/hr (0.08 mL/kg 100% ethanol, 0.8 mL/kg of 10% ethanol, 0.16 mL/kg of 100 proof ethanol) and is based on an average rate of ethanol metabolism in the non-drinker. Chronic alcoholics should be expected to metabolize ethanol more rapidly and should have their maintenance infusion rates increased by a factor of 2-2.5 times. If the patient is undergoing hemodialysis to enhance elimination of the toxic alcohol, the hourly maintenance rate must be increased by 2-3 times to account for the removal of ethanol by dialysis.

   3. **Ethanol levels** should be checked frequently and the infusion rate adjusted according to the above guidelines.

C. **Adverse effects and toxicity.** Ethanol is irritating to the veins and a concentration no higher than 10% should be used in the peripheral vessels. Otherwise, central venous access should be used if higher ethanol concentrations are to be administered. In children, hypoglycemia, sedation with loss of protective airway reflexes, and hyponatremia may occur with ethanol therapy. These should be monitored for closely.

XI. **Flumazenil.** Flumazenil (ROMAZICON®) is a competitive antagonist to benzodiazepines that binds to CNS specific receptors and blocks the activation of GABAnergic synapses.

A. **Uses and indications.** Flumazenil is effective in reversing the sedation caused by benzodiazepines. It is most safely used to rapidly reverse the benzodiazepine induced sedation that is employed in many surgical and orthopedic procedures. This agent has also been used, but is cautioned against, in the setting of undiagnosed coma. Many different disease processes can present with coma; such as, metabolic, structural, and drug toxicities, and the inappropriate use of flumazenil can lead to deleterious consequences (see below). Since patients with significant benzodiazepine toxicity can be well managed with supportive care and still have excellent outcomes, the empirical use of flumazenil in the unknown comatose patient is not recommended.

B. **Flumazenil is not recommended to reverse the respiratory compromise** due to benzodiazepine toxicity, because the duration of action of the sedating agent is often longer than that of the reversal agent. In the setting of drug toxicity, where pharmacokinetics are altered, the duration of drug effect is even less predictable. Under these circumstances, the patient will require constant observation and frequent readministration of the reversal agent in the event of resedation and loss of protective respiratory reflexes. In a busy emergency department or an intensive care unit, the use of staff resources in this manner is not practical. Thus, if either the airway or breathing is compromised in benzodiazepine toxicity, it is recommended to manage these with intubation.

C. **Dosage**
1. **Reversal of anesthesia:** 0.2 mg IV is administered over 15 sec. and the patient is observed for 45 sec. This can be repeated 4 times at these time intervals, until the desired level of arousal is achieved. The maximum dose is 1.0 mg, and most patients respond to 0.6-1.0 mg. Repeat doses of 1.0 mg (0.2 mg/min.) may be administered for resedation, but no more than 3.0 mg/hr. should be used.
2. **Benzodiazepine toxicity:** 0.2 mg IV is administered over 30 sec. and the patient is observed for 30 sec. If no effect is seen, then 0.3 mg can be given with the same time intervals. Doses of 0.5 mg can be repeated at 1.0 min intervals in the non responsive patient for a total dose of 3.0 mg. Most patients respond to 1-3 mg, and if no effects are seen 5.0 min. after 5.0 mg, then the diagnosis of benzodiazepine should be questioned.

D. **Adverse effects and toxicity.** The most significant side effects observed in the use of flumazenil has been in the setting of mixed drug overdose. The administration of flumazenil to patients that have ingested benzodiazepines with other agents, have resulted in seizures, dysrhythmias, and death. In these mixed overdoses, the benzodiazepine served as a protective measure against the toxic effects of the other agents that they ingested. By using flumazenil, this protective effect is removed and the patient manifests toxicity of the other drugs. Seizures are most notable in mixed tricyclic antidepressant ingestions, and dysrhythmias have been reported in mixed chloral hydrate ingestions.

E. **Other side effects** of flumazenil include the precipitation of benzodiazepine withdrawal and resedation phenomenon. Flumazenil has produced withdrawal seizures and sympathetic discharge in dependent patients. The duration of effect of flumazenil is dependent on several factors, including the dose administered, the duration of effect of the benzodiazepine, and the state of hepatic function. In patients with significant liver disease, the duration of effect of flumazenil is prolonged. When the benzodiazepine has a longer duration of effect than flumazenil, the patient must be observed for the complete duration before being discharged home or left unmonitored.

XII. Glucagon

A. **Uses and indications.** Glucagon is the antidote for β-adrenergic blocker toxicity because of its ability to promote inotropic and chronotropic actions despite blocked adrenergic receptors. These effects are achieved by increasing intracellular cAMP concentrations through the activation of adenylate cyclase through a receptor other than the b-adrenergic site. Glucagon has been demonstrated to be effective in managing calcium channel blocker toxicities, and is to be administered in all symptomatic patients.

B. **Dosage.** The therapeutic response of glucagon is variable, and a total dose of 10 mg IV should be given before moving onto another agent. An initial adult dose can be 2 mg (50-150 µg/kg in pediatrics), and then 4 mg every five minutes if no response is observed. If a desired effect is observed, then a maintenance glucagon infusion is needed due to its short duration of activity. The dose of the infusion is equivalent to the total amount of glucagon needed to achieve the desired effect, given continuously over an hour in a saline solution. The infusion can be tapered as the patient's status improves.

C. **Adverse effects and toxicity.** Some of the observed complications from glucagon therapy include nausea, vomiting, and hyperglycemia. The manufacturer distributes glucagon with a phenol diluent. Due to the large amount of glucagon that may be needed in the management of these cases, resuspend glucagon with either normal saline or sterile water to prevent potential phenol toxicity.

XIII. Hydroxocobalamin.
Hydroxocobalamin is an investigational agent used to treat cyanide toxicity. It combines with the cyanide molecule to form cyanocobalamin (Vitamin B12) which is non toxic and can be safely excreted by the kidney. Hydroxocobalamin is not yet FDA approved, although animal studies suggest that it is a safe and effective agent. It is presently employed as the principle antidote for cyanide poisoning in France.

XIV. Folinic acid (Leucovorin)

A. **Uses and indications.** Folinic acid (Leucovorin), is the biologically active form of folic acid, and is an essential cofactor for many enzymatic reactions. It is indicated in overdoses of methanol, and folate antagonists such as methotrexate (MTX), pyrimethamine, or trimethoprim. In methanol poisoning, folinic acid may enhance the metabolism of methanol's toxic end product, formic acid to carbon dioxide and water. The toxic manifestations of folate antagonists may be averted with folinic acid by allowing cellular reactions to continue. This form of rescue therapy has limited methotrexate induced bone marrow, gastrointestinal, and renal toxicity. Folic acid may be used in methanol toxicity, though it is not preferred. This is because of the time it takes for it to be converted to folinic acid.

B. Dosage

1. **Methanol toxicity:** In adults, folinic acid 50 mg IV every 4-6 hours until resolution of metabolic acidosis.
2. **Methotrexate toxicity:** The goal of folinic acid rescue therapy for methotrexate toxicity in the patient not receiving MTX therapy, is to achieve a serum folinic acid concentration that is comparable to that of the MTX concentration. The initial parenteral dose of folinic acid should be equal to the amount of exposed MTX. The usual beginning maintenance dose of folinic acid is 10 mg/m^2 (IV or PO), every six hours. However, this dose will be dependent upon the anticipated MTX level at the time of rescue, and may have to be increased in patients with inadequate renal function and delayed drug elimination. The parenteral route should be used if more than 50 mg of folinic acid is needed. In large MTX exposures, either more frequent dosing (every 2 to 3 hours), or a continuous infusion of leucovorin should be considered because of its short half life of less than 4 hours. Serum methotrexate levels should be monitored at 12, 24 and 48 hours post exposure so that folinic acid therapy can be adjusted accordingly. Generally, folinic acid therapy should be continued if the serum MTX level is above 0.5 μM at 48 hours post exposure, and maintained until the level is below 0.05 μM. The recommended folinic acid dose in adults for pyrimethamine induced bone marrow suppression is 3-9 mg/day IM for three days or more.

C. Adverse effects and toxicity. The oral administration of folinic acid is non toxic in man. If the intravenous route is used, then the rate of administration should be limited to 160 mg/min. because of the calcium content of the infusate. There have been some rare reports of adverse reactions associated with the parenteral administration of both folic and folinic acids. Hypersensitivity has been noted with both of these agents, and a variety of central nervous system effects, including altered sleep patterns, irritability, excitability, and hyperactivity have been reported with folate use. If a patient reports a history of such occurrences, the physician should be cautious in readministering the agent.

XV. Methylene blue

A. Uses and indications. Methylene blue (tetramethylthionine chloride) is an antidote for patients suffering from methemoglobinemia. It acts as an electron carrier for the hexose monophosphate pathway that facilitates the reduction of methemoglobin to hemoglobin. At high levels of methemoglobinemia (greater than 70%) methylene blue reduces the methemoglobin half-life from an average of 15-20 hours to 40-90 minutes. Methylene blue therapy is indicated in patients with either manifestations of toxicity or a level greater than 30%. Symptoms may appear to lower levels in patients with anemia, pulmonary disease or processes that reduce cerebral or coronary perfusion. Asymptomatic cyanosis is not an indication for antidotal therapy. Some of the toxins that induce methemoglobin formation include nitrates, aniline dyes, and local anesthetics.

B. Dosage. Methylene blue may be given at a dosage of 1-2 mg/kg as a 1% (10 mg/mL) solution over 5 minutes. This dosage may be repeated in 60 minutes, if necessary, to a total maximum of 7 mg/kg.

C. Adverse effects and toxicity
   1. **Large intravenous doses** (greater than 7 mg/kg) may result in nausea, vomiting, diaphoresis, dizziness, abdominal and chest pain, and cyanosis from increased methemoglobin formation. Oxygen saturation and methemoglobin levels should be followed frequently by blood gas analysis on a co-oximeter.
   2. **Skin discoloration.** Methylene blue may cause a bluish discoloration of the skin, tears, and urine.
   3. **Methylene blue** should be administered cautiously to glucose-6-phosphate dehydrogenase (G6PD) deficient patients due to their susceptibility for hemolysis.

XVI. 4-Methyl pyrazole
   A. **Uses and indications:** 4-Methyl pyrazole (4-MP) is a specific inhibitor of alcohol dehydrogenase that appears to be effective in the management of methanol and ethylene glycol toxicity. This form of therapy is advantageous because of its simplicity in use, long duration of activity, and limited adverse effects. However, this form of therapy offers no benefits in the correction of any metabolic derangements and may prolong the duration of treatment. 4-MP is currently under investigation in Europe, and is not approved for use in the United States.
   B. **Adverse effects and toxicity:** Some of the side effects noted in human trials include dermatitis and gastrointestinal symptoms.

XVII. N-Acetyl-L-Cysteine
   A. **Uses and indications.** N-Acetyl-L-Cysteine (Mucomyst®, NAC) is an antidote that limits acetaminophen and possibly carbon tetrachloride induced hepatotoxicity. The indications for NAC use in acetaminophen are ever changing, but the current standard for acute toxicity, is if the acetaminophen level is in the toxic range by the Rumack-Matthew nomogram **(Figure 6-1).** NAC is also recommended for acetaminophen poisoning in the following instances: if the estimated ingestion exceeds 150 mg/kg, if the time of ingestion is not known and there is a measurable serum acetaminophen level, and if there is evidence of hepatotoxicity. The efficacy of NAC is greatest if given within 8 hours of ingestion, and is of less benefit after 24 hours.
   B. **Dosage.** NAC is only approved for oral administration in the United States. The **loading dose** is 140 mg/kg (diluted in soda pop or juice to a 5% solution) and the **maintenance dose** is 70 mg/kg every 4 hours for an additional 17 doses. Once NAC therapy has been decided upon, it is necessary to continue the full course of treatment even if subsequent acetaminophen levels fall below the toxic range.
      1. **If the patient vomits** within one hour of administration, an additional loading dose may be given. NAC is foul-smelling, foul-tasting and a stomach irritant. Disguising the taste and smell in chilled juice may be helpful. At times it may be necessary to administer NAC through a nasogastric tube.
      2. **Activated charcoal** is able to adsorb NAC, however, this has not been shown to diminish the efficacy of NAC in the management of acetaminophen toxicity. Charcoal is useful in the following situations with acetaminophen overdoses: mixed drug ingestions, and if the patient presents soon after the ingestion. The charcoal can be administered by several ways. One if to remove the charcoal by gastric lavage before the

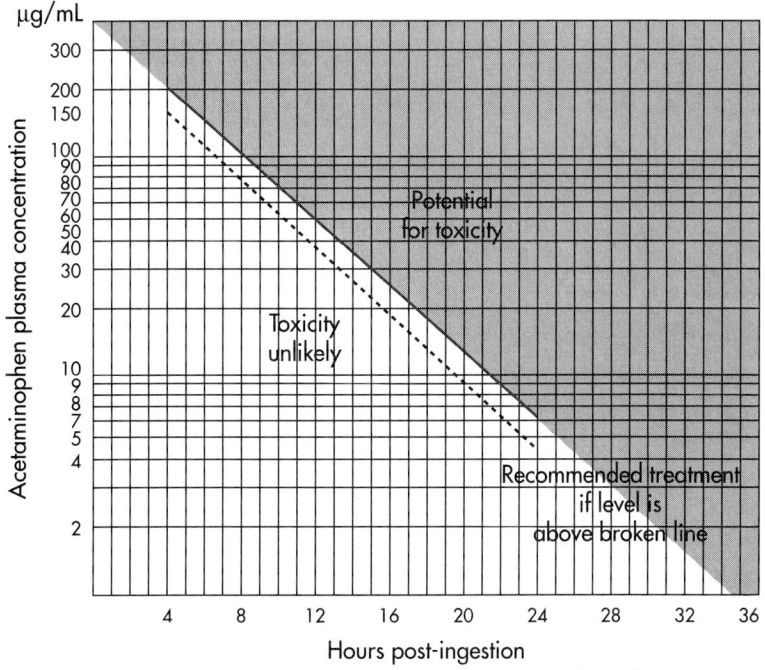

Figure 6-1. Nomogram: plasma or serum acetaminophen concentration vs time post acetaminophen ingestion. This nomogram has been developed to estimate the probability that plasma levels in relation to intervals post ingestion will result in hepatotoxicity. Cautions for the use of this chart: (1) The time coordinates refer to time post ingestion. (2) The graph relates only to plasma levels following a single acute overdose ingestion. (3) The broken line, which represents a 25% allowance below the solid line, is included to allow for possible errors in acetaminophen plasma assays and estimated time from ingestion of an overdose. (Adapted from Rumack and Matthew: *Pediatrics* 55:871-876, 1975.)

administration of NAC. Another, is to stagger the dosing intervals of charcoal and NAC by two hours. This will allow the stomach to clear the previous agent before the next one is administered.

3. **Parenteral administration of NAC** has been used in Europe and Canada. It has been especially useful in patients with persistent vomiting and in situations where the gut cannot be used. The intravenous route is currently being studied in the United States and is not yet approved.
4. **Adverse effects and toxicity.** Adverse reactions such as fever, rhinitis, nausea and vomiting are rare with the oral dose. Anaphylactoid reactions have been reported with the intravenous route.

XVIII. Naloxone

A. **Uses and indications.** Naloxone is an antidote for opioid toxicity. It is a semisynthetic opioid antagonist derived from thebaine. It is thought to competitively block opiates at the mu, kappa and sigma receptors. Unlike its predecessor, levallorphan and nalorphine, naloxone is a pure antagonist and lacks any agonist properties of respiratory or CNS depression.

1. **Natural and synthetic opioid poisonings** such as morphine, codeine, heroin, meperidine, propoxyphene, and fentanyl can be reversed with naloxone. It is also effective against the partial agonists such as pentazocine, butorphanol and nalbuphine.
2. **Clonidine poisoning.** Naloxone appears to have a variable response in reversing the sedation and respiratory compromise seen in clonidine toxicity. The mechanism is not well defined, though it may be that receptors activated by clonidine and naloxone are located in close proximity in the midbrain, and the effects of naloxone are carried over. In the setting of symptomatic clonidine toxicity, naloxone should be used in addition to standard practices for stabilization. The dosing is the same as that for opioid toxicity.

B. **Dosage.** The dosing of naloxone in the overdose setting is empirical, and begins with 2.0 mg IV, IM, SC, or intralingually. In the opioid dependent patient, a lesser dose may be used to prevent the precipitation of withdrawal symptoms. If no response is observed after the initial dose, then 4.0 mg may be given and repeated once for a total of 10.0 mg. Some opioids such as propoxyphene, pentazocine, fentanyl, and codeine may require large amounts of naloxone to reverse their toxic effects. If there is no response after 10.0 mg, then the diagnosis of opioid toxicity is in question.

1. **Maintenance.** If there is a response with the above loading dose, then a maintenance infusion can be established by administering 2/3 of the naloxone loading dose per hour.
2. **Adults and children.** In the setting of toxicity, the dosing regimen is the same for both adults and pediatrics. If intravenous access is not available, then naloxone may be administered by the endotracheal or intraosseous route.

C. **Adverse effects and toxicity.** Naloxone has few adverse side effects. Hypertension and dysrhythmias have been rarely encountered. Naloxone can produce an opioid withdrawal syndrome in drug dependent individuals. This withdrawal syndrome is not life-threatening, is usually short-lived, and should not be managed with more opioids in this setting. **The half-life of naloxone** is only 30-60 minutes, while that of most opioids is much longer. A maintenance infusion can extend the duration of effect of naloxone, however, close monitoring of the patient is still required for delayed toxic manifestations due to ongoing drug absorption in the setting of toxicity.

XIX. **Oxygen**

A. **Uses and indications.** Oxygen (O_2) is a basic and universal medication that should be administered whenever there is a question of adequate tissue oxygenation. Oxygen is effective as part of the supportive care approach in virtually all poisonings, and as a specific antidote for poisonings due to carbon monoxide, cyanide, and hydrogen sulfide. This group of toxins affect either oxygen transport or utilization. Administration of supplemental O_2 also accelerates the elimination of carbon monoxide ($T_{1/2}$ of COHgb at room air is 5-6 hours and at 100% O_2 this is reduced to 90 mins.).

B. **In poisonings by CO, CN, or H_2S,** the maximum achievable O_2 concentration should be administered, preferably 100%. This level of oxygen delivery is best approximated by high flow rates with an endotracheal tube

or a tight-fitting oxygen reservoir ("nonrebreathing") mask. Hyperbaric oxygen (HBO) therapy allows delivery of oxygen at higher tensions to allow for improved tissue oxygenation, and decreased half life of COHgb ($T_{1/2}$ = 20-30 mins. at 3 atm). This aggressive treatment appears to be of clinical benefit to patients. Proposed indications for HBO therapy of CO toxicity are as follows:
1. **COHgb level >25%** and regardless of symptoms
2. **Neurologic manifestations:** coma, altered mental status, focal deficits, and seizures;
3. **Pregnancy:** controversial, would consider HBO at COHgb levels even less than 25%;
4. **Cardiac manifestations:** syncope, electrocardiographic changes consistent with ischemia/infarction, angina, hypotension;
5. **Pulmonary edema**

C. Stabilization. Patients should not be transferred to facilities for HBO therapy if they have not been stabilized. Prior to HBO therapy, devices containing an air bladder cuff should be replaced with sterile water. Otherwise, the cuff will deflate at high atmospheric pressures.

D. Adverse effects and toxicity.
1. **Loss of respiratory drive:** Oxygen may depress respirations and cause CO_2 retention in patients with hypoxia-dependent respiratory drive (e.g. patients with chronic obstructive pulmonary disease).
2. **Retinopathy.** In neonates, arterial pO_2 >100 mmHg is associated with an increased risk for the development of retinopathy of prematurity (retrolental fibroplasia). This risk must be weighed against the expected benefits of supplemental oxygen and mandates careful monitoring of arterial blood gases in the newborn.
3. **Oxygen toxicity** is a function of both inspired pO_2 and duration of exposure. Oxygen tensions of up to 1/2 atmosphere (380 torr) appear to be well-tolerated indefinitely. Respiratory toxicity (mucous membrane irritation, cough, tracheobronchitis, and pulmonary congestion, transudates, exudates, or atelectasis) develops after prolonged exposures to oxygen tensions between 1/2 and 2 atmospheres. Neurologic toxicity (nausea, vertigo, mood changes, paresthesias, muscle twitches, loss of consciousness, and seizures) is seen at oxygen tensions greater than 2 atmospheres, and usually occurs before the onset of pulmonary toxicity.
4. **Barotrauma.** When the body is subjected to increased atmospheric tension, air cavities in the body (ear, sinuses, lungs) are subject to damage. A pretreatment chest radiograph should be obtained to identify pulmonary blebs, and occult pneumothoraces. Pulmonary blebs are not a contraindication for HBO therapy, but knowledge of their existence prepares the physician for potential complications. A pneumothorax should be decompressed before HBO therapy.

XX. **Penicillin G**
A. Uses and Indications. High dose penicillin therapy is believed to be effective in limiting hepatic uptake of the amatoxins in *Amanita Phalloides* exposures. In retrospective studies, improvement in survival appears to be associated with penicillin use. However, since multiple other drug therapies were used in conjunction with penicillin, the true efficacy of this agent remains in question. If considered, penicillin should be adminis-

tered early. *Silibinin and silimaryn* are also believed to limit hepatocellular uptake of the amatoxin; however, they are not available in the United States.

    B. Dosage: Penicillin G300,000 to 1,000,000 units/kg/day IV.

    C. Adverse effects and toxicity: Penicillin therapy should be avoided in patients that demonstrate sensitivity to this agent.

XXI. Physostigmine. Physostigmine is a reversible cholinesterase inhibitor that prolongs the duration of acetylcholine and causes cholinergic symptoms. These include salivation, lacrimation, urination, diarrhea, emesis, bronchorrhea, bradycardia, abdominal cramps, and miosis. This agent is effective in reversing many of the manifestations of anticholinergic toxicity.

    A. Uses and indications: Physostigmine's use in the clinical setting is restricted to treat significant CNS toxicity due to drugs with sole anticholinergic properties (e.g. diphenhydramine, benztropine). The anticholinergic CNS manifestations that physostigmine is effective for, include psychomotor agitation, coma, and seizures. A 12 lead electrocardiogram must be obtained prior to drug administration. If there is evidence of cardiac conduction disturbances, then physostigmine is contraindicated.

    B. Dosage: Once the decision has been made to use physostigmine, the patient should be placed on a cardiac monitor, and atropine be made available at the bedside.

        1. Adults. Start with 1-2 mg IV (1 mg/min).

        2. Pediatrics. Start with 0.01 mg/kg.

    C. After the administration of the agent, the patient should be observed for signs of improvement, or cholinergic toxicity (i.e. bradycardia, abdominal pain, etc.). In either situation, further therapy should be withheld. However, if there is no change, then the dose can be repeated in 20 mins. The maximum dose in adults is 2-4 mg, and in pediatrics 0.5 mg.

    D. The therapeutic effects of physostigmine lasts for about 45-60 mins., and the dose can be repeated if the clinical situation warrants it.

    E. Adverse effects and toxicity

        1. Cholinergic toxicity: Cholinergic manifestations with significant consequences may occur when physostigmine is used in the patient without anticholinergic toxicity, or when there are other drug effects associated with the drug toxin. The use of physostigmine in tricyclic antidepressant toxicity has resulted in seizures, bradycardia, and refractory asystole.

        2. Seizures: related to rapid IV administration of physostigmine.

        3. Contraindications. Physostigmine is contraindicated in the setting of the following active diseases: asthma, cardiac, gangrene, diabetes, pregnancy, hyperthyroidism, and mechanical obstruction of either the bowel or urinary tract. Similarly, patients with sensitivity to cholinesterase inhibitors, angle closure glaucoma, and narrow angles are not to receive physostigmine.

XXII. Pralidoxime

    A. Uses and indications. Pralidoxime (2-PAM) is a cholinesterase reactivator used in the management of organophosphate pesticide exposures. These pesticides are strong inhibitors of carboxylic esterase enzymes including acetylcholinesterase and pseudocholinesterase and act by inhibiting the enzyme through phosphorylation. Pralidoxime removes the phos-

phoryl group from the inhibited enzyme, thereby regenerating acetylcholinesterase. The clinical benefits of pralidoxime include, the need for less atropine, reversal of nicotinic symptoms, and limiting the occurrence of late neurologic manifestations of toxicity. Pralidoxime should be administered as soon as possible after exposure, in order to achieve the greatest benefit. However, in symptomatic patients that present days after exposure, pralidoxime may still be effective and should be administered. The distinction in use of pralidoxime between organophosphate and carbamate pesticides no longer exists. Thus, regardless of the pesticide, pralidoxime should be administered when the following are present:
1. **Muscarinic manifestations.** When atropine is needed to manage the cholinergic symptoms, pralidoxime can reactivate the cholinesterase enzyme, and result in lesser amounts of atropine needed.
2. **Nicotinic manifestations.** Pralidoxime is most effective at nicotinic sites, while atropine works mostly at muscarinic sites. 2PAM is indicated in organophosphate/carbamate exposures when nicotinic symptoms of muscle fasciculations, weakness, hypertension, tachycardia, and respiratory depression are present.
3. **CNS:** Pralidoxime may also have a CNS therapeutic effect, both immediately as well as in preventing long term neurological sequelae. Due to its quarternary nitrogen structure, pralidoxime would not be expected to cross the blood-brain barrier. However, clinicians have observed this beneficial effect, and its mechanism remains to be determined.

B. Dosage
1. **Adults.** Initially as 1-2 gms. IV over 30 mins. (200 mg/min.) in 250 mL of normal saline. Clinical improvement usually occurs in 10-45 mins, and the initial dose can be repeated if no change is observed. Pralidoxime is continued as 1-2 gms IV q 8 hrs for a minimum of 24 hours. Further therapy will depend on the patient's clinical status.
2. **Pediatrics.** Initially as 25-50 mg/kg IV, administered as a 5% solution in normal saline over a period of 5 to 30 mins. Therapy is continued every 8 hrs and re-evaluated at 24 hours.

C. Adverse effects and toxicity. Rapid intravenous administration can cause nausea, vomiting, blurred vision, tachycardia, muscle rigidity, hypertension and laryngospasm.
1. **Renal failure.** Dosage should be reduced in patients with renal failure, since 80-90% pralidoxime is excreted unchanged in the urine.
2. **Myasthenia gravis.** Caution should be used in myasthenia gravis patients in order to prevent a myasthenic crisis.

XXIII. **Phytonadione (Vitamin K$_1$)**
A. Uses and indications. Phytonadione is used to treat hypoprothrombinemia in moderate to severe coumarin poisonings. Phytonadione (Vitamin K$_1$) is a fat-soluble vitamin needed for the synthesis of coagulation factor 2 (Prothrombin), factor 7 (Proconvertin), factor 9 (Christmas), and factor 10 (Stuart-Power). The therapeutic effects of vitamin K1 are delayed and may take up to 6 hours to occur. It is important that vitamin K1, the active form of vitamin K, is used in coumarin exposures. This is because the conversion pathway for vitamin K is blocked by the anticoagulant. Therapy should begin only when there is an elevation of the patient's prothrombin time; otherwise, vitamin K1 should be withheld.

B. Dosage
 1. **Adult.** Initially 10-25 mg SC. The dose can be repeated in 6-8 hrs, if there is no improvement in the prothrombin time.
 2. **Pediatrics.** Initially 1.0 mg SC.

C. The intravenous administration of vitamin K1 is associated with significant complications (see below), and should not exceed 1 mg/min. If there is a hemorrhagic emergency, factor replacement with blood products is indicated, and not IV vitamin K1. Otherwise, vitamin K1 should be administered subcutaneously.

D. Adverse effects and toxicity. Anaphylactoid shock: Although vitamin K1 is relatively non toxic, hypotension and death have resulted from the IV administration of this agent. The subcutaneous route is not recommended because intramuscular administration can result in painful hematomas in the coagulopathic patient.

XXIV. Protamine sulfate

A. Uses and indications. Protamine sulfate is used to reverse the anticoagulant effects of heparin toxicity. It is a protein derived from fish sperm and complexes directly with heparin to form a stable product that lacks anticoagulant properties. Protamine acts rapidly, usually within 5.0 mins of its IV administration. This agent should not be used in the setting where there is only minor bleeding that can be controlled with compression and discontinuation of heparin therapy.

B. Dosage. One milligram neutralizes approximately 100 units of heparin. The appropriate dose can be calculated but should not exceed 50 milligrams and can be infused intravenously as 10 mg/mL over 5 minutes. Subsequent therapy is guided by partial thromboplastin times.

C. Adverse effects and toxicity. Anaphylactic/anaphylactoid reactions can occur with the administration of protamine. Patients at risk are those that may have developed sensitivity through prior heparin reversal, or use of insulin containing protamine.

XXV. Pyridoxine

A. Uses and indications. Pyridoxine (Vitamin B6) is used to control the intractable seizures of hydrazine toxicity (e.g. isoniazid/INH, monomethylhydrazine/MMH), and to enhance the elimination of the toxic metabolites of ethylene glycol. Monomethylhydrazine is found in the false morel *(Gyromitra esculenta)* mushroom, and in rocket propellent used in the aerospace industry.

 1. **Seizures.** Pyridoxine is a water soluble vitamin used in the transamination of amino acids and synthesis of gamma amino butyric acid (GABA) within the CNS. Isoniazid and MMH interfere with the normal synthesis of pyridoxine and lower the CNS GABA neurotransmitter level. Clinically, this results in intractable seizures. Pyridoxine should be administered when seizures are present. Its role as a prophylactic measure in the overdose setting is of limited value since many patients do not take enough to cause seizures, and hospitals often have a limited supply of pyridoxine available.
 2. **Pyridoxine** is also a cofactor in the metabolism of ethylene glycol toxic metabolites and may hasten the removal of these products.
 3. **In the treatment of refractory seizures,** pyridoxine should not be used as the sole agent. Diazepam has been found to act synergistically

with pyridoxine as an anticonvulsant, and should be administered. Other standard anticonvulsant drug therapies should be utilized as indicated.

B. Dosage
  1. **INH toxicity**: A gram for gram single intravenous infusion over 30 minutes is used. If an unknown quantity of INH has been ingested, either 70 mg/kg or 5 gms IV, of pyridoxine is initially recommended.
  2. **Monomethylhydrazine toxicity**: 25 mg/kg IV is recommended.
  3. **Ethylene glycol**: Adults: 50 mg IV/IM q 6 hrs, until the resolution of metabolic acidosis.

C. Adverse effects and toxicity. Neuropathy: High dose pyridoxine is associated with incoordination, ataxia, and sensory dysfunction. The dose at which these occur is not well defined, but when 70-357 mg/kg have been administered, no adverse effects were noted.

XXVI. Sodium bicarbonate

A. Uses and indications. Sodium bicarbonate has a variety of applications in the field of toxicology, the most notable of which is in the treatment of the cardiotoxic effects of tricyclic antidepressants (TCA). The mechanisms responsible for this are two folds. One is the ability of sodium to reactivate the fast sodium channels of the myocardial cells that are competitively blocked by the TCA. Another is the alkalinizing effect of the bicarbonate which favors the unbinding of the TCA moiety from the myocardial cell. Clinical improvements from sodium bicarbonate therapy in TCA toxicity include enhanced cardiac conduction and inotropy. Recommendation for use of sodium bicarbonate in TCA toxicity is when the QRS >0.1 sec. There is no current evidence for the use of sodium bicarbonate in either prophylactic or therapeutic measures for TCA induced CNS toxicity.

B. Respiratory symptoms. Sodium bicarbonate is also used to ameliorate the respiratory symptoms associated with the inhalational exposure to chlorine gas. Some of these manifestations include cough, dyspnea, burning sensation, chest pain, and bronchospasm. When chlorine gas comes in contact with the water of mucous membranes, hydrochloric acid is formed and corrosive damage occurs. The administration of aerosolized sodium bicarbonate is believed to neutralize the hydrochloric acid and provide symptomatic relief.

C. Renal elimination. Another use for sodium bicarbonate is to enhance the renal elimination of salicylate, chlorpropamide, phenobarbital, and chlorphenoxy herbicides.

D. Dosages
  1. **TCA cardiotoxicity loading**: 1-2 mEq/kg IV. **Maintenance.** 2-4 mL/kg/hr IV, of a 150 mEq/L solution of sodium bicarbonate (150 mL 8.4% sodium bicarbonate in 1.0 liter D5W). The serum pH should be maintained between 7.45-7.55, and therapy is continued for the duration of cardiac conduction abnormalities.
  2. **Chlorine gas.** Inhalational therapy with humidified 3.75% sodium bicarbonate. This solution is prepared by mixing 2.0 mL of 7.5% sodium bicarbonate with 2.0 mL normal saline. This therapy can be administered as needed depending on symptoms.

E. Adverse effects and toxicity
   1. **Hypokalemia.** Alkalinization of the serum causes the intracellular shift of potassium and a resultant hypokalemia. Serum potassium should be monitored and replaced as needed.
   2. **Serum alkalinization.** The overuse of IV sodium bicarbonate can result in an excessively high serum pH. This creates an unphysiologic environment and the potential for cardiac, neurologic, and metabolic complications. The serum pH should be monitored closely during therapy, and adjusted accordingly.

XXVII. **Thiamine (Vitamin B$_1$)**
   A. Uses and indications. Thiamine is a water soluble vitamin B complex that is essential as a cofactor of many enzymatic processes. It is effective in the treatment of thiamine deficient states (i.e. beriberi, Wernicke's encephalopathy), and may enhance the elimination of the toxic products of ethylene glycol metabolism.
   B. Dosage. Adults: Ethylene glycol: 100 mg IV/IM q 6 hrs until resolution of metabolic acidosis.
   C. Adverse effects and toxicity
      1. **Anaphylactoid.** The newer formulation of thiamine have resulted in a significantly lower incidence of hypotension, anaphylactoid, and hypersensitivity reactions. The frequency of these occurrences with the use of IV thiamine is so low, that is does not warrant significant concern.
      2. **Others.** Pain at the injection site and dermatis have been noted with thiamine use. The former is due to the too rapid administration of this agent.

Suggested Readings

Bayer MJ, Rumack B, Wanke L: *Toxicologic emergencies,* Brady/Prentice-Hall, Bowie, 1985.

Boehnert M, Lacouture PG, Guttmacher A, et al: Massive iron overdose treated with high dose deferoxamine infusion, *Vet Hum Toxicol* 28:291-292, 1985.

Chen HC: Naloxone in shock and toxic coma, *Am J Emerg Med* 2:444-452, 1984.

Decker WJ: Antidotes: Some ineffective, insufficiently tested, outmoded and potentially dangerous therapeutic agents, *Vet Hum Toxicol* 25(suppl 1):10-15, 1983.

Ellenhorn M, Barceloux D: *Medical toxicology,* Elsevier, New York, 1988.

Joe G, McKinney H, Wythe E: Antidotes-1984, *Clin Toxicol Update* 6:3, 1984.

Leiken J, Vogel S, Graff J, et al: Use of Fab fragments of digoxin specific antibodies in the therapy of massive digoxin poisoning, *Ann Emerg Med* 14:175-178, 1985.

Meredith T, Caisley J, Volans G: Emergency drugs. Agents used in the treatment of poisoning, *Br Med J* 289:742-748, 1984.

Robthoam JL, Lietman PS: Acute iron poisoning. A review, *Am J Dis Child* 134:875-879, 1980.

Smith TW, Butler VP Jr, Haber E, et al: Treatment of life threatening digitalis intoxication with digoxin specific Fab fragments. Experience in 26 cases, *N Engl J Med* 307:1357-1362, 1982.

Spivey WH: Flumazenil and seizures: Analysis of 43 cases, *Clin Therap* 14:292-305, 1992.

Spoerke DG, Smolinske SC, Wruk KM, et al: Infrequently used antidotes: Indications and availability, *Vet Hum Toxicol* 28:69-75, 1986.

Sullivan JB: Immunotherapy in the poisoned patient. Overview of present applications and future trends, *Med Toxicol* 1:47-60, 1986.

Sullivan JB, Russell FE: Isolation quantitation and subclassing of IgG antibody to Crotalidae venom by affinity chromatography and protein electrophoresis. *Toxicon* (suppl 3):429-432, 1983.

7

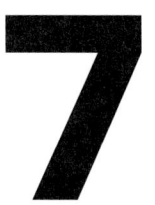

Cardiac Arrhythmias and Antiarrhythmic Drugs

Ernest A. Kopecky, B.Sc., Ph.D. (candidate)

The vital importance of rapid recognition, diagnosis, and treatment of patients presenting with chest pain in the emergency department is paramount in order to decrease the extent of cardiac muscle damage. This chapter presents a concise synopsis of the life-threatening arrhythmias, both adult and pediatric, utilizing a quick-reference format, and subdividing each arrhythmia into three aspects: clinical definition, salient features of the ECG, and medical management. The first section is devoted to the crucial pharmacokinetic profile and dosing regimen of each of the predominant antiarrhythmic drugs. Understanding and achieving the principal goals of clinical pharmacology **(Table 7-1)** requires a thorough knowledge of the pharmacokinetic parameters involved in the function and metabolism of each antiarrhythmic agent. Optimal drug administration requires not only comprehension of the mechanisms involved in drug absorption, metabolism, and elimination but also a detailed insight into the pharmacokinetic profile of the therapeutic agent. Pharmacokinetics encompass dosing, dosage forms, dosing frequency, and the route of administration of each preparation, which in turn are related to the plasma concentration–time relationships in the body.

Classification

Classifying drugs enables the clinician to readily access information needed to treat a particular dysrhythmia. Drug classification by site of action **(Table 7-2)** is advantageous in the emergency department when an ECG is readily available to aid in identifying the pathologic site in the heart.

Classification by drug class **(Table 7-3)** is a descriptive, physiologic approach, separating the antiarrhythmic drugs according to predominant electrophysiologic effect on the action potential.

Table 7-1. Goals of Therapeutic Pharmacology

1. Correct hypoxemia
2. Reestablish spontaneous circulation
3. Optimize cardiac function
4. Suppress sustained ventricular arrhythmias
5. Correct acidosis
6. Relieve pain
7. Treat congestive heart failure (CHF)

From Textbook of advanced cardiac life support, 1990, American Heart Association.

Ch 7. Cardiac Arrhythmias and Antiarrhythmic Drugs

Table 7-2. Classification by Site of Action

SA node and atrium	AV node	Ventricle	Accessory pathways
β-Blockers	Digoxin	Lidocaine	Disopyramide
Digoxin	β-Blockers	Procainamide	Amiodarone
Disopyramide	Verapamil	Disopyramide	Flecainide
Quinidine	Diltiazem	β-Blockers	
Amiodarone	Encainide	Amiodarone	
Procainamide	Flecainide	Mexiletine	
Verapamil	Propafenone	Quinidine	
		Phenytoin	
		Tocainide	

Class I

Class I antiarrhythmic drugs are used to slow the rate of rise of phase 0 of the action potential by blocking the sodium channels in the membrane and eliciting a decrease in the entry of sodium into the membrane. At clinical levels, there is a negligible effect on the resting membrane potential, a decrease in excitability and conduction velocity, and a reduction in automaticity. Class I agents also function as membrane stabilizers.

I. Class Ia drugs

This group of drugs slows conduction, prolongs the refractory period, prolongs the action potential duration, and exhibits the following effects in the ECG tracing: prolongs the PR, QRS, and QT intervals.

A. Quinidine sulfate

1. Application
   a. **Ventricular arrhythmias:** ventricular ectopy and tachycardias.
   b. **Junctional arrhythmias:** junctional ectopy and tachycardias.
   c. **Supraventricular arrhythmias:** atrial ectopy, paroxysmal atrial tachycardia (PAT), atrial fibrillation, and atrial flutter.
   d. ↑PR, QRS, QT.
   e. ↑HR—reflex increase in sympathetic activity.

2. Pharmacokinetics
   a. Apparent **volume of distribution (V_d)**, 2.3 L/kg.
   b. **Protein binding (PB),** 70%-95%.
   c. **Half-life ($T_{1/2}$),** 4-8 hours.
   d. **Therapeutic range,** 2-6 µg/ml (7.3-21.9 µmol/L).
   e. **Bioavailability,** 75%.
   f. **Elimination**—hepatic 80%; renal 10%-20% unchanged.

3. Adverse effects
   a. **Cardiovascular system (CVS):** ↓ myocardial contractility, hypotension, impaired conduction/asystole, arrhythmias (torsades de pointes [1%-2%] due to ↑HR, and ventricular arrhythmias), and peripheral vasodilation.
   b. **Thrombolytic**—antibody-mediated thrombocytopenia.
   c. **GI:** intolerance, diarrhea.
   d. Drug fever.

4. Drug interaction
   a. **Digoxin:** increases serum digoxin levels by 100%.

Table 7-3. Classification by Drug Class

Class Ia	Class Ib	Class Ic	Class II	Class III	Class IV
Quinidine	Lidocaine	Flecainide	β-Blockers	Bretylium tosylate	Calcium channel blockers
Procainamide	Mexiletine	Encainide	Propranolol	Amiodarone	Verapamil
Disopyramide	Phenytoin	Propafenone	Atenolol	Sotalol	Diltiazem
Moricizine	Tocainide		Metoprolol		
			Sotalol		

5. **Dosing**
    a. **Adult**
       (1) 330 to 750 mg—dilute 10 ml preparation in 50 ml D5W and administer at 1 ml/min or give an initial 600 mg IM, then 400 mg q2h.
       (2) **Premature atrial contractions (PACs) and premature ventricular contractions (PVCs):** 200-300 mg TID or QID or loading dose of 12 mg/kg, then maintain at 6 mg/kg q4-6h.
       (3) **Paroxysmal supraventricular tachycardias (PSVTs):** 400-600 mg q2-3h.
       (4) **Conversion of atrial fibrillation:** 200 mg PO q2-3h × 5-8 doses to a maximum of 3-4 gm in any regimen.
       (5) **Maintenance level:** 200-300 mg TID or QID.
       (6) **Extended release preparations** are administered q8-12h.
    b. **Pediatric:** 15-60 mg of base/kg/day PO ÷ q4-6h to 500 mg/dose maximum.

B. **Procainamide**
    1. **Application**
       a. **Ventricular arrhythmias:** ventricular ectopy and tachycardias.
       b. **Junctional arrhythmias:** junctional ectopy and tachycardias.
       c. **Supraventricular arrhythmias:** atrial ectopy, PAT, atrial fibrillation, and atrial flutter.
       d. ↑PR, QRS, QT (less QT prolongation than quinidine).
       e. ↑HR—reflex increase in sympathetic activity.
    2. **Pharmacokinetics**
       a. **Vd,** 1.5-2.5 L/kg.
       b. **PB,** 15%-25%.
       c. **$T_{1/2}$,** 2-4 hours.
       d. **Therapeutic range,** 4-10 µg/ml (17.0-42.5 µmol/L).
       e. **Bioavailability,** 75%-95%.
       f. **Elimination**—hepatic 40%; renal 60% unchanged.
    3. **Adverse effects**
       a. **CVS:** arrhythmogenic, vasodilation if given IV.
       b. **GI:** intolerance.
       c. Lupus-like syndrome.
    4. **Dosing**
       a. **Adult:** Infuse at 20-30 mg/min to a maximum of 17 mg/kg; maintenance levels, set the rate at 1-4 mg/min.
       b. **Pediatric:** 12-15 mg/kg/hr IV over ≤75 minutes to a maximum of 2 gm/day IV loading dose; infuse at 20-80 µg/kg/min or administer at 15-60 mg/kg/day PO ÷ q4-6h to a maximum of 500 mg/dose PO for maintenance levels.

C. Disopyramide
    1. **Application**
       a. **Ventricular arrhythmias.**
       b. ↓SA node discharges.
       c. ↓HR, PR, QRS, QT.
    2. **Pharmacokinetics**
       a. **V_d,** 0.5-1.5 L/kg.
       b. **PB,** 35%-95%.
       c. **$T_{1/2}$,** 6-9 hours.

- d. **Therapeutic range,** 2-5 µg/ml.
  - e. **Bioavailability,** 90%.
  - f. **Elimination**—renal 50% unchanged; hepatic 25%-35%.
 3. **Adverse effects**
    - a. **CVS:** marked inotrope, ventricular arrhythmias (prolonged QT), ↓ myocardial contractility.
    - b. **Anticholinergic** effects cause dry mouth, constipation, urinary retention, and blurred vision.
 4. **Dosing**
    - a. **Adult:** Loading dose is 2 mg/kg IV infusion over 15 minutes to be repeated at 1-2 mg/kg slow IV infusion over 45 minutes, or give 400-800 mg in four divided doses with a single load of 300 mg followed by 100 mg q6h for maintenance levels, then 150-200 mg q6h if necessary.
    - b. **Pediatric:** No clinical value.
- D. Moricizine
  1. **Application**
     - a. **Type Ia.**
     - b. **Ventricular** and supraventricular arrhythmias.
     - c. ↓Premature **ventricular complexes.**
     - d. ↓Nonsustained **ventricular tachycardia.**
  2. **Pharmacokinetics**
     - a. **$T_{1/2}$:** 2-5 hours, 10 hours in cardiac patients, 47 hours in renal insufficiency.
     - b. **Therapeutic range,** 0.1-0.3 µg/ml.
     - c. **Bioavailability,** 38% due to extensive first-pass effect.
     - d. **Elimination**—hepatic 60%; renal 40%.
  3. **Adverse effects**
     - a. **CNS:** dizziness, headache.
     - b. **GI and GU:** nausea, vomiting, urinary retention.
  4. **Dosing**
     - a. **Adult:** 200 mg PO q8h and increase every 3 days by 150 mg/day to maximum of 900 mg/day.
     - b. **Pediatric:** No clinical value.

II. Class Ib drugs

Class Ib agents cause a minor slowing of conduction, elicit no change in refractoriness, and shorten the action potential duration. There are no significant ECG changes caused by this class of drugs.

- A. Lidocaine
  1. **Application**
     - a. **Ventricular** arrhythmias.
     - b. ± ↓**QT** interval.
  2. **Pharmacokinetics**
     - a. **V_d,** 1-2 L/kg.
     - b. **PB,** 65%-75%.
     - c. **$T_{1/2}$,** 0.3-2 hours (100 minutes).
     - d. **Therapeutic range,** 1.5-5 µg/ml (5.7-21.3 µmol/L).
     - e. **Bioavailability,** 65%-75% with extensive first-pass extraction.
     - f. **Elimination,** hepatic 90% dealkylated.
  3. **Adverse effects**
     - a. **CNS:** drowsiness, paresthesias, convulsions with toxic doses.
     - b. **Respiratory:** arrest.

4. Dosing
  a. **Adult:** 1.0-1.5 mg/kg is given initially, followed by 0.5-0.75 mg/kg after 5-10 minutes to a maximum loading dose of 3 mg/kg; a drip can be started at 2-4 mg/min upon converting the rhythm.
  b. **Pediatric:** 0.05 ml/kg/dose (1 mg/kg/dose) IV/endotracheal tube (ETT) given over 2 minutes and repeated every 5 minutes × 2; infuse at 20-50 µg/kg/min (total initial dose = 300 mg or 3 mg/kg, whichever is less).

B. Mexiletine
1. Application
  a. **Ventricular arrhythmias:** ventricular tachycardia.
2. Pharmacokinetics
  a. V_d, 5-9 L/kg.
  b. **PB,** 75%.
  c. $T_{1/2}$, 9-12 hours.
  d. **Therapeutic range,** 0.5-2 µg/ml.
  e. **Bioavailability,** 90%.
  f. **Elimination**—hepatic 90%; renal 10% unchanged.
3. Adverse effects
  a. **GI:** anorexia, nausea.
  b. **CNS:** tremor, visual blurring, dizziness, confusion.
4. Dosing
  a. **Adult:** 400 mg loading dose is given, followed by 200 mg TID to start 8 hours after the loading dose to a maximum of 1200 mg/day given in 3-4 divided doses.
  b. **Pediatric:** 6-8 mg/kg PO loading dose to 1200 mg/day; 6-16 mg/kg/day PO divided TID or QID to a maximum of 600 mg/day PO divided QID.

C. Phenytoin
1. Application
  a. **Noncardiac.**
  b. **Anticonvulsant.**
  c. **Digitalis**-induced arrhythmias and long QT syndromes.
  d. ↓QT interval.
2. Pharmacokinetics
  a. V_d, 0.5-1 L/kg.
  b. **PB,** 90%.
  c. $T_{1/2}$, 18-36 hours.
  d. **Therapeutic range,** 10-20 µg/ml (39.6-79.2 µmol/L).
  e. **Bioavailability,** variable.
  f. **Elimination,** hepatic 95%.
3. Adverse effects
  a. **Nystagmus,** ataxia, lethargy.
  b. **GI:** intolerance.
4. Dosing
  a. **Adult:** 10-15 mg/kg PO or slow IV loading that is not to exceed 50 mg/min IV; for maintenance dose, give 300 mg/day single dose PO or IV, or 100 mg/kg PO or IV q6-8h.
  b. **Pediatric:** 15-20 mg/kg slow IV mixed with NS for a loading dose + simultaneously administer 3 mg/kg/dose × 1, then 6 hours later, 2 mg/kg/dose PO × 1; 5-6 mg/kg/day PO divided q12h for maintenance is given again 6 hours later.

D. Tocainide
  1. **Application**
     a. **Ventricular arrhythmias:** ventricular tachycardia.
     b. ↓QT interval.
  2. **Pharmacokinetics**
     a. **V_d,** 2-3 L/kg.
     b. **PB,** 2%-22%.
     c. **$T_{1/2}$,** 11-15 hours.
     d. **Therapeutic range,** 4-10 µg/ml.
     e. **Bioavailability,** 100%.
     f. **Elimination**—hepatic 60%; renal 40% unchanged.
  3. **Adverse effects**
     a. **GI:** nausea, vomiting.
     b. **CNS:** lightheadedness, dizziness, vertigo, nervousness.
  4. **Dosing**
     a. **Adult:** 400 mg q8h is given initially, followed by 1200-1800 mg/day in divided doses q6-8h to a maximum of 2400 mg ÷ QID q6h; geriatric adjustment is required.
     b. **Pediatric:** No clinical value.

III. Class Ic drugs

Marked slowing of conduction, slight elongation of refractoriness, and no significant effect on the action potential duration are the predominant characteristics exemplified by these drugs. ECG effects are a marked prolongation of the PR and QRS intervals.

A. Encainide
  1. **Application**
     a. **Ventricular arrhythmias:** ventricular tachycardia.
     b. ↑PR, QRS, ↑QT interval
  2. **Pharmacokinetics**
     a. **V_d,** 2.7 L/kg.
     b. **PB,** 70%.
     c. **$T_{1/2}$,** 3 hours.
     d. **Therapeutic range,** 250-1400 ng/ml in absence of metabolites.
     e. **Bioavailability,** 7%-82%.
     f. **Elimination,** hepatic >99% except in poor metabolizers.
  3. **Adverse effects**
     a. **CNS:** headache, dizziness, blurred vision.
     b. Taste perversion, rash, asthenia.
  4. **Dosing**
     a. **Adult:** 25-50 mg q8h to a maximum dose of 200 mg/day.
     b. **Pediatric:** No clinical value.

B. Propafenone
  1. **Application**
     a. ↓Conduction.
     b. ↑PR, QRS, QT.
     c. **Oral treatment** of ventricular arrhythmias: sustained ventricular tachycardia.
  2. **Pharmacokinetics**
     a. **V_d,** 3 L/kg.
     b. **PB,** 95%.
     c. **$T_{1/2}$,** 3-5 hours.

d. **Therapeutic range,** 500-1000 ng/ml.
   e. **Bioavailability,** 5%-12% (dose dependent) due to extensive first-pass effect.
   f. **Elimination,** hepatic >99%.
3. **Adverse effects**
   a. **CVS:** ↓cardiac contractility.
   b. **CNS:** dizziness, altered taste, psychosis.
   c. **GI:** constipation.
4. **Dosing**
   a. **Adult:** 150 mg q8h (450 mg/day) to 300 mg q12h (600 mg/day) to a maximum of 300 mg q8h (900 mg/day).
   b. **Pediatric:** 200-600 mg/m^2/day PO in divided doses TID or QID to a maximum of 900 mg/day, or the usual adult dose of 450-600 mg/day PO divided q8-12h.

Class II Drugs

Class II drugs compose the β-adrenoceptor antagonists commonly referred to as β-blockers, which exert their effect through a competitive inhibition of the β-adrenoceptor site. The predominant effect is the depression of phase 4 depolarization.

A. Propranolol
  1. **Application**
     a. **Prophylactic treatment** of paroxysmal atrial tachycardia.
     b. ↓Automaticity.
     c. ↓HR.
  2. **Pharmacokinetics**
     a. **V$_d$,** 3-4 L/kg.
     b. **PB,** 25%-50%.
     c. **T$_{1/2}$,** 3-6 hours.
     d. **Therapeutic range,** 50-100 ng/ml (192.8-385.5 nmol/L).
     e. **Bioavailability,** 85%-95% high first-pass effect.
     f. **Elimination,** hepatic >95%.
  3. **Adverse Effects**
     a. **CVS:** negative inotrope, ↓ contractility, hypotension, bradycardia to asystole.
     b. **CNS:** nightmares, insomnia.
     c. **Respiratory:** bronchospasm.
  4. **Dosing**
     a. **Adult:** 0.1 mg/kg slow IV push at 2- to 3-minute intervals administered to a maximum rate of 1 mg/min; the PO maintenance dose is 180-320 mg/day given in divided doses.
     b. **Pediatric: Arrhythmias,** 0.01-0.15 mg/kg/dose IV q6-8h prn to a maximum of 3 mg/dose IV; **Wolff-Parkinson-White** syndrome, 2-10 mg/kg/day PO ÷ TID or QID.

B. Esmolol
  1. **Application**
     a. **Prolongation** of sinus node recovery time.
     b. **Prolongation** of the atrium–His bundle (AH).
     c. ↓HR.
     d. **Atrial fibrillation** and atrial flutter.

e. **Prevention** of automatic and reentrant SVTs.
f. **Ventricular** arrhythmias.
g. **Digitalis-induced** arrhythmias.
2. **Pharmacokinetics**
   a. **T$_{1/2}$,** 10.9 hours.
3. **Adverse effects**
   a. **CVS:** hypotension and bradycardias.
   b. **CNS:** dizziness, headache, and somnolence.
4. **Dosing**
   a. **Adult:** Loading dose is 0.5 mg/kg/min over 1 minute, followed by a 4-minute maintenance infusion at 0.05 µg/kg/min; if no response, repeat the loading dose and give a maintenance dosage of 100 µg/kg/min to a maximum of 200 µg/kg/min; titrate by repeating the loading dose and increasing every 4 minutes by 50 µg/kg/min for maintenance.
   b. **Pediatric:** No clinical value.

Class III Drugs

Class III agents primarily operate by extending the duration of the action potential, causing an increase in the absolute and effective refractory periods.

A. Bretylium tosylate
   1. **Application**
      a. Ventricular fibrillation and ventricular tachycardia
      b. ↓HR
      c. ↑QT
   2. **Pharmacokinetics**
      a. **V$_d$,** 5-6 L/kg.
      b. **PB,** <10%.
      c. **T$_{1/2}$,** 6-10 hours.
      d. **Therapeutic range,** 0.5-1.5 µg/ml.
      e. **Bioavailability,** 15%-30%.
      f. **Elimination,** renal 80% unchanged.
   3. **Adverse effects**
      a. **CVS:** orthostatic hypotension, arrhythmogenic.
      b. **GI:** nausea, vomiting, diarrhea.
      c. **Endocrine:** parotitis with long-term oral treatment.
   4. **Dosing**
      a. **Adult:** Initially administered at 5-10 mg/kg IV push over 1-2 minutes; loading dose is 5 mg/kg, followed by a continuous infusion of 1-2 mg/min (2 gm in 500 ml D5W at 30 ml/hr).
      b. **Pediatric:** 5.0 mg/kg IV, which is repeated at 10 mg/kg if first dose is not effective, with a maximum of three repeated doses.

B. Amiodarone
   1. **Application**
      a. **Recurrent** ventricular tachycardia and ventricular fibrillation.
      b. **Wolff-Parkinson-White** syndrome arrhythmias.
      c. ↑HR, QT.
      d. **Prolongs** action potential duration and end-refractory period.
      e. **Slows** phase 4 depolarization.

- f. **Slows conduction.**
- g. **Weak** β-blocker.
- h. **Weak** calcium channel blocker.

2. **Pharmacokinetics**
   - a. **V$_d$,** very large L/kg.
   - b. **PB,** high.
   - c. **T$_{1/2}$,** 20-50 days.
   - d. **Therapeutic range,** 0.5-3 µg/ml.
   - e. **Bioavailability,** 20%-50%.
   - f. **Elimination,** hepatic via deethylation.

3. **Adverse effects**
   - a. **CVS:** bradycardia, hypotension, arrhythmogenic.
   - b. **CNS:** central and peripheral neuropathies, tremor, ataxia, corneal microdeposits.
   - c. **Respiratory:** pulmonary interstitial fibrosis.
   - d. **Endocrine:** hyperthyroid and hypothyroid states.
   - e. **MSK:** muscle weakness.
   - f. **Skin:** blue-grey facial discoloration.
   - g. **Liver** abnormalities.

4. **Dosing**
   - a. **Adult:** 800-1600 mg/day loading dose and a maintenance dose of 200-400 mg/day.
   - b. **Pediatric:** 10 mg/kg/day PO single dose or BID × 7-10 days loading to a maximum of 800-1600 mg/day; 5 mg/kg/day PO single dose to a maximum 200-400 mg/day for maintenance.

C. Sotalol
   1. **Application**
      - a. **Class II and III.**
      - b. **WPW syndrome,** AV nodal reentrant SVT, SV arrhythmias, ventricular arrhythmias.
      - c. **Prolongs action potential** duration and end-refractory period.
      - d. Competitive β-**blocker.**
      - e. ↓Phase 4 **depolarization.**
      - f. ↓AV **conduction.**
      - g. ↑QT, ↓HR.
   2. **Pharmacokinetics**
      - a. **V$_d$,** 1.5 L/kg.
      - b. **PB,** negligible.
      - c. **T$_{1/2}$,** 13 hours.
      - d. **Therapeutic range,** 1-2 µg/ml (3.7-7.4 µmol/L).
      - e. **Bioavailability,** 95%.
      - f. **Elimination,** renal 100%.
   3. **Adverse effects**
      - a. **CVS:** left ventricular failure, torsades de pointes, hypotension, ↑QT interval.
      - b. **CNS:** fatigue, lethargy.
   4. **Dosing**
      - a. **Adult:** 80 mg BID given initially to 160-320 mg ÷ bid to a maximum of 480 mg/day.
      - b. **Pediatric:** 2-10 mg/kg/day PO ÷ bid to 480 mg/day.

Class IV Drugs

Class IV antiarrhythmic drugs, commonly known as calcium channel blockers, cause a decrease in the rate of rise of phase 4 spontaneous depolarization, and slow conduction in calcium current–dependent tissues. This occurs by decreasing the amount of calcium readily available for cell membrane displacement and concomitantly decreasing the inward current carried by calcium.

A. Verapamil
  1. **Application**
     a. **IV:** PSVT, control of ventricular response in atrial fibrillation or atrial flutter not associated with accessory pathway syndromes.
     b. **Slows** AV node conduction.
     c. ↑**Refractory period** in AV node.
     d. ↑PR interval.
  2. **Pharmacokinetics**
     a. V_d, 4-5 L/kg.
     b. **PB,** 90%.
     c. $T_{1/2}$, 3-7 hours.
     d. **Therapeutic range,** ≅100 ng/L.
     e. **Bioavailability,** 15%-30%.
     f. **Elimination,** hepatic.
  3. **Adverse effects**
     a. **CVS:** ↓contractility, hypotension, bradycardia/asystole.
     b. **GI:** nausea, vomiting, constipation.
  4. **Dosing**
     a. **Adult:** 2.5-5 mg initially IV over 2 minutes and repeated at a dosage of 5-10 mg every 15-30 minutes to a maximum dose of 20 mg.
     b. **Pediatric:** Birth to 2 years of age, 0.1-0.2 mg/kg/dose IV; 2-15 years of age, 0.1-0.3 mg/kg/dose IV which may be repeated × 1 in 30 minutes prn to a maximum 10 mg/dose IV—maintained ECG monitoring; the maintenance dose is 2-10 mg/kg/day PO ÷ TID/QID to maximum dose of 240-480 mg/day.

Cardiac Arrest Drugs: Advanced Cardiac Life Support (ACLS)

ACLS is a composite of basic life support (BLS), ECG rhythm recognition, interpretation and monitoring, the use of specialized equipment and techniques, intravenous therapy, and stabilization utilizing antiarrhythmic agents. The clinician should have detailed knowledge of the pharmacokinetic and pharmacodynamic principles of each of these ACLS drugs. Rapid pharmacologic control of life-threatening dysrhythmias is paramount for increasing the patient's probability for survival.

A. Oxygen
  1. **Application**
     a. **Hypoxemic patients.**
     b. ↑ **Arterial O_2** tension (PaO_2) and ↑ arterial O_2 content.
     c. **Acute chest pain** due to cardiac ischemia.
     d. **If breathing,** titrate according to PaO_2 and O_2 saturation values.

2. **Delivery devices**
   a. **Nasal cannula**—low-flow system, normal tidal volume with flows 1-6 L/min delivers 24%-44% oxygen.
   b. **Face mask**—at 8-10 L/min, oxygen concentration is 40%-60%.
   c. **Face mask with oxygen reservoir**—at 6 L/min, $[O_2]$ = 60%; at 10 L/min, $[O_2]$ = 100%.
   d. **Venturi mask**—high-flow system used for chronic hypercarbia and moderate to severe hypoxemia; 24%, 28%, 35%, 40% oxygen concentrations with O_2 flow rates of 4, 4, 8, and 8 L/min, respectively.
3. **Adverse effects**
   a. **Respiratory depression** due to sudden ↑ in PaO_2; titrate to desired PaO_2 level.
4. **Oxygen delivery**
   a. **Bag-valve resuscitator.**
   b. **Manually triggered O_2**—powered breathing device.
   c. **Positive pressure ventilator** with 100% oxygen.
5. **Rate**
   a. **Adult:** 10-15 L/min at 100% concentration depending on route of administration.
   b. **Pediatric:** 5-15 L/min at 100% concentration depending on route of administration; humidify to prevent drying and thickening of pulmonary secretions.

B. Epinephrine
1. **Application**
   a. **Circulatory shock** and cardiopulmonary resuscitation (CPR)—ACLS.
   b. ↑ **Systemic vascular resistance**.
   c. ↑ **Arterial BP,** HR, automaticity, myocardial contraction.
   d. ↑ **Myocardial oxygen** requirements.
   e. ↑ **Coronary** and cerebral blood flow.
   f. **Potent β- and α-adrenoceptor agonist.**
   g. ↑ **Blood glucose,** lactic acid, and respiration.
2. **Pharmacokinetics**
   a. **V_d,** unknown.
   b. **PB,** 50%.
   c. **$T_{1/2}$,** few minutes.
   d. **Bioavailability,** 0% oral and 10% aerosol.
   e. **Elimination,** renal.
3. **Adverse effects**
   a. **Do not mix** epinephrine in same bag containing alkaline solution (i.e., $NaHCO_3$).
   b. 20 µg/min or 0.3 µg/kg/min produces hypertension in non-CPR situations.
   c. **CVA:** may exacerbate ventricular ectopy and myocardial ischemia.
   d. **Acute:** anxiety, palpitations, tremor, headache, fear, dizziness.
4. **Dosing**
   a. **Adult:** 0.5-1.0 mg IV push in a 1:10,000 dilution every 3-5 minutes; 1 mg to 500 ml NS or D5W given at 1 µg/min initial infusion and titrate to produce effect (2-10 µg/min).
   b. **Pediatric**
      (1) **Resuscitation**—0.1 ml/kg IV/ETT; minimum 1 ml: infuse at 0.1-1 µg/kg/min IV.

(2) **Bradycardia**—0.01 mg/kg (1:10,000) IV/IO (intraosseous route) or 0.1 mg/kg (1:1000) ET.

C. Atropine
  1. **Application**
     a. **Abolition** of reflex vagal cardiac slowing or asystole.
     b. **Sinus node** automaticity.
     c. **AV** conduction.
     d. **Symptomatic** bradycardia and asystole.
     e. **Pulseless** idioventricular rhythms (potential).
     f. **Competitive antagonism** of acetylcholine and muscarinic cholinergic receptors.
  2. **Pharmacokinetics**
     a. **V_d,** 2-4 L/kg.
     b. **PB,** 50%.
     c. **$T_{1/2}$,** biphasic: 2-4 hours and 13-38 hours.
     d. **Bioavailability,** 80% orally.
     e. **Elimination,** renal unchanged.
  3. **Adverse effects**
     a. **CVS:** tachycardia and ventricular fibrillation after IV administration, bradycardia.
     b. **Xerostomia,** mydriasis, urinary retention, respiratory failure, convulsions.
     c. **CNS:** delirium, coma, flushed and hot skin, ataxia, blurred vision.
  4. **Dosing**
     a. **Adult:** 0.5-1.0 mg IV push every 3-5 minutes to a maximum of 0.04 mg/kg (3 mg).
     b. **Pediatric:** 0.2 ml/kg IV/ETT; minimum 1 ml every 5 minutes (0.02 mg/kg; minimum 0.1 mg) to a maximum of 20 ml (2 mg) total or 0.4 ml/kg.

D. $NaHCO_3$
  1. **Application**
     a. **Documented preexisting metabolic acidosis** with or without hyperkalemia.
     b. **Determine necessity** by measuring arterial pH and P_{CO_2}.
  2. **Adverse effects**
     a. ↑ **Intracellular acidosis** during CPR.
     b. ↑ **Cerebrospinal fluid** and central venous acidosis during CPR.
  3. **Dosing**
     a. **Adult:** 1 mEq/kg initial IV push over 30-60 seconds; subsequently, 0.5 mEq/kg every 10 minutes.
     b. **Pediatric:** 2-3 ml/kg IV initially; subsequent doses require ABG monitoring and are given at 1-2 ml/kg every 10-20 minutes of arrest time.

E. Morphine
  1. **Application**
     a. ↑ **Venous capacitance.**
     b. ↓ **Systemic vascular resistance,** intramyocardial wall tension, myocardial oxygen requirements.
     c. **Ischemic** chest pain.
     d. **Acute cardiogenic** pulmonary edema.
     e. **MI-associated** pain and anxiety.
  2. **Pharmacokinetics**
     a. **V_d,** 3 L/kg.
     b. **PB,** 35%.

c. $T_{1/2}$, 2-3 hours.
d. **Bioavailability,** 20%-33% orally.
e. **Elimination,** renal 90%.

3. **Adverse effects**
   a. **Narcosis,** reversed by naloxone: adult: 0.4-2.0 mg IV.
   b. **CVS:** hypotension and HR variances.
   c. **Acute:** respiratory depression, coma, hypothermia.
   d. **CNS:** dysphoria, drowsiness, pupillary constriction.
   e. **GI:** nausea, constipation.

4. **Dosing**
   a. **Adult:** 1-3 mg IV every 5 minutes; 15-30 mg IM q4h as analgesia.
   b. **Pediatric:** 0.1-0.2 mg/kg IV loading dose; 0.01-0.02 mg/kg/hr IV continuous infusion for maintenance.

F. Dopamine

1. **Application**
   a. **Stimulates norepinephrine** at low dosage of 1-2 µg/kg/min.
   b. **Stimulates β$_1$- and α-adrenergic receptors** at 2-10 µg/kg/min.
   c. ↑ Carbon monoxide.
   d. **Stimulates α-adrenergic effects** at 10 µg/kg/min resulting in renal mesenteric, peripheral arterial, and venous vasoconstriction with marked increase in systemic vascular resistance and preload.
   e. **Hemodynamically significant hypotension** (systolic BP <90 mm Hg) in absence of hypovolemia.

2. **Adverse effects**
   a. **Do not administer** with volumetric infusion pumps.
   b. **CVS:** may exacerbate supraventricular and ventricular arrhythmias.
   c. **GI:** nausea, vomiting.
   d. **Serious acute hypertension** in patients with pheochromocytoma.
   e. **Do not add** to $NaHCO_3$ or alkaline IV solutions.

3. **Dosing**
   a. **Adult:** 1 or 2 ampules (400 mg/ampule) IV in 250 ml D5W, which equals 1600 or 3200 µg/ml to a final dosage of 5-20 µg/kg/min, the initial infusion rate is 2.5-5 µg/kg/min (use lowest rate to minimize side effects).
   b. **Pediatric:** Infuse at 5-20 µg/kg/min IV to a maximum of 25 µg/kg/min.

G. Isoproterenol

1. **Application**
   a. Positive chronotropic and inotropic activity
   b. ↓ Mean BP
   c. ↑ Myocardial oxygen requirements
   d. Vasodilatory effects

2. **Pharmacokinetics**
   a. V_d, 0.7 L/kg.
   b. **PB,** 65%.
   c. $T_{1/2}$, 2 hours.
   d. **Bioavailability**—0% orally; 80%-100% by inhalation.
   e. **Elimination**—renal 50% free, 50% methylated.

3. **Adverse effects**
   a. **CVS:** cardiac arrest, ischemic heart disease, ventricular tachycardia and fibrillation, palpitations exacerbate tachycardic arrhythmias due to digitalis toxicity or hypokalemia, flushing, angina, sweating.
   b. **CNS:** tremor, headache, nausea.

Cardiac Arrest Drugs: Advanced Cardiac Life Support (ACLS)

4. **Dosing**
   a. **Adult:** Infuse initially at 2-10 µg/min titrated until HR is 60 beats/min by mixing 1 mg in 500 ml D5W (2 µg/ml concentration).
   b. **Pediatric:** 0.3 ml/kg (3 µg/kg) IV/ETT to a maximum of 100 µg; for a continuous infusion, set the dosage at 0.05-1.0 µg/kg/min IV.

H. Digitalis (digoxin)
  1. **Application**
     a. ↑ **Myocardial contraction.**
     b. ↑ **Rate** of atrial conduction.
     c. **Control ventricular response** to atrial flutter and fibrillation, PAT, PSVT.
     d. **Direct** and indirect effects on SA and AV nodes.
  2. **Pharmacokinetics**
     a. **V_d,** 7.3 L/kg.
     b. **PB,** 30%.
     c. **$T_{1/2}$,** 20-50 hours.
     d. **Therapeutic range,** 0.5-2 ng/ml.
     e. **Onset of action,** 5-30 minutes.
     f. **Peak effect,** 1.5-3 hours.
     g. **Bioavailability,** 75% orally.
     h. **Elimination,** renal unchanged.
  3. **Adverse effects**
     a. **CVS:** atrial and ventricular premature complexes, ventricular bigeminy, ventricular tachycardia, accelerated junctional rhythm or nonparoxysmal junctional tachycardia, PAT with 2:1 AV block, AV block.
     b. **GI:** anorexia, nausea, vomiting, diarrhea.
     c. **CNS:** agitation, visual disturbances, psychosis, lassitude.
     d. **Toxicity:** frequent with hypokalemia, hypomagnesemia, +/− hypocalcemia.
     e. **Toxicity treatment:** stop drug, correct signs and symptoms, treat arrhythmias, cardiovert with very low energy levels (10-20 J), antidigoxin antibodies for massive digoxin overdose or refractory digitalis toxicity.
     f. **Drug interaction: quinidine** increases the digitalis blood levels 2- to 4-fold; **diuretics** may cause potassium depletion → digoxin toxicity; **amiodarone and spironolactone** ↑ digoxin blood levels.
  4. **Dosing**
     a. **Adult:** Loading dose is 5-8 µg/kg of lean body weight (LBW) for therapeutic effect; 0.75-1.5 mg given slowly IV with a maintenance dosage of 0.25-0.75 mg/day; acute oral digitalizing, 1.5-2 mg over 24 hours.
     b. **Pediatric:**
        (1) **Digitalizing dose:** 3 doses—1st STAT, 2nd in 6 hours, 3rd in next 6 hours with a total digitalizing dose of 1.0 mg (when terminating a tachycardia, a total digitalization dose is ÷ 1/2, 1/4, 1/4).

	IV	PO
<37 wk gestation	0.005 mg/kg/dose	0.007 mg/kg/dose
≥37 wk-2 yr	0.012 mg/kg/dose	0.017 mg/kg/dose
>2 yr	0.01 mg/kg/dose	0.013 mg/kg/dose

        (2) **Maintenance dose**

	IV	PO
<37 wk gestation	0.003 mg/kg/day ÷ q12hr	0.004 mg/kg/day ÷ q12hr
≥37 wk-2 yr	0.007 mg/kg/day ÷ q12hr	0.01 mg/kg/day ÷ q12hr or

		0.01 mg/kg/day ÷ BID/single
>2 yrs	—	0.008 mg/kg/day ÷ BID/single

The maintenance dose limit is 0.25 mg/day.

Life-threatening Arrhythmias

This section subdivides each arrhythmia into three aspects: clinical definition, salient features of the ECG, and medical management. A separate section is devoted to the crucial pharmacokinetic profile of each of the predominant antiarrhythmic drugs.

I. **Normal sinus rhythm**
   A. **Definition:** Regular discharge of the SA node producing atrial depolarization at a rate of 60-100 beats/min.
   B. Salient features

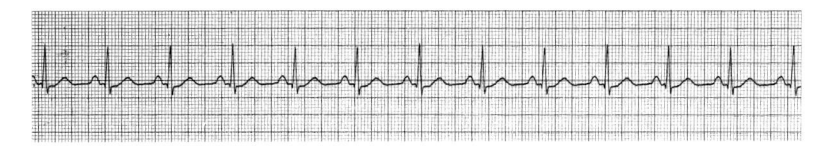

   1. **Rate:** 60-100 beats/min.
   2. **Rhythm:** regular.
   3. **P wave:** upright in leads I, II, a VF.

II. **Ventricular fibrillation (VF), pulseless ventricular tachycardia (VT), pulseless electrical activity (PEA), and asystole**
   A. Definition
   1. **VF. Complete absence** of properly formed ventricular complexes with baseline waver and no attempts at forming evident QRS deflections.
   2. **VT**
      a. **Three or more** consecutive ectopic ventricular complexes (wide QRS complexes >0.12 seconds) recurring at a rapid rate culminating in severe circulatory compromise.
      b. **Pressure gradients** are created between intrathoracic and extrathoracic veins, which aid circulation despite the absence of effective cardiac contraction.
      c. **VT is divided into sustained,** greater than 30 seconds in duration, and nonsustained, which is less than 30 seconds in duration.
   3. **PEA**
      a. **Electrical activity** without effective mechanical contraction.
      b. Usually **represents terminal arrhythmias** in end-stage heart disease.
      c. **Etiologic mechanisms** may include a tension pneumothorax and hypovolemia.
   4. **Asystole. Complete absence** of electrical and controlled mechanical activity.
   B. Salient features
      1. **VF**

Life-threatening Arrhythmias 221

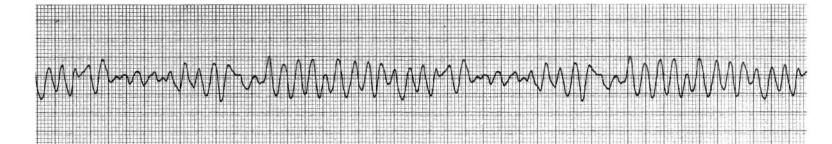

- a. **Disorganized ventricular complexes** with loss of organized cardiac contraction.
- b. **Rate:** rapid but not readily countable.
- c. **Rhythm:** irregular.
- d. **No P wave,** QRS, ST segment, or T wave.
- e. **May appear** as asystole in one lead.

2. **VT**

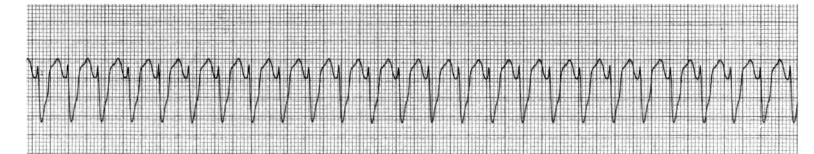

- a. **Very wide** QRS >140 msec.
- b. **Left axis** deviation $<-30°$.
- c. **For RBBB-like** QRS pattern: V_1, monophasic R or QR or RS pattern; V_6, R/S ratio <1 and monophasic R or QS or QR pattern.
- d. **For LBBB-like** QRS pattern: V_1, R wave width >30 msec or R to S interval >60 msec; V_6, QR or QS pattern.
- e. **Rate:** between 100 and 200 beats/min.
- f. **Rhythm:** usually regular
- g. **P wave** in rapid VT is not present or recognizable.
- h. **Fixed** QRS - P wave relationship.

3. **PEA**

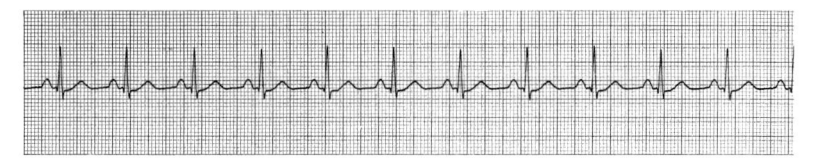

- a. **ECG** appears normal; however, the patient has no discernible pulse or blood pressure.

4. **Asystole**

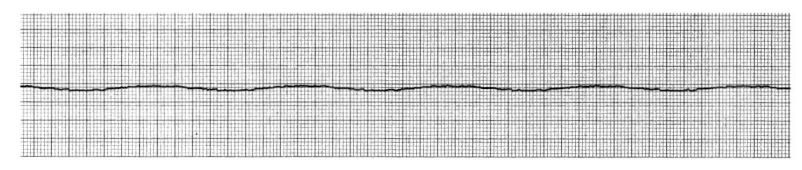

- a. **Rate:** 0.
- b. **P wave** may occur.

C. Management
  1. **Preliminary treatment**
     a. **Assess** level of consciousness.

Ch 7. Cardiac Arrhythmias and Antiarrhythmic Drugs

   b. **Assess** airway, breathing, and circulation (ABC).
   c. **Begin CPR** until defibrillator is available.
   d. **Place** patient on bed board.
   e. **Start** 100% oxygen and telemetry.
   f. **Assess** rhythm.
  2. **Management of ventricular fibrillation and pulseless ventricular tachycardia (VF and VT) (Fig. 7-1).**
  3. **Management of pulseless electrical activity (PEA) and asystole (Fig. 7-2).**

III. Wolff-Parkinson-White syndrome (WPW)
  A. Definition
   1. **Preexcitation syndrome** defined as an early depolarization of ventricular parenchymal myocardium utilizing alternative atrium-to-ventricle conduction pathways that replace the usual AV node–bundle of His–Purkinje system pathway.
   2. Due to accessory pathways or Kent bundles.
  B. Salient features

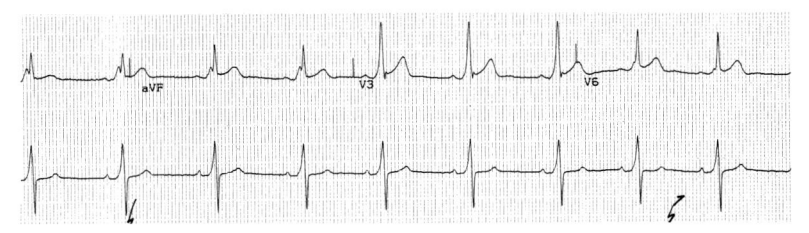

   1. **Characterized by** a delta wave or slurred initial uptake of the QRS associated with a PR interval of 0.12 seconds or less.
   2. **Patterns:** type A, accessory pathway in the left AV groove; type B, accessory pathway in the right AV groove.
   3. **Do not confuse** with ischemic heart disease, conduction system disease, right ventricular hypertrophy, and vice versa.
   4. **Use delta wave** morphology to predict the pathway location.
  C. Management of WPW syndrome
   1. **Vagal maneuvers.**
   2. **Cardiovert at 50 J.**
   3. **Laboratory:** CBC, ABGs, CXR, 12-lead ECG, and 24-hour Holter.
   4. **Quinidine gluconate,** 15 mg/kg in 150 ml D5W over 4-6 hours loading dose, followed by 8 mg/kg/hr infusion (↓25% in patients with CHF); **OR quinidine sulfate,** 400 mg PO q2-4 hr × 2 doses for loading, followed by **quinidine gluconate,** 330 mg IM or PO q8h; **OR quinidine gluconate,** 330 mg IM or PO q2-4h × 2 doses, then 330 mg IM or PO q8h.
   5. **Then Procainamide,** IV loading dose of 20 mg/min until maximum total dose of 1 gm, then 2-6 mg/min IV maintenance; or PO loading dose of 750-1000 mg, then 0.5-1 gm PO q4-6h (50 mg/kg/day in 6-8 doses); **OR Propranolol,** 1-5 mg IV in 1 mg aliquots/min, then 60-80 mg PO TID; **OR Propafenone,** 150-300 mg PO q8h with a maximum of 1200 mg/day; **OR Adenosine** (may ↑ bypass tract conduction), 6 mg rapid IV over 1-2 seconds followed by a saline flush, then repeat 12 mg IV after 2-3 minutes to maximum of 30 mg total dose.

IV. Ventricular ectopy

Life-threatening Arrhythmias 223

A. Definition: Abnormal impulse generation from enhanced automaticity; for example, multifocal PVCs.

B. Salient features

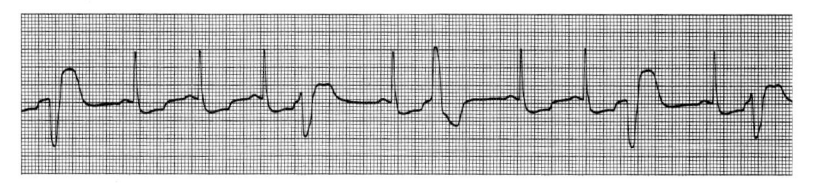

1. **Modified grading system**
   a. **<30** uniform ventricular premature beats (VPBs)/hr.
      (1) <1/min.
      (2) >1/min.
   b. **>30** uniform VPBs/hr.
   c. **Multiform** VPBs.
   d. **Couplets** (two consecutive VPBs).
   e. **Triplets** (three or more consecutive VPBs).
   f. **R-on-T phenomenon.**
2. In the presence of PVCs in patients with acute heart disease (i.e., MI or in patients with severe chest pain), start lidocaine immediately.

C. Management of ventricular ectopy **(Fig. 7-3).**

V. Sinus tachycardia

A. Definition
   1. **An increased sinus node discharge rate** manifested as a sinus rhythm with a heart rate >100 beats/min.
   2. **A response to stimuli** rather than a cause; hence, treat the underlying cause.

B. Salient features

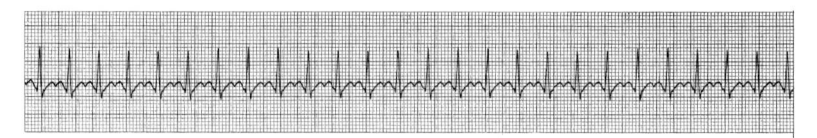

   1. **Rate:** >100 beats/min.
   2. **Rhythm:** regular.
   3. **P waves** present upright in leads I, II, and a VF.

C. Management of sinus tachycardia **(Fig. 7-4).**

VI. Multifocal atrial tachycardia (MAT)

A. Definition: Multiple atrial sites possessing automatic pacemaker activity producing multiple, irregular, rapid, but discrete P waves.

B. Salient features

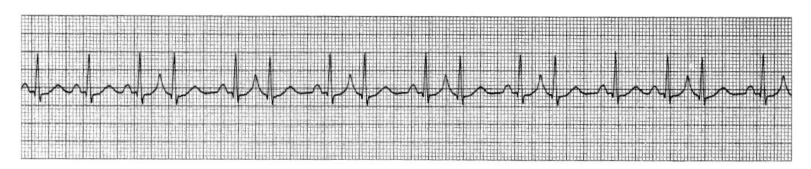

   1. **P waves** cause irregularly irregular QRS complexes mimicking atrial fibrillation—MAT is distinguished by the definable P waves.
   2. **Varying PR interval** with an atrial rate of 100-200 beats/min.

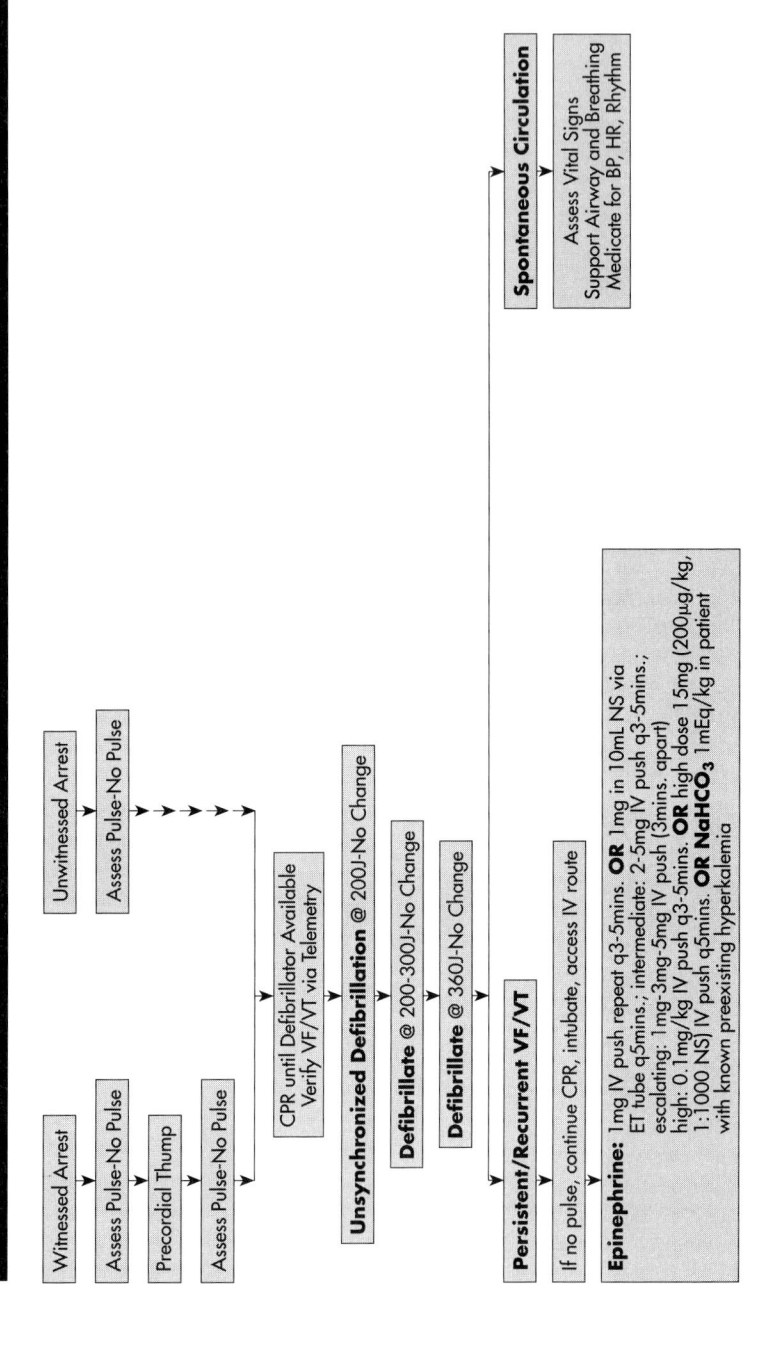

Figure 7-1. Algorithm for Ventricular Fibrillation and Pulseless Ventricular Tachycardia (VF & VT)

Witnessed Arrest
→ Assess Pulse-No Pulse
→ Precordial Thump
→ Assess Pulse-No Pulse

Unwitnessed Arrest
→ Assess Pulse-No Pulse

→ CPR until Defibrillator Available
Verify VF/VT via Telemetry

Unsynchronized Defibrillation @ 200J-No Change

Defibrillate @ 200-300J-No Change

Defibrillate @ 360J-No Change

Persistent/Recurrent VF/VT

If no pulse, continue CPR, intubate, access IV route

Epinephrine: 1mg IV push repeat q3-5mins. **OR** 1mg in 10mL NS via ET tube q5mins.; intermediate: 2-5mg IV push q3-5mins.; escalating: 1mg-3mg-5mg IV push (3mins. apart) high: 0.1mg/kg IV push q3-5mins. **OR** high dose 15mg (200µg/kg, 1:1000 NS) IV push q5mins. **OR NaHCO₃** 1mEq/kg in patient with known preexisting hyperkalemia

Spontaneous Circulation
→ Assess Vital Signs
Support Airway and Breathing
Medicate for BP, HR, Rhythm

Life-threatening Arrhythmias

- **Defibrillate** @ 360J within 30-60secs. post medication
- **Lidocaine:** 1.5mg/kg IV push q3-5mins. to total loading dose 3mg/kg
- **Defibrillate** @ 360J within 30-60secs. post medication
- **Bretylium** 5mg/kg IV push & repeat in 5mins. @ 10mg/kg **OR** repeat **Lidocaine** and **Defibrillate**
- **MgSO$_4$**, 1-2mg IV in Torsades or suspected hypomagnesemic states or severe refractory VF **OR Procainamide** 30mg/min. in refractory VF (max 17mg/kg total)
- **NaHCO$_3$:** 1mEq/kg IV if: known preexisting bicarbonate responsive acidosis, OD on tricyclic antidepressants, and intubated and continued long arrest interval (LAI); to: alkalinize urine in drug OD; upon: return to spontaneous circulation after LAI or hypoxic lactic acidosis
- **Defibrillate** @ 360J within 30-60secs. post medication
- Repeat **Bretylium** 10mg/kg (700mg) IV push q5-10mins. to max 30mg/kg total **OR** repeat **Lidocaine** as above
- **Defibrillate** @ 360J within 30-60secs. post medication
- Repeat **Bretylium OR Lidocaine-Defibrillate** @ 360J & consider **Procainamide** 1g IV over 30mins., then 1-4mg/min. **OR Internal Defibrillation**
- If indicated, **Lidocaine infusion** @ 2-4mg/min. (2g in 500mL D5W @ 30mL/hr.=2mg/min. **and/OR Bretylium infusion** @ 1-4mg/min. (2g in 500mL D5W @ 30mL/hr.-2mg/min.)

226 Ch 7. Cardiac Arrhythmias and Antiarrhythmic Drugs

Figure 7-2. Algorithm for Pulseless Electrical Activity (PEA) and Aystole

Witnessed Arrest → Assess Pulse-No Pulse → Precordial Thump → Assess Pulse-No Pulse

Unwitnessed Arrest → Assess Pulse-No Pulse

↓

CPR until Defibrillator Available
Verify VF/VT via Telemetry

Unsynchronized Defibrillation @ 200J-No Change

Defibrillate @ 200-300J-No Change

Defibrillate @ 360J-No Change

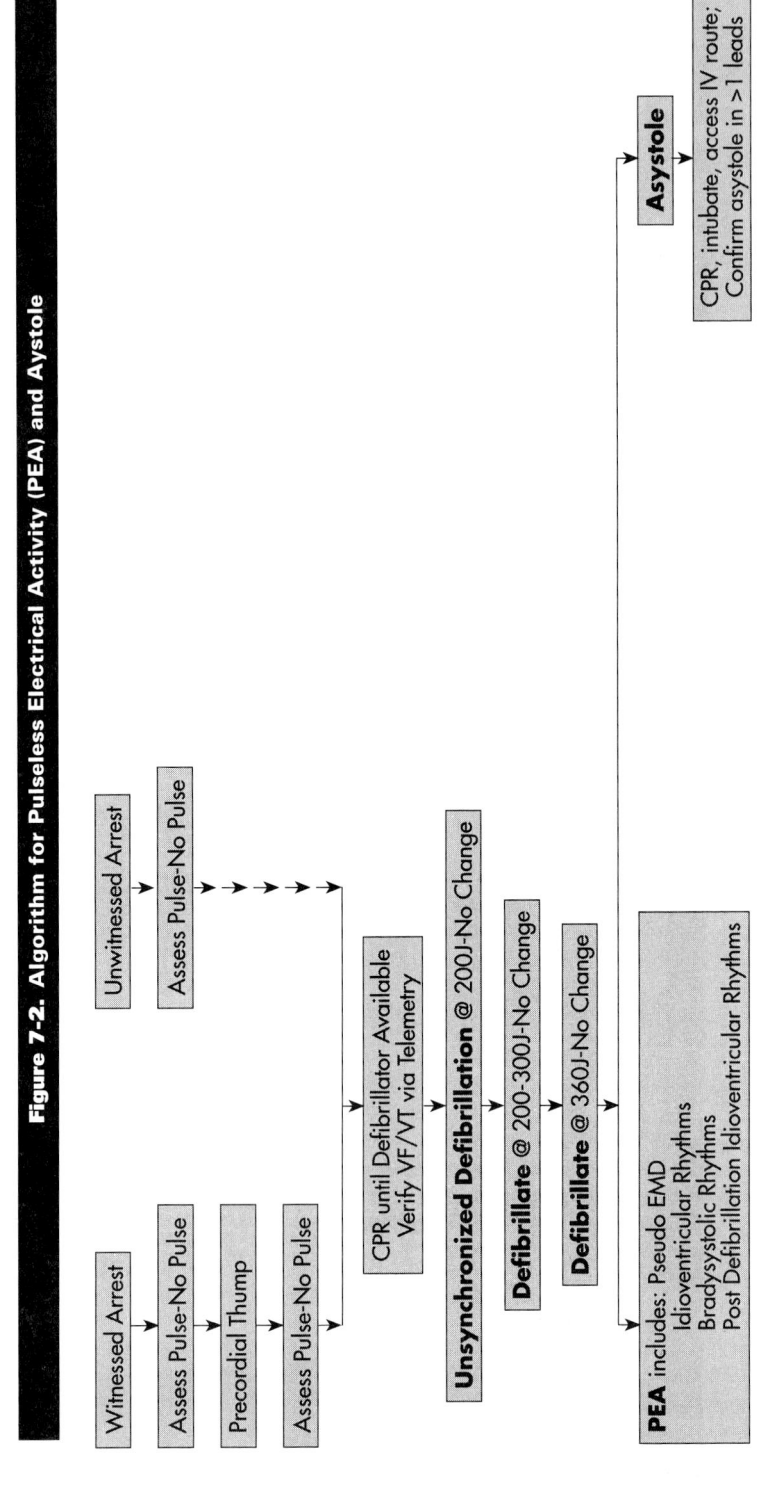

PEA includes: Pseudo EMD
Idioventricular Rhythms
Bradysystolic Rhythms
Post Defibrillation Idioventricular Rhythms

Asystole
CPR, intubate, access IV route;
Confirm asystole in >1 leads

Life-threatening Arrhythmias

→ Determine etiology & treat:
- Hypoxia
- Hyperkalemia
- Hypokalemia
- Preexisting Acidosis
- Drug OD
- Hypothermia

↓

TCP-perform early and simultaneously with drugs

↓

Epinephrine: 1mg IV push q3-5mins., if no change: intermediate: 2-5mg IV push q3-5mins.; escalating: 1mg-3mg-5mg IV push (3mins. apart); high: 0.1mg/kg IV push q3-5mins. **OR NaCO$_3$** 1mEq/kg in patient with known preexisting hyperkalemia; high dose: 15mg (200μg/kg; 1:1000 NS) IV push q5mins.

↓

Atropine: 1mg IV q3-5mins. to total 0.04mg/kg
- shorter dosing intervals in asystolic arrest
NaCO$_3$ 1mEq/kg

Consider Termination of Efforts

→ CPR, intubate, access IV route, assess BF via Dopler U/S

↓

Determine etiology & treat:
- Hypovolemia (volume infusion)
- Hypoxia (ventilate)
- Cardiac Tamponade (pericardiocentesis)
- Tension Pneumothorax (needle decompression)
- Hypothermia
- Massive PE (Sx & thrombolytics)
- Drug OD
- Hyperkalemia (NaCO$_3$ 1mEq/kg)
- Acidosis (NaCO$_3$ 1mEq/kg)
- Massive Acute MI

↓

Epinephrine: 1mg IV push q3-5mins., if fails: intermediate: 2-5mg IV push q3-5mins. escalating: 1mg-3mg-5mg IV push (3mins. apart) high: 0.1mg/kg IV push q3-5mins. **OR** if known, preexisting hyperkalemia, **NaHCO$_3$** 1mEq/kg

↓

If relative or absolute bradycardia (<60bpm), **Atropine** 1mg IV q3-5mins. to total 0.04mg/kg - shorten dosing interval in cardiac arrest

Figure 7-3. Algorithm for Ventricular Ectopy

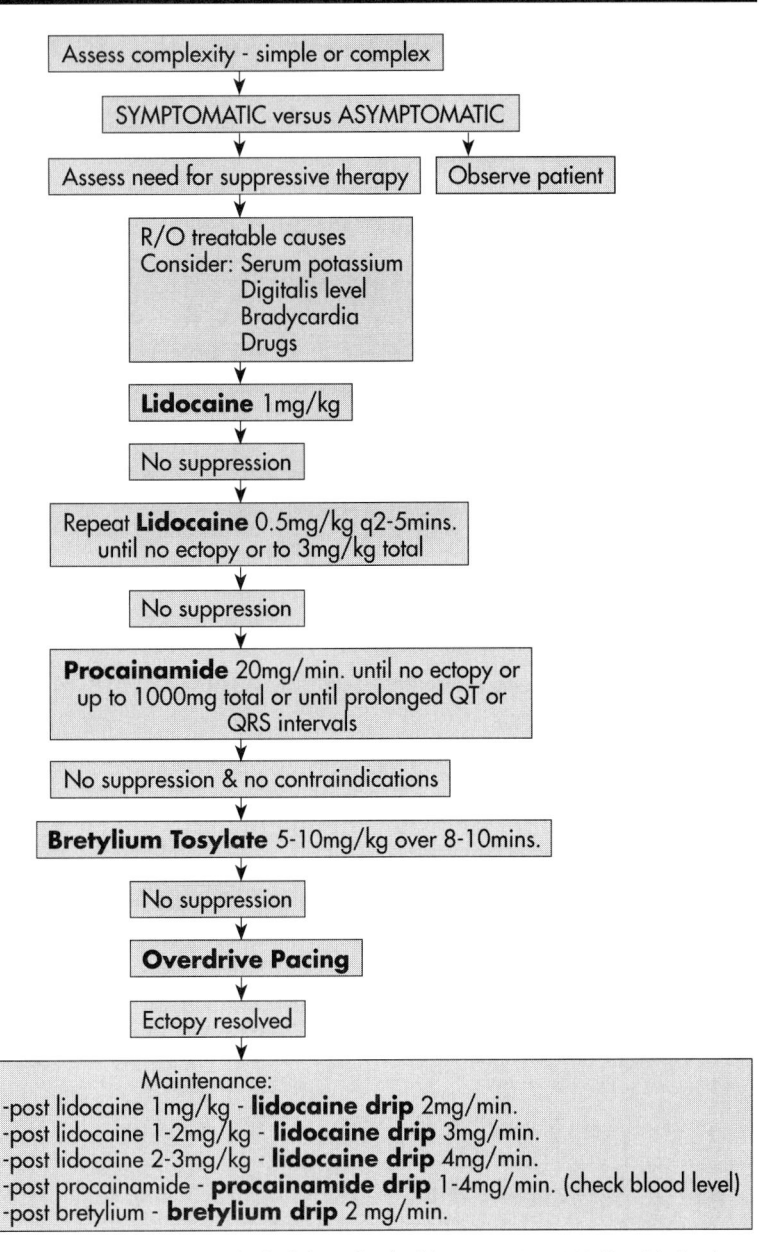

```
Assess complexity - simple or complex
             ↓
   SYMPTOMATIC versus ASYMPTOMATIC
             ↓                          ↓
Assess need for suppressive therapy   Observe patient
             ↓
   R/O treatable causes
   Consider: Serum potassium
             Digitalis level
             Bradycardia
             Drugs
             ↓
   **Lidocaine** 1mg/kg
             ↓
       No suppression
             ↓
   Repeat **Lidocaine** 0.5mg/kg q2-5mins.
   until no ectopy or to 3mg/kg total
             ↓
       No suppression
             ↓
   **Procainamide** 20mg/min. until no ectopy or
   up to 1000mg total or until prolonged QT or
              QRS intervals
             ↓
   No suppression & no contraindications
             ↓
   **Bretylium Tosylate** 5-10mg/kg over 8-10mins.
             ↓
       No suppression
             ↓
     **Overdrive Pacing**
             ↓
       Ectopy resolved
             ↓
   Maintenance:
   -post lidocaine 1mg/kg - **lidocaine drip** 2mg/min.
   -post lidocaine 1-2mg/kg - **lidocaine drip** 3mg/min.
   -post lidocaine 2-3mg/kg - **lidocaine drip** 4mg/min.
   -post procainamide - **procainamide drip** 1-4mg/min. (check blood level)
   -post bretylium - **bretylium drip** 2 mg/min.
```

(Reproduced with permission. Textbook of advanced cardiac life support. 1987, 1990, Copyright American Heart Association.)

Figure 7-4. Algorithm for Sinus Tachycardia

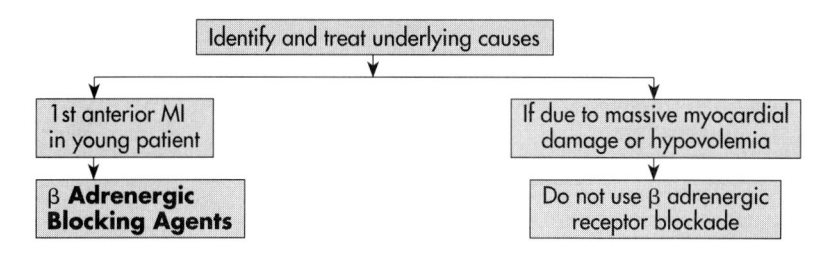

```
                    Identify and treat underlying causes
                    ↓                               ↓
    1st anterior MI                      If due to massive myocardial
    in young patient                     damage or hypovolemia
    ↓                                                ↓
    β Adrenergic                         Do not use β adrenergic
    Blocking Agents                      receptor blockade
```

3. **Nonconducted P waves** and an isoelectric baseline.

   C. Management of MAT
   1. **In stable patient,** diagnose arrhythmic mechanism.
   2. **Treat underlying causes** and decrease firing rate of the atrial automatic foci. Treat with **Verapamil,** 2.5-5 mg IV initially over 2 minutes, then 5-10 mg every 15-30 minutes to maximum dose of 20 mg; OR $MgSO_4$ for MAT 1-2 g (as 10% solution) IV over 15 minutes then 1 g IM q4-6h based on response and Mg^{2+} blood levels **OR quinidine sulfate** 200-300 mg TID or QID.

VII. Torsades de pointes (TDP)

A. **Definition:** An acquired or congenital polymorphic VT occurring in the presence of, or rarely in the absence of, a prolonged QT interval.

B. Salient features

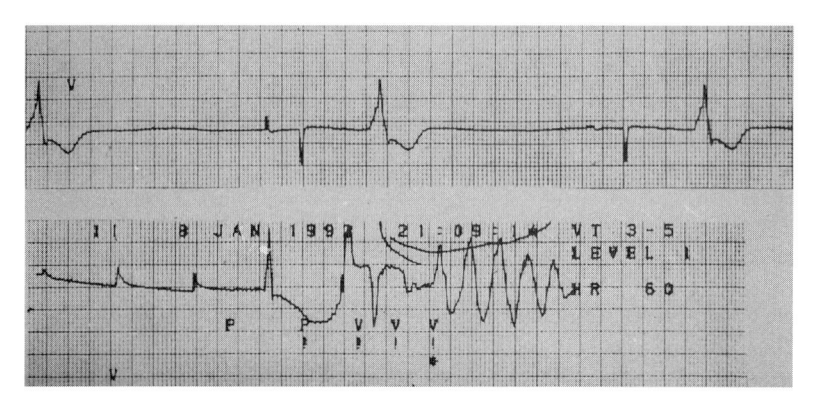

1. **Note the spindle-shaped groupings** of VT beats ("twisting of the points") with a prolonged QT interval.
2. **Treated with drugs** that decrease the QT interval, and by overdrive pacing or isoproterenol infusion in ED cases.

C. Management of torsades de pointes
1. **Distinguish TDP** from polymorphic VT.
2. **Distinguish if congenital** or acquired.
3. **Correct underlying cause** and consider discontinuing quinidine, procainamide, disopyramide, moricizine, lidocaine, amiodarone, phenothiazine, and tricyclics.

4. **Treatment. Magnesium sulfate** (drug of choice), 1-2 gm IV bolus over 1-2 minutes or **infuse** at 1-2 gm IV over 1 hour. **Isoproterenol** (may worsen ischemia), 2-10 μg/min, **OR phenytoin,** 100-300 mg IV in 50 mg aliquots every 5 minutes.
5. **Sustained episodes. Transcutaneous pacing,** then **transvenous Pacemaker OR cardioversion.**

VIII. Tachycardias
A. Definition: An operating heart rhythm with a rate of at least 100 beats/min.
B. Salient features: Look ahead to the specific arrhythmia.
C. Management **(See Fig. 7-5).**

IX. Atrial fibrillation and atrial flutter
A. Definition
1. **Atrial fibrillation**
   a. **Total irregularity** of the arterial pulse produced by an ineffective atrial contraction.
   b. **Categorized as** paroxysmal atrial fibrillation without disease; paroxysmal atrial fibrillation with underlying heart disease; atrial fibrillation related to specific systemic problems.
   c. **Types of atrial fibrillation**
      Type I: discrete atrial electrogram separated by discrete isoelectric intervals.
      Type II: discrete atrial electrogram not separated by discrete isoelectric intervals.
      Type III: absence of both discrete atrial electrograms and isoelectric intervals of any sort.
      Type IV: electrogram varies among types I to III.
2. **Atrial flutter**
   a. **More organized rhythm** than seen in atrial fibrillation.
   b. **A micro-reentry phenomenon** or due to the presence of an automatic focus low in the atrium.
   c. **Type I antiarrhythmics** will decrease the rate to ≅ 200 beats/min.
B. Salient features
   1. **Atrial fibrillation**

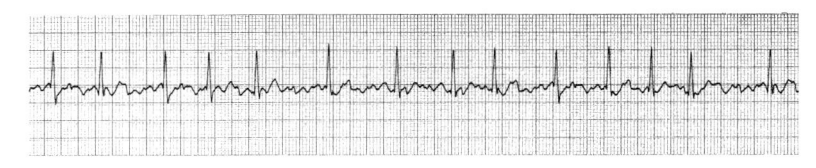

   a. **Atrial rate:** range 400-600 beats/min.
   b. **Rhythm**: irregularly irregular without P waves due to lack of atrial electrical activity.
   c. **QRS complex normal** unless aberrant ventricular conduction.
   d. **P waves** are not evident and may be replaced with f waves.
   e. **Fibrillatory activity** may be course or fine.
   f. If **antegrade conduction** down a collateral pathway, rate ≅ 300 beats/min.

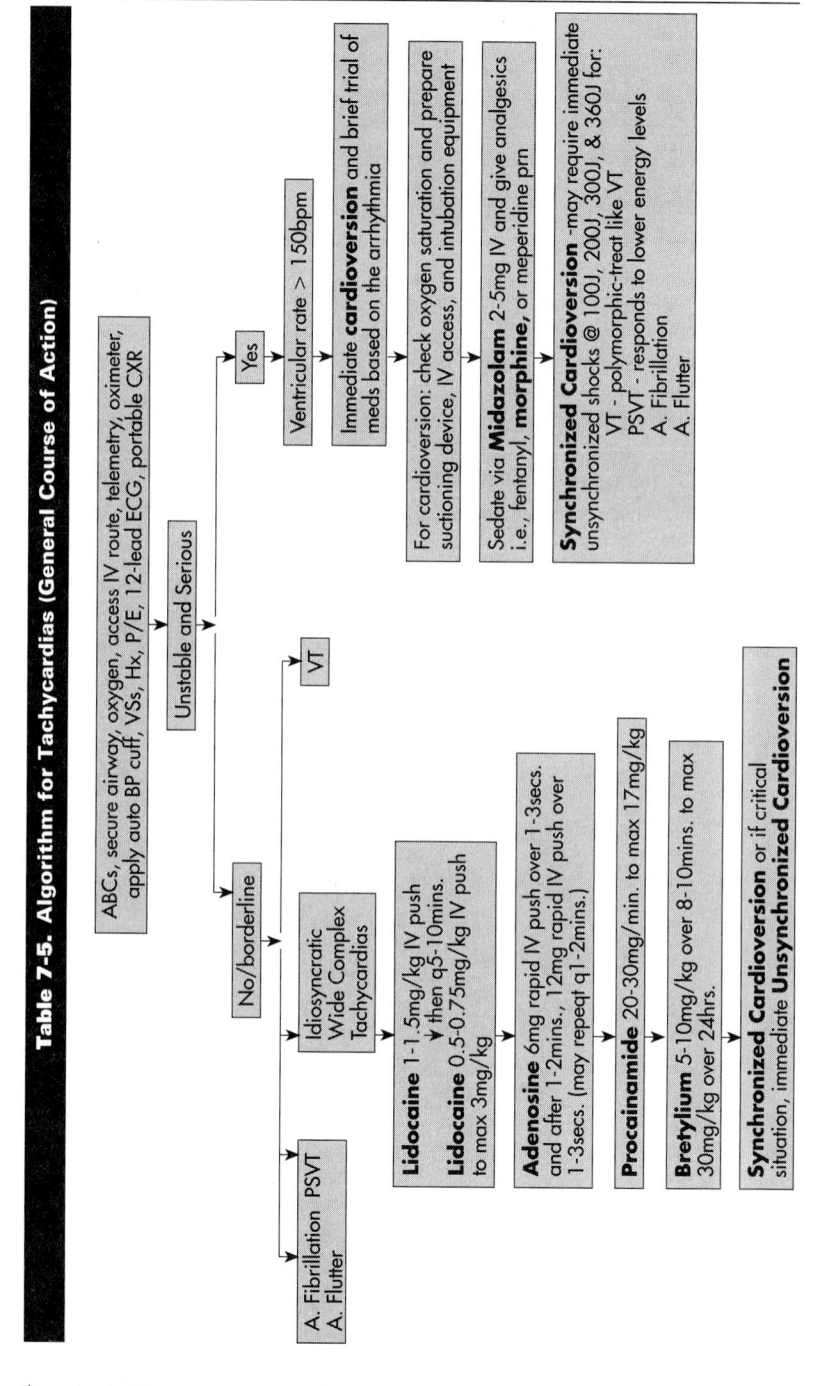

Table 7-5. Algorithm for Tachycardias (General Course of Action)

ABCs, secure airway, oxygen, access IV route, telemetry, oximeter, apply auto BP cuff, VSs, Hx, P/E, 12-lead ECG, portable CXR

Unstable and Serious

No/borderline

- A. Fibrillation PSVT
- A. Flutter

- Idiosyncratic Wide Complex Tachycardias
- VT

Lidocaine 1-1.5mg/kg IV push ↓ then q5-10mins.
Lidocaine 0.5-0.75mg/kg IV push to max 3mg/kg

Adenosine 6mg rapid IV push over 1-3secs. and after 1-2mins., 12mg rapid IV push over 1-3secs. (may repeat q1-2mins.)

Procainamide 20-30mg/min. to max 17mg/kg

Bretylium 5-10mg/kg over 8-10mins. to max 30mg/kg over 24hrs.

Synchronized Cardioversion or if critical situation, immediate **Unsynchronized Cardioversion**

Yes

Ventricular rate > 150bpm

Immediate **cardioversion** and brief trial of meds based on the arrhythmia

For cardioversion: check oxygen saturation and prepare suctioning device, IV access, and intubation equipment

Sedate via **Midazolam** 2-5mg IV and give analgesics i.e., fentanyl, **morphine**, or meperidine prn

Synchronized Cardioversion -may require immediate unsynchronized shocks @ 100J, 200J, 300J, & 360J for:
- VT - polymorphic-treat like VT
- PSVT - responds to lower energy levels
- A. Fibrillation
- A. Flutter

(Reproduced with permission. JAMA October 28, 1992, 268:16, 2223. Copyright 1992, American Medical Association.)

2. Atrial flutter

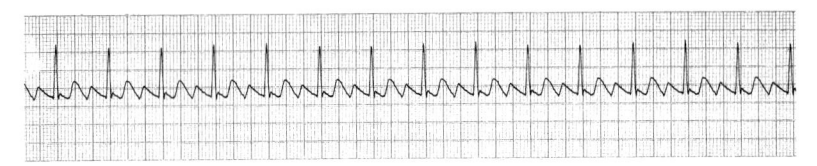

- a. **Rate:** range 200-350 beats/min.
- b. **Rhythm:** regular.
- c. **PR interval:** regular but may vary.
- d. **QRS interval** appears normal.
- e. **Categories: Type I,** 230-350 beats/min; restoration to normal sinus rhythm is possible with overdrive pacing. **Type II,** 340-430 beats/min; unresponsive to pacing.
- f. **Occurs with** 2:1 AV block, 1:1 AV conduction, and with aberrations.
- g. **Suspect** if rate 140-180 beats/min even in absence of characteristic "saw-tooth" wave pattern evident in leads II, III, aVF, and V_1.
- h. **Saw-tooth flutter** usually has an inverted appearance secondary to the low atrial focus in the area of the AV junction—if upright, indicative of a higher atrial focus.

C. Management of atrial fibrillation and atrial flutter

1. **Initial laboratory workup:** CBC, electrolytes, cardiac enzymes with creatine kinase (CK) and CK–myocardial bands (CK-MB), PT/PTT, ABGs, CXR, ECG, M-mode echocardiogram (to discern chamber size and appearance).
2. **Diagnosis of atrial fibrillation or atrial flutter. Controlled ventricular response:** no emergency treatment required.
3. **Diagnosis of atrial fibrillation or atrial flutter. Rapid ventricular response:** Unstable onset <12 months or refractory to drugs.
   - a. **Treatment. Midazolam** 2-5 mg IV for sedation.
   - b. **Synchronized cardioversion** at 200 J for atrial fibrillation and 25-50 J for atrial flutter.
   - c. **Rate control: Digoxin**—load with 0.25-0.5 mg IV, then 0.25 mg IV push q4h prn until ventricular rate 60-90 beats/minute at rest or until 15-20 µg/kg given; then 0.125-0.25 mg IV q2-6h prn to 0.75-1.5 mg total or 0.125-0.375 mg PO or IV qd +/− synergistic effect:
     - (1) **verapamil,** 3-5 mg IV initially, then 5-10 mg or 2.5-10 mg IV over 2-3 minutes (may give **calcium gluconate,** 1 gm IV over 3-6 minutes prior to verapamil), then 40-120 mg PO q8h or **verapamil SR** at 120-140 mg PO qd **OR diltiazem,** 90-360 mg/day PO
     - (2) *****propranolol,** 0.5-1 mg by slow IV over 5 minutes to total 5 mg or 1-5 mg (0.15 mg/kg) given IV in 1 mg aliquots per minute, then 40-80 mg PO TID-QID **OR esmolol,** 500 µg/kg IV loading dose, then 50 mg/min—if no effect, reload and ↑ maintenance dose by 25-50 µg/min **OR metoprolol,** 5-15 mg IV loading dose, then 25-100 mg/day PO **OR atenolol,** 5-10 mg IV loading dose, then 25-100 mg/day PO.
   - d. **Pharmacological conversion** after rate control and anticoagulation if >3 days duration: **quinidine gluconate,** 15 mg/kg in 150 ml D5W IV over 4-6 hours loading followed by 0.8 mg/kg/hr infusion (reduce dose by 25% in CHF patients) **OR quinidine sulfate,** 400 mg PO q2-4h ×

2 doses loading followed by **quinidine gluconate,** 324 mg IM or PO q8h **OR quinidine gluconate,** 330 mg IM or PO q2-4h × 2 doses, then 330 mg IM or PO q8h **OR procainamide,** IV loading dose 1000 mg (15 mg/kg) at 20 mg/min IV then 2-6 mg/min IV maintenance or PO loading dose 750-1000 mg then 250-1000 mg PO q6h (50 mg/kg/day in 4-6 divided doses) **OR amiodarone,** 5 mg/kg IV over 3-20 minutes; 200 PO QID-BID; **Propafenone,** 150-300 mg PO q8h (max 1200 mg/day): **sotalol,** (0.4-1.5 mg/kg IV or 160-320 mg/day PO BID (investigational) **OR drug combinations:** quinidine 400-600 mg, diazepam 5 mg, and propranolol 40 mg IV—may repeat in 2-3 hours.

e. **Anticoagulation** if Hx of rheumatic HD, prosthetic valve, embolism, mitral valve disease, cardiomyopathy, and/or thyrotoxicosis: **Heparin** IV bolus 5,000-10,000 U (100 U/kg IBW), then 1000-2000 U/hr. (20 U/kg/hr if <70 years, 15 U/kg/hr if ≥70 years. [25,000 U in 250 or 500 ml D5W (50-100 U/ml)]; adjust q4-6h to PTT 1.5-2.5 × control values of 45-75 seconds × 7-10 days. Draw PTT 6 hours after bolus and q4-6h until PTT 1.5-2.5 × control, then qd or q12h. - Check PT at start of warfarin then qd—**warfarin,** 5 mg PO qd × 2-3 days, then titrate based on the rate of rise of PT 4 mg (2-15 mg/day) PO qd. Goal = 1.2-1.5 × control. Adequately heparinize prior to warfarin administration.

f. **Symptomatic meds—lorazepam,** 2 mg PO TID prn for anxiety.

g. **Contraindications:** *IV β blockers not to be given in close proximity to IV verapamil; Do not cardiovert if process is chronic and patients blood has not been anticoagulated.

4. **Diagnosis of atrial fibrillation or atrial flutter. Rapid ventricular response:** Stable.

  a. Start **quinidine gluconate** and **procainamide** 2-3 days prior and **anticoagulate** (3 weeks if chronic A. Fib; not required if onset <3 days); NPO × 6 hours; dig level ≤2.4; normal serum K

  b. **Quinidine gluconate,** 15 mg/kg in 150 ml D5W IV over 4-6 hours, then 0.8 mg/kg/hr infusion (reduce dose 25% in CHF cases) **OR procainamide,** 10-15 mg/kg slow IV to max rate of 20 mg/min.

X. Paroxysmal supraventricular tachycardia (PSVT)

A. Definition

1. Repeated episodes of atrial tachycardia (AT) with abrupt onset and a duration of seconds to hours.
2. A general term referring to several arrhythmias, with different electrophysiologic mechanisms, encompassing atrioventricular nodal reentry, concealed atrioventricular bypass tract, sinus node reentry, intraarterial reentry, and automatic atrial tachycardia.

B. Salient features

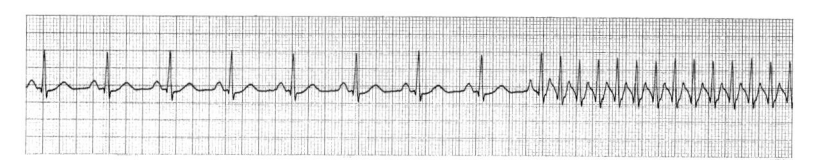

1. **Rate:** 75-250 beats/min.
2. **Atrial activation** begins at end of QRS complex caused by AV nodal reentry.

3. **RP interval** <50% RR interval.
4. **Ratio** of PR/RP >1.
5. **P waves** are difficult to identify—may be lost in preceding T wave.
6. **QRS interval** is normal but can be prolonged.

C. Management of PSVT (Fig. 7-6).

XI. Ventricular tachycardia

A. Definition: Refer to **Section II.A. 2.**

B. Salient features: Refer to **Section II.B. 2.**

C. Management of hemodynamically unstable, sustained ventricular tachycardia with pulse

1. **If pulse present and patient has** chest pain, dyspnea, ischemia, CHF, ventricular rate >150 beats/min, systolic BP <90 mm Hg, infarction: administer **100% oxygen,** establish IV access, sedate with **midazolam** (see note), 2-5 mg IV, and use **synchronized cardioversion** (see note) 50 J, 100 J, 200 J, 300 J, 360 J.

    NOTE: If patient unconscious, or has pulmonary edema or hypotension, use **unsynchronized cardioversion** and omit sedation.

2. **If recurrent,** add **lidocaine,** 1-1.5 mg/kg IV push, and repeat IV bolus 0.5-0.75 mg/kg IV push every 5-10 minutes until VT resolved or maximum total dose of 3 mg/kg has been given. Consider: **infusion** at 2 mg/min (2 gm in 500 ml D5W at 30 ml/hr = 2 mg/min) and increase rate 1 mg/min to maximum of 4 mg/min. **Synchronized cardioversion** at 360 J, and if recurrent VT, cardiovert at last successful energy level. **Procainamide** (see note), 20-30 mg/min until conversion, hypotension, or maximum total dose of 17 mg/kg. **Bretylium tosylate,** 5-10 mg/kg IV over 8-10 minutes, **then infuse** at 1-2 mg/min to maximum dose of 30 mg/kg over 24 hours. Then, **synchronized cardioversion** (see note).

    NOTE: If patient unconscious, or has pulmonary edema or hypotension, use **unsynchronized cardioversion** and omit sedation and procainamide.

3. **Note:** If no pulse, treat as **ventricular fibrillation.**

D. Management of stable, sustained ventricular tachycardia with pulse

1. **Patient with pulse** exhibits chest pain, ventricular rate <150 beats/min, CHF, systolic BP <90 mm Hg, infarction. Administer **100% oxygen,** establish IV access. If no pulse treat as ventricular fibrillation.

    a. **Treatment. Lidocaine,** 1-1.5 mg/kg IV bolus and repeat bolus 0.5-0.75 mg/kg IV bolus (40 mg) every 5-10 minutes until VT resolved or maximum total dose of 3 mg/kg given. If converted, start **IV drip** of 2 mg/min (2 gm in 500 ml D5W at 30 ml/hr = 2 mg/min); ↑ drip at 1 mg/min to maximum of 4 mg/min.

    b. **Procainamide,** 20-30 mg/min IV infusion until converted, hypotension, 50% wider QRS complex, or maximum total dose of 17 mg/kg; upon arrhythmia suppression, continue **procainamide infusion** at 1-4 mg/min.

    c. **Bretylium,** 5-10 mg/kg IV continuous infusion over 8-10 minutes; if converted, complete loading dose of 5 mg/kg and start a continuous infusion at 1-2 mg/min.

    (1) If there is **no conversion,** chest pain, dyspnea, infarction, use **synchronized cardioversion** if HR <150-160 beats/min and patient remains stable.

    (2) If there is **no pulse,** treat as ventricular fibrillation.

XII. Sinus bradycardia and atrioventricular blocks

A. Definition

1. **Sinus rhythm** with a rate of <60 beats/min and a decrease in the rate of atrial depolarization due to slowing of the sinus node—**sinus bradycardia.**
2. **Failure** of some or all of the atrial impulses to reach the ventricles as a result of impaired conduction—**atrioventricular block.**

B. Salient features

1. **Sinus bradycardia**

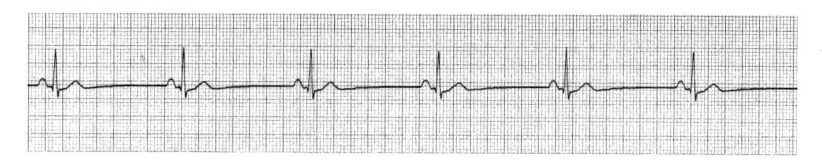

    a. **Rate:** <60 beats/min.
    b. **Rhythm:** regular.
    c. **P waves** are upright in leads I, II, and a VF.
    d. **Caused by drugs** with negative chronotropic effects (i.e., β-blockers).
    e. **Prevalent during** first hour after onset of symptoms due to autonomic dysfunction.
    f. **Common mechanisms:** sinus bradycardia, junctional escape rhythm, and 2° and 3° AV block.
    g. **Clinically, distinguish** absolute from relative bradycardia.

2. **AV blocks: 1° AV block.**

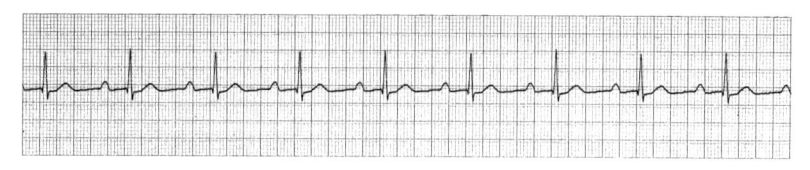

    a. **PR** >0.21 seconds.
    b. **Mainly** due to a delay in the AV node.
    c. **PR prolongation** is due to delayed conduction along the atrial bundle of His (AH) interval; causes include digitalis, calcium channel blockers, ischemia, and degenerative disease.
    d. **Conduction delay** along bundle of His (BH) and/or BB to produce 1° AV block.

3. **AV blocks: 2° AV block—Mobitz type I (Wenckebach)**

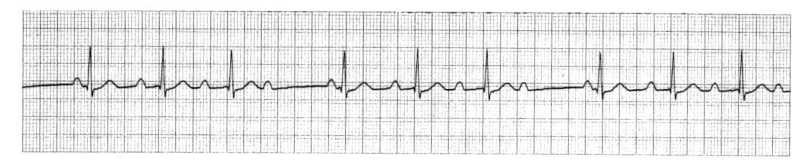

    a. **Constant** PP interval.
    b. **Progressive PR prolongation** until P wave is blocked.
    c. **Progressive** shortening of the RR interval.
    d. **QRS morphology** is normal or aberrant.
    e. **Anywhere in the** conducting system—mainly AV node; causes include digitalis, calcium blockers, ischemia, and degenerative disease.

Figure 7-6. Algorithm for PSVT

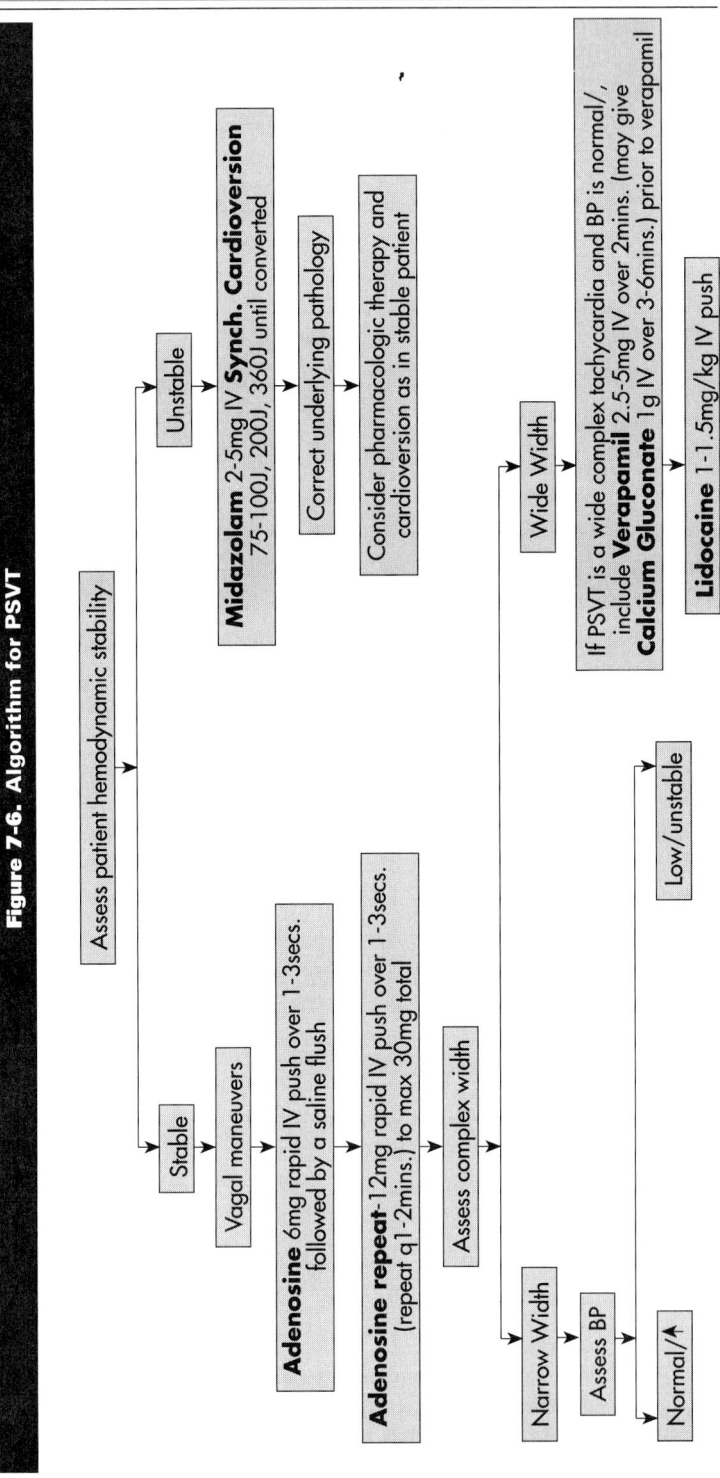

Assess patient hemodynamic stability

Stable
- Vagal maneuvers
- **Adenosine** 6mg rapid IV push over 1-3secs. followed by a saline flush
- **Adenosine repeat**-12mg rapid IV push over 1-3secs. (repeat q1-2mins.) to max 30mg total
- Assess complex width

Narrow Width
- Assess BP
  - Normal/↑
  - Low/unstable

Wide Width
- If PSVT is a wide complex tachycardia and BP is normal/↑, include **Calcium Gluconate** 1g IV over 3-6mins.) prior to verapamil **Verapamil** 2.5-5mg IV over 2mins. (may give
- **Lidocaine** 1-1.5mg/kg IV push

Unstable
- **Midazolam** 2-5mg IV **Synch. Cardioversion** 75-100J, 200J, 360J until converted
- Correct underlying pathology
- Consider pharmacologic therapy and cardioversion as in stable patient

Life-threatening Arrhythmias

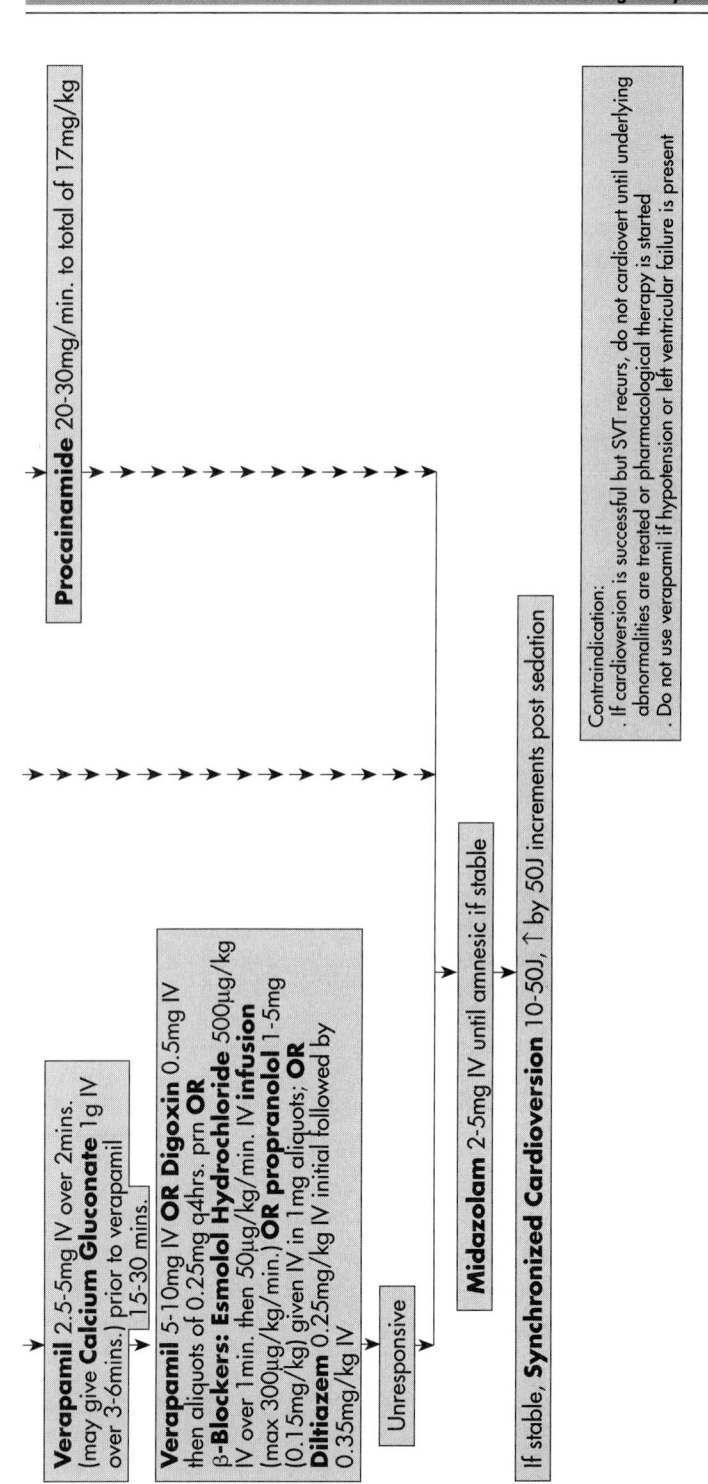

Verapamil 2.5-5mg IV over 2mins. (may give **Calcium Gluconate** 1g IV over 3-6mins.) prior to verapamil 15-30 mins.

↓

Verapamil 5-10mg IV **OR Digoxin** 0.5mg IV then aliquots of 0.25mg q4hrs. prn **OR** β-**Blockers: Esmolol Hydrochloride** 500μg/kg IV over 1min. then 50μg/kg/min. IV infusion (max 300μg/kg/min.) **OR propranolol** 1-5mg (0.15mg/kg) given IV in 1mg aliquots; **OR Diltiazem** 0.25mg/kg IV initial followed by 0.35mg/kg IV

↓

Unresponsive

↓ ➤➤➤➤➤➤➤➤➤➤➤➤➤➤➤➤➤➤➤➤➤➤

Procainamide 20-30mg/min. to total of 17mg/kg

➤➤➤➤➤➤➤➤➤➤➤➤➤➤➤➤➤➤➤➤➤➤

↓

Midazolam 2-5mg IV until amnesic if stable

↓

If stable, **Synchronized Cardioversion** 10-50J, ↑ by 50J increments post sedation

Contraindication:
. If cardioversion is successful but SVT recurs, do not cardiovert until underlying abnormalities are treated or pharmacological therapy is started
. Do not use verapamil if hypotension or left ventricular failure is present

4. AV blocks: 2° AV block—Mobitz type II

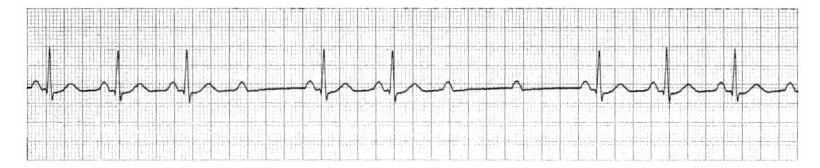

a. **Constant** PP interval.
b. **Constant** PR interval.
c. **Occasional** blocked P waves.
d. **QRS morphology** usually aberrant; normal at times.
e. **Only** in heart block (HB) and BB prolongation of His bundle–ventricle (HV) interval; caused mainly by degenerative disease.
f. **2:1 AV block** exhibits retrograde P waves, which suggest a block in the BB.

5. AV blocks: 3° AV (complete) block

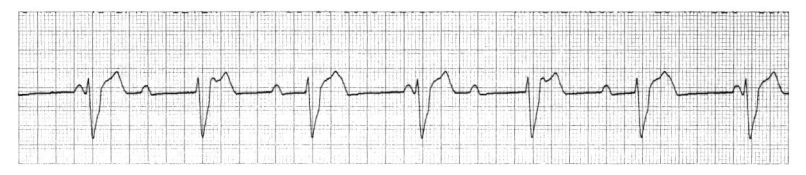

a. **No P wave** is conducted.
b. **QRS morphology** is normal or aberrant.
c. **Occurs in the proximal AV node** and the distal bundle of His branches; causes include congenital, digitalis, ischemia, and degenerative disease.

C. Management of sinus bradycardia and atrioventricular blocks **(Fig. 7-7)**

1. **Contraindications**
   a. **Lidocaine** is lethal if the bradycardia is a ventricular escape rhythm.
   b. **Transcutaneous pacing (TCP)** may be painful and fail to produce effective mechanical contractions.
   c. **Never treat 3° heart block** and ventricular escape beats with lidocaine.
   d. **Isoproterenol**—use extreme caution; low dose may be helpful but at high dose may be harmful.

Pediatric Cardiac Arrhythmias: Management Algorithms

Pediatric Advanced Life Support utilizes similar principles and techniques maintained in adult advanced cardiac life support. Cardiopulmonary arrest in infants and children is often the result of a progressive deterioration in circulatory and respiratory function rather than attributable to a sudden event. The rapid identification and treatment of underlying chest pathology is an absolute necessity to prevent cardiorespiratory arrest. Pediatric arrhythmias are an indication of an injured or critically ill child. This section is composed of seven treatment figures specifically designed, with pediatric protocols and drug dosages, to treat the predominant arrhythmias seen in the pediatric population.

Management algorithms focus on the treatment of dysrhythmias and the restoration of normal sinus rhythm, emphasizing pharmacologic regimens. The clinician should not underestimate the importance of properly assessing and diagnosing the dysrhythmia through correctly interpreting the ECG. Initially establishing hemodynamic stability or instability is paramount in the treatment of arrhythmias. Humidified oxygen should be administered to all seriously ill patients exhibiting respiratory or cardiopulmonary distress. Inadequate oxygen delivery secondary to respiratory defects or cardiopulmonary compromise can quickly lead to metabolic acidosis, organ failure, and more clinically grave arrhythmias indicative of deteriorating patient stability. Pediatric bag-valve devices, oxygen masks, oropharyngeal and nasopharyngeal airways, and endotracheal intubation may be used to oxygenate patients.

I. **Management of ventricular tachycardia with pulse** (Fig. 7-8).
II. **Management of ventricular fibrillation, pulseless ventricular tachycardia, asystole, and PEA** (Fig. 7-9).
III. **Management of Wolff-Parkinson-White syndrome (WPW)** (Fig. 7-10).
IV. **Management of supraventricular tachycardia (SVT)**
    Adenosine is the drug of choice for converting supraventricular tachycardias in stable children with an established intravenous access route. Cardioversion should not be delayed to gain intravenous access for adenosine administration. This endogenous nucleoside slows conduction time through the AV node and interrupts the reentry circuits that involve the AV node and operate in the underlying mechanism associated with the majority of SVT episodes in infants and children. Adenosine is metabolized by erythrocyte adenosine deaminase and must be given in higher doses if peripheral venous administration is chosen versus central line administration (Fig. 7-11).
V. **Management of paroxysmal supraventricular tachycardia (PSVT)** (Fig. 7-12).
VI. **Management of atrial fibrillation and atrial flutter** (Fig. 7-13).
VII. **Management of sinus bradycardia**
    Cardiac output in infants younger than 6 months is dependent on heart rate. A child of any age with a bradycardic ECG associated with poor systemic perfusion should be expeditiously treated with epinephrine. Atropine is used to treat bradycardias with concomitant poor perfusion or hypotension. The parasympatholytic properties of the drug accelerate the atrial pacemakers and increase AV conduction. Tachycardia may follow after the administration of a vagolytic dose of atropine and is well tolerated in children (Fig. 7-14).

Acknowledgments

The author would like to thank Thom Benson, R.N., Dr. Jewel Gold, and especially Dr. S. Belo for their assistance in obtaining sample ECG rhythms for this chapter.

Suggested Readings

Adgey AA, et al: Acute phase of myocardial infarction, *Lancet* 2:501, 1971.
American Heart Association: *Textbook of advanced cardiac life support,* ed 2, Dallas, 1990, American Heart Association.
American Heart Association: Guidelines for cardiopulmonary resuscitation and emergency care, *JAMA* 269(16):2171-302, 1992.
Alderman EL: Analgesics in the acute phase of myocardial infarction, *JAMA* 229:1646-8, 1974.

Ayres, SM: Mechanisms and consequences of pulmonary edema: cardiac lung, shock lung, and principles of ventilator therapy in adult respiratory distress syndrome, *Am Heart J* 103:97-112, 1982.

Berenyi KG, Wolk M, Killip T: Cerebrospinal fluid acidosis complicating therapy of experimental cardiopulmonary arrest, *Circulation* 52:319-24, 1975.

Brown DC, Lewis AJ, Criley JM: Asystole and its treatment: the possible role of the parasympathetic nervous system in cardiac arrest, *Am Coll Emerg Phys J* 8:11448, 1979.

Chan PD, Brenner M: *Current clinical strategies: critical care medicine—medical and surgical,* Fountain Valley, 1993, Current Clinical Strategies Publishing International.

Chan PD, Gennrich JL, Pham T: *Current clinical strategies: pediatrics,* Newport Beach, 1992, Current Clinical Strategies Publishing International.

Chung EK: *Digitalis intoxication,* Baltimore, 1969, Williams and Wilkins.

Cohen ML, Lindsay BD: Cardiac arrhythmias. In Woodley M, Whelan WH, editors: *Manual of medical therapeutics: the Washington manual,* ed 27, St. Louis, 1992, Little, Brown.

Coon GA, Clinton JE, Ruiz E: Use of atropine for bradyasystolic prehospital cardiac arrest, *Ann Emerg Med* 10:462-7, 1981.

Criley JM, Blaufuss AH, Kissel GL: Cough induced cardiac compression: self-administered form of CPR, *JAMA* 236:1246-50, 1976.

Dorian P, Myers MG: Antiarrhythmatic drugs. In Kalant H, Roschlau WHE, editors: *Principles of medical pharmacology,* ed 5, Toronto, 1989, B.C. Decker.

Gallagher JT et al: The preexcitation syndromes, *Prog Cardiovasc Dis* 20:285-327, 1978.

Greenburg MI et al: Endotracheal administration of atropine sulphate, *Ann Emerg Med* 11:546-8, 1982.

Hasegawa EA: The endotracheal administration of drugs, *Heart Lung* 15:60-83, 1986.

Horowitz LN et al: Torsades de pointes: electrophysiologic studies in patients without transient pharmacological or metabolic abnormalities, *Circulation* 63:1120-8, 1981.

Iseri LT et al: Magnesium and potassium therapy in multifocal atrial tachycardia, *Am Heart J* 110:789-794, 1985.

Iseri LT, Humphrey SB, Siner EJ: Pre-hospital bradyasystolic cardiac arrest, *Ann Intern Med* 88:741-5, 1978.

Josephson ME, Sudes SF: *Clinical cardiac electrophysiology,* Philadelphia, 1979, Lea and Febiger.

Kinball JT, Killip T: Aggressive treatment of arrhythmias in acute myocardial infarction: procedures and results, *Prog Cardiovasc Dis* 10:483, 1968.

Klein GJ, Hackel DB, Gallagher JT: Anatomic substrate of impaired antegrade conduction over an accessory AV pathway in the Wolff-Parkinson-White syndrome, *Circulation* 61:1249-56, 1980.

Krogh CME, editor: *Compendium of pharmaceuticals and specialties,* ed 28, Ottawa, 1993, CK Productions.

Levine JH, Michael JR, Guarnieri T: Treatment of multifocal atrial tachycardia with verapamil, *N Engl J Med* 312:21-44, 1985.

Lown B, Wolf M: Grading system for ventricular ectopy, *Circulation* 44:130-42, 1971.

Madias JE, Madia NE, Hood WB Jr: Precordial ST-segment mapping. 2. Effects of oxygen inhalation on ischemic injury on patients with acute MI, *Circulation* 53:411-7, 1976.

Marriott HJL: *Practical electrocardiography,* ed 7, Baltimore, 1983, Williams and Wilkins.

Myerburg RJ et al: Outcome from resuscitation from bradyarrhythmic or asystolic prehospital arrest, *J Am Coll Cardiol* 4:1118, 1984.

Ornato JP et al: Treatment of presumed asystole during pre-hospital cardiac arrest, *Am J Emerg Med* 3:395-9, 1985.

O'Rourke GW, Greene NM: Autonomic blockade and the resting heart rate in man, *Am Heart J* 80:469-79, 1970.

Otto CW, Yakaitis RW: The role of epinephrine in CPR: a reappraisal, *Ann Emerg Med* 13:840-3, 1984.

Packer M, Gotlieb SJ, Kessler PD: Hormone-electrolyte interactions in the pathogenesis of lethal cardiac arrhythmias in patients with control of arrhythmias, *Am J Med* 80(suppl 4A):23-9, 1986.

Rahi RH et al: Recent life changes, myocardial infarction, and abrupt coronary death. Studies in Helsinki, *Arch Intern Med* 133:221, 1974.

Rose RM et al: Occurrence of arrhythmias during the first hour in acute myocardial infarction, *Circulation* 50(suppl 3):111-21, 1974 (abstract).

Rosenbaum FF et al: The potential variations of the thorax and the esophagus in anomalous AV excitation (Wolff-Parkinson-White syndrome), *Am Heart J* 29:281-326, 1945.

Rudikoff MT et al: Mechanisms of blood flow during CPR, *Circulation* 61:345-52, 1980.

Shefler AG, editor: *The HSC handbook of paediatrics,* ed 8, Toronto, 1992, Mosby–Year Book.

Smith J, editor: *The hospital for sick children 1993 drug formulary,* Toronto, 1993, Graphic Centre, HSC.

Smith TW et al: Digitalis glycosides: mechanisms and manifestations of toxicity, Part I, *Prog Cardiovasc Dis* 26:413-58, 1984.

Smith TW et al: Treatment of life-threatening digitalis intoxication with digoxin-specific FAB antibody fragments, *N Engl J Med* 307:1357-62, 1982.

Steen PA et al: Efficacy of dopamine, dobutamine, and epinephrine during emergence from cardiopulmonary bypass in man, *Circulation* 57:378-84, 1978.

Stueven HA et al: Atropine in asystole: human studies, *Ann Emerg Med* 13:845, 1984.

Todres D: The role of morphine in acute myocardial infarction, *Am Heart J* 81:566-670, 1971.

Tonkin AM et al: Initial forces of ventricular depolarization in the Wolff-Parkinson-White syndrome analysis based upon location of the accessory pathway by epicardial mapping, *Circulation* 52:1030-6, 1975.

Waldo AL, Maclean WAH: *Diagnosis and treatment of cardiac arrhythmias following open heart surgery,* Mt. Kisco, 1980, Futura.

Ward JM, McGrath RL, Weil JV: Effects of morphine on the peripheral vascular response to sympathetic stimulation, *Am J Cardiol* 29:659-66, 1972.

Weil MH et al: Difference in acid-base state between venous and arterial blood during cardiopulmonary resuscitation, *N Engl J Med* 315:153-6, 1986.

Weiner N: Atropine, scopolamine, and related antimuscarinic drugs. In Gilman AG, Goodman LS, Gilman A, editors: *The pharmacologic basis of therapeutics,* New York, 1980, Macmillan.

Wells JL et al: Characterization of atrial fibrillation in man: studies following open heart surgery, *PACE Pacing Clin Electrophysiol* 1:426-38, 1978.

Vlay SC: Ventricular arrhythmias. In Vlay SC, editor: *Manual of cardiac arrhythmias: a practical guide to clinical management,* Boston, 1988, Little, Brown.

Vlay SC: Pharmacology of antiarrhythmatic drugs. In Vlay SC, editor: *Manual of cardiac arrhythmias,* Boston, 1988, Little, Brown.

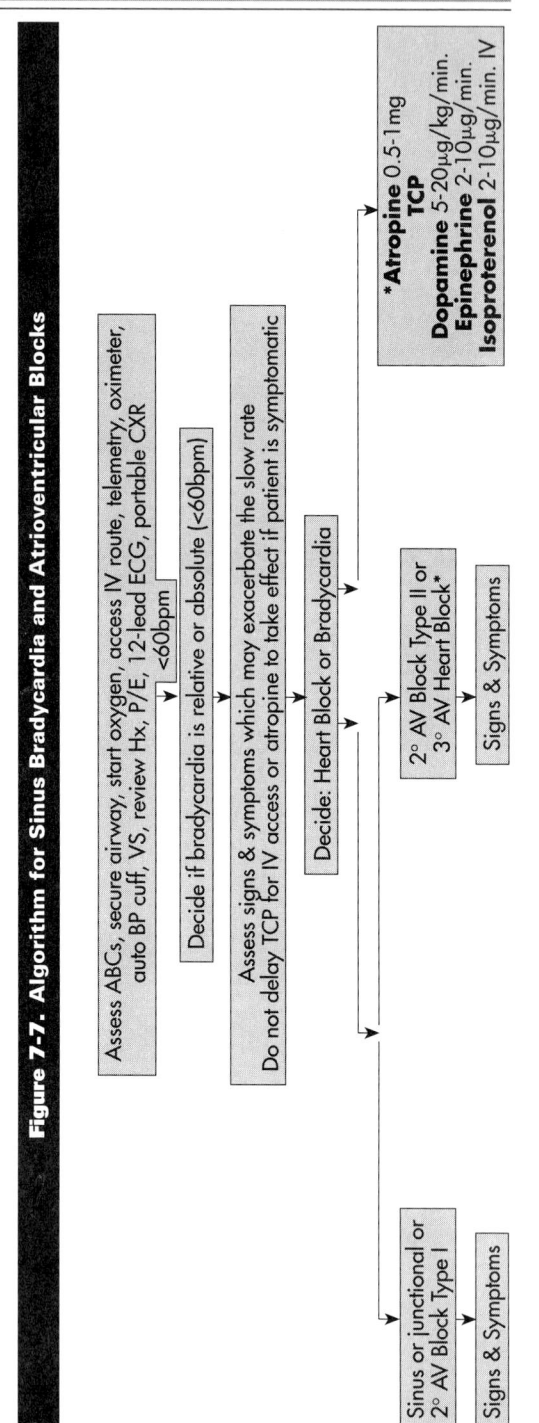

242 Ch 7. Cardiac Arrhythmias and Antiarrhythmic Drugs

Figure 7-7. Algorithm for Sinus Bradycardia and Atrioventricular Blocks

Assess ABCs, secure airway, start oxygen, access IV route, telemetry, oximeter, auto BP cuff, VS, review Hx, P/E, 12-lead ECG, portable CXR

<60bpm

Decide if bradycardia is relative or absolute (<60bpm)

Assess signs & symptoms which may exacerbate the slow rate
Do not delay TCP for IV access or atropine to take effect if patient is symptomatic

Decide: Heart Block or Bradycardia

- Sinus or junctional or 2° AV Block Type I
  - Signs & Symptoms

- 2° AV Block Type II or 3° AV Heart Block*
  - Signs & Symptoms

*__Atropine__ 0.5-1mg
TCP
Dopamine 5-20µg/kg/min.
Epinephrine 2-10µg/min.
Isoproterenol 2-10µg/min. IV

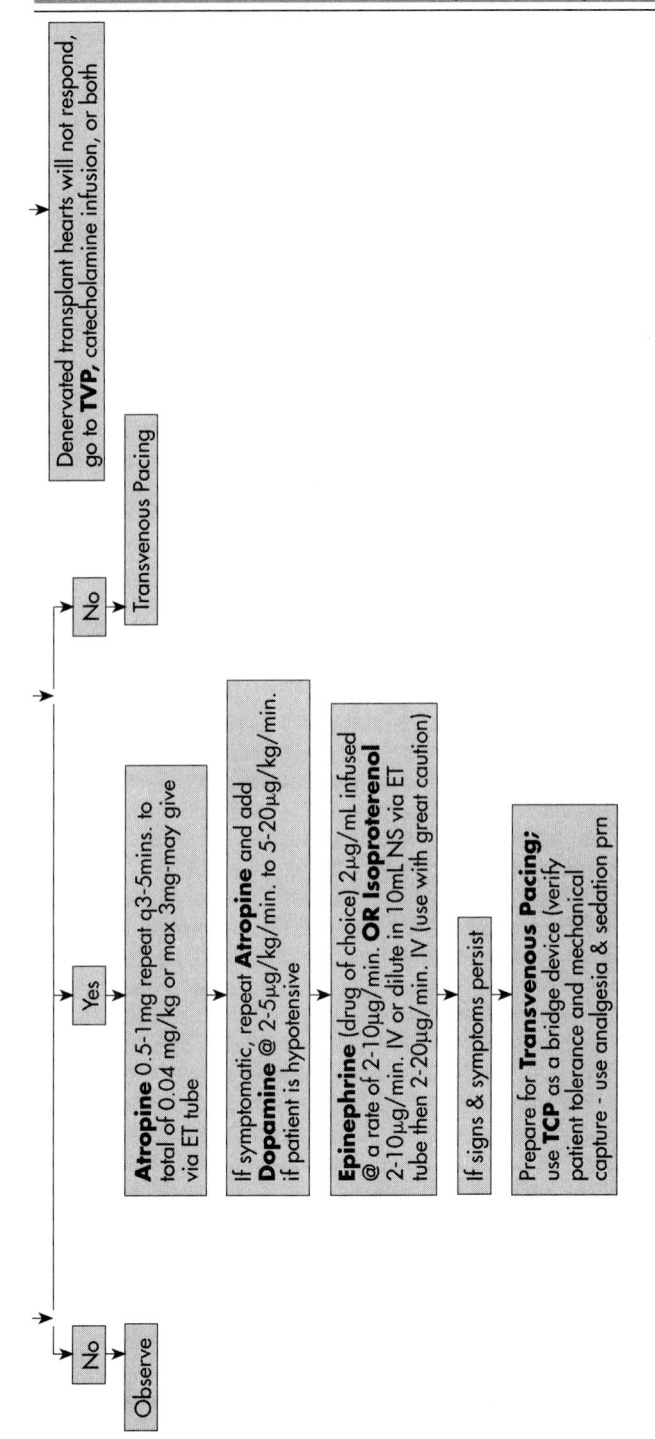

Pediatric Cardiac Arrhythmias: Management Algorithms

Denervated transplant hearts will not respond, go to **TVP**, catecholamine infusion, or both

→ No → Transvenous Pacing

→ Yes → **Atropine** 0.5-1mg repeat q3-5mins. to total of 0.04 mg/kg or max 3mg-may give via ET tube

If symptomatic, repeat **Atropine** and add **Dopamine** @ 2-5µg/kg/min. to 5-20µg/kg/min. if patient is hypotensive

Epinephrine (drug of choice) 2µg/mL infused @ a rate of 2-10µg/min. **OR Isoproterenol** 2-10µg/min. or dilute in 10mL NS via ET tube then 2-20µg/min. IV (use with great caution)

If signs & symptoms persist

Prepare for **Transvenous Pacing**; use **TCP** as a bridge device (verify patient tolerance and mechanical capture - use analgesia & sedation prn

→ No → Observe

(Reproduced with permission. *JAMA* October 28, 1992, 268:16, 2221. Copyright 1992, American Medical Association.)

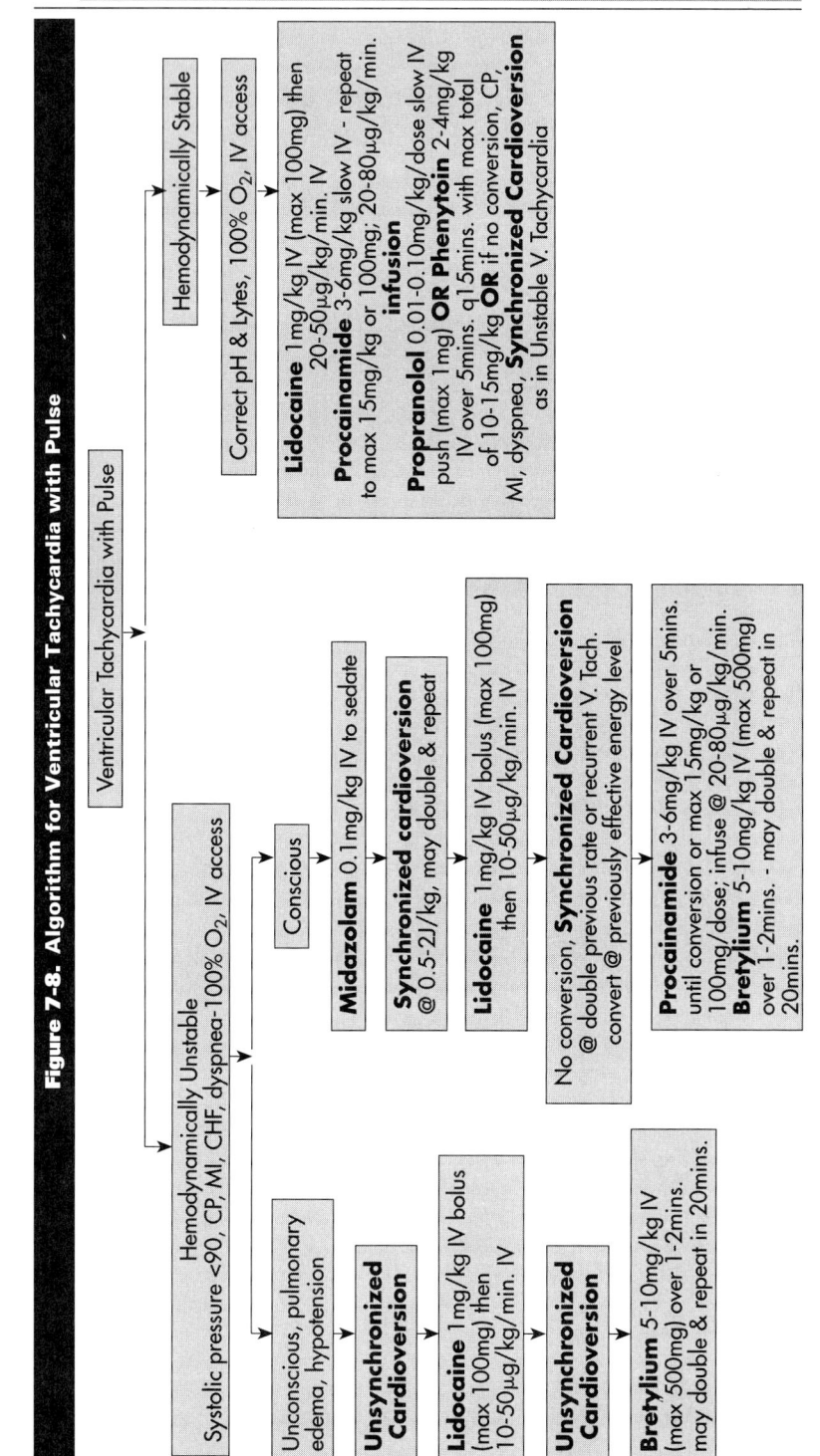

Figure 7-8. Algorithm for Ventricular Tachycardia with Pulse

Ventricular Tachycardia with Pulse

Hemodynamically Unstable
Systolic pressure <90, CP, MI, CHF, dyspnea-100% O₂, IV access

Unconscious, pulmonary edema, hypotension

- **Lidocaine** 1mg/kg IV bolus (max 100mg) then 10-50μg/kg/min. IV
- **Unsynchronized Cardioversion**
- **Bretylium** 5-10mg/kg IV (max 500mg) over 1-2mins. may double & repeat in 20mins.

Conscious

- **Midazolam** 0.1mg/kg IV to sedate
- **Synchronized cardioversion** @ 0.5-2J/kg, may double & repeat
- **Lidocaine** 1mg/kg IV bolus (max 100mg) then 10-50μg/kg/min. IV

No conversion, **Synchronized Cardioversion** @ double previous rate or recurrent V. Tach. convert @ previously effective energy level

- **Procainamide** 3-6mg/kg IV over 5mins. until conversion or max 1.5mg/kg or 100mg/dose; infuse @ 20-80μg/kg/min.
- **Bretylium** 5-10mg/kg IV (max 500mg) over 1-2mins. - may double & repeat in 20mins.

Hemodynamically Stable

Correct pH & Lytes, 100% O₂ IV access

Lidocaine 1mg/kg IV (max 100mg) then 20-50μg/kg/min. IV
Procainamide 3-6mg/kg slow IV - repeat to max 15mg/kg or 100mg; 20-80μg/kg/min. **infusion**
Propranolol 0.01-0.10mg/kg/dose slow IV push (max 1mg) **OR Phenytoin** 2-4mg/kg IV over 5mins. q15mins. with max total of 10-15mg/kg **OR** if no conversion, CP, MI, dyspnea, **Synchronized Cardioversion** as in Unstable V. Tachycardia

Pediatric Cardiac Arrhythmias: Management Algorithms

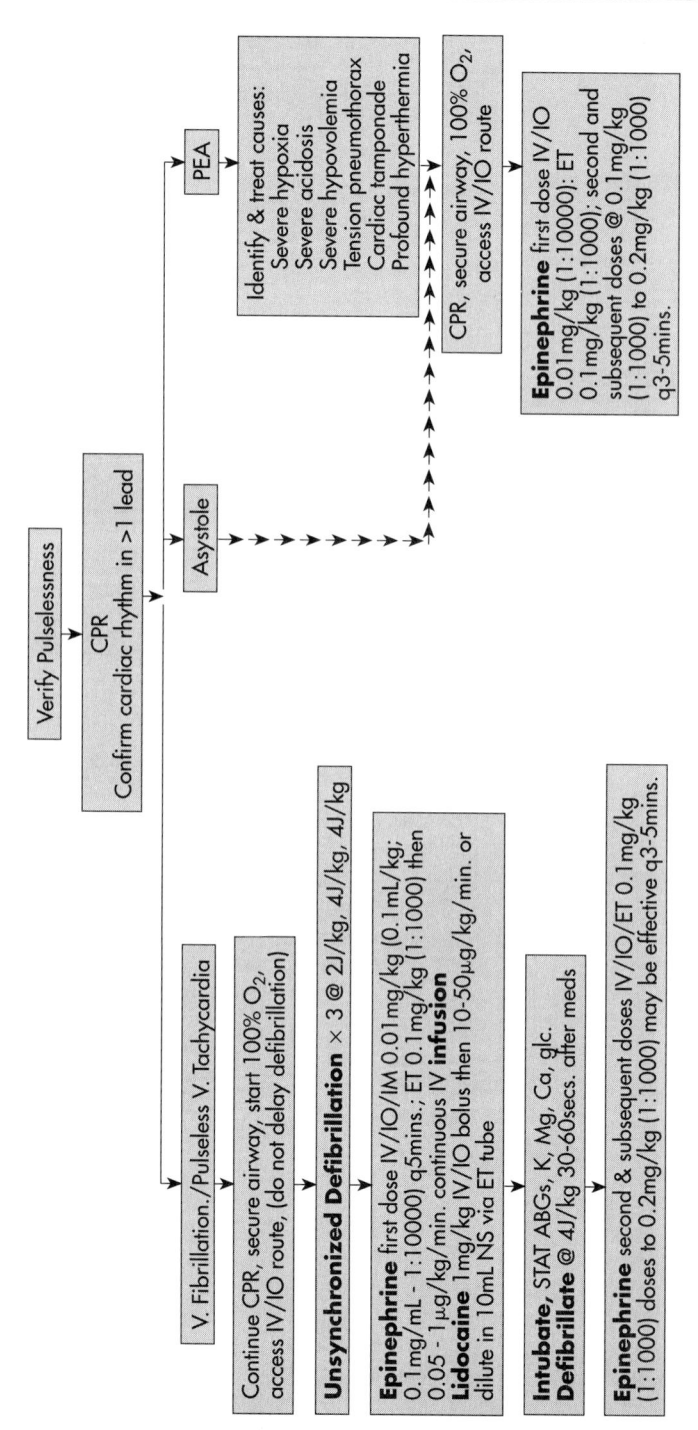

Figure 7-9. Algorithm for V. Fibrillation, Pulseless V. Tachycardia, Asystole, and PEA

Verify Pulselessness
↓
CPR
Confirm cardiac rhythm in >1 lead
↓
- V. Fibrillation./Pulseless V. Tachycardia
- Asystole
- PEA

V. Fibrillation./Pulseless V. Tachycardia:

Continue CPR, secure airway, start 100% O_2, access IV/IO route, (do not delay defibrillation)

Unsynchronized Defibrillation × 3 @ 2J/kg, 4J/kg, 4J/kg

Epinephrine first dose IV/IO/IM 0.01mg/kg (0.1mL/kg 0.1mg/mL - 1:10000) q5mins.; ET 0.1mg/kg (1:1000) then 0.05 - 1µg/kg/min. continuous IV **infusion**
Lidocaine 1mg/kg IV/IO bolus then 10-50µg/kg/min. or dilute in 10mL NS via ET tube

Intubate, STAT ABGs, K, Mg, Ca, glc.
Defibrillate @ 4J/kg 30-60secs. after meds

Epinephrine second & subsequent doses IV/IO/ET 0.1mg/kg (1:1000) doses to 0.2mg/kg (1:1000) may be effective q3-5mins.

Asystole / PEA:

Identify & treat causes:
- Severe hypoxia
- Severe acidosis
- Severe hypovolemia
- Tension pneumothorax
- Cardiac tamponade
- Profound hyperthermia

CPR, secure airway, 100% O_2, access IV/IO route

Epinephrine first dose IV/IO 0.01mg/kg (1:10000): ET 0.1mg/kg (1:1000); second and subsequent doses @ 0.1mg/kg (1:1000) to 0.2mg/kg (1:1000) q3-5mins.

Continued on next page

246 Ch 7. Cardiac Arrhythmias and Antiarrhythmic Drugs

→ **Defibrillate** @ 4J/kg 30-60secs. after medication

→ **Lidocaine** 1mg/kg IV/IO bolus and **Defibrillate**; consider **Bretylium** first dose @ 5mg/kg; consider **Bicarbonate** 1mEq/kg IV/IO

→ **Difibrillate** @ 4J/kg 30-60secs. after meds

→ Repeat **Bretylium** 10mg/kg IV bolus q5-10mins until a max of 30mg/kg

→ **Difibrillate** @ 4J/kg 30-60secs. after meds

→ Repeat **Bretylium OR Defibrillate**; consider **Procainamide** 3-6mg/kg slow IV over 5mins. to max of 100mg/dose

---

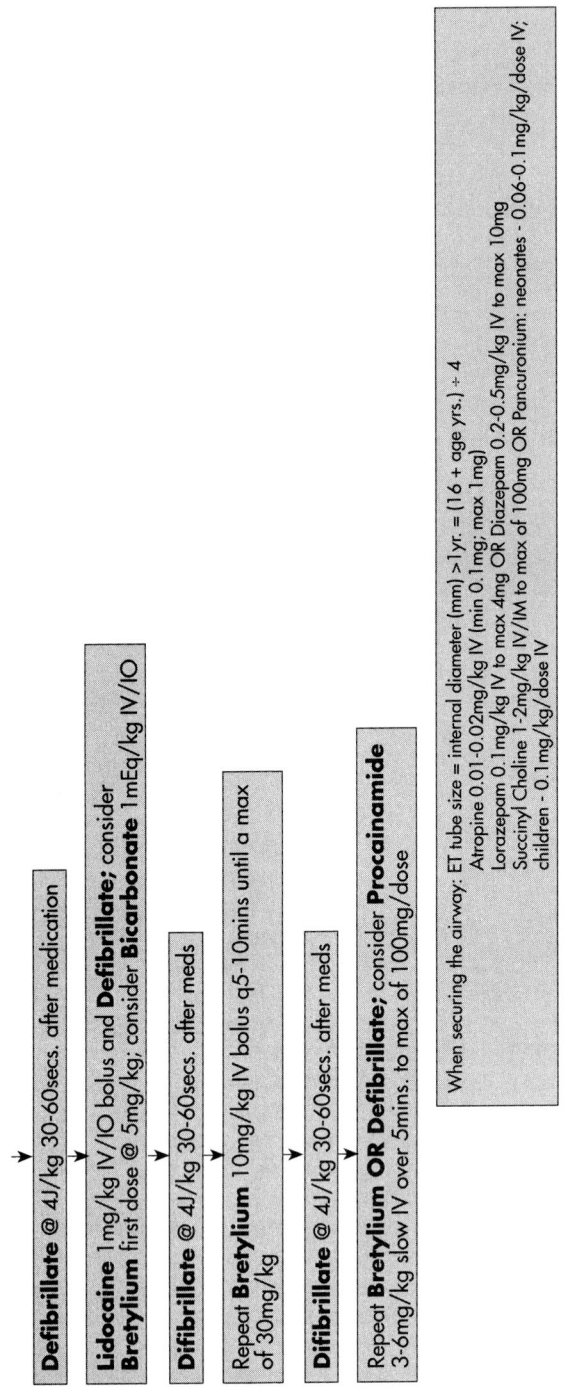

When securing the airway: ET tube size = internal diameter (mm) >1yr. = (16 + age yrs.) ÷ 4
Atropine 0.01-0.02mg/kg IV (min 0.1mg; max 1mg)
Lorazepam 0.1mg/kg IV to max 4mg OR Diazepam 0.2-0.5mg/kg IV to max 10mg
Succinyl Choline 1-2mg/kg IV/IM to max of 100mg OR Pancuronium: neonates - 0.06-0.1mg/kg/dose IV; children - 0.1mg/kg/dose IV

(Reproduced with permission. *JAMA* October 28, 1992, 268:16, 2266. Copyright 1992. American Medical Association.)

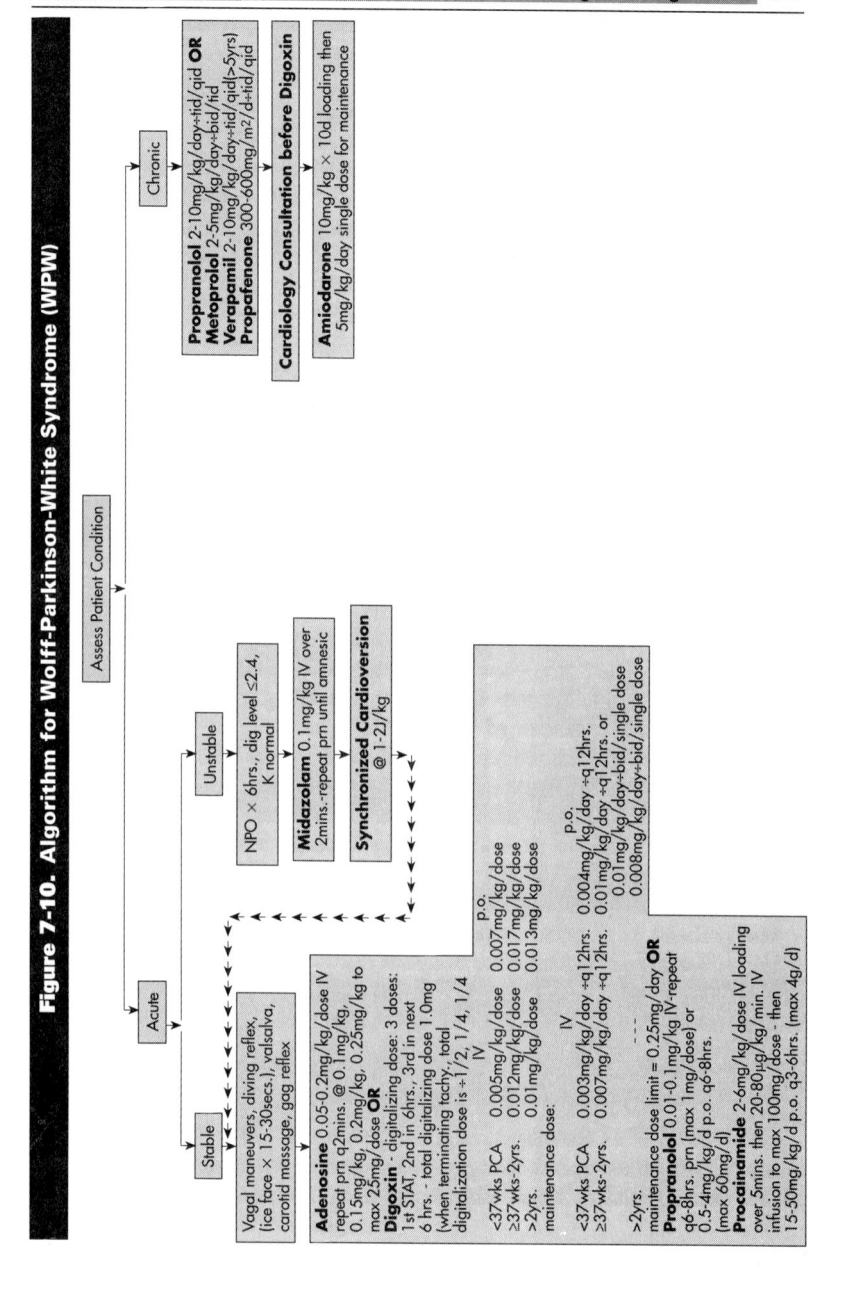

Figure 7-10. Algorithm for Wolff-Parkinson-White Syndrome (WPW)

Assess Patient Condition

Acute

Stable

Vagal maneuvers, diving reflex, (ice face × 15-30secs.), valsalva, carotid massage, gag reflex

Adenosine 0.05-0.2mg/kg/dose IV repeat prn q2mins. @ 0.1mg/kg, 0.15mg/kg, 0.2mg/kg, 0.25mg/kg to max 25mg/dose **OR**

Digoxin - digitalizing dose: 3 doses: 1st STAT, 2nd in 6hrs., 3rd in next 6 hrs. - total digitalizing dose 1.0mg (when terminating tachy., total digitalization dose is ÷1/2, 1/4, 1/4

	IV	p.o.
<37wks PCA	0.005mg/kg/dose	0.007mg/kg/dose
≥37wks-2yrs.	0.012mg/kg/dose	0.017mg/kg/dose
>2yrs.	0.01mg/kg/dose	0.013mg/kg/dose

maintenance dose:

	IV	p.o.
<37wks PCA	0.003mg/kg/day ÷q12hrs.	0.004mg/kg/day ÷q12hrs.
≥37wks-2yrs.	0.007mg/kg/day ÷q12hrs.	0.01mg/kg/day÷bid/single dose
>2yrs.	---	0.008mg/kg/day÷bid/single dose

maintenance dose limit = 0.25mg/day **OR**
Propranolol 0.01-0.1mg/kg IV repeat q6-8hrs. prn (max 1mg/dose) or 0.5-4mg/kg/d p.o. q6-8hrs. (max 60mg/d)
Procainamide 2-6mg/kg/dose IV loading over 5mins. then 20-80μg/kg/min. IV infusion to max 100mg/dose - then 15-50mg/kg/d p.o. q3-6hrs. (max 4g/d)

Unstable

NPO × 6hrs., dig level ≤2.4, K normal

Midazolam 0.1mg/kg IV over 2mins.-repeat prn until amnesic

Synchronized Cardioversion @ 1-2J/kg

Chronic

Propranolol 2-10mg/kg/day÷tid/qid **OR**
Metoprolol 2-5mg/kg/day÷bid/tid
Verapamil 2-10mg/kg/day÷tid/qid(>5yrs)
Propafenone 300-600mg/m2/d÷tid/qid

Cardiology Consultation before Digoxin

Amiodarone 10mg/kg × 10d loading then 5mg/kg/day single dose for maintenance

Ch 7. Cardiac Arrhythmias and Antiarrhythmic Drugs

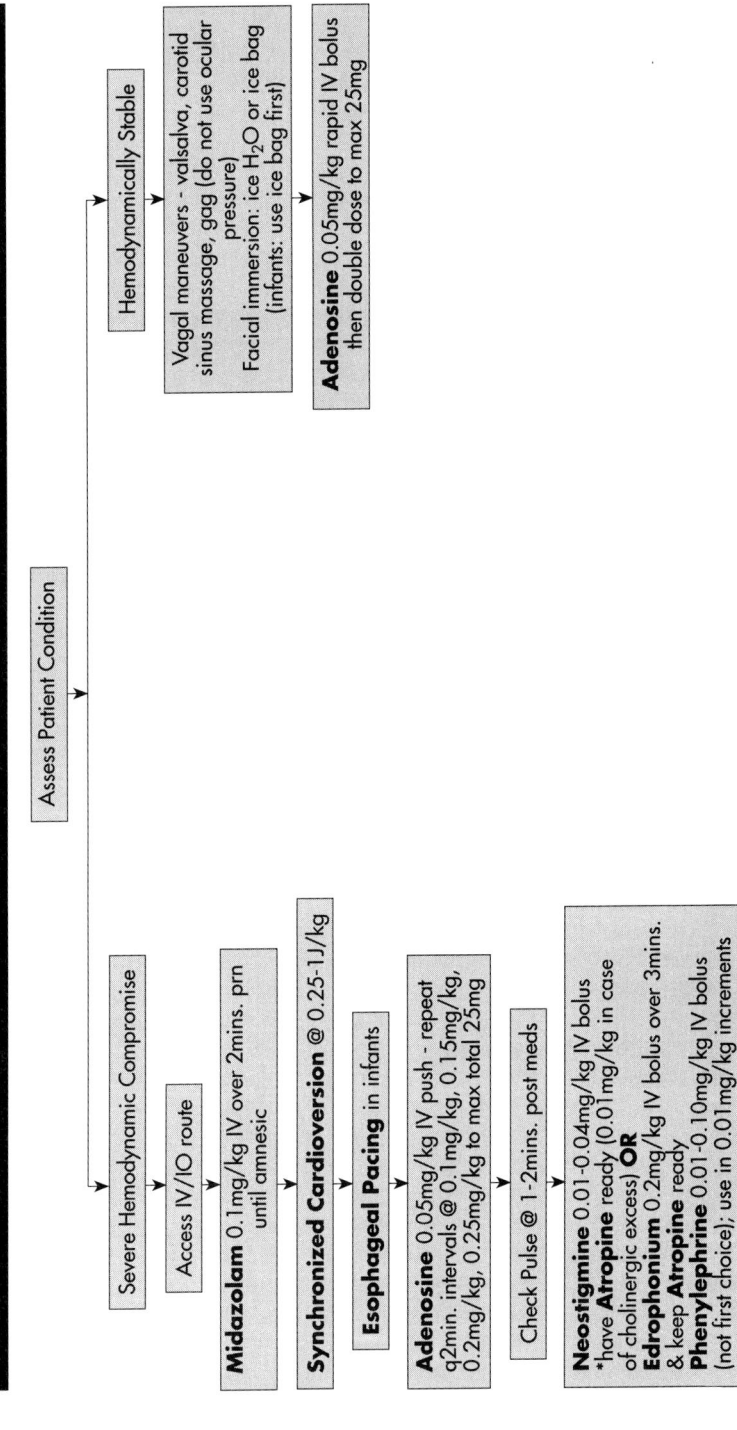

Figure 7-11. Algorithm for Supraventricular Tachycardia (SVT)

Assess Patient Condition

Hemodynamically Stable

Vagal maneuvers - valsalva, carotid sinus massage, gag (do not use ocular pressure)
Facial immersion: ice H$_2$O or ice bag (infants: use ice bag first)

Adenosine 0.05mg/kg rapid IV bolus then double dose to max 25mg

---

Severe Hemodynamic Compromise

Access IV/IO route

Midazolam 0.1mg/kg IV over 2mins. prn until amnesic

Synchronized Cardioversion @ 0.25-1J/kg

Esophageal Pacing in infants

Adenosine 0.05mg/kg IV push - repeat q2min. intervals @ 0.1mg/kg, 0.15mg/kg, 0.2mg/kg, 0.25mg/kg to max total 25mg

Check Pulse @ 1-2mins. post meds

Neostigmine 0.01-0.04mg/kg IV bolus
*have **Atropine** ready (0.01mg/kg in case of cholinergic excess) **OR**
Edrophonium 0.2mg/kg IV bolus over 3mins. & keep **Atropine** ready
Phenylephrine 0.01-0.10mg/kg IV bolus (not first choice); use in 0.01mg/kg increments

Pediatric Cardiac Arrhythmias: Management Algorithms 249

Figure 7-12. Algorithm for Paroxysmal Supraventricular Tachycardia (PSVT)

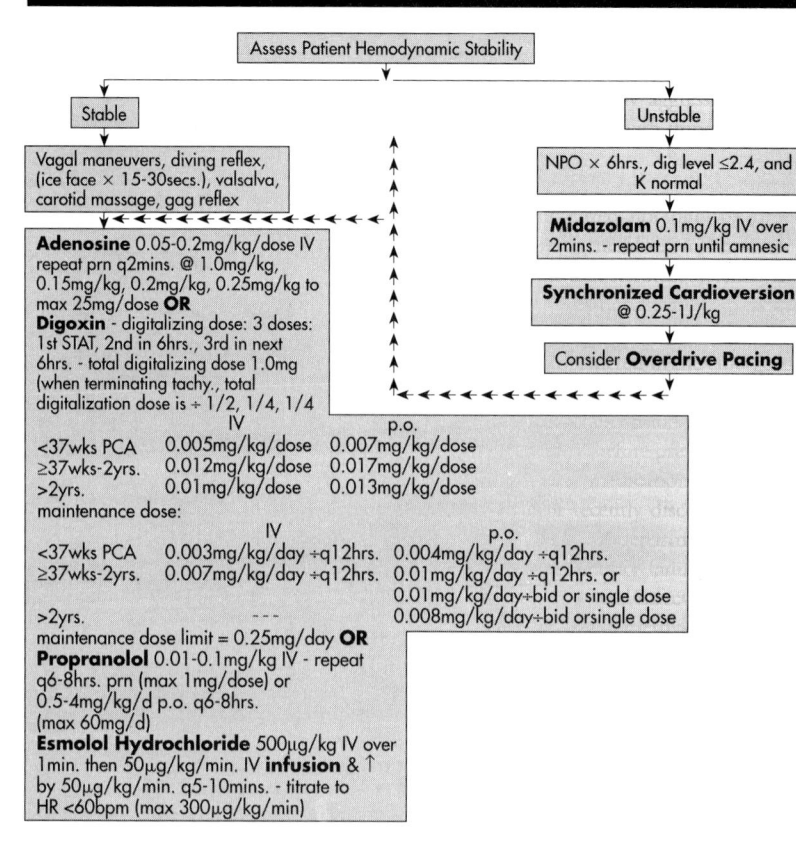

Assess Patient Hemodynamic Stability

Stable

Vagal maneuvers, diving reflex, (ice face × 15-30secs.), valsalva, carotid massage, gag reflex

Adenosine 0.05-0.2mg/kg/dose IV repeat prn q2mins. @ 1.0mg/kg, 0.15mg/kg, 0.2mg/kg, 0.25mg/kg to max 25mg/dose **OR**
Digoxin - digitalizing dose: 3 doses: 1st STAT, 2nd in 6hrs., 3rd in next 6hrs. - total digitalizing dose 1.0mg (when terminating tachy., total digitalization dose is ÷ 1/2, 1/4, 1/4

	IV	p.o.
<37wks PCA	0.005mg/kg/dose	0.007mg/kg/dose
≥37wks-2yrs.	0.012mg/kg/dose	0.017mg/kg/dose
>2yrs.	0.01mg/kg/dose	0.013mg/kg/dose

maintenance dose:

	IV	p.o.
<37wks PCA	0.003mg/kg/day ÷q12hrs.	0.004mg/kg/day ÷q12hrs.
≥37wks-2yrs.	0.007mg/kg/day ÷q12hrs.	0.01mg/kg/day ÷q12hrs. or 0.01mg/kg/day÷bid or single dose
>2yrs.	---	0.008mg/kg/day÷bid or single dose

maintenance dose limit = 0.25mg/day **OR**
Propranolol 0.01-0.1mg/kg IV - repeat q6-8hrs. prn (max 1mg/dose) or 0.5-4mg/kg/d p.o. q6-8hrs. (max 60mg/d)
Esmolol Hydrochloride 500µg/kg IV over 1min. then 50µg/kg/min. IV **infusion** & ↑ by 50µg/kg/min. q5-10mins. - titrate to HR <60bpm (max 300µg/kg/min)

Unstable

NPO × 6hrs., dig level ≤2.4, and K normal

Midazolam 0.1mg/kg IV over 2mins. - repeat prn until amnesic

Synchronized Cardioversion @ 0.25-1J/kg

Consider **Overdrive Pacing**

250 Ch 7. Cardiac Arrhythmias and Antiarrhythmic Drugs

Figure 7-13. Algorithm for Atrial Fibrillation and Atrial Flutter

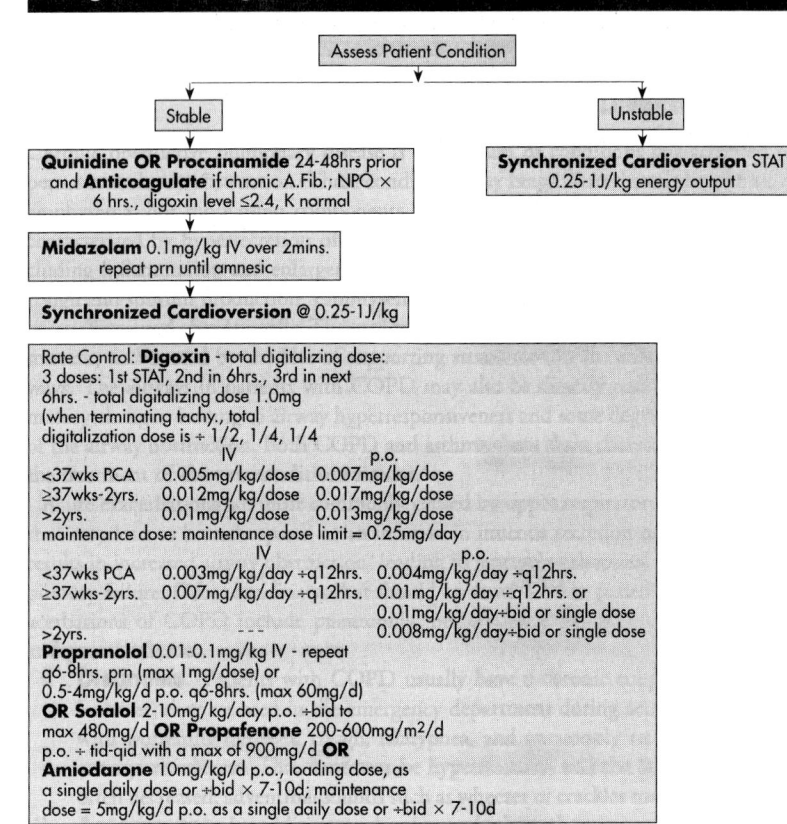

Assess Patient Condition

Stable

Quinidine OR Procainamide 24-48hrs prior and **Anticoagulate** if chronic A.Fib.; NPO × 6 hrs., digoxin level ≤2.4, K normal

Midazolam 0.1mg/kg IV over 2mins. repeat prn until amnesic

Synchronized Cardioversion @ 0.25-1J/kg

Rate Control: **Digoxin** - total digitalizing dose: 3 doses: 1st STAT, 2nd in 6hrs., 3rd in next 6hrs. - total digitalizing dose 1.0mg (when terminating tachy., total digitalization dose is ÷ 1/2, 1/4, 1/4

	IV	p.o.
<37wks PCA	0.005mg/kg/dose	0.007mg/kg/dose
≥37wks-2yrs.	0.012mg/kg/dose	0.017mg/kg/dose
>2yrs.	0.01mg/kg/dose	0.013mg/kg/dose

maintenance dose: maintenance dose limit = 0.25mg/day

	IV	p.o.
<37wks PCA	0.003mg/kg/day ÷q12hrs.	0.004mg/kg/day ÷q12hrs.
≥37wks-2yrs.	0.007mg/kg/day ÷q12hrs.	0.01mg/kg/day ÷q12hrs. or 0.01mg/kg/day÷bid or single dose
>2yrs.	---	0.008mg/kg/day÷bid or single dose

Propranolol 0.01-0.1mg/kg IV - repeat q6-8hrs. prn (max 1mg/dose) or 0.5-4mg/kg/d p.o. q6-8hrs. (max 60mg/d)
OR Sotalol 2-10mg/kg/day p.o. ÷bid to max 480mg/d **OR Propafenone** 200-600mg/m^2/d p.o. ÷ tid-qid with a max of 900mg/d **OR Amiodarone** 10mg/kg/d p.o., loading dose, as a single daily dose or ÷bid × 7-10d; maintenance dose = 5mg/kg/d p.o. as a single daily dose or ÷bid × 7-10d

Pharmacological Conversion:
Procainamide 2-6mg/kg/dose IV loading over 5mins. then 20-80μg/kg/min. IV **infusion** to max 100mg/dose or 2g/24h; then 15-50μg/kg/d po q3-6h to max 4g/d

Unstable

Synchronized Cardioversion STAT 0.25-1J/kg energy output

Figure 7-14. Algorithm for Sinus Bradycardia

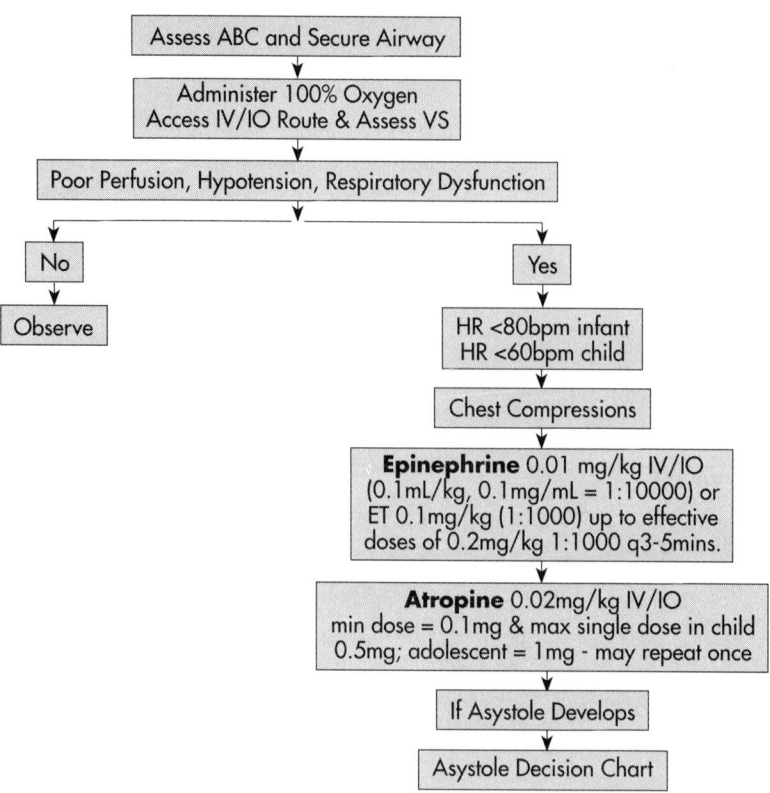

```
Assess ABC and Secure Airway
              ↓
   Administer 100% Oxygen
  Access IV/IO Route & Assess VS
              ↓
Poor Perfusion, Hypotension, Respiratory Dysfunction
         ↓                    ↓
        No                   Yes
         ↓                    ↓
      Observe         HR <80bpm infant
                      HR <60bpm child
                            ↓
                     Chest Compressions
                            ↓
              Epinephrine 0.01 mg/kg IV/IO
              (0.1mL/kg, 0.1mg/mL = 1:10000) or
              ET 0.1mg/kg (1:1000) up to effective
              doses of 0.2mg/kg 1:1000 q3-5mins.
                            ↓
              Atropine 0.02mg/kg IV/IO
              min dose = 0.1mg & max single dose in child
              0.5mg; adolescent = 1mg - may repeat once
                            ↓
                 If Asystole Develops
                            ↓
                 Asystole Decision Chart
```

Cardiac output in infants younger than 6 months is heart rate dependent. A child of any age presenting a bradycardic ECG associated with poor systemic perfusion should be expeditiously treated with epinephrine. Atropine is used to treat bradycardias with concomitant poor perfusion or hypotension. The parasympatholytic properties of the drug accelerate the atrial pacemakers and increase AV conduction. Tachycardia may follow after the administration of a vagolytic dose of atropine and is well tolerated in children. (Reproduced with permission. *JAMA* October 28, 1992, 268:16, 2266. Copyright 1992, American Medical Association.)

8 Emergency Neurologic Therapeutics

Marc Kamin, M.D.
Thomas D. Sabin, M.D.

Neurologic emergencies constitute some of the most perplexing problems for the emergency physician. Therapy of several common emergency situations is reviewed in this chapter. Standard textbooks of neurology should be consulted for a more detailed account of the clinical aspects of these conditions. The most current therapeutic regimens and options are presented, with the realization that therapy must be individualized in some cases.

Seizures

Seizures are associated with a wide variety of neurologic and medical diseases **(Table 8-1)**. Common ways a patient with seizures may present to the emergency physician include (1) a first seizure, (2) recurrent seizures in a patient with epilepsy, and (3) status epilepticus.

I. New-onset seizures
  A. When a child or adult is seen after their first unprovoked seizure, the emergency physician should do the following:
   1. **Obtain a thorough history** from the patient, witnesses, and/or family to verify the diagnosis. Seizures can be confused with cardiac arrhythmias, syncope (organic or psychogenic), the hyperventilation syndrome, or breath-holding spells. Evidence of focal onset of the seizure should be sought. A history of headache, fever, and a stiff neck should arouse suspicion of a central nervous system (CNS) infection.
   2. **Perform a physical examination** including a neurologic examination. This examination includes a search for evidence of head trauma, ear infection, neck stiffness, heart murmur, and signs of a focal neurologic deficit.
   3. **Obtain a laboratory evaluation** including a complete blood cell count, serum levels of glucose, electrolytes, calcium, and magnesium, and an electrocardiogram in older patients. Computerized axial tomographic (CAT) scanning of the brain should be performed if there are focal neurologic signs or there is a suspicion of CNS infection or hemorrhage. Lumbar puncture is performed when appropriate.
      a. **Patients with normal** physical, neurologic, and laboratory examinations after the seizure may be released from the emergency department with no treatment. They should have no historical, physical, or laboratory findings to suggest more than an idiopathic seizure disorder. Even a newly diagnosed focal seizure may not be treated immediately. Follow-up by a neurologist or internist is mandatory, and the patient should be warned not to drive. A decision about treatment with anticonvulsants depends on further neurologic evaluation and results of an electroencephalogram (EEG). If

Table 8-1. Common Causes of Seizures in Patients Seen in an Emergency Department

Adult
Idiopathic
Alcohol or drug withdrawal
Reduction of or abrupt withdrawal of anticonvulsant drugs
Head trauma
Cerebral anoxia
Intracranial infection
  Abscess
  Subdural empyema
Intracerebral hemorrhage
Toxic-metabolic
  Hypoglycemia
  Hypocalcemia
Brain tumor
Subdural hematoma
Cortical vein thrombosis

Children
All of the above
Benign febrile
Degenerative diseases
Inborn errors of metabolism
Congenital malformations

---

abnormalities on the initial evaluations are found or there is evidence of focal onset of the seizure, a neurologic consultation should be obtained.

b. **When intracranial infection,** brain tumor, or a stroke syndrome is associated with a first seizure, adults and children should be treated with anticonvulsants in the emergency department to prevent seizure recurrence. **Table 8-2** outlines the commonly used anticonvulsant drugs including their loading doses and maintenance dosages. Oral loading with phenytoin usually suffices. Phenytoin, 15 to 18 mg/kg, is given as one dose, or over a period of 1 hour if a large number of capsules is required.

c. **In the acutely ill patient,** a slow intravenous infusion of the same loading dose may be given at a rate of 25 to 50 mg/min through an intravenous line containing normal saline solution. In the emergency department it must be administered by a nurse or doctor with electrocardiographic (ECG) monitoring. The most serious side effects are hypotension, cardiac conduction defects, respiratory depression, and cardiovascular collapse. Hypotension may be overcome by discontinuing the administration and restarting at a slower rate when vital signs are more stable. Intramuscular injection of phenytoin is ineffective. If phenytoin cannot be used, phenobarbital can be administered parenterally. A total dose of 10 to 15 mg/kg is usually required for loading with maintenance dosages of 2 to 3 mg/kg/day. An initial dose of 240

Table 8-2. Commonly Used Anticonvulsant Drugs and Routes of Administration

Name	Loading dose	Maintenance dosage
Phenytoin (Dilantin)	15-18 mg/kg IV or PO	5 mg/kg/day in one or two divided doses, PO, IV
Phenobarbital	15-20 mg/kg IV, IM, PO	5 mg/kg in children, 1-2 mg/kg in adolescents and adults IV, IM, PO
Carbamazepine (Tegretol)	Not clinically useful	400-1200 mg/day or more in three or four divided doses with monitoring of blood levels, PO
Valproic acid (Depakene, Depakote)	1000 mg per rectum in selected cases	15-60 mg/kg/day in three divided doses, PO
Ethosuximide (Zarontin)	Not clinically useful	250-750 mg/day, PO
Primidone (Mysoline)	Not clinically useful	150-300 mg/day in children, 300-1250 mg/day in adults, in three divided doses, PO
Felbamate (Felbatol)	Not clinically useful	3600 mg/day monotherapy or add-on in adults with partial seizures, 45 mg/kg/day in children with Lennox-Gastaut syndrome
Gabapentin (Neurontin)	Not clinically useful	Up to 1800 mg/day as add-on in adults with partial seizures

mg is administered intravenously immediately at a rate of 50 to 100 mg/min, followed by 120 mg every 4 hours until therapeutic blood levels are attained. Respiratory depression and hypotension are the most serious side effects.

B. Uncomplicated alcohol withdrawal seizures, even if multiple, need not be treated unless there is evidence of status epilepticus. These patients must be admitted to the hospital to observe for more serious signs of alcohol withdrawal.

C. Seizures secondary to metabolic disturbances such as hyponatremia are treated by correcting the underlying biochemical abnormality.

D. A young child with a first febrile convulsion represents a dilemma for the emergency physician. Even with a normal neurologic examination, these children must have a lumbar puncture to exclude the possibility of CNS infection. When all examinations in the emergency department are normal, these children need not be treated. Any decision to treat is made after pediatric consultation and an EEG is obtained. The use of prophylactic antibiotics is controversial.

II. Recurrent seizures. When faced with the situation of recurrent grand mal or focal seizures in a patient already taking anticonvulsant medication, measurement of blood levels is essential to emergency room management. **Table 8-3** outlines

Table 8-3. Therapeutic Levels of Commonly Used Anticonvulsants

Drug	Therapeutic level
Phenytoin (Dilantin)	10-20 µg/ml
Phenobarbital	20-45 µg/ml
Primidone (Mysoline)	7-15 µg/ml primidone, active metabolite is phenobarbital found at levels of 10-40 µg/ml
Valproic acid (Depakene, Depakote)	50-100 µg/ml
Carbamazepine (Tegretol)	4-12 µg/ml
Ethosuximide (Zarontin)	40-100 µg/ml

the accepted therapeutic levels of the more commonly used anticonvulsant drugs. These are guidelines, and effectiveness may be obtained slightly below or above these levels. Intercurrent metabolic or new structural brain abnormalities must be considered. If noncompliance is not the causative factor, then a dosage adjustment of the currently used drugs is warranted. Required dosage adjustments can be made empirically or determined by the following formula: volume of distribution (Vd) × weight in kilograms × change in blood level desired, equals amount of additional dose in milligrams. The values for Vd of phenobarbital, phenytoin, and carbamazepine are 0.8, 0.6, and 0.8, respectively. The volume of distribution for valproic acid is approximately 0.2 in adults and 0.4 in children. This formula does not always produce the expected blood level because of differences in body habitus and metabolism. Antiepileptic drugs are typically titrated to toxicity before their effectiveness is ruled out. The most important treatment is good neurologic follow-up. Multiple recurrent seizures are best treated by admission to the hospital for further evaluation and dosage adjustment.

III. Status epilepticus

A. Grand mal status epilepticus is a life-threatening condition that develops in children and adults. It manifests as constant or frequently repetitive seizures with no intervening period of normal consciousness. The most common causes of grand mal status are abrupt withdrawal of antiepileptic medication, alcohol withdrawal, anoxic encephalopathy, and ischemic cerebrovascular disease.

B. The treatment of generalized tonic-clonic status epilepticus in adults and children is similar. As in all life-threatening emergencies, the airway must first be protected. Blood pressure and ECG are monitored. Venous access is obtained, and blood is drawn for glucose, electrolytes, calcium, and anticonvulsant drug levels, as well as a toxic drug screen. Intravenous dextrose (50 ml of a 50% solution) and thiamine (100 mg) are administered if patients are alcoholic, diabetic, or malnourished. Diazepam (Valium) is usually administered first at a rate of 2 mg/min. A total dose of 5 to 10 mg in children and 10 to 20 mg in adults can be infused. Side effects of respiratory depression or hypotension may be seen. Lorazepam, a benzodiazepine with a longer duration of action, is being used more frequently but is not approved by the Food and Drug Administration (FDA) as a treatment for status epilepticus. It is administered at 0.05 to 0.2 mg/kg at 2 mg/min, with a maximum dose of 8 mg. If diazepam is used, because it has only a 20-minute duration of activity, a loading dose of phenytoin should be administered at the same time through a different intravenous line. The loading dose of phenytoin is 18 mg/kg given at a rate of 50 mg/min. If the seizures are not controlled by the end of the phenytoin infusion, a phenobarbital trial is begun. Respiratory depression, especially if diazepam has been used, is a complication of high-dose phenobarbital therapy. In adults phenobarbital can be infused at 100 mg/min to a total loading dose of 10 mg/kg. In children the loading dose is 5 to 20 mg/kg. Some authors recommend using midazolam at this stage. A loading dose of 0.2 mg/kg is followed by a maintenance dosage of 0.1 to 0.4 mg/kg/hr. If the seizures are not controlled within an hour of onset of therapy, general anesthesia is the most effective method of terminating grand mal status epilepticus at this point. Phenobarbital coma, a form of generalized anesthesia, can be induced in the intensive care unit. A loading dose of 12 mg/kg is followed by a maintenance dosage of 5 mg/kg/hr. An EEG pattern of burst suppression is the level of coma at which the best results have been reported.

C. **Petit mal** (3-Hz spike and wave pattern) or temporal lobe status epilepticus may result in the confusing clinical picture of a persistently altered state of consciousness. A high index of suspicion is necessary for diagnosis, and EEG confirmation is essential. Nonconvulsive status epilepticus resulting from petit mal or psychomotor seizures may be treated initially with intravenous diazepam, 5 to 10 mg. Because of the risks of respiratory depression, diazepam may only be necessary when the patient's condition is so serious that immediate cessation of the seizures is required. Institution of appropriate oral anticonvulsant therapy in nonemergent cases will also terminate the pattern. Drugs useful in petit mal status include valproic acid (Depakote) and ethosuximide (Zarontin). Temporal lobe status can also be treated with increasing doses of carbamazepine or phenytoin. Focal motor status or epilepsia partialis continua most commonly occur in an awake patient. Focal motor status epilepticus in a conscious patient is not a medical emergency unless respiratory decompensation is occurring. These patients are admitted to the hospital and treated with oral loading doses of phenytoin or intramuscular phenobarbital, followed by carbamazepine if necessary.

Head Injury

Patients with closed or penetrating head trauma are frequently encountered in the emergency department. Closed head trauma includes mild concussion with or without brief periods of altered consciousness (usually less than 10 minutes), subdural and epidural hematomas, and cerebral contusions.

I. **Mild head injury.** One of the most important decisions to be made by the emergency physician is when to admit a patient with mild head trauma to the hospital. Some authors recommend admission for any patient that has lost consciousness. An approach recommended by Barnett of the Cleveland Clinic is as follows. Those patients that are stunned or had a brief period of altered consciousness with mild headache and who are neurologically normal and alert need not be admitted or have a CAT scan of the brain. A responsible party must be available to monitor the level of alertness and be able to return the patient to an emergency department within 15 minutes.

II. **Severe brain injury.** All other patients with head trauma are to be admitted. Patients with a severe headache, seizures, clinical signs of a skull fracture, nausea or vomiting, altered state of consciousness, or focal neurologic signs require an emergency CAT scan after their airway and circulation are secure. Skull roentgenograms may reveal foreign bodies or air-fluid levels in cranial sinuses. Significant head trauma also requires cervical spine radiographs to be done. Patients should be handled as though a cervical spine fracture were present until it is ruled out. A Philadelphia collar, not a soft cervical collar, should be used to stabilize the neck. Lateral cervical spine radiographs must include the seventh cervical vertebrae to be complete.

A. **More severely injured** patients with a persistent altered state of consciousness may have cerebral edema. This is characterized by an increased amount of intracellular and extracellular water in the brain. In these patients maintenance of an airway is crucial either via a nasal airway or nasotracheal intubation with assisted ventilation. Hypercarbia is avoided because it dilates cerebral vasculature, increases cerebral blood flow, and can aggravate cerebral edema. Restoration of blood volume if bleeding or hypotension occurred should be performed by using isotonic fluids. Hypotonic fluids may aggravate cerebral edema. Prophylactic anticonvulsants are not widely used at this time. Evidence of other traumatic injuries should be sought.

B. **Expanding cerebral lesions** such as an epidural hematoma or worsening cerebral edema may cause rising intracranial pressure and lead to the herniation syndrome. The herniation syndrome presents with progressive obtundation and sometimes focal neurologic signs. Pupils are initially small but eventually dilate bilaterally or on the side of an expanding lesion. Disorders of respiration such as Cheyne-Stokes or central hyperventilation occur as the level of consciousness decreases. Cerebral herniation can rapidly progress to fatal brain stem compression. This neurologic emergency must be treated immediately before further studies are obtained. Treatment for increasing intracranial pressure includes the following:

  1. **Assisted hyperventilation** to reduce the carbon dioxide pressure (PCO_2) to 25 to 30 mm Hg.

  2. **An immediate dose of mannitol, 1 gm/kg,** given over 5 to 10 minutes. This is accompanied by 20 mg of furosemide intravenously. Mannitol should not be given if the serum osmolality is greater than 320 mOsm/L. Steroid therapy is not effective for this type of increased intracranial pressure.

C. **A neurosurgical consultation** should be obtained immediately in all patients with severe head injury for subsequent appropriate management, including intracranial pressure monitoring and/or surgery.

Cerebrovascular Disease

I. **Transient ischemic attack.** Transient ischemic attacks (TIAs) are transient neurologic deficits lasting less than 24 hours that occur within a specific vascular territory. Most TIAs last less than 15 minutes. **Tables 8-4** and **8-5** outline the symptoms and differential diagnosis of TIAs. Patients with transient neurologic signs or symptoms for the first time with no obvious cause should be admitted to the hospital. Patients with neurologic signs in the emergency department, those with an increasing frequency of attacks, and those with a suspected embolus should also be admitted immediately. The cause of the TIA must be determined promptly because TIA is a predictor for a completed stroke in the near future. Treatment includes daily aspirin, correction of metabolic abnormalities, or carotid endarterectomy in patients with >70% stenosis. Patients with repetitive TIAs from carotid stenosis or dissection of the carotid or vertebral arteries are commonly managed with intravenous heparin.

Table 8-4. Common Symptoms of Transient Ischemic Attacks

Carotid TIA
Hemiparesis or monoparesis
Hemihypesthesia or monohypesthesia
Aphasia
Monocular visual loss (amaurosis fugax)
Hemianopsia
Vertebrobasilar TIA
Monoparesis, hemiparesis, or quadraparesis
Paresthesia, hypesthesia in various combinations over one or both sides of the body or face
Crossed motor and sensory deficits
Hemianopsia
Ataxia
Vertigo

Table 8-5. Differential Diagnosis of Transient Ischemic Attacks

Atheromatous embolus
Hypoglycemia
Cerebral embolism of cardiac origin
Hypoperfusion syndrome
Seizure
Migraine
Hypertensive encephalopathy
Nonatherosclerotic arteriopathies
Hematologic disorders

II. **Thromboembolic stroke**
   A. **The acute onset** of a fixed neurologic deficit in a specific vascular distribution lasting more than 24 hours in the carotid circulation and more than 72 hours in the vertebral circulation is commonly referred to as a stroke. Pathophysiologic mechanisms associated with stroke are outline in **Table 8-6**. All these patients are admitted to the hospital, unless the deficit occurred several days or weeks earlier and there are minimal signs or symptoms.
   B. **Diagnosis.** The role of the emergency physician is to confirm the diagnosis of stroke by determining the pathophysiology if possible, defining the vascular territory, and initiating basic treatment. Appropriate history, physical examination, and laboratory examination including CAT scanning of the brain should allow the emergency physician to arrive at the correct diagnosis in the majority of cases. Initial therapeutic efforts include maintaining vital signs, correcting obvious metabolic derangements, and minimizing the amount of brain tissue destroyed. Blood glucose levels should be maintained in the normal range. Recent evidence suggests that hyperglycemia may contribute to acidosis in marginal areas of perfusion. Hypotension, congestive heart failure, and cardiac arrhythmias should be promptly corrected. Hypertension in a stroke patient, in whom autoregulation of blood flow is deranged, should not

Table 8-6. Classification of Cerebrovascular Disease

Arterial
Occlusion of lumen with distal infarction
  Thrombosis
  Embolus
  Arteriopathies (infective, inflammatory)
  Trauma and mechanical compression
  Dissection
  Spasm
    Migraine
    Subarachnoid hemorrhage
    Angiography
Hypoperfusion with infarction in border zone territories
  Hypotension
  Arrhythmia
  Cardiac valvular lesion
Venous
Aseptic thrombotic occlusion
Septic thrombotic occlusion

---

be treated too aggressively; rapid lowering of blood pressure can quickly produce extension of an infarction. Systolic blood pressure of 180 to 200 mm Hg and diastolic blood pressure up to 110 mm Hg are acceptable. Higher levels of blood pressure are best treated with nitroprusside, beginning at a rate of 0.5 µg/kg/min and increasing the rate in increments of 0.5 to 1.0 µg/kg/min until the blood pressure is in a safer range. Anticoagulation is not used in completed thrombotic or lacunar infarction. It is often used when the stroke is embolic or when the stroke is evolving in the hospital. In cases of a stroke in evolution, a bolus of heparin is given followed by a maintenance dosage. In cases of cardiac emboli, anticoagulation may be instituted early in small infarcts or may be delayed 24 to 48 hours in larger infarcts. It is usually initiated at a maintenance level to maintain the partial thromboplastin time at one and one-half times control. Two to 5 days after a large cerebral infarction, brain swelling with progressive obtundation and signs of the herniation syndrome may develop. This is treated emergently with osmotic agents such as mannitol (1 gm/kg) or glycerol, and hyperventilation as described in the section on head injury. Dexamethasone is ineffective in this setting.

III. **Other causes of stroke.** There are less common but treatable causes of stroke. These include hypercoagulable states, subacute bacterial endocarditis, and cerebral vasculitis. Abnormal clotting profiles, fever, heart murmurs, or laboratory evidence of inflammation help the physician make these diagnoses. Treatment with fresh frozen plasma, antibiotics, and corticosteroids can be effective.

IV. **Intracranial hemorrhage**

   A. **Intracranial hemorrhage** can be divided into two broad categories, intracerebral and extracerebral **(Table 8-7).** The diagnosis of intracranial hemorrhage is based on a clinical history of sudden onset of severe headache (with or without head trauma), stiff neck, typical focal neurologic signs, and obtundation. In most cases, CAT scanning of the brain, clotting studies, and lumbar puncture when appropriate will confirm the diagnosis. When increased intracranial pressure or focal neurologic signs are present, lumbar puncture should not be considered until a CAT scan of the brain is obtained. Lumbar puncture in the presence of large focal lesions can result in herniation.

B. **Treatment.** A treatment schematic for intracranial hemorrhage is shown in **Figure 8-1**.
   1. **General measures. Immediate steps** include routine care of the acutely ill patient, including maintenance of the airway and stabilization of the circulation. When signs of increased intracranial pressure are present with obtundation, hyperventilation with assisted ventilation to P_{CO_2} of 25 to 30 mm Hg is indicated. A herniation syndrome is treated with mannitol and furosemide as described earlier. These patients commonly have systemic hypertension on admission to the emergency department. Systolic blood pressure should be reduced to 180 to 190 mm Hg and the diastolic blood pressure to 100 mm Hg. Nitroprusside at an initial rate of 0.5 μg/kg/min, with subsequent rate increases in increments of 0.5 to 1.0 μg/kg/min, is used for blood pressure reduction. Clotting disorders are corrected as soon as possible with fresh frozen plasma.
   2. **The diagnosis** of intracerebral or extracerebral hemorrhage determines the next therapeutic measures.
      a. **Intracerebral hemorrhages** commonly arise in hypertensive patients or those with clotting disorders. They are treated more conservatively, with most efforts directed at reducing intracranial pressure. Parenchymal hemorrhages with signs of progressively increasing intracranial pressure may be surgically removed depending on their location. Cerebellar hemorrhages are usually rapidly evacuated because of possible direct brain stem compression. They can be treated conservatively with close observation in awake and stable patients.
      b. **Extracerebral hemorrhages** include epidural and subdural hematomas and subarachnoid hemorrhage.
         (1) **Subdural hematoma** either of traumatic or spontaneous nature can be difficult to diagnose. A high degree of suspicion is necessary, especially in older patients with subtle focal neurologic findings and a remote or absent history of trauma. The diagnosis is confirmed by CAT scanning of the brain. Treatment is generally surgical. Smaller subdural hematomas can be treated conservatively and will resolve.

Table 8-7. Classification of Intracranial Hemorrhage

Intracerebral	Extracerebral
Hypertensive	Subarachnoid
Hemorrhagic infarction	Subdural
Arteriovenous malformation	Traumatic
Clotting disorder	Spontaneous
Liver disease	Clotting disorder
Leukemia	Epidural
Thrombotic thrombocytopenia purpura	
Anticoagulant therapy	
Hemorrhage into tumor	

Cerebrovascular Disease 261

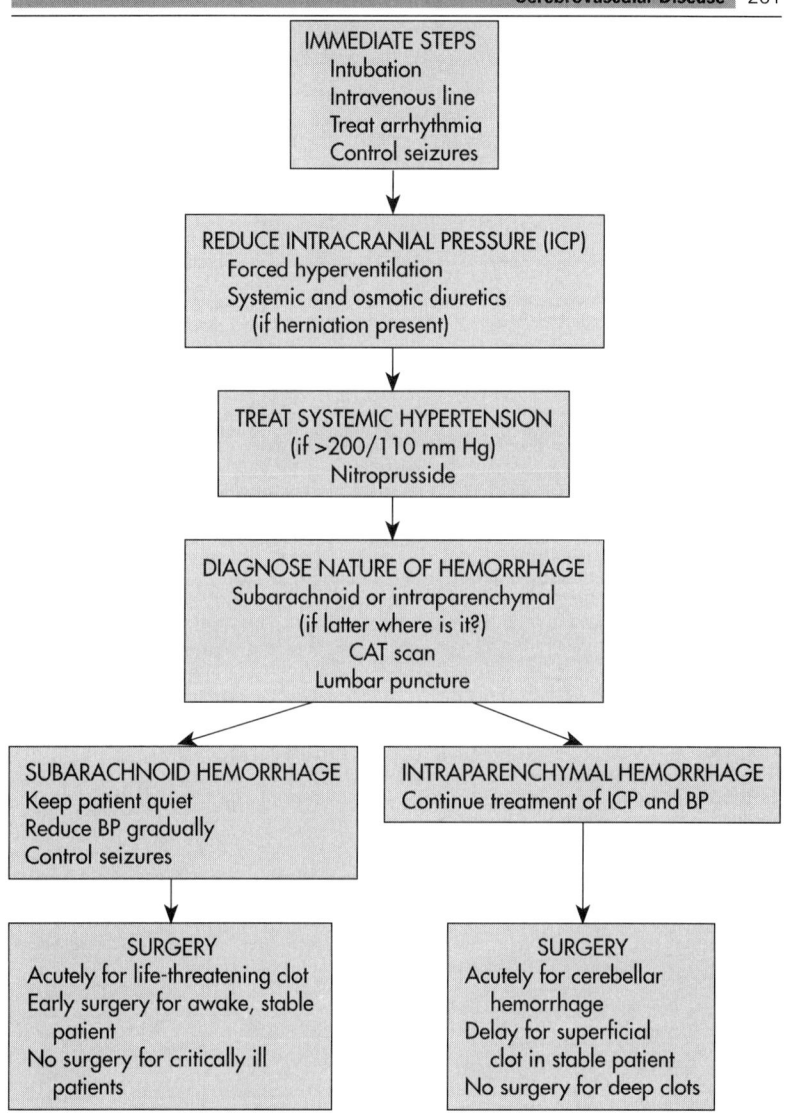

```
┌─────────────────────────────────┐
│       IMMEDIATE STEPS           │
│         Intubation              │
│       Intravenous line          │
│       Treat arrhythmia          │
│       Control seizures          │
└─────────────────────────────────┘
              │
              ▼
┌─────────────────────────────────┐
│  REDUCE INTRACRANIAL PRESSURE   │
│             (ICP)               │
│     Forced hyperventilation     │
│   Systemic and osmotic diuretics│
│      (if herniation present)    │
└─────────────────────────────────┘
              │
              ▼
┌─────────────────────────────────┐
│   TREAT SYSTEMIC HYPERTENSION   │
│       (if >200/110 mm Hg)       │
│          Nitroprusside          │
└─────────────────────────────────┘
              │
              ▼
┌─────────────────────────────────┐
│  DIAGNOSE NATURE OF HEMORRHAGE  │
│  Subarachnoid or intraparenchymal│
│      (if latter where is it?)   │
│             CAT scan            │
│          Lumbar puncture        │
└─────────────────────────────────┘
          ↙             ↘
┌──────────────────────┐  ┌──────────────────────┐
│ SUBARACHNOID         │  │ INTRAPARENCHYMAL     │
│ HEMORRHAGE           │  │ HEMORRHAGE           │
│ Keep patient quiet   │  │ Continue treatment   │
│ Reduce BP gradually  │  │ of ICP and BP        │
│ Control seizures     │  │                      │
└──────────────────────┘  └──────────────────────┘
          │                         │
          ▼                         ▼
┌──────────────────────┐  ┌──────────────────────┐
│      SURGERY         │  │      SURGERY         │
│ Acutely for life-    │  │ Acutely for cerebellar│
│ threatening clot     │  │ hemorrhage           │
│ Early surgery for    │  │ Delay for superficial│
│ awake, stable        │  │ clot in stable patient│
│ patient              │  │ No surgery for deep  │
│ No surgery for       │  │ clots                │
│ critically ill       │  │                      │
│ patients             │  │                      │
└──────────────────────┘  └──────────────────────┘
```

Fig. 8-1. Management scheme for intracranial hemorrhage.

- **(2) Epidural hematoma** as a result of trauma is a neurosurgical emergency and requires immediate evacuation.
- **(3) Once subarachnoid hemorrhage** (SAH) is diagnosed in the emergency department, procedures to reduce the chance of further bleeding are instituted. The patient must be kept quiet in a darkened room. Blood pressure is reduced as described previously. In younger patients blood pressures of 160/90 are tolerable. Blood pressure will commonly stabilize in the normal range with bed rest and mild sedation. Prophylactic anticonvulsants such as phenytoin,

Table 8-8. Hunt-Hess Scale

Grade	Clinical description
0	Asymptomatic
I	Mild headache
II	Moderate to severe headache, nuchal rigidity, can have oculomotor palsy
III	Confusion, drowsiness, or mild focal signs
IV	Stupor or hemiparesis
V	Coma, moribund, and/or extensor posturing

5 mg/kg/day, are instituted. Nimodipine, 60 mg every 4 hours, reduces the incidence of ischemic events and improves overall outcome in patients with Hunt-Hess grade I-III SAH **(Table 8-8).** Antifibrinolytics are no longer widely used. Angiography is usually performed early to locate the source of bleeding. Early operation for patients in good clinical condition is advocated. Patients with Hunt-Hess grade 0, I, and sometimes II SAH are operated on within the first few days of diagnosis. This eliminates rebleeding and makes delayed-onset vasospasm easier to treat with volume expansion. In more severe cases, 2 to 3 weeks of observation before surgery is common practice.

Headache

Headache is the most common reason for visits to a primary care physician. The major pathophysiologic categories of headache are displayed in **Table 8-9** and commonly used medications for the treatment of acute headache are displayed in **Table 8-10.** An exhaustive review of headache signs and symptoms is beyond the scope of this section on therapeutics. Instead we intend to focus on the differentiation of muscle contraction and migrainous syndromes from headaches encountered in urgent and life-threatening situations in the emergency department.

I. **Diagnosis**
  A. **The diagnosis of headache rests on a clinical history and a neurologic examination.** The most common types of headache encountered are migraine and muscle contraction headaches. Muscle contraction or tension headaches are daily aching pains all over the head or in a hat-band distribution. They are present on awakening and continue all day, typically for weeks at a time. Classic migraines are typically unilateral, throbbing headaches preceded or accompanied by a neurologic symptom (aura). The aura may be visual scotoma, flashing lights, sensory disturbances, or even aphasia. The aura evolves over a period of 30 minutes. The headache may be accompanied by autonomic symptoms such as nausea, vomiting, photophobia, sweating, and diarrhea. Common migraine presents with a more generalized headache and no neurologic signs or symptoms. Migraines may begin abruptly or gradually, lasting hours to days, with days or weeks of pain-free intervals. Cluster headaches are brief (15 to 30 minutes), intense episodes of boring or throbbing pain around one eye. This is accompanied by ipsilateral lacrimation and nasal stuffiness. They occur more frequently in males, occurring several times a day and often awakening the patient from sleep. A persistent bitemporal or unilateral

Table 8-9. Headache Commonly Encountered in an Emergency Department

Headaches Whose Cause is Unknown or Controversial
Migraine
  Classical
  Common
Muscle contraction
Cluster
Headaches with a Structural Cause
Extracranial
  Nasal sinus
  Temporal arteritis
  Temporomandibular joint disease
Intracranial
  Meningeal
    Infectious—bacterial, fungal, viral
    SAH
  Subdural
    Empyema
    Hematoma
  Intraparenchymal
    Hemorrhage
    Tumor
    Abscess
    Ischemic vascular
  Obstructive hydrocephalus
  Cerebral venous occlusion

headache in a patient older than 55 years should raise the possibility of temporal arteritis. Associated symptoms include transient or permanent visual loss, jaw claudication, myalgias, and arthralgias.

B. **Migraineurs** are not spared from SAH, meningitis, or brain tumors. We have seen grave errors based on the assumption that any headache in a migraineur is a migraine headache. Recent and gradual onset of headache and fever with or without a stiff neck must arouse suspicion of a meningeal process. As the old dictum goes, if one thinks of a lumbar puncture it is best to do it. The sudden onset of "the worst headache in my life" is commonly associated with a diagnosis of SAH, although migraine headache can present that way. Sentinel hemorrhages or "leaks" from an aneurysm may occur days to weeks before more catastrophic bleeding. They present as abrupt headaches, possibly focal in nature, lasting hours or days with few associated symptoms. The diagnosis of SAH cannot be excluded by a normal CAT scan of the brain. Lumbar puncture must be done if SAH is suspected. Headache associated with intracerebral hemorrhage is usually accompanied by other neurologic signs and symptoms. Subdural hematoma may present as a mild headache with subtle neurologic signs; a high index of suspicion is necessary to make this diagnosis. The headache of increased intracranial pressure seen with obstructive hydrocephalus, brain tumor, or idiopathic intracranial hypertension typically is diffuse and worse on awakening. The headache of increased intracranial pressure may worsen with sudden head movement, coughing, sneezing, or straining.

Table 8-10. Headache Preparations Effective in the Acute Treatment of Headache

Drug	Preparation	Dosage and route of administration	Headache type
Ergotamine	Cafergot	1 suppository, repeat in 1 hr	Migraine
	Ergomar	2 mg SL, repeat in ½ hr	Migraine, cluster
	Medi-haler	0.36 mg/puff, 1-6 puffs/day	Migraine, cluster
Dihydroergotamine	DHE-45	0.5-0.75 mg IV, 1 mg IM	Migraine, cluster
Metoclopramide	Regland	10 mg IV	Migraine
Sumatriptan	Imitrex	6 mg SC	Migraine
Meperidine	Demerol	75-100 mg IM	Migraine
Xylocaine	Lidocaine	1 ml 4% solution, 1-3× intranasal	Cluster
Oxygen	—	8-10 L of 100% O_2 over 10-15 min	Cluster
Diazepam	Valium	5 mg PO TID	Muscle contraction
Cyclobenzaprine	Flexeril	5-10 mg PO TID	Muscle contraction
Nonsteroidal antiinflammatory	—	750 mg naproxen, 600 mg ibuprofen	Muscle contraction

II. Treatment
A. Migraine.
Once a migraineur comes to the emergency department, prophylactic or other abortive measures have probably failed.
1. **Patients should be placed in a dark room** with a cold compress on the forehead.
2. If in the judgment of the emergency department physician the pain is "mild," a large dose of a **nonsteroidal antiinflammatory drug** may help (naproxen 750 mg).
3. **A dose of an antiemetic,** like metaclopramide 10 mg or promethazine 50 mg, is utilized if nausea is a prominent symptom.
4. **Although narcotic analgesics** are not widely approved, in more severe cases an intramuscular injection of meperidine, 75 to 100 mg, with promethazine 50 mg or hydroxyzine 50 mg may produce enough pain relief in many patients to allow them to return home. The danger of this treatment is that patients may become habituated to this method of relieving headaches. It should only be used after a thorough physical examination, a diligent search of medical records, and contact with the family physician. The patient must be followed-up by the family physician or a neurologist.
5. **Persistent vomiting** may result in dehydration, and treatment with dextrose and normal saline solution will be necessary.
6. **Parenteral dihydroergotamine** (DHE-45) is also useful in this setting; DHE-45, 1.0 mg, is administered intramuscularly in evolving headaches. If the headache is established, metoclopramide, 10 mg intravenously, followed by DHE-45, 0.75 mg intravenously, are administered. If the attack has not subsided in 30 minutes, another 0.5 mg of DHE-45 can be given. Side effects of dihydroergotamine include aggravation of angina, nausea, vomiting, muscle cramps, and signs of peripheral vasoconstriction. DHE-45 is contraindicated in patients with Prinzmetal's angina, peripheral vascular disease, coronary artery disease, hypertension, impaired renal or hepatic function, and sepsis. Acute dystonic reactions are a complication of parenteral metoclopramide.
7. **Sumatriptan,** a 5-hydroxytryptamine ($5\text{-}HT_1$) receptor subtype agonist is effective for the acute treatment of classic and common migraine. A 6 mg dose can be self-administered during the headache. Although not frequently effective, the dose can be repeated in 1 hour with a maximum 24-hour dose of 12 mg. Sumatriptan can cause coronary vasospasm. In susceptible individuals it is recommended the first dose be administered in the physician's office. Other side effects include tingling and dizziness. Sumatriptan is contraindicated in basilar and hemiplegic migraine.
8. In cases where the headache has persisted for several days, **admission to the hospital** is warranted. Treatment with repetitive dosing of DHE-45 or parenteral steroids can relieve the headache.

B. Muscle contraction headache
1. **Mild muscle contraction** headache will respond to reassurance; a short course of muscle relaxants such as diazepam, 5 mg three times daily, or cyclobenzaprine, 10 mg three times daily; or nonsteroidal antiinflammatory drugs.
2. **More severe exacerbations** can be treated with one or two doses of narcotic-containing compounds. Potentially habituating medications like barbiturates, caffeine, and benzodiazepines should not be prescribed for longer than 2 weeks.

3. The most important therapy for these patients is **good long-term follow-up.**
C. Cluster headache
   1. **Ergotamine** is effective for the fully developed headache. It may be administered sublingually, 2 mg, by rectal suppository, or in aerosolized form, 1 to 3 puffs of 0.36 mg of ergotamine per puff.
   2. **An intramuscular injection of DHE-45,** 1.0 mg, or 6 mg of sumatriptan subcutaneously can also be effective.
   3. **Inhalation of 100% oxygen by mask,** 8 to 10 L/min, at the onset of the attack may produce relief in some patients. Intranasal application of 1 ml of a 4% Lidocaine solution, repeated once or twice, can also terminate the headache.
D. Temporal arteritis. An erythrocyte sedimentation rate and consultation by an ophthalmologist or neurologist should be obtained immediately. Steroid treatment prevents potentially irreversible visual loss and relieves other symptoms.

Vertigo

Patients with an acute attack of vertigo will commonly go to the emergency department for evaluation. Vertigo is an illusion of movement of one's environment or one's self, with symptoms of rotation or swaying. Frequently patients complain of nausea, vomiting, and inability to walk. **Table 8-11** outlines common causes of acute vertigo.

I. **Acute labyrinthitis.** Acute labyrinthitis is characterized by a sudden onset of vertigo, nausea, and vomiting. Patients may selectively lie on one side to reduce the vertiginous sensation. Spontaneous nystagmus is seen most easily with gaze toward the involved labyrinth. There is a conspicuous absence of headache, as well as brain stem signs like diplopia, dysarthria, or dysphagia. The acute vertigo usually lasts for hours and stops spontaneously. Symptomatic therapy involves a variety of vestibular sedatives **(Table 8-12).** They include antihistamines, anticholinergics, phenothiazines, and benzodiazepines—all of which have some vestibular suppressant effect. Treatment of a severe attack commonly begins with promethazine, diphenhydramine, or scopolamine (0.6 to 1.0 mg), intramuscularly or intravenously. When vomiting is prominent, prochlorperazine is a good adjunctive treatment. Milder symptoms can be treated with oral promethazine or prochlorperazine. The most common side effects of these drugs are sedation and dry mouth.

II. **Positional vertigo.** Positional vertigo is characterized by brief vertiginous episodes lasting 30 to 60 seconds that are precipitated by turning the head or assuming a certain position. It is most commonly a benign disorder associated with labyrinthine dysfunction but can have a central cause. Attacks may last several weeks. Diazepam or clonazepam are effective prophylactic treatments. Chronic attacks can be treated with labyrinthine conditioning exercises.

III. **Meniere's disease.** Meniere's disease is characterized by repeated episodes of vertigo lasting minutes to hours, associated with tinnitus and progressive sensorineural hearing loss. The onset of the attacks may cause the patient to fall. There is no headache, and there should be no brain stem neurologic signs other than nystagmus. The same vestibular sedatives used for acute labyrinthitis are effective for the acute attack of Meniere's disease. A low-salt diet and diazepam, 5 mg three times daily, may be an effective prophylactic in some patients.

Table 8-11. Common Causes of Acute Vertigo

Labyrinthine	Central
Acute labyrinthitis	Vascular
Positional	Vertebrobasilar insufficiency
Meniere's disease	Posterior fossa stroke or hemorrhage
Middle ear infection	Infectious
Drug induced or toxic	Herpes zoster
	Multiple sclerosis

Table 8-12. Commonly Used Vestibular Sedatives

Generic name	Trade name	Usual adult dose	Route of administration
Meclizine	Antivert	12.5-25 mg q6h	PO
Promethazine	Phenergan	25 mg	PO, IM, IV
Dimenhydrinate	Dramamine	25-50 mg q6h	PO
Diphenhydramine	Benadryl	25-50 mg q6h	PO, IM, IV
Scopolamine	TransdermScop	0.5 mg	Cutaneous patch
Clonazepam	Klonopin	0.5 mg BID/TID	PO
Prochlorperazine	Compazine	10 mg q4-6h	IM, PO
Diazepam	Valium	5 mg TID	PO

IV. **Vertebrobasilar insufficiency.** The most common symptom of vertebrobasilar insufficiency is transient dizziness or vertigo. It older patients it is commonly orthostatic; however, it can be due to cardiac arrhythmias, atherosclerotic narrowing of the vertebral or basilar arteries, or rarely emboli. When there are no other symptoms, the diagnosis can be difficult. Diplopia, dysarthria, ataxia, and crossed sensory or motor deficits support a diagnosis of vascular insufficiency. Treatment of the vertigo is symptomatic.

V. **Cerebellar hemorrhage.** Cerebellar hemorrhage is an important cause of acute vertigo. It is usually accompanied by headache, nausea, vomiting, obtundation, and other brain stem signs. Stiff neck can be seen with a cerebellar hemorrhage or infarction. Patients initially seen with an acute onset of headache and vertigo should be assumed to have a posterior fossa hemorrhage or infarction until proven otherwise. A CAT scan of the brain must be obtained immediately. Emergency evacuation of a clot is sometimes necessary.

VI. **Other conditions associated with vertigo**
   A. **Vertigo can be a consequence of middle ear infection** with secondary involvement of the labyrinth. Diagnosis is made after inspection of the ear canal, and treatment is with the appropriate antibiotics.
   B. **Alcohol, other sedative drugs,** streptomycin, and rarely monosodium glutamate are among the substances that can cause toxic labyrinthitis. Diagnosis depends on a good clinical history.
   C. **Vertigo with ear pain** and herpetic vesicles in the external ear canal is diagnostic of Ramsay-Hunt syndrome or herpes zoster infection of the eighth

cranial nerve. After appropriate neurologic examination and neuroimaging, vestibular sedatives may be given. Corticosteroid treatment is controversial and generally not used.

D. Acute vertigo may be the initial symptom in 7% to 10% of cases of **multiple sclerosis**. The diagnosis should be suspected in patients 25 to 45 years of age, especially when other brain stem signs are present. Treatment is complex, and patients should be admitted to the hospital for evaluation.

Oncologic Emergencies

Malignant and occasionally benign tumors produce a variety of neurologic complications necessitating visits to the emergency department. Primary or metastatic tumors to the brain may present with a stroke syndrome in a vascular territory or with an intracerebral hemorrhage. Enlarging unilateral cerebral lesions can produce a herniation syndrome. Midline tumors obstructing the outflow of cerebrospinal fluid, such as a colloid cyst of the third ventricle, may result in rapidly progressive obstructive hydrocephalus with headache, papilledema, and no localizing neurologic findings. Computerized tomographic scanning with and without contrast enhancement usually confirms this diagnosis. Clotting studies should be obtained immediately to diagnose potentially treatable causes of stroke. Lumbar puncture should generally be avoided when there is evidence of increased intracranial pressure.

I. Increased intracranial pressure. Brain tumors cause increased intracranial pressure by direct mass effect and vasogenic edema incited by the tumor. Dexamethasone rapidly reduces the vasogenic edema and is effective via oral or parenteral routes. If symptoms are not progressing quickly, oral dosages of 4 mg every 6 hours are given. More significant symptoms such as hemiparesis and decreased level of consciousness should be treated more aggressively with an initial intravenous bolus of dexamethasone, 10 mg, followed by 4 mg intravenously every 6 hours. A herniation syndrome requires an intravenous dehydrating agent such as mannitol or glycerol. Mannitol, 1 gm/kg, accompanied by furosemide, 20 mg, are administered. This can be repeated every 4 to 6 hours. After 3 to 5 days of this treatment, a rebound increase in intracranial pressure may occur. Neurosurgical consultation is obtained immediately for definitive treatment if appropriate. Obstructive hydrocephalus may progress rapidly to herniation. Mannitol should be administered, but ventricular shunting is the treatment of choice.

II. Seizure. The initial symptom of a primary or metastatic brain tumor may be a focal or secondarily generalized seizure, or status epilepticus. This is particularly true in patients older than 50 years who have a first seizure. The emergency treatment of seizures or status epilepticus secondary to brain tumors is no different from that outlined earlier. When a metastatic or primary brain tumor is first discovered, prophylactic phenytoin (Dilantin), 5 mg/kg/day is instituted.

III. Spinal cord compression. Symptoms such as back pain for several weeks, followed by paresthesias and weakness involving both legs, and urinary retention occurring over a period of days should alert the emergency physician to the possibility of spinal cord compression. This may be a complication arising in a patient with a known malignancy or the initial symptom of a neoplasm of the spinal column. Other causes of spinal cord compression include trauma, epidural abscess, collections of inflammatory tissue from rheumatoid arthritis, hematoma, or degenerative disc disease. Radicular pain aggravated by coughing or sneezing, or local bone pain made worse by lying down or percussion, may define the spinal level. Emergency neurosurgical consultation should be obtained in all cases. In cases consistent with progressive cord compression, an emergency myelogram or magnetic resonance imaging of the spinal cord must be performed. These tests should reliably confirm the level and nature of the lesion. Dexamethasone, 10 mg intravenously, can be administered before the diagnosis is confirmed when there is a strong clinical suspicion of a malignant cause; otherwise it is administered as soon as the diagnosis is made. In certain cases of malignancy where surgery is inadvisable, radiation therapy is given on an emergency basis. In many cases, especially when a benign process is suspected or no definitive diagnosis is available, neurosurgical intervention is obtained and decompression of the spinal cord is done as soon as possible.

IV. **Metabolic/infectious conditions.** Malignant tumors can give rise to electrolyte disturbances such as hyponatremia or hypercalcemia that result in confusion, obtundation, or seizures. Treatment of these conditions is covered in any standard medical textbook. Fungal or carcinomatous meningitis should also be considered when there is a new onset of confusion with a headache in a patient with a malignancy. Diagnosis is made by lumbar puncture.

Treatment of the Acutely Agitated Patient

When an acutely agitated patient is seen in the emergency department, a long list of differential diagnoses should be generated including both organic and psychiatric causes **(Table 8-13).** Treatable sources of agitation should be sought by history, physical, and laboratory examination.

In some instances "chemical restraints" may be necessary in addition to physical ones. Chemical restraints may increase the difficulty of diagnosis, obscure the clinical course of the patient, or result in paradoxical agitation. Diazepam, 5 to 10 mg intravenously, may be given before CAT scanning or lumbar puncture.

When rapid control of severely agitated patients is required, the drugs of choice are the major tranquilizers. Haloperidol is the drug of choice, although it is somewhat more likely to have Parkinsonian side effects. Drugs such as chlorpromazine and thioridazine should be avoided because of their anticholinergic side effects. A procedure known as rapid neuroleptization can be useful. A dose between 2 mg and 10 mg, or even up to 30 mg in a severely agitated patient, is administered initially intramuscularly. A dose of 5 mg intramuscularly may then be given hourly or every 4 to 8 hours until control is achieved. Side effects include hypotension and laryngospasm. The latter is treated with diazepam, 5 to 10 mg intravenously. Haloperidol should be avoided in alcohol and benzodiazepine withdrawal, and in hepatic failure; benzodiazepines, up to 30 mg/day, are the drugs of choice in these conditions. Appropriate anticholinesterase drugs should be used in cases of anticholinergic toxicity.

Dystonic Reactions to Drugs

Early in the course of treatment with the major tranquilizers or related drugs, patients may develop involuntary movements or postures known as dyskinesias or dystonias. The drugs commonly associated with these reactions include phenothiazines, thioxanthines, and butyrophenones. Antiemetics such as prochlorperazine and metoclopromide may also cause this condition.

The typical reaction is a dystonic or twisting movement of axial muscles of the tongue, neck (torticollis), trunk, or eye muscles (oculogyric crisis). It may occur after a

Table 8-13. Causes of Acute Agitation

Endocrine	**Metabolic**
Hypoglycemia/hyperglycemia	Electrolyte disturbance
Hypocalcemia	Hypoxemia
Thyroid storm	Wernicke's encephalopathy
Infectious	**Psychiatric**
Meningitis	Mania
Encephalitis	Schizophrenia
Sepsis	**Drugs and Toxins**
Vascular	Psychotropic
Stroke	Anticholinergic
Vasculitis	Antiparkinson
SAH	Drug withdrawal
Hypertensive encephalopathy	Cocaine, phencyclidine
Epilepsy	**Head Trauma**
Ictal state	**Increased Intracranial Pressure**
Postictal state	

few doses of the medication or even after the first dose. These patients have been misdiagnosed as hysterical because of the bizarre nature of the movements. Treatments include anticholinergic drugs such as benztropine, 1 mg intravenously or intramuscularly, or antihistamines such as diphenhydramine, 50 mg intravenously. Oral forms of the medication are continued for 2 days.

Anticholinesterase Drugs and Myasthenia Gravis

Myasthenia gravis, an autoimmune disease of neuromuscular transmission, is characterized by fatigable weakness. The disease most commonly affects bulbar musculature and may present as an acute or subacute onset of diplopia, ptosis, dysarthria, or dysphagia, in addition to weakness of the extremities or respiratory muscles. **Table 8-14** outlines other disorders that can cause neuromuscular paralysis and should be considered in the differential diagnosis of myasthenia gravis.

I. Diagnosis. Correct diagnosis depends on a high degree of suspicion. In the emergency department, the condition may be quickly diagnosed with a short-acting parenteral anti-acetylcholinesterase, edrophonium chloride. The edrophonium test is only performed when there is a readily measurable neurologic sign such as ptosis or an ocular muscle weakness. It should not be performed on patients in respiratory distress or with unknown cardiac status. Electrocardiographic monitoring is recommended in older patients. Edrophonium, 10 mg, is drawn into a tuberculin syringe; 2 mg is administered intravenously and the patient observed for changes in strength. If there is no change after 1 minute, the remaining 8 mg is given. The dosage is staged to avoid cholinergic weakness in sensitive patients. Patients should be observed for at least 20 minutes for signs of improvement. Cholinergic side effects such as excess tearing, nausea, and diarrhea may occur, and atropine, 0.4 mg, should be available if bradycardia or hypotension develops.

II. Treatment. Treatment of myasthenia gravis includes oral anticholinesterase medications and corticosteroids. Pyridostigmine, an anticholinesterase drug, is

Table 8-14. Disorders Associated with Neuromuscular Weakness

Peripheral Neuropathy
Guillain-Barré syndrome
Critical illness
Chronic inflammatory demyelinating polyneuropathy
Toxins
   1. Organophosphates
   2. Thallium, arsenic, lead
Drugs
   1. Vincristine
   2. Platinum
Metabolic
   Acute intermittent porphyria
Neuromuscular Junction
Myasthenia gravis
Cholinergic crisis
Tick paralysis
Eaton-Lambert syndrome
Myopathy
Polymyositis
Acute rhabdomyolysis
Anterior Horn Cell
Amyotrophic lateral sclerosis
Poliomyelitis

---

administered in a dosage of 60 to 120 mg every 4 hours in patients with mild disease. Prednisone or methylprednisolone is used for patients with more severe forms of the disease.

III. Myasthenic versus cholinergic crisis

A. **A patient may initially be seen in myasthenic crisis with serious muscle weakness and respiratory decompensation.** Maintenance of an airway and stabilization of vital signs is most important. Clinical suspicion must be present to make the diagnosis in a patient with new onset of shortness of breath and weakness. The edrophonium test may confirm the diagnosis. More commonly a myasthenic patient will have worsening weakness because of an intercurrent infection or use of a mediation with neuromuscular junction–blocking effects such as aminoglycoside and polymyxin antibiotics.

B. **A difficult question** arises when the patient is already on an anticholinesterase drug and has worsening weakness. This may be due to worsening disease or an overdose of the medication, known as cholinergic crisis. Valuable time in securing an adequate airway should not be lost trying to remember the nuances of neuromuscular junction pharmacology. The dilemma may be resolved with an edrophonium test. A patient undertreated with anticholinesterase medication may improve or show no response. Patients in cholinergic crisis will worsen and subsequently have fasciculations and crampy abdominal pain. Cholinergic crisis is treated by hospitalizing the patient and discontinuing the anticholinesterase drug until the symptoms subside. Myasthenic crisis also necessitates admission to the hospital, but treatment is with intravenous corticosteroids or plasmapheresis.

Drug Therapy Guidelines of the Management of Stroke

Drugs Used to Manage Cerebrovascular Emergencies

Anticoagulants
- **Heparin** is given 5000 to 10,000 U IV (100 U/kg; loading dose should be reduced if patient is 65 years of age or older), then 700 to 1200 U/h (10 to 20 U/kg/h) IV. The dose should be adjusted every 6 to 12 hours until partial thromboplastin time is 1.2 to 1.4 × control. **Warfarin** (Coumadin) therapy can begin immediately following heparin therapy and consists of an initial dose of 10 to 15 mg orally every day for 3 days followed by 4 mg orally every day in order to maintain PT time at 1.2 to 1.4 × control.

Antihypertensives
- **Nitroprusside:** A constant infusion should be titrated gradually at an initial dose of 0.25 mcg/kg/min IV. The dose can be increased at increments of 0.25 mcg/kg/min up to a maximum of 10 mcg/kg/min.
- **Labetalol:** Begin with a 20 mg IV bolus (0.25 mg/kg), then 20 to 40 mg boluses every 10 to 15 minutes titrated to desired BP; this is followed by an infusion of 0.5-2 mg/min as required.

Anticonvulsants
- **Lorazepam** 4 to 8 mg IV at 1 to 2 mg/min slow IV infusion, or
- **Diazepam** 5 to 10 mg IV at 1 to 2 mg/min slow IV infusion.

Vasospasm-Reducing Agents
- **Nimopidine:** (60 mg) is administered every 4 hours, continuing treatment for up to 21 consecutive days after the initial event.

Anti-Platelet Drugs
- **Aspirin (dose regimen still controversial):** High-dose therapy (325 mg to 1300 mg/day) for prevention of TIA and stroke in nonvalvular atrial fibrillation versus low-dose aspirin therapy (30 to 80 mg/day) for prevention of TIA in patients with normal sinus rhythm.
- **Ticlopidine**

Osmotic Agents
- **Mannitol:** 1 to 2 g/kg of 20% solution given over 5 to 10 minutes and additional 0.5 to 1 g/kg every 4 to 6 hours will reduce ICP. It should be stressed that the use of mannitol is somewhat controversial. It represents only a temporizing measure and may lead to a rebound intracerebral hyperosmolar state, which may worsen cerebral edema.

Initial Stabilization and Management of Thrombotic, Nonhemorrhagic Cerebral Infarction

- Stabilize airway, breathing, or circulation abnormalities
- Treat systemic hypertension only if: a) systolic blood pressure is >220 mm Hg or >120 mm Hg diastolic on three repeated measurements made at 15-minute intervals; b) mean arterial pressure is greater than 140 mm Hg; or c) patient is in danger of sustaining myocardial, aortic, or renal damage associated with elevated blood pressure
- Administer anticonvulsants if patient has seizures
- Obtain neurosurgery consultation if diagnosis of cerebellar infarction is confirmed

Initial Stabilization and Management of Subarachnoid Hemorrhage

- Stabilize airway, breathing, or circulation
- Obtain neurosurgery consultation
- Reduce elevated blood pressure to pre-SAH levels
- Begin nimodipine 60 mg orally every four hours in patients with Hunt and Hess grades 1, 2, and 3
- Administer anticonvulsants if seizures occur
- Administer analgesics and sedatives as needed
- Consider emergency angiography, invasive hemodynamic monitoring, and early surgery in patients with aneurysmal SAH

Initial Stabilization and Management of Intracerebral Hemorrhage

- Stabilize airway, breathing, or circulation
- Obtain neurosurgery consultation promptly if need for surgical intervention may be required (e.g., cerebellar hemorrhage, acute hydrocephalus, AVM)
- Treat systemic hypertension immediately if: a) the systolic or diastolic pressure exceeds 220 mm Hg or 120 mm Hg, respectively, on three repeated measurements made at 15-minute intervals, or b) arterial dissection or cardiac failure has been identified
- If increased intracranial pressure is suspected, treatment with intravenous mannitol may help. In selected patients, hyperventilation should be considered

Suggested Readings

Biller J et al: Management of aneurysmal subarachnoid hemorrhage, *Stroke* 9:1300-1305, 1988.

Bosker G et al: Diagnostic challenge and therapeutic strategies in focal neurologic lesions, *Emergency Medicine Report* 9:65-72, 1988.

Earnest MP: Emergency diagnosis and management of brain infarctions and hemorrhages. In Earnest MP, editor: *Neurologic emergencies,* New York, 1983, Churchill Livingstone.

Hughes RAC, Bihari D: Acute neuromuscular respiratory paralysis, *J Neurol Neurosurg Psychiatry* 56:334-343, 1993.

Johnston RA: The management of acute spinal cord compression, *J Neurol Neurosurg Psychiatry* 56:1046-1054, 1993.

Kopitnik TA, Samson DS: Management of subarachnoid hemorrhage, *J Neurol Neurosurg Psychiatry* 56:947-959, 1993.

Marshall RS, Mohr JP: Current management of ischemic stroke, *J Neurol Neurosurg Psychiatry* 56:6-16, 1993.

Miller JD: Head injury. *J Neurol Neurosurg Psychiatry* 56:440-447, 1993.

Pickard JD, Czosnyka M: Management of raised intracranial pressure, *J Neurol Neurosurg Psychiatry* 56:845-858, 1993.

Raskin NH: *Headache,* ed 2, New York, 1988, Churchill Livingstone.

Sabin TD: Neurologic emergencies. In Schwartz GR et al, editors: *Principles and practices of emergency medicine,* Philadelphia, 1986, WB Saunders.

Sabin TD: Neurology. In Noble J, editor: *Textbook of general medicine and primary care,* Boston, 1987, Little, Brown.

Samuels MA, et al: *Manual of neurologic therapeutics with essentials of diagnosis,* ed 3, Boston, 1986, Little, Brown.

Shorvon S: Tonic clonic status epilepticus, *J Neurol Neurosurg Psychiatry* 56:125-134, 1993.

Taylor D, Lewis S: Delirium, *J Neurol Neurosurg Psychiatry* 56:742-751, 1993.

Wolfson RJ, et al: Vertigo. In Schwartz GR et al, editors: *Principles and practices of emergency medicine,* Philadelphia, 1986, WB Saunders.

9
Noninfectious Pulmonary Diseases

Louis J. Perretta, M.D., F.A.C.E.P.

A knowledge of pulmonary emergencies and their treatment is essential for all physicians practicing in an emergency department. With some conditions the challenge will be in making the diagnosis; with other conditions the diagnosis will be obvious, and the challenge will be in choosing the proper agent(s) to treat the condition. A thorough knowledge of the pathophysiology of pulmonary diseases will increase a clinician's chance of making a correct diagnosis and choice of treatment.

The following chapter will examine pulmonary emergencies, exploring the assessment, pathophysiology, and most importantly the therapy that is most appropriate. In addition, the chapter will outline a method for the rapid sequence intubation of an awake patient with respiratory failure. This will include a listing and description of the pharmacologic agents used in rapid sequence intubation to sedate and paralyze the patient.

Reactive Airway Diseases: Acute Asthma

Asthma is a condition that causes widespread narrowing of the tracheobronchial tree. Asthma is a common disease, estimated to affect 4% to 5% of the population in the United States, amounting to about 10 million people. The disease is chronic in nature but characterized by acute exacerbations that may resolve spontaneously or with therapy. Pulmonary function is usually normal between exacerbations.

Asthma is caused by an increased responsiveness of the trachea and bronchi to various stimuli, resulting in reduced airflow and bronchospasm. It is recognized that fatal asthma is associated with marked inflammatory changes in the airways; however, more recent data show that inflammation is present as well in patients with mild asthma. Asthma represents a special type of inflammation of the airway, leading to contraction of airway smooth muscle, microvascular leakage, and bronchial hyperresponsiveness. Asthma is distinguished from chronic obstructive pulmonary disease (COPD) (e.g., emphysema, chronic bronchitis) by the reversibility of airflow obstruction and return to normal pulmonary function between exacerbations. With COPD, there is a fixed or permanent airflow obstruction with abnormal pulmonary function between exacerbations. It may be difficult to distinguish exacerbations of COPD and asthma, but fortunately the acute therapy for these conditions is similar **(Tables 9-1, 9-2, 9-3)**.

I. **Diagnosis.** Patients with asthma may have the classic symptoms of wheezing, cough, shortness of breath, and chest tightness, alone or in combination. These symptoms are episodic, frequently occurring at night, in early morning, or with exercise. It is critical to consider other diagnostic possibilities in these patients, including nonasthmatic diseases such as pulmonary embolism, cardiac asthma (left ventricular failure), central airway obstruction, and asthma-related complications such as pneumothorax or pneumomediastinum.

Table 9-1. Recommended Drugs and Dosages for Acute Asthma in Adults

Inhaled β_2-agonists
Albuterol 2.5 mg (0.5 ml of a 0.5% solution diluted in 2-3 ml NS)
Metaproterenol 15 mg (0.3 ml of a 5% solution diluted in 2-3 ml NS)
Isoetharine 5 mg (0.5 ml of a 1% solution diluted in 2-3 ml NS)
Albuterol MDI

Subcutaneous β-agonists
Epinephrine 0.3 mg subcutaneous
Terbutaline 0.25 mg subcutaneous

Corticosteroids
Methylprednisolone 125 mg IV push (ED administration for acute episodes)
Methylprednisolone 60-80 mg IV push every 6-8 hours (for inpatient hospitalization)
Prednisone or methylprednisolone 60 mg PO in ED, followed by 60-120 mg/day in divided doses tapered over several days (in place of IV corticosteroids or in patients discharged after acute episodes)

Methylxanthines
Aminophylline IV at a rate of 0.6 mg/kg/hr by continuous infusion. In patients not on methylxanthines, a loading dose of 6 mg/kg should be given. Adjust the infusion rate for factors affecting metabolism such as liver disease, congestive heart failure, and certain medications (erythromycin, ciprofloxacin, and cimetidine).
Theophylline can be given orally; daily dose (mg) = total dose of aminophylline in 24 hours × 0.8

NS, Normal saline solution; *MDI*, metered dose inhaler; *ED*, emergency department.

II. **Assessment.** It is important to assess the severity of an exacerbation of asthma. A comparison of this episode to previous attacks should be made, as well as a history of precipitating causes, medications, previous or current steroid use, other medical problems, frequency of hospitalization, need for mechanical ventilation, and recent emergency department visits. Patients at risk for a fatal attack of asthma are characterized by a circadian variation in lung function, psychologic factors, the concurrent use of three or more medications, recurrent hospitalization, recurrent emergency department visits, or a previous history of life-threatening attack. In addition to these factors, it is suggested that certain aeroallergens may precipitate asthmatic attacks that could be severe or fatal.

   A. **On physical examination,** respiratory distress at rest, difficulty in speaking more than two- to three-word sentences, diaphoresis, and accessory muscle use (including intercostal, supraclavicular, and abdominal retractions) are all indicative of a severe episode. In mild asthma, there may be no wheezing or diminished breath sounds, but cough may be the only symptom. The presence or intensity of wheezing does not correlate well with the severity of an asthma attack. In patients with diminished breath sounds and poor air movement, there may be no wheezing and only a "silent chest" on auscultation. The findings of a respiratory rate greater than 30 breaths/min, a pulse greater than 120 beats/min, and a pulsus paradoxicus of greater than 18 mm Hg also indicate a severe attack. The presence of subcutaneous emphysema in the neck suggests a pneumomediastinum, while the absence of breath sounds on one side or pleuritic chest pain suggests a pneumothorax.

Table 9-2. Recommended Drugs and Dosages for Acute Asthma in Children

Inhaled β_2-agonists

Albuterol 0.1-0.15 mg/kg/dose up to 5 mg (minimum dose is 1.25 mg/dose) every 20 minutes as needed. May use by continuous nebulization 0.5 mg/kg/hr in severe cases that are unresponsive to therapy every 20 minutes (maximum dose of 15 mg/hr).

Metaproterenol 0.1-0.03 ml of a 5% solution (50 mg/ml); not to exceed 15 mg.

Systemic β-agonists

Epinephrine HCl 0.01 mg/kg sucutaneous up to 0.3 mg of the 1:1000 solution every 20 minutes up to three doses. The inhaled selective β-agonists are preferred.

Terbutaline 0.01 mg/kg up to 0.3 mg subcutaneous every 2 to 6 hours as needed. The inhaled selective β-agonists are preferred.

Methylxanthines

Aminophylline 6 mg/kg loading dose IV if there is no previous theophylline use and 3 mg/kg if there is a history of recent theophylline use. The guidelines for continuous infusions are by age:

1-6 months	0.5 mg/kg/hr
6 mo-1 year	1.0 mg/kg/hr
1-9 years	1.5 mg/kg/hr
10-16 years	1.2 mg/kg/hr

Corticosteroids

Methylprednisolone can be given IV or PO giving a 1-2 mg/kg bolus. In patients with severe asthma that is not resolving, this dose can be repeated every 6 hours. Patients may be discharged on 1-2 mg/kg/day in divided doses every 12 hours.

B. Laboratory assessment should include the measurement of a peak expiratory flow rate (PEFR). It has been shown that the PEFR correlates well with the forced expiratory volume in 1 second (FEV_1). The PEFR in the emergency department should be used to monitor the response to therapy during an acute attack. Measurement of PEFR has limitations in that it is effort dependent, determined by the patient's willingness and ability to exhale maximally each time the PEFR is measured. In addition, PEFR measures only large airway function. In patients with mild asthma, where abnormalities are seen in the small airways, PEFR measurement alone may underestimate the severity of their illness.

C. Pulse oximetry can be helpful in assessing oxygenation; however, unless capnometry is also available, arterial blood gas values are needed to determine the arterial carbon dioxide tension($PaCO_2$). A normal or increased $PaCO_2$ value with a severe, prolonged asthmatic attack may be a sign of impending respiratory failure. Laboratory assessment should include a complete blood cell count (CBC), serum theophylline level (if indicated), and serum potassium level in patients with moderate to severe asthma. Eosinophils are suggested to play an important role in the pathogenesis of asthma, and eosinophilia in the peripheral blood has been correlated with the severity of asthma. A chest radiograph is also indicated in moderate to severe attacks if the history or physical examination suggests pneumonia, pneumothorax, pneumomediastinum, or another condition that has a similar presentation to asthma (e.g., congestive heart failure [CHF]).

Table 9-3. Treatment Sequence for Acute Exacerbation of Acute Asthma in Adults

Initial Assessment
History/physical exam
Peak expiratory flow rate (PEFR)
Pulse oximetry or arterial blood gas (ABG) in severe cases

Initial Treatment
Inhaled β_2-agonist in three doses over 60-90 minutes
Supplemental oxygen
Systemic corticosteroid for patients not responding to initial inhaled β-agonist

Secondary Assessment
Further history, repeat exam, and PEFR
Chest radiograph, theophylline level in certain patients

Disposition
Complete response with no wheezing or shortness of breath; may be discharged with inhaled β_2-agonist MDI to be taken as needed, and provide any needed education on its use. Consider systemic corticosteroids (oral) in patients with history of steroid use or recent steroid use.

Incomplete response with mild wheezing and persisting shortness of breath. Patients should continue treatment with inhaled β_2-agonists for the first three treatments within 90 minutes, and every hour thereafter if no improvement. Consider IV corticosteroids in most patients. If they show improvement, they can be discharged.

Poor response with continued marked diffuse wheezing and shortness of breath. Patients should continue treatment with inhaled β_2-agonists for the first three treatments within 90 minutes, and every hour thereafter if no improvement. Give IV corticosteroids and consider for hospital admission.

Respiratory failure in patients with extreme respiratory distress, impaired consciousness, arterial carbon dioxide pressure ($PaCO_2$) >45-50 mm Hg, and severe wheezes or no air movement at all. These patients need admission to the ICU and should be receiving frequent inhaled β_2-agonists and systemic corticosteroids. They may need intubation and mechanical ventilation using rapid sequence intubation.

III. Therapy. The goal of therapy in an acute asthmatic attack is to reduce bronchospasm and ensure adequate oxygenation. Asthma includes bronchospasm, as well as a generalized inflammatory reaction within the airways. The medications used to treat asthma can be divided into two groups: the bronchodilators (e.g., methylxanthines, β-adrenergic agonists, and anticholinergics) and the antiinflammatory agents (e.g., corticosteroids, cromolyn sodium). The primary treatment of an acute asthmatic attack is with bronchodilators of the selective β_2-agonist class. Antiinflammatory agents do not have immediate effects in an acute attack but exert their effects 10 to 12 hours later.

    A. Oxygen. Hypoxia that is seen in advanced asthma is generally relieved with oxygen administered at low flow rates (2 to 4 L/min) by nasal cannula. A pulse oximeter is helpful in determining the amount of oxygen to give. The $PaCO_2$ is usually low during asthma attacks. However, it should be monitored closely in severe attacks or prolonged attacks lasting several hours where rising $PaCO_2$ values may identify impending respiratory failure.

B. Intubation/respiratory failure. Intubation and ventilatory support, although infrequent, become necessary when respiratory failure occurs or is imminent. Respiratory failure occurs in patients with continued severe respiratory distress, mental status changes, exhaustion, and a progressive increase in $PaCO_2$ values. A rise in the $PaCO_2$ value greater than 50 to 55 mm Hg despite aggressive therapy, associated with acute respiratory acidosis, refractory hypoxemia despite oxygen administration, or oxygen suppression of ventilation, indicates the need for intubation and controlled ventilatory support.

C. Bronchodilators

1. **β-Adrenergic agonists.** These agents induce bronchodilation of the small airways by stimulating smooth muscle $β_2$-receptors, causing the smooth muscle around these airways to relax. They are the most effective and rapid bronchodilators available, and are the primary agents used to treat acute attacks of asthma or bronchospasm in the emergency department. The selective $β_2$-agents (isoetharine, metaproterenol, terbutaline, albuterol, and salmeterol) produce fewer cardiac side effects than the nonselective agents (epinephrine, isoproterenol). Salmeterol, a new $β_2$-agonist, is structurally similar to albuterol, but it has an extended duration of action and a more potent bronchodilator effect than albuterol.

    a. **In acute airway obstruction,** bronchospasm may be rapidly relieved with a subcutaneous injection of epinephrine or terbutaline in young, healthy patients with no history of cardiac disease or hypertension. Selective $β_2$-agents such as metaproterenol and albuterol are also effective in relieving bronchospasm rapidly when administered by nebulizer. These agents can be administered by nebulizer, metered dose inhaler (MDI), and parenteral or oral routes, but the nebulized preparation is the preferred method of delivery for acute asthmatic attacks. Use of a spacer with the MDI enhances the delivery of the agent into the lung. It has been argued that this route is more cost-effective than administration by nebulizer.

    b. Although **$β_2$-agonists** are the treatment of choice for acute exacerbations of asthma, their long-term regular use may be associated with a worsening of control of asthma in some patients. Aerosolized or inhaled therapy may be more effective than oral therapy in treating bronchospasm and also associated with fewer systemic adverse effects. These effects include cardiovascular stimulation, anxiety, and skeletal muscle tremor. Cardiac arrhythmias and myocardial ischemia resulting from $β_2$-agonist therapy are seen more frequently in patients who are elderly or who have preexisting cardiovascular disease. An additional complication of frequently inhaled $β_2$-agonist therapy is a decrease in serum potassium, magnesium, and phosphorus levels, which could contribute to cardiac instability.

2. **Methylxanthines.** The methylxanthines cause their therapeutic effects by relaxing bronchial smooth muscle. Their mechanism of action involves the inhibition of phosphodiesterase, an enzyme responsible for the breakdown of cyclic adenosine monophosphate (AMP). Cyclic AMP ultimately causes smooth muscle relaxation.

    a. **$β_2$-agonists.** Although methylxanthines are recommended for patients hospitalized with asthma, they do not significantly enhance the bronchodilator response to β_2-agonists when the β_2-agonists are given repetitively at short intervals. However, when the frequency and dose of β_2-agonists are decreased, the methylxanthines may lead to increased bronchodilation. Theophylline and aminophylline (86% anhydrous theophylline) are available for oral and parenteral use in the United States.

    b. **Methylxanthines** have historically been used to treat patients with acute exacerbations of asthma. Currently, with the β_2-adrenergic agonists occupying the primary role in the treatment of acute asthmatics, methylxanthines have fallen to the third or fourth line of treatment, behind corticosteroids and anticholinergics. A recent metaanalysis examining the use of aminophylline in severe acute asthma showed that despite widespread practice, there was no difference between the control and the aminophylline-treated groups. Other studies have confirmed that methylxanthines do not add any further benefit to patients even with severe disease exacerbations and, indeed, may have significantly major adverse effects.

    c. **Monitoring.** The use of aminophylline requires careful monitoring of serum theophylline levels because of a large variability in clearance among patients. Because of the low therapeutic index, the serum levels for optimal bronchodilation are close to levels that cause toxicity. Toxicity is also more likely in patients with impaired cardiac or hepatic function, as well as by concomitant administration of other medications. These include ciprofloxacin and other quinalone antibiotics, erythromycin, and cimetidine.

3. **Anticholinergic agents.** Optimal bronchodilator therapy should lead to maximal bronchodilation while minimizing unwanted side effects. Anticholinergic agents act through different receptor and biochemical pathways than the β-adrenergic agonists or methylxanthines; they work by inhibiting cholinergic muscarinic receptors in the respiratory tract. This combination therapy may be more effective than individual therapy alone for several reasons. There is an increase in the maximal response to bronchodilator therapy in patients relatively resistant to the effects of β_2-agonists. In addition, the duration of effect is increased and lower doses of both agents may be used, decreasing the frequency and severity of unwanted side effects. The use of anticholinergic agents alone is not recommended because β_2-agonists are more effective as single agents for the treatment of acute exacerbations of asthma. Anticholinergic agents should not be used in the routine treatment of acute asthmatic exacerbations but may be considered for patients who are deteriorating and not responding to conventional therapy (β_2-agonists, steroids, and methylxanthines).

4. **Magnesium.** There have been studies and case reports to suggest that intravenous magnesium sulfate effectively treats bronchospasm in patients with acute asthma. It has been theorized that magnesium relaxes bronchial smooth muscle and produces dilation of the airways. Despite this, magnesium administration does not decrease the duration of treatment in the emergency department or the need for hospitalization. The dose for magnesium is 1 to 2 gm infused over 20 to 30 minutes. Although there are no large clinical trials showing the beneficial effects of intravenous magnesium

in patients with acute bronchospasm, a trial of magnesium should be considered in patients who are not responding to otherwise conventional therapy (β_2-agonists, steroids, and methylxanthines), and in patients who are deteriorating or not responding to aggressive conventional therapy. Hypotension and bradycardia can occur with rapid intravenous administration of magnesium. It is also important not to delay aggressive airway management with mechanical ventilation in patients with impending respiratory failure.

D. Antiinflammatory agents
 1. **Corticosteroids.** Asthma is a disease characterized not only by bronchospasm and hyperactive airways, but also by a generalized inflammatory reaction within the airways. It is because of this that steroids, systemic and aerosolized, are important adjuncts in the treatment of asthmatic patients. Aerosolized steroids are used primarily in the outpatient management of asthma, but steroid administration should be considered in the emergency department for patients with severe asthma or who poorly respond to β_2-agonist inhalation therapy. Steroids should also be considered in (1) patients with a long duration of symptomatic asthma before presentation, (2) patients chronically using multiple antiasthmatic medications at the time of presentation, (3) patients with long-term or recently discontinued use of oral steroids, (4) patients with frequent emergency department visits for their asthma, (5) patients with a history of respiratory failure caused by asthma, and (6) children with asthma induced by viral infection.
 2. **The recommended dose** initially is 80 to 125 mg of methylprednisolone administered intravenously in adults, and 1 to 2 mg/kg of methylprednisolone administered orally or parenterally in children. The time to peak effect may be 6 to 12 hours. The adverse effects associated with short-term, high-dose systemic therapy include abnormalities in glucose metabolism, increased appetite, fluid retention, weight gain, mood alteration, hypertension, and peptic ulcer disease.
 3. **Oral steroids.** A short course of oral steroids on discharge from the emergency department may reduce the rate of recurrent severe symptoms and prevent early relapse and return to the emergency department. It is suggested that systemic corticosteroids (methylprednisolone) given orally are as effective as intravenous administration. The dosage of methylprednisolone is 60 to 120 mg/day in three divided doses and tapered over several days. A recent retrospective study examined the relationship between the eosinophil count and relapses in patients who were not taking oral corticosteroids. The findings suggested than an initial eosinophil count may be useful in predicting the risk of relapse and need for oral corticosteroids in patients with moderately severe acute asthma. Inhaled steroids such as beclamethasone, flunisolide, and triamcinalone, administered through an MDI, are effective in controlling mild asthma and should also be considered in patients discharged from the emergency department. Some significant adverse effects of inhaled corticosteroids, including thrush, dysphonia, coughing, and wheezing, can be prevented by using a spacer with the MDI.
 4. **Cromolyn sodium.** Despite currently being the best nonsteroidal antiinflammatory drug for the treatment of asthma, cromolyn sodium has no role in the treatment of acute exacerbations of asthma. It is generally ac-

cepted that cromolyn sodium works to prevent the inflammation leading to bronchospasm by preventing mediator release from mast cells.

Chronic Obstructive Pulmonary Disease

Chronic obstructive pulmonary disease is a spectrum of conditions characterized by permanent airway obstruction. These conditions may range from chronic bronchitis to emphysema, but most often components of both are present. Chronic bronchitis is characterized by hypersecretion of mucus and structural changes in the bronchi, including inflammation and enlargement of the mucous glands, usually causing a daily cough and sputum production. Emphysema is a destructive process involving the lung parenchyma and alveolar walls. The expiratory airflow obstruction seen is chronic, permanent, and caused by the loss of supporting structures for the small peripheral airways. The airways in patients with COPD may also be directly narrowed by inflammatory changes, leading to airway hyperresponsiveness and some degree of reversibility of the airway obstruction. Both COPD and asthma share these characteristics, making the treatment of the two conditions similar.

Acute exacerbations are most commonly caused by upper respiratory tract infections that may lead to bronchospasm or an increase in mucous secretion or plugging. This results in increased airway obstruction, leading to worsening dyspnea, fatigue, and respiratory failure. Other conditions that should be considered in patients with acute exacerbations of COPD include pneumonia, pulmonary embolus, pulmonary edema, and pneumothorax.

I. Diagnosis. Patients with COPD usually have a chronic cough and dyspnea; however, they are seen in the emergency department during acute exacerbations with worsening dyspnea, cough, tachypnea, and commonly retractions and accessory muscle use. The chest may be hyperresonant and the breath sounds are often decreased; adventitial sounds such as wheezes or crackles may also be found.

II. Assessment. In addition to history and physical examination, chest radiographs may be helpful in evaluating patients with an acute exacerbation to rule out other diagnostic possibilities and complications such as pulmonary embolism, cardiac asthma (left ventricular failure), pneumonia, and pneumothorax. Peak expiratory flow evaluation should be performed in all patients with an exacerbation of COPD. The PEFR can be used to follow the treatment course of the patient while in the emergency department. In addition, pulse oximetry should be performed to evaluate the adequacy of oxygenation. Patients with stable COPD will have a certain degree of hypoxemia secondary to perfusion of poorly ventilated areas of the lungs. During acute exacerbations, pulse capnometry and the ability to follow $PaCO_2$ values may be necessary in patients with worsening airway obstruction, increased dead space ventilation, and respiratory muscle fatigue. Acute respiratory failure is preceded by a rising $PaCO_2$ and acute respiratory acidosis.

III. Therapy. Despite the fixed airflow obstruction of COPD, most patients having an exacerbation have a reversible obstruction amenable to bronchodilator therapy. Since both COPD and asthma share the disease characteristics of airway obstruction and hyperresponsiveness, acute exacerbations in both can be treated with β_2-agonists, corticosteroids, and anticholinergics.

    A. Oxygen. Patients with acute exacerbations of COPD should have noninvasive pulse oximetry monitoring to establish the degree of hypoxemia. The goal of oxygen therapy in these patients would be to receive concentrations of oxygen sufficient to raise the arterial oxygen pressure (PaO_2) to 60 mm Hg or 90% oxygen saturation. In certain patients, an oxygen saturation above 90% to 92% may result in an elevation of $PaCO_2$, with depression of mental status, hypoventilation, and further impairment of gas exchange. Intubation and mechanical ventilation should be performed in patients with respiratory failure.

B. Bronchodilators

1. **β-Adrenergic agonists.** Nebulized $β_2$-adrenergic agonists are the first-line treatment for patients with acute dyspnea secondary to an exacerbation of COPD. Metaproterenol, albuterol, and terbutaline are three selective $β_2$-agents; all three are available in an MDI, while metaproterenol and albuterol are also available in solution for nebulizer therapy. The preferred method of delivery for acute exacerbations of COPD is by nebulizer.

2. **Anticholinergic agents.** The inhalation form of the anticholinergic agents—atropine as a solution for a nebulizer and ipratropium in an MDI—can be used as second-line treatment for patients who are not responding to, or worsening with, $β_2$-agonist therapy. Anticholinergic agents have a slower onset of action, and both local and systemic adverse effects. These include drying of respiratory secretions, along with cardiac and central nervous system stimulation. Atropine should be used with caution because it is readily absorbed from the respiratory and gastrointestinal tracts, and should not be used in patients with narrow-angle glaucoma or prostatic hypertrophy. On the other hand, ipratropium, a quaternary anticholinergic agent, has a low bioavailability when inhaled and lacks the side effects that are seen with atropine. In the majority of patients with COPD, the inhaled quaternary agents are as effective as other bronchodilators, with fewer side effects. The regular use of ipratropium bromide (MDI) appears to be quite effective in patients with COPD and partially reversible airflow obstruction. This drug may also be used with $β_2$-agonists. A recent study showed that the duration of emergency department treatment was decreased with the addition of ipratropium MDI to $β_2$-agonist therapy in patients with COPD exacerbations.

3. **Methylxanthines.** The administration of aminophylline should be considered in patients with severe COPD not responding to $β_2$-agonists. Aminophylline can be given intravenously, but serum levels need to be monitored closely to maintain optimal bronchodilation and to avoid toxicity.

C. Antiinflammatory agents: corticosteroids. Given the underlying nature of chronic airway obstruction, it would be expected that corticosteroids would provide little benefit to patients with emphysema who have a fixed airway obstruction secondary to tissue destruction. However, COPD may include some conditions in which airway inflammation and bronchial hyperresponsiveness may precipitate the acute exacerbation. In one study, patients hospitalized for an acute exacerbation of COPD and respiratory failure were given standard bronchodilator therapy, plus methylprednisolone or placebo. Methylprednisone dose was 0.5 mg/kg every 6 hours for 3 days. The group given methylprednisolone showed significant improvement when compared with the placebo group. Corticosteroids should be administered to patients with an exacerbation of COPD leading to respiratory failure or when there is an incomplete response to $β_2$-agonists. The doses used are the same as for the treatment of acute asthma.

D. Antibiotics. Antibiotics should be administered to patients with acute exacerbations of COPD, manifest by increasing dyspnea and increased purulent sputum. The duration of symptoms, risk of serious infection, and deterioration in lung function can be reduced with a 7- to 10-day course of a broad-spectrum antibiotic. In the absence of pneumonia, either amoxicillin, 250 mg PO TID, or trimethoprim-sulfamethoxazole, 160 mg/800 mg PO BID (one double-strength tablet), can be given.

Pulmonary Embolism

Venous thrombosis and pulmonary embolism (PE) are some of the most common cardiopulmonary disorders and are among the leading causes of morbidity and death in hospitalized patients. In some parts of the world, such as North America and Europe, death from PE occurs more frequently with advancing age. The diagnosis of PE is difficult, particularly with patients who are elderly or have underlying cardiopulmonary disease. Pulmonary embolism that is not treated, has a high mortality rate, which decreases significantly with anticoagulation therapy. Traditionally, anticoagulation therapy was the principal pharmacologic therapy for PE, but thrombolytic therapy has begun to play a more important role in the treatment of patients with massive PE, PE with shock, and severe deep venous thrombosis. Other acceptable nonpharmacologic therapies include pulmonary embolectomy and interruption of the inferior vena cava. The clinical challenge in patients with suspected PE is to confirm the diagnosis, which requires a thorough knowledge of the pathophysiology of PE and the diagnostic studies used.

I. Diagnosis

A. Predisposing factors for the development of venous thrombosis or PE include posttraumatic and postoperative immobility, pregnancy, a previous history of venous thrombosis, use of oral contraceptives, stroke, neoplasia, systemic lupus erythematosis, polycythemia vera, inflammatory bowel disease, shock, CHF, and a previous history of deep venous thrombosis or PE. In addition, deficiencies of procoagulants (protein C, protein S, and antithrombin III) or inhibitors to the clotting mechanism may lead to the development of thromboembolism. One autopsy study showed that the danger of postoperative PE continues for more than a month after surgery. Pulmonary embolism is highly unlikely in patients younger than 40 years with signs and symptoms suggestive of PE when there are no predisposing factors, no evidence of deep venous thrombosis, and the chest x-ray is normal.

B. Patients with venous thrombosis may initially complain of a swollen extremity, with or without pain. The swelling is more commonly in the lower extremities and is localized or unilateral. The clinical presentation of acute PE can be nonspecific, with signs and symptoms ranging from subtle to severe, with hypotension and sudden death being the most severe. The most common presenting symptoms of PE are dyspnea, pleuritic chest pain, apprehension, and cough, while the most common presenting signs include tachypnea (>20 breaths/min), tachycardia (>100 beats/min), and inspiratory crackles.

II. Assessment

A. When PE is suspected on the basis of clinical signs, symptoms, and presence of predisposing factors, ancillary laboratory data and diagnostic studies should be obtained. A chest radiograph and an electrocardiogram may be helpful in differentiating PE from other conditions, or reinforcing the clinical suspicion that PE is present. Nonspecific chest radiographic findings such as atelectasis are found in about 45% of patients with angiographically proven PE. Infiltrates and pleural-based consolidations or effusions may also be seen on a chest radiograph. It may take anywhere from a few hours to a few days after symptom onset for these radiographic abnormalities to appear. The electrocardiogram will demonstrate sinus tachycardia most often, with right heart strain (right atrial enlargement, right ventricular hypertrophy, right axis deviation) and the classic $S_1Q_3T_3$ (deep S wave in lead I with a deep Q wave and inverted T wave in lead III) occurring only in a small number of cases.

B. **The use of pulse oximetry** or arterial blood gas values may be helpful in assessing hypoxemia. The findings of hypoxemia and predisposing factor occur in all patients with PE. In patients with proven PE, 95% have a PaO_2 less than 90 mm Hg in addition to a predisposing factor. An arterial blood gas would be helpful in evaluating the PaO_2. A recent study, however, showed that there was no difference in the room air PaO_2 or the alveolar-arterial oxygen gradient between patients with PE diagnosed at angiography and patients with suspected PE who had normal angiograms.

C. **Deep venous thrombosis (DVT).** In evaluating patients for acute DVT, it is important to realize that clots in the lower extremities that have a high likelihood of embolizing are located in the popliteal and femoral venous system. Most pulmonary emboli originate in the lower extremities, but if the process is confined to the tibial-soleal system in the calf, the chance of subsequent embolic episodes is low. Deep venous thrombosis can occur spontaneously, after prolonged bed rest, or in association with certain clinical disorders including neoplasms, hypercoagulable states, and estrogen use. Unfortunately, the presence or absence of clinical signs indicating DVT (extremity pain, tenderness, swelling, and edema) does not correlate well with the presence or absence of active DVT.

  1. **Noninvasive studies.** There are a number of noninvasive studies used to diagnose DVT including I^{125} fibrinogen scanning, impedance plethysmography (IPG), Doppler ultrasonography, and duplex ultrasonography. The I-125 fibrinogen scan works because of the tendency for clots to consume fibrinogen as they propagate. It is limited, however, in that it requires an active thrombotic process for uptake of the labeled fibrinogen, is limited to the veins between the middle calf and middle thigh, and numerous conditions lead to false-positive tests (e.g., superficial thrombophlebitis, skin ulcers, active arthritis, cellulitis, and lymphedema). Both IPG and Doppler ultrasonography are highly sensitive for diagnosing DVT in the thigh. The technique of venous duplex scanning, providing both ultrasonic venous imaging and Doppler ultrasonography, may be more accurate than IPG or Doppler ultrasound alone. Anticoagulant therapy should be initiated in patients with noninvasive studies that are positive for DVT. If initial noninvasive studies are negative for DVT, patients should be reexamined by using serial impedance plethysmography or duplex ultrasonography every other day for the next 7 to 10 days. If the serial studies are negative, patients can be safely observed without anticoagulation therapy. If they are positive, patients should either be started on anticoagulant therapy or have the diagnosis confirmed with ascending venography.

  2. **Ascending venography.** The most reliable technique for diagnosing DVT is ascending venography (sensitivity and specificity ~100%). This is an invasive study that involves the injection of contrast material into the

venous system. Although ascending venography is highly accurate, it exposes the patient to the risks of an invasive study. The noninvasive studies either alone or in combination provide a sound alternative to ascending venography in most medical centers. It is important to have a thorough understanding of the operation and accuracy of the noninvasive studies in one's own medical center before allowing noninvasive studies to replace ascending venography in diagnosing DVT.

3. **The diagnosis** of DVT is ruled out when the venogram is normal. However, in one study venography was negative in about a third of the patients with documented PE. Confirming DVT would certainly provide an indication for anticoagulation therapy. A negative venogram, however, does not exclude the diagnosis of PE. A high index of suspicion for PE should be maintained, despite a negative venogram, in patients with certain predisposing conditions. These include malignancy, CHF, COPD, postpartum states, and the use of oral contraceptives.

D. **Ventilation-perfusion scanning.** Ventilation-perfusion (V/Q) scanning, when available, should be the primary screening examination used to diagnose PE when the patient's history is suggestive of PE. A normal perfusion scan would exclude the diagnosis of PE. According to a recent multicenter study involving more than 900 patients prospectively, almost all patients with proven PE had abnormal V/Q scans ranging from low to high probability. The high-probability scans were associated with PE 88% of the time. The clinical assessment alone was more often correct in excluding PE than in identifying PE. However, in the majority of patients studied, the clinical assessment was noncommittal. Combining the clinical assessment and V/Q scan interpretations improved the chances of reaching a correct diagnosis.

1. **A high-probability scan** usually indicates PE; however, less than half of all patients with PE have a high-probability scan. In patients with low-probability scans (single or multiple subsegmental perfusion defects with matching ventilation defects) and normal scans, the diagnosis of acute PE is very unlikely. A high-probability scan, defined as multiple segmental or larger perfusion defects with mismatching ventilation defects or a perfusion defect larger than the matching ventilation or chest x-ray defect, confirms the diagnosis of PE sufficiently to begin treatment. Intermediate probability scans and low-probability scans combined with a strong clinical suspicion that PE is present are not helpful in establishing a diagnosis. In this situation, additional diagnostic testing for patients with "inconclusive" scans should begin with bilateral lower leg venography, plethysmography, or a duplex study, depending on the expertise available at your own medical center. Pulmonary angiography should be considered to establish the diagnosis with a high degree of accuracy in patients with "inconclusive" scans and negative peripheral extremity examinations. However, unless the patient is hemodynamically unstable, warranting consideration of thrombolytic therapy, or empiric heparinization is absolutely contraindicated (e.g., active GI or CNS bleeding), angiography usually does not need to be performed on an emergency basis.

2. **Cardiogenic shock and right-sided heart failure.** A small subset of patients with PE are first seen in cardiogenic shock and right-sided heart failure. These patients may be too unstable to undergo either lung scanning

or pulmonary angiography; in these circumstances, a portable two-dimensional and Doppler echocardiogram may be helpful in establishing the diagnosis of PE. Typical features of right-sided heart failure caused by PE include right ventricular dilation with visualization of right atrial, right ventricular, or proximal pulmonary artery thrombi.

III. **Therapy.** Supportive care for patients with PE includes supplemental oxygen to correct hypoxemia. When hypotension secondary to reduced cardiac output is present, intravenous "normal saline" challenges with 500 to 1000 ml should be tried first, with vasopressors being used if there is no response to the fluid challenge. In patients with severe, massive PE associated with hypotension, thrombolytic therapy, or surgical intervention should be considered.

   A. **Prophylaxis: anticoagulation.** In any patient where anticoagulation therapy is being considered, the risk of anticoagulation should be assessed. Anticoagulants should be used with great caution or avoided if there is a history of recent GI bleeding, intracranial bleeding, or pericarditis. Heparin is safe to use during pregnancy because it does not cross the placenta, while warfarin (Coumadin) administration is not advised because it does cross the placenta.

   Heparin exhibits anticoagulant effects by binding to antithrombin III, which then rapidly binds the active sites of thrombin and other coagulation enzymes. Heparin also inhibits platelet function and increases the permeability of vessel walls. The "therapeutic threshold" for heparin would be an activated partial thromboplastin time (APTT) that is 1.5 times the control. Rapidly exceeding the therapeutic threshold reduces the rate of recurrent thromboembolism from 25% to 2%. The treatment of DVT should begin with an initial 5000 U of heparin administered as a bolus intravenously after a baseline APTT is obtained. Thereafter, patients should be given approximately 30,000 U per 24 hours, with a goal of maintaining APTT at 1.5 to 2.5 times the control value. In cases in which thrombosis is more extensive or PE is present, an initial bolus of 10,000 U can be given with the same drip rate to maintain APTT at 1.5 to 2 times the control value. Alternatives to intravenous heparin include adjusted dose subcutaneous heparin, 17,500 U every 12 hours, with subsequent doses adjusted to maintain APTT at 1.5 to 2.5 times the control value. This may be as safe and effective as intravenous therapy. An alternative to the dosing schedule for heparin listed above would be to use a weight-based nomogram that would achieve therapeutic threshold rapidly without needing to give excessive heparin doses. This nomogram starts with an initial bolus of 80 U/kg and follows with an infusion at 18 U/kg/hr. The APTT should be obtained 6 hours after the bolus, and adjusting the heparin infusion should be based on the scale in the **box** on page 289. If any adjustments are made on the infusion rate, the APTT should be obtained 6 hours after the adjustment is made. The APTT can be obtained every 24 hours after two consecutive APTTs are therapeutic (APTT 46 to 70). Warfarin or Coumadin therapy is used several days before stopping heparin therapy and is continued for 3 months or indefinitely if risk factors are still present.

   B. Thrombolysis
      1. **The indication** for thrombolytic therapy is massive PE with or without shock. Massive PE is defined as 40% or greater obstruction in the pulmonary vascular bed. In more severe cases, thrombolytic therapy can lyse

Weight-Based Nomogram for Heparin Dosing

Initial dose	80 U/kg bolus, then 18 U/kg/hr
APTT <35 sec (1.2× control)	80 U/kg bolus, then 22 U/kg/hr
APTT 35 to 45 sec (1.2-1.5× control)	40 U/kg bolus, then 20 U/kg/hr
APTT 46 to 70 sec (1.5-2.3× control)	No change
APTT 71 to 90 sec (2.3-3× control)	Decrease infusion to 16 U/kg/hr
APTT >90 sec (>3× control)	Hold infusion for 1 hour, then decrease infusion to 15 U/kg/hr

the embolus, bringing about a more rapid resolution of the pulmonary vascular obstruction and preventing long-term complications. Short-term improvement was well documented with the use of urokinase and urokinase-streptokinase, with a greater reperfusion of the obstructed pulmonary artery when compared with heparin therapy alone.

2. **Recommendations.** Specifically, thrombolysis for PE is recommended for patients with obstruction of blood flow to a lobe or multiple pulmonary segments and for patients with hemodynamic compromise, regardless of the degree of obstruction. Currently, the three thrombolytic agents approved for use in the treatment of PE by the Food and Drug Administration (FDA) are streptokinase, urokinase, and recombinant tissue plasminogen activator (rt-PA). The dosages for these agents are as follows:

   a. **Streptokinase:** 250,000 IU intravenously as a loading dose over 30 minutes, followed by 100,000 U/hr intravenously for 24 hours.

   b. **Urokinase:** 4400 U/kg intravenously over 10 minutes, followed by 4400 U/kg/hr intravenously for 12 to 24 hours.

   c. **rt-PA:** 100 mg as a continuous peripheral intravenous infusion administered over 2 hours.

3. **After the administration** of the thrombolytic agent of choice, heparin should be started as described above. The contraindications to thrombolytic therapy and anticoagulation, both absolute and relative, are listed in the chapter on the treatment of acute myocardial infarction.

C. **Inferior vena caval interruption.** Inferior vena caval interruption is indicated for patients at high risk for fatal PE; these include patients with a major bleeding complication from anticoagulation, those with a contraindication to anticoagulation, or patients in whom emboli recur despite adequate anticoagulation therapy. Vena caval interruption is achieved by surgically placing a transvenous filter in the inferior vena cava.

D. **Pulmonary embolectomy.** This procedure should only be considered in patients with angiographically proven PE who remain in shock despite thrombolytic therapy, or patients with severe PE where thrombolytics would be appropriate but contraindicated.

Respiratory Distress Syndrome

Respiratory distress syndrome (RDS) is characterized by a diffuse pulmonary endothelial injury, leading to a marked increase in capillary permeability. This results in pulmonary edema that is not caused by an imbalance in the Starling forces but by an increase in the capillary permeability in the lungs (noncardiogenic pulmonary edema). The major causes of RDS include sepsis, trauma, gastric aspiration, and diffuse pneumonia. Conditions associated with RDS include inhalation injuries, nonpulmonary infections (bacteremia, sepsis, toxic shock syndrome), nonpulmonary inflammation or injury (pancreatitis, fat embolism, multiple organ system trauma), erythrocyte transfusions, and certain drug overdoses (heroin, barbiturates, salicylates, methadone).

I. **Diagnosis.** It is important to distinguish RDS from cardiogenic causes of pulmonary edema. Respiratory patterns are characterized by small tidal volumes and a rapid respiratory rate. Severe hypoxemia is seen despite increases in the fraction of inspired oxygen (FIO_2). Initially $PaCO_2$ is low or normal, but as RDS progresses, hypercapnia becomes extreme and less responsive to increasing minute ventilation. The chest radiograph reveals diffuse infiltrates in the absence of cardiomegaly. A Swan-Ganz catheter should be utilized to determine the pulmonary capillary wedge pressure (PCWP) and to monitor closely the patient's fluid status. A low or normal PCWP would rule out a cardiogenic cause of pulmonary edema and support the diagnosis of RDS.

II. **Therapy.** One of the major goals of therapy includes the identification and treatment of the underlying disorder and the prevention of complications such as barotrauma and secondary infection. Since sepsis is so often associated with RDS, any therapy that is considered to be beneficial for sepsis may also be beneficial in RDS. Empiric antibiotic treatment should be instituted until infection and sepsis as a cause can be excluded.

   A. **Oxygen.** Hypoxia should be corrected to maintain adequate tissue oxygenation and to minimize the risk of oxygen toxicity caused by administering high concentrations of inspired oxygen (FIO_2 >0.5) for a prolonged period. Because RDS is associated with a reduction in lung compliance, high airway pressure is required to maintain normal ventilation and open collapsed alveoli. Mechanical ventilation with positive end-expiratory pressure (PEEP) is needed in many cases to maintain adequate oxygenation with a low FIO_2. High levels of PEEP (>10 cm H_2O) may cause hemodynamic compromise requiring invasive hemodynamic monitoring. Patients on PEEP should also be carefully monitored for barotrauma (pneumothorax, pneumomediastinum) with frequent examinations and chest radiographs.

   B. **Hypovolemia.** Noncardiogenic pulmonary edema will worsen unless intravascular volume is maintained at the lowest level necessary for adequate tissue perfusion. This should be monitored with a Swan-Ganz catheter.

Acute Respiratory Failure/Rapid Sequence Intubation

I. **Intubation,** with either mechanical or assisted ventilation, is seldom necessary in patients with the pulmonary conditions described in this chapter. Patients who decompensate during treatment or are initially seen in acute respiratory failure require rapid, safe airway management and adequate assisted ventilation.

   A. **Selecting patients** who require this method of invasive airway intervention requires careful clinical assessment. Patients in severe respiratory distress who have mental status changes, exhaustion, significant hypoxemia, or progressively rising $PaCO_2$ values should be considered candidates for invasive airway intervention and mechanical ventilation. The following section will outline the procedure and agents used to perform rapid sequence intubation, as well as provide guidelines for initiating mechanical ventilation.

B. Rapid sequence intubation (RSI) allows a physician to quickly secure airway access in a controlled manner and ensures full patient compliance with the ventilations that follow. It involves the induction of general anesthesia and neuromuscular blockade to permit optimal intubation in the "unfasted" patient, with maximal protection against aspiration of stomach contents. When RSI is performed, it is assumed that the patient has a full stomach, full resuscitation facilities are available, and that a surgical airway can be established (cricothyrotomy) if attempts at intubation fail.

C. Positive pressure ventilation before RSI should be avoided if the patient is awake and breathing because it can cause vomiting and lead to aspiration of gastric contents. In the event that the paralyzed patient cannot be intubated during RSI, the physician must be prepared to perform a cricothyrotomy to establish a surgical airway. At least one secure intravenous line should be established. The agents needed to perform RSI along with the doses are listed in **Table 9-4**.

D. Continuous cardiac and pulse oximeter monitoring are essential once the decision to perform RSI is made. An end-tidal carbon dioxide monitor may be helpful in confirming placement of the endotracheal tube in the patient with a palpable pulse and a blood pressure. The necessary equipment should also be at the bedside, including adequate suction, endotracheal tubes, a stylet, a laryngoscope with both straight and curved blades, a cricothyrotomy tray, and

Table 9-4. Drugs and Dosages for Rapid Sequence Intubation

Neuromuscular Blocking Agents

Succinylcholine, 1.5 mg/kg IV push. This achieves paralysis and intubating conditions in 30-60 seconds. The effect lasts for about 5-7 minutes. Do not use in patients with recent massive burns or crush injuries. Use with caution or avoid in patients with head injuries and elevated intracranial pressure. Fasciculations are common and prevented by using a pretreating dose of a competitive neuromuscular blocker such as pancuronium or vercuronium.

Vercuronium, 0.25 mg/kg IV push, achieves paralysis and intubating conditions in 60 seconds, but the effect lasts for greater than 90 minutes. A pretreating dose, 0.01 mg/kg, may also be used to avoid fasciculations when using succinylcholine. This agent can be safely used in patients with elevated intracranial pressure.

Pancuronium should only be used as a pretreating competitive neuromuscular blocker in a dose of 0.01 mg/kg, to prevent fasciculations when using succinylcholine.

Induction Agents

Thiopental, 3-5 mg/kg IV push, has an onset of 20-40 seconds and lasts about 5-10 minutes.

Midazolam, 0.07-0.3 mg/kg IV push, has an onset of less than 1 minute and duration of 30-60 minutes.

Ketamine, 1-2 mg/kg IV push, has an onset of 1 minute and a duration of 5-15 minutes. This is the preferred agent to use in patients with bronchospasm and status asthmaticus.

a bag-valve mask that can deliver 100% oxygen. A complete knowledge of airway anatomy, pharmacology, and the ability to establish a surgical airway (cricothyrotomy) are necessary prerequisites for performing RSI.

II. Rapid sequence intubation can be divided into the following phases:

A. **Preoxygenation/preparation** (3 to 5 minutes before intubation). This phase includes preparation of the patient, as well as securing all the equipment. Patient preparation involves placing the patient on 100% oxygen. The patient can be preoxygenated for 5 minutes; however, preoxygenation time can be compressed by having the conscious patient take three full breaths of 100% oxygen.

B. **Premedication** (2 to 3 minutes before intubation). During this phase, patients are premedicated with lidocaine (1 mg/kg) and pancuronium or vercuronium (0.01 to 0.02 mg/kg). Lidocaine is used to help prevent harmful reflex responses that cause hypertension, cardiac arrhythmias, and increased intracranial pressure. Pancuronium or vercuronium is used to prevent fasciculations after succinylcholine is administered. Atropine (0.02 mg/kg) is recommended in pediatric patients and is used to prevent bradycardia.

C. **General anesthesia/paralysis** (1 minute before intubation). General anesthesia is induced with either thiopental (4 mg/kg) by rapid intravenous push, midazolam (0.1 to 0.3 mg/kg) by intravenous push, or ketamine (0.5 to 1 mg/kg) by intravenous push. Ketamine is the preferred agent in patients with asthma and severe bronchospasm, or patients with hypotension or hypovolemia. Immediately after giving one of these agents, administer succinylcholine (1 to 1.5 mg/kg) or vercuronium (0.25 mg/kg). If vercuronium is used, the defasciculating agent used in the premedication phase (pancuronium, vercuronium) is not necessary.

D. **Intubation.** About 30 seconds after administration of the neuromuscular blocker, spontaneous respiration begins to cease. At that time an assistant should apply pressure over the cricoid cartilage (Sellick maneuver) to occlude the esophagus. At this time monitor for adequacy of blockade, and when the jaw and mandible are completely relaxed, intubate the trachea under direct visualization. The Sellick maneuver should be maintained until tube placement has been confirmed by auscultation and end-tidal carbon dioxide detector. Endotracheal tube placement should also be confirmed with a chest radiograph. After intubation, it may be necessary to consider longer acting sedation and/or paralysis. When using vercuronium, be sure to use a generous amount of induction agent to avoid waiting too long to achieve optimal intubating conditions. Succinylcholine is the most reliable agent and leads to complete relaxation within 30 to 60 seconds. It is also much shorter acting than vercuronium, with paralysis lasting only 5 to 7 minutes with succinylcholine and about 60 minutes with vercuronium.

E. **Mechanical ventilation.** A variety of mechanical ventilators are effective for the patient in respiratory failure. With certain pulmonary conditions, such as bronchospasm or RDS, high pulmonary inflation pressures may be necessary; therefore, volume-cycled ventilators are preferred in patients with these conditions. The physiology of asthma is primarily airway obstruction mostly during the expiratory phase. Therefore, adequate time should be allowed for expiration to minimize air trapping. Increasing the inspiratory/expiratory ratio (1:3 or greater) and decreasing the ventilatory rate would provide for longer expiratory times. The use of PEEP in asthma is controversial, with one study suggesting that PEEP is detrimental when there is severe airflow obstruction. If PEEP is used at all, peak airway pressures should be maintained below 50 cm H_2O to minimize the risk of barotrauma.

Suggested Readings

Barnes PJ: New approach to the treatment of asthma, *N Engl J Med* 321:1517, 1989.

Chapman KR: Therapeutic algorithm for chronic obstructive pulmonary disease, *Am J Med* 91(suppl 4A):17S, 1991.

Chapman KR et al: Effect of a short course of prednisone in the prevention of early relapse after the emergency room treatment of acute asthma, *N Engl J Med* 324:788, 1991.

Goldhaber SZ et al: Diagnosis, treatment, and prevention of pulmonary embolism: report of the WHO/International Society and Federation of Cardiology Task Force, *JAMA* 268:1727, 1992.

Guidelines for the diagnosis and management of asthma, Expert Panel Report, National Asthma Education Program, National Institutes of Health, Publication Number 91-3042, August 1991.

Hirsch J: Heparin, *N Engl J Med* 324:1565, 1991.

Hull RD et al: Continuous intravenous heparin compared with intermittent subcutaneous heparin the initial treatment of proximal-vein thrombosis, *N Engl J Med* 315:1109, 1986.

McFadden ER, Gilbert IA: Asthma, *N Engl J Med* 327:1928, 1992.

PIOPED Investigators: Value of the ventilation/perfusion scan in acute pulmonary embolism, *JAMA* 263:2753, 1990.

Raschke RA et al: The weight-based heparin dosing nomogram compared with a "standard care" nomogram, *Ann Intern Med* 119:874, 1993.

Skobeloff EM et al: Intravenous magnesium sulphate for the treatment of acute asthma in the emergency department, *JAMA* 262:1210, 1989.

Weiss EB, Segal MS, Stein M, editors: *Bronchial asthma: mechanisms and therapeutics,* ed 2, Toronto, 1985, Little Brown.

10

Drug Therapy for Gastrointestinal Emergencies

Marc Smith, M.D., F.A.C.E.P.

Esophageal Foreign Bodies

Esophageal foreign bodies such as coins and other hard items are commonly seen in children between 6 months and 6 years of age. The elderly with poorly fitting dental prostheses are another group at risk because they typically ingest food that has not been thoroughly masticated. Psychiatric patients form the third large group of patients at risk; there is no limit to the type of foreign body that is encountered within this group. Patients with a prior history of esophageal problems are also at increased risk.

The esophagus has three distinct anatomic sites where foreign bodies lodge. The uppermost (and most common site of impaction) is the cricopharyngeus muscle, which is attached to the cricoid cartilage and composed of striated muscle. The next site of impaction occurs where the esophagus passes behind the aortic arch, where the muscular lining of the esophagus is composed of mixed striated and smooth muscle fibers. The third common site of impaction is the lower esophageal sphincter (LES), which is also known as the gastroesophageal junction.

I. **Signs and symptoms.** Esophageal foreign bodies may cause pain (which may or may not be localized to the site of the obstruction), vomiting, an inability to swallow and/or handle secretions (drooling or constantly spitting), and a foreign body sensation. Extrinsic compression of the posterior trachea by the esophageal foreign body may produce partial compromise of the airway. Thus these patients may initially have symptoms of partial airway obstruction such as coughing, choking, or stridor. Perforation, which occurs more commonly with sharp objects, button battery ingestion, greater than 24 hours since time of impaction, prior esophageal disease, and iatrogenic use of papain-containing compounds, can produce mediastinitis, aortoesophageal fistula, pericardial tamponade, abscesses, empyema, pneumothoraces, mucosal ulcerations, and hematemesis secondary to esophageal vessel injury. Because of these complications, patients may rarely present in a moribund state, requiring vigorous resuscitation.

II. **Diagnosis.** History and physical examination usually provide the diagnosis. In cases where the diagnosis is not clear, additional studies may aid the physician. With radiopaque objects, plain radiographs are diagnostic. Typically, coins lodged within the esophagus at the cricopharyngeus lie in the coronal plane, while those in the trachea lie within the sagittal plane. Radiolucent objects lodged within the esophagus may be delineated with the addition of oral contrast administered under fluoroscopy. The type of oral contrast is chosen based on the inherent risks involved: if perforation is suspected, a water-based contrast agent is used, with barium being used in all other cases since aspiration is the other primary risk of these agents. With a partial obstruction, the addition of a small piece of cotton that has been soaked in contrast material will increase the sensitivity of the study when oral contrast alone has not delineated the foreign body. The cotton will usually "hang up" on the object in question, with the cotton fibers retaining contrast material, allowing elucidation of the location of the foreign body. When available, xeroradiography, computed tomography (CT), and magnetic resonance imaging (MRI) play a role in the evaluation of possible esophageal foreign bodies. Esophagoscopy remains the "gold standard" in evaluation of esophageal foreign bodies because it allows the skilled endoscopist to diagnose and remove the foreign body, survey the site for damage caused by the foreign body impactions, and evaluate the site for underlying disease. Endoscopy is, however, not available in all locations.

III. **Treatment.** All esophageal foreign bodies must be removed. The methods used to remove the foreign body depend on the type of object involved, age and condition of the patient, availability of resources and specialists, and the skills of the physician caring for the patient. Foreign bodies lodged at the cricopharyngeus or aortic arch do not respond to pharmacologic maneuvers and must be removed manually. This can be accomplished either by an endoscopist using a bronchoscope or by the emergency physician or radiologist using a Foley catheter under direct fluoroscopy. In order for the Foley catheter technique to be safely performed, the object must be smooth and impacted for less than 24 hours, with the patient being without signs or symptoms of esophageal perforation and without a prior history of esophageal disease. Venous access should be established, anxiolytics should be administered as necessary (with appropriate monitoring), and suction, oxygen, laryngoscope, McGill forceps, endotracheal tubes and stylettes, and a cricothyrotomy kit should be available at the bedside. An appropriate-sized Foley catheter (12 to 16 French) first has the balloon checked for patency and symmetry with a small amount of contrast material. Topical anesthetics are applied to the nasopharynx and/or posterior oropharynx. The patient is placed on the fluoroscopy table in a head-down, prone or left lateral decubitus position, with the catheter being introduced through either the nares or oropharynx and then slowly advanced under direct fluoroscopy to a site just distal to the foreign body. The balloon is then slowly inflated with the contrast material. Should the patient experience pain with the inflation, the esophagus is being dilated past its normal size. The balloon should be deflated, repositioned distally, and slowly reinflated—5 ml of contrast is usually sufficient. The balloon is slowly retracted with gentle pressure until the hypopharynx, where the decreased friction on the object causes it to "pop" into the oropharynx, where the patient can either spit it out or it can be retrieved by the physician using fingers or forceps. Foreign body aspiration is a risk at this juncture. If resistance to retraction of the balloon catheter is encountered, efforts should cease and the patient immediately referred to a skilled endoscopist. If the balloon slips past the foreign body proximally, it can be slipped distally again and reinflated with several more milliliters of contrast. Foreign bodies will sometimes be passed into the stomach with these maneuvers.

A. **Smooth foreign bodies lodged at the LES are susceptible to pharmacologic manipulation** with agents that relax the smooth muscle of the LES. **Glucagon** (dosage: adult, 1 mg; pediatric, 0.1 mg/kg), administered intravenously over 1 to 2 minutes, will usually be effective within 15 minutes. A second dose (adult, 2 mg; pediatric, 0.1 mg/kg) may be administered 20 minutes after the first dose. Peristalsis (and subsequent passage of the foreign body) may be promoted by judicious sips of water. Glucagon may cause vomiting, most commonly during rapid IV injection. Slow injection and concomitant use of antiemetics decrease the potential risk of rupture of the totally obstructed esophagus. **Nitroglycerin** (dosage: adult, 0.4 mg sublingual (SL) every 5 minutes to a maximum of 3 mg; pediatric, not established) and **nifedipine** (dosage: adult, 10 mg chew and swallow or SL; pediatric, 0.25 to 0.5 mg/kg PO/IV) have also been shown to promote passage of foreign bodies impacted at the LES. They may be used individually or concomitantly with glucagon. While tempting, nasogastric tubes should not be used in the attempt to push objects through the LES because of the possibility of further damaging the esophagus. The use of papain is condemned because of the small but significant risk of esophageal rupture that is caused by its use. Sharp esophageal foreign bodies, button batteries lodged within the esophagus, and failure to remove a smooth esophageal foreign body require immediate consultation with an endoscopist for further management. All cases of successful removal of the foreign body should be referred for further evaluation of intrinsic esophageal or extrinsic disease. A low threshold for evaluation of esophageal perforation must be maintained because of the high morbidity and mortality of this complication. Foreign bodies that have passed into the stomach usually pass without sequelae; however, sharp foreign bodies (pins, etc.) may cause perforation and dictate emergent referral to an endoscopist. Patients may be monitored through careful examination of their stools or, in the case of radiopaque objects, serial radiographs. Admonitions of the signs and symptoms of intestinal hemorrhage, intestinal obstruction, and perforations should accompany the discharge of these patients.

B. Patients who initially have pharyngodynia after ingesting fish seldom have bones impacted in their mucosa. Of those who do have retained fish bones, the vast majority (93%) are lodged in the base of the tongue, posterior pharyngeal wall, or tonsil, and are easily removed under direct visualization by using a tongue blade, a good light source, and a forceps (Knight LC, Lesser THJ: *Arch Emerg Med* 6:13, 1989). Patients in whom a bone has not been identified and who are without fever, localized swelling, hematemesis, inability to swallow, or signs and symptoms consistent with esophageal perforation may be referred to an endoscopist for further evaluation in 24 to 48 hours.

Acid and Alkaline Ingestions

Acids produce a coagulation necrosis that limits their penetration of the gastroesophageal mucosa, while alkalis produce a liquefaction necrosis that results in a much higher perforation rate. **Table 10-1** lists the determinants of toxicity for ingestions. Pediatric ingestion is usually accidental, while adult ingestion is usually intentional.

I. Signs and symptoms. These include dysphagia, drooling, stridor, chest pain, abdominal pain, vomiting, hematemesis, melena, respiratory distress, peritonitis, shock, and oropharyngeal erythema and burns. The absence of visible oropharyngeal burns does not reliably exclude the diagnosis of corrosive ingestion. Acids produce their primary effect at the antrum and pylorus, while alkalis produce primarily esophageal injuries. There is, however, considerable crossover in the injury spectrum. HF can produce systemic hypocalcemia leading to cardiopulmonary arrest.

II. Treatment. Endoscopy is mandatory in all patients with a history of corrosive ingestion who are symptomatic or have oropharyngeal burns. Diluents adminis-

Table 10-1. Determinants of Toxicity

Factor	Severe toxicity
pH	<2, >12
Normality	Greater concentrations
Viscosity	Greater viscosity increases contact time
Contact time	Areas subject to increased contact time—narrow areas and sphincters
State	Solids have longer transit times than liquids
Volume	Large volumes
Heat	Exothermic reactions
Underlying toxicity	Cyanide, hydrofluoric acid, oxalic acid
Pyloric condition	Spasm

tered as first aid have no proven efficacy, are potentially harmful, and are not recommended. The patient should be made NPO. Emesis and activated charcoal are potentially dangerous and ineffective. Lavage is contraindicated. Steroids have been shown in animal trials to reduce stricture formation when administered within the first 48 hours; no large human trials have been completed. Steroids should not be administered if there is a possibility of perforation (or with active infection or a history of peptic ulcer disease) and should be administered ideally after endoscopy has documented that the extent of the injury is limited to transmucosal lesions. **Methylprednisolone** (dosage: older than 2 years, 40 mg IV every 8 hours; younger than 2 years, 20 mg IV every 8 hours) is the recommended corticosteroid. Antibiotics should be reserved until perforation has occurred or secondary infection has manifested itself.

Gastroesophageal Reflux

Gastroesophageal reflux disease (GERD) is a common disorder affecting up to 10% of Americans. Agents and conditions that decrease LES pressure, decrease esophageal motility, and increase gastric emptying times contribute to the development of GERD (see **box** on page 298).

I. **Signs and symptoms.** While the pain is characteristically described as a burning, retrosternal chest pain with radiation upward, sometimes associated with a bitter, acid taste in the mouth, it commonly mimics ischemic heart disease. It may be described as a dull, squeezing, or pressure-type pain and may be associated with nausea, vomiting, diaphoresis, and radiation of the pain to the neck, jaw, shoulders, and arms. Meals, especially large meals, often exacerbate the pain associated with GERD, as does any position that places the esophagus in a dependent position, such as lying down. Exercise may aggravate GERD, thereby further mimicking ischemic heart disease. Pain is typically relieved by the upright position and antacids. Pain from GERD may be relieved by nitrates, adding to the diagnostic confusion. While patients in whom the diagnosis of GERD is easily made may be safely discharged from the emergency department, many patients need to be admitted to first eliminate ischemic heart disease as the cause of their pain.

II. **Treatment.** Outpatient management of GERD is oriented toward elimination of symptoms. Patients with mild symptoms are managed with dietary and medication modification (elimination of items in the **box** below), elevation of the head and shoulders 6 to 10 inches from the horizontal plane while in bed (through the use of blocks placed under the head of the bed, special beds, or a special wedge placed under the head and shoulders), avoidance of food 3 hours before bedtime, and the use of antacids 1 hour after mealtimes, at bedtime, and as needed. Patients who have severe symptoms or who fail to improve within 2 to 3 weeks despite the conservative regimen above should begin pharmacologic therapy (see **Table 10-2** for dosage). Histamine receptor antagonists (H_2 blockers) used BID or QID are effective as initial therapy. Sucralfate is a reasonable alternative therapy, especially in patients who are medically frail or on multiple medications. Omeprazole, a "proton pump inhibitor," should be reserved for those individuals who fail H_2-blocker therapy. Metoclopramide and bethanecol are useful adjuncts in therapy, with metoclopramide increasing LES tone and acting as a prokinetic agent, while bethanecol acts as a prokinetic agent. Cisapride, a new prokinetic agent, is as effective as H_2 blockers when used as an isolated agent. Surgery (fundoplication without vagotomy) is reserved for those with severe symptoms who fail aggressive medical management.

Agents Related to GERD

Alcohol
Anticholinergics
Birth control pills
Caffeinated beverages
Calcium channel blockers
Chocolate
Diabetic gastroparesis
Fatty foods
Gastric outlet obstruction
Nicotine
Nitrates
Pregnancy

Table 10-2. Agents Used to Treat GERD

Agent	Dose
Antacids	30 ml 1 hour pc and qhs
H_2 blockers	
Cimetidine	400-800 mg BID or 300-400 mg QID
Ranitidine	150 mg BID or 150 mg QID
Famotidine	20-40 mg BID
Nizatidine	150 mg BID
Omeprazole	20 mg QD
Metoclopramide	5-20 mg QID
Bethanechol	25 mg QID
Sucralfate	1 g QID
Cisapride	10-20 mg QID

Gastrointestinal Bleeding

Patients with gastrointestinal (GI) bleeding commonly present to the emergency department with complaints of hematemesis, hematochezia, or melena, though the chief complaint may reflect end-organ hypoperfusion (weakness, dizziness, syncope, angina, shortness of breath, hypotension, cardiopulmonary arrest). Upper GI bleeding is usually due to duodenal or gastric ulcers, but gastritis, Mallory-Weiss tears, varices, vascular malformations, esophagitis, and duodenitis are all important causes. While minor lower GI bleeding is usually due to anal fissures or hemorrhoids, major bleeding has diverse causes that tend to be age specific. Swallowed maternal blood (during delivery or secondary to cracked nipples) and hemorrhagic disease of the newborn can present in the first few days of life. Necrotizing enterocolitis affects neonates (usually premature) within the first 2 weeks of life. Meckel's diverticulum presents with painless rectal bleeding in patients younger than 2 years, while intussusception presents in the same age group, but with abdominal pain. Polyps usually present in children 2 to 5 years of age. Diverticular disease, arteriovenous malformations, ulcerative colitis, and carcinoma should be considered as possible causes in all patients, once they reach young adulthood. Rapid evaluation occurs concurrently with immediate resuscitation and stabilization in an attempt to minimize morbidity and mortality.

The history obtained from the patient can often point toward a likely cause of the bleeding. A history of hematemesis, with or without melena, usually points to a site of bleeding proximal to the ligament of Treitz. Prosthetic abdominal aortic grafts may erode into bowel, creating an aortoenteric fistula. A history of forceful vomiting that preceded the hematemesis heightens the suspicion of a Mallory-Weiss tear, while a history of portal hypertension (usually secondary to chronic alcohol abuse) increases the probability of variceal bleeding. While a prior history of variceal bleeding should always make one consider this as the probable cause, the continued abuse of alcohol makes alcoholic gastritis and peptic ulcers highly probable causes also. Nonsteroidal antiinflammatory drugs, alcohol, and smoking all increase the rate of gastritis and peptic ulcer disease. Weight loss and changing bowel habits indicate possible carcinoma, while known diverticular disease points to diverticuli as the likely source of hematochezia.

I. **Signs and symptoms.** The physical examination often reveals vital signs consistent with hypovolemia (tachycardia, hypotension, and tachypnea); when these are absent, orthostatic vital signs should be obtained to aid in assessing volume status, realizing that pediatric and geriatric patients may be orthostatic at a euvolemic baseline. Color, warmth, mental status, and capillary filling time should be assessed, and thorough cardiac, pulmonary, and abdominal examinations should be performed. Rectal examination, with gross evaluation and examination for occult blood, should be done. Bright red blood per rectum should be evaluated with bedside anoscopy; if this is negative, proctosigmoidoscopy should be performed. Hematochezia or melena in the absence of hematemesis, or a history of hematemesis, necessitates passage of a nasogastric or orogastric tube to evaluate the site of bleeding and the degree of blood loss. Careful passage of gastric tubes has not been shown to increase bleeding from Mallory-Weiss tears or esophageal varices.

II. **Treatment.** Treatment should be initiated as soon as the possibility of a major GI bleed is recognized, with the history and physical examination occurring concurrently with the stabilization of the patient. If the airway is clear and the patient is breathing without undue distress, he should be placed on high-flow oxygen and a cardiac monitor while establishing a minimum of two large-bore IV lines and beginning fluid resuscitation with balanced salt solution (2 L in adults; 20 ml/kg in children, repeat up to a total of 60 ml/kg; 10 ml/kg in neonates, repeat up to a total of 30 ml/kg). Blood should be obtained from the first IV start for a complete blood cell count, chemistry profile, prothrombin time (PT), partial thromboplastin time (PTT) (INR as appropriate), as well as for type and crossmatch. While packed erythrocytes should be available within 30 minutes of receipt of the clot tube in the blood bank, the patient with persistent hypotension (despite adequate fluid resuscitation), myocardial ischemia, altered sensorium, or significant anemia should not await their arrival; O-negative packed erythrocytes or type-specific blood should be transfused. A foley catheter should be placed to help assess the adequacy of resuscitation. Patients with upper GI bleeding should receive histamine receptor antagonists (H_2 blockers) IV (cimetidine 300 mg or ranitidine 50 mg or famotidine 20 mg). Iced saline lavage does not help and places the patient at risk of hypothermia. Immediate consultation with a gastroenterologist skilled in endoscopy is mandatory, with surgical consultation also prudent (should the hemorrhage be uncontrollable). Upper GI bleeding can usually be accurately diagnosed endoscopically and often be treated at the same time with a plethora of emerging tools. Angiography can define the site of lower GI bleeding and stop the hemorrhage through embolization of the bleeding vessel. Angiography plays a secondary role in the treatment of upper GI bleeding. Radionuclide imaging can define the general area of bleeding. Colonoscopy is difficult in the patient with acute lower GI bleeding but is effective and accurate in defining the bleeding site 2 to 3 days after the cessation of hemorrhage (in a prepared colon). Vasopressin and Sengstaken-Blakemore tubes should only be used after the endoscopist has determined that the site of bleeding is variceal in nature; they have no role in the emergency department.

Intussusception

Intussusception, the telescoping or prolapse of one portion of intestine into the immediately adjoining segment, is an abdominal emergency almost entirely limited to infants and toddlers, 3 to 24 months of age (usually 3 to 12 months), with a male/female ratio of 2:1. The usual site of intussusception is just proximal to the ileocecal valve, causing the terminal ileum to prolapse into the ascending colon. The incidence increases in the spring and fall, with concomitant viral infections common; hypertrophy of the Peyer's patches is felt to be the "lead point" in these circumstances.

I. **Signs and symptoms.** The clinical presentation often leads to the diagnosis. Patients initially have colicky abdominal pain that lasts for short periods, with pain-free intervals of up to 30 minutes between attacks. During the pain, patients will cry, pull their knees to their chest, and clutch their abdomen. Vomiting usually occurs. While the early abdominal exam will usually be unremarkable except for the intermittent colic, a sausage-shaped mass can be palpated later in the right upper quadrant of the abdomen. Eventually the examination of the abdomen is only significant for peritonitis. The hallmark "currant jelly stool" (stool containing red blood and mucus) is passed by only 60% of patients. Lethargy, fever, shock, and death invariably follow in the untreated patient. Surgical consultation should be obtained immediately in all patients in whom the diagnosis of intussusception is entertained.

   A. **The patient presenting with intussusception** must first be assessed for shock, and if present, this is the focus of initial emergency treatment. Oxygen administration, vigorous volume replacement with isotonic crystalloid, Foley catheterization, nasogastric intubation, and continuous monitoring in the patient with shock is mandatory. Blood for type and cross, complete blood cell count, and chemistry profile should be sent with the initiation of intravascular access. If peritonitis is clinically present, empiric coverage with broad-spectrum antibiotics should be initiated. If severe shock is present, control of the airway should be a high management priority with a controlled orotracheal intubation. Immediate surgical consultation is mandatory because definitive reduction of the intussusception will be required, as well as possible resection of nonviable bowel.

B. In patients without shock or peritonitis in whom the intussusception has been present for only a short period, reduction of the intussusception with a barium enema should be attempted. Adequate sedation and analgesia of the child is mandatory because crying and tensing the abdomen will decrease the success rate and increase the possibility of perforation. Adequate hydration increases the probability of successful reduction. The barium should be hung no more than 1 m above the abdomen, with no more than three separate attempts at reducing the intussusception, each no longer than 3 minutes. No pressure should be applied to the enema, and no manipulation of the abdomen should be performed during the procedure because these maneuvers increase the rate of perforation of the intestine. Successful reduction is noted by the reflux of barium into the terminal ileum. Failure to reduce the intussusception with barium or any extravasation of barium into the peritoneal cavity warrants immediate surgery.

Hypertrophic Pyloric Stenosis

Hypertrophic pyloric stenosis (HPS) is the most common disorder of infancy requiring surgical correction. Developing postnatally, the disorder almost always occurs between 1 week and 3 months of age, and prototypically appears in 2- to 3-week-old infants. Demonstrating an inheritable factor, the patient is at an increased risk of acquiring HPS if one of their parents had HPS. Boys are more commonly affected (5:1), with the firstborn boy most commonly afflicted. Vomiting, usually projectile, causes the caregivers to seek medical attention, and usually occurs with or immediately after feeding, although it may sometimes be delayed for several hours. Constipation commonly accompanies HPS because of the lack of milk retention.

I. Signs and symptoms. Clinically, the infant shows signs and symptoms of dehydration, with poor capillary refill, dry mucous membranes, absent tearing, poor skin turgor, and tachycardia. The infant usually has insufficient weight gain for age, and may be below birth weight. Palpation of the stomach may reveal the elongated, thickened pylorus as an "olive," palpable lateral to the rectus abdominus just below the edge of the liver. Peristaltic waves are visible in the abdomen before vomiting occurs.

II. Treatment. Careful attention should be paid to correcting the volume status, with the immediate dispatch of a blood chemistry profile to detect electrolyte abnormalities, usually a hypokalemic, hypochloremic metabolic alkalosis with either normal or depressed serum sodium levels. Volume and electrolyte correction is mandatory before surgery. Abdominal ultrasound in the hands of an experienced ultrasonographer will usually demonstrate HPS. When the ultrasound is negative, an upper GI series is performed to exclude the possibility of a false-negative ultrasound. Once the diagnosis has been made and the infant stabilized, a pyloromyotomy is performed in the operating room.

Volvulus

Volvulus results from the twisting of a segment of bowel about its mesenteric axis, producing an obstruction of the lumen of the bowel, with possible compromise of the vascular supply leading to ischemic bowel. Three distinct types of volvulus, involving different types of patients, exist: sigmoid volvulus, cecal volvulus, and malrotation with midgut volvulus.

Sigmoid volvulus is a disease almost exclusively limited to the debilitated elderly and patients who are severely compromised secondary to severe neurologic or psychiatric disease. The severe, chronic constipation that afflicts these patients leads to lengthening of the sigmoid colon, which, attached to a narrow mesenteric stalk, predisposes to torsion and volvulus.

I. **Signs and symptoms.** Clinically, the patient is first seen with crampy, left lower quadrant abdominal pain associated with abdominal distention and tympany. Delay in presentation, quite common in this patient population, leads to generalized abdominal pain, vomiting, and obstipation, as well as marked fluid sequestration within the lumen of the bowel, with subsequent dehydration and hypovolemia. Rapid replacement of fluid and electrolyte deficits in these patients is mandatory. Strangulation is suggested by fever, peritonitis, and an elevated leukocyte count with a left shift, with the patient appearing clinically toxic. History and physical examination suggest the diagnosis, with an upright radiograph confirming the diagnosis by demonstrating a loop of colon with two air-fluid levels arising out of the left pelvis. Decompression and detorsion of the nonstrangulated sigmoid volvulus is accomplished by the passage of a rectal tube through the sigmoidoscope. While highly successful, this treatment occasionally fails, in which case a barium enema may reduce the volvulus. Failure to reduce the volvulus and all cases of suspected strangulation require immediate surgical intervention to reduce the volvulus. Patients who have had a successful reduction and are good operative candidates should be referred for elective removal of the redundant loop of sigmoid colon because of the high incidence of recurrence.

   A. **Cecal volvulus,** an entity most commonly seen in young adults, is secondary to congenital poor fixation of the cecum, allowing it to twist on itself and obstruct. The patient has crampy abdominal pain, nausea, vomiting, and abdominal distention as the small intestine sequesters fluid within its lumen. Examination of the abdomen reveals high-pitched rushes on auscultation, with tympany evident on percussion. The upright abdominal film demonstrates the classic "stair-stepping" seen with small bowel obstruction, as well as the massively distended cecum with a single air-fluid level within it. Because of its poor fixation, the cecum may appear anywhere within the abdominal cavity in this presentation. Vascular access with prompt rehydration, dispatch of specimens to the laboratory in preparation for surgery, nasogastric suction, and prompt surgical referral for operative intervention should proceed expeditiously once the diagnosis has been made.

   B. **Malrotation and midgut volvulus** are preceded by abnormal rotation and fixation of the midgut (duodenum, small intestine, and the right half of the colon) during embryonic development. While torsion can occur at any time (including adulthood), it commonly occurs in neonates and is heralded by the acute onset of abdominal pain, bilious vomiting, and shock. Physical examination reveals an infant in shock with poor capillary refill, rapid heart rate, grunting respirations, distended abdomen, and diffuse abdominal tenderness. Vascular access should be established immediately in two sites, with blood sent for a complete blood cell count, chemistry profile, and type and crossmatch. Vigorous fluid hydration with isotonic crystalloid should begin immediately. Oxygen (100%) should be administered, and endotracheal intubation should be considered. Nasogastric suction should be started, and a Foley catheter should be placed to help monitor adequacy of rehydration. Early surgical consultation is advised. Broad-spectrum antibiotics should be initiated. While abdominal radiographs may demonstrate the classic "double-bubble" sign of a markedly dilated duodenum and stomach, they may demonstrate only small bowel obstruction or be entirely normal. Air-contrast studies, upper GI series, and ultrasound may all help delineate the lesion in a stable patient. Detorsion in the operating suite should occur within 1 hour (of initial onset of symptoms) in the unstable patient; otherwise, irreversible ischemia will lead to bowel necrosis, with subsequent high morbidity and mortality.

Pancreatitis

Pancreatitis is the acute inflammation of the pancreas, with a pathologic spectrum ranging from minimal edema to hemorrhagic necrosis of the gland. While many etiologic factors have been implicated in pancreatitis, no adequate explanation of the pathophysiology is currently available. The myriad biologic insults that result in pancreatitis **(Table 10-3)** demonstrate the limited ability of the pancreas to cope with any insult. The most common causes of pancreatitis in the Western world are biliary tract disease and ethanol abuse, with the leading cause dependent on the practice setting.

I. Signs and symptoms. Clinically, the patient initially has abdominal pain localized to the midepigastric region and characterized as a constant, dull pain, that frequently radiates to the back. The pain ranges from mild to severe, with the patient constantly trying to find a position of comfort (unsuccessfully) on the stretcher. Partial relief of the pain is sometimes reported by the patient by assuming the knee-chest position while sitting. Examination of the abdomen reveals abdominal tenderness greatest in the midepigastric region, often with voluntary guarding. The degree of patient distress, however, may exceed the findings of the abdominal exam. Nausea, vomiting, diaphoresis, abdominal distention, low-grade fever, tachycardia, and hypotension are common. Cullen's and Turner's signs are uncommon.

   A. While the diagnosis is often suspected based on history and physical examination, laboratory evaluation is usually required. The serum amylase level is often used but lacks the sensitivity and specificity of the serum lipase level. When pancreatitis is suspected, measurement of the serum lipase level is the diagnostic test of choice. Amylase is secreted by many other organs including the salivary glands, small intestine, fallopian tubes, kidney, liver, and tumors of the lung, esophagus, and ovaries. Amylase isoenzyme assay can identify the site of origin of a serum amylase elevation but is not readily available in the emergency department. An elevated amylase level is considered reliable if it exhibits the typical rise and fall with clinical symptoms. The amylase/creatinine clearance ratio has been shown to be of little value. Serum lipase levels remain elevated longer than amylase, which makes this test useful when symptoms have been present for several days. Persistent elevation of amylase, however, suggests the development of complications such as a pseudocyst. Since the lipase levels remain elevated, they are less useful than amylase levels as a marker of compli-

Table 10-3. Etiologic Factors in Acute Pancreatitis

Noninfectious

Ethanol ingestion*	Biliary tract disease (Cholelithiasis)*
Methanol ingestion	Penetrating duodenal ulcer
Duodenal diverticulosis	Papillitis
Trauma	Hyperlipidemia
Hereditary	
Diabetes mellitus	ERCP
Postoperative	Pregnancy
Cystic fibrosis	Tumor
Hypercalcemia	Scorpion bite
Hemochromatosis	SLE
Vasculitis	Porphyria
Renal transplantation	Hypothermia
Regional enteritis	SMA syndrome
Shock	Renal failure
TTP	Pancreas divisum

Infectious

Mumps	Hepatitis A and B
Typhoid	Mycoplasma
Coxsackie group B	Mononucleosis
Parasitic	Echovirus
Rubella	Influenza A

Drugs

Acetaminophen	Azathioprine
Cimetidine	Estrogens
Furosemide	Indomethacin
Opiates	Salicylates
Steroids	Sulfonamides
Tetracycline	Thiazides
Valproic acid	Warfarin
Idiopathic	Multiple other drugs

*These categories account for 90% of all pancreatitis.
ERCP, Endoscopic retrograde cholangiopancreatography; *SLE*, systemic lupus erythematosus; *SMA*, superior mesenteric artery; *TTP*, thrombotic thrombocytopenic purpura.

cations. Hypocalcemia occurs with severe or hemorrhagic pancreatitis and may require replacement therapy.

B. Plain films of the abdomen may demonstrate a localized ileus with air-fluid levels in the area of the pancreas ("sentinel loop") in one third of patients, but this is neither sensitive or specific. Pancreatic calcifications suggest chronic pancreatitis. Major complications occur in up to 10% of patients with pancreatitis and only half are apparent clinically. In patients with severe or complicated pancreatitis, abdominal ultrasound is the test of choice to identify pseudocyst formation. If infectious or hemorrhagic complications such as infected pseudocyst, abscess or pancreatic hemorrhage are suspected, abdominal CT scan is the test of choice. Ranson et al. (*Surg Gynecol Obstet* 138:69, 1974) defined criteria **(Table 10-4)** that aid in assessing the outcome of patients with pancreatitis. Patients with more criteria have higher mortality, as noted in **Table 10-5** (Ranson JHC: *Am J Gastroenterol* 77:663, 1982).

Table 10-4. Ranson's Criteria for Acute Pancreatitis

On admission	Within 48 hours
Age >55 years	Hematocrit fall >10%
WBC >16,000/mm^3	BUN rise >5 mg/dl
Blood glucose >200 mg/dl	Serum calcium <8 mg/dl
Serum LDH >350 IU/L	Arterial Po$_2$ <60 mm Hg
Serum AST >250 SFU	Base deficit >4 mEq/L
	Fluid sequestration >6 L

WBC, white blood cell count; *LDH*, lactate dehydrogenase; Po$_2$, oxygen pressure; *AST*, aspartate aminotransferase; *BUN*, blood urea nitrogen.

Table 10-5. Mortality Associated with Pancreatitis

Mortality (%)	No. of positive factors
1	<3
15	3-4
40	5-6
100	7-11

II. **Treatment.** Fluid resuscitation with balanced electrolyte solution and control of pain and nausea are the principal goals of initial management. Morphine should not be used because it causes spasm of the sphincter of Oddi and may exacerbate the pain. While nasogastric suction has been a mainstay of therapy, it has been shown to be of no benefit. The patient should be made NPO, and the state of hydration should be carefully followed. Patients with new onset pancreatitis, severe pancreatitis, and those with an unclear diagnosis all require prompt surgical evaluation. No medication has been shown to be efficacious in the treatment of pancreatitis. Peritoneal lavage has been shown to be efficacious in the treatment of severe pancreatitis. Patients with mild recurrent pancreatitis secondary to chronic alcohol abuse who are well hydrated, able to keep down oral fluids, and whose pain can be easily managed with oral narcotics are candidates for discharge, as long as close follow-up can be arranged; all others should be admitted for observation and treatment.

Cholecystitis

Cholecystitis is the acute inflammation of the gallbladder, usually associated with obstruction of the neck of the gallbladder or the cystic duct by a gallstone. Acalculous cholecystitis is not associated with gallstones and usually occurs in hospitalized patients as a complication of any major illness or surgery. Passage of small gallstones through the cystic duct into the common bile duct is heralded by pain commonly referred to as biliary colic. Common risk factors for gallstones include obesity, female gender, increasing age, heredity, and the use of estrogen compounds.

I. **Signs and symptoms.** The patient with acute cholecystitis or biliary colic usually is first seen at night or in the early morning hours with complaints of abdominal pain localized to the midepigastrium or the right upper quadrant, often starting in the midepigastrium and then migrating to the right upper quadrant.

The pain is a severe, dull, steady pain that is unrelenting in acute cholecystitis but resolves with the passage of the stone(s) in biliary colic. Nausea, vomiting, and temperature elevation are more common with acute cholecystitis, with flatulence common to both.

  A. The physical examination reveals localized tenderness in the right upper quadrant in both entities, with the tenderness in acute cholecystitis being much more pronounced. In addition, splinting of the musculature of the right upper quadrant, as well as a positive Murphy's sign (arrest of inspiration with deep palpation beneath the right costal margin), is seen in acute cholecystitis but not in biliary colic. Laboratory evaluation may reveal a leukocytosis, as well as a mild elevation of the serum alkaline phosphatase level. Higher elevations are usually indicative of a common duct stone, with an elevated serum amylase level suggestive of a gallstone pancreatitis.

  B. Imaging. While plain radiographs usually do not aid in determining the diagnosis (unless calcified gallstones are visible), other imaging techniques are extremely useful. Ultrasound is a safe, effective, noninvasive means of evaluating possible gallbladder disease, allowing the delineation of stones, sludge, thickened gallbladder walls, impacted stones with ductal dilatation, as well as identifying pericholecystic abscesses. If this test is inconclusive but the clinical suspicion is high for acute cholecystitis, nuclear scintigraphy should be performed to evaluate gallbladder functioning. If the ultrasound is negative but the clinical suspicion is high for biliary colic and cholelithiasis, an oral cholecystogram should be done to evaluate the gallbladder for gallstones.

II. Treatment. The patient undergoing evaluation for right upper quadrant pain in the emergency department should be made NPO, hydrated, and offered analgesics. Morphine causes spasm of the sphincter of Oddi and is contraindicated, with meperidine having the same problem but to a much smaller degree. Ketorolac (30 to 60 mg IM/IV [not licensed for IV use in the United States, but extremely effective]), a parenteral nonsteroidal antiinflammatory drug (NSAID), has been used with great efficacy in the emergency department for management of pain in patients with biliary colic and acute cholecystitis.

  A. Surgical consultation. All patients with acute cholecystitis should have immediate surgical consultation. Antibiotic choice should be made in conjunction with the surgical consultant because many excellent choices are available. Laparoscopic removal, when possible, significantly reduces the associated morbidity. Patients with biliary colic who have had resolution of their pain within the emergency department are candidates for outpatient management.

  B. Laparoscopic removal has emerged as the definitive treatment of patients with cholelithiasis, but a small group of patients with cholesterol stones <20 mm in diameter who have normal hepatic function and who are not good surgical candidates may be managed with **chenodiol** (13 to 16 mg/kg/day in BID dosing starting with 250 mg BID and increasing 250 mg/week until maximal dosing achieved or diarrhea results) or **ursodiol** (8 to 10 mg/kg/day in BID or TID dosing). Ursodiol appears to have fewer side effects, with careful monitoring of liver function tests necessary. Serial ultrasounds or oral cholecystograms are necessary to evaluate treatment success. Treatment should not be extended beyond 18 months. Monoctanoin, a semisynthetic esterified glycerol, may be infused via a nasobiliary tube placed endoscopically to achieve dissolution of cholesterol stones. A total of 2 to 10 days of therapy are usually required for stone dissolution or size reduction.

Hepatitis

Hepatitis is an acute inflammation of the liver that can result from exposure to toxins (especially ethanol), side effects of certain medications, and fungal, bacterial, parasitic, and viral infections. While many viruses can cause hepatitis, the viral hepatitides (A,B,C,D,E) deserve special mention.

I. **Hepatitis A** is transmitted through fecal-oral contamination and seafood (particularly shellfish) contaminated with untreated sewage. Outbreaks are commonly associated with infected food workers who contaminate food through poor sanitary practices, as well as infected water supplies during periods of natural disaster. Most cases are subclinical, with the majority of clinical cases being mild. No carrier state is known. The incubation period ranges from 15 to 50 days, and the mortality rate is approximately 0.1%. Diagnosis is made by a positive serum IgM titer to the hepatitis A virus. Pooled gamma globulin, given prophylactically to contacts via an IM injection (dose 0.02 ml/kg), protects against clinical disease.

II. **Hepatitis B** is transmitted through sexual contacts, percutaneous exposure, and mucous membrane exposure to contaminated fluids. While most cases are subclinical, the clinical cases can become quite severe, with fulminant hepatic failure occurring in about 1%, with a mortality rate of 0.4% to 1.0%. The carrier rate ranges from 0.1% to 0.5%, with an incubation period ranging from 25 to 160 days. Diagnosis is made by serology, with hepatitis B surface antigen (HB_sAg) first appearing in the sera, followed by the antibody to hepatitis B core antigen (anti-HB_c), and eventually the antibody to hepatitis B surface antigen (anti-HB_s). Because anti-HB_c is elevated during a period when both HB_sAg and anti-HB_s are nonexistent, it is mandatory to evaluate this marker to make the diagnosis in some cases. Chronic active hepatitis develops in up to 10% of patients. Hepatitis B immune globulin (HBIG), given in an IM injection at a dose of 0.06 ml/kg, protects the person who is anti-HB_s negative from the development of clinical disease after exposure. Efficacy of HBIG is greatest if administered within 24 hours of exposure, with declining efficacy out through 7 days. Active immunization is also available against hepatitis B through the use of two different recombinant DNA vaccines, each of which entails three IM injections over a 6-month period. To ensure maximal immune response, the injection should be given in the deltoid muscle of adults and children, with the anterolateral thigh muscle being the site for infants and neonates.

III. **Hepatitis C** virus is transmitted by parenteral exposure, as well as through sexual contacts. Diagnosis is made by serology. Chronic active hepatitis develops in up to 60% of those exposed. Pooled gamma globulin offers theoretical protection against an exposure, but this is unproven. Interferon alpha (3 million units given subcutaneously three times a week for 12 weeks or 5 million units given subcutaneously daily for 6 months) has been advocated by some to prevent progression to chronic liver disease.

IV. **Hepatitis D** virus is transmitted percutaneously. It can only exist as a co-infection with hepatitis B virus and has a mortality rate up to 20%. The disease is often mistaken as a severe case of hepatitis B and can only be diagnosed serologically. The incubation period is unclear but probably approximates that of hepatitis B. It is rare in the United States, confined almost exclusively to IV drug abusers. Immunization against hepatitis B protects against hepatitis D.

V. **Hepatitis E** is spread by fecal-oral contamination, with an incubation period ranging from 10 to 56 days. It is rare in the United States and has a mortality rate of 1% to 2%. No treatment is available.

VI. **Signs and symptoms.** The patient with hepatitis usually complains of malaise, anorexia, fatigue, dark urine, nausea, and low-grade fevers. Vomiting, clay-colored stools, cephalgia, myalgias, and a loss of taste for cigarettes in a smoker all suggest the disease. Jaundice may be the factor that actually prompts the patient to seek medical evaluation. A careful history that includes risk factors for viral hepatitis, exposure to potential hepatotoxins, history of ethanol use, and present or recent use of medications usually elucidates the cause of the inciting event(s). Physical examination reveals icterus, usually with hepatomegaly that is tender to palpation and percussion. Asterixis, fetor hepaticus, and any alteration in mental status are all hallmarks of severe disease in the patient with acute hepatitis. Rectal examination is important to exclude GI bleeding. Laboratory evaluation should include a complete blood cell count, coagulation parameters (PT and activated PTT), and a chemistry profile to include liver function tests. For patients who are stuporous or comatose, blood glucose levels should be determined at the bedside. Plasma ammonia levels and arterial blood gases should be evaluated in severe cases. A lymphocytosis is usually present. Serum alanine aminotransferase (ALT) and aspartate aminotransferase levels (AST) usually show moderate to marked elevations (10 to 100 times the normal values). A PT that is prolonged 3 seconds or more in a patient without preexisting hepatic disease is a hallmark of severe disease, as are elevated plasma ammonia levels and a serum bilirubin level greater than 20 mg/dl without concomitant intravascular hemolysis.

VII. **Treatment.** Patients who are hypoglycemic should receive 50% **dextrose** (glucose), 50 ml, and 100 mg of thiamine IV. Fluid and electrolyte imbalance, if not severe, can usually be treated in the emergency department. Nausea and vomiting can be managed with a variety of antiemetics: **prochlorperazine** (Compazine), 5 to 10 mg PO/IM QID or 25 mg PR BID; **promethazine** (Phenergan), 25 to 50 mg PO/IM/IV/PR q4 to 6 hours; **trimethobenzamide** (Tigan), 250 mg PO QID or 200 mg IM/PR QID; or **droperidol** (Inapsine), 0.625 to 2.5 mg IM/IV. Any of these antiemetics can cause dysphoric or dystonic side effects that are readily treated with dephenhydramine (Benadryl), 25 to 50 mg IV/IM. Patients with intractable nausea and vomiting require admission. Correction of clotting abnormalities with fresh frozen plasma is necessary when bleeding is present and PT is prolonged. Hepatic encephalopathy is managed with **lactulose** enema (300 ml diluted to 1 L with normal saline). It should be retained 30 to 60 minutes. Heavy caloric intake may shorten the recovery period but is often impossible to achieve in an anorectic, nauseous patient.

Appendicitis

Appendicitis is the most common surgical emergency. While many cases present classically, the diagnosis of appendicitis is fraught with peril in the atypical presentation, making it one of the leading causes of malpractice dollars lost in emergency medicine. Atypical presentations are common in the young and the old, and it remains a disease that plagues the pregnant patient in whom the diagnosis presents unique challenges.

I. **Signs and symptoms.** The classic presentation of appendicitis is the patient who has a history of crampy midepigastric or periumbilical pain associated with anorexia, nausea, and vomiting. The pain eventually shifts to the right lower quadrant where it becomes a dull, steady, severe pain. A low-grade fever is common, with the elevation of the fever not correlating with the presence of perforation unless generalized peritonitis is present. Physical examination reveals tenderness in the right lower quadrant, typically over McBurney's point (2 inches from the anterior iliac spine on a line drawn through the umbilicus and the anterior iliac spine), with localized rebound at the site increasing the probability of the diagnosis. Diarrhea or constipation may occur. Hyperesthesia over McBurney's point and voluntary guarding are not consistently present. The iliopsoas test (passive extension of the right hip or active flexion against resistance) and obturator test (passively internally rotating the flexed right thigh) indicate acute inflammation in the area of the tested muscles and are consistent with, but not diagnostic of, acute appendicitis. Variant positioning of the appendix may cause pain in the left lower quadrant or the right upper quadrant, as well as within the pelvis, where it may present on physical examination as rectal or cervical motion tenderness. Urinary symptoms accompanied by pyuria may obfuscate the diagnosis in patients in whom the inflamed appendix overlies a ureter; in this case, flank pain may be the initial complaint. All females in whom the diagnosis is suspected should have a pelvic exam in their evaluation, while all males must have a rectal exam and careful examination of their genitalia to exclude epididymitis.

II. **Treatment.** Management within the emergency department is focused on intravenously rehydrating the often dehydrated patient (now made NPO) while expeditiously evaluating the patient with focused laboratory studies. Patients with a history and physical examination consistent with acute appendicitis should have a complete blood cell count and urinalysis; female patients of childbearing age should have a pregnancy test. A leukocytosis with left shift is commonly seen. A mild pyuria, with or without erythrocytes and/or bacteria may also be seen. A positive pregnancy test is suggestive of ectopic pregnancy. Repeated abdominal examinations will demonstrate progression of disease and are a valuable diagnostic aid. Patients with atypical presentations may need to have radiographs to exclude bowel obstruction as the cause of the pain, as well as serum amylase levels to exclude pancreatitis and liver function tests to exclude cholecystitis. All patients with suspected appendicitis should have immediate surgical consultation. In selected patients with an unclear diagnosis after surgical consultation, graded compression ultrasound, barium enema, radiolabeled autologous leukocyte scans, CT, and MRI will establish the diagnosis of appendicitis. The advent of advanced laparoscopy surgery has allowed the skilled surgeon to evaluate the cause of the pain and to treat it appropriately, often by using the laparoscope. Once the decision has been made to operate, prophylactic antibiotics should be initiated. While antibiotic choice is the decision of the surgeon, the selected antibiotic(s) should provide coverage against Enterobacteriaceae and gram-negative anaerobes. Delay in diagnosis and treatment substantially increases morbidity and mortality.

Rectal Foreign Bodies

I. **The diagnosis** of rectal foreign body (RFB) is usually based on the history of the patient. Morbidity and mortality is associated with perforation. Digital examination, anoscopy, sigmoidoscopy, plain radiographs, and radiographic contrast enemas may aid in delineating the size, shape, and position of the foreign body. Patients with suspected perforation, excessive bleeding, sharp objects, lacerations deeper than the superficial mucosa, fragile objects that produce sharp edges on breakage, inability to remove the object in the emergency department within a reasonable period, and inability to reach the object secondary to proximal migration all warrant immediate surgical referral for admission. The vast majority of the objects encountered can be removed in the emergency department.

II. **Treatment.** A comfortable, relaxed patient is the key to successful removal within the emergency department, making the judicious use of IV benzodiazepines, IV narcotics, or both an important adjunct in this procedure. With the patient in the left lateral decubitus position, the RFB can sometimes be removed by the examining finger(s), aided by steady pressure in the suprapubic area. If the examining finger(s) cannot adequately grasp the RFB, further exposure can be achieved through the use of an anoscope or vaginal speculum. A tenaculum or forceps can then be used to grasp the object and apply gentle traction, removing the anoscope or speculum at the same time. Objects that are difficult to grasp can often be removed by a Foley catheter that is first passed distal to the object and then inflated with water, allowing the physician to apply gentle traction. Two catheters may occasionally be needed. If a suction effect occurs proximal to the object, this can be overcome through the instillation of air through the lumen of the catheter. After all successful removals, anoscopy, sigmoidoscopy, or both is mandatory to exclude the possibility of perforation. If perforation is suspected, broad-spectrum antibiotic coverage against gram-negative anaerobes should be promptly administered, abdominal plain films should be obtained in search of free air, and a surgeon consulted.

Rectal Prolapse

Rectal prolapse is most commonly seen in the young and the elderly. In the young, it may be associated with cystic fibrosis, constipation, or paraplegia. In the elderly, neurologic conditions, pregnancy, diarrhea, and hemorrhoids have been associated with rectal prolapse. Diagnosis is made by physical examination. **Treatment:** Reduction is made through the application of firm, gentle pressure to the mass. Sedation may be necessary. A dressing is then placed, and the buttocks taped together. All cases should be referred for surgical evaluation, although many cases of minor prolapse, especially in the pediatric population, are managed nonsurgically.

Hemorrhoids

Hemorrhoids are common in patients older than 40 years. Constipation, portal hypertension, and a low-bulk diet have all been implicated in the development of hemorrhoids. Internal hemorrhoids originate above the pectinate line and are covered with mucosa, while external hemorrhoids start below the pectinate line and are covered with skin. Internal hemorrhoids commonly are associated with rectal bleeding on defecation. Diagnosis is made with anoscopy. While bleeding is usually minimal, brisk bleeding should prompt immediate evaluation of cardiovascular status and appropriate resuscitation should be administered. If the bleeding hemorrhoid can be visualized, it should be clamped and ligated. Thrombosed internal hemorrhoids are managed conservatively with stool softeners, analgesics, topical anesthetics, and sitz baths. Thrombosed external hemorrhoids are painful and present as a bluish nodule that is exquisitely tender beneath the skin. For mild symptoms, conservative therapy is recommended with stool softeners, analgesics, topical anesthetics, and sitz baths. For moderate to severe pain, the thrombosis is excised. The skin is first prepared, with local analgesia obtained through subcutaneous infiltration. A radial incision is then made to expose the clot, which can then be removed with direct manipulation. It is preferable to excise a small ellipse of skin to prevent premature closure. After satisfactory removal of the offending clot(s), a small dressing is placed over the site, with a large amount of gauze placed on top of that. The buttocks are then taped together, holding the dressing in place and creating a pressure dressing at the same time. This will usually not be required beyond the first 12 hours. The patient is then instructed to rest, preferably in bed, for the next 12 hours, to minimize bleeding. Oral narcotics, stool softeners, sitz baths QID, and hemorrhoidal creams will ease the postoperative course. A follow-up examination in 2 days should be performed.

Perirectal Abscesses

I. **Emergency department.** Only very small, localized perianal abscesses not involving the rectal sphincter or rectum in immunocompetent patients may be managed in the emergency department. All others should be admitted for evaluation and surgical drainage under general anesthesia. Perirectal abscesses can be very misleading because these abscesses are often more extensive than originally appreciated, which leads to attempts to drain them under local anesthesia in the emergency department. With inadequate analgesia, it is often impossible to fully explore these abscesses and break down all loculations, leading to increased morbidity and mortality in this patient group. When in doubt, consult and admit appropriately.

II. **Treatment.** Liberal use of parenteral analgesics is recommended. Nitrous oxide has also been used effectively. With good lighting and surgical exposure, the area is prepared with Betadine, draped, and local analgesia is obtained through subcutaneous infiltration of long-acting local anesthetics with epinephrine. A linear incision over the central part of the abscess is made to the full length of the abscess cavity. Having entered the abscess cavity, the physician must ensure that all loculations are broken down through blunt use of hemostats or the gloved finger. This blunt dissection is poorly tolerated by patients. Once drainage has ceased, the wound is loosely packed and a dressing placed. The patient may then be discharged with oral narcotics for pain control, sitz baths to begin in 24 hours on a thrice daily regimen, and follow-up in 48 hours to replace the packing. Replacement packing should not be placed as deeply, allowing gradual advancement of granulation tissue.

Abdominal Hernia

Hernias are defects that allow the protrusion of abdominal contents. These defects may be either external (through to the outside where it can be examined) or internal (through an internal opening and confined to body cavities). Reducible hernias are defined as those in which the affected tissue can be returned to its correct site without surgical manipulation, while irreducible (or incarcerated) hernias are those in which the affected tissue cannot be returned to its anatomic site without surgical manipulation. Strangulated hernias are incarcerated hernias in which the process of herniation has produced vascular compromise of the herniated tissue. Common types of hernias include inguinal (direct and indirect), femoral, umbilical, epigastric, and incisional.

I. **Signs and symptoms.** The typical emergency department presentation is that of the patient who seeks evaluation of a mass. These patients typically have reducible hernias and merely require education regarding their problem and surgical referral.

II. **Treatment.** If the hernia is not easily reducible, adequate sedation and analgesia should be obtained through the judicious use of narcotics and anxiolytics. While awaiting the onset of medication effects, local cooling measures should be applied to reduce blood flow and edema. Inguinal and femoral hernias should then be placed in 20 to 30 degrees of Trendelenburg. Gentle, continuous pressure on the herniated tissue, directed back toward the site of herniation will then usually reduce these hernias. Incarcerated hernias that are chronically incarcerated and nonpainful may be referred for elective repair, while those in which the incarceration is acute require inpatient admission for reduction and surgical repair. Patients with strangulated hernias are usually ill appearing, with peritonitis, fever, and a leukocytosis with a left shift. Attempts at reduction are contraindicated, and immediate surgical consultation is required. Rapid replacement of intravascular volume deficits and administration of broad-spectrum antibiotics to cover bowel flora should be initiated. Blood for blood cultures, complete blood cell count, chemistry profile, and type and crossmatch should be obtained when intravascular access is achieved. Nasogastric suction is indicated if obstruction is present, and supplemental oxygen should be administered.

Suggested Readings

Corcetti JP, Avran DA: Acute pancreatitis. In Panzer RJ, Black ER, Griner PF, editors: *Diagnostic strategies for common medical problems,* Philadelphia, 1991, American College of Physicians.

Knight LC, Lesser THJ: Fish bones in the throat. *Arch Emerg Med* 6:13, 1989.

Panzer RJ: Complications of acute pancreatitis. In Panzer RJ, Black ER, Griner PF, editors: *Diagnostic strategies for common medical problems,* Philadelphia, 1991, American College of Physicians.

Ranson JHC: Etiologic and prognostic factors in human pancreatitis: a review. *Am J Gastroenterol* 77:663, 1982.

Ranson JHC, Rifkind KM, Roses DF, et al: Prognostic signs and the role of operative management in acute pancreatitis. *Surg Gynecol Obstet* 138:69, 1974.

Webb WR, Koutras P, Ecker RR, et al: An evaluation of steroids and antibiotics in caustic burns of the esophagus. *Ann Thorac Surg* 9:95-102, 1970.

11

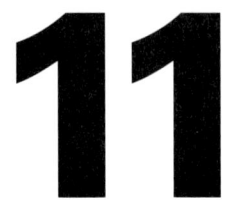

Acute Food-Related and Toxic Plant Emergencies

George R. Schwartz, M.D., F.A.C.E.P.

This chapter will focus on three aspects of food-related factors in emergency medicine: malnutrition and vitamin deficiency, food toxicities (e.g., sulfites, monosodium glutamate [MSG]), and food poisoning by exotoxin and bacterial infection. These latter groups may rapidly cause severe electrolyte disorders and dehydration, which place excessive strain on the reduced physiologic reserve and can cause serious morbidity or death.

Malnutrition and Vitamin Deficiency Syndromes

Symptoms that may result from vitamin deficiency are frequently ascribed to other causes. Malabsorption, poor dentition, hypochlorhydria, and decreased intestinal secretions further tend to reduce absorption. Drugs and/or medications may also interact with nutrients.

I. **Elderly population.** Malnutrition is widespread among the elderly population. As the mean age of the elderly population increases, these problems will tend to increase, despite some simple partial solutions (e.g., dental work, hearing aids, visual aids). Many of our elderly, either living independently or in institutions, are in states of malnutrition.

II. **Symptoms and signs.** It is well known that severe chronic malnutrition is accompanied by marked physical and psychologic changes: apathy, emotional instability, retardation, memory impairment, and even psychotic illness.

  A. **When deficiency syndromes do arise,** replacement of a single vitamin is inadequate since we are dealing with problems with the entire diet (including, usually, protein and trace minerals) as well as possible other problems already mentioned (e.g., malabsorption, poor dentition, depression, medications, alcoholism).

  B. **The symptoms and signs** in **Table 11-1** represent "full-blown" syndromes. These conditions do not suddenly appear. Instead, there is a slow and insidious progression, although severe stress or infection may rapidly precipitate some signs or symptoms. Profound deficiencies may also occur in patients maintained for a considerable time on intravenous fluids particularly after surgery for a gastrointestinal disorder.

  C. **Many chronic conditions** (e.g., Wernicke's encephalopathy, dementia) will not respond well to dietary change since the physiologic failure has given way to permanent anatomic change through deterioration and cell death. Similarly, chronic calcium deficiency in the elderly can lead to widespread osteoporosis and, although not easily reversed, treatment should certainly begin with calcium and estrogens as needed for women.

  D. **Despite the resistance of some symptoms,** others may clear rapidly when the deficiency is corrected. For example, the confabulation and disorienta-

Table 11-1. Signs and Symptoms of Vitamin and Nutritional Deficiency

Protein-Calorie Malnutrition
Pallor
Fatigue
Coldness
Inanition
Contractures
Anemia
Impaired immunity
Hypoproteinemia and edema
Hypotension
Autonomic nervous system hyporesponsiveness
Organ wasting (including heart)

Niacin Deficiency
Dermatitis*
Mental confusion
Gastrointestinal disturbance (e.g., pancreatic disorders)
Depression
Lethargy
Diarrhea
Weight loss

B$_{12}$ Deficiency
Anemia (macrocytic)
Myelopathy
Peripheral neuropathy
Optic atrophy
Impaired vibration sense
Ataxia
Footdrop
Fatigue, difficulty concentrating
Exaggerated deep tendon reflexes
Paresis, paresthesias
Limb pain, cramps
Disorientation and mental confusion
Depression
Memory impairment

Thiamine Deficiency
Peripheral neuropathy
Paresthesias
Weakness, muscle tenderness
Mental confusion
Memory changes
Beriberi heart disease (severe cardiac failure)
Wernicke's encephalopathy
Footdrop, wristdrop
Decreased deep tendon reflexes
Pulmonary and peripheral edema

Ascorbic Acid Deficiency
Petechial hemorrhage
Follicular hyperkeratosis
Aching limbs
Bleeding or swollen gums
Joint effusions, hemorrhages
Dyspnea
Edema
Neuropathy
Depression
Confusion
Ocular hemorrhages
Coiled hairs, hair loss
Dry eyes
Abdominal colic

Folic Acid Deficiency
Macrocytic anemia
Diarrhea
History of chronic medication (anticonvulsant use)
Anorexia
Irritability
Confusion
Dementia
Depression

*Hyperkeratotic hyperpigmentation on backs of hands, elbows, and neck.

tion of Korsakoff's psychosis may respond to thiamine within hours. Ocular abnormalities are present in over 90% of cases (nystagmus, sixth nerve palsies, sluggish pupils) and will similarly respond very rapidly, although nystagmus may be permanent. The emotional abnormalities (anxiety, insomnia, later depression, some psychosis) usually respond well. Ataxia, on the other hand,

Table 11-2. Vitamin A, D, and E Syndromes

Hypovitaminosis A

Symptoms:
  Associated with malabsorption, diarrhea, gastroenteritis, or protein deficiency with infection
  Night blindness
  Conjunctival xerosis
  Corneal xerosis, ulcers
  Keratomalacia (leading to blindness)

Treatment:
  If eye lesions are occurring, treatment is urgent. An intramuscular injection of 100,000 units of water-miscible vitamin A will rapidly restore vitamin A levels. Oral supplementation is adequate in most cases. Oil-based vitamin A should not be given parenterally.

Hypervitaminosis A

Symptoms:
  Headache
  Malaise, anorexia
  Vomiting
  Pleural effusion, ascites
  Possible papilledema in adults
  Alopecia
  Weight loss
  Dermatitis
  Skeletal pain
  Liver enlargement, cirrhosis

Laboratory findings:
  Elevated vitamin A levels
  Hypercalcemia
  Abnormal liver function tests
  Bone resorption on x-ray in chronic cases

Treatment:
  Simply eliminating the excessive vitamin is usually satisfactory. However, with hypercalcemia, normal saline intravenously over several days is effective.

Vitamin D Deficiency

May be associated with decreased intake or can be related to anticonvulsant medications (e.g., hydantoins, barbiturates)

Symptoms:
  Bone pain
  Hyperparathyroidism
  Senile osteomalacia and fractures
  Muscle weakness

Laboratory findings:
  Low-serum vitamin D level (<10 ng/mL), hypoparathyroidism, hypocalcemia

---

takes a month or two for maximum resolution, and one fourth to one half of the patients will have ongoing balance difficulties. The confusion states take weeks to clear, and some memory loss remains unless treatment is started immediately after a short illness.

Table 11-2. Vitamin A, D, and E Syndromes—cont'd

Vitamin D Intoxication
Symptoms:
  Metastatic calcification
  Hypercalcemia
  Renal insufficiency
  Anorexia
  Anemia
  Dermatitis
Laboratory findings:
  Elevated serum calcium, increased calcium in urine
  Serum vitamin D elevated (usually above 50 ng/mL)
  X-ray evidence of periosteal thickening or metastatic calcification
  Urine may show proteinuria
  ECG may show arrhythmias
Treatment:
  Fluids, saline diuresis
  Stop vitamin D intake
  Treat severe hypercalcemia with calcitonin or mithramycin
  Cholestryamine orally (8 g b.i.d.) may aid in decreasing hypercalcemia*

Vitamin E Excess
Long-term excess can cause:
  Nausea
  Vomiting, gastrointestinal upset
  Weakness and fatigue
  Creatinuria
  Visual blurring
Evaluation:
  Blood levels (normal 0.5 to 2.0 mg/dL)
Treatment:
  Simple discontinuance†

*See Jibani M and Hodges NH: Prolonged hypercalcemia after industrial exposure to vitamin D, *Br Med J* 290:748, 1985, for more information.
†See Bierie JG, Corash C, and Hubbard US: Medical uses of vitamin E, *N Engl J Med* 308:1063, 1983, for more information.

E. **Excess.** While the water-soluble vitamins will rarely cause problems in excess, marked abnormalities have occurred from excess vitamins A and D. **Table 11-2** illustrates the vitamin A, D, and E syndromes of deficiency and excess. Some older people might take, or their guardians might provide, an excessive amount of vitamins in a well-meaning attempt to strengthen bones or increase vision.

Food Poisoning

I. **Elderly.** Food poisoning assumes much greater importance in the elderly since dehydration and electrolyte imbalance, which are caused by profuse diarrhea or a period of intense vomiting, can more easily precipitate a lethal arrhythmia or cause mental changes, confusion, and severe hypotension in older patients, as well as leading to renal failure. High mortality rates underscore the need to admit elderly patients with infectious colitis into the hospital since these diseases are far more serious in such patients. The so-called "benign self-limiting" food poisoning can be lethal in the already physiologically compromised elderly patient.

II. **Etiology.** "Food poisoning" following the ingestion of certain foods has multiple etiologies.

   A. **Bacterial toxins.** It may be caused by bacterial toxins that are ingested preformed or that are elaborated in the intestine by bacteria contaminating the particular food. For example, the ingestion of food (such as salads, ham and other cold meat products, and cream-filled desserts) contaminated with enterotoxin is responsible for staphylococcal food poisoning. Botulism, staphylococcal food poisoning, cholera *(Vibrio cholerae),* and food poisoning from *Clostridium perfringens* and *Bacillus cereus* are considered true intoxications, since clinical illness is produced in each case by a toxin.

   B. **Infection.** Food poisoning may also be caused by a direct *infection* or invasion of the intestine by bacteria, as classically occurs in *Salmonella* food poisoning following ingestion of contaminated food—particularly poultry, milk and dairy products, egg products, and water. Other causes of food poisoning by direct bacterial infection include shigellosis (bacillary dysentery), *Campylobacter fetus* (enteritis), *Streptococcus faecalis,* and *Yersinia enterocolitica.*

   C. *E. coli* produces gastroenteritis both by elaboration of an enterotoxin, as the cause of *E. coli* "traveler's diarrhea," and by direct bacterial invasion. Furthermore, in certain bacterial infections, it is unclear whether the acute gastrointestinal symptoms are caused by toxin or by direct infection, as with *Vibrio parahaemolyticus.*

   D. **Viruses and protozoa.** Food poisoning may also be caused by viruses and protozoa, such as *Entamoeba histolytica,* the etiologic agent in amebiasis, and *Giardia lamblia.* Food poisoning produced by marine organisms, plants, and mushrooms is discussed later in this chapter. Food poisoning may also occur from toxic contaminants (PCBs, heavy metals, radioactivity), from natural toxic substances (e.g., akee fruit), or from toxic substances added to foods (e.g., MSG or sulfites).

Botulism

Botulism is a serious disease caused by the toxin elaborated by the spore-forming anaerobic bacillus *Clostridium botulinum.* The toxin is generally conceded to be the most poisonous substance yet discovered. As an example of its toxicity, as few as 950 molecules of toxin can be lethal for white mice, and the amount of toxin that can cause human death has been estimated to be between 0.1 and 1 μm of toxin. The toxins are good antigens, but natural immunity in people rarely occurs because the lethal dose is less than that needed to elicit antibody production. Botulism is considered to be a rare disease, and outbreaks must be reported to the Centers for Disease Control (CDC) in Atlanta, Georgia.

I. **Outbreaks.** From 1899 to 1977, 766 outbreaks involving 1,961 cases were reported in the United States. There were 99 deaths. The Canadian experience from 1919 through 1973 was reported by Dolman. He found 62 authenticated outbreaks involving 181 persons, with 83 deaths. The incidence of fatality has been substantially reduced over the past two decades from greater than 60% to less than 20%. This reduction is primarily because of better respiratory care of victims, though it is possible that milder cases are being recognized. Prompt administration of antitoxin is probably also a factor.

II. **There is good reason to suspect that botulism is far more common than is generally realized and is underdiagnosed, particularly in the elderly.** The diagnosis is difficult to make, particularly in isolated cases. One analysis of eight cases of botulism caused by contaminated smoked fish showed that the attending physicians failed to reach the diagnosis initially in each instance. An outbreak of botulism occurred in New Mexico in 1978, and more than half the affected group were not correctly diagnosed initially in the emergency department. Since death may occur rapidly from respiratory paralysis, cases unassociated with a large outbreak are likely to be unrecognized, especially in older people with preexistent disease. The mode of death appears natural. Conversely, since there is a range of disease—from very mild (associated with only a slight headache and perhaps some malaise and nausea) to lethal—very mild weakness may never come to medical attention.

III. **Mode of toxin action.** The action of the toxin prevents the release of the neurotransmitter acetylcholine at the neuromuscular and other cholinergic junctions. The C. botulinum toxin is protein in nature, and there are at least seven immunologically distinct types. In human beings, almost all disease results from the types identified as type A, type B, and type E, though there have been recent reports of a type F. It is impossible to determine in the acute situation the type of toxin involved in a case of botulism. As a result, the initial treatment requires use of a trivalent (A, B, and E) antiserum, which will be described in more detail in the section on treatment.

IV. **Geographic considerations.** Despite the difficulty in differentiating toxin type, some epidemiologic information is of interest and might perhaps have increasing relevance in the future. Of the outbreaks reported in the United States, approximately 40% were tested for type of toxin; 26% were type A, 7.8% were type B, and 4.2% were type E. Although outbreaks were reported from 44 states, 5 states (California, Oregon, Washington, Colorado, and New Mexico) accounted for more than half the cases. This may relate to the altitude, particularly in Colorado and New Mexico. A large part of these two states has an altitude greater than 5,000 feet, with a resultant reduction in the temperature at which water boils. At 5,000 feet, water boils at approximately 95° C (203° F)—as compared with 100° C (212° F) at sea level. Any chef can tell you this difference is important in food preparation. At 10,000 feet, water boils at about 90° C (194° F). Temperature makes a substantial difference when it comes to killing spores of *C. botulinum* in foods. A large-scale test demonstrated that type A and type B spores can be totally destroyed by boiling for 6.5 hours at 100° C. At 95° C, the time required for killing spores is doubled (13 hours). Using a pressure cooker can make a substantial difference. Heating to 120° C (248° F) resulted in spore death within 3 minutes. Although spores are resistant to heat, toxin is readily inactivated by heat. Boiling for 5 minutes, even at high altitude, ensures destruction of the toxin. More than 90% of reported botulism outbreaks caused by type A occurred west of the Mississippi River. Two thirds of the reported type B outbreaks occurred in eastern states. Most of the type E outbreaks in the United States occurred in Alaska or in the Great Lakes region. No type A or type B has been reported from Alaska.

V. **Types of food implicated**
   A. **Home-processed foods.** Botulism is much more likely to result from home-processed foods—particularly those that are smoked, pickled, or home-canned—than from commercially processed foods. Despite the

widely publicized outbreaks that have resulted from commercially prepared foods, of 766 outbreaks in the United States over a 78-year period, only 66 could be traced to commercial foods.* Home-canned vegetables (e.g., tomatoes, beans) have been frequently implicated. If the pH of the food is lower than 4.5, toxin formation is unlikely though there have been some reports of toxin production from pickled herring kept at a pH of 4 to 4.2. Cases have been reported from smoked fish, ham, and other meats. The word botulism actually arises from the Latin *botulus,* which means sausage. In Alaska, a recent outbreak involved stored beaver tail and beaver flippers. The incidence of botulism appears to be higher among Eskimos because of their storage method and ingestion of uncooked seal and whale meat.

B. Spoilage of the food may be obvious, but relying on gross signs is inadequate because of the lethality of very small amounts of the toxin. Although toxin-containing foods are the principal cause of the clinical syndrome of botulism, wound botulism has been reported in association with soil-contaminated deep wounds suitable for growth of the anaerobic *C. botulinum.*

VI. Clinical signs and course. The following facts have been noted concerning botulism outbreaks:

A. In many outbreaks, initial cases are incorrectly diagnosed as flu, viral syndrome, or stroke. Early recognition and diagnosis are most difficult. It is important to note that in neither of the preceding cases was the correct diagnosis made on initial physician contact.

B. Symptoms usually appear within the first 24 hours but may be delayed as long as 48 hours or even longer than 72 hours. My experience with a local outbreak exhibited a range of 8 to 80 hours for patients to develop initial symptoms.

C. Earliest symptoms involve vague malaise, headache, weakness, dizziness, blurred vision, and sometimes dry mouth.†

D. Progression is variable, but, most commonly, initial symptoms appear, and in severe cases, progression over the subsequent 6 to 8 hours leads to respiratory paralysis. Of 34 cases studied locally, 11 required mechanical ventilation. Botulism can be mild; symptoms may rarely progress beyond nausea and mild visual problems, or perhaps fatigue. Mild cases usually clear in 1 week.

E. An important early symptom is blurring of vision. Patients usually do not complain of classic diplopia. Instead, they say, "Everything is blurred," or "I can't get the image into focus," or "My eyes are tired or wandering."

F. Progression of more severe cases includes increasing problems with vision, slurred speech, dryness of mouth, diffuse weakness, difficulty in swallowing, and difficulty in walking, usually described as "staggering." The rapidity of the course is highly individual over a 24-hour period. Most significantly, the sensorium and intellectual functioning remain intact, and memory is not impaired. The neurologic symptoms are usually bilateral and symmetric and are motor, not sensory. The cerebrospinal fluid is normal.

---

*The CDC reports have been confusing in this statistic. In a report by a CDC representative in 1969, the statement appears that "since 1910 . . . only a few outbreaks have been ascribed to commercially prepared foods." In a 1977 report, the figure is given of 66 such outbreaks. This seems larger than "a few." No definitions of "commercially prepared foods" are given that might account for this apparent difference.

†In the largest series of botulism patients from a single outbreak (in Michigan, 1977), dry mouth was found in all those affected, and 86% had difficulty with focusing or diplopia. This outbreak was type B in origin.

G. Nausea and vomiting may occur, but large studies have demonstrated that in only 30 to 40% of cases of botulism were nausea and vomiting prominent. With detailed questioning, nausea was found as a symptom in 60 to 70% of patients. In contrast, visual difficulty was reported in more than 90% of the patients. Constipation and urinary disturbance were found in less than 50% of the patients. The visual disturbance results from abducens nerve palsy.

H. More severe cases show early third cranial nerve involvement. Pupils may become fixed and dilated.

I. *As a general rule, the earlier the onset, the more severe the case.*

VII. Clinical differentiation. Early cases are difficult to diagnose as are mild cases that do not progress. No laboratory test can readily be used to diagnose botulism in the emergency department. Common conditions that figure in the differential diagnosis include Guillain-Barré syndrome, cardiovascular accident or transient ischemic attack, tick paralysis, heavy metal poisoning (particularly lead), psychiatric conditions, drug abuse, alcohol intoxication, or untoward reaction to medication—anticholinergic type, myasthenia gravis, phenytoin toxicity, atropine poisoning, encephalitis, carbon monoxide poisoning, electrolyte abnormalities, and amyotrophic lateral sclerosis.

A. Diagnosis rests on clinical grounds. Confirmation comes from observing botulism in a mouse (sensitive to 900 molecules) that has been injected with toxin from the patient's serum or with the suspected food. It is worthwhile to test for toxin even weeks after the onset of clinical illness because of the high sensitivity of the mouse to the toxin as well as the reports of circulating toxin even 2 weeks after onset. *C. botulinum* and toxin also may be identified in the patient's feces.

B. Put all specimens in *leak-proof* containers, and remember that the *C. botulinum* toxin is the most powerful toxin known. In case of a spill, neutralize the specimens with a strong alkaline solution if available. Suitable specimens may include serum, stool, vomitus, food samples, food containers, or wound material. The specimens should be refrigerated. Label carefully! Include, in particular, any drugs the patient is taking. Call the CDC for further information.

VIII. Medical treatment

A. Immediate care. Immediate attention must be given to airway and respiratory function. When deaths occur initially, they almost always result from respiratory paralysis. Careful gastric lavage should be performed. Emesis can be initiated if there is a good gag reflex. In addition, charcoal should be instilled through the tube after emesis and lavage. A cathartic is unlikely to be helpful but can be used and may speed the flow of the charcoal. Similarly, colonic enemas can be used. If there is **difficulty with breathing** and arterial blood gases and if vital capacity deteriorates or initially shows hypoxia, hypercapnia, or a measurement of less than 100 mL, a tracheostomy should be considered. Certainly, with borderline cases, a trial of ventilatory assistance can be instituted prior to any surgical procedure. In the large 1977 Michigan outbreak of type B botulism, the presence of ptosis, dilated and sluggishly reacting pupils, and paresis of the medial recti was associated with the need for artificial ventilatory support in 8 of 11 patients. These aspects of third nerve dysfunction became apparent after approximately 12 hours. Tracheostomy is best performed as a slow, careful procedure under ideal conditions, since a ventilator may be necessary for months.

B. Antitoxin therapy. Trivalent antitoxin is available from the CDC and should be administered to all patients with suspected botulism. Each vial of equine antiserum contains 7,500 IU of type A, 5,500 IU of type B, and 8,500 IU of type E antitoxins. One to two vials are administered intravenously initially and again in 4 hours. One vial of antiserum may be given intramuscularly in 24 hours; repeated injections may be indicated, depending on the clinical condition. Desensitization may be necessary because the antitoxin is a horse serum derivative. In cases of known reactions to horse serum, 100 mg of hydrocortisone can be injected prior to the use of antiserum. Allergic reactions can be treated with antihistamines or steroids, or both. Of 30 patients in the 1978 New Mexico outbreak who received antitoxin, one developed serum sickness.

C. Penicillin. Penicillin is indicated in the management of patients with wound botulism, because this form of botulism is caused by active infection with *C. botulinum*. Since botulinum food poisoning is usually caused by toxin and not by the organism, penicillin probably serves no role in management of these patients; however, it is often used on an empiric basis and may occasionally treat a *C. botulinum* intestinal infection. Penicillin therapy is usually continued for 1 week.

D. Guanidine hydrochloride. Guanidine hydrochloride has been used experimentally to chemically compete with the toxin. No dramatic results have been observed with guanidine, and its use is no longer routinely recommended.

E. Respiratory function. Continued meticulous maintenance of respiratory function is a most important aspect of treatment. A patient's improvement is best followed by a periodic assessment of vital capacity and arterial blood gases *off* ventilatory support. In cases of preexisting pulmonary disease, the baseline state may require estimation.

F. Hospitalization. In severe cases, patients may be hospitalized for as long as 3 to 6 months. Weaning from the ventilator may be difficult. With long-term hospitalization, release from the hospital must follow a graded rehabilitation program. Muscle wasting, lack of conditioning, orthostatic hypotension, and syncope frequently follow prolonged bed rest and muscle inactivity. There may be some minor dysphagia or malaise 6 to 12 months after the onset of illness.

Food Poisoning Caused by Microorganisms

I. *Shigellosis*. The *Shigella* species are aerobic, gram-negative, nonmotile bacteria. There are four main species, all of which can cause human disease. Asymptomatic carriers are common.

A. When bacillary dysentery occurs, the cause can be the ingestion of as few as 200 organisms. If a "suboptimal" number of bacteria are ingested, or if there is some immunity, an individual can have a subclinical infection or a nonsymptomatic carrier state. The range of clinical illness is very broad. Although the condition is found more often in the tropics, it is endemic throughout the world. Epidemics have been traced to a variety of foods con-

Symptoms and Signs of Shigella Poisoning

1. Severe diarrhea: mucous, blood stools
2. Abdominal colic and tenderness
3. Tenesmus
4. Fever to 40° C (104° F) and malaise
5. Pain often relieved by defecation
6. Bowel sounds active and high pitched
7. Possible syncope and hypotension with *Shigella dysenteriae;* if this species is responsible for the illness, it usually is more severe
8. Outpouring of polymorphonucleocytes into the intestines and stool; sometimes sheets of white blood cells can be seen microscopically
9. Rise in fever and white blood cell count
10. Hypotension and circulatory collapse (more common in the elderly)

taminated by feces, but, most commonly, milk, eggs, and dairy products are implicated.

B. The incubation period is usually about 48 hours; however, it may be as short as 8 hours, or symptoms can be postponed for a week. It appears that there is some small intestinal colonization, but the large intestine is the preferred area. Bacterial growth depends on factors of immunity and existing flora, as well as the number of *Shigella* organisms. Usually, within 1 week after recovery, the organism is not found in the feces. Occasionally, sequelae are reported, including neuropathy, arthritis, and skin eruptions. Sepsis in the acute stage is rare, but serious.

C. Diagnosis. Table 11-3 shows a differential diagnosis of shigellosis with a comparison of amebic dysentery. The following features are helpful in diagnosis:
   1. Stool culture
   2. A rise in serum agglutinin titer in 50% of the cases—however, not useful in diagnosis or treatment because of the delay
   3. White blood cell count usually greater than 10,000 with a left shift

D. Treatment. For management of shigellosis, give supportive treatment by preventing dehydration and maintaining electrolytes. The diarrheal condition is usually self-limited. However, shock with dehydration and acidosis may occur, requiring intensive treatment.
   1. **Antibiotics** are useful in moderate to severe cases for shortening the clinical course. Treatment regimens consist of (1) ciprofloxacin, 500 mg orally twice a day for 3 to 5 days; or (2) ampicillin (susceptible strains), 500 mg orally four times a day for 3 to 5 days; or (3) trimethoprim/sulfamethoxazole (SMX), one double-strength tablet orally twice a day for 3 to 5 days.
   2. **Antidiarrheal agents** (e.g., diphenoxylate hydrochloride and atropine [Lomotil], paregoric, or opiates) must be used cautiously because they may prolong the clinical course. Nonproductive tenesmus would be the best indication for using such agents.
   3. **For amebic colitis,** antimicrobial therapy is needed—usually metronidazole followed in 1 week by diiodohydroxyquin (to eradicate cysts). (See **Table 11-3 and 11-4.**)

Table 11-3. Acute Differentiation of Shigellosis from Amebic Dysentery in Elderly Patients*

Amebic dysentery	Shigella
Usually slower in progression with mild to moderate diarrhea	Rapid onset with severe explosive diarrhea with cramps and tenesmus
Temperature usually less than 101° F	Temperature usually more than 101.5° F (though hypothermia may be present)
Usually moderate symptoms that tend to wax and wane (only rarely presenting with a fulminant course with explosive diarrhea)	Rapid dehydration can lead to hypotension and shock (which is the reason for the estimated 10 to 20% mortality rate in the elderly)
Blood in stool on microscopic examination	Gross blood in stool
Fecal smear shows mononuclear cells and trophozoites	Fecal smear shows many leukocytes
Other systemic manifestations outside of the gastrointestinal tract (e.g., amebic liver abscesses, lung abscesses, central nervous system [CNS] symptoms, intestinal perforation, peritonitis)	Some systemic manifestations (e.g., meningitis, pyelonephritis, and osteomyelitis) have been reported but are rare. Other manifestations—e.g., arthritis or Reiter's syndrome—occur days to weeks after the acute syndrome. Abdominal pain is common, however.

*A therapeutic trial with antibiotics is necessary if shigellosis is suspected since the mortality is so much higher in the elderly.

Table 11-4. Antimicrobial Therapy for Food-Related Gastroenteritis

Shigellosis
Ciprofloxacin, 500 mg PO BID for 3-5 days; or
Ampicillin (susceptible strains) 500 mg PO QID × 3-5 days; or
Trimethoprim/SMX double-strength tablet PO BID × 3-5 days.

Salmonellosis
Ceftriaxone, 1-2 gm IV q12 h × 14 days; or
Ciprofloxacin, 500 mg PO BID × 14 days; or
Trimethoprim/SMX double-strength tablet PO BID × 14 days; or
Ampicillin, 2 gm IV q6h × 14 days; or
Chloramphenicol, 500-1000 mg IV q6h × 14 days.

Enteropathic *E. coli* (Traveler's Diarrhea)
Ciprofloxacin, 500 mg PO BID × 5-10 days; or
Trimethoprim/SMX double-strength tablet PO BID × 5-7 days.

Vibrio cholerae
Tetracycline, 500 mg PO QID × 5-7 days; or
Ciprofloxacin, 500 mg PO BID × 5-7 days.

Campylobacter enteritis
Ciprofloxacin, 500 mg PO BID × 5-10 days; or
Erythromycin, 250 mg PO QID × 5-10 days.

Antibiotic-Associated Pseudomembranous Colitis
(Clostridium difficile)
Metronidazole, 250 mg PO or IV QID × 10-14 days; or
Vancomycin, 125 mg PO QID × 10 days (500 PO QID × 10-14 days if recurrent).

Giardia lamblia
Quinacrine HCl, 100 mg PO TID × 5 days; or
Metronidazole, 250 mg PO TID × 7 days.

Entamoeba histolytica **(Amebiasis)**
Asymptomatic cyst carrier
  Iodoquinol, 650 mg PO TID × 20 days; or
  Paramomycin, 25-30 mg/kg/day in 3 doses × 7 days; or
  Diloxanide sulfate, 500 mg PO TID × 10 days.
Mild to moderate intestinal disease
  Metronidazole, 750 mg PO TID × 10 days; or
  Tinidazole, 2 gm/day PO × 3 days followed by:
    Iodoquinol, 650 mg PO TID × 20 days or
    Paromomycin, 25-30 mg/kg/day PO in 3 divided doses × 7 days.
Severe intestinal disease
  Metronidazole, 750 mg PO TID × 10 days; or
  Tinidazole, 600 mg PO BID × 5 days followed by:
    Iodoquinol, 650 mg PO TID × 20 days or
    Paromomycin, 25-30 mg/kg/day PO in 3 divided doses × 7 days.

II. ***Salmonellosis.*** The salmonellae, named for Dr. Salmon who described them in 1885, are gram-negative motile bacteria. The most common form of salmonella-induced human disease is the syndrome of *Salmonella* gastroenteritis. The range of gastroenteritis can be mild to severe, with the latter being associated with abdominal pain, colitis, and signs of a systemic inflammation (fever, elevated white blood cell count, malaise, and so on).

A. Typhoid fever is caused by *Salmonella typhosa* and differs from the common gastroenteritis primarily by its severity, prolonged course, and hematogenous dissemination of the bacillus with accompanying diffuse manifestations. A persistent carrier state can result.

B. **The primary reservoir is the vertebrate intestine,** and the passage is from person to person by fecal contamination of foodstuffs. Most commonly, meat, poultry, dairy, and egg products have been implicated. However, other items, including creamy foods and prepared salads, have been implicated. Sterilization of contaminated foods is not always achieved by cooking, especially in large stuffed turkeys and in cooked eggs. The disease may also be transmitted by pets, since salmonellae can cause disease in animals. Dogs, cats, birds, and turtles have been commonly implicated.

1. **Growth medium.** To produce clinical disease in humans, at least 100,000 to 1 million bacteria of the nontyphoid salmonellae are usually required. To achieve these levels, a growth medium (i.e., food) is necessary, because simple contamination usually does not involve transfer of so many organisms. Subsequently, intestinal multiplication occurs. The need for a "minimum dose" makes direct fecal-oral transmission uncommon and in the United States water-borne transmission is uncommon because of over-all water sanitation.

2. **The clinical disease results from an infection.** There appears to be no production of toxin. Thus, prevention must focus on overall sanitation and identification of asymptomatic carriers. Prevention is important not only in terms of human comfort but also in view of studies that have demonstrated that salmonellosis costs at least $500 to $1,000 per case for diagnosis, treatment, and follow-up, and unquestionably more in the elderly.

3. **Antacids.** Because *Salmonella* bacteria are killed at a pH level of 2, the use of an antacid may increase susceptibility, as will conditions of reduced stomach acidity (including subtotal gastrectomy, vagotomy, and gastroenterostomy). It was noted that mortality was higher also in *E. coli* colitis in those who had achlorhydria.

C. *Salmonella* **gastroenteritis is a reportable infectious disease.** Estimates have been made that the incidence reported by the CDC (10 cases per 100,000 population) represents one tenth to one hundredth of the actual incidence. The incidence is highest in the summer.

D. **Increased intercountry tourism,** as well as intercountry trade involving foods, has resulted in increased risks of acquiring *Salmonella* gastroenteritis. There are more than 2,500 species of *Salmonella,* some of which are found in one country and not in another. Mass tourism tends to make a more uniform distribution (one of the aspects of a "world community"). The largest outbreak of *Salmonella* food poisoning in recorded history occurred in the United States in March, 1985. This situation demonstrates the impact of large companies with wide food distribution. More than 14,000 cases were reported (almost all confirmed) with at least four associated deaths. The source was a large dairy, and contaminated low-fat milk was the vehicle for transmission of the *Salmonella typhimurium.* Lawsuits involving at least $100 million have been filed.

E. **Increase.** Some epidemiologists believe *Salmonella* infections are increasing, in part, because of the widespread use of antibiotics in animal feed and the development of drug-resistant bacteria. These can be passed widely by contaminated beef or chicken.

Food Poisoning Caused by Microorganisms 325

Symptoms and Course of Salmonella Poisoning

1. General incubation period is 8 to 48 hours.
2. Complaints of general malaise, headache, mild abdominal pain, and fever of 37.78° to 38.33° C (100° to 101° F) are common initially.
3. Despite some nausea and vomiting that may occur, major symptoms are cramps and diarrhea; tenesmus is common and may help in diagnosis.
4. Rarely, bloody diarrhea is present; shigellosis and amebic dysentery are more often associated with bloody stools.
5. Occasionally, abdominal symptoms are so severe as to suggest appendicitis or some other acute intraabdominal process.

F. Although most acute symptoms subside within 2 to 5 days, occasionally a prolonged course of weeks occurs. Death from *Salmonella* gastroenteritis is uncommon and occurs primarily in infants and the aged and persons with severe underlying disease.

G. Gastroenteritis vs. typhoid fever. Although arbitrary divisions have been made between "gastroenteritis" and the systemic disease "typhoid fever," the division may not be clinically clear-cut. *Salmonella* bacteria other than *S. typhosa* (the cause of typhoid fever) may produce gastrointestinal symptoms, as well as sustained fever, and even positive blood cultures. In addition, it is possible to be infected by *Salmonella* bacteria and have few gastrointestinal signs and symptoms but manifest chills, fever, anorexia, and even some hepatosplenomegaly. Spiking fever, headache, abdominal cramps, and rose spots on the torso are useful diagnostically.

H. The presence of bacteremia may result in a localized internal abscess, and even endocarditis, septic arthritis, or osteomyelitis can occur. Such severe infections usually show striking signs and a marked leukocytosis, though in typhoid fever leukopenia occurs after the first 1 to 2 weeks. The elderly are much more susceptible to endocarditis due to preexisting valvular disease.

I. Diagnosis. Diagnosis and differentiation from shigellosis, enterotoxic *E. coli,* and amebic dysentery may be difficult. Often less common causes of acute diarrheal disease, such as that produced by *Vibrio parahaemolyticus* or viral agents, can also cause difficulty in diagnosis.

  1. Clinically, definitive diagnosis rests on isolation of the organism from the stool. If the contaminated food is available, it can be cultured. Excretions from pets can be tested as well if they appear to be possible sources.

  2. A fecal smear may show inflammatory leukocytes but, usually, somewhat less than with shigellosis and amebic dysentery. Bloody diarrhea is uncommon in *Salmonella* enterocolitis.

  3. Blood cultures. If there are systemic signs, blood cultures may show bacteremia. Although immunologic tests of various titers may show increases, the time delays usually render such tests of limited value.

J. Treatment. The cornerstone of treatment is prompt correction of dehydration and fluid and electrolyte imbalances. Intravenous fluids are often necessary, depending on clinical symptoms.

  1. Antimotility agents (e.g., Lomotil and similar agents) that inhibit activity of the bowel substantially may also increase the severity of the disease. Experimental animals pretreated with antimotility agents showed increased susceptibility to *Salmonella* infection. If symptoms are severe and no contraindications are present, a low dose of morphine or atropine can be used to partially relieve symptoms.

2. **In cases of limited *Salmonella* gastroenteritis,** the use of antibiotics does not appear to be generally helpful. In fact, there is some evidence that the excretion of the organism occurs for a longer period of time after antibiotics have been used.

3. **Antibiotics.** If the patient shows high fever, chills, or other evidence of severe systemic infection, antibiotics are indicated. Treatment regimens consist of (1) ceftriaxone, 1 to 2 gm intravenously every 12 hours for 14 days; or (2) ciprofloxacin, 500 mg orally twice a day for 14 days; or (3) trimethoprim/SMX, one double-strength tablet orally twice a day for 14 days; or (4) ampicillin, 2 gm intravenously every 6 hours for 14 days; or (5) chloramphenicol, 500 to 1000 mg intravenously every 6 hours for 14 days. The course of antibiotics is for 10 days to 2 weeks. In cases in which there is evidence of an abscess, endocarditis, osteomyelitis, or other evidence of persistent internal infection, antibiotics may have to be continued for 4 to 6 weeks, and surgical drainage may be needed.

III. Enteropathic *E. coli* (traveler's diarrhea)

A. **Method of acquisition.** Dairy and meat products or contaminated water are common vehicles for infection. There is some suggestive evidence that bismuth salicylate may be effective prophylactic therapy against traveler's diarrhea (30 to 60 mL every 4 hours). However, this may increase susceptibility to other forms of food poisoning. In addition, other prepared foods (salads, sauces) may harbor bacteria from fecal contamination. A general rule is to eat cooked foods shortly after preparation and to wash and peel raw fruits and vegetables thoroughly.

B. **Symptoms and course of illness.** Acute diarrhea may begin 8 to 12 hours after ingestion of contaminated food or water, though there may be a delayed onset of up to several days. Common symptoms include abdominal cramps, tenesmus, and profuse watery diarrhea, though there is a wide range of clinical illness.

1. **There appear to be two types of *E. coli*** associated with food poisoning. One type does not produce a toxin, and symptoms result from intestinal infection. The other type is more commonly associated with the epidemic diarrhea of travelers, and this type does produce an enterotoxin. In the latter type, symptoms result from infection as well as from the effect of the toxin upon the colon. In general, *E. coli* produces a clinical disease that is usually milder than *Salmonella* disease or shigellosis, but in severe cases it may be indistinguishable from them. In fact, one strain of *E. coli* can cause severe hemorrhagic colitis and produce a toxin similar to one produced by *Shigella dysenteriae*. This is the type associated with high institutional mortality, e.g., in nursing homes.

2. ***E. coli* is of particular concern in the aged,** who have limited tolerance to an electrolyte imbalance because of their overall condition, an underlying illness, or the taking of medications that can affect electrolytes (e.g., diuretics).

C. **Diagnosis.** Diagnosis may be possible by isolating the organism in food or water and by culturing a stool. Serologic diagnosis through testing for rises in titer against *E. coli* can be done, but such tests are not readily available. Smear of stool is important. Polymorphonucleocytes can be present, though

usually less than with shigellosis. Bloody diarrhea is also less common, but has been associated with severe outbreaks.
  D. **Treatment.** Supportive treatments are generally satisfactory for mild cases. Moderate to severe cases require antibiotic treatment and intensive fluid and electrolyte stabilization. The disease generally lasts in its acute form for only 2 or 3 days. However, nonspecific symptoms and malaise usually continue for at least 1 week. **Doxycycline** (100 mg orally per day) has shown a demonstrable benefit when used prophylactically. Treatment regimens consist of (1) ciprofloxacin, 500 mg orally twice a day for 5 to 10 days; or (2) trimethoprim/SMX, one double-strength tablet orally twice a day for 5 to 7 days. Bactrim (trimethoprim-sulfamethoxazole) has also been used successfully. In the usual case, however, the disease is treated effectively with clear liquids and intravenous fluids if the diarrhea is severe enough to produce dehydration or electrolyte imbalance. The over 80 age group is at much higher risk, and must be hospitalized for aggressive treatment.
  E. **Other causes of traveler's diarrhea.** While *E. coli* is the most common cause, traveler's diarrhea may also be caused by other microorganisms including rotavirus (up to 10% of cases), *Salmonella* or *Shigella* (15 to 20%), and parasites (0 to 5%). Rotavirus infection is generally self-limiting.
    1. ***G. lamblia*** infection generally occurs days to weeks after the exposure and is characterized by foul-smelling, watery stools. A stool smear and culture will help in diagnosing this parasite. This condition is usually not severe, but it occasionally requires treatment with metronidazole (250 mg 3 times daily for 5 days). Quinacrine may also be used.
    2. ***E. histolytica*** is a parasite that invades the mucous membranes of the intestines, resulting in ulcerations, hemorrhage, and diarrhea. In severe cases, the parasite may cause perforation of the intestines or may invade other organs, particularly the liver or lung. Diagnosis rests on physical examination, stool examination, and possible liver function tests and liver scan. Treatment of confirmed cases is mandatory and should include metronidazole and iodoquinol.
IV. ***C. perfringens* conditions.** *C. perfringens* is a nonmotile, gram-positive, spore-forming rod. Disease is caused by growth of bacteria and toxin formation. It is now considered to be one of the most common types of food poisoning.
  A. **Method of acquisition.** Meat and poultry products are commonly implicated, as are gravies and creamy (dairy or mayonnaise-containing) foods.
  B. **Symptoms and course of illness.** Because large numbers of organisms (usually greater than 10^6 organisms per gram) are generally necessary to cause significant disease, most food poisoning resulting from *C. perfringens* is relatively mild. The incubation period is more than 8 hours and usually less than 24 hours. The disease is associated with cramps and diarrhea. Diarrhea is generally not as profuse as that found with *Shigella, Salmonella,* or *E. coli;* characteristically, it is not bloody. There may be mild nausea, but vomiting is uncommon.
  C. **Diagnosis.** Diagnosis is made by detection of the organism in food and stool.
  D. **Treatment.** Symptomatic therapy is generally all that is required.
V. ***B. cereus* conditions.** *B. cereus* is a slightly curved gram-positive rod found singly and in chains. The organism is motile. Disease arises from infection and some toxin production.

A. Method of acquisition. Food, particularly meat, dairy, and poultry products, has been discovered to be contaminated with this organism. Dried foods (e.g., mixes, potatoes) may be contaminated. Growth does not ordinarily occur until hydration.

B. Symptoms and course of illness. Average incubation period is 8 to 12 hours. Average duration of illness is approximately 24 hours. Symptoms in order of magnitude are diarrhea, abdominal cramps, nausea, and vomiting. Fever is generally absent or is below 37.78° C (100° F).

C. Treatment. Supportive therapy with intravenous fluids is usually sufficient even for relatively severe cases. Antinauseants may be given. There is no evidence that antibiotics are of value.

VI. Cholera. Cholera is caused by *V. cholerae,* a curved, motile, gram-negative rod. This condition is included because it can be rapidly fatal. Fortunately, however, it is rare in the United States at this time. During worldwide cholera pandemics, the United States has had many cases (e.g., 150,000 deaths in 1832 and 1849 and 50,000 deaths in 1866). In the United States, cholera is still endemic along the Gulf Coast with cases being reported particularly from Texas and Louisiana, where association with contaminated water and seafood has been found. While uncommon, this disease poses a great threat to the elderly due to the massive, rapid fluid-electrolyte shifts.

A. Method of acquisition. In the epidemic form, the *Vibrio* organisms are usually water-borne or come from seafood. Person-to-person transmission is usually in the nonepidemic form. Occasionally, it may come from a restaurant in which a worker is infected. Food can also become contaminated, particularly when "night soil" (human excrement) is used as a fertilizer.

B. Symptoms and course of illness. The illness develops usually within 8 to 48 hours after ingestion. With it comes a severe enteritis associated with passage of copious amounts of non-foul-smelling diarrhea usually containing mucus and occasionally blood. The disease arises in association with an exotoxin that causes a severe disorder of the intestinal tract and results in marked intestinal secretions. Frequently, the first stool is more than 1,000 mL with a characteristic appearance of "rice water." The symptoms arise directly from the gastrointestinal fluid and electrolyte losses. Prostration and a shocklike state may occur rapidly. The patient may die within 12 to 24 hours if intravenous fluids or oral electrolytes are not provided. The illness characteristically lasts 1 to 7 days. With adequate fluid and electrolyte repletion, recovery is rapid. Hypokalemia is a particular problem in those older people taking diuretics.

C. Diagnosis. Clinical suspicion of cholera is important, particularly in endemic or epidemic areas. Persons with decreased stomach acidity (because of surgical operations and antacids) are at higher risk. Also, those with type O blood are at higher risk for unknown reasons. The organism may be identified by culture, and one may look for the organisms on a Gram stain slide. At medical centers familiar with cholera, a fluorescent antibody technique may identify the organism positively within 1 hour.

D. Treatment. The patient in a shock state must be treated with intravenous fluids. Oral fluids may be used when intravenous fluids are not available. A glucose-containing electrolyte solution may be given orally.

1. Generally, acidosis, severe potassium losses, and dehydration occur. Those experienced in treating cholera use weight as a measure of de-

hydration and consider the case to be severe if there is greater than a 10% body weight loss and mild if the loss is less than 5%.
2. **In severely ill patients,** the use of tetracycline has caused a highly significant reduction in total stool volume and duration of diarrhea and has resulted in a more rapid disappearance of the organism from the stool. The dose administered should be approximately 1 g of tetracycline by mouth initially, then at least 500 mg every 6 hours for a total of 3 days. Treatment regimens consist of (1) tetracycline, 500 mg orally four times a day for 5 to 7 days; or (2) ciprofloxacin, 500 mg orally twice a day for 5 to 7 days. The usual stool composition per liter in adults is sodium (135 mEq), potassium (15 mEq), bicarbonate (45 mEq), and chloride (100 mEq).
3. **Cholera may be prevented** by cooking all foods thoroughly, boiling water, and immunization, which seems to offer up to 75% protection for up to 18 months. Even when clinical disease develops, cholera appears to be less severe in the vaccinated patient.

VII. *Campylobacter enteritis*
   A. **Method of acquisition.** Raw milk most frequently has been implicated in the transmission of *Campylobacter* enteritis.
   B. **Diagnosis.** Diagnosis rests on isolating the organism *(Campylobacter fetus* subspecies *jejuni)* from a fecal specimen. **The common symptoms** include diarrhea (in more than 90%), abdominal pain (in more than 80%), frequently with fever, headache, nausea, or vomiting. Bloody diarrhea is less common, but blood in the stool is present in about one fourth of cases.
   C. **Treatment.** Treatment is supportive but must include identifying and stopping the offending food. In elderly patients, this ordinarily benign, self-limiting condition may develop into a severe illness. When symptoms are severe and dehydration is a concern, treatment regimens for *campylobacter* enteritis consist of (1) ciprofloxacin, 500 mg orally twice a day for 5 to 10 days; or (2) erythromycin, 250 mg orally four times a day for 5 to 10 days.

VIII. *Listeriosis.* Caused by the gram-positive bacillus *Listeria monocytogenes,* listeriosis can result in septicemia and meningitis as well as focal infectious symptoms. Milk and cheese products have been increasingly involved in its spread throughout the population. There is an increased susceptibility in immunocompromised patients. Ampicillin is usually the antibiotic of choice in treatment. Recent outbreaks (1985) may indicate an increasing problem.

IX. *Staphylococcal* **food poisoning.** Enterotoxic staphylococci are found widely on the skin and mucous membranes of many individuals. Most staphylococci (a gram-positive, clustered coccus) cannot elaborate this particular toxin.
   A. **When foodstuffs are contaminated,** a lack of refrigeration and a warm environment are ideal conditions for bacterial growth and toxin elaboration. Foods usually implicated are those with a high fat content such as creamy cakes, custards, creamed soups, mayonnaise, and so on. However, cases resulting from meat products have also been reported. Milk has been rarely implicated. The ideal food as a culture medium is pancake batter, which has a pH close to 7, a high moisture content, and is frequently left without refrigeration for hours. Also beware of turkey stuffing and the "too-beautiful" cooked and dressed turkey too large to fit into a refrigerator and handled by many persons during its preparation.
      1. **Staphylococcal food poisoning is common.** The toxin is preformed and is remarkably "heat stable." Therefore, even if food is subsequently

cooked, a period of hours is necessary for toxin destruction. In fact, in one test, autoclaving for 15 minutes did not result in substantial reduction in potency.
2. **There are at least four different types of toxin,** but all may be elaborated by the same organism and, with minor variation, all have the same unfortunate effect.

B. Symptoms and course of illness. Symptoms usually begin within ½ hour to 6 hours after ingestion and may begin slowly or violently. Severe nausea and vomiting are common. The affected individual vomits repeatedly, then has dry heaves and may even vomit blood—probably representing a vomiting-induced Mallory-Weiss syndrome. After vomiting, abdominal cramps may become severe and diarrhea may develop. However, the diarrhea is usually relatively mild, and the individual scarcely notices this symptom.
1. **Patients appear markedly "gray" and severely ill.** Severe dehydration can result, and intravenous therapy must be started. Although the acute stage usually lasts less than 12 hours, many patients complain of severe nausea and malaise for 1 to 2 days. Hospitalization is often needed.
2. **Milder cases** do occur and may not be diagnosed as staphylococcal food poisoning unless a careful history is taken.
3. **Initial studies** were conducted with paid volunteers. Despite increased pay, few, if any, said they would volunteer again. Thus, current studies are done with primates, but monkeys are far less susceptible than humans. Toxin is not formed in appreciable amounts below 12.78° C (55° F) or above 48.89° C (120° F). If the food is acidic, toxin is produced very slowly, depending on temperature and acidity. If there is contaminated food with a pH of 7, or greater than 30% moisture content, appreciable amounts of toxin are produced in 4½ hours at 32.22° C (90° F). Given the same food, but changing the temperature, the same amount of toxin was produced in 10 hours at 18.33° C (65° F) and in 9 hours at 46.11° C (115° F). *Thus, the conclusion is that to prevent staphylococcal food poisoning, "keep it hot, keep it cold, or eat it within 2 hours."* Frequently, institutions such as nursing homes must prepare large quantities of food in advance, increasing the risk.
4. **Simple diagnosis** can be made by a Gram stain of the suspected food, which will show abundant staphylococci if contaminated (although this, of course, is not a test for the toxin). A culture can verify type, but the time period necessary for culturing renders the findings primarily of scholarly interest.

C. Treatment. To manage a staphylococcal food poisoning, give intravenous fluids. To prevent retching, use 10 mg compazine intramuscularly. Also, propantheline bromide, 15 mg or 30 mg intramuscularly, is effective. Medications that reduce stomach acid secretion are also useful such as H_2 blockers (e.g., cimetidine or ranitidine). Monitor electrolytes and urine output.
1. **Fatalities** have been reported because of mineral imbalance and dehydration. In the elderly, the severe retching may worsen existing heart disease, and myocardial infarction has been reported.

2. **No antibiotics.** Since the disease is caused by a preformed toxin, antibiotics are of no value. No suitable antitoxin is available for routine use.
3. **Physicians should document** their findings carefully since many restaurant outbreaks result in legal action.
4. **Duration.** Although the acute stage generally is over within 2 days, weakness and malaise can often last for weeks.

Trichinosis

The worm *Trichinella spiralis* enters the body through pork or other meat that has been inadequately cooked. For many reasons, the United States does not routinely inspect for trichinosis, although an enzyme assay being developed will allow such testing in the future—a necessity for exporting pork to many countries.

Trichinosis in humans causes weakness, swelling, and muscle pain along with general malaise and a low-grade fever. The duration of the acute illness is usually 3 weeks, although chronic indolent cases have been reported as well as rapidly developing cases leading to death.

According to the CDC, only 60 cases were reported in 1984. Autopsy studies have demonstrated that up to 4% of Americans harbor *Trichinella* worms in their muscles. Thus, very few cases are actually diagnosed. Symptoms are usually ascribed to "flu." The condition is rarely progressive. More often, the worms become encapsulated and do not cause later clinical disease. The risk of having trichinosis increases with age.

Shellfish-Associated Food Poisoning

Shellfish may be associated with typhoid fever, hepatitis, cholera, *Campylobacter* gastroenteritis, *V. parahaemolyticus* infection, and viral gastroenteritis. Of the latter type, the most common cause at this time appears to be the Norwalk virus. One study demonstrated widespread outbreaks of clam- and oyster-associated gastroenteritis with the Norwalk virus implicated as the cause.

Of 103 outbreaks affecting 1,017 persons in New York State, the most common symptoms were diarrhea (84%), nausea (52%), abdominal cramps (58%), and vomiting (30%). Illness lasted only 48 hours in most people but up to a week in a minority. There is no specific treatment. The elderly are the group at highest risk for serious morbidity and mortality from shellfish ingestion. Cooking thoroughly reduces the risk and steaming for at least 4 to 6 minutes after the shell opens will reduce the number of cases dramatically. Elderly people should be advised to have their shellfish "well done."

Food Additives

There are well over a thousand food additives generally recognized as safe (GRAS), most of which are benign. Certain substances may trigger reactions in sensitive people. For example, sulfites are commonly added to fruit and vegetable salads and to potatoes to prevent darkening. Acute attacks of asthma have been triggered by such substances.*
Another substance that is widely used is MSG, which acts as a flavor enhancer. Depending on dosage, many people will develop tingling, flushing, diaphoresis, nausea,

---

*Because of their dangers, sulfites were removed from the "GRAS" list for use in restaurants and salad bars in August of 1985.

vomiting, or headache. Some more sensitive individuals respond with behavioral changes including anger and depression. Asthma, chest pain, arrhythmias, balance difficulties, and diarrhea are also common symptoms.

The subject of additives is generally beyond the scope of emergency medicine unless reactions occur that bring people to emergency facilities.

However, when outbreaks of food poisoning or food reactions occur, the emergency facility is often in the best position to detect early "epidemics." It is prudent then to be in touch with the CDC through their reports and the state health department. When there are occasional toxicities (e.g., heavy metal contamination, polychlorinated biphenyls [PCBs]), special testing can be initiated in the emergency department.

Food Poisoning Caused by Chemicals Naturally Present in Foods and Plants

As has been previously discussed, the difference between what is therapeutic and what is toxic may be just a question of dosage. Foods are composed of many chemical substances that are essential for life, such as carbohydrates, proteins, minerals, and vitamins. However, many foods contain chemical substances that are part of their nature but that do not appear to be involved in nutritional processes. In many cases, the chemicals exert modest effects, and even ingestion of large quantities will not exert apparent toxic effects.

I. **Examples.** For example, lettuce contains the chemical lactucin, which exerts sedative effects when it is concentrated. Another example is spinach, which has a high oxalic acid content; however, even with larger ingestions, which might produce feelings of malaise and bloating, a spinach overdose would only rarely present as a clinical problem. Conversely, there are common foods that can cause severe poisoning because of their being underripe, because too much has been eaten, or because the patient has been taking a pharmacologic agent that interacts in some way with a chemical or chemicals in a food. For example, the "vomiting sickness" of Jamaica has been traced to eating the unripe akee fruit. The toxic substance has been termed "hypolycin" because it acts to rapidly lower blood sugar.

   A. **The common potato plant** ordinarily has leaves that contain belladonna-type actions. When some potatoes are unripe, belladonna poisoning can occur. In fact, deaths have been linked to eating potatoes. Even recently there have been outbreaks. Dr. Mary McMillan and Dr. S.C. Thompson reported on 78 cases of potato poisoning in 1979. Symptoms included severe circulatory impairment in three who needed hospitalization.

   B. **Occasionally, outbreaks can also occur from glands** of animals inadvertently allowed to remain in the food. For example, one large outbreak of thyrotoxicosis occurred among residents of southwestern Minnesota and adjacent areas of South Dakota and Iowa. The cause was ground beef prepared from neck trimmings containing large amounts of bovine thyroid hormone. Of these 121 cases, almost 25% were in patients over age 60.

   C. **Alcohol** is an example of toxicity of a common food in which overdosage may be lethal. However, there are many more. Severe toxicity with sympathomimetic effects can come from an overdose of nutmeg because of the content of myristin, and a prized fish of Japan called "fugu" contains a toxin that exerts cholinergic effects. Overdose can cause cholinergic poisoning.

D. Tyramine. As an example of food-drug interactions, the presence of tyramine in aged cheese, pickled herring, Chianti wine, and some other aged foods can cause hypertensive crises in patients who are taking monoamine oxidase inhibitors for treatment of depression.

II. Plant poisonings. The number of plants that can exert toxic actions is vast. For purposes of emergency treatment, it is useful to identify the major type of chemical actions caused by the poisoning. **Table 11-5** identifies common plants and their chemical actions. **Table 11-6** offers symptoms and signs associated with plant intoxications, and **Table 11-7** was prepared by the Food and Drug Administration (FDA) to alert health professionals and consumers to some herbal remedies that can be dangerous.

III. Mushroom poisoning. Although the *Psilocybe* mushroom has gained notoriety, and poisoning from ingestion of these mushrooms can induce severe vomiting, abdominal cramps, and marked hallucinations, the poisoning is relatively benign because of a large tolerance of the body to psilocybin. The mushroom *Amanita muscaria* has also been eaten for its hallucinatory effects, and the Vikings were said to have consumed them prior to going into battle because of the rage-like reaction induced. With overdose, muscarine causes parasympathomimetic symptoms that occur usually within 30 minutes after ingestion and cause profuse salivation, lacrimation, bradycardia, and other cholinergic responses. Treatment involves atropine, which can be given at a dose of 0.5 to 1 mg intramuscularly or intravenously (when symptoms warrant). This dose can be repeated every 30 minutes.

A. Important questions in the assessment of mushroom poisoning are the following:

1. When were the mushrooms eaten? When did symptoms appear (time course)? Rationale: Symptoms that begin immediately or within the first hour usually herald a relatively minor poisoning. Emesis, charcoal, and a cathartic should be used. Delayed symptoms are characteristic of the amatoxin-containing mushrooms. The nature of the symptoms may indicate seriousness of the ingestion (e.g., hallucinations, muscarinic effects, sweating, delirium).
2. How many mushrooms were eaten? What types were they? Rationale: If different types were ingested, it is difficult to arrive at identification by symptoms. In addition, of course, there is a dose-related effect.
3. Did anyone who ate the mushrooms not get sick? Rationale: People often blame mushrooms because of the widespread awareness of their toxicity, whereas another food poisoning or virus might be the cause of symptoms.
4. Did the patient consume alcoholic beverages? Rationale: Some mushrooms have a disulfiram-type effect with added alcohol. As with Antabuse, there can be extreme nausea, vomiting, and headache.

B. The most severe mushroom poisoning comes from those containing peptide toxins (phallotoxins or amatoxins). They can be deadly at low doses. Symptoms may be delayed several hours to as long as 24 hours after ingestion. Severe abdominal pain, diarrhea, and vomiting are present. Amatoxins cause liver, brain, and renal tubule cell injury, which may lead to death. Early treatment consists of the following:

1. Supportive treatment, with monitoring of vital signs and urine output. Renal failure may occur. Urine output must remain high. Early diuresis may be necessary.
2. Large doses of steroids have been used empirically.

Table 11-5. Chemical Actions of Some Poisonous Plants*

Digitalis-like; Cardiotoxic
Foxglove
Oleander
Lily-of-the-valley

Atropine-like; Anticholinergic
Jimsonweed
Larkspur
Nightshade
Tomato and potato leaves, green potatoes
Mandrake
Henbane

Sympathomimetic; Pressors
Ephedra (Mormon's tea)
Mistletoe
Nutmeg

LSD-hallucinogenic Effects
Yohimbe
Morning glory seeds

Parasympathetic (Cholinergic)
Poinsettia

Strychninelike
Hemlock (conium fruit)
Water hemlock (cicutoxin)

Nicotine Effects
Wild tobacco
Tree tobacco
Indian tobacco
Cultivated tobacco made into tea

*Sometimes used in herbal teas and prescribed by folk healers for symptoms in the elderly.

---

3. Hemodialysis or peritoneal dialysis should be used early, when available, because of the small molecular size of the peptide toxins. Dialysis may have substantial benefit if used early.
4. Penicillin, chloramphenicol, and sulfamethoxazole have been used in animals to decrease binding of the toxin to albumin. This might be of value if dialysis is used subsequently. Also, thioctic acid (50 to 150 mg every 6 hours) has been used in Europe but has not been well tested.

C. If severe poisoning has occurred, all these measures should be instituted as early as possible, along with activated charcoal and catharsis. The characteristic course has been divided into three stages: 1) the first 24 hours (acute symptoms), 2) some remission (24 to 36 hours), and 3) severe stage (with clinical liver damage, renal failure, and seizures), which can lead to death in up to 80% of cases.

D. A specimen of the ingested mushroom can prove valuable in identification. For quick emergency department testing, rub some of the mushroom cap over newsprint and allow to dry. A drop of concentrated hydrochloric acid is applied to the paper. A bluish-green color indicates amatoxins. The mushroom should then be sent for chemical analysis. A negative "newsprint" test does not mean that amatoxins may not be present. Only a positive test is useful.

Table 11-6. Signs and Symptoms of Common and/or Serious Plant Intoxications*

	Dieffenbachia/Philodendron	Colchicum/Gloriosa	Euphorbia/Hippomane	Actaea/Anemone/Ranunculus	Convallaria/Digitalis/Nerium	Aconitum	Solanum	Pieris/Rhododendron/Veratrum	Conium/Laburnum/Nicotiana/Sophora	Cicuta	Taxus	Gelsemium	Brugmansia/Datura	Amaryllis/Narcissus/Wisteria	Ilex	Abrus/Ricinus	Prunus	Phytolacca	Podophyllum	Karwinskia
Mouth and Throat																				
Burning/irritation	++	++	D	++	+	+	D	+	+											
Increased salivation	+		D	++		+			+	+										
Dry mouth											D	+	++							
Dysphonia/dysphagia		+		D			±				+	+	+							
Gastrointestinal Tract																				
Nausea		+			+	±		D	+	+				+	+	DD				
Vomiting		+	+		+	±	D	D	+	±	D			++	++	DD	D	++	+	
Diarrhea		++	+		+		D	D	+					±	±	DD		D	+	
Abdominal pain		++	++		+			D			D			+			D	+		
Decreased bowel sounds									+				++						±	
Cardiovascular																				
Tachycardia					+								+							
Bradycardia					±			++			D									
Arrhythmias					++	++					D									
Conduction defects					++															

Continued on next page

Ch 11. Acute Food-Related and Toxic Plant Emergencies

Cardiovascular, cont'd																			
Hypertension														+					
Hypotension	+																		
Nervous and Neuromuscular																			
Dizziness			±					++			D								
Weakness/lethargy					+			+			+	+							
Syncope			±		+						D						D		
Delirium/psychosis			±											+					
Tremors/convulsions			±					D±				±					D±	±	
Depression/coma								D			D						D±		
Headache								+						+					
Paresthesias				±	++			D											
Muscle weakness/paralysis	±							D			+	+					D±	±	DD
Visual																			
Mydriasis					+						+	+		+					
Visual disturbances					+			D			+								
Cutaneous								+				+					D		
Increased sweating													++						
Dry skin											D	++							
Flushing/rash											D	+							
Cyanosis																	D±		
Miscellaneous																			
Hyperthermia	+					+						+							
Painful/bloody micturition	+																		

*Key: + = Commonly occurs; ++ = pronounced or persistent; ± = occasionally reported; D = delayed onset; DD = occurs significantly.

Table 11-7. Common Dangerous Herbal Remedies

Botanical name of plant source	Common names	Remarks
Arnica montana L.	Arnica; arnica flowers; wolfsbane; leopard's bane; mountain tobacco; flores arnicae	Aqueous and alcoholic extracts of the plant contain choline, plus two unidentified substances that affect the heart and vascular systems. Arnica, an active irritant, can produce violent toxic gastroenteritis, nervous disturbances, change in pulse rate, intense muscular weakness, collapse, and death.
Atropa belladonna L.	Belladonna; deadly nightshade	Poisonous plant that contains the toxic solanaceous alkaloids hyoscyamine, atropine, and hyoscine.
Solanum dulcamara L.	Bittersweet twigs; dulcamara; bittersweet; woody nightshade; climbing nightshade	Poisonous. Contains the toxic glycoalkaloid solanine; also solanidine and dulcamarin.
Sanguinaria canadensis L.	Bloodroot; sanguinaria; red puccoon	Contains the poisonous alkaloid sanguinarine and other alkaloids.
Cytisus scoparius L.	Broom-top; scoparius; spartium; Scotch broom; Irish broom; broom	Contains toxic sparteine, isosparteine, and other alkaloids; also hydroxytyramine.
Aesculus hippocastanum L.	Buckeye; aesculus; horse chestnut	Contains a toxic coumarin glucoside, aesculin (esculin). A poisonous plant.
Acorus calamus L.	Calamus; sweet flag; sweet root; sweet cane; sweet cinnamon	Oil of calamus, Jammu variety, is a carcinogen (causes cancer). FDA regulations prohibit marketing of calamus as a food or food additive.
Heliotropium europaeum L.	Heliotrope	A poisonous plant. It contains alkaloids that produce liver damage. Not to be confused with garden heliotrope (*Valeriana officinalis* L.).

Continued on next page

Table 11-7. Common Dangerous Herbal Remedies—cont'd

Botanical name of plant source	Common names	Remarks
Conium maculatum L.	Hemlock; conium; poison hemlock; spotted hemlock; spotted parsley; St. Bennet's herb; spotted cowbane; fool's parsley	Contains the poisonous alkaloid conine and four other closely related alkaloids. Often confused with water hemlock (*Cicuta maculata* L.). Not to be confused with the conifer hemlock, hemlock spruce, etc. (*Tsuga canadensis* L. Carr.).
Hyoscyamus niger L.	Henbane; hyoscyamus; black henbane; hog's bean; poison tobacco; devil's eye	Contains the alkaloids hyoscyamine, hyoscine (scopolamine), and atropine. A poisonous plant.
Exagonium purga (Wenderoth) Bentham. *Ipomoea jalapa* Nutt. and Coxe. *Ipomoea purga* (Wenderoth) Hanye. *Exagonium jalapa* (Wenderoth) Baillon.	Jalap root; jalap; true jalap; jalapa; Vera Cruz jalap; high John root	A large twining vine of Mexico, this plant has undergone many name changes. The drug is a powerful, drastic cathartic. Purgative powers of jalap reside in its resin. In overdoses, jalap may produce dangerous hypercatharsis.
Datura stamonium L.	Jimsonweed; datura; stamonium; apple of Peru; Jamestown weed; thornapple; tolguacha	Contains the alkaloids atropine, hyoscyamine, and scopolamine. Illegal drug for nonprescription use. A poisonous plant.
Convallaria majalis L.	Lily of the valley; convallaria; may lily	Contains the toxic cardiac glycosides convallatoxin, convallarin, and convalamarin. Poisonous plant.
Lobelia inflata L.	Lobelia; Indian tobacco; wild tobacco; asthma weed; emetic weed	A poisonous plant that contains the alkaloid lobeline plus a number of other pyridine alkaloids. Overdoses of the plant or extracts of the leaves or fruits produce vomiting, sweating, pain, paralysis, depressed temperatures, rapid but feeble pulse, collapse, coma, and death.

Table 11-7. Common Dangerous Herbal Remedies—cont'd

Botanical name of plant source	Common names	Remarks
Mandragora officinarum L.	Mandrake; mandragora; European mandrake	The plant is a poisonous narcotic similar in its properties to belladonna. Contains the alkaloids hyoscyamine, scopolamine, and mandragorine.
Podophyllum peltatum L.	Mandrake; May apple; podophyllum; American mandrake; devil's apple; umbrella plant; vegetable mercury	A poisonous plant, it contains podophyllotoxin, a complex polycyclic substance, and other constituents.
Phoradendron flavescens (Pursh.) Nutt. *Viscum flavescens* (Pursh.)	Mistletoe; viscum; American mistletoe	Poisonous. Contains the toxic pressor amines β-phenylethylamine and tyramine.
Phoradendron juniperinum Engelm.	Mistletoe; viscum; juniper mistletoe	May be poisonous. Little is known about its properties.
Viscum album L.	Mistletoe; viscum; European mistletoe	Poisonous. Contains the toxic pressor amines β-phenylethylamine and tyramine.
Ipomoea purpurea (L.) Roth.	Morning glory	Contains a purgative resin. In addition, morning glory seeds contain amides of lysergic acid but with a potency much less than that of LSD.
Vinca major L. and *Vinca minor* L.	Periwinkle; greater periwinkle; lesser periwinkle	Contains pharmacologically active, toxic alkaloids such as vinblastine and vincristine that have cytotoxic and neurologic actions and can injure the liver and kidneys.
Hypericum perforatum L.	St. Johnswort; hypericum; klamath weed; goatweed	A primary photosensitizer for cattle, sheep, horses, and goats. Contains hypericin, a fluorescent pigment, as a photosensitizing substance.
Euonymus europaea L.	Spindle-tree	Violent purgative.

Continued on next page

Table 11-7. Common Dangerous Herbal Remedies—cont'd

Botanical name of plant source	Common names	Remarks
Dipteryx odorata (Aubl.) Willd. *Coumarouna odorata* (Aubl.) *Dipteryx oppositifolia* (Aubl.) Willd. *Coumarouna oppositifolia* (Aubl.)	Tonka bean; tonco bean; tonquin bean	Active constituent of seed is coumarin. Dietary feeding of coumarin to rats and dogs causes extensive liver damage, growth retardation, and testicular atrophy. FDA regulations prohibit marketing of coumarin as a food or food additive.
Euonymus atropurpurea Jacq.	Wahoo bark; euonymus; burning bush; wahoo	The poisonous principle has not been completely identified. Laxative.
Eupatorium rugosum Houtt. *E. ageratoides* L.f. and *E. urticaefolium*	White snakeroot (also called snakeroot, righweed)	Poisonous plant. Contains a toxic, unsaturated alcohol called *tremetol* combined with a resin acid. Causes "trembles" in cattle and other livestock. Milk sickness is produced in humans by ingestion of milk, butter, and possibly meat from animals poisoned by this plant.
Artemisia absinthium L.	Wormwood; absinthium; absinth; absinthe; madderwort; wermuth; mugwort; mingwort; warmot; magenkraut; harba absinthii	Contains a volatile oil (oil of wormwood) that is an active narcotic poison. Oil of wormwood is used to flavor *absinthe*, an alcoholic liqueur illegal in this country because its use can damage the nervous system and cause mental deterioration.
Corynanthe yohimbe Schum. *Pausinystalia yohimbe* (Schum.) Pierre	Yohimbe; yohimbi	Contains the toxic alkaloid yohimbine (quebrachine) and other alkaloids.

Prepared by the Food and Drug Administration, Washington, D.C.

Miscellaneous Food Poisoning

Table 11-8 summarizes some other food poisonings and their treatment.

Anaphylaxis

I. **Symptoms and signs.** Food-mediated anaphylaxis can result from ingestion of shrimp, peanuts, fish, and many other comestibles. The clinical response to ingested antigens, much like the reaction to a drug or physical stimulus, may range from a local hive to the systemic inflammatory cascade associated with anaphylaxis. Once exposed to an inciting antigen or stimulus, most patients will develop signs and symptoms of anaphylaxis within 30 to 60 minutes. Less commonly, patients will not manifest symptoms after several hours. The majority of patients follow a uniphasic course, i.e., they develop signs and symptoms of anaphylaxis, recover with appropriate therapy, and remain asymptomatic.

Biphasic reactions, which occur in 20 percent of patients, are characterized by a second wave of signs and symptoms seen with the first episode that recur 4 to 8 hours after the initial remission of anaphylaxis. A smaller percentage will rebound at 24 to 48 hours, and in a few patients anaphylaxis will be continuous and protracted, lasting as long as 24 to 48 hours. There are no tests or clinical features that help distinguish among patients at risk for a biphasic or protracted response.

A. **Complications.** Whatever the clinical course, the leading causes of death from anaphylaxis are airway obstruction and intractable hypotension. Although it has been widely held that the rapidity of symptom onset predicts reaction severity, this correlation has not been confirmed in a recent controlled trial. However, the severity of a reaction is increased by several factors: quantity of antigen, the route and rapidity of administration (intravenous or intramuscular exposure posing a much greater risk than oral administration), patients with a history of asthma or cardiac disease, and patients using beta-adrenergic blockers. Patients with a history of atopy are not at increased risk of anaphylaxis or increased severity of reaction.

B. **Manifestations.** Ninety percent of patients with anaphylaxis will have manifestations of a cutaneous response, which can include pruritis, urticaria or angioedema. In addition, patients often feel anxious or may have a sense of impending doom. Tachycardia and tachypnea may be present, and nearly all patients are afebrile. Blood pressure response varies depending on the severity of the reaction and may be normal, slightly elevated, or low. Patients may experience perioral tingling, hoarseness, dyspnea, change in voice, or stridor, all of which are signs of upper airway involvement.

Lower airway signs and symptoms include wheezing, cough, and chest tightness. Cardiovascular involvement is suggested by the presence of hypotension, arrhythmias, syncope, chest pain, and shock. Because of histamine effects on gut smooth muscle contraction, gastrointestinal symptoms such as nausea, vomiting, diarrhea, colicky abdominal pain, cramping, and bloating may be encountered. Gynecologic and genitourinary manifestations of anaphylaxis include uterine cramping, bleeding, and urinary incontinence secondary to visceral smooth muscle contraction. Finally, dizziness, confusion, and seizures may reflect neurologic involvement, which usually reflects cere-

Table 11-8. Other Food Poisonings and Their Treatments*

Name	Food involved	Symptoms/signs	Treatment
Chinese restaurant syndrome (MSG syndrome)	Monosodium glutamate	Flushing, diaphoresis, weakness, headaches, pruritus, hypotension, depression, lethargy, arrhythmias, asthma, balance difficulties, vomiting	No specific treatment; IV fluids as needed
Cyanide poisoning	Pits from apricots, cherries, cassava, unripe millet, bitter almonds	Metabolic poisoning, loss of consciousness, cyanosis, convulsions	Amyl nitrite, oxygen
Cycad poisoning	Cycad starch and leaves (eaten in Philippines, Malay)	Neurologic symptoms, weakness, paresthesias	No specific treatment
Diascorism	Toxic yam with diascorine	Convulsions, deaths have occurred	Anticonvulsants
Ergotism	Grain with ergot fungus	Hypertension, vasoconstriction, CNS symptoms	Vasodilation by amyl nitrite inhalation or papaverine infusion
Favism	Fava bean	Glucose-6-phosphate dehydrogenase deficiency (inherited) produces hemolysis, severe anemia	Supportive: monitor urinary output, transfusions as needed; deferoxamine may arrest hemolysis
Fish poisoning (ichthyosarcotoxism) (ciguatera toxin)	Ciguatera (sea bass, snapper, barracuda)	Fish usually good as food contains a toxin that causes weakness, paresthesia, GI symptoms, hypotension, and, in fatal cases, respiratory paralysis (probably formed due to ingestion of dinoflagellate by the fish)	Gastric lavage, respiratory support as needed; charcoal

Table 11-8. Other Food Poisonings and Their Treatments*—cont'd

Name	Food involved	Symptoms/signs	Treatment
Fish poisoning, cont'd	Puffer fish	Far Eastern fish contains a neurotoxin that can cause paralysis (tetrodotoxin) and death	
	Tuna, mackerel, mahi mahi, (scromboid)	Bacteria act on histidine in flesh, producing a toxin with GI symptoms; headache and allergic manifestation (histamine-like)	Antihistamines, cimetidine, supportive and symptomatic treatment
Hemagglutination	Castor bean, partially cooked bean flakes, kidney bean flour, legume seeds	Nausea, vomiting, respiratory impairment, anemia; deaths reported from castor beans	No specific treatment
Lathyrism	Some beans, peas	Muscular weakness, partial paralysis, spinal cord impairments	No specific treatment
Licorice poisoning	Licorice	Weakness, myopathy, hypokalemia	IV treatment for fluid-electrolyte imbalance
Paralytic shellfish poisoning	Mussels and clams, usually along Pacific coast June to October—associated with "red tides"	Paresthesias, neurologic symptoms, respiratory paralysis	Supportive, particular attention to respiratory function
Sulfite sensitivity	Added to foods as antioxidant, found in mixes, wines	Asthma, urticaria	Bronchodilators
Tartrazine (Yellow dye #5) sensitivity	Orange-yellow colored foods	Urticaria, asthma, anaphylaxis	Supportive and symptomatic

*Of the food poisonings listed, the fish and shellfish contain poisons generally not present in a dangerous amount (the puffer fish is an exception). Ergotism is due to a fungus contaminant. In contrast, yam poisoning, cyanide poisoning, hemagglutination reaction, cycad poisoning, lathyrism, and favism result from chemicals that are natural constituents of the foods.

bral hypoperfusion or hypoxemia secondary to cardiovascular instability and/or respiratory compromise.

II. **Diagnosis.** Because there are no timely, pathognomonic laboratory tests associated with anaphylaxis, establishing the diagnosis depends on recognition of systemic features such as skin, airway, cardiovascular, and gastrointestinal signs that are temporally related to exposure to an inciting agent. Past history of allergic reactions, as well as response to therapy, should be sought. Moreover, the time and route of exposure should be ascertained. A history of asthma, cardiovascular disease, beta-adrenergic blocker use, or ACE inhibitor use may help identify an etiologic diagnosis or predisposing risk factor.

Although elevated histamine levels are measurable in acute anaphylactic and anaphylactoid reactions, the half-life of histamine is very short. From a practical point of view, serum samples would have to be drawn within 10 to 60 minutes of the event in order to be clinically useful. As a result, this test is impractical for almost all cases occurring in the Emergency Department. Tryptase, on the other hand, has a half-life of several hours, and increased levels are highly correlative with the diagnosis of anaphylaxis. Consequently, serum obtained up to 6 hours after the event may help establish the diagnosis. As a result, this test may be useful in rare instances when the diagnosis remains in question.

   A. **Laboratory evaluation.** From a practical perspective, histamine and tryptase levels are not indicated in the vast majority of patients with anaphylaxis. However, pulse oximetry should be performed on all patients, and arterial blood gases should be considered for all patients with respiratory problems. Furthermore, cardiac monitoring should be instituted during the initial phase for all patients exhibiting signs of cardiac involvement, patients with underlying cardiac disease, and patients older than 50 years of age who are experiencing a moderate to severe reaction.

   B. **Differential diagnosis.** As a rule, food-mediated anaphylaxis usually does not present a diagnostic dilemma. Nevertheless, other clinical entities should be considered in the differential diagnosis of anaphylaxis. For example, if signs of upper airway obstruction are present, foreign body aspiration, supraglottitis, croup, status asthmaticus, or globus hystericus should all be considered; none of these diagnoses are associated with concomitant cutaneous reactions. Disorders with cutaneous and/or pulmonary manifestations include: carcinoid syndrome and mastocytosis (flushing, wheezing, hypotension, and diarrhea), monosodium glutamate syndrome (flushing, headache, and nausea without hives or angioedema), and scombroid poisoning (urticaria, headache, nausea, vomiting, and sweating, which occur after ingestion of spoiled mackerel or tuna; the histidine in spoiled fish degrades to histamine and is exogenously ingested).

III. **Management.** Patients with anaphylactic reactions require prompt, priority-based management. Because airway obstruction can occur rapidly secondary to angioedema or laryngeal edema, immediate assessment and stabilization of the airway are essential. Directly visualized oral tracheal intubation is the preferred method of airway control and should be performed early (i.e., before edema formation obscures visualization of the airway).

Because it is impossible to determine how quickly a reaction will progress or how severe it will become, every patient with an allergic reaction requires a quick, careful history with aggressive probing for the type and site of allergen exposure and for a history of prior reactions, asthma, cardiovascular disease, or angioedema. Moreover, rapid assessment of the airway is critical. In this regard, complaints of a change in voice, increasing bronchospasm, stridor, and perioral or lingual angioedema herald potential upper airway obstruction and mandate preparation for possible intubation.

A. Intubation. In a decompensating, awake patient, oral intubation with local anesthesia is the preferred method for securing an airway. Upper airway angioedema may make intubation difficult; consequently, some patients may require a smaller endotracheal tube and fiberoptic bronchoscopic nasal intubation, although airway edema and excessive secretions may limit the usefulness of this procedure. Emergent cricothyroidotomy or temporizing percutaneous jet ventilation may be necessary. Monitor vital signs and insert a large bore intravenous cannula.

B. Pharmacologic management

1. **Epinephrine.** Epinephrine is the most important pharmacotherapeutic agent used in the management of systemic anaphylaxis. All other drugs should be considered second-line therapy. The alpha agonist effects of epinephrine will promote resolution of angioedema, urticaria, and hypotension by reversing peripheral vasodilatation. In addition, the beta effects lead to bronchodilation, cardiac inotropy, and increased cyclic adenosine monophosphate (cAMP) production, which stabilizes mast cell membranes and prevents mast cell degranulation.

   Although the efficacy of epinephrine in the management of anaphylactic or anaphylactoid reactions is well established, there is some controversy regarding dosing of intravenous epinephrine for refractory anaphylaxis or shock. Epinephrine doses for mild to moderate reactions, however, are well-established. For mild reactions (e.g., urticaria and wheezing), the subcutaneous administration of 0.3 to 0.5 mL of a 1:1000 concentration of epinephrine every 10 to 20 minutes is recommended. Asthmatics may exhibit a sluggish beta-receptor response and may require higher doses of epinephrine.

   The pediatric dose is 0.01mL/kg of 1:1000 concentration epinephrine, up to a maximum of 0.5 mL. A moderate reaction, characterized by hypotension, angioedema, signs of impending upper airway obstruction, or poor response to the subcutaneous route, suggests the need for intramuscular administration of epinephrine. Upper airway obstruction may respond to nebulized racemic epinephrine 2.25% diluted in 2.5 mL of normal saline.

2. **Intravenous epinephrine.** Intravenous epinephrine may be used for anaphylaxis, but should be reserved for the severe, refractory cases characterized by hypotension that are unresponsive to intramuscular epinephrine and vigorous fluid resuscitation, or imminent or actual airway obstruction. The data regarding intravenous epinephrine for anaphylaxis are anecdotal, but poor outcomes from excessively vigorous intravenous epinephrine dosages have led to cautious recommendations. When epinephrine is infused slowly, beta-receptor effects predominate, whereas alpha effects predominate with rapid rates of infusion. In addition, beta receptors respond to lower doses of epinephrine than alpha receptors. Therefore, a low, slow dose of epinephrine favors beta-receptor effects and minimizes undesirable increases in systolic blood pressure.

   For anaphylactic patients who are in extremis, some experts recommend infusing one mL of 1:10,000 epinephrine (i.e., one mL of the "crash cart" 10 mL vial), diluted in 10 mL of normal saline and infusing slowly over 5 to 10 minutes. An epinephrine drip can be administered as well and then titrated to effect. Endotracheal instillation of epinephrine (using the same dose as the aforementioned intravenous formulation) is an alternative if intravenous access cannot be obtained.

Although epinephrine is the first-line agent for anaphylaxis, there are relative contraindications to its use. When administered intravenously, epinephrine should be given with extreme caution to patients over age 35, patients with underlying cardiovascular disease, pregnant women, and patients using beta blockers. Malignant hypertension, myocardial infarction, and fetal demise have all been reported. Patients who are on beta blockers are particularly susceptible to extreme blood pressure responses because the alpha receptor remains the only site available for epinephrine binding. In elderly patients, or patients with cardiovascular disease, consider a test dose of epinephrine of 0.1 to 0.15 mL of 1:1000 administered subcutaneously.

3. **Volume repletion.** Rapid infusion of crystalloid fluids in conjunction with epinephrine administration is an important aspect of clinical management. Hypotension that fails to respond to volume repletion and epinephrine administration is an indication for use of pressor agents such as dopamine.

4. **Glucagon.** Fortunately, when epinephrine is contraindicated, glucagon, a 29 amino acid polypeptide, may be an effective pharmacotherapeutic option. This agent has positive inotropic and chronotropic cardiac effects that are mediated independently of alpha and beta receptors. Instead, glucagon is thought to enhance cAMP synthesis within the myocardium and gastrointestinal and genitourinary tracts, which leads to positive inotropy, chronotropy, and smooth muscle relaxation.

Although the usefulness of glucagon in the treatment of anaphylaxis is anecdotal (i.e., no well-controlled trials justifying its routine use are available) glucagon administration should be considered in an anaphylactic patient taking beta-blockers, individuals with known coronary artery disease, pregnant women (glucagon is a Category B drug), and patients not responding to traditional therapy with epinephrine (i.e., epinephrine-resistant hypotension and airway obstruction).

A reasonable initial dose of glucagon is 1 mg intravenously in an adult, or 0.5 mg intravenously in a child, although a bolus dose of 3 to 5 mg intravenously may be required. Glucagon can be administered subcutaneously, intramuscularly, or intravenously and is generally well tolerated. Side effects include nausea, vomiting, hypokalemia, hyperglycemia, and rare reports of erythema multiforme and Stevens-Johnson syndrome. To sustain therapeutic efficacy in the patient, a glucagon drip of 1 to 5 mg/hr may be required.

5. **Antihistamines and corticosteroids.** Antihistamines, such as diphenhydramine, and corticosteroids are second-line therapeutic agents for anaphylaxis. They are particularly useful adjuncts after epinephrine, glucagon, and/or crystalloid infusion have stabilized cardiorespiratory status. Dose and route of administration are dictated by the severity of the reaction, but in most cases, these agents should be administered intramuscularly initially, at a dose of 50 mg, and then orally every 6 to 8 hours for 24 to 48 hours following the initial reaction. Anticholinergic side effects, including sedation, should be monitored.

H$_2$ antagonists such as cimetidine are helpful in acute reactions as well. They confer no benefit when used alone, but in combination with H$_1$ antagonists, they provide greater relief from urticaria. Corticosteroids exert multiple effects, although their benefits are not seen until 4 to 6 hours after administration. They have both anti-inflammatory and antichemotactic effects, and may stabilize the mast cell membrane, blunting the biphasic and protracted anaphylactic reactions. Other agents that should be considered, especially for persistent bronchospasm, include aminophylline, terbutaline, and nebulized beta-agonist therapy (i.e., albuterol).

Suggested Readings

Carter AO et al: A severe outbreak of *Escherichia coli* 0157:H7: associated hemorrhage colitis in a nursing home, *N Engl J Med* 317:24, 1987.

Centers for Disease Control: Botulism in the United States, 1899-1977: handbook for epidemiologists, clinicians and laboratory workers, Atlanta, Georgia, May 1979.

Chia JK et al: Botulism in an adult associated with food borne intestinal infection with *Clostridium botulinum, N Engl J Med* 315:239, 1986.

Dolman CE: Human botulism in Canada (1919-1973), *Can Med Assoc J* 110:191, 1974.

Eisbruch A, Lweinski U, Djaidett M: Severe opisthotonos and trismus associated with water intoxication, *J R Soc Med* 77:158, 1984.

Fleming DW et al: Pasteurized milk as a vehicle of infection in an outbreak of listeriosis, *N Engl J Med* 312:404, 1983.

Gangarosa EJ: Botulism in the United States, 1899-1967, *J Infect Dis* 119:308, 1969.

Gill G: Treatment of hyponatremic seizures with intravenous 29.2% saline, *Br Med J* 292:625, 1986.

Goldman JM, Ahn Y, Wheeler MF: Vitamin D and hypercalcemia, *JAMA* 254:1719, 1985.

Goldman MB, Luchins DJ, Robertson GL: Mechanisms of altered water metabolism in psychotic patients with polydipsia and hyponatremia, *N Engl J Med* 318:7, 1988.

Gupta KL, Dworkin B, Gambert SR: Common nutritional disorders in the elderly: atypical manifestations, *Geriatrics* 43:87-97, 1988.

Hedberg CW et al: An outbreak of thyrotoxicosis caused by the consumption of bovine thyroid gland in ground beef, *N Engl J Med* 316:993, 1987.

Helweg-Larsen P et al: Famine disease in German concentration camps: complications and sequels, *Acta Psychiatr Neurol Scand Suppl* 83, 1952.

Hessov IB, Elsborg L: Nutritional studies on long-term surgical patients with special reference to the intake of vitamin B$_{12}$ and folic acid, *Int J Vitam Nutr Res* 46:427, 1976.

Holmberg SD et al: Drug resistant *Salmonella* from animals fed antimicrobials, *N Engl J Med* 311:617, 1984.

Hughes RE et al: Clinical manifestations of ascorbic acid deficiency in man, *J Clin Nutr* 24:432, 1971.

Koenig MG et al: Type B botulism in man, *Am J Med* 42:208, 1967.

Kolata G: Testing for trichinosis, *Science* 227:621, 1985.

Lind J: *A treatise on the scurvy,* ed 3, London, 1772, S Crowder, D Wilson, G Nicholls, T Cadell, T Becket.

Lindenbaum J et al: Neuropsychiatric disorders caused by cobalamin deficiency in the absence of anemia or macrocytosis, *N Engl J Med* 318:26, 1988.

McMillan M, Thompson JG: An outbreak of suspected solanine poisoning in schoolboys, *Q J Med* 48:227, 1979.

Morgan AG et al: Nutritional survey in the elderly, *Int J Vitam Nutr Res* 43:465, 1973.

Morley JE: Nutritional status of the elderly, *Am J Med* 81:679-695, 1986.

Morse DL et al: Widespread outbreaks of clam and oyster associated gastroenteritis, *N Engl J Med* 314:678, 1986.

Munro HN: Nutrition and the elderly: a general overview, *J Am Coll Nutr* 3:341-350, 1984.

Nairns RG: Therapy of hyponatremia: does haste make waste? *N Engl J Med* 314:1573, 1986.

Roos D: Neurological symptoms and signs in a selected group of partially gastrectomized patients with particular reference to B_2 deficiency, *Acta Neurol Scand* 50:719, 1974.

Schwartz GR: *In bad taste: the MSG syndrome,* Santa Fe, 1988, Health Press.

Terris M, Goldberger ON: *Pellagra,* New Orleans, 1964, Louisiana State University Press.

Victor M, Adams RD, Collins GH: *The Wernicke-Korsakoff syndrome,* Oxford, 1971, Blackwell Scientific Publications.

Vir SC, Love AHG: Nutritional evaluation of B groups of vitamins in institutionalized aged, *Int J Vitam Nutr Res* 47:213, 1977.

Winick M, editor: *Hunger disease: studies by the Jewish physicians in the Warsaw ghetto,* New York, 1979, John Wiley & Sons.

This chapter is modified from Schwartz GR. Acute Nutritional Emergencies. In: Bosker et al: Geriatric Emergency Medicine. St. Louis: Mosby, 1990, 336–356.

12 Metabolic Emergencies

Dan A. Henry, M.D.
Gideon Bosker, M.D., F.A.C.E.P.

Rapid and Systematic Assessment of Metabolic and Acid-Base Disorders

Metabolic problems are frequently encountered within the province of the emergency department. Manifestations of such disorders in the adult patient are legion. In cases of acute renal or pulmonary failure, ingestion of toxins, and diabetic coma, the nature of the metabolic derangement can frequently be diagnosed from the history, physical examination, and laboratory data base. However, when a metabolic disturbance is expressed as a focal neurologic lesion, coma, seizure disorder, cardiac arrest, myopathy, or nonspecific symptom complex, the diagnosis may be much more difficult. In such cases, if a systematic approach to metabolic problems is not employed, the disease may go undiagnosed and, hence, untreated.

To ensure rapid institution of appropriate therapy for derangements of metabolic homeostasis, the emergency physician must be familiar with myriad disorders and be able to distinguish among them using a paucity of quickly available laboratory data.

I. **Metabolic emergencies: importance of early diagnosis**
   A. **Metabolic derangements** can serve as diagnostic clues to the presence of the following:
      1. Toxic ingestions
      2. Hemodynamic compromise
      3. Respiratory failure
      4. Postictal states
      5. Others (SIADH, Addisonian crisis, hypothyroidism, etc.)
   B. **Therapeutic decisions** depend upon rapid diagnosis:
      1. Choice of IV fluids
      2. Oral therapy
      3. Dextrose therapy
      4. ETOH therapy (i.e., in ethylene glycol ingestion)
      5. Insulin therapy
      6. Others (dialysis, hemoperfusion with charcoal, etc.)
   C. **Disposition and triage** of patients depends upon early recognition of the nature and severity of metabolic disturbance:
      1. ICU, CCU versus dialysis
      2. Invasive versus noninvasive monitoring

II. **Clinical conditions: metabolic problems.** The metabolic disorders that are associated with systemic disease states in the emergency department include the following:

1. Shock (lactic acidosis, rhabdomyolysis, hyperkalemia, hyperphosphatemia, alcohol or drug ingestion, respiratory alkalosis, or acidosis)
2. Cardiopulmonary arrest (hypokalemia or hyperkalemia, lactic acidosis, hypocalcemia in electromechanical [EM] dissociation, etc.)
3. Seizures (hyponatremia, hypocalcemia, hypomagnesemia, hypoglycemia, hyperosmolar states, rhabdomyolysis, etc.)
4. Coma (diabetic or alcoholic ketoacidosis, hyperosmolar nonketotic coma, hyponatremia, hypoglycemia, hyperammonemia, etc.)
5. Respiratory failure (hypercapnia, CO_2 narcosis, etc.)
6. Toxic ingestion (methanol, ethylene glycol, paraldehyde, ethanol, etc.)

III. **Emergency department battery (EDB).** The emergency department battery (EDB) is a conceptual, quasialgorithmic scheme that is intended to guide the emergency department physician in the diagnosis and evaluation of acute metabolic emergencies. The EDB framework (EDB-6, EDB-9, EDB-15, EDB-18, EDB-20—number represents how many lab tests are included in the battery) is organized in hierarchical fashion to facilitate the diagnosis of increasingly complex and/or unusual metabolic derangements. The laboratory tests in the EDBs include only those available on a STAT basis.

A. **EDB-6 = Na, K, Cl, CO_2, Glucose, BUN.** This is the minimal and initial diagnostic data base for the evaluation of metabolic disorders in coma, seizures, acute renal failure, nonketotic hyperosmolar coma, prerenal azotemia, high anion gap (i.e., organic acid) acidoses, adrenocortical insufficiency, toxic ingestions, and in nonspecific presentations. **NOTE:** The EDB-6 is almost always used in conjunction with other lab tests (especially ABGs) in order to fully elucidate the exact nature of a metabolic disturbance. Creatinine is usually measured to assess renal function.

B. **EDB-9 = EDB-6 + pH, P_{CO_2}, P_{O_2}.** The EDB-9 is needed for nearly all of the entities listed under EDB-6 plus all cases of suspected mixed acid-base disorders **(Table 12-1),** respiratory distress, as well as for nonmetabolic disorders such as asthma, pulmonary embolism, and pulmonary edema.

C. **EDB-15 = EDB-9 + U_{Na}, U_{Cl}, $U_{ketones}$, $U_{glucose}$, U_{osm}, P_{osm}.** The EDB-15 is needed for many of the conditions listed under EDB-6 and EDB-9, as well as for the *complete* and *rapid* evaluation (or confirmation) of diabetic ketoacidosis, alcoholic ketoacidosis (false negative nitroprusside reaction for ketones is common), and SIADH (syndrome of inappropriate ADH can easily be di-

Table 12-1. Nine Categories of Acid-Base Disturbance as Defined by the P_{CO_2} and Bicarbonate Levels

P_{CO_2}	Bicarbonate (mEq/L) <21	21-26	>26
>45	Combined metabolic and respiratory acidosis	Respiratory acidosis	Metabolic alkalosis and respiratory acidosis
35-45	Metabolic acidosis	Normal	Metabolic alkalosis
<35	Metabolic acidosis and respiratory alkalosis	Respiratory alkalosis	Combined metabolic respiratory alkalosis

agnosed as U_{osm} is inappropriately concentrated with respect to P_{osm}). It is also needed for distinguishing acute tubular necrosis (ATN) from prerenal azotemia and a differentiating "saline-responsive" versus "saline-resistant" (U_{Cl}) metabolic alkalosis. Finally, it is needed as a clue (P_{osm}) to the presence of ETOH, methanol, or ethylene glycol ingestions.

D. **EDB-18 = EDB-15 + Ca, PO$_4$, Mg.** This EDB is used for many of the conditions listed under other EDBs (i.e., DKA, ETOH withdrawal, renal failure, etc.) and especially when myoirritability (i.e., positive Chvostek's or Trousseau's syndrome), EM dissociation, rhabdomyolysis (i.e., elevated PO_4 and decreased Ca), lactic acidosis (elevated PO_4), starvation, metastatic cancer (elevated Ca), cardiomyopathy, or hypophosphatemia is present or suspected.

E. **EDB-20 = EDB-18 + U_{Cr}, P_{Cr}.** This EDB is used for renal disorders, assessment of volume status, and in other conditions when a renal failure index (RFI) may be helpful.

IV. Diagnostic tools for rapid evaluation of metabolic disorders

A. Arterial blood gas interpretation

B. **BUN/Cr ratio.** When ratio >15:1, this suggests *prerenal azotemia* (i.e., dehydration or prerenal hypoperfusion on some other basis).

C. **Use of the renal failure index (RFI) and fractional excretion of sodium FE_{Na}**

$$RFI = \frac{U_{Na}}{U_{Cr}/P_{Cr}}$$

If RFI <1: prerenal causes
If RFI >1: ATN, vascular or postrenal causes

D. Interpretation of urinary electrolytes

1. **U_{Na}.** In general, a healthy (i.e., non-ATN) kidney is able to conserve sodium. Therefore, in the oliguric patient (anuria is seen almost *only* in postrenal *obstruction*) who has an elevated BUN and Cr, a *prerenal* picture will be characterized by a low U_{Na} (i.e., < 20 mEq/L), whereas the ATN picture will be characterized by high U_{Na} (i.e., > 40). NOTE: Diuretics can make a prerenal picture look like ATN because they increase U_{Na} excretion (in such cases use RFI or FE_{Na} to refine diagnosis).

2. **U_{Cr}.** In general, a healthy kidney is able to concentrate creatinine (Cr) in the urine, whereas a diseased (i.e., ATN, etc.) kidney will excrete Cr at about the same concentration as it is in the plasma.

    Therefore, a *prerenal* picture is characterized by:

    $$U_{Cr}/P_{Cr} > 20:1$$

    whereas an ATN picture is characterized by:

    $$U_{Cr}/P_{Cr} = 1:1$$

3. **U_{Cl}.** Value lies in distinguishing among etiologies in metabolic alkalosis. *Volume contraction* (i.e., nasogastric suction, diuretic therapy, dehydration) alkalosis will be characterized by avid NaCl reabsorption, and, therefore, the U_{Cl} will be low (i.e., <10 mEq/L). Metabolic alkalosis caused by *hyperadrenal* states (i.e., increased serum cortisol and/or mineralocorticoids that caused increased Na for K and H^+ exchange distally) is usually characterized by U_{Cl} > 10 mEq **(Table 12-2).**

Table 12-2. Value of the Determination of Urinary Chloride Concentration in the Differential Diagnosis of Metabolic Alkalosis

Saline responsive (U_{Cl} < 10 mEq/L)	Saline resistant (U_{Cl} > 10 mEq/L)
• Loss of gastric secretions (i.e., vomiting or nasogastric suction) • Diuretic therapy	• Primary aldosteronism • Cushing's disease • Adrenocorticotropic-hormone (ACTH) producing tumors • Severe potassium depletion • Steroid therapy

4. **U_{osm}.** In general, a diseased kidney will not be able to concentrate well, and so in the oliguric patient with elevated BUN and Cr, an isosmotic urine suggests ATN, and a concentrated urine (i.e., >550 osm) suggests *prerenal* causes. Also, the U_{osm} is probably the most important test for ascertaining the diagnosis of SIADH. If the $U_{osm} > P_{osm}$ in the patient who is severely hyponatremic and hypoosmolar, this virtually confirms the diagnosis of SIADH. Actually, any U_{osm} that is not maximally dilute (i.e., 50 to 85 mOsm/L) in a patient with hyponatremia and hypoosmolarity is suggestive of SIADH.

E. **Serum osmolality.** Serum osmolality can be both calculated and measured. If calculated:

$$S_{osm} = 2 \times Na^+ + Glucose/18 + BUN/3$$

where serum sodium (Na^+) is measured in mEq/L, and glucose and BUN in mg/dL.

If:

$$\text{MEASURED } S_{osm} \neq \text{CALCULATED } S_{osm}$$

then molecules (i.e., other than Na, BUN, and glucose) with significant osmotic properties are present in the serum. In general, these might be ETOH (a 25 mOsm difference between calculated and measured serum osmolality would be compatible with an ETOH level of 100 to 120 mg/dL), methanol, ethylene glycol, or mannitol. Therefore, patients whose serum osmolality cannot be explained by ETOH level should be suspected of having ingested one of the above-mentioned toxins.

F. **Winter's formula.** Winter's formula is a quick way to measure appropriateness of respiratory response (i.e., hyperventilation or hypoventilation) to a metabolic disturbance.

As a rule:

$$\text{If } P_{CO_2} = 1.5 \text{ (total serum } CO_2) + 8.3,$$
appropriate respiratory compensation is present.

$$\text{If } P_{CO_2} < 1.5 \text{ (total serum } CO_2) + 8.3, \text{ then a}$$
primary respiratory alkalosis is superimposed on metabolic disturbance.

If $P_{CO_2} > 1.5$ (total serum CO_2) + 8.3, then a primary respiratory acidosis is superimposed on metabolic disturbance.

G. **Bypassing Henderson-Hasselbalch equation**
A simple method reported that allows you to *estimate* serum bicarbonate (HCO_3^-) concentration from the arterial blood gas (ABG) values, pH, P_{CO_2} is shown in **Table 12-3**.

V. **Anion gap**

$$Na^+ - (Cl^- + HCO_3^-) = AG$$

A. NOTE: This is one of the most important diagnostic tools for evaluation of acute metabolic emergencies. **The anion gap is a calculation of diagnostic convenience.** There is, of course, no true anion gap since positive and negative charges in the blood must be equal. However, the principal cation of the blood, sodium (Na), exceeds the sum of the principal anions, chloride and bicarbonate, by about 12 ± 2 mEq/L in normal persons. The additional, or so-called unmeasured, anions include albumin (which is an anion at physiologic pH) and other metabolites such as sulfate, phosphates, and small amounts of organic acids. When metabolic acids are generated and added to the body fluid, the hydrogen ion of the acid destroys bicarbonate, and if the anion associated with the proton (i.e., hydrogen) is any other than chloride, the sum of chloride and bicarbonate must fall, thereby increasing the anion gap.

B. **Differential diagnosis of elevated and reduced anion gap.** The most important thing about the anion gap is for the emergency physician to get into the habit of using this simple and revealing calculation on a routine basis. Failure to employ this diagnostic tool may allow any of the following to go undetected:
   1. Organic acidoses
   2. Toxin-induced acidoses
   3. Severe alkalemia
   4. Mixed acid-base disturbances

   A reduced anion gap may also be an important finding and is frequently the first clue in the ED that cirrhosis, lithium toxicity, hypercalcemia, hypermagnesemia, or multiple myeloma is present **(Table 12-4)**.

C. Anion gap and alkalemia
   1. NOTE: This is a relatively new, but relevant, discovery.

   $$\text{Anion gap} = Na^+ - (Cl^- + HCO_3^-) = AG$$

   2. **When investigating the cause** of an elevated anion gap (AG), the ED clinician routinely seeks evidence for the presence of lactic acidosis, ASA ingestion, advanced renal failure, methanol, paraldehyde, or ethylene glycol ingestion, diabetic ketoacidosis (DKA), or alcoholic ketoacidosis.
   3. **Changes in unmeasured anions.** Frequently, however, consideration is not given to the possibility that changes in unmeasured anions, originating from plasma proteins, may have contributed to the increase in anion gap. It is now well established that increases in unmeasured anions may result from alkalemia-induced elevations in the net negative charge of plasma proteins.

D. Anion gap, serum proteins, and alkalemia

$$AG = Na^+ - (Cl^- + HCO_3^-)$$

Table 12-3. Estimating Bicarbonate Ion Concentration

Range	$[HCO_3^-]/P_{CO_2}$ estimate	Examples $[HCO_3^-]/P_{CO_2}$ from pH	Estimated $[HCO_3^-]$
Severe acidemia ($7.00 > $ pH)	0.20	if pH = 6.89 $\frac{[HCO_3^-]}{P_{CO_2}} = 0.02$	$[HCO_3^-]$ = 20% of P_{CO_2}
Mild — moderate acidemia ($7.00 \leq$ pH ≤ 7.40)	(pH − 7) + 0.20	if pH = 7.25 $0.25 + 0.20 = 0.45$ $\frac{[HCO_3^-]}{P_{CO_2}} = 0.45$	$[HCO_3^-]$ = 45% of P_{CO_2}
Alkalemia (pH > 7.40)	2[(pH − 7) − 0.10]	if pH = 7.60 $0.60 + 0.10 = 0.50$ $2 \times 0.50 = 1.00$ $\frac{[HCO_3^-]}{P_{CO_2}} = 1.00$	$[HCO_3^-]$ = 100% of P_{CO_2}

From Kamens DR et al: Circumventing the Henderson-Hasselbalch equation, JACEP 8:462, 1979.

Table 12-4. Differential Diagnosis of Metabolic Acidosis

Normal anion gap (hyperchloremic)	Increased anion gap
Gastrointestinal Loss of HCO₃	**Increased Acid Production**
• Diarrhea	• Diabetic ketoacidosis
• Ureterosigmoidostomy	• Lactic acidosis
• Anion-exchange resin	• Starvation
• Small bowel drainage	• Alcoholic ketoacidosis
Renal Loss of HCO₃⁻	• Inborn errors of metabolism
• Carbonic anhydrase inhibitors	**Ingestion of Toxins**
• Renal tubular acidosis (RTA)	• Salicylate overdose
Miscellaneous	• Paraldehyde poisoning
• Dilutional acidosis	• Methanol ingestion
• Hyperalimentation acidosis	• Ethylene glycol ingestion
	Acute or Chronic Renal Failure

The anion gap largely reflects organic sulfates, phosphates, and negatively charged serum proteins, of which albumin is the most important.

$$\text{Alkalemia}$$
$$\text{Albumin} - H \rightarrow \text{Albumin}^- + H^+$$

$$\text{Albumin}^- \uparrow \rightarrow \uparrow \text{ANION GAP}$$

E. Anion gap: some pearls
  1. **Recognize that a normal measured serum** HCO_3^- does *not* mean that there is not a *metabolic acidosis* present. If there is a preexisting metabolic alkalosis (i.e., vomiting, diuretics, ETOH'ism, metabolic compensation for respiratory acidosis, etc.), the serum HCO_3^- will be elevated *at first* and then can *fall to a normal range* (or perhaps lower) in the presence of a superimposed metabolic acidosis.
  2. **The presence of a preexisting metabolic alkalosis** can be detected using the AG.

$$\Delta AG = AG \text{ (calculated)} - AG \text{ (normal, i.e., 12)}$$

$$\Delta HCO_3^- = HCO_3^- \text{ (expected—i.e., 24 mEq)} - HCO_3^- \text{ (measured)}$$

If:

$$\Delta AG > HCO_3^-$$

suspect a metabolic acidosis that has been superimposed on a preexisting metabolic *alkalosis*.

F. Anion gap: extended data base (i.e., further lab workup in ED). Extended data base for evaluation of elevated anion gap
  1. DKA: urine ketones, serum ketones, serum K^+, serum PO_4, glucose, lactate level, ABG

2. Alcoholic ketosis
   a. Urine ketones (but note that the nitroprusside reagent, Acetest, may be entirely negative because this kind of acidosis is characteristically a B-OH butyric acidosis; serum ketones are usually positive)
   b. Glucose (especially important, since this syndrome may be accompanied by hypoglycemia, i.e., hypoglycemic ketoacidotic coma) **(Table 12-5)**
   c. Urine glucose (almost always negative in this kind of ketoacidosis)
3. Lactic acidosis
   a. Lactate level, K^+; may need to draw CN^-, methemoglobin, or carboxyhemoglobin level for "unexplained" cases of lactic acidosis
   b. In cases of quickly resolving LA, consider generalized motor seizures as likely etiology and initiate workup as needed
4. Salicylate overdose: salicylate level, ABGs, and lactate level (if acidosis is very severe; salicylates may uncouple oxidative phosphorylation and lead to LA)
5. Ethylene glycol ingestion: blood level, serum osmolality, urinalysis, and renal workup
6. Methanol: blood level, serum osmolality
7. Paraldehyde
8. Alkalemia: work up various etiologies

G. Low anion gap: differential diagnosis. Causes of low anion gap
1. Reduced concentration of unmeasured anions
   a. Dilution
   b. Hypoalbuminemia
2. Systematic underestimation of serum sodium
   a. Hypernatremia (severe)
   b. Hyperviscosity
3. Systematic overestimation of serum chloride
   a. Bromism
4. Retained nonsodium cations
   a. Paraproteinemia
   b. Hypercalcemia, hypermagnesemia, lithium toxicity

H. Anion gap and metabolic acidosis: causes of lactic acidosis (most common cause of elevated AG)
1. Inadequate oxygen delivery
   a. Cardiac arrest
   b. Shock states
   c. Profound anemia
   d. Hypoxemia
2. Failure to utilize oxygen
   a. Phenformin
   b. Ethanol
   c. Diabetic ketoacidosis
   d. Leukemia and lymphoma
   e. INH overdose
3. Others
   a. Hepatic cirrhosis
   b. Pregnancy
   c. Pancreatitis
   d. Seizures
   e. CRF

Table 12-5. Laboratory Summary of Nondiabetic Alcoholic Patients with Hypoglycemic Ketoacidotic Coma

Case	Arterial pH	Serum Acetest for ketones	Urine Acetest for ketones	Serum glucose (mg/dL) Initial	Serum glucose (mg/dL) Discharge	Serum bicarbonate (mEq/L) (normal 24-30) Initial	Serum bicarbonate (mEq/L) (normal 24-30) Discharge	Lactic acid, arterial (mEq/L) (normal 0.5-1.5)	Serum β-hydroxy-butyrate (mEq/L) (normal <.05)	Anion gap (Na + K − [Cl + HCO$_3^-$])	Serum bilirubin (mg/dL)	Serum insulin (µU/mL)	SGOT (IU/L) (normal <17)
1	7.16	+	+	25	105	14	21	2.6	9.8	27	1.0	..	55
2	7.18	+	+	21	120	15	20	2.3	..	21	0.8	3	40
3	7.23	−	−	27	125	17	24	..	7.3	22	0.7	..	35
4	7.19	−	−	21	110	13	22	2.2	8.5	29	1.1	5	30
5	7.18	+	+	19	105	15	23	2.4	5.9	24	0.9	2	31
Mean	7.19	..	..	23	..	15	..	2.4	7.9	25	0.9	3	38

From Platia EZ and Hsu TH: Hypoglycemic coma with ketoacidosis in nondiabetic adults, West J Med 131(4):272, 1981.

Some "Clinical Pearls" For Metabolic Emergencies

I. Refractory ventricular fibrillation: Consider hypokalemia.
II. Diuretic therapy in a patient with altered mental status: Consider hyponatremia with/without SIADH.
III. Diuretic therapy in a patient with muscle weakness: Consider hypokalemia.
   A. *Complications and side effects of diuretic therapy*
   1. Volume depletion
   2. Hypokalemia, hyperkalemia
   3. Hyponatremia (SIADH) **(Table 12-6)**
   4. Acidosis, alkalosis
   5. Hyperuricemia
   6. Carbohydrate intolerance
   7. Hypercalcemia
   8. Hypersensitivity reactions
   9. Gastrointestinal disorders
IV. Hypothermia may be the first clue to the presence of hypoglycemia.
V. Hypothermia in combination with hypoglycemia and hypotension (in the non-exposed patient): Consider Addisonian crisis.
VI. Hypothermia in combination with bradycardia and hyponatremia: Consider hypothyroidism.
VII. Decreased anion gap in a patient with carcinoma: Consider hypercalcemia.
VIII. Hyperphosphatemia in a patient with shock: Consider superimposed lactic acidosis.
IX. Hypocalcemia, hyperphosphatemia, and hyperuricemia in a patient with crush injury, muscle aches, or after strenuous exercise: Consider rhabdomyolysis.
X. Increased anion gap in a patient with elevated serum osmolality: Consider ETOH ketoacidosis, ethylene glycol, methanol, or paraldehyde ingestion.
XI. Focal neurologic lesions in the diabetic: Consider both nonketotic hyperosmolar states and hypoglycemia.
XII. Acidosis and hypercapnia in patients with COPD: Remember the acidosis may represent an underlying and potentially correctable *metabolic acidosis*—you have to look for it!
XIII. Unexplained symptom complex consisting of neurologic, hematologic (thrombocytopenia, decreased O_2 delivery by RBCs, etc.), cardiac (cardiomyopathy), and/or respiratory (failure) disturbances in ETOH abusers, diabetics, and starved individuals: Consider hypophosphatemia.

Metabolic Acidosis: Anion Gap

In all these circumstances, the patient has an unmeasured anion HA that has lowered the serum bicarbonate level and resulted in an anion gap as described below:

$$H^+ \text{Anion}^- + NaHCO_3 \leftrightarrows Na^+ \text{Anion}^- + H_2O + CO_2$$

I. **Lactic acidosis.** Lactic acid is normally produced from pyruvate as follows:

$$\text{Pyruvate}^- + NADH + H^+ \leftrightarrows \text{LDH Lactate} + NAD^+$$

Table 12-6. Differential Diagnosis of Hyponatremia with Normal Hydration

	Inappropriate ADH secretion	Hypopituitarism	Hypothyroidism	Diuretic-induced	Chlorpropamide-induced	Polydipsic vomiting
Creatinine clearance	Normal or ↑	Normal or slightly ↓	Normal or slightly ↓	Normal or slightly ↓	Normal or ↑	Normal or ↓
Serum K	Normal	Normal	Normal	↓	Normal	↓
Serum HCO_3^-	Normal	Normal	Normal	↑ Early ↓ Later	Normal	↔
Urine Na^+	↑	↑	↓	↑ Early ↓ Later	↑	↓
Urine osmolality	↑	↑	↑		↑	
Metapyrone response	Normal	↓	Normal	Normal	Normal	Normal
H_2O load response	↓	↓	Delayed	Normal	Delayed	Normal
Correction	H_2O restriction	Cortisol	Thyroid	Withdraw diuretics or ↑ K^+ intake	Withdraw chlorpropamide	NaCl, KCl, and H_2O restriction

From Berti T et al: Clinical disorders of water metabolism, Kidney Int 10(117), 1976. Reprinted from Kidney International with permission.

The lactate is released into the bloodstream from organs such as muscle, gut, brain, skin, and erythrocytes. It is metabolized to pyruvate by lactic dehydrogenase (LDH) and eventually to glucose by the liver, kidney, and heart. Normally the rate of production and metabolism of lactate are in balance. The concentration of lactate can increase if there is (1) excess production that is seen when oxygen delivery is inadequate to meet energy requirements, (2) decreased utilization of lactate, or (3) high NADH levels, since more pyruvate would be metabolized to lactate.

A. Differential diagnosis. Some of the conditions associated with lactic acidosis are shown in **Table 12-7.** Type A conditions refer to tissue hypoperfusion or acute hypoxia, with a resulting increase in lactate production, and Type B conditions refer to common disorders including ingestion of drugs and toxins, as well as hereditary and miscellaneous disorders. It is important to note that an elevated lactate level may be part of the metabolic acidosis due to salicylates and methanol (see below). Most cases of lactic acidosis in the ED will be due to Type A disorders. Carbon monoxide poisoning is a cause of lactic acidosis that can be difficult to diagnose. The arterial blood gas values may be misleading unless it directly measures oxygen saturation. Some blood gas analyzers calculate oxygen saturation, and if you suspect carbon monoxide poisoning, you need to directly measure carbon monoxide levels or oxygen saturation.

B. Symptoms and signs. In addition to symptoms pertinent to the underlying disorder causing lactic acidosis, hyperventilation, abdominal pain, and disturbances in consciousness are frequently present. Laboratory abnormalities often include hyperphosphatemia (intracellular release), leukocytosis, and hyperuricemia. Hyperkalemia is often not present, which is in contrast to inorganic acidosis.

Table 12-7. Causes of Lactic Acidosis

Type A
Poor tissue perfusion
Shock
  Hypovolemic
  Cardiogenic
  Septic
Acute hypoxemia
Carbon monoxide poisoning
Severe anemia

Type B
Common disorders
  Diabetes mellitus
  Renal failure
  Liver failure
Ingestion of drugs or toxins
  Phenformin
  Ethanol
  Methanol
  Salicylates
  Isoniazide
  Cyanide
  Nitroprusside

C. Treatment. The most important therapy for lactic acidosis is to treat the underlying disorder. In patients with hypovolemic shock, volume expanders are essential to therapy. Vasoconstricting drugs such as norepinephrine and high-dose dopamine are not advisable unless volume repletion fails to elevate blood pressure. In severe heart failure, dobutamine and/or nitroprusside are of potential benefit, but these agents should not be used if the patient is hypotensive. The use of alkali therapy in lactic acidosis is very controversial. The argument for its use is concern that acidemia may impair cardiac function (decreased inotropy). The argument against its use is that bicarbonate therapy can actually increase lactate production and worsen cardiac performance and acidemia, and may cause fluid overload, hypernatremia, and metabolic alkalosis. I currently do not recommend bicarbonate therapy.

II. Ketoacidosis

A. Diabetic ketoacidosis. See page 383.

B. Alcoholic ketoacidosis (AKA). AKA is usually seen in chronically malnourished alcoholics. On admission to the ED, about two thirds of patients have elevated blood alcohol levels and may be intoxicated.

1. **Symptoms.** Nausea, vomiting, and abdominal pain are the most common symptoms seen in uncomplicated AKA. Other findings may be seen in patients with AKA but usually imply another underlying process. These include altered mental status resulting from hypoglycemia, alcohol intoxication, seizures, and stroke; rebound abdominal tenderness resulting from pancreatitis and sepsis; and hypothermia resulting from hypoglycemia and sepsis. Laboratory abnormalities include the anion gap metabolic acidosis that is predominantly due to ketoacids; however, a concomitant lactic acidosis is often present. As a result of an altered redox state, most of the ketoacids are in the form of β-hydroxybutyrate. The nitroprusside reaction (Acetest) predominantly measures acetoacetate. It therefore may underestimate the level of ketoacids. About 90% of patients will have a positive urine and serum nitroprusside reaction. The cases with negative nitroprusside reactions are usually milder. In addition to the anion gap metabolic acidosis, patients often have other acid-base abnormalities. These include primary metabolic alkalosis caused by vomiting and volume depletion, and respiratory alkalosis caused by alcohol withdrawal, sepsis, cirrhosis, or pain. Some of the patients with AKA will actually have alkalemia. A mild osmolar gap (see below) may also be present. Hyponatremia, hypokalemia, hypomagnesemia, and hypocalcemia are common. The serum phosphorus concentration may be elevated or decreased on presentation. Hyperphosphatemia is due to intracellular release, and with severe AKA it may be significantly elevated. Even if initially elevated, the level will usually fall rapidly to hypophosphatemic levels after treating the AKA (see Hypophosphatemia).

2. **The treatment of AKA** is to administer saline and dextrose solution to restore extracellular volume and glycogen stores, and treat concomitant metabolic abnormalities. Initially intravenous fluids are given at 500 ml/hr for 4 hours, followed by administration at 250 ml/hr for the next 4 hours. This should be adequate to correct the fluid deficit. During rehydration therapy, it is essential to monitor the concentrations of serum electrolytes, phosphorus, magnesium, and glucose, as well as the acid-base balance.

C. Starvation ketoacidosis. This is usually mild and occurs within the first 24 to 48 hours of fasting. Therapy is to infuse glucose or feed the patient.

III. **Renal failure.** Patients with both acute and chronic renal failure usually develop a metabolic acidosis because of an inability of the kidney to completely retain the bicarbonate that is lowered by body metabolism. The acidosis is often initially nonanion gap, since the kidney is able to excrete unmeasured anions such as phosphates and sulfates. As kidney failure worsens, an anion gap usually appears resulting from accumulation of poorly defined unmeasured anions.

IV. **Ingestions**
  A. **Methanol.** Methanol can produce inebriation similar to the other alcohols but has profound toxicity as a result of its metabolites. It is metabolized in the liver by alcohol dehydrogenase and aldehyde dehydrogenase to formaldehyde and then formic acid.
   1. **Clinical manifestations** usually occur 12 to 24 hours after ingestion and include nausea, vomiting, abdominal pain, headache, CNS depression, and cardiovascular collapse. The damaging effect on the retina, ranging from blurring of vision to blindness and occasionally papilledema, can be helpful in the diagnosis of methanol toxicity. Patients have a profound anion gap metabolic acidosis caused not only by formic acid but also by lactic acid as a result of interference with carbohydrate metabolism. These patients have an osmolar gap (see below) as a result of methanol ingestion.
   2. **The purpose of treatment** is to remove methanol and its metabolites. Ethanol is used to bind alcohol dehydrogenase, thereby decreasing the metabolism of methanol to its toxic metabolites. Hemodialysis is used to remove methanol and correct the metabolic acidosis. The goal of ethanol therapy is to achieve a blood ethanol concentration of 100 to 200 mg/dl. A loading dose of 0.6 gm/kg of 100% ethanol in D_5W can be given over 15 to 20 minutes, followed by a maintenance dose of 0.1 to 0.15 gm/kg/hr. Since hemodialysis removes ethanol, the ethanol infusion will need to be increased by about 50% during hemodialysis to maintain a level of 100 to 200 mg/dl.
  B. **Ethylene glycol.** Used in antifreeze, ethylene glycol is like other alcohols in that it produces inebriation and CNS depression. It is similar to methanol in that its metabolites are toxic. It is rapidly absorbed from the gastrointestinal tract and metabolized in the liver by alcohol dehydrogenase and aldehyde dehydrogenase to glycolaldehyde, glycolic acid, and oxalic acid.
   1. **Clinical manifestations** initially resemble alcohol intoxication, but over the next 12 to 24 hours manifestations may include congestive heart failure and even pulmonary edema secondary to myocardial depression, oliguric renal failure secondary to calcium oxalate deposition, or seizures secondary to CNS precipitation.
   2. **Treatment** is similar to the treatment of methanol ingestion, where ethanol is infused and hemodialysis is used to remove ethylene glycol and correct the metabolic acidosis (see above). Oliguric renal failure should be treated with mannitol, but it should be used cautiously in patients with fluid overload because it may cause pulmonary edema.
  C. **Salicylates.** Intoxication in the adult is often not due to an intentional overdose; instead, it is often seen in patients who are either on long-term salicylate therapy or ingest additional amounts due to increasing pain. Salicylates are rapidly absorbed from the stomach and upper gastrointestinal tract. They are metabolized by the liver to salicylic acid and other metabolites. Salicylic acid causes toxicity by both a direct CNS effect and an uncoupling of oxidative phosphorylation. The metabolic acidosis is a high anion gap due to sali-

cylic acid and accumulation of varying amounts of lactic acid and other poorly defined acids that are generated as a result of uncoupling of oxidative phosphorylation.

1. **Clinical manifestations** can include (1) hyperventilation, (2) mental status changes ranging from stupor to coma, (3) hyperthermia (more common in infants), (4) gastrointestinal bleeding (local effects and an antiplatelet effect), (5) adult respiratory distress syndrome, and (6) tinnitus and even deafness. The CNS manifestations are dependent on salicylic acid levels and on arterial pH. Salicylic acid is a CNS toxin, but it only enters the brain as a nonionized acid. Acidemia increases the amount of nonionized diffusible salicylic acid and can adversely affect CNS function significantly. Respiratory alkalosis, anion gap metabolic acidosis, or mixed anion gap metabolic acidosis and respiratory alkalosis are the various acid-base disturbances, with about 50% of adults having the mixed disorder. In some patients a respiratory acidosis may exist if the patient also took a CNS depressant. Other abnormalities may include hypoglycemia, hyperthermia, hypouricemia secondary to the uricosuric effect of salicylates, and elevated prothrombin time secondary to decreased synthesis of factor VII. Diagnosis is made by measuring the blood concentration of salicylates.

2. **Treatment modalities** include charcoal, bicarbonate, and hemodialysis. Bicarbonate therapy is important to minimize tissue deposition and also to increase salicylate elimination. When sodium bicarbonate is administered, it initially remains largely confined to the extracellular space for a period of hours. The relative extracellular alkalemia not only decreases salicylate movement into cells but also promotes movement out of cells, especially in the CNS. This increase in extracellular concentration of salicylates causes an increase in filtered load, and along with alkalization of the urine, enhances renal clearance. The major limiting factors in administering sodium bicarbonate is the development of systemic alkalemia or pulmonary edema due to salicylate-induced adult respiratory distress syndrome. The pulmonary edema may be preexisting or develop when administering fluids and bicarbonate. Patients with preexisting alkalemia secondary to primary respiratory alkalosis need to be followed closely; if the pH is greater than 7.50, bicarbonate should not be given. The purpose of alkali therapy is to increase pH to 7.50 and urinary pH to 7 to 8. Dialysis is indicated in severe toxicity when (1) patients are unresponsive to conservative measures, or (2) conditions are present that contraindicate alkali therapy (systemic alkalemia, renal failure, pulmonary edema).

V. **Approach to a patient with an anion gap metabolic acidosis** (Tables 12-4, 12-7, and 12-8). When patients present to the emergency department and are found to have an anion gap metabolic acidosis, the diagnoses of diabetic ketoacidosis (positive serum ketones and plasma glucose level >300 mg/dl) and uremia are usually easily made. In patients with a possible toxic ingestion, the osmolar gap is a useful test. Osmolar gap refers to the difference between the measured serum osmolality and calculated serum osmolality (2Na + BUN/2.8 + Glucose/18). When ethanol is present, the calculated osmolality includes ethanol. The osmotic contribution of ethanol is ethanol concentration in milligrams per deciliter divided by 4.6. An osmolar gap greater than 10 after correcting for ethanol implies the presence of molecule(s) that contribute significantly to the osmolality but are not included in the calculations.

In the past, the presence of an anion gap metabolic acidosis and an osmolar gap of more than 10 mmol/kg was a good marker for recent toxic alcohol ingestion. Recently alcoholic ketoacidosis (after eliminating the contribution of ethanol) and lactic acidosis have been reported to cause an osmolar gap. The following approach[1] is recommended for patients with an anion gap metabolic acidosis, an increased osmolar gap, and a suspected recent toxic alcohol ingestion. The contribution of ethanol should be considered in all patients. If toxicology screens are readily available, an ethanol drip should be started and hemodialysis should be withheld, unless the toxicology screen is positive for methanol, ethylene glycol, or isopropanol. If toxicology screens are unavailable, ethanol administration and hemodialysis should be considered when the osmolar gap is greater than 25 mmol/kg. For milder osmolar gap elevations, the decision about ethanol infusion and dialysis is less clear because there is considerable overlap in the osmolar gap in patients with lactic acidosis, alcoholic ketoacidosis, and ingestion of small volumes of toxic alcohol. If a clinical diagnosis of lactic acidosis or alcoholic ketoacidosis can be made, the underlying condition should be treated appropriately. If the clinical picture is inconsistent with lactic acidosis or alcoholic ketoacidosis, ethanol treatment should be initiated and hemodialysis considered. The diagnosis of lactic acidosis can be made by measuring levels, but if elevated it is important that salicylates and methanol be considered since they can also cause a lactic acidosis due to interference with oxidative phosphorylation.

Metabolic Acidosis: Non-Anion Gap

I. **Causes**
   A. **Acid loads.** Diabetic ketoacidosis (DKA) can present as a non-anion gap acidosis in about 10% of cases. The ketoacids lower the bicarbonate concentration, and instead of accumulating are readily excreted in the urine and replaced with chloride. Most patients with the disorder have intact renal function and are able to excrete unmeasured anions. The diagnosis of DKA should be considered in any diabetic with a metabolic acidosis (see DKA). Early renal failure

Table 12-8. Metabolic Acidosis: Hyperchloremic, Normal Anion Gap

Acid loads
   Ketoacidosis with urinary losses of ketone (presentation and recovery)
   Early renal failure
Gastrointestinal losses of HCO_3^-
   Diarrhea
   Small bowel or pancreatic drainage or fistula
   Ureterosigmoidoscopy
   Long or obstructed ileal loop conduit
Renal losses of HCO_3^-
   Carbonic anhydrase inhibitors
   Renal tubular acidosis

---

[1]Reproduced with permission from Schilling JR et al: Increased osmolal gap in alcoholic ketoacidosis and lactic acidosis, *Ann Intern Med* 113:580-2, 1990.

typically is non anion gap since unmeasured anions do not accumulate with mild decreases in renal function.
- **B. Gastrointestinal losses of HCO_3.** Diarrhea is the most common cause of non anion gap acidosis. The acidosis is a result of the HCO_3 level in diarrheal fluid being greater than the plasma HCO_3 level. Small bowel or pancreatic drainage or fistulas contain fluids high in bicarbonate, and the fluid loss can lead to a non anion gap metabolic acidosis. Ureterosigmoidostomy (rarely done today) can cause a non anion gap metabolic acidosis secondary to intestinal exchange of Cl with HCO_3. Ureteroileostomy does not usually cause this; if seen, the patient should be evaluated for an obstructed ileal loop, since that would cause increased exposure time to the intestinal mucosa.
- **C. Renal losses of HCO_3.** Carbonic anhydrase inhibitors (i.e., acetazolamide) are an important cause. They work by blocking proximal tubule bicarbonate absorption. Renal tubular acidosis (RTA) is divided into Type I (distal), Type II (proximal), and Type IV (hyperkalemic distal RTA). Type I distal RTA is characterized by inability of the distal tubule to maintain a gradient for acid excretion. Patients with hypokalemic distal RTA are unable to increase their urine pH >5.3 when systemically acidemic. Some of the causes of distal RTA include toluene ingestion and treatment with amphotericin B. Type II (proximal RTA) is similar to carbonic anhydrase inhibitors in that there is a deficiency in bicarbonate reabsorption. Some of the causes include lead, multiple myeloma, and Fanconi's syndrome. Type IV or hyperkalemic distal RTA is most commonly seen in diabetic patients with underlying renal disease. In these patients the cause is hyporeninemic hypoaldosteronism. It usually presents as asymptomatic hyperkalemia but may occur after the use of drugs that can affect serum potassium levels. These drugs include potassium-sparing diuretics, angiotensin-converting enzyme inhibitors, nonsteroidal antiinflammatory drugs, and digoxin.

II. Treatment. In patients with non anion gap metabolic acidosis, the treatment should be directed at the underlying disorder. In most patients with non anion gap acidosis secondary to diarrhea, the kidney will be able to make bicarbonate to replace the deficit, and bicarbonate therapy is not required. I feel it is usually indicated in Type I and II RTA and in diarrheal disorders if plasma HCO_3 <10 mEq/L or pH <7.2, since the kidney's response will take time. The amount of $NaHCO_3$ needed to raise plasma HCO_3 to a given level can be estimated by the following formula:

$$NaHCO_3 \text{ dose} = (\text{desired } [HCO_3^-] - \text{observed } [HCO_3^-]) \times 50\% \text{ body weight (kg)}$$

The 50% of body weight is the estimated volume of distribution of HCO_3, but it can increase to greater than 100% of body weight in some patients with severe metabolic acidosis (HCO_3^- <5 mEq/L). In addition, the formula does not take into account continued loss of HCO_3, addition of acid during the time of correction, or the kidney response during correction. Therefore, bicarbonate therapy is empiric in patients with non anion gap metabolic acidosis and pH K^+, and HCO_3 levels need to be frequently monitored. Bicarbonate therapy should be given cautiously if the patient is hypokalemic since the increase in pH may cause a further decrease in K (see hypokalemia). If using bicarbonate, initially give two ampules of $NaHCO_3$ over 5 minutes, and then infuse 1000 ml D_5W with 2 to 3 ampules of $NaHCO_3$ at 200 to 250 ml/hr. If the patient is 70 kg and the volume of distribution is 50% of body weight (i.e., 35 L), then administration of 100 mEq of NaHCO$_3$ should increase plasma HCO$_3$ by 2 to 3 mEq/L.

Metabolic Alkalosis

An elevated serum bicarbonate level is either due to a primary metabolic alkalosis or secondary to chronic respiratory acidosis. Arterial blood gas measurements are required to differentiate the two possibilities. If the patient has secondary (compensatory) metabolic alkalosis, the pH should be acidemic and the plasma HCO$_3$ level should be increased about 3.5 mEq/L or pH decreased 0.03 for every 10 mm Hg increase in arterial carbon dioxide pressure (PaCO$_2$). If a patient has a primary metabolic alkalosis, the pH should be alkalemic and PaCO$_2$ increased 4 to 7 mm Hg for every 10 mEq/L increase in HCO$_3$. Some patients with lung disease can have both a primary respiratory acidosis and primary metabolic alkalosis, especially if on diuretics or vomiting.

I. **Causes.** Primary metabolic alkalosis requires a process to generate HCO$_3$ and also process(es) to maintain the metabolic alkalosis. Processes that generate HCO$_3$ include loss of H$^+$ in urine, emesis, or administration of alkali. Factors that maintain alkalosis include chloride depletion, increased reabsorption of chloride/bicarbonate, renal insufficiency, mineralocorticoid excess, and hypokalemia causing increased tubular reabsorption of bicarbonate. Metabolic alkalosis is classified based on urinary chloride concentrations as either chloride responsive or chloride resistant **(Table 12-9)**. The cause of metabolic alkalosis is usually evident from history and physical examination, and urinary electrolyte concentrations are not usually required.

II. **Symptoms.** The symptoms of metabolic alkalosis are usually due to a combination of alkalemia, other metabolic abnormalities (e.g., hyponatremia, hypophosphatemia, hypokalemia), volume depletion, and concomitant medical conditions (if present). They are similar to those seen with hypocalcemia and may include mental confusion, muscle cramps or weakness, cardiac arrhythmias, and neuromuscular irritability including tetany.

III. **Treatment.** Most patients with chloride-responsive metabolic alkalosis are volume depleted and require volume replacement, usually in the form of NaCl solution. Hypokalemia is invariably present in these patients, and treatment usually requires significant quantities of potassium chloride. As volume and potassium are restored, the patient excretes bicarbonate in the urine and the plasma bicarbonate level returns to normal. In patients who are fluid overloaded, acetazolamide may be effective by blocking proximal tubular reabsorption of sodium bicarbonate. In dialysis patients, dialysis with a low-bicarbonate dialysate may be indicated, since the kidney will not be able to excrete the bicarbonate. Intra-

Table 12-9. Causes of Metabolic Alkalosis

Chloride responsive (U$_{Cl}$ <15 mEq/L)	Chloride resistant (U$_{Cl}$ >15 mEq/L)
Vomiting	Excess mineralocorticoid activity
Nasogastric suctioning	Hyperaldosteronism
Correction of chronic hypercapnia	Cushing's syndrome
Diuretic therapy*	Bartter's syndrome

*If actively taking diuretics, U$_{Cl}$ may be >15 mEq/L.

venous HCl acid is rarely indicated in the management of metabolic alkalosis. Indications include severe metabolic alkalosis (pH >7.55) in a markedly symptomatic patient in CHF, or in a patient in renal failure when a low-bicarbonate dialysate bath is not available. In the rare situation where dilute HCl is given, the amount required is based on the formula below:

$$H^+ \text{ deficit (mEq/L)} = 0.2 \times \text{Body weight (kg)} \times (\text{measured [HCO}_3^-] - \text{desired [HCO}_3^-])$$

The solution is usually 0.1 HCl, which contains 150 mEq/L of hydrogen ion (H^+). The goal is to lower the plasma bicarbonate level halfway to normal over 12 hours. It is important to follow arterial blood gas and serum electrolyte values frequently during the administration of HCl solution.

Respiratory Alkalosis

Respiratory alkalosis results from an increased rate of pulmonary CO_2 excretion. The causes of respiratory alkalosis are included in **Table 12-10**. In evaluating patients, the serum bicarbonate and pH values are useful to differentiate acute from chronic respiratory alkalosis. In acute respiratory alkalosis the serum HCO_3 level decreases 1 to 2 mEq/L, and the pH increases 0.08 for every 10 mm Hg decrease in the Pa_{CO_2}. In chronic respiratory alkalosis the serum bicarbonate level can fall up to 4 mEq/L, and the pH increases 0.03 for every 10 mm Hg decrease in Pa_{CO_2}. Since this adaptation takes 48 to 72 hours, many patients, depending on duration, will have a decrease in bicarbonate level between 2 and 5 mEq/L and an increased pH between 0.03 and 0.08 for every 10 mm Hg decrease in Pa_{CO_2}. In addition, the underlying cause for the respiratory alkalosis may cause other acid-base abnormalities. Salicylates are a classic example where metabolic acidosis may be accompanying.

I. **Symptoms** are due to the respiratory alkalosis and any underlying disease(s). Symptoms produced by respiratory alkalosis include lightheadedness, altered consciousness, and paresthesias of the extremities and circumoral area. These symptoms are in part due to decreased ionized calcium levels. As pH increases, there is increased binding of ionized Ca^{++} to proteins, causing a decreased serum ionized

Table 12-10. Causes of Respiratory Alkalosis

Central Stimulation
Anxiety
Head trauma
Brain tumors
Fever
Pregnancy
Salicylates
Gram-negative septicemia
Pulmonary Disease
Pneumonia
Interstitial lung disease
Pulmonary embolus
Pulmonary edema
Asthma
Pleural effusion

Ca^{++} level. In addition, some of the symptoms are due to decreased cerebral flow as a result of respiratory alkalosis. Laboratory tests in patients with primary respiratory alkalosis often reveals a decreased serum PO_4 level.

II. **Treatment** is to treat the underlying cause of respiratory alkalosis and any accompanying abnormalities.

Respiratory Acidosis

Respiratory acidosis is characterized by acidosis and an elevated $PaCO_2$. Respiratory acidosis is also present if the $PaCO_2$ is higher than the expected compensation for patients with metabolic alkalosis or metabolic acidosis. In evaluating a patient with respiratory acidosis, it is essential to differentiate acute from chronic respiratory acidosis. Acute respiratory acidosis often requires immediate intubation unless the underlying process can be readily reversed. Chronic respiratory acidosis usually does not require immediate intubation. The serum bicarbonate or pH values help in making the distinction. In acute respiratory acidosis, the bicarbonate level increases about 1 mEq/L or pH decreases 0.08 for every 10 mm Hg increase in $PaCO_2$; in chronic respiratory acidosis, the HCO_3 increases 3.5 mEq/L or pH decreases 0.03 for every 10 mm Hg increase in $PaCO_2$.

I. **Clinical manifestations** include headache, agitation, and blurred vision and may progress to somnolence. Other manifestations may be due to any accompanying hypoxemia or other medical conditions.
II. **Treatment** of respiratory acidosis is covered in Chapter 9.

Hyponatremia

Hyponatremia refers to a decrease in the concentration of the serum sodium. Since sodium is the most prevalent osmotically active solute, patients are initially classified on the basis of their serum osmolality as high, normal, or low. An estimate of the serum osmolality is 2[Na] + [Glucose]/18 + [BUN]/2.8.

I. **Classification**
   A. **High serum osmolality.** The causes include hyperglycemia and administration of mannitol. These substances are osmotically active and cause a movement of water from the intracellular to extracellular space. This increase in extracellular water results in a dilution of the serum sodium concentration. Hyperglycemia causes the sodium level to decrease 1.3 to 1.6 mEq/L for each 100 mg/dl rise in the serum glucose level above normal. The treatment is to lower the serum glucose (see section on Hyperglycemia).
   B. **Normal serum osmolality or pseudohyponatremia.** The causes include hypertriglyceridemia and hyperproteinemia. These substances increase the nonaqueous portion of plasma (normally 5% to 7% of plasma volume) but are included in the plasma Na (mEq Na/L plasma). The amount of Na in the aqueous phase is normal, but since the plasma Na concentration includes the aqueous and nonaqueous phases, the measured Na level is low. Therefore, osmolality is normal since osmolality measures milliosmoles per liter of water and does not include the nonaqueous phase. No therapy is indicated except treating the underlying condition.
   C. **Low serum osmolality.** The causes of hyponatremia associated with a decreased osmolality are divided on the basis of their volume status into decreased extracellular fluid (ECF) volume, normal ECF volume, and volume excess usually with edema.

1. **Decreased ECF volume.** This results when there is a relatively greater loss of sodium than water. In the ED most patients have extrarenal losses caused by vomiting or diarrhea. As a result of volume depletion, the patients retain salt and retain H_2O because of nonosmotic release of antidiuretic hormone (ADH). Hyponatremia develops when there is increased free water intake relative to free water excretion. Urinary sodium is usually less than 20 mEq/L due to the effect of volume depletion stimulating Na^+ retention, and U_{osm} is usually elevated due to increased ADH levels. In patients with metabolic alkalosis (usually due to vomiting), urinary chloride levels should also be measured because these patients may be losing bicarbonate in the urine, accompanied by a loss of Na or K (see Metabolic Alkalosis). Renal sodium losses are seen in patients on hydrochlorothiazide and, most importantly, in patients with Addison's disease (see p. 390). In patients actively taking diuretics and with Addison's disease, urinary sodium levels are usually elevated >20 to 30 mEq/L. This sodium loss is inappropriate for the decreased volume status of the patient. Patients with diuretic-induced hyponatremia often have accompanying hypokalemia and metabolic alkalosis.

2. **Clinically normal ECF volume.** The causes include the syndrome of inappropriate secretion of antidiuretic hormone (SIADH), hypothyroidism, isolated glucocorticoid deficiency, or water intoxication. SIADH is seen in CNS disorders, pulmonary disorders, and carcinoma (especially small cell), as well as during treatment with certain drugs such as chlorpropamide and carbamazepine. The criteria for SIADH includes (1) hyponatremia and hypoosmolality, (2) U_{osm} inappropriately high for hyponatremia, (3) urine Na^+ concentration greater than 20 mEq/L, (4) normovolemia, and (5) normal renal, adrenal, and thyroid function. Hypothyroidism and glucocorticoid deficiency can also cause hyponatremia. Isolated glucocorticoid deficiency would be seen in patients on long-term steroid therapy who discontinue steroids, or in patients with hypopituitarism. These patients do not have Addison's disease since mineralocorticoid activity should still be intact. Some patients compulsively drink massive amounts of water in a short period and may present to the ED after drinking water at a rate greater than the kidney can excrete. U_{osm} is often difficult to interpret in these patients. One would anticipate a U_{osm} <100 mOsm/kg, but in most of these patients it is >100 mOsm/kg. An ADH-independent inability to minimally dilute the urine has been described in these patients, but in addition, some of these patients after developing hyponatremia have nausea and/or vomiting that may temporarily increase ADH and U_{osm}. The history is very important in making the diagnosis of compulsive water drinking. Since these patients have clinically normal ECF and are able to maintain sodium homeostasis, they usually have a urinary sodium >20 mEq/L.

3. **Expanded ECF.** These patients usually have edema and include patients with congestive heart failure, liver disease, renal failure, and nephrotic syndrome. Patients with congestive heart failure, liver disease, and some patients with nephrotic syndrome have a decreased effective circulating volume, which causes a sodium- and water-retaining state. Urinary Na is usually low (unless on a diuretic), and U_{osm} is increased. As can be seen, the urinary values are identical to what is seen in volume-depleted patients.

II. Symptoms.
The symptoms are in part related to the rapidity and duration of the decrease in serum sodium concentration. It is not uncommon to have an asymptomatic patient with chronic hyponatremia with a Na level <110 mEq/L. Symptoms may include confusion progressing to coma, seizures, weakness, and vomiting.

III. Treatment of hyponatremia without associated neurologic deficits

A. **Hyponatremia with decreased ECF.** These patients need repletion of their ECF with isotonic saline solution. Infusion of isotonic saline results in these patients receiving salt in excess of H_2O (isotonic saline 154 mEq/L). In addition, repletion of ECF causes an increase in free water excretion. Patients with Addison's disease need glucocorticoid and mineralocorticoid replacement (see Addison's disease).

B. **Hyponatremia with normal ECF.** These patients need treatment of the underlying cause and water restriction, since the hyponatremia results from free water intake greater than free water excretion.

C. **Hyponatremia with expanded ECF.** The therapy is to treat the underlying cause and to decrease Na and water intake, since these patients are volume overloaded. Normal saline solution should not be used in these patients because the saline will be retained and exacerbate the underlying fluid overload. In patients with CHF or renal failure, loop diuretics can be very effective in increasing urine volume and free water excretion. This is potentially hazardous in patients with decompensated liver disease or nephrotic syndrome because intravascular volume depletion may result.

IV. Treatment of hyponatremia with associated neurologic deficits.
There is no consensus on how rapidly or to what level the serum Na should be raised in patients with neurologic deficits manifested by stupor, coma, or seizures. The following are general guidelines: (1) initial therapy should raise the serum sodium level 1 to 2 mEq/hr for 2 to 3 hours; (2) sodium levels should not increase more than 12 mEq in 24 hours (some authors say 20 mEq/day); (3) aggressive therapy should stop when the Na level is 125 to 130 mEq/L; and (4) avoid hypernatremia during the correction. The initial increase in serum sodium levels is indicated in these patients to decrease cerebral edema. In spite of these recommendations, sodium levels (especially in volume-depleted patients and compulsive water drinkers) often rise more rapidly than anticipated. In patients who clinically respond as the sodium levels increase, it is important to stop aggressive therapy to avoid the development of hypernatremia. The concern about increasing sodium levels too rapidly is that central pontine myelinolysis, manifested by paralysis, could develop. In the ED, initial therapy is based on the cause of hyponatremia.

A. **Hyponatremia with decreased ECF.** Normal saline solution is still appropriate therapy in these patients since restoration of intravascular volume will correct the hyponatremia. The rate of rise in serum Na level is not predictable in these patients because as the patient's volume is repleted, urine volume increases resulting in increased free water excretion and rapid correction of hyponatremia.

B. **Hyponatremia with normal ECF.** In patients with compulsive water drinking, therapy depends in part on the patient's urine volume. If the patient is excreting >300 ml/hr of urine, water restriction alone should cause a rapid increase in serum Na concentration. If urine output is <300 ml/hr, then 1 ml/kg/hr of 3% saline solution is indicated for 2 to 3 hours. In most of these patients, complete recovery is expected even if they had seizures. Patients with SIADH have a normal total body sodium, and the hyponatremia is due to increased total body water. An estimate of the increase in total body water is calculated with the following formula:

$$\text{Free water excess} = (0.6 \times BW)(S_{Na}/140)$$

Since the problem is an excess of total body water, one approach is to diurese the patient with intravenous furosemide or bumetanide and replace the Na and K losses with a hypertonic solution (usually 3% saline, i.e., 513 mEq/L), resulting in a pure loss of water. The advantage of this approach is that it prevents fluid overloading the patient and it causes a loss of free water, which is the patient's problem. In patients with neurologic deficits, infuse 1 to 2 ml/kg/hr of 3% saline solution and diurese the patient with furosemide, 40 mg, or bumetanide, 1 mg. An infusion of 1 ml/kg of 3% saline solution should cause the sodium concentration to increase about 1 mEq/L. One hour after the diuretic is given, obtain a urinary sodium concentration and begin replacement of sodium and potassium losses with 3% saline solution and supplemental potassium.

$$\text{Sodium losses} = U_{Na} \times V$$
$$\text{Amount of 3\% saline solution to replace Na losses} =$$
$$\frac{\text{Sodium losses}}{513 \text{ mEq/L}} = \frac{U_{Na} \times V}{513 \text{ mEq/L}}$$

Replace the urinary sodium losses during the previous 2 hours with hypertonic saline solution given over the next 2 hours. The advantage of this method is that the rise in Na concentration will be due to water losses and that it will depend on the patient's urine volume, which is mainly dependent on dose and frequency of intravenous diuretics.

C. Hyponatremia with expanded ECF
  1. **CHF.** Severe hyponatremia in a patient with CHF usually implies severe left ventricular dysfunction. Since these patients are salt and water loaded, therapy should be to increase free water losses with diuresis. These patients often do not respond to intravenous furosemide or bumetanide and often require inotropic support with dobutamine. Invasive hemodynamic monitoring in a critical care unit is usually required.
  2. **Renal failure.** In a volume-overloaded nondialyzed patient, therapy should be to diurese with high-dose loop-acting diuretics (100 to 400 mg furosemide or 2 to 5 mg bumetanide). Dialysis may be necessary if the patient does not respond to diuresis. Dialysis is indicated if the patient is on chronic dialysis.
  3. **Liver disease with ascites.** These patients are very difficult to treat. Diuresis is very difficult in these patients because they are in an active sodium- and water-retaining state. In addition, diuresis may decrease intravascular volume, resulting in hypotension and/or renal decompensation. In order to raise the sodium concentration 1 mEq/L/hr, the sodium deficit formula (misnomer in this case) can be used: Na deficit = Volume of distribution × Change in sodium level. For example, in an 80 kg patient where the goal is to raise the Na 1 mEq/L/hr, the volume of distribution is about 0.7 × 80 kg. Therefore the patient would require about 56

mEq/hr of sodium, which is about 100 ml/hr of 3% saline solution. The hypertonic saline solution is only indicated for 2 to 3 hours, and if possible any further rise in Na concentration should be by an increase in free water loss.

Hypernatremia

When hypernatremia is seen in the ED, it frequently is associated with a disease where physical immobility or altered mental status prevents the patient from having access to water. The classification of hypernatremia is similar to hyponatremia, where patients are classified on the basis of their volume status.

I. **Causes**
   A. **Sodium and water losses.** These patients have a disorder associated with a loss of salt and water and an inability to adequately replace water losses. Some of the causes include diarrhea, vomiting, diuretics, hyperglycemia, and sweating. It is seen typically in an elderly patient with dementia or a recent stroke who has losses of salt and free water secondary to diuretics, diarrhea, or a febrile illness and does not replace those losses of salt and especially water. Patients with nonrenal losses will usually have low urinary sodium levels and concentrated urine because they are in a volume-depleted state and are appropriately trying to conserve sodium and water. The urinary sodium levels and osmolality are identical to the values seen with hyponatremia due to volume depletion, with serum sodium levels depending on the amount of water intake.
   B. **Losses of water.** These patients have water losses as a result of diabetes insipidus (DI). Possibilities include central DI, partial central DI, nephrogenic DI, and partial nephrogenic DI. One important cause of nephrogenic DI in the ED is lithium toxicity. Most of these patients will have polyuria and normal serum sodium levels or mild hypernatremia, unless an underlying condition limits their access to water in the setting of hypernatremia. Some patients will have hypernatremia during hospitalization if they receive normal saline solution and continue to lose free water because of their DI.
   C. **Salt and water overload.** Hypernatremia is a rare condition since most of these patients have hyponatremia as a result of decreased ability to excrete free water. In the ED hypernatremia may be seen after hypertonic sodium bicarbonate administration during cardiac arrest, dialysis against a high-sodium concentrate dialysate, a sea water drowning, or an attempted suicide with ingestion of salt tablets.

II. **Symptoms.** The most prominent manifestations are neurologic and occur as a result of cellular dehydration. The brain attempts to compensate for the cellular dehydration by forming poorly defined osmoles known as organic osmolytes. These may be present within 4 hours. Because of these osmolytes, brain water is often not severely decreased. Manifestations include restlessness, irritability, and lethargy progressing to coma, seizures, and death, with a mortality rate as high as 60%.

III. **Treatment.** The goal of treatment is to restore the serum sodium concentration to normal. However, due in part to an accumulation of organic osmolytes in the brain, therapy should be slow. Therapy that is too rapid may result in marked cerebral edema and a deterioration in mental status. There is no consensus on how rapidly to lower the serum sodium level, but in general, serum sodium concentration should be lowered about 10 to 15 mEq/24 hours. In patients with a pure loss of water, the water deficit to lower the sodium level to 140 mEq/L is calculated as follows:

$$\text{Water deficit} = (0.6 \times \text{BW}) ((\text{Serum Na}/140) - 1)$$

A. Volume depletion. These patients often have clinically significant volume depletion (hypotension, renal failure, decreased urine output); however, the deficit is predominantly free water. Initially isotonic saline solution is given until hemodynamics are stabilized, and subsequently D_5W, $D_5W\frac{1}{4}NS$, or $D_5W\frac{1}{2}NS$ is appropriate. The water deficit formula can help in estimating the rate of infusion of free water.

> Example: Wt 70 kg, Na 168 mEq/L.
> Water deficit = (0.6 x 70 kg) ((168/140) − 1) = 8.4 L

So 8.4 L of water should lower the Na 28 mEq/L, or 300 ml to lower the Na 1 mEq/L. Since the goal is about ½ mEq/L/hr, this would be 150 ml of free water per hour (i.e., 200 ml $D_5\frac{1}{4}NS$ or 150 ml D_5W). The formulas are not always adequate, especially if free water loss is ongoing. Frequent monitoring of electrolytes is indicated.

B. Water losses. Most of these patients will have polyuria and not hypernatremia since free water intake should be able to match free water excretion. If these patients have hypernatremia, they can be very difficult to manage because they usually have large urine volumes causing massive water losses. If appropriate therapy is not instituted immediately, ongoing water losses may result in a further increase in the serum sodium concentration. In these patients with hypernatremia, send urine for Na and U_{osm}. Before the results of the urinary electrolytes are known, replace ongoing urinary losses with D_5W or D_5W ¼ NS hourly, milliliter for milliliter. This will prevent a further rise in the serum sodium level. Treat the water deficit with D_5W to decrease the serum sodium level about ½ mEq/L/hr. It is also imperative to attempt to decrease urinary free water losses, and 1-deamino-8-D-arginine vasopressin (DDAVP) should be administered intranasally, intravenously, or subcutaneously. Measure U_{osm} 1 hour after DDAVP administration to see if there is an increased U_{osm}, implying central diabetes insipidus.

C. Sodium and water excess. In these patients diuresis of excess sodium is indicated along with 5% dextrose infusion.

Hypokalemia

Potassium is the major intracellular cation in the body, with more than 90% located intracellularly and only 1.4% found in the extracellular space. The high intracellular potassium concentration is due to sustained activity of the Na-K pump, which transports potassium into cells and sodium out of cells. Normally any leak of potassium out of cells is balanced by the Na-K pump. A variety of factors modify the transcellular distribution of potassium. These factors are important in the differential diagnosis and treatment of disorders of potassium.

I. Factors affecting transcellular distribution
  A. Acid-base homeostasis. A low pH promotes potassium exit from cells, and a high pH promotes potassium entry into cells. The change in potassium concentration with a low pH depends on many factors including whether the acidosis is metabolic or respiratory and whether the metabolic acidosis is organic or mineral. Organic acidosis (e.g., lactic, β-hydroxybutyrate, acetoacetate)

causes less of a change in potassium concentration than mineral acids (i.e., hydrochloric acid). Infusion of organic acids is not accompanied by a significant change in potassium concentration, while mineral acids increase potassium levels (average 0.7 mEq/L/0.1 pH unit).

B. Insulin. Insulin promotes cellular potassium uptake by a mechanism independent of glucose transport, with higher insulin levels promoting greater transport.

C. Catecholamines. Catecholamines have varying effects on the serum potassium level depending on whether they are β-adrenergic or α-adrenergic. The $β_2$-agonists promote cellular potassium uptake, while nonselective β-blocking agents interfere with this uptake. The α-adrenergic agonists increase plasma potassium levels by promoting potassium release from liver and probably from muscle.

D. Aldosterone. Aldosterone has a role in transcellular potassium distribution in addition to its effect on increasing urinary potassium losses.

E. Osmolality. An increase in serum osmolality causes water movement from the intracellular to extracellular fluid, increasing intracellular potassium. The serum potassium level increases because of solvent drag of potassium from the water movement, and increased intracellular potassium increases the transcellular gradient promoting potassium exit from cells. This increase in osmolality is particularly important in diabetics with hyperglycemia.

II. Causes

A. Pseudohypokalemia. Pseudohypokalemia is seen in a setting of many leukocytes, which are metabolically active and take up potassium if they are allowed to stand.

B. Transcellular shift. Any condition that is associated with endogenous release of catecholamines can cause a transient hypokalemia. This may be seen in many acute illnesses including congestive heart failure, delirium tremens, and myocardial infarction. One important disorder causing transcellular shift is hypokalemic periodic paralysis, often due to underlying hyperthyroidism. It is usually seen in people of Asian descent, and precipitating events that have been implicated include carbohydrate intake, exertion, and epinephrine administration. These patients often are seen with acute flaccid paralysis.

C. Hypokalemia with potassium deficit. Hypokalemia secondary to deficits in total body potassium is due to either poor potassium intake, treatment of megaloblastic anemia, gastrointestinal losses, or renal losses.

1. Inadequate intake. This is an unusual isolated cause of hypokalemia since the kidney can significantly lower potassium excretion. However hypokalemia may be seen in patients with anorexia nervosa because there is often accompanying vomiting, diuretic use, or laxative abuse. Alcoholics not only may have decreased intake of potassium but also may have stool losses because of diarrhea or urinary losses of potassium from magnesium deficiency (see below).

2. Gastrointestinal losses. These are usually due to diarrhea, which is often accompanied by concomitant metabolic acidosis due to loss of bicarbonate. Laxative abuse is often a very difficult diagnosis to make because patients often deny taking laxatives. Ureterosigmoidostomy (rarely done) and obstructed ileal loop can cause hypokalemia resulting from absorption of sodium chloride with secretion of potassium and bicarbonate into the lumen.

3. Renal losses. Type I RTA (distal) and Type II RTA (proximal) are both associated with a decreased serum bicarbonate. Carbonic anhydrase inhibitors (acetazolamide) can cause hypokalemia and metabolic acidosis mimicking Type II RTA. Bartter's syndrome includes severe hypokalemia, metabolic alkalosis, renal potassium and chloride wasting, normotension, hyperreninemia, and hyperaldosteronism. The syndrome is rare and usually the patients are on diuretics (some surreptitiously). Primary aldosteronism secondary to adrenal hyperplasia or adenoma is usually associated with mild metabolic alkalosis. In addition, patients are usually hypertensive. Glucocorticoid excess may also be associated with hypokalemia. The hypokalemia seen in vomiting is predominantly due to renal potassium losses as a result of bicarbonaturia. Hypomagnesemia is often associated with hypokalemia due to renal potassium losses. Diabetic ketoacidosis is associated with potassium depletion, but due to acidemia, lack of insulin, and increased osmolality, these patients usually have normal or elevated potassium levels. If hypokalemia is seen in DKA, profound potassium depletion is usually present and insulin therapy is potentially very hazardous, since profound hypokalemia may result (see DKA).

III. **Manifestations.** These usually do not occur unless the serum potassium level is less than 3.0 mEq/L, but in patients with heart disease (especially patients on digitalis), potassium levels less 3.5 mEq/L may be associated with cardiac abnormalities. Symptoms of hypokalemia include neuromuscular disturbances (weakness, fatigue, paresthesias, hyporeflexia, rhabdomyolysis), gastrointestinal disturbances (constipation, ileus), cardiovascular disturbances (U waves, T wave flattening, ST segment depression), renal disturbances (nephrogenic DI, rarely hypokalemic nephropathy), and metabolic disturbances (glucose intolerance).

IV. **Treatment**
   A. The **deficit of potassium** is very difficult to estimate on the basis of a serum potassium level. This is because potassium is predominantly located in cells, and a variety of factors (see above) affect the transcellular distribution. An asthmatic patient receiving epinephrine or inhaled β-agonist may have a decrease in serum potassium concentration secondary to intracellular movement but no potassium deficit. A diabetic patient in ketoacidosis with a serum potassium of 3.0 mEq/L has a profound deficit (200 to 400 mEq), but serum potassium concentration is only slightly decreased because the increased glucose levels, decreased insulin levels, and acidemia decrease potassium movement into cells. A rough estimate of the potassium deficit is that for every 1 mEq/L decrease in serum potassium concentration, the deficit is 100 to 400 mEq/L. Most patients with hypokalemia have mild hypokalemia and can be treated orally with potassium chloride.
   B. **Intravenous therapy** is indicated in patients with mild hypokalemia who cannot take oral replacement or in patients with severe hypokalemia. In mild hypokalemia, intravenous potassium should not be infused at a rate greater than 10 mEq/hr. In patients with severe hypokalemia (K^+ <2.5 mEq/L) or hypokalemia associated with cardiac arrhythmias, extreme muscle weakness, or rhabdomyolysis, aggressive intravenous therapy is indicated. It should be administered in a glucose-free solution because glucose increases insulin levels and may cause potassium levels to fall further. Therapy can be given at rates of 20 to 30 mEq/hr and rarely 40 mEq/hr with ECG monitoring and frequent (every 1 to 2 hours) monitoring of the serum potassium concentration. Once the emergency has resolved, the rate should be decreased to 10 to 20 mEq/hr. When infusing potassium at a concentration greater than 60 mEq/L, it should be infused through a central vein, since it is a venous irritant.

Hyperkalemia

I. Causes

A. Pseudohyperkalemia. This is seen when a tight tourniquet is around an exercising extremity. Hemolysis at the time of blood drawing can also raise the serum potassium level. However, it is important not to assume the entire elevation in the potassium level is due to hemolysis, especially if there is an underlying condition that may be associated with hyperkalemia. Leukocytosis in the range of 70,000 to 100,000 per cubic millimeter and platelet counts greater than 1 million per cubic millimeter can increase the potassium concentration as a result of releasing potassium during clotting. If this is suspected, then measurement of serum potassium needs to be repeated by placing the blood sample in a heparinized container.

B. Transcellular shift. Acidosis causing a transcellular shift is more likely with mineral acids (HCl) than organic acids. Succinylcholine increases muscle potassium permeability, resulting in potassium moving into the ECF space. The rise in potassium concentration is only 0.5 mEq/L but may be significant if the potassium concentration is already elevated. β_2-Adrenergic blockers usually cause the potassium level to rise only 0.1 to 0.2 mEq/L. Insulin deficiency may contribute to hyperkalemia associated with hyperosmolality in diabetic patients by not being able to promote a potassium shift back into cells. Digitalis intoxication as a result of blocking Na-K-ATPase can cause severe hyperkalemia unresponsive to all measures, and requires treatment with digoxin antibodies. Hyperkalemic periodic paralysis is a rare autosomal dominant disorder.

C. Potassium excess. This is due to iatrogenic causes, a decrease in renal function, a deficiency of aldosterone, or a defect in tubular potassium secretion. It can also be seen in conditions where rapid endogenous intracellular release of potassium occurs from cell lysis (tumor lysis syndrome, rhabdomyolysis, hemolysis) or when there is excessive intake. Since the body is able to closely regulate the serum potassium level, increased intake does not usually cause potassium concentration to rise unless there is some defect in potassium excretion.

1. **Renal failure.** As a result of adaptive mechanisms, most patients with chronic renal failure do not develop a problem with hyperkalemia. Hyperkalemia may result when potassium intake is increased or the patients are given a drug which interferes with potassium excretion. Acute renal failure, especially if oliguric, is a common setting for the development of severe hyperkalemia. The highest risk patients are those with renal failure due to rhabdomyolysis or tumor lysis syndrome as a result of intracellular release.

2. **Deficiency of aldosterone.** This may be due to Addison's disease (see Endocrine) but is more commonly due to the syndrome of hyporeninemic hypoaldosteronism (SHH). SHH is usually seen in patients with underlying renal disease (usually diabetics). It is usually the explanation for the increased potassium level with renal disease when the GFR is not low enough (<10 to 15 ml/min) to explain the hyperkalemia. It may present as an asymptomatic elevation of the potassium level, but significant elevations of the potassium level can result in these patients, especially if they are given drugs interfering with potassium excretion (see below).

3. **Primary renal tubular potassium secretory defects.** These can be seen in systemic lupus erythematosus, sickle cell disease, and obstructive uropa-

thy. The initial manifestion of obstructive uropathy may be hyperkalemia. In patients with obstructive uropathy, SHH has also been described.
 4. **Drugs.** These cause hyperkalemia by either directly interfering with potassium excretion, opposing the action of aldosterone, or decreasing levels of aldosterone. Triamterene and amiloride are potassium-sparing diuretics that directly block potassium excretion, while spironolactone antagonizes the action of aldosterone. Angiotensin-converting enzyme (ACE) inhibitors cause a decrease in angiotensin II levels. Since angiotensin II normally stimulates aldosterone, this may result in an increase in serum potassium levels. In most patients this is not a problem because the decline in aldosterone is not enough to affect the serum potassium level. However, in patients with renal disease with low-baseline levels of aldosterone (see SHH), this drop in aldosterone may result in hyperkalemia. It is also a concern if the ACE inhibitors are combined with potassium-sparing diuretics, since both drugs can cause an increase in serum potassium levels. Other drugs include the nonsteroidal antiinflammatory agents, heparin, and cyclosporine.
II. **Manifestations.** These usually begin when the serum potassium level is >6.5 mEq/L but can occur at lower levels if the patient has underlying cardiac disease. The life-threatening manifestations involve the cardiac effects. Usually the earliest manifestation is peaking of the T waves. Subsequently other changes include first-degree AV block, flattening of P waves, QRS widening, and eventually loss of R waves and widening of the S and T waves, so they blend together forming a sine-wave configuration. Ventricular arrhythmias including ventricular fibrillation may occur. The sequence of changes is not predictable, and patients may progress over minutes from a normal ECG to ventricular fibrillation or asystole. Cardiac arrhythmias are more likely in patients with underlying cardiac disease or in patients taking cardiac medications. Neuromuscular effects are not usually seen until the serum potassium level is >7.0 mEq/L.
III. **Treatment.** The following are various therapies available to treat hyperkalemia:
 A. **Calcium** will antagonize the cardiac and neuromuscular effects of hyperkalemia. Calcium gluconate (10 ml of a 10% solution or 93 mg elemental calcium) given over a few minutes will usually have an effect within minutes and last about 30 minutes. Calcium administration is potentially hazardous in renal failure due to calcium phosphate precipitation, especially if the phosphate concentration is >8 mg/dl. Calcium therapy is also dangerous in the setting of digitalis intoxication (increased incidence of digitalis toxic arrhythmias). Even in renal failure, however, calcium administration is still indicated if there are significant ECG changes or neuromuscular effects.
 B. **Insulin** infusion will cause the serum potassium level to decrease as a result of intracellular shift. Various regimens have been used: (1) infuse 10 units of insulin in 500 ml $D_{10}W$ over 1 hour, checking plasma glucose levels every 30 minutes; or (2) infuse 10 units of insulin by intravenous push with one ampule (50 ml) of $D_{50}W$ (25 gm), checking glucose levels at 30 minutes and 1 hour. Both insulin and glucose should be given simultaneously since in an acute situation, failure to administer glucose may result in hypoglycemia. If the patient has diabetes with glucose level >500 mg/dl, an intravenous bolus of 10 units of insulin followed by 0.1 units/kg/hr is indicated (see Diabetes).
 C. **Sodium bicarbonate** administration as a result of increasing pH may cause a transcellular shift of potassium from the ECF to the ICF. If bicarbonate is used, one ampule (50 mEq HCO_3/50 ml) is infused over 5 minutes.

D. **Nebulized albuterol** has also been recently used for hyperkalemia in patients on dialysis. The β_2-adrenergic drug promotes ECF to ICF flux of potassium. In one study, patients receiving 10 mg and 20 mg of albuterol had a fall in potassium levels of 0.5 mEq/L and 0.9 mEq/L, respectively, at 60 minutes.

E. **Dialysis** can be very effective in lowering the potassium level as a result of dialyzing against a 0 or 1 mEq/L dialysate. It should be reserved for patients in whom conservative methods are ineffective. The treatment depends on the level of potassium, the degree of neuromuscular and cardiac effects, and the underlying disorders causing the hyperkalemia. If the potassium level is 5.5 mEq/L in an asymptomatic patient with mild renal insufficiency receiving potassium-sparing diuretics, discontinuing the medication is appropriate. In contrast, a potassium level of 5.5 mEq/L in a patient with acute oliguric renal failure caused by rhabdomyolysis requires therapy to remove potassium from the body, since potassium will continue to be released from the damaged muscle.

In general, levels greater than 6.0 mEq/L, even if asymptomatic, need more aggressive therapy including active removal from the body. Usually the patients are given sodium polystyrene sulfonate (Kayexalate), a cation exchange resin. About 1 gm of Kayexalate (1.5 mEq Na) will exchange with 1 mEq of potassium. The preferred route of administration is oral, and it is given with sorbitol. Usually 30 to 50 gm of Kayexalate in 100 to 200 ml of a 20% sorbitol solution is given every 3 to 4 hours until the potassium level has normalized. If the patient cannot take Kayexalate orally, a retention enema (50 gm in 50 ml of 70% sorbitol solution added to 100 to 200 ml of water) is indicated. It should be retained for 30 to 60 minutes and can be given again at 3- to 4-hour intervals. In patients with symptomatic hyperkalemia or ECG changes, more aggressive therapy is indicated.

In unstable patients, it is important to first stabilize the myocardium with calcium and administer agents that cause potassium to move intracellularly. Insulin and nebulized albuterol can be used at the same time. On average, the potassium level should be decreased by 1.2 mEq/L after 1 hour. Once the patient is stable, Kayexalate (orally or rectally) needs to be given to remove potassium from the body. Some patients need to be retreated with intravenous medications because the acute effects may have dissipated before the resin is effective. The serum potassium level needs to be followed every 1 hour until the level is decreasing. The potassium level should subsequently be followed every 2 to 4 hours.

Disorders of Calcium

The measurement of the total serum calcium includes the measurement of ionized calcium (Ca^{++}) and bound calcium. In interpreting a total serum calcium level one needs to know the serum albumin level, since about 45% of calcium is bound to protein (mainly albumin). In order to correct the serum Ca level for a decreased albumin level the following formula is used: Corrected Ca^{++} = Serum Ca + 0.8(4.5 gm/dl − Patient's albumin level). This is only a rough estimate, and if available an ionized Ca^{++} should be used.

I. **Hypocalcemia**

A. **Causes.** The most common cause of a low total calcium level is a low serum albumin level. Ideally a measurement of an ionized Ca should be done, but if not available a corrected calcium level can be estimated by using the above formula. Other causes include hypomagnesemia, alcoholism, gastrointestinal disease (vitamin D malabsorption), renal insufficiency, rhabdomyolysis, pancreatitis, hypoparathyroidism, severe hyperphosphatemia, and treatment with diphenylhydantoin.

B. Clinical manifestations. These depend on the underlying cause(s), duration, severity, accompanying electrolyte abnormalities, and pH. Many patients with chronic renal failure have significant decreases in Ca^{++} levels and are asymptomatic. The main clinical manifestations of hypocalcemia are neuromuscular, where patients usually have circumoral and acral paresthesias. This may progress to carpopedal spasm and rarely laryngeal involvement. Latent tetany may be detected by Chvostek's or Trousseau's sign. Chvostek's sign refers to a facial twitch on tapping the branches of the facial nerve, but this can be seen in 25% of adults. Trousseau's sign is carpal spasm produced after 3 minutes of inflation of a blood pressure cuff above systolic pressure. Both signs may not be seen in patients with clinically significant tetany. Acidemia protects against tetany, and treating acidemia may precipitate severe tetany. Alkalemia appears to potentiate tetany. Central nervous system manifestations include seizures, delirium, dementia, and papilledema. Cardiac manifestations include prolonged QT interval and rarely ventricular fibrillation and heart block. Hypotension and heart failure have also been reported.

C. Treatment. Most patients with hypocalcemia do not usually require intravenous calcium. Most patients with a low serum calcium level have hypoalbuminemia but a normal ionized calcium level. In addition, most patients with a low ionized calcium level are asymptomatic, and acute treatment is also not indicated. In patients with acute symptomatic hypocalcemia manifested by seizures, cardiac arrhythmias, or tetany, intravenous calcium is indicated. Initially one to two ampules of calcium gluconate (each ampule is 10 ml containing 93 mg of elemental calcium) is given as a slow intravenous push over a few minutes. Usually one to two ampules will be effective in stopping the acute symptoms. This can be followed by 15 mg/kg of calcium as a continuous infusion over 4 to 6 hours. Ideally ionized Ca^{++} levels should be followed, but if not available total calcium levels can be followed. After the acute intravenous infusion the patient should be followed, and subsequent therapy will depend on the underlying cause. In any patient with hypocalcemia, especially in an alcoholic patient, magnesium depletion should be suspected and treated if present. Treatment of hypocalcemia caused by magnesium depletion requires treatment of the magnesium deficiency to be effective (see Magnesium).

II. Hypercalcemia. Hypercalcemia refers to an elevation of the ionized calcium level above 1.29 mmol/L or total calcium level above 10.5 mg/dl. The measured total calcium includes both ionized and bound calcium, with the ionized Ca^{++} level clinically more important.

A. Causes. These include hyperparathyroidism, malignancy, hypervitaminosis D, milk-alkali syndrome, sarcoidosis, thiazide diuretics, immobilization, familial hypocalciuric hypercalcemia, hyperthyroidism, and Addison's disease. In dialysis patients, hypercalcemia may be due to vitamin D therapy, calcium intake, aluminum-induced osteomalacia, or severe secondary hyperparathyroidism. Symptomatic hypercalcemia in the ED is usually due to malignancy. The most common malignancies are multiple myeloma, and cancers of the lung, breast, prostate, or kidney.

- **B. Clinical manifestations.** Since calcium is important in many physiologic processes, the manifestations may involve many organ systems. The clinical presentation depends on the absolute level, rate of development, and underlying cause. It may involve the kidney (nephrogenic diabetes insipidus, stones, acute decline in glomerular filtration rate), the gastrointestinal tract (nausea, vomiting, constipation, peptic ulcer disease), the neuromuscular system (weakness, lethargy, confusion, coma), the cardiovascular system (shortened QT interval, cardiac arrhythmia, digitalis toxicity, hypertension), or the skeletal system (pseudogout, arthralgias, bone pain).
- **C. Evaluation.** Most patients seen in the ED with symptomatic hypercalcemia have an underlying malignancy. If the cause is not known, the history will usually provide information on calcium carbonate ingestion (milk-alkali syndrome), thiazide diuretics, immobilization, vitamin D ingestion, and family contribution (familial hypocalciuric hypercalcemia). Multiple myeloma should be considered if the patient has anemia, a peripheral blood smear showing rouleaux, renal failure, or lytic lesions on radiographic studies.
- **D. Therapies.** Current therapies decrease calcium by either (1) enhancing urinary excretion of Ca, (2) reducing intestinal absorption, (3) decreasing bone resorption, or (4) extracellular removal by dialysis.
  1. **Volume expansion.** Most patients with symptomatic hypercalcemia are volume depleted as a result of decreased fluid intake, vomiting, and increased urinary losses due to hypercalcemia-induced nephrogenic DI. Volume depletion decreases urinary calcium excretion secondary to a combination of a decreased GFR and an enhanced calcium reabsorption. Initial therapy consists of 1 to 2 L of 0.9% saline solution, followed by 250 ml/hr of 0.9% saline solution until volume is repleted. Volume repletion should increase GFR and increase calcium excretion, resulting in a decrease in serum calcium levels.
  2. **Saline diuresis with furosemide.** This can increase calcium excretion by (1) enabling more saline solution to be administered, and (2) directly inhibiting calcium reabsorption. After the patient is volume repleted, 20 to 40 mg of furosemide can be given intravenously with the patient receiving 250 ml/hr of 0.9% saline solution alternating with 0.45% saline solution. It is mandatory not to initiate furosemide therapy until after the patient is volume expanded. Careful following of intake and output, as well as serum electrolyte, and Mg^{++} levels, is required.
  3. **Calcitonin.** Calcitonin can be very effective, especially in carcinoma or severe hyperparathyroidism, by inhibiting bone resorption. Initially 4 to 8 units/kg are given subcutaneously every 6 to 12 hours. It can lower the serum calcium level by 2 to 3 mg/dl. Calcitonin or mithramycin should be considered as initial therapy if the patient is volume overloaded or if the patient with renal failure does not rapidly respond to hydration and furosemide.
  4. **Glucocorticoids.** These decrease the serum calcium level in patients with tumors by a direct lytic effect on the tumor and by inhibiting osteoclastic activity. Tumors likely to respond include multiple myeloma, lymphomas, and breast cancer.
  5. **Dialysis.** This is only a temporary measure but may be necessary in a patient with renal failure due to hypercalcemia who does not respond to other measures, or in a patient who is fluid overloaded.

E. **Treatment.** In most patients in the ED with symptomatic hypercalcemia, initial treatment consists of volume expansion with saline solution followed by saline diuresis with furosemide. It is imperative to know the cause of hypercalcemia because subsequent therapy will depend on the underlying cause. In patients with renal insufficiency and hypercalcemia, lowering of the calcium level may improve GFR. These patients may not respond to volume expansion and therefore should be closely followed. They are likely to become fluid overloaded, and additional measures including calcitonin administration and hemodialysis may be indicated.

Disorders of Phosphorus

The total phosphorus content in a 70 kg adult is 700 to 800 gm, of which 80% is in bone, 9% in skeletal muscle, and 11% in soft tissue. Almost all blood phosphorus exists as phosphate anions (PO_4^{-3}, HPO_4^{-2}, $H_2PO_4^{-}$). The laboratory usually measures elemental phosphorus (P) in milligrams/deciliter, with normal values considered to be from 2.5 to 4.5 mg/dl. Phosphate is the major intracellular anion, and similar to potassium its concentration in the blood can change rapidly as a result of intracellular shifts.

I. **Hypophosphatemia**
   A. **Causes.** These include inadequate intake, decreased intestinal absorption, transcellular shifts, and decreased renal reabsorption. One of the most common causes of hypophosphatemia is respiratory alkalosis, which causes an intracellular shift. The respiratory alkalosis may be due to pain, sepsis, alcoholic withdrawal, hepatic encephalopathy, or salicylate intoxication. Alcoholics often have hypophosphatemia as a result of poor intake, use of antacids, vomiting, and the presence of respiratory alkalosis. In addition, hypomagnesemia is often seen in alcoholics and can increase urinary excretion of phosphorus. In alcoholics, the serum phosphorus level may initially be low, normal, or high but usually falls rapidly secondary to the administration of glucose-containing fluids, causing an intracellular shift. The treatment of DKA with insulin often leads to severe hypophosphatemia (see DKA). Administration of glucose-containing fluids to malnourished patients often causes an intracellular shift. Other causes include phosphate-binding antacid therapy.
   B. **Clinical manifestations.** Many organ systems are involved because phosphorus is the major intracellular anion. Manifestations include erythrocyte dysfunction with hemolysis, leukocyte dysfunction, platelet dysfunction, muscle weakness including the respiratory muscles, rhabdomyolysis, CNS dysfunction (metabolic encephalopathy), osteolysis, metabolic acidosis secondary to decreased titratable acid, and cardiomyopathy.
   C. **Treatment.** This depends on the clinical manifestation, severity, underlying cause, and whether the patient can take oral replacement fluids. In addition, it is important to decide if there is just an intracellular shift (acute hyperventilation) or a true deficiency. If there is a deficiency of phosphorus, then replacement is indicated. In most patients oral therapy is adequate, but patients with severe hypophosphatemia (serum P <1 mg/dl) require intravenous therapy. When administering intravenous fluids, it is important to be careful about the quantity administered, since hyperphosphatemia and hypocalcemia can result from too rapid administration. In moderate to severe cases, 2.5 to 7.5 mg/kg of elemental P is administered over 6 to 8 hours, with frequent monitoring of P levels in the blood. Intravenous phosphate is usually given as potassium or

sodium phosphate. One ml of potassium phosphate contains 3 mmol phosphate and 4.4 mEq potassium; 1 ml of sodium phosphate contains 3 mmol phosphate and 4 mEq sodium. Since 1 mmol is 31 mg phosphate, each milliliter of sodium and potassium phosphate is 93 mg of phosphate. Most of the time, 3 to 5 ml of potassium phosphate is required. Subsequent dosages depend on serum level and clinical manifestations. Once the patient's phosphate level is >1.5 to 2 mg/dl, the patient can be changed to oral therapy. In patients with mild hypophosphatemia (1 to 2.5 mg/dl), oral therapy with either Neutra-Phos, 500 mg 2 to 3 times a day, or Fleets Phospho-Soda, 5 ml (129 mg/ml) 2 to 3 times daily, is appropriate. It is important to note that many patients (especially alcoholics) with phosphate depletion do not have a low serum phosphate level on initial blood work. A second serum phosphorus level is indicated, especially after a patient has received glucose-containing solutions.

II. **Hyperphosphatemia.** This refers to a serum phosphorus level >5 mg/dl and is usually due to acute or chronic renal insufficiency, but can also be seen with hypoparathyroidism, tumor lysis syndrome, and rhabdomyolysis. Transient hyperphosphatemia secondary to transcellular shifts can also be seen with acidosis (lactate and alcoholic ketoacidosis). Acute treatment of hyperphosphatemia is not indicated, but therapy of accompanying hypocalcemia may be indicated.

Magnesium

The normal concentration of magnesium is 1.5 to 2.2 mEq/L. Only about 2% of magnesium present in the body is in the extracellular fluid compartment. The intracellular body stores of magnesium include bone, 67%; muscle, 20%; and nonmuscle tissues, 11%.

I. **Hypomagnesemia**
   A. The **causes** include (1) decreased intake, (2) decreased intestinal absorption (short bowel syndrome), chronic diarrhea, steatorrhea) and (3) renal losses (diuretics, amphotericin B, cisplatin, aminoglycosides, cyclosporine, hyperaldosteronism, diabetic ketoacidosis). In the ED alcoholism is the most common cause, and hypomagnesemia in these patients is due to a combination of decreased intake, diarrhea, and possibly renal losses secondary to alcohol.
   B. **Clinical manifestations** of hypomagnesemia are often due to a combination of magnesium and calcium deficiency, since calcium deficiency is often also present. The hypocalcemia is due to a combination of decreased parathyroid hormone (PTH) release and PTH resistance. Clinical manifestations include cardiac abnormalities (ventricular tachycardia including a variant torsades de pointes, prolongation of QT interval, asystole, increased sensitivity to digitalis) and neuromuscular abnormalities (tetany usually associated with accompanying hypocalcemia, tremors, seizures, confusion, muscle weakness).
   C. **Treatment** of hypomagnesemia usually requires parenteral magnesium given in 1 or 2 gm doses. Acute intravenous therapy is indicated for treatment of seizures, tetany, and ventricular arrhythmias. In a patient with a high likelihood of magnesium deficiency (especially anorexia nervosa) who initially is seen with ventricular arrhythmias (especially torsades de pointes), therapy should be instituted before results of the serum magnesium level are available. If the patient is subsequently found to have a normal magnesium level, the increase in magnesium will not be harmful if the patient has normal renal function, since it will only be a temporary elevation. Usually 2 to 4 ml of a 50%

solution (8 to 16 mEq) is given over 10 minutes. Subsequently 2 ml (8 mEq) can be given intravenously every 3 to 4 hours for the first 24 hours. In non-life-threatening situations (alcoholic prophylaxis), 2 ml can be given intravenously every 3 to 4 hours.

II. **Hypermagnesemia.** Hypermagnesemia is usually asymptomatic but levels above 5 mg/dl can be symptomatic.
   A. **Clinical manifestations** are usually neuromuscular (absent reflexes, paralysis, lethargy), cardiovascular (bradycardia, heart block, cardiac arrest, hypotension), or respiratory depression.
   B. **Mild hypermagnesemia** is treated by decreasing intake of magnesium. In patients with respiratory depression and life-threatening arrhythmias intravenous Ca gluconate 100-200 mg (each 10 cc vial of calcium gluconate contains 93 mg) is indicated. In dialysis patients this should be followed by dialysis against a Mg free dialysate.

Endocrine Emergencies

Diabetic Ketoacidosis (DKA)

Diabetic ketoacidosis is a common disease in the ED, and therapy is usually initiated in the ED. It usually is seen in Type I diabetics but can also be seen in Type II diabetics if severely stressed, due in part to increased counterregulatory hormones such as glucagon, cortisol, or catecholamines. The most common precipitating factor is lack of insulin (not taking or insufficient amount). Infections precipitating DKA include urinary tract infections (pyelonephritis, perinephric abscess, or renal abscess), skin infections, (cellulitis, ulcer, abscess), dental abscess, osteomyelitis, and pneumonia. Other causes include surgery, myocardial infarction, and pregnancy.

I. **Clinical presentation.** Most patients have polyuria, polydipsia, and anorexia. They often have vague abdominal pain, nausea, and vomiting. Physical examination usually reveals rapid deep (Kussmaul) respirations, and their breath may have a fruity odor secondary to ketone production. Patients usually have orthostatic hypotension, but shock is unusual. Dry mucous membranes are usually present. Abdominal examination may reveal tenderness with guarding. Mental status may range from normal to stuporous to comatose.

II. **Laboratory**
   A. **Glucose.** Glucose concentration is usually in the range of 400 to 800 mg/dl. Higher glucose levels can be seen especially if patients have developed renal insufficiency or have underlying renal insufficiency, since this decreases their ability to excrete glucose in the urine.
   B. **Sodium.** Patients are usually sodium depleted as a result of osmotic diuresis. The serum sodium level is usually low because hyperglycemia causes an osmotic movement of water from the intracellular to extracellular space (see Hyponatremia). If the sodium level is normal or elevated in the setting of hyperglycemia, this indicates a profound degree of water loss. This is more commonly seen in nonketotic hyperosmolar coma (see below).
   C. **Potassium.** Patients are usually profoundly potassium depleted as a result of urinary losses due to osmotic diuresis, ketoacid excretion as a potassium salt, and vomiting (if present). The serum level is usually normal to high due to

transcellular shifts involving increased serum osmolality, insulin deficiency, and acidemia. A low serum potassium level implies profound potassium deficiency (see Treatment).
- **D. Acid-base disorders.** Most patients have an anion gap metabolic acidosis. The anion gap is usually highest in patients with the greatest amount of volume depletion. Other patients may have non-anion gap and anion gap acidosis (see Acid Base) where the sum of the bicarbonate level and change in anion gap is less than 25 mEq/L. As many as 10% of patients have a pure hyperchloremia or non-anion gap metabolic acidosis. These patients usually have normal renal function and are able to excrete most of the caducities; therefore, they do not have an anion gap since they do not retain significant caducities. A general rule should be that any patient with diabetes and a metabolic acidosis should be evaluated for possible DKA. Most patients have appropriate respiratory compensation, but some patients with underlying lung disease, drug overdose, or altered mental status do not compensate appropriately.
- **E. Phosphorus.** The serum phosphorus level is usually normal or elevated on presentation but can abruptly fall after insulin therapy.
- **F. Amylase.** Many patients have hyperamylasemia, but this is not due to pancreatitis; instead it is of salivary origin. Many patients are falsely given a diagnosis of pancreatitis because they have abdominal pain and elevated amylase levels. If the diagnosis of pancreatitis is clinically suspected, a serum lipase level is needed.
- **G. Triglycerides.** Hypertriglyceridemia is often seen in patients with uncontrolled diabetes. Clinically significant elevations are usually evident as grossly lipemic serum. The hypertriglyceridemia may result in pancreatitis (usually levels >1000 to 2000 mg/dl), eruptive xanthoma, and lipemia retinalis. The lipase should be measured in these patients to evaluate for possible pancreatitis. It is also important to check serum calcium levels, since they may be low if there is concomitant pancreatitis.
- **H. Serum ketones.** When testing for serum ketones, acetoacetate is measured by a nitroprusside reaction and normally β-hydroxybutyrate is more prevalent. Lower levels of acetoacetate can be seen with altered reduced states such as lactic acidosis (see Metabolic Acidosis).

III. Treatment
- **A. Fluid replacement.** Patients are usually deficient of 6 to 8 L of water and 6 to 10 mEq/kg of sodium. Lesser degrees or no fluid deficit may be seen in patients with chronic renal failure or congestive heart failure. In most patients initial fluid replacement should be 1 L of 0.9% saline solution rapidly administered, and 0.9% saline solution should be continued until the patient is hemodynamically stable. After the first 1 to 2 L of 0.9% saline solution is given, therapy should usually be changed to 0.45% saline solution at 250 to 300 ml/hr, since continued administration of 0.9% saline solution will usually result in hypernatremia. Once the serum glucose level decreases to 200 to 250 mg/dl, the fluid should be changed to $D_5\frac{1}{2}NS$, $D_5\frac{1}{4}NS$, or D_5W.
- **B. Hyperglycemia.** Fluid repletion can cause the glucose level to fall as much as 50% as a result of dilution and increased urinary excretion. In most patients, insulin therapy can be instituted immediately after the diagnosis of DKA. In patients with a history of diuretic use or excessive vomiting, do not administer insulin without knowing the serum potassium level. If the patient is hypokalemic, insulin can cause a life-threatening decrease in potassium (see below). When insulin therapy is initiated, usually 10 units of regular insulin is

given intravenously, followed by infusing 50 units in 250 ml of 0.9% saline solution at 0.1 units/kg/hr. The goal is to cause the glucose level to fall at 100 to 150 mg/dl per hour. When the glucose level decreases to 200 to 250 mg/dl, insulin can usually be decreased to 2 to 3 units/hr. If there is no fall in glucose after 5 to 7 units of insulin per hour, the insulin drip rate should be increased 2 to 3 units/hr until the glucose level decreases. In addition, the patient should be evaluated extensively for a precipitating cause of DKA such as a silent MI or a possible infection involving the genitourinary tract, skin, dentition, bone, and lungs.

C. **Potassium.** The treatment of the potassium deficit is very important in the management of DKA. The following approach is based on the initial potassium concentration:
   1. K^+ >5.5 mEq/L—recheck the potassium level 30 minutes after insulin therapy is started and begin potassium replacement at 10 mEq/hr when K^+ <5.5 mEq/L.
   2. K^+ 4.5 to 5.4 mEq/L—administer potassium at 10 to 15 mEq/hr.
   3. K^+ 3.5 to 4.4 mEq/L—administer potassium at 10 to 20 mEq/hr.
   4. K^+ <3.5 mEq/L—administer 20 to 30 mEq/hr of KCl until the potassium level is >3.5 mEq/L and then decrease to 10 to 20 mEq/hr.

D. **Metabolic acidosis.** Some physicians feel that if the patient is in shock, has a pH <7.0, or has severe hyperkalemia, bicarbonate therapy is indicated. Minimal further decreases in serum bicarbonate level or increases in $PaCO_2$ can have a profoundly adverse effect on pH. For example, if the patient has a bicarbonate level of 4 mEq/L and $PaCO_2$ is 14 mm Hg, the pH is 7.08. If the bicarbonate level decreased to 2 mEq/L and $PaCO_2$ remained at 14 mm Hg, the pH would be 6.78. Some physicians recommend adding two ampules of bicarbonate to 0.45% saline solution until the pH is >7.1 and the bicarbonate level is >10 mEq/L. Other physicians feel it may not be indicated since it is hard to demonstrate that a low pH is detrimental. In addition, after insulin is administered, ketogenesis will be inhibited and caducities will be converted to bicarbonate. My recommendation is not to give bicarbonate.

E. **Phosphorus.** On admission, a high serum phosphate level is usually seen, but after treatment of DKA as a result of intracellular shift, the phosphate level decreases. Since hyperphosphatemia is often initially seen, it is important to *not* routinely administer phosphate without documenting a decreased phosphate level. If intravenous phosphate is given, follow the guidelines in the section on Hypophosphatemia.

Hyperosmolar Hyperglycemic Syndrome

Most patients who come to the ED and have hyperglycemia do not require admission. According to a position statement by the American Diabetes Association,[1] guidelines for inpatient care for a diabetic include "either blood glucose >19.6 mmol/L (>350 mg/dl), serum osmolality >295 mOsm, and impaired mental status, or blood glucose >39.2 mmol/L (>700 mg/dl)." Patients requiring admission often have hyperosmolar hyperglycemic syndrome (HHS).

I. **Clinical presentation.** This tends to occur in older patients, with a mortality rate as high as 50%. Many have no history of diabetes or a history of mild di-

---
[1]From *Diabetes Care* 13(12):1990, copyright 1990 by the American Diabetes Association.

abetes controlled by diet. After it is treated, many patients can be controlled by diet or oral agents. It is usually precipitated by either infection, pancreatitis, stroke, myocardial infarction, surgery or medications (glucocorticoids, diuretics, β-blockers). Hyperglycemia causes an osmotic diuresis, resulting in losses of water, sodium, and potassium. Because of inadequate thirst, altered mental status, or underlying medical conditions, patients do not replace their urinary losses and become severely volume depleted and often hypernatremic. This volume depletion leads to decreased renal function, which limits the ability to excrete glucose and further exacerbates the hyperglycemia. The hyperglycemia and frequent hypernatremia contribute to an abnormal mental status that further limits intake. The history often reveals progressive polyuria and polydipsia over days to weeks. There may also be signs or symptoms of a precipitating event. On admission, most patients are severely volume depleted, with hypotension and often evidence of poor tissue perfusion—cyanosis, absent pulses, and cool extremities. Mental status ranges from alert to comatose.

II. Laboratory

A. **Serum osmolality.** This usually exceeds 350 mOsm/kg, and it can be measured or calculated by the following formula: Serum osmolality = 2[Na] + [BUN]/2.8 + [Glucose]/18. Glucose levels are usually >600 mg/dl but can be >2000 mg/dl. The serum sodium level is variable but is usually normal or elevated. When corrected for hyperglycemia, almost all patients are hypernatremic. The following formula is used to calculate corrected sodium concentration: [Corrected Na] = [Serum Na] + 1.6 ([Glucose] − 100)/100).

B. **Potassium.** Even though patients are usually potassium depleted, the serum potassium level may be high as a result of a transcellular shift due to hyperglycemia.

C. **Acid-base balance.** Most patients have a mild metabolic acidosis without significant ketonemia. It is due to a combination of lactic acidosis (decreased peripheral perfusion), uremia, and mild ketosis.

III. Therapy

A. **Fluid replacement.** The volume deficits of HHS usually exceed those of DKA, probably due to a longer time before recognition. The deficits are often 6 to 8 L. Patients are usually hypernatremic, and therefore the water deficit is more significant than the sodium deficit. Since these patients are usually profoundly volume depleted and often hypotensive, the initial therapy with 1 to 2 L of 0.9% saline solution is indicated until the patient is hemodynamically stable. The 0.9% saline solution is hypertonic (308 mOsm/L) but is relatively hypotonic for these patients. Continued therapy with 0.9% saline solution should be avoided because it may result in worsening hypernatremia. After the patient is no longer hypotensive, therapy should be changed to 0.45% saline solution. The rate should be based on the clinical status of the patient. It is important to follow urine output closely. Occasionally urine output will be significant secondary to the osmotic diuresis. Once volume is restored, patients that are still hypernatremic can be changed to D_5W solution to replace the water deficit (see Hypernatremia). It is important to replace the water deficit slowly to decrease the incidence of cerebral edema. Similar to DKA, patients with HHS can be changed to glucose-containing solutions once glucose levels are 200 to 250 mg/dl.

B. **Hyperglycemia.** The glucose level will significantly fall after volume repletion because of dilution and urinary losses. Insulin therapy is not as essential in the management of these patients and should not be administered until a serum potassium level is available. Insulin therapy should be started only if the potassium level is >3.5 mEq/L (see Potassium below). Regular insulin therapy is similar to that in DKA except that these patients usually require less insulin. Initially give 0.1 units/kg/hr, followed by 2 to 5 units/hr, and decreasing to 1 to 2 units/hr when glucose levels decrease to 200 to 250 mg/dl.

- **C. Potassium.** Potassium replacement is essential in the management of these patients, but the rate is less than with DKA because these patients are usually older and on admission often have more severe renal insufficiency. In patients with potassium levels >5.5 mEq/L, potassium replacement should be delayed until potassium levels are <5.5 mEq/L. Then potassium should be initially administered at 10 mEq/hr. If potassium levels are <3.5 mEq/L, the patient should have potassium repleted at 10 to 20 mEq/hr and insulin started after potassium levels are >3.5 mEq/L. When insulin is started, potassium should be administered at 10 to 15 mEq/hr.
- **D. Phosphorus.** Treatment is similar to that of DKA, but often these patients will need intravenous therapy because of altered mental status that makes oral therapy impossible (see Phosphorus).

IV. Complications. Hypotension has been described in patients with renal failure when, as a result of decreasing the glucose level, there is movement of water intracellularly, resulting in intravascular depletion. In most patients the administration of saline solution will prevent this problem. Cerebral edema is almost universal in the management of HHS and is due to treatment of the hyperosmotic state. Once the patient is volume repleted, it is important to decrease sodium levels slowly to decrease cerebral edema (see Hypernatremia). As a result of volume depletion, low cardiac output, hemoconcentration, and any underlying vascular disease, thrombosis has also been described.

Hypoglycemia

I. Causes. Hypoglycemia most commonly occurs in diabetic patients receiving treatment with insulin or oral agents. The hypoglycemia results from either (1) missing meals, (2) increased physical activity, (3) a change in insulin or oral sulfonylurea dose, or (4) the development of renal failure. In patients who develop renal failure, insulin has a longer half-life. Sulfonylureas are also partly excreted by the kidney. Other causes of hypoglycemia include cortisol deficiency (Addison's disease and panhypopituitarism), alcoholism, starvation, acute hepatitis, salicylate intoxication, insulinoma, myxedema, and surreptitious insulin injection or sulfonylurea ingestion. Fingerstick evaluation of glucose levels can be falsely low in patients with sepsis. Even though they should be treated as if they have hypoglycemia, the definitive diagnosis of hypoglycemia requires blood glucose confirmation.

II. Clinical manifestations. Hypoglycemia should always be suspected in any patient (especially diabetics) with a change in mental status. Symptoms of mild hypoglycemia are related in part to release of catecholamines, a compensatory reaction to increase the blood glucose level. Symptoms include anxiety, diaphoresis, tremulousness, tachycardia, weakness, and hunger. More severe symptoms include seizures, obtundation, coma, and focal neurologic signs. Patients with long-standing diabetes may have decreased catecholamine and glucagon response to hypoglycemia, and may have severe symptoms. β-blockers block most symptoms except diaphoresis, since that is a cholinergic response.

III. Diagnosis and treatment

A. Diabetic. Mild symptoms warrant fingerstick measurement of the glucose concentration and administration of oral glucose, juice, and foods such as crackers, fruit, and cheese. Severe symptoms require administration of glucose, 25 gm intravenously (50 ml of 50% solution), or glucagon, 1 mg intramuscularly. Glucagon is obviously indicated if unable to get intravenous access. When glucose levels are documented >100 mg/dl, intravenous glucose (100 ml $D_{10}W$/hr) should be administered and glucose levels followed hourly. Patients with long-standing diabetes who develop severe symptoms should have family members taught how to administer glucagon. Indications for admission are as follows: "blood glucose (<50 mg/dl) and the treatment of hypoglycemia has not resulted in prompt recovery of sensorium; or coma, seizures, or altered behavior (e.g., disorientation, ataxia, unstable motor coordination, dysphasia) due to documented or suspected hypoglycemia; or the hypoglycemia has been treated but a responsible adult cannot be with the patient for the ensuing 12h; or the hypoglycemia was caused by a sulfonylurea drug."

B. Nondiabetic. Nondiabetic patients are treated similarly to diabetics. It is important to administer thiamine, 25 to 50 mg, when giving glucose to suspected alcoholics. If the diagnosis is unknown, blood should be obtained, before giving glucose, for insulin, C-peptide, proinsulin, insulin antibodies, and cortisol levels. If hypothyroidism is suspected, thyroid function tests should be ordered. If Addison's disease is suspected, immediate therapy should be started with hydrocortisone, 300 mg (see Addison's disease). Patients with surreptitious insulin injection may have insulin antibodies and low levels of C-peptide (not part of injected insulin). Oral hypoglycemics will mimic an insulinoma with insulin, C-peptide, but no insulin antibodies in the serum. Measurement of sulfonylurea levels is essential for diagnosis in these patients.

Hyperthyroidism

I. Clinical manifestations.
Patients with hyperthyroidism usually have symptoms of tachycardia, weight loss, diarrhea, nervousness, and sweating. Other symptoms may include atrial fibrillation, hypokalemic periodic paralysis, and high-output congestive heart failure. Physical examination may reveal systolic hypertension, wide pulse pressure, tachycardia, exophthalmos, lid lag, stare, goiter, myopathy, and pretibial myxedema.

II. Differential diagnosis.
The causes of hyperthyroidism include Graves' disease, toxic adenoma or toxic multinodular goiter, thyroiditis, iodine induced (rare), surreptitious thyroid hormone ingestion, and hydatiform mole.

III. Outpatient diagnosis and management.
Most patients with hyperthyroidism do not require admission to the hospital. Indications to admit include possible thyroid storm (see below), atrial fibrillation, congestive heart failure, hypokalemic periodic paralysis, or pregnancy. If hyperthyroidism is clinically suspected, patients should have thyroid function tests including serum thyroxine (T_4), triiodothyronine resin uptake (T_3RU), T_3 radioimmunoassay (T_3RIA), and suprasensitive thyroid-stimulating hormone levels (TSH). Propranolol, 20 to 40 mg every 6 to 8 hours, can be started. Propranolol will blunt some of the manifestations of hyperthyroidism and decrease T_3 levels by blocking the conversion of T_4 to T_3 (active form of thyroid hormone). Patients should be scheduled for

follow-up to review the results of the thyroid function tests, and a thyroid scan should be scheduled. Propylthiouracil (PTU) or methimazole should not be given until after the thyroid scan, since they may interfere with uptake.

IV. **Thyroid storm.** Thyroid storm is a sudden, severe, life-threatening exacerbation of hyperthyroidism with associated organ decompensation. Symptoms may include severe fever, mental confusion (delirium, agitation, stupor, coma), tachycardia, rapid atrial fibrillation (including cardiovascular collapse), abdominal pain, or diarrhea. It is usually precipitated by infection, surgery, discontinuing antithyroid medication, and iodine therapy. Any hyperthyroid patient who develops a fever should be suspected of having thyroid storm. The fever may be due to thyroid storm, an infection, or an infection that has precipitated thyroid storm. Patients with suspected thyroid storm should have therapy initiated in the ED. Therapy includes drugs to block synthesis and release of thyroid hormone, conversion of T_4 to T_3, and peripheral manifestations of thyroid hormone.

    A. Stabilization. Patients may require fluids as a result of increased insensible losses from fever, sweating, and increased metabolism. Salicylates raise free hormone levels and should not be used as an antipyretic. Acetaminophen is the preferred antipyretic.

    B. β-Blockers. In patients with severe sinus tachycardia or rapid atrial fibrillation, intravenous β-blockers are appropriate. In atrial fibrillation secondary to hyperthyroidism, digoxin is not as effective as β-blockers. Regimens available include the following: (1)Propranolol, 1 mg intravenously every 5 minutes until rate is controlled, followed by oral propranolol, 40 to 80 mg every 6 to 8 hours; (2) Esmolol infusion until rate is controlled, followed by oral propranolol. The infusion can be discontinued once the oral propranolol is effective; and (3) Metoprolol 5 mg intravenously every 5 minutes until rate is controlled, followed by 50 to 75 mg orally every 6 to 8 hours. Even if the patient is in heart failure, controlling ventricular rate with intravenous β-blockers may be crucial in treating the patient.

    C. Propylthiouracil (PTU) or methimazole. These both inhibit iodination of thyroid hormone. In addition, PTU blocks conversion of T_4 to T_3 and therefore is a better agent. Propylthiouracil is given initially (orally or by nasogastric tube) in a dose of 300 to 400 mg, followed by 200 to 300 mg every 4 hours. If methimazole is given, the initial dose is 30 to 40 mg, followed by 20 to 30 mg orally every 8 hours.

    D. Iodide therapy. Iodide inhibits the release of thyroid hormone and should be administered 1 to 2 hours after PTU or methimazole. If administered before PTU, it may acutely increase production of thyroid hormone. Iodide can be given in the form of saturated solution of potassium iodide (SSKI) (5 drops PO or by nasogastric tube) every 8 hours, or sodium iodide (1 gm in 1000 ml of 0.9% saline solution intravenously over 12 hours) every 12 hours.

    E. Dexamethasone in a dosage of 2 mg intravenously every 6 hours is indicated because it provides glucocorticoid support and blocks the release and conversion of T_4 to T_3.

Myxedema Coma

I. **Clinical manifestations.** Myxedema coma is a manifestation of severe hypothyroidism that may require therapy in the ED. Patients with myxedema coma usually have all the features of severe hypothyroidism but are distinguished from severe hypothyroidism by the following: the patient is hypothermic, hypotensive, and partially or completely obtunded. Some patients may not be hypothermic, especially if there is a concurrent infection. On physical examination, there are often features of hypothyroidism, including dry skin, periorbital swelling, bradycardia, and slow relaxation phase of the deep tendon reflexes. Occasionally a pericardial effusion or heart failure is seen. Laboratory may reveal hyponatremia, macrocytosis, and hypoglycemia. Blood gas measurements are essential since carbon dioxide retention may be seen. The coma may be precipitated by a medication (narcotics or sedatives), infection, surgery, exposure to cold, or trauma. Laboratory should be sent for thyroid function tests (T_4, T_3RU, TSH), CBC, and serum cortisol, electrolytes, and glucose levels. Because of the high mortality rate if untreated, therapy should be administered if there is any suspicion of myxedema coma.

II. **Thyroid hormone and steroid replacement.** Intravenous levothyroxine is indicated and 200 to 500 µg is given, followed by 100 µg intravenously daily. In addition, hydrocortisone, 100 mg intravenously every 6 to 8 hours, is administered. The steroids are indicated because the patient may have accompanying ACTH or adrenal deficiency, or impaired ACTH or adrenal response to stress.

III. **Supportive therapy**
   A. **Hypothermia.** This is one of the classic manifestations of myxedema coma but may be overlooked if the thermometer is not adequately shaken down or does not register below 30° C. It will usually respond to thyroxine therapy and should not be treated with active warming, since active warming increases oxygen consumption and promotes peripheral vasodilation and further heat loss.
   B. **Hypotension.** The potential contributing factors to hypotension include hypothermia, hypoadrenocorticism, infection, and bleeding. It should be treated with isotonic saline solution, intravenous levothyroxine, steroids (hydrocortisone, 100 mg intravenously every 6 to 8 hours), and if no response, pressor agents. Hypotension is usually poorly responsive to pressor agents unless thyroxine is administered.
   C. **Hypoventilation and respiratory acidosis.** This may be due to respiratory muscle weakness, upper airway obstruction from macroglossia, or respiratory center impairment. Most cases of myxedema coma require ventilatory support.
   D. **Hypoglycemia.** If present it suggests the presence of accompanying cortisol deficiency but can be seen without cortisol deficiency due to impaired gluconeogenesis.
   E. **Hyponatremia.** This is commonly seen, but it is not usually severe enough to explain the mental status. If mild it should be treated with fluid restriction, since these patients are felt to be euvolemic. If severe it should be treated with hypertonic saline solution and furosemide (see Hyponatremia).

Adrenal and Pituitary Emergencies

I. **Adrenocortical hypofunction (Addison's disease)**
   A. **Causes.** These include idiopathic autoimmune adrenalitis, metastatic cancer, hemorrhage resulting from trauma or use of anticoagulants, granulomatous disease (tuberculosis, cryptococcosis, or histoplasmosis), and HIV disease.
   B. **Clinical manifestations.** These result from the deficiencies of glucocorticoids and mineralocorticoids. Glucocorticoids are important in maintaining a nor-

mal blood pressure, and mineralocorticoids are important in maintaining sodium and potassium homeostasis by reabsorbing sodium and excreting potassium. Patients' symptoms range from nonspecific symptoms such as weakness, fatigue, anorexia, nausea, increased pigmentation (due to increased ACTH), arthralgias, and postural dizziness to adrenal crisis. Symptoms of adrenal crisis may include shock, high fever, and abdominal pain. Signs may include hypotension, increased pigmentation, hyponatremia, hyperkalemia, metabolic acidosis, hypoglycemia, and renal insufficiency.

The diagnosis of Addison's disease should be suspected in any patient with volume depletion and hyponatremia, especially if associated with hyperkalemia. The urinary sodium concentration in Addison's disease should be >20 mEq/L as a result of mineralocorticoid deficiency decreasing sodium reabsorption. In contrast, most other causes of volume depletion have a urinary sodium concentration <20 mEq/L as a result of urinary sodium retention. Patients who are seen in the ED with adrenal crisis often have an acute precipitating event that normally would result in increased glucocorticoid and mineralocorticoid response. Precipitating events include infection, trauma, myocardial infarction, diarrhea, and increased sweating especially during summer months.

C. Treatment. In patients with suspected acute adrenal crisis with hypotension, immediate therapy is essential. Patients should have blood drawn for cortisol and aldosterone levels, and immediate therapy consisting of (1) volume repletion with 0.9% saline solution with dextrose added, with the deficit usually 2 to 3 L; and (2) glucocorticoid and mineralocorticoid replacement with a bolus of 200 to 300 mg of hydrocortisone, followed by 100 mg intravenously every 6 to 8 hours. In many patients the diagnosis of Addison's disease is often delayed because hypotension may respond to volume repletion without glucocorticoids and mineralocorticoids. The diagnosis is then considered when hypotension returns after volume repletion is stopped. In patients with suspected adrenal insufficiency who are not in adrenal crisis, a Cortrosyn stimulation test for primary adrenal insufficiency should be undertaken. Blood should be drawn for plasma cortisol and aldosterone levels, and then synthetic ACTH cosyntropin (Cortrosyn), 0.25 mg, is administered intravenously or intramuscularly with plasma cortisol measured at 60 minutes. After this test hydrocortisone can be administered.

II. Glucocorticoid deficiency. This is a more common disease in the ED than Addison's disease. Glucocorticoid deficiency is usually seen in a patient treated with glucocorticoids at pharmacologic dosages who subsequently discontinues therapy. This results in adrenocortical atrophy through its suppressive effect on release of ACTH. The clinical manifestations are due to glucocorticoid deficiency. The patient should not have symptoms of mineralocorticoid deficiency since the renin-angiotensin system can be activated, maintaining mineralocorticoid activity. The manifestations of glucocorticoid deficiency may include hypotension, abdominal pain, and hyponatremia. The stressed patient seen in the ED with a history of steroid use in the past 6 to 12 months should be considered to be adrenal insufficient, since often a detailed history of steroid dosage is not available. Usually 100 mg of hydrocortisone is given every 6 to 8 hours, but since mineralocorticoids are not required, methylprednisolone (20 mg intravenously every 6 to 8 hours) could also be given.

III. Pituitary hypofunction. This may involve the posterior pituitary (see DI) or anterior pituitary. The anterior pituitary produces thyroid-stimulating hormone

(TSH), corticotropin (ACTH), growth hormone (GH), and gonadotropins (FSH and LH). The causes of anterior hypofunction include hemorrhage ("pituitary apoplexy"), postpartum pituitary necrosis (Sheehan's syndrome), complicating radiation therapy, tumor, immunologic causes, sarcoid, and hemochromatosis.

- **A. Clinical manifestations** depend on the patient's age, extent of hormonal deficiencies, and rapidity of onset. Pituitary apoplexy may have an acute presentation with symptoms of severe headache, visual loss, and ophthalmoplegia, and may have signs of meningeal irritation. These patients may have symptoms related to glucocorticoid deficiency but, as a result of the long half-life of T_4, will not initially have symptoms of hypothyroidism.
- **B. The other causes** may result in varying insufficient amounts of anterior pituitary hormones. Patients with Sheehan's syndrome often are seen with failure to have menses (gonadotropin deficiency) and no other manifestation. Other patients may come to the ED with long-standing, nonspecific complaints such as weakness, lassitude, arthralgias, or an acute illness. These symptoms are related to deficiency of ACTH (see Glucocorticoid Deficiency) and TSH (see Hypothyroidism). The patients with nonspecific complaints are often very hard to diagnose and require a high level of suspicion for a possible endocrinopathy. Tests for the more chronic patient may include obtaining blood specimens for measuring T_4, TSH, prolactin, FSH, LH, cortisol, and ACTH concentrations. If immediate therapy with glucocorticoids is essential, serum for TSH, T_4, and cortisol levels can be obtained before initiating therapy with glucocorticoids and possibly thyroxine.

Pheochromocytoma

Pheochromocytomas are rare catecholamine-secreting tumors that arise from enterochromaffin systems. They comprise about 0.1% of cases of hypertension. They arise 90% of the time from the adrenal gland, and 10% are bilateral and 10% malignant.

- **I. Clinical manifestations.** Most patients who are seen in the ED with a pheochromocytoma are difficult to diagnose. Pheochromocytoma should be suspected if symptoms of headache, palpitations, or inappropriate perspiration are present. Patients may have a history of normotension, hypertension, or paroxysms of an increase in blood pressure superimposed on normotension or hypertension. These paroxysms last from minutes to usually less than an hour. Their blood pressure may also increase after antihypertensive therapy with β-blockers because catecholamines act unopposed on α-receptors. An increase in blood pressure has also been reported after therapy with imipramine and desipramine. In the ED patients may present with isolated hypertension or with a hypertensive crisis that may be accompanied by angina, myocardial infarction, stroke, or congestive heart failure. The ECG may reveal subendocardial ischemia, left ventricular hypertrophy from long-standing hypertension, or sinus tachycardia. Laboratory findings may include polycythemia as a result of contracted blood volume. Lactic acidosis secondary to profound vasoconstriction has also been reported. Another clue to the diagnosis is marked lability of blood pressure. These patients are usually intravascularly depleted; thus if there is decreased production of endogenous catecholamines or use of vasodilating drugs, this may cause a profound drop in blood pressure. More common than a pheochromocytoma is acute hypertension due to essential hypertension, cocaine, or amphetamines.
- **II. Treatment.** In patients who come to the ED with hypertension and suggestive symptoms (perspiration, palpitations, pallor, headaches) but do not have a

hypertensive emergency, tests should be ordered including urine levels of catecholamines, vanillylmandelic acid (VMA), and metanephrines. These tests may also be positive in patients with catecholamine excess due to cocaine or amphetamines. Some physicians do an abdominal computed tomography (CT) scan when the diagnosis is strongly suspected since it is positive in 90% to 96% of cases. If a history is strongly suggestive of a pheochromocytoma, begin therapy with an α-blocker (prazosin, terazosin, doxazosin, or phenoxybenzamine) or labetolol, which is both an α-blocker and β-blocker. Patients need frequent follow-up as they are being worked up. In the patient with a hypertensive emergency, therapy with nitroprusside, labetalol, and phentolamine have been used. It is important not to give a β-blocker without prior adequate α-blockade because of the effect of catecholamines on unopposed α-receptors. In the unstable patient who is not responding to medical therapy, emergent surgery has rarely been done.

Acute Renal Failure

In patients with an elevated serum creatinine level in the ED, the possibilities are acute renal failure, chronic renal failure, and acute renal failure superimposed on chronic renal failure. A previous creatinine level (if available) is helpful in differentiating the possibilities. Without a previous creatinine level, it is very hard to differentiate acute from chronic renal failure. An element of chronic renal failure is *suggested* if there is a history of nocturia, hematuria, edema, proteinuria, or underlying illnesses such as hypertension or diabetes. Laboratory tests revealing hypocalcemia, hyperphosphatemia, or anemia are also suggestive of chronic renal failure but can also be seen in acute renal failure. An ultrasound revealing small kidneys or radiographic evidence of renal osteodystrophy shows there is an element of chronicity but does not exclude an acute component. The causes of acute renal failure are classified as prerenal, renal, or postrenal.

Prerenal Azotemia

Prerenal azotemia refers to a decreased renal blood flow usually associated with a decreased effective circulating volume. As a result of a decreased renal blood flow, there is a functional decline in renal function. Nonsteroidal antiinflammatory drugs can cause deterioration of renal function in all patients with a decreased effective circulating volume. Their inhibition of prostaglandins, which are renal vasodilators, can cause unopposed vasoconstriction and a decline in renal function. Causes of prerenal azotemia are as follows:
  Gastrointestinal disease (vomiting, bleeding, diarrhea)
  Renal losses (diuretics, hyperglycemia, Addison's disease)
  Third spacing (small bowel obstruction, pancreatitis)
  Sepsis
  Liver disease with ascites
  Congestive heart failure (severe)
  Pericardial effusion with tamponade
  Hypotension secondary to medications
  Renal vascular disease
  Patients with unilateral renal artery stenosis involving one kidney or bilateral involving both kidneys may worsen their renal function after their blood pressure has been lowered by antihypertensive agents. This is more likely with angiotensin-converting enzyme inhibitors because they not only lower filtration pressure by lowering systemic

pressure, but they also lower efferent arteriolar pressure by inhibiting production of angiotensin II, which normally constricts the efferent arteriole.

Intrinsic Renal Disease

Intrinsic renal disease can be due to arteriolar disease, glomerular disease, acute tubular necrosis, interstitial disease, and tubular deposition.

I. **Arteriolar diseases.** Many of the patients often have concomitant glomerular disease.
   A. **Malignant hypertension**
   B. **Thrombotic thrombocytopenia purpura (TTP).** The pentad for TTP is microangiopathic hemolytic anemia, thrombocytopenia, neurologic manifestations, renal manifestations, and fever. Patients may not have all components present especially on initial presentation.
   C. **Hemolytic uremic syndrome (HUS)** is similar to TTP but without neurologic involvement, and it is usually found in pediatric patients.
   D. **Renal artery embolus.** Risk factors include recent myocardial infarction with mural thrombus, atrial fibrillation, and congestive cardiomyopathy. Flank pain is not always present.
   E. **Renal artery thrombus.** These patients often have underlying renal vascular disease and have developed collaterals. Acute thrombosis may not present as flank pain since collaterals may maintain a small amount of renal function.
   F. **Atheroembolic renal disease.** These patients typically are seen after an invasive arteriographic procedure such as an abdominal aortogram or a coronary arteriogram. Other symptoms and signs include livedo reticularis, abdominal pain, hypereosinophilia, hypertension, and eosinophiluria.
   G. **Polyarteritis nodosa.** These patients have a medium vessel vasculitis. When it involves the kidney, hypertension is a prevalent feature. These patients may have underlying hepatitis B antigenemia.

II. **Glomerular disease** may be part of a systemic disease or localized to the kidney. The following are various systemic diseases that can also affect the kidney:
   1. Wegener's granulomatosis
   2. Goodpasture's syndrome
   3. Cryoglobulinemia
   4. Poststreptococcal glomerulonephritis
   5. Endocarditis secondary to *Staphylococcus* or *Streptococcus* causing immune complexes
   6. HIV nephropathy
      (The diagnosis of HIV nephropathy may be after AIDS is diagnosed or in patients with HIV disease. In intravenous drug abusers, focal sclerosis, amyloid, and hepatitis B–associated glomerular disease are part of the differential diagnosis.)

III. **Acute tubular necrosis** may be due to all the causes of prerenal azotemia if the underlying cause is not promptly treated. Other causes include the following:
   A. **Rhabdomyolysis.** This should be suspected in alcoholics, after crush injuries, after electrocution, in phencyclidine intoxication, with cocaine use, in seizure disorders, with lovastatin therapy, in severe hypokalemia, in severe hypophosphatemia, and in heat stroke. Associated findings may include hypocalcemia, hyperphosphatemia, and hyperuricemia. One characteristic finding of rhabdomyolysis is that the dipstick on urinalysis is positive for blood, but on microscopic examination there are no erythrocytes. This is due

to filtered myoglobin reacting to the dipstick. This can also be seen with hemoglobin, but with hemolysis the serum will be pinkish.
- B. **Hemolysis due to intravascular destruction** such as microangiopathic hemolytic anemia (TTP, HUS, prosthetic valves) and immune hemolytic anemia.
- C. Drugs
  Chemotherapeutic drugs such as cisplatin, methotrexate, and interleukin
  Cyclosporine often associated with hypertension
  Amphotericin B toxicity
  Radiocontrast

IV Interstitial disease
- A. **Allergic interstitial nephritis** is usually due to drugs, including penicillins, sulfonamides, cimetidene, cephalosporins, and allopurinol. Patients usually do not have a fever and rash. Other signs include eosinophilia and pyuria (often eosinophiluria).
- B. **Polycystic disease** may present as asymptomatic elevation of serum creatinine levels, bleeding into cysts, infected cysts, hypertension, or a palpable mass. Recently renal function has been reported to decline after ACE inhibitor therapy. There is often a family history of renal disease since it has autosomal dominant transmission.

V. Tubular obstruction
- A. **Multiple myeloma (MM).** Most patients with renal involvement with MM have light chains in the urine. Precipitating causes for renal failure in these patients include volume depletion (precipitation of light chains), hypercalcemia, and hyperuricemia. Patients are occasionally misdiagnosed as having chronic renal failure because they are often anemic. Myeloma should be ruled out in most patients who are seen with unexplained renal failure. The urine dipstick is typically negative with myeloma since it measures albumin, and the protein found in the urine is usually light chains. A serum and urine electrophoresis are necessary for diagnosis.
- B. **Oxalate deposition secondary to ethylene glycol intoxication.** These patients should also have severe anion gap metabolic acidosis (see Metabolic Acidosis).
- C. **Tumor lysis syndrome.** This occurs after treatment of rapidly proliferating neoplasms such as leukemia or high-grade lymphomas.
- D. **Infections.** Severe parenchymal infections can rarely cause renal failure.

Renal Failure

Postrenal causes should always be excluded in patients with renal failure. A postvoid residual only diagnoses prostate and urethral disorders, but ultrasound is necessary to diagnose ureteral obstruction. Some patients only have one functioning kidney, and unilateral obstruction can cause acute renal failure. **Ureteral obstruction** can be caused by extrinsic compression from a tumor, papillary necrosis (diabetes, analgesic abuse, sickle cell anemia), clots, stones, ureteral pelvic junction blockage, retroperitoneal fibrosis, or tumors of the ureter or bladder. **Bladder outlet obstruction** can be caused by prostatic hypertrophy, prostatic carcinoma, bladder carcinoma, urethral structure, stones, clots, and neurogenic bladder.

- I. **Anuria.** The differential diagnosis of anuria includes aortic occlusion or dissection, renal artery embolus or thrombus, acute cortical necrosis, severe acute tubular necrosis (ATN), acute rapidly proliferating glomerulonephritis, or obstructive uropathy. Some of the patients with anuria only have one kidney. Acute exacer-

bations of patients with chronic renal failure (CRF) can be due to any of the causes previously mentioned but usually are due to the following causes:
- **A.** **Volume depletion** (overdiuresis, gastrointestinal losses).
- **B.** **Nephrotoxic drugs** (nonsteroidal antiinflammatory drugs (NSAIDs), angiotensin-converting enzyme inhibitors, cyclosporine).
- **C.** Urinary tract infection.
- **D.** Renal vein thrombosis.
- **E.** Obstructive disease.
- **F.** Worsening hypertension.

II. **Evaluation of a patient with acute renal failure (ARF).** Rapid diagnosis and treatment of the underlying cause of acute renal failure is important. All patients need laboratory evaluation including serum levels of electrolytes, calcium, and phosphate, and a urinalysis. The serum calcium level is usually in the normal range with ARF but can be low, especially with acute rhabdomyolysis. A high Ca^{++} level may be the underlying reason for the acute decline in renal function (see Hypercalcemia).

- **A.** **Urinalysis** in acute tubular necrosis ranges from relatively unremarkable, with few leukocytes and erythrocytes, to an active urinary sediment consisting of renal tubular cells and tubular cell casts ("muddy" brown). Interstitial nephritis usually has pyuria (often eosinophiluria) but can also have erythrocytes and even gross hematuria. Rhabdomyolysis and hemoglobin may result in a positive urine dipstick for blood secondary to myoglobin or hemoglobin; however, no erythrocytes are seen on microscopic examination of the urine. The serum is clear with myoglobin but is pink with hemolysis. Acute glomerulonephritis usually has an active urinary sediment, with protein, erythrocytes, leukocytes, and occasionally reticuloendothelial cell (REC) casts present. Prerenal azotemia usually has an unremarkable urinary sediment except hyaline and granular casts may be seen. Postrenal azotemia usually has an unremarkable urinalysis. Other tests that may be useful, depending on the patient, include the following:

- **B.** **Fractional excretion of sodium** (FE_{Na}). This refers to the fraction of filtered sodium that is excreted.

$$FE_{Na} = \frac{U_{Na} \times P_{Cr} \times 100}{P_{Na} \times U_{Cr}}$$

In order to perform the test, a spot urine for creatinine and sodium concentrations, and a blood sample for plasma creatinine and sodium concentrations are required. The FE_{Na} for various conditions is shown below.

1. **Prerenal.** Because of sodium-retaining state most patients have FE_{Na} <1, but if patients are on diuretics, may be >1.
2. **Renal.** Acute tubular necrosis has an FE_{Na} usually >1 and typically >3. Acute interstitial nephritis, rhabdomyolysis, and glomerulonephritis often have FE_{Na} <1.
3. **Postrenal.** Usually FE_{Na} >1, but early on can also be <1.

- **C.** **Postvoid residual** is essential in patients with obstructive symptoms but also in any patient with acute renal failure. The postvoid residual only evaluates obstruction at the level of the urethra and prostate. A postvoid residual <100 ml makes obstruction at the urethra or prostate an unlikely explanation for renal failure.

D. **Renal ultrasound.** Ultrasonography is essential for evaluating kidney size and for evaluating obstructive uropathy. It is mandatory in patients with known malignancies, especially cervical, uterine, and prostatic, as well as lymphoma. Some patients have obstructive disease and a normal ultrasound. If obstructive disease is strongly suspected, a retrograde pyelogram is indicated.
   E. **Nuclear medicine flow scan.** This is helpful in the anuric patient to demonstrate flow to the kidney or when renal thromboembolic disease is suspected.
III. **Treatment of acute renal failure**
   A. **Prerenal azotemia.** Most patients with prerenal azotemia are intravascularly depleted due to diarrhea, vomiting, hemorrhage, third spacing, or sepsis. Aggressive fluid resuscitation is essential in the management of these patients because all causes of prerenal azotemia can lead to acute tubular necrosis. In addition, some patients with profound intravascular depletion may actually have ATN when initially seen, but this is not known until there is no response to fluid repletion. Depending on the clinical situation, rapid fluid infusion is indicated until the patient is hemodynamically stable. If there is still no increase in urine output in hemodynamically stable patients, then it is important to consider invasive hemodynamic measurements, such as with a Swan-Ganz catheter. If this is not available, subsequent fluids should be administered as a bolus of 250 to 300 ml of normal saline solution, reassessing volume status after each bolus. Obviously if the patient is anuric due to ATN, continuous fluid resuscitation will result in fluid overload.
   B. **Congestive heart failure.** If the patient has pulmonary edema and there is no urine output, intravenous furosemide or bumetanide is indicated. If there is no response to furosemide or bumetanide, or the patient is hypotensive, intravenous dopamine or dobutamine is indicated to increase cardiac output. The patient can then have invasive hemodynamic monitoring after admission.
   C. **Pericardial tamponade.** Pericardiocentesis is indicated if the patient is hemodynamically unstable. This should be suspected in the patient with known malignancy, especially of the lung or breast. Patients usually have a narrowed pulse pressure, pulsus paradoxus, tachycardia, jugular venous distention, peripheral edema, and cardiomegaly on chest x-ray.
   D. **Liver disease with ascites.** In these patients with renal failure and no decreased urine output, the diagnostic possibilities are worsening prerenal azotemia due to diarrhea, vomiting, hemorrhage, pancreatitis (alcoholic), or infection (especially spontaneous bacterial peritonitis), intrinsic renal disease, postobstructive renal disease, and hepatorenal syndrome. If prerenal azotemia is suspected, intravenous fluids including normal saline solution, fresh frozen plasma, and albumin are indicated. If the prerenal azotemia is felt due to severe liver disease, albumin, 12.5 to 25 gm, is a good volume expander. Hepatorenal syndrome is a consideration if there is no response to fluids and there is no other explanation. Patients with hepatorenal syndrome have a U_{Na} <10 mEq/L, similar to prerenal azotemia. It is important not to administer too much fluid during fluid resuscitation because it can cause variceal bleeding.
IV. **Intrinsic renal disease.** The following is a list of potential causes of intrinsic renal disease seen in the ED and their treatment:
   A. **Rhabdomyolysis or hemolysis.** These patients need treatment of any volume depletion because volume repletion minimizes the damage of these pigments on the tubules. Some physicians feel bicarbonate therapy to alkalinize the

urine is important. Administer 1 L of D_5W with two ampules $NaHCO_3$ added to it; follow urine pH and attempt to increase urine pH > 6.5 to 7. One potential risk of giving bicarbonate is that if the patient has ATN, bicarbonate infusion may lead to metabolic alkalosis, since the patient will not be able to excrete the administered bicarbonate.

- **B. Renal artery embolus.** If diagnosed by nuclear medicine scan or angiogram, heparin therapy is indicated.
- **C. TTP and HUS.** These patients require fresh frozen plasma and plasmapheresis.
- **D. Glomerular disease.** Acute glomerulonephritis requires treatment of the underlying cause, usually with steroids, cytotoxic agents, and occasionally plasmapheresis.
- **E. Allergic interstitial nephritis.** Therapy requires discontinuation of the offending drug and often a short course of steroids.
- **F. Postrenal causes** are treated by removing the obstruction. Since most obstructions are at the prostate, a Foley catheter is appropriate, but ureteral obstruction requires stent placement or percutaneous nephrotomy. These patients often have a postobstructive diuresis and can rapidly become volume depleted if fluids are not monitored carefully. The postobstructive diuresis is usually matched with intravenous replacement.

V. Complication of ATN. The complications of metabolic acidosis, hypocalcemia, hyperphosphatemia, and hyperkalemia have previously been covered. Fluid overload is often very hard to treat, and patients may need large doses of intravenous furosemide (200 to 400 mg) or bumetanide (2 to 5 mg) before a response occurs. It is very important to consult a nephrologist. Indications for early dialysis include severe fluid overload not responding to diuresis, hyperkalemia not responding to medical measures, and metabolic acidosis, when the patient cannot receive bicarbonate because of fluid overload. Other indications include mental status changes that are felt to be due to uremia and pericarditis.

Suggested Readings

Berger W, Keller U: Treatment of diabetic ketoacidosis and nonketotic hyperosmolar diabetic coma, *Baillieres Clin Endocrinol Metab* 6:1-22, 1992.

Buonocore CM, Robinson AG: The diagnosis and management of diabetes insipidus during medical emergencies, *Endocrinol Metab Clin North Am* 22:411-23, 1993.

Burger AG, Philippe J: Thyroid emergencies, *Baillieres Clin Endocrinol Metab* 6:77-93, 1992.

Comi RJ: Approach to acute hypoglycemia, *Endocrinol Metab Clin North Am* 22:247-62, 1993.

Gaillard RC: Pituitary gland emergencies, *Baillieres Clin Endocrinol Metab* 6:57-75, 1992.

Gough JE, Jones JL, Garrison HG: Fingerstick detection of hypoglycemia can prevent dangerous doses of dextrose, *N C Med J* 53:466-7, 1992.

Hoffman JR et al: The empiric use of hypertonic dextrose in patients with altered mental status: a reappraisal, *Ann Emerg Med* 21:20-4, 1992.

Holmwood, KI, Williams DR, Roland JM: Use of the accident and emergency department by patients with diabetes, *Diabet Med* 9:386-8, 1992.

Kecskes SA: Diabetic ketoacidosis, *Pediatr Clin North Am* 40:355-63, 1993.

Mallette LE: The hypercalcemias, *Semin Nephrol* 12:159-90, 1992.

Molitch ME: Endocrine emergencies in pregnancy, *Baillieres Clin Endocrinol Metab* 6:167-91, 1992.

Rizzoli R, Bonjour JP: Management of disorders of calcium homeostasis, *Baillieres Clin Endocrinol Metabol* 6:129-42, 1992.

Roberge RJ, Martin TG, Delbridge TR: Intentional massive insulin overdose: recognition and management, *Ann Emerg Med* 22:228-34, 1993 (clinical conference).

Spencer E, Pycock C, Lytle J: Pheochromocytoma presenting as acute circulatory collapse and abdominal pain, *Intensive Care Med* 19:356-7, 1993.

Tohme JF, Bilezikian JP: Hypocalcemic emergencies, *Endocrinol Metab Clin North Am* 22:363-75, 1993.

Vallotton MB: Endocrine emergencies: disorders of the adrenal cortex, *Baillieres Clin Endocrinol Metabol* 6:41-56, 1992.

Yaxley L, Greenwood RH: Use of Lucozade and glucagon by ambulance staff in hypoglycaemia, *Br Med J* 305:185, 1992.

Parts of this chapter appeared in Isley WL, Hamburger S, Bosker G. Overview of Endocrine and Metabolic Emergencies. In Bosker et al: Geriatric Emergency Medicine. St. Louis: Mosby, 1990, 295–314.

13

Antimicrobial Agents: Uses, Indications, and Interactions

David A. Talan, M.D., F.A.C.E.P.

General Principles

I. **Factors that affect the choice of a specific antimicrobial agent**
   A. **Determining the likely pathogen(s).** The choice of an antimicrobial is dictated by the prediction or knowledge of the infectious pathogen(s). From the perspective of outpatient and emergency care, culture and sensitivity results will not usually be available within the time frame of the initial visit.
      1. **Gram stain** of specimens is frequently helpful to determine the presumptive cause of certain bacterial infections (i.e., meningitis, septic arthritis, and urethritis). This test is occasionally helpful for other infections, but its utility is often limited by contamination with underlying flora or inability to obtain appropriate specimens.
      2. **Rapid antigen tests** are most useful for evaluation of pharyngitis and some cases of meningitis; however, in the future, these tests will have much broader utility for outpatient medicine. When rapid tests are not helpful, the likely pathogen(s) must be predicted based on the known epidemiology of the infection and a knowledge of the host, as well as the circumstances, appearance, and location of the infection. This will be discussed further in Chapter 14 for specific infectious diseases.
   B. **In vitro activity of antimicrobial agents to treat the predicted pathogen(s).** One of the most important factors in determining which antibiotic to use is the known activity of the drug in vitro. In general, most drugs are specific to one class of infectious agents (i.e., fungi, viruses, or bacteria). Of drugs active against one class of pathogens, there may be further specificity. This is particularly important for bacteria. Certain antibiotics may be active against gram-positive bacteria and not gram-negative bacteria (e.g., vancomycin). Others may only be active against anaerobic but not aerobic bacteria (e.g., metronidazole).

   The in vitro activity of an antibiotic against certain bacteria is determined by the **minimal inhibitory concentration** (MIC). This value represents the lowest concentration of antibiotic that will inhibit visible growth of bacteria incubated overnight. The methods for determining and interpreting MIC values are best standardized for aerobic bacteria. When the MIC of an antibiotic for specific bacteria is less than the expected serum and tissue levels of that antibiotic, the likelihood that the clinical infection will be cured is optimized. The microbiology laboratory will report that a bacteria is "sensitive" or "resistant" based on whether the MIC is above or below a standardly agreed on, achievable serum level of antibiotic.
   C. **Tissue penetration.** Although an antibiotic may be active in vitro, if it does not achieve adequate tissue levels it will not be effective. Most antibacterials penetrate most tissues well. An important example of an antibiotic class that

has limited effectiveness because of poor tissue penetration is the aminoglycoside class for treatment of gram-negative central nervous system (CNS) infection. Certain tissues are more difficult to penetrate (i.e., bone and prostate) and generally require longer courses of therapy for cure.

D. Clinical efficacy. In vitro activity and adequate tissue penetration are generally necessary but not sufficient requirements for clinical cure. The likelihood that the infection will be cured is also dependent on the host's ability to fight the infection. **Host factors** that are detrimental include malignant disease, corticosteroid use, diabetes, asplenia, chronic renal and hepatic disease, acquired immunodeficiency syndrome (AIDS), and extremes of age. Protected sites of infection such as abscesses and foreign bodies should be drained or removed, respectively.

  1. **Clinical research studies** are also helpful in determining absolute and relative antimicrobial effectiveness and in choosing antimicrobial therapy. The generalization of the results greatly depends on the similarity of study patients, their infections, and local organism resistance patterns to those in one's own setting. Clinical experience and consultation with the hospital infectious diseases specialist are also valuable to understand which antimicrobials work best in a specific local environment.
  2. **Knowledge of the local bacterial resistance patterns in one's own community and hospital are critically important in choosing an appropriate antibiotic.** This information can generally be obtained from the hospital microbiology department.

E. Compliance. Compliance with oral antimicrobials is greatly influenced by the frequency with which drugs must be taken. Drugs that are prescribed to be taken once or twice per day have compliance rates as low as 70%, compared with drugs prescribed to be taken three or four times per day that may have compliance rates as low as 40%. Other factors that have been associated with poor compliance include low income, less formal education, and crowded living conditions. In general, if all other factors are equal, it is best to prescribe drugs that can be taken less frequently. **Table 13-1** lists the oral antibacterials by

Table 13-1. Standard Dosing Frequencies for Oral Antibacterial Antibodies

QD	BID	TID	QID
Cefadroxil	Cefadroxil	Amoxicillin	Ampicillin
Cefixime	Cefuroxime axetil	Amoxicillin/clavulanic acid	Penicillin
Azithromycin	Cefprozil	Cefaclor	Cephalexin
Lomefloxacin	Loracarbef	Metronidazole	Cephradine
	Cefpodoxime		Carbenicillin
	Ciprofloxacin		Tetracycline
	Norfloxacin		Erythromycin
	Ofloxacin		
	Enoxacin		
	Clarithromycin		
	Trimethoprim/sulfamethoxazole		
	Doxycycline		
	Bacampicillin		

their standard and preferred dosing frequency. These dosing recommendations are based on Food and Drug Administration (FDA) approved indications. Alternative dosing frequencies for specific indications may exist, and treatment options are discussed under specific antibiotics below and in Chapter 14.

F. Cost. The immediate cost of an antibiotic is determined by the cost of the prescribed dose. The overall cost of treatment must also take into account drug efficacy and the cost of treatment failure, along with the cost of drug treatment, treating complications, time off from work, and additional office visits or hospital days. The use of more expensive antibiotic must be justified by improved efficacy or safety. The charge to the patient for parenteral antibiotics is significantly affected by the charge to mix and administer the medication. In many hospitals, this drug administration charge is $50 to $70 per dose. **The wholesale price** of antibiotics is published annually in the *Red Book* (Medical Economics Data, Oradell, N.J.). Community and hospital pharmacies may negotiate prices differently from the published wholesale prices. It is best to obtain specific price information at one's local pharmacy in order to make definitive price comparisons.

G. Antibiotic use in pregnancy. Certain antimicrobials may be dangerous in pregnancy. For some antimicrobials the prenatal risks are known, but for many the teratogenic potential is not fully understood. In certain circumstances, treatment options in pregnancy are further limited by a history of drug allergy (e.g., penicillin allergy in a pregnant patient with active syphilis). In some circumstances it may be prudent to consider desensitization procedures so as to be able to give the most efficacious therapy.

1. **The antimicrobials that are *contraindicated in pregnancy*** include the **quinolones** (arthropathy in immature animals), **erythromycin estolate** (increased risk of cholestatic jaundice), **nalidixic acid** (arthropathy in immature animals and increased intracranial pressure in newborn infants), **nitrofurantoin** at term (hemolytic anemia in newborn infants), **tetracycline** (fetal tooth discoloration and bone growth inhibition, hepatic and renal dysfunction in pregnant female), **sulfonamides** at term (hemolysis in newborn infant with glucose-6-phosphate dehydrogenase [G-6-PD] deficiency, kernicterus in newborn infant), **metronidazole** in the first trimester (carcinogenic in rats and mice, possibly mutagenic), **griseofulvin** (embryotoxic, teratogenic, and carcinogenic in animals), **amantadine** (teratogenic and embryotoxic in rats), **ribavirin** (mutagenic, teratogenic, and possibly carcinogenic in animals), **dehydroemetine/emetine** (cardiotoxic), **furazolidone** at term (hemolysis in newborn infants and carcinogenic in rats), **lindane** (potential CNS toxicity in newborn infants), **oxamniquine** (embryocidal in animals), and **primaquine** (hemolysis in G-6-PD deficiency).

2. If there is a strong clinical indication, **antimicrobials that can be used with caution in pregnancy** include **aminoglycosides** (possible toxicity of cranial nerve VIII in fetus), **clindamycin, chloramphenicol** (gray-baby syndrome), **imipenem-cilastatin** (toxic in some pregnant animals), **metronidazole** in the last two trimesters, **nitrofurantoin** (hemolytic anemia), **sulfonamides** and **trimethoprim** in the first and second trimesters (folate antagonism, teratogenic in some animal studies), and **vancomycin** (possible auditory and renal toxicity in fetus).

3. **All antituberculous medications** can be used with caution in pregnancy; however, the use of streptomycin is discouraged because of eighth cranial

nerve toxicity in the fetus and the availability of alternative therapies. The antiviral drugs acyclovir, ganciclovir, vidarabine, and zidovudine can be used with caution, although their toxicity is largely unknown. The antimalarials (chloroquine, hydroxychloroquine, and mefloquine) and the antihelminthics (mebendazole and thiabendazole) can also be used with caution during pregnancy.
   4. **For standard antibacterial therapy during pregnancy,** penicillins, cephalosporins, aztreonam, and nonestolate erythromycin are considered safe.
   5. **Most antimicrobials are secreted in breast milk;** therefore, breast-feeding should be limited during antibiotic therapy. Certain agents such as tetracyclines and quinolones are contraindicated in children and in pregnant and nursing mothers.
H. **Antimicrobial use in hepatic and renal failure.** Antimicrobials are generally metabolized and excreted by the liver or kidneys. **Certain agents that are primarily excreted by the kidneys may accumulate in renal failure; therefore, dosage adjustment is required. These agents include aminoglycosides, vancomycin, trimethoprim, and the sulfonamides.** For emergency treatment, a standard loading dose of aminoglycosides should still be given to initiate therapy; however, subsequent dosing must be adjusted (see p. 415). Generally an initial loading dose of aminoglycoside is safe and rarely associated with adverse effects. The potential benefit of continuation of nephrotoxic agents such as aminoglycosides that are rapidly bactericidal against aerobic gram-negative bacilli must be weighed against the risk of renal dysfunction, particularly in the face of hypoperfusion, parenteral iodinated contrast, diabetes, rhabdomyolysis, and preexisting renal disease. All parenteral penicillins and cephalosporins (except ceftriaxone and cefoperazone) require some change in dosage with severe renal insufficiency (creatinine clearance <10 ml/min). Hepatic dysfunction may also cause increases in levels of antimicrobials excreted by the liver; however, no standard guidelines for dose adjustment in this situation exist.

Specific Antimicrobials

I. Penicillins
   A. General information. Penicillins are beta-lactam antibiotics that act by binding to penicillin-binding proteins on the bacterial cell wall and inhibiting peptidoglycan synthesis. The activity of penicillins varies considerably with class, including natural penicillins, aminopenicillins, carboxypenicillins, ureidopenicillins, and beta-lactamase–resistant semisynthetic penicillins. Specific activities are described below. Beta-lactamase inhibitor penicillins will be discussed on p. 412.
   B. Penicillin allergy/sensitivity. Anaphylactic reactions to penicillin are uncommon, occurring in only 0.2% of courses of treatment, with 0.001% resulting in fatality. Most cases of anaphylaxis occur in patients without a history of an allergic reaction. Whereas many patients state a history of penicillin allergy, immediate sensitivity is demonstrated with skin testing in only 7% to 35% of patients, and only those with positive skin tests appear to be at increased risk of a major allergic reaction. When taking an allergic history, it is important to distinguish major allergic reactions (e.g., anaphylaxis and immediate urticaria) from minor allergic reactions (e.g., delayed rash). Patients with minor penicillin allergy do not appear to have an increased risk for ma-

jor reactions and can be prescribed related beta-lactam drugs such as cephalosporins. In many cases, patients with a history of minor penicillin allergy can be rechallenged safely with penicillin without recurrence of allergic symptoms; however, it is safest to avoid penicillin if there is any history of allergy and there is an equally acceptable nonpenicillin alternative therapy.

1. **Patients with a history of major allergic reactions to penicillins should not receive beta-lactams (i.e., penicillins, cephalosporins, imipenem) unless there is no acceptable alternative therapy.** In this situation the patient should be desensitized under closely monitored intensive observation by one of the recommended desensitization protocols.
2. **The rate of cross-allergy to cephalosporins** for patients with major allergy to penicillin is small but finite. Recent studies suggest that the rate of cross-allergy is approximately 1%. In general, cephalosporins should not be administered to patients with a history of major penicillin allergy. If alternative therapies are unacceptable, a cephalosporin antibiotic may be administered to the patient under close supervision. Note that the monobactam antibiotic, aztreonam (see page 411), has not been reported to display cross-allergy to patients with penicillin sensitivity.

C. **Adverse reactions.** Relatively frequent adverse reactions to all penicillins include rash (more common with ampicillin and amoxicillin than with other penicillins), diarrhea (most common with ampicillin and amoxicillin-clavulanic acid), and nausea and vomiting (especially with amoxicillin-clavulanic acid in children). Less frequent adverse reactions include hemolytic anemia, neutropenia, pseudomembranous colitis, thrombocytopenia, platelet dysfunction, cholestatic jaundice, hepatic damage, interstitial nephritis, muscle irritability, hallucinations, and seizures (especially with high doses or renal insufficiency). For more specific reactions see sections on individual drugs.

D. **Bacterial resistance.** The most important mechanism of bacterial resistance to penicillin is the production of beta-lactamase, an enzyme that destroys the penicillin ring. This mechanism of resistance is important for the following commonly encountered bacteria:
   1. *Staphylococcus aureus.* More than 90% of isolates are resistant to all penicillins except the beta-lactamase–stable penicillins—methicillin, nafcillin, oxacillin, and related compounds.
   2. *Haemophilus influenzae.* Approximately 20% to 30% of U.S. isolates produce beta-lactamase and are resistant to ampicillin and amoxicillin. Other penicillins are not significantly more active.
   3. **Aerobic gram-negative bacilli.** As many as 50% of community-acquired *Escherichia coli* and essentially all *Pseudomonas aeruginosa* isolates are resistant to ampicillin because of beta-lactamase production. The carboxylpenicillins and ureidopenicillins (antipseudomonal penicillins) generally are less susceptible to this mechanism of resistance.
   4. *Bacteroides fragilis.* Approximately 90% of these anaerobic isolates produce beta-lactamase and are resistant to penicillin.
   5. *Neisseria gonorrhoeae.* Depending on the geographic area, as many as 10% to 40% of these isolates are penicillinase-producing *N. gonorrhoeae* (PPNG).

E. Specific penicillins
   1. **Natural penicillins** are active against most aerobic gram-positive and gram-negative cocci that do not produce beta-lactamase such as *Streptococcus* species and some strains of *N. gonorrhoeae,* respectively. They are

also active against anaerobic cocci, *Clostridium* species, enterococci, and various spirochetes. These drugs do not have significant activity against *S. aureus, H influenzae,* and gram-negative bacilli.

  a. **Parenteral agents**

   (1) **Aqueous penicillin G (generic)** is available as a potassium or sodium salt (1.7 meq K$^+$/million units). With high doses in the presence of hyperkalemia or renal failure, the more expensive sodium preparation should be considered. **Dosage:** Adult, 1-4 million units IM/IV q 4-6h; Children, 100,000-250,000 U/kg/d q 4-6h.

   (2) **Procaine penicillin (Wycillin)** is only for intramuscular use; accidental intravenous use has been associated with serious reactions. This preparation provides serum and tissue levels for at least 12 hours. Doubling the dose at a single injection site will not double the serum level. Therefore, two injection sites are used when large doses are given (e.g., previously standard treatment of gonorrhea with two IM injections of 2.4 million units each). Presently, this preparation has limited usefulness in the outpatient setting. **Dosage:** Adult, 600,000-1 million U IM q 12-24h; Children, 25,000-50,000 U/kg/d divided q 12-24h.

   (3) **Benzathine penicillin (Bicillin L-A)** is only for intramuscular use. A dose of 1.2 million units provides low but detectable serum levels for 15-30 days. Its use is generally limited to treatment of syphilis, streptococcal pharyngitis, and prophylaxis of rheumatic fever. Some preparations combine 300,000 units of procaine and 900,000 units of benzathine penicillin **(Bicillin C-R)**. **Dosage:** Adults, 1.2 million units IM (pharyngitis, prophylaxis of rheumatic fever), 2.4 million units IM (primary and early secondary syphilis); Children, 50,000 U/kg (one dose).

  b. **Oral preparations. Phenoxy penicillin (Betapen-VK, Ledercillin VK, Pen Vee K, Veetids, generic)** (Penicillin VK) is resistant to gastric acid hydrolysis and is administered orally. Typical indications for oral penicillin include streptococcal pharyngitis and dental infections. **Dosage:** Adults, 250-500 mg PO q6h; Children, 25-50 mg/kg/d PO divided q6h.

2. **Aminopenicillins. Ampicillin and amoxicillin** have similar activity to natural penicillins (see above). They also provide coverage against many non-beta-lactamase–producing isolates of Enterobacteriaceae and *H. influenzae.* These drugs should not be used for presumed resistant infections due to gram-negative bacilli. Indications: otitis media, sinusitis, bronchitis, pneumonia, typhoid fever, and community-acquired lower urinary tract infections.

  a. **Ampicillin (Omnipen, Polycillin, generic)** can be administered intravenously, intramuscularly, or orally. **Parenteral dosage:** Adults, 1-2 gm q6h IM/IV (for severe infections up to 12 gm/day); Children (over 1 month), 100-400 mg/kg/d, in divided doses q4-6h. **Oral dosage:** Adults, 250-500 mg PO q6h; Children (over 1 month), 50-100 mg/kg/d in four doses.

  b. **Amoxicillin (Amoxil, Polymox, Wymox, Trimox, Biomox, generic)** is a congener of ampicillin with similar activity but is significantly better absorbed orally. Peak serum levels are approximately twice those achieved with a similar dose of ampicillin. Food does not decrease ab-

sorption, and there is less diarrhea than with ampicillin. Ampicillin appears to be more effective than amoxicillin for treatment of shigellosis. **Dosage:** Adults, 250-500 mg PO q8h; Children, 20-40 mg/kg/d PO in divided doses q8h (as tablets or pediatric suspension).
  c. **Bacampicillin (Spectrobid)** is an ester form of ampicillin that is better absorbed and achieves significantly higher serum levels than ampicillin. Although more expensive than ampicillin and amoxicillin, it can be dosed twice daily. **Dosage:** Adults, 400-800 mg PO BID, Children, 25-50 mg/kg/d divided q12h.
II. **Carboxypenicillins and ureidopenicillins.** These "antipseudomonal" penicillins have similar activity to ampicillin with an extended spectrum that includes *P. aeruginosa* and other gram-negative bacilli including many strains of *B. fragilis.* These drugs should not be used to treat *S. aureus* infections, and they have variable activity against enterococci. When treating a compromised host with a serious infection presumed to be caused by *P. aeruginosa,* the combination of a beta-lactam antipseudomonal agent with an aminoglycoside should be strongly considered to provide potential synergy, broad coverage, and to avoid emergence of resistance. These agents do not penetrate the cerebrospinal fluid (CSF) well, and therefore, third-generation cephalosporins are preferred for treatment of gram-negative bacillary meningitis. **Indications:** moderate-to-severe or potentially resistant gram-negative infections, as well as mixed aerobic and anaerobic infections such as intraabdominal sepsis. **Adverse effects** are similar to other penicillins but also include hypokalemia due to the nonabsorbable anion effect and prolongation of bleeding time resulting from inhibition of platelet aggregation (both anticoagulant effects are particularly seen with carbenicillin). All these agents contain sodium that may provoke hypervolemia: ticarcillin, 5.7 mEq/gm; carbenicillin, 4.2 mEq/gm; mezlocillin, 2.17 mEq/gm; and azlocillin and piperacillin, 1.85 mEq/gm.
  A. **Carboxypenicillins. Carbenicillin (Geopen) and ticarcillin (Ticar)** have activity against *P. aeruginosa;* however, for more resistant strains, ureidopenicillins, antipseudomonal third-generation cephalosporins, aminoglycosides, or quinolones may be more consistently active. These agents are not active against enterococci or *Klebsiella.* **Dosage** of carbenicillin: Adults, 30-40 gm/d; Children, 100-600 mg/kg/d in divided doses IV q4-6h. **Dosage** of ticarcillin: Adults and children, 200-300 mg/kg/d in divided doses IV q4-6h. Dosages must be adjusted for renal dysfunction.
  B. **Ureidopenicillins. Azlocillin (Azlin), mezlocillin (Mezlin), and piperacillin (Pipracil)** have similar activity to the carboxypenicillins; however, they are also active against enterococci, *Klebsiella,* and more resistant strains of *P. aeruginosa.* **Dosage:** Adults, 8-18 gm/d; Children, 200-300 mg/kg/d, in divided doses IV q4-6h.
  C. **Indanyl carbenicillin (Geocillin)** is an oral drug that is stable in gastric acid. It is used for treatment of urinary tract infection due to *P. aeruginosa* and other resistant gram-negative bacilli. This drug does not provide adequate serum levels and should not be used for systemic infections. Quinolones (see p. 412) have largely replaced oral carbenicillin for resistant urinary tract infections and prostatitis. **Dosage:** Adults, 1-2 gm PO q6h; Children, 50-65 mg/kg/d in divided doses PO q6hr.
III. **Beta-lactamase–resistant penicillins** are semisynthetic drugs that are the drugs of choice (along with first-generation cephalosporins) for treatment of *S. aureus* infections. They also have activity against *Streptococcus pyogenes* (group A

beta-hemolytic streptococcus). These drugs should not be used for gram-negative infections. **Indications:** empiric therapy of uncomplicated skin and soft tissue infections, staphylococcal coverage for treatment of endocarditis, osteomyelitis, or septic arthritis. Some *S. aureus* isolates are resistant to these agents when tested in vitro against methicillin and are referred to as methicillin-resistant *S. aureus* (MRSA). The MRSA isolates are resistant to other agents in this class. The parenteral drug of choice to treat MRSA is vancomycin (see p. 421). Methicillin is no longer used because of a higher risk for interstitial nephritis, cholestatic jaundice, and neutropenia compared with other agents in this class.

- **A. Nafcillin (Nafcil, Unipen, generic)** is administered intravenously and is cleared by the liver. Therefore it does not require a change in dosage with renal dysfunction. **Dosage:** Adults, 1-2 gm IV q4-6h; Children, 100-200 mg/kg/d IV in divided doses q4-6h.
- **B. Oxacillin (Bactocil, Prostaphlin, generic)** requires dosage adjustment with renal dysfunction. **Dosage:** Adults, 1-2 gm IV q4-6h; Children, 100-200 mg/kg/d IV in divided doses q4-6h. Oxacillin also is available in oral preparations. However, dicloxacillin is the preferred oral preparation (see below).
- **C. Dicloxacillin (Dycill, Dynapen, Pathocil, generic)** is similar to oxacillin and is the preferred oral preparation. **Cloxacillin** is recommended by some authorities. **Dosage** of dicloxacillin: Adults, 250-500 mg PO q6h; Children, 25 mg/kg/d in divided doses q6h (suspension available).

IV. Cephalosporins

- **A. General information.** Cephalosporins are beta-lactam antibiotics that, like penicillin, inhibit bacterial cell wall synthesis. Cephalosporins are grouped according to activity by generation. All cephalosporins are active against streptococci, but inactive against enterococci. The activity of first-generation agents against *S. aureus* is excellent and generally decreases with successive generations. Most community-acquired, enteric gram-negative bacteria are susceptible to first-generation cephalosporins. Gram-negative coverage expands with second- and third-generation drugs to include *H. influenzae* and *N. gonorrhoeae* (including beta-lactamase–producing strains), *Neisseria meningitidis,* and more "resistant" aerobic gram-negative bacilli. Third-generation agents are unique for excellent coverage of resistant, aerobic gram-negative bacilli including nosocomial pathogens and for activity of certain of these agents against *P. aeruginosa.* The first-generation and most second-generation cephalosporins are not active within the CSF; however, all third-generation drugs yield high CSF levels when the meninges are inflamed. Significant anaerobic coverage is not present among cephalosporins except for some agents within the second-generation group.
- **B. Cross-sensitivity to penicillin.** Some patients with penicillin allergy may also be sensitive to cephalosporins. Although cross-sensitivity rates have been estimated at 5% to 10%, prospective studies suggest that the true rate of cross-reactivity in patients with a history of major allergy is approximately 1%. Cephalosporins should not be used if there is a history of anaphylaxis or immediate urticaria to penicillins; however, they may be used if there is only a history of minor allergy (i.e., delayed rash) (see pp. 403-404).
- **C. Adverse reactions.** Relatively frequent adverse reactions include thrombophlebitis with intravenous use, serum sickness with prolonged parenteral administration, and diarrhea. Less common adverse reactions include gastrointestinal disturbance, hypoprothrombinemia and clinical bleeding with methythiotetrazole (MTT) side chain cephalosporins (cefamandole, cefote-

tan, cefoperazone, and moxalactam), platelet dysfunction, coagulopathy, rash and arthritis (serum sickness) with cefaclor, pseudocholelithiasis with ceftriaxone, hemolytic anemia, hepatic dysfunction, nephrotoxicity, interstitial nephritis, seizures, and toxic epidermal necrolysis. A disulfiram-like reaction to alcohol may be seen in patients getting MTT side chain drugs.

D. **First-generation cephalosporins** are among the drugs of choice to treat infections due to *S. aureus*. They also have activity against streptococci and community-acquired, aerobic gram-negative bacilli such as *E. coli* and *Klebsiella* species. They are inactive against more resistant or nosocomial gram-negative organisms. The first-generation agents do not possess significant antianaerobic activity and do not sufficiently penetrate the meninges to treat meningitis. **Indications:** empiric therapy of uncomplicated skin and soft tissue infections, community-acquired upper and lower urinary tract infections, and prophylaxis for open fractures and other nonbite wounds at high risk for infection.

1. **Parenteral agents. Cefazolin (Ancef, Kefzol, Zolicef, generic) and cephapirin (Cefadyl)** can be administered intramuscularly or intravenously. They all have similar activity. **Cefazolin** is generally preferred because it produces higher serum levels and can be administered every 8 hours. The combination of cephalothin and aminoglycosides has been associated with nephrotoxicity. **Dosage:** Cefazolin—Adults, 1-2 gm IV q6-8h; Children, 25-100 mg/kg/d in divided doses q6-8h. Cephapirin, cephradine, and cephalothin—Adults, 1-2 gm IM/IV q4-6h; Children, cephapirin 40-80 mg/kg/d IV q4-6h; cephalothin 80-160 mg/kg/d IV q4-6h; cephradine 50-100 mg/kg/d IV q4-6h.

2. **Oral agents**
   a. **Cephalexin (Keflex, Biocef, Keftab, generic)** and **cephradine (Anspor, Velosef, generic)** have similar activity and pharmacokinetics. **Dosage:** Adults, 250-500 mg PO q6h; Children, 50-100 mg/kg/d PO in divided doses q6h (indication for twice-daily dosing in pharyngitis, skin infections, and uncomplicated cystitis in patients older than 15 years).

   b. **Cefadroxil (Duricef, Ultracef)** has similar in vitro activity to cephalexin and cephradine but has a longer duration of action. Although cefadroxil is more expensive than these agents, it offers greater convenience. Cefadroxil can be administered once or twice a day. The regimen of once daily is acceptable for pharyngitis; however, twice-daily dosing is preferred for other indications. **Dosage:** Adults, 500-1000 mg PO BID or 1000-2000 mg PO QD; Children, 30 mg/kg/d PO divided BID or QD.

   c. **Cefaclor (Ceclor) and loracarbef (Lorabid)** are considered to have some characteristics of second-generation cephalosporins in that they have similar activity to other first-generation agents yet have good activity against *H. influenzae*, although generally less activity than second-generation agents listed below. Loracarbef is from a new cephalosporin-related class of drugs, carbacephems. **Indications:** refractory otitis media or sinusitis, and lower respiratory tract infections. **Dosage:** Adults—cefaclor, 250-500 mg PO TID, loracarbef, 200-400 mg BID; Children—cefaclor, 40 mg/kg/d divided q8-12h (indication for BID dosing for otitis and pharyngitis), loracarbef, 15-30 mg/kg/d

divided q12h. Note: the higher dosages are recommended for otitis, sinusitis, and pneumonia.

E. **Second-generation cephalosporins** have extended activity against aerobic gram-negative bacilli compared with first-generation agents. Some agents of this group also possess significant activity against anaerobes. **Indications:** Certain second-generation cephalosporins are particularly useful for treatment of bacterial pneumonia due to *Streptococcus pneumoniae, S. aureus,* or organisms potentially resistant to first-generation drugs such as *H. influenzae* and certain Enterobacteriaceae. The agents with anaerobic activity are often used for mixed aerobic-anaerobic infections (e.g., intraabdominal sepsis or infected diabetic foot ulcers).

1. **Parenteral agents**
    a. **Cefamandole (Mandol)** has increased activity against *H. influenzae* and other aerobic gram-negative bacilli compared with first-generation cephalosporins. It is an MTT side chain cephalosporin and has been associated with bleeding (see p. 407). It does not reliably penetrate the CSF and should not be used to treat meningitis. Other cephalosporins are now preferred for most indications. **Dosage:** Adults, 1.5-12 gm/d IV; Children, 50-150 mg/kg/d IV, in divided doses q4-8h.
    b. **Cefonicid (Monocid)** has a similar spectrum of activity to cefamandole but has a longer half-life (4 hours), so it is administered daily or every 12 hours. It only has an adult indication. **Dosage:** 0.5-2 gm IM/IV QD.
    c. **Cefoxitin (Mefoxin), cefotetan (Cefotan),** and **cefmetazole (Zefazone)** are more resistant to beta-lactamases. They are more active than cefamandole against anaerobes such as *B. fragilis, N. gonorrhoeae,* and certain Enterobacteriaceae. Cefotetan possesses the MTT side chain and has been associated with bleeding (see p. 407). **Dosage:** Adults—cefoxitin, cefotetan, and cefmetazone, 3-12 gm/d IM/IV divided q4-6h, 2-6 gm/d IM/IV divided q12h, and 4-8 mg/d IM/IV divided q6-12h, respectively; Children, cefoxitin 80-160 mg/kg/d divided IM/IV q4-6h. Cefotetan and cefmetazole do not have pediatric indications.
    d. **Cefuroxime (Zinacef)** retains activity against staphylococci comparable to first-generation cephalosporins, yet has a broad activity against Enterobacteriaceae *(E. coli, Klebsiella, Enterobacter,* and *Proteus)* and *N. gonorrhoeae.* **Indications:** Cefuroxime is recommended for broad-spectrum coverage of community-acquired pneumonia and for serious pediatric sepsis in which ampicillin-resistant *H. influenzae* is a concern. Third-generation cephalosporins are now generally preferred for pediatric sepsis, especially bacterial meningitis, because of superior in vitro activity against *H. influenzae* and favorable clinical outcome. **Dosage:** Adults, 0.75-1.5 gm IM/IV q8h; Children, 50-100 mg/kg/d IM/IV divided q8h.
2. **Oral agents. Cefuroxime axetil (Ceftin)** and **cefprozil (Cefzil)** have activity similar to parenteral cefuroxime including activity against *S. aureus, H. influenzae, Moraxella catarrhalis,* as well as many Enterobacteriaceae. **Indications:** refractory or potentially resistant cases of otitis media and sinusitis, lower respiratory tract infections, and animal bite infections (active against *Pasteurella multocida,* an option in penicillin-sensitive patients). Note: Cefuroxime axetil is an alternative agent for treatment of early Lyme disease. **Dosage:** Adults—Cefuroxime axetil and cefprozil, 250-500 mg

PO BID; Children—cefuroxime axetil, 125-250 mg PO BID (as crushed tablet, no suspension), and cefprozil, 7.5-15 mg/kg q12h. Note: the higher dosages are recommended for otitis, sinusitis, and pneumonia.

F. Third-generation cephalosporins are less active than second-generation cephalosporins against gram-positive cocci but more active against aerobic gram-negative bacilli, including nosocomially acquired, multiply resistant strains. These agents are highly active against *H. influenzae* and *N. gonorrhoeae,* including beta-lactamase–producing strains. **Indications:** All third-generation cephalosporins penetrate the CSF well and are utilized for treatment of bacterial meningitis. Third-generation cephalosporins are particularly useful for treatment of gram-negative sepsis, and some of these agents have excellent activity against *P. aeruginosa.* In this setting they are often combined with an aminoglycoside to provide synergistic coverage. Third-generation cephalosporins have moderate activity against anaerobes, usually limited to oral species. Although these agents have inferior in vitro activity against *S. aureus* compared with first-generation agents (MIC 2-4 µg/ml vs 1 µg/ml), they achieve relatively high serum levels (100-200 mg/ml) and are clinically effective in treating most such infections.

Moxalactam (Moxam) has been associated with serious bleeding disorders, and its usage is no longer advised.

1. Parenteral agents
   a. Cefotaxime (Claforan), ceftizoxime (Cefizox), and **ceftriaxone (Rocephin)** have similar in vitro activity, with excellent activity against aerobic gram-negative bacilli including many resistant strains except *P. aeruginosa.* These agents have superior activity against gram-positive cocci compared with the other third-generation cephalosporins. **Indications:** Almost all penetrate the CSF well and are the drugs of choice for empiric treatment of bacterial meningitis in children and adults. In this context, it should be noted that cephalosporins do not have activity against *Listeria monocytogenes* or sufficient activity against staphylococci to treat meningitis. Also, third-generation cephalosporins are not consistently active against penicillin-resistant *Streptococcus pneumoniae;* vancomycin should be added if this infection is documented or strongly suspected. Other indications include community-acquired pneumonia, potentially resistant urinary tract infection, gonorrhea and pelvic inflammatory disease, and serious pediatric sepsis.

   (1) **Ceftriaxone is unique** because of its long serum half-life of 8 hours, thus allowing administration once or twice a day. This property is advantageous for initiation and/or continuation of outpatient therapy for certain cases of pyelonephritis, pneumonia, skin and soft tissue infection, and possibly pediatric occult bacteremia.

   (2) **Dosage**
   Cefotaxime: Adults, 1-2 gm IM/IV q4-8h; Children, 100-200 mg/kg/d IM/IV divided q4-8h.
   Ceftizoxime: Adults, 1-4 gm IM/IV q8-12h; Children, 150-200 mg/kg/d IM/IV divided q8-12h.
   Ceftriaxone: Adults, 1-2 gm IM/IV q12-24h; Children, 50-100 mg/kg/d IM/IV divided q12-24h.

   b. Ceftazidime (Fortaz, Tazicef, Tazidime, Ceptaz) and **cefoperazone (Cefobid)** are the two third-generation cephalosporins with significant activity against *P. aeruginosa.* Of the two, ceftazidime is the most active

against *P. aeruginosa;* however, cefoperazone has superior activity against gram-positive cocci. Cefoperazone has the MTT side chain associated with prothrombin deficiency and bleeding (see p. 407).
- **(1) Indications:** Nosocomial pneumonia, urosepsis, and bacterial meningitis presumed secondary to resistant gram-negative bacilli (e.g., *P. aeruginosa*). When treating an immunocompromised patient, the addition of an aminoglycoside is recommended.
- **(2) Dosage**
  Ceftazidime: Adults, 1-2 gm IM/IV q8-12h; Children, 90-150 mg/kg/d IM/IV q8-12h.
  Cefoperazone: Adults, 1-4 gm IV q6-12h; Children, 100-150 mg/kg/d IM/IV divided q6-12h.

2. **Oral agents**
   a. **Cefixime (Suprax)** has similar in vitro activity to cefotaxime, ceftizoxime, and ceftriaxone, but it is not active against *S. aureus.* Cefixime is active against upper and lower respiratory tract pathogens *(H. influenzae* and *Moraxella),* including beta-lactamase–producing strains, as well as streptococci. Because of inconsistent activity against *S. pneumoniae,* it is not recommended as first-line therapy for infections such as otitis media. It is unique in that its long serum half-life of 4 hours allows administration once a day. **Indications:** Refractory acute otitis media and sinusitis. It is the preferred single-dose **oral** therapy for uncomplicated gonorrhea. **Dosage:** Adults, 400 mg PO QD (400 mg as a single dose for uncomplicated gonorrhea); Children, 8 mg/kg/d (suspension available).
   b. **Cefpodoxime (Vantin)** has extended activity against Enterobacteriaceae, *H. influenzae,* and *M. catarrhalis,* but retains excellent activity against *S. aureus* and *S. pneumoniae.* Therefore it is similar to oral second-generation cephalosporins. **Indications:** refractory or potentially resistant cases of otitis media and sinusitis, lower respiratory tract infections, animal bite infections (active against *P. multocida,* an option in penicillin-sensitive patients) and single-dose therapy (200 mg) for uncomplicated gonorrhea. **Dosage:** Adults, 200-400 mg PO BID; Children, 10 mg/kg/d PO divided q12h, maximum 400 mg/d). Note: the higher dosages are recommended for otitis, sinusitis, and pneumonia.

V. **Aztreonam (Azactam)** is a monobactam that is highly active against aerobic gram-negative bacilli, including *P. aeruginosa.* It is inactive against gram-positive cocci and anaerobes. Aztreonam, like third-generation cephalosporins and quinolones, is an alternative agent to aminoglycosides. It is not nephrotoxic or ototoxic. It may be used in patients with penicillin allergy because there is no apparent cross-sensitivity. **Dosage:** Adults, 1-2 gm IV q6-8h.

VI. **Imipenem (Primaxin)** is a carbepenem that is given with cilastatin, an inhibitor of renal metabolism of imipenem. Imipenem has the broadest activity of any antibiotic, including activity against gram-positive cocci, multiply resistant aerobic gram-negative bacilli including *P. aeruginosa,* and anaerobes. It is not active against MRSA. In general, imipenem is reserved for directed therapy against identified multiply resistant pathogens. Its empiric use is discouraged. Of note are adverse CNS effects such as seizures that occur most commonly in patients with CNS disorders and those with impaired renal function. **Dosage:** Adults, 500-1000 mg IV q6-8h. (An IM formulation is also available.)

VII. Beta-lactamase–inhibitor antibiotics

VII. Beta-lactamase–inhibitor antibiotics that are currently available are penicillin antibiotics with another beta-lactam molecule. These beta-lactamase–inhibitor molecules block the action of the beta-lactamases that confer resistance to *S. aureus, H. influenzae, M. catarrhalis, N. gonorrhoeae, B. fragilis,* and many *E. coli* and other Enterobacteriaceae to penicillins. These are among the most active antianaerobic drugs. The utility of antibiotics that are beta-lactamase inhibitors is their very broad spectrum that includes anaerobes, *S. aureus,* and many aerobic gram-negative bacteria. **Indications:** Empiric therapy of ear, sinus, respiratory, abdominal/pelvic, and complicated skin/bite infections. There is inadequate experience to recommend their use for treatment of meningitis. The adverse effects of these agents reflect those of the parent penicillin compound. Oral clavulanic acid appears to add to the frequency of gastrointestinal side effects of amoxicillin.

A. Parenteral agents

1. **Ampicillin/sulbactam (Unasyn)** has the activity of ampicillin (see p. 405) against streptococci including enterococci, certain anaerobes, and community-acquired Enterobacteriaceae, as well as the extended spectrum noted above because of the addition of the beta-lactamase inhibitor, sulbactam. **Indications:** Gynecologic, abdominal and lower respiratory tract, and complicated skin/bite infections. **Dosage:** Adults, 1.5-3.0 gm IM/IV q6h. Dosage must be adjusted for renal dysfunction.

2. **Ticarcillin/clavulanic acid (Timentin)** and **piperacillin/tazobactam (Zosyn)** have the activity of ticarcillin and piperacillin (see page 406) against many aerobic gram-negative bacilli, some strains of *P. aeruginosa,* and *B. fragilis.* In general, piperacillin has superior antipseudomonal activity compared with ticarcillin. These agents have the extended spectrum noted above because of the addition of the beta-lactamase inhibitors, clavulanic acid, and tazobactam. **Indications:** Gynecologic, abdominal, lower respiratory tract, and complicated skin/bite infections (especially if there is some concern for *P. aeruginosa*). **Dosage:** Adults—ticarcillin/clavulanate, 3.1 gm IV q4-6h; piperacillin/tazobactam, 3.375 gm q6h. Dosage must be adjusted for renal dysfunction.

B. Oral Agents

1. **Amoxicillin/clavulanic acid (Augmentin)** has a similar spectrum of activity as ampicillin/sulbactam (see above). **Indications:** Complicated skin/bite infections, refractory or potentially resistant cases of otitis media and sinusitis, and outpatient treatment of pyogenic pneumonia. It causes gastrointestinal upset more frequently than amoxicillin alone; however, this effect may be somewhat ameliorated if taken with food. **Dosage:** Adults, 250-500 mg PO TID; Children, 20-40 mg/kg/d divided TID (as oral suspension and chewable tablets).

2. **Note:** The 250 mg and 500 mg Augmentin tablets contain the same amount of clavulanic acid, 125 mg. Therefore, two 250 mg tablets are not equal to a 500 mg tablet and should not be substituted to avoid increased gastrointestinal toxicity.

VIII. Quinolones are derivatives of nalidixic acid that inhibit the enzyme DNA gyrase. As a class they have unique potent activity against many aerobic gram-negative bacteria including even beta-lactamase–producing *H. influenzae, N. gonorrhoeae,* and *M. catarrhalis,* as well as the Enterobacteriaceae. Certain of the quinolones are unique as oral agents with potent activity against *P. aeruginosa.* Some quinolones are active against *S. aureus* and some strains of MRSA.

Quinolones are active against all common bacterial diarrheal pathogens including *Campylobacter.*
- **A. Streptococci and anaerobes.** The currently available quinolones do not have consistent activity against streptococci or anaerobes. Empiric treatment of community-acquired lower respiratory tract infections and uncomplicated skin and soft tissue infections with quinolones alone is discouraged because of inconsistent activity against *S. pneumoniae* and *S. pyogenes.*
- **B. Quinolones are contraindicated** in persons 18 years of age or younger, and pregnant and nursing mothers because of interference with articular cartilage development demonstrated in young animals. Absorption is inhibited by concomitant administration of calcium- or magnesium-containing antacids. As a class, quinolones should be administered with caution to patients taking theophylline preparations, caffeine, or warfarin, since quinolones may increase the serum levels of these drugs, causing toxicity. Excitation of the CNS (and rarely seizures) is an uncommon but characteristic side effect of quinolones, which may be more common with concomitant administration of nonsteroidal antiinflammatory drugs.
- **C. Parenteral agents. Ciprofloxacin (Cipro)** and **ofloxacin (Floxin)** are available for intravenous use. Their in vitro activity is identical to the oral preparation. These agents have broad activity against aerobic gram-negative bacteria (see above) including *P. aeruginosa.* They are active against *S. aureus* and some strains of MRSA. Ciprofloxacin has slightly superior gram-negative activity, while ofloxacin has slightly superior gram-positive activity. The utility of the intravenous preparation is as an alternative to aminoglycosides (along with third-generation cephalosporins, aztreonam, and imipenem) to treat resistant, aerobic gram-negative infections. Note that serum levels achieved with oral administration of these drugs are similar to those achieved with intravenous dosing.
    1. **Adverse reactions and drug interactions (also see general comments above):** Quinolone use may lead to increased theophylline and Coumadin levels. Nonsteroidal antiinflammatory drugs may increase the risk of CNS stimulation and seizures.
    2. **Dosage:** Ciprofloxacin and ofloxacin, 200-400 mg IV q12h. Dosage must be adjusted for renal dysfunction.
- **D. Oral agents**
    1. **Ciprofloxacin (Cipro)** has identical activity to the parenteral preparation (see above). It is the most active oral agent against *P. aeruginosa.*
        a. **Indications:** Complicated urinary tract infections and prostatitis (it appears to be more efficacious than trimethoprim-sulfamethoxazole in this setting), empiric therapy of severe or prolonged bacterial diarrhea, single-dose treatment of gonococcal urethritis (note that it is incompletely effective with longer courses against *Chlamydia trachomatis* and is not active against *Treponema pallidum*—i.e., incubating syphilis), long-term therapy of osteomyelitis, and empiric treatment of animal bite infections in patients with major beta-lactamase allergy because it is active against *P. multocida* and *S. aureus.* **Adverse reactions and drug interactions (also see general comments above):** as above for parenteral quinolones.
        b. **Dosage:** Adults, 250-750 mg PO BID.
    2. **Ofloxacin (Floxin)** is similar to ciprofloxacin in activity, although activity against *S. aureus* may be somewhat superior and activity against *P.*

aeruginosa may be somewhat inferior to ciprofloxacin. It is the only quinolone that has activity against *C. trachomatis* that is clinically equivalent to the tetracycline or azithromycin.

  a. **Indications:** for concomitant treatment of *N. gonorrhoeae* (single dose for uncomplicated gonorrhea) and *C. trachomatis* (tetracycline and doxycycline are less expensive for *Chlamydia* treatment, and the quinolones are not effective against incubating syphilis), and salpingitis (with metronidazole or clindamycin). Other indications are similar to those mentioned for ciprofloxacin. **Adverse reactions and drug interactions (also see general comments above):** as above for parenteral quinolones.
  b. **Dosage: Adults,** 200-400 mg PO BID.
 3. **Norfloxacin (Noroxin), Lomefloxacin (Maxaquin)** and **Enoxacin (Penetrex)** have broad activity against aerobic gram-negative bacteria and the bacterial diarrheal pathogens; however, unlike ciprofloxacin and ofloxacin, they do not have reliable activity against *Staphylococcus aureus* and *Pseudomonas aeruginosa.* Lomefloxacin is administered once daily.
  a. **Indications:** Complicated urinary tract infections, prostatitis, single dose therapy of uncomplicated gonorrhea, and empiric treatment of bacterial diarrhea (in adults) as mentioned above for ciprofloxacin. **Adverse reactions and drug interactions (also see general comments above):** as above for parenteral quinolones.
  b. **Dosage:** Adults, Norfloxacin, 400 mg PO BID, loracarbef, 400 mg qd, enoxacin, 200-400 mg PO BID.
 4. **Drug Interactions:** as above for parenteral quinolones.

IX. **Aminoglycosides** act by inhibition of protein synthesis and are rapidly bactericidal for most aerobic gram-negative bacilli. They also act synergistically with ampicillin, penicillin, or vancomycin for treatment of streptococcal (particularly enterococcal) endocarditis. Aminoglycosides are ineffective against anaerobes.
  A. **Indications.** Aminoglycosides are standard parenteral therapy for presumed sepsis due to aerobic gram-negative bacilli. Gentamicin is least expensive and, depending on local sensitivity patterns, may be as effective as the other agents. Amikacin is generally reserved for treatment of isolates known or suspected to be resistant to other aminoglycosides. Previous hospitalization, nursing home residence, or concurrent antibiotic use would suggest a more "resistant" infection that might require a more active aminoglycoside. In this setting, an aminoglycoside is often combined with a beta-lactam antibiotic, such as a third-generation cephalosporin or an antipseudomonal penicillin for synergistic activity. Aminoglycosides do not penetrate the blood-brain barrier and must be administered intrathecally to treat meningitis. An aminoglycoside would also be combined with nafcillin and penicillin, or vancomycin for empiric treatment of bacterial endocarditis (for coverage of gram-negative organisms or enterococci). Streptomycin is the treatment of choice for plague, tularemia, and brucellosis, and is occasionally useful for treatment of certain cases of tuberculosis.
  B. **Adverse reactions.** The major adverse effects of aminoglycosides are nephrotoxicity and otoxicity (both vestibular and auditory). Toxicity is associated with excessive doses and prolonged treatment, and rarely occurs with a single loading dose. These agents should be avoided in patients with a prior history of non–end-stage renal dysfunction or ear disease. Neuro-

muscular blockade occurs rarely, and aminoglycosides should not be administered to patients receiving anesthetics, neuromuscular blocking agents, massive transfusions, citrated anticoagulated blood, or those with neuromuscular diseases such as myasthenia gravis. If neuromuscular blockade occurs, calcium salts may reverse it. Toxicity does not appear to be significantly different between aminoglycosides.

C. Dosage (with normal renal function). Gentamicin, tobramycin, netilmicin, and amikacin are administered intramuscularly or intravenously. In order to rapidly achieve therapeutic serum levels, it is necessary to administer an initial loading dose: 1.5-2.0 mg/kg for gentamicin, tobramycin, and netilmicin, and 5.0-7.5 mg/kg for amikacin. The maintenance dosages must be adjusted for renal dysfunction (see below). Note that more recent protocols have utilized q24h dosing with daily doses of the aminoglycosides and have noted similar efficacy without increased toxicity compared to standard q8-12h regimens.

1. **Maintenance dosage**
   a. **Gentamicin (Garamycin, generic)**. Adults, 3-5 mg/kg/d divided q8h; Children, 3.0-7.5 mg/kg/d divided q8h; Neonates, 5.0-7.5 mg/kg/d divided q8h; Premature or full-term neonates <1 week, 5 mg/kg/d divided q12h.
   b. **Tobramycin (Nebcin, generic)**. Adults, 3-5 mg/kg/d divided q8h; Children, 6.0-7.5 mg/kg/d divided q8h; Premature and full-term neonates <1 week, 4 mg/kg/d divided q12h.
   c. **Netilmicin (Netromycin)**. Adults, 3.0-6.5 mg/kg/d divided q8h; Children, 5.5-8.0 mg/kg/d divided q8-12h; Neonates (<6 weeks), 4.0-6.5 mg/kg/d divided q12h.
   d. **Amikacin (Amikin)**. Adults, Children, and Neonates: 15 mg/kg/d divided q8-12h (note: with neonates, a 10 mg/kg loading dose is recommended dosage with renal dysfunction).

2. **Aminoglycoside maintenance dosages** must be reduced with renal impairment. In general, either the dose is reduced or the interval between doses is increased proportionately to the decrease in glomerular filtration rate (GFR). The GFR is estimated with the following formula:

$$\text{GFR} = \frac{(140 - \text{age in years}) \times \text{weight (kg)}}{72 \times \text{serum creatinine (mg/d)}}$$

If the GFR is 10 to 50 ml/min, the interval for the standard dose of gentamicin, tobramycin, and netilmicin is 12 hours, and for amikacin 12 to 18 hours. If the GFR is less than 10 ml/min, the dosing interval is over 24 hours. Optimal maintenance dosing is best established by determining the peak and trough serum aminoglycoside levels.

X. Sulfonamides act by inhibition of folic acid synthesis. Sulfisoxazole is the preferred sulfonamide because of its low cost and high solubility. Other preparations such as sulfamethoxazole, sulfacytine, sulfadiazine, and triple-sulfa (a combination of three sulfonamides to increase solubility) offer no therapeutic advantage.

A. Indications. The sulfonamides are among the drugs of choice to treat uncomplicated urinary tract infections. The combination of trimethoprim with sulfamethoxizole (see below) is preferred because of better activity and less frequent dosing. Sulfonamides are also used for treatment of nocardiosis, toxoplasmosis (with pyrimethamine), and *Pneumocystis carinii* pneumonia (with trimethoprim). Sulfonamides are alternative agents for treatment of *C. trachomatis* genital infection (e.g., during pregnancy when tetracyclines are contraindicated) and chancroid (with trimethoprim).

B. Adverse reactions. Sulfonamides are contraindicated in the last trimester of pregnancy and during nursing because of the risk of neonatal kernicterus. Rashes are common including erythema multiforme and rarely Stevens-Johnson syndrome. Agranulocytosis and aplastic anemia have been rarely noted. Sulfonamides may induce hemolysis in patients with G-6-PD deficiency. Older, less soluble preparations were more often associated with crystalluria.

C. Drug interactions. Transient hypoglycemia may result from protein displacement of oral hypoglycemics. Transient hypothrombinemia may result from protein displacement or inhibition of metabolism of oral anticoagulants. Sulfonamides may inhibit phenytoin metabolism and increase serum phenytoin levels.

D. Dosage. Adults, 0.5-1.0 gm PO or IV q6h; Children, 30-60 mg/kg/d PO or IV divided q6h. Sulfonamides are excreted by the kidney; therefore their dosage should be reduced with renal dysfunction. If the GFR (see p. 415) is between 10 and 50 ml/min, the dosing interval should be q8-12h, and if the GFR is <10 ml/min, the interval should be q18-24h.

XI. Trimethoprim (Proloprim, Tripex, generic) inhibits folic acid synthesis and is active against many aerobic gram-negative bacteria excluding *P. aeruginosa*. Trimethoprim is most often used in combination with sulfamethoxazole (see below); however, it is effective alone for treatment of urinary tract infections. **Dosage:** Adults, 100 mg PO q12h or 200 mg PO q24h. The use of trimethoprim in patients with a creatinine clearance of less than 15 ml/min is not recommended. For patients with a creatinine clearance of 15-30 ml/min, the dosage should be 50 mg PO q12h. Trimethoprim has also been used in combination with dapsone for prevention and treatment of *P. carinii* pneumonia.

XII. Trimethoprim-sulfamethoxazole (Bactrim, Septra, generic). Trimethoprin-sulfamethoxazole (TMP/SMZ) is a fixed combination of trimethoprim and sulfamethoxazole in a ratio of 1:5. This antibiotic blocks sequential steps in folic acid synthesis. It is active against many aerobic gram-negative bacteria excluding *P. aeruginosa*. It has good in vitro activity against many aerobic gram-positive bacteria excluding enterococci; however, there is less clinical experience with its use against these bacteria.

A. Indications. TMP/SMZ is the antibiotic of choice for treatment of cystitis, uncomplicated pyelonephritis, *P. carinii* pneumonia (also for prophylaxis), and shigellosis. It is standard therapy for prostatitis, but quinolones appear to be more effective. TMP/SMZ is effective for treatment of otitis media and sinusitis, although activity against streptococci is not optimal. It has also been effective in treatment of listeriosis, nocardiosis, and typhoid fever. TMP/SMZ is an alternative treatment for animal bite infections in patients with major beta-lactam allergy because it is active against *P. multocida* and *S. aureus*. TMP/SMZ penetrates the CSF and has effectively treated meningitis.

B. Adverse reactions. Oral TMP/SMZ may cause nausea and vomiting. Both trimethoprim and sulfamethoxazole may produce depression of all bone marrow cell lines and hemolytic anemia, especially in patients with G-6-PD deficiency. Large doses may lead to macrocytic anemic in patients who are already folate deficient. Patients with human immunodeficiency virus

(HIV) infection have a higher rate of skin rash, fever, leukopenia, and elevated serum transaminase levels than non-HIV-infected patients.
  C. **Drug interactions** are the same as those mentioned above for sulfonamides. Folate deficiency may be aggravated in patients on phenytoin, and TMP/SMZ may increase serum phenytoin levels. It may displace methotrexate from protein binding sites and increase free methotrexate levels. TMP/SMZ has been reported to increase the prothrombin time of patients taking warfarin. In elderly patients receiving diuretics, primarily thiazides, an increased incidence of thrombocytopenia has been reported.
  D. **Dosage.** TMP/SMZ comes in two strengths: as an oral preparation, 80 mg/400 mg and 160 mg/800 mg (double strength), and as an intravenous 5 ml ampule containing 80 mg TMP and 400 mg SMZ.
     A. **For bacterial infections:** Adults, one double-strength tablet or two single-strength tablets PO q12h; Children, 8 mg/kg/d (based on trimethoprim component) divided q12h (suspension available). Intravenous dosage for adults and children: 8-10 mg/kg/d divided q12h.
     B. **For *P. carinii* pneumonia:** Adults and children, 15-20 mg/kg/d (based on trimethoprim component) divided q6h (as oral or parenteral preparation).
     C. **TMP/SMZ dosage should be altered in patients with renal dysfunction:** for patients with a creatinine clearance (see p. 415) of 15-30 ml/min, one half the usual regimen is recommended. TMP/SMZ is not recommended for use if the creatinine clearance is less than 15 ml/min.
XIII. **Clindamycin (Cleocin, generic)** inhibits protein synthesis by ribosomal binding. It is active against most gram-positive cocci including *S. aureus* and *S. pyogenes,* and has significant activity against most gram-positive and gram-negative anaerobes, including most strains of *Clostridia* species and *B. fragilis.* However, resistance of *Bacteroides* species is increasing.
  A. **Indications.** Clindamycin is an alternative to penicillins and cephalosporins in patients with major beta-lactam allergy for treatment of infections due to *S. aureus, S. pyogenes,* and/or anaerobes (e.g., routine cellulitis, necrotizing infections, and head and neck infections). It covers most pathogens of human bite infections excepting *Eikenella corrodens.* Clinical studies have demonstrated that it is superior to penicillin for treatment of lung abscess and anaerobic pneumonia. Clindamycin provides broad anaerobic coverage for treatment of abdominal and pelvic infections, and also has fair activity against *C. trachomatis.* It does not penetrate the CSF well.
  B. **Adverse reactions.** The most common adverse reactions are rash and diarrhea. Pseudomembranous colitis, secondary to *Clostridia difficile,* appears to occur relatively more frequently with this antibiotic when either administered orally or intravenously. It should be prescribed with caution in patients with a history of gastrointestinal disease, particularly colitis.
  C. **Drug interactions.** Clindamycin may enhance the effects of neuromuscular blocking agents.
  D. **Dosage**
     1. **Parenteral.** Adults, 600-1200 mg/d IM/IV divided q6-8h (for more serious infections 1200-2700 mg/d IM/IV divided q6-8h); Children (over 1 month of age), 20-40 mg/kg/d IM/IV divided q6-8h; Neonates, 15-20 mg/kg/d IM/IV divided q6-8h.
     2. **Oral.** Adults, 150-450 mg PO q6h; Children, 8-20 mg/kg/d PO divided q6-8h.

XIV. **Erythromycin** is a macrolide antibiotic that inhibits protein synthesis by ribosomal binding. It is active against aerobic gram-positive bacteria such as *S. pyogenes, S. pneumoniae,* and *S. aureus;* however, occasionally some of these bacteria may demonstrate in vitro resistance. Erythromycin is active against some gram-negative bacteria such as *N. gonorrhoeae, N. meningitidis,* and *Bordetella pertussis.* It has relatively poor activity against *H. influenzae.* In general, erythromycin has poor anaerobic activity, although many *Clostridium perfringens* isolates are susceptible. Erythromycin is also active against *Mycoplasma pneumoniae, Legionella pneumophila, Ureaplasma urealyticum, T. pallidum, C. trachomatis, Corynebacterium diphtheriae,* and *M. catarrhalis.*

A. Indications. Erythromycin is the preferred antibiotic for outpatient treatment of pneumonia in young adults so as to cover for *M. pneumoniae, Chlamydia pneumoniae* (TWAR), and early pneumococcal infection. Intravenous erythromycin might be added to a broad-spectrum regimen for empiric treatment of severe pneumonia if *L. pneumophila* was suspected. It is the drug of choice to treat diphtheria, pertussis, neonatal *Chlamydia* infection, and campylobacteriosis. Erythromycin is an alternative to penicillin to treat streptococcal and staphylococcal infections, and syphilis, and is an alternative to tetracycline for treatment of chlamydial genital infections.

B. Adverse reactions. Gastrointestinal side effects are very common, including cramps, nausea, vomiting, and diarrhea. These may occur with oral or intravenous use, are dose related, and are more common in children and young adults than in older patients. No erythromycin preparation appears to be significantly less problematic with regard to gastrointestinal side effects. Cholestatic jaundice occurs rarely, in particular with the estolate preparation. This reaction appears more common in pregnancy. Therefore the estolate preparation should not be used during this period. Transient hearing loss has been rarely reported with large doses.

C. Drug interactions. Erythromycin can interfere with the hepatic metabolism of several drugs, thereby causing an increase in drug levels that sometimes leads to toxicity. These drugs include theophylline, warfarin, methylprednisolone, carbamazepine, and cyclosporin. Erythromycin can increase bioavailability of digoxin by decreasing inactivation by gut flora.

D. Dosage

1. **Parenteral (Erythromycin lactobionate, generic).** Adults, 1-4 gm/d divided q6h; Children, 15-50 mg/kg/d divided q6h.

2. **Oral preparations.** The base preparation **(E-Mycin, ERYC, Ery-Tab, Erythromycin Base Filmtab, Erythromycin Delayed Release Capsules, PCE Disperstab, Ilotycin, generic)** and various salts are available, including erythromycin estolate **(Ilosone, generic)** ethylsuccinate **(E.E.S., EryPed, Wyamycin E),** and stearate **(Erythrocin Stearate, Wyamycin S, generic).** The most common preparations that are available are 250 mg tablets or capsules, and suspensions of 125 and 250 mg/5 ml. The standard dosing interval is q6h; however, twice the dose can be given q12h for most infections. Adults, 1-2 mg/d PO divided q6-12h; Children, 30-50 mg/kg/d PO divided q6-12h.

   a. **Erythromycin ethylsuccinate and sulfisoxazole (Pediazole)** are active against most otitis media pathogens, including ampicillin-resistant *H. influenzae,* and is useful for treatment of acute or refractory otitis media in children.

b. Dosage: Children, 50 mg/kg/d based on the erythromycin component (200 mg erythromycin per 5 ml of suspension) divided q6h.

XV. **Clarithromycin (Biaxin) and Azithromycin (Zithromax)** are new macrolide and azalide antibiotics related to erythromycin but with significantly better bioavailability, higher tissue levels, less gastrointestinal side effects, and an extended antibacterial spectrum that also includes *H. influenzae.* These agents are indicated for respiratory tract infections and are active against atypical pathogens such as *M. pneumoniae, C. pneumoniae,* and *Legionella* species, as well as the common pyogenic pathogens *S. pneumoniae* and *H. influenzae.* Both drugs have similar activity to erythromycin against gram-positive bacteria and are alternative agents for skin and soft tissue infections. Azithromycin also has activity against *C. trachomatis* and is indicated for single-dose oral therapy of uncomplicated chlamydial genital infections. Its long tissue half-life (2-4 days) also allows for shorter durations of therapy (5 days) for other indications. Both agents have activity against *P. multocida* and are alternative therapies for animal bite infections.

  A. **Drug interactions:** Clarithromycin should be used with caution in patients taking theophylline preparations, digoxin, ergot alkaloids, triazolam, terfenadine and astemizole, and drugs metabolized by the cytochrome P450 system. Azithromycin is not known to produce any clinically significant drug-drug interactions.

  B. Dosage:
    1. **Clarithromycin**—Adults, 250-500 mg PO BID.
    2. **Azithromycin**—Adults, First day 500 mg, then 250 mg QD for 4 days; for chlamydial infections, 1 gm PO (single dose).

XVI. **Chloramphenicol (Chloromycetin, generic)** inhibits protein synthesis by ribosomal binding. It has broad-spectrum activity against aerobes and anaerobes but has largely been replaced by other less toxic antibiotics. Chloramphenicol has excellent activity against the most common meningopathogens, *H. influenzae, N. meningitidis,* and *S. pneumoniae.* It is also active against *Salmonella typhi* and rickettsial species.

  A. **Indications.** Chloramphenicol is an alternative to penicillin and cephalosporins for treatment of bacterial meningitis in patients with a serious sensitivity to these agents. It would be used for empiric and directed treatment of presumed Rocky Mountain spotted fever and other rickettsial infections because it would also treat most common causes of serious bacterial sepsis. Chloramphenicol remains one of the drugs of choice for treatment of typhoid fever. It is an alternative therapy for treatment of brain abscess.

  B. **Adverse reactions.** Chloramphenicol may cause dose-related (usually >4 gm/d), reversible bone marrow suppression and rare idiosyncratic aplastic anemia (estimated to occur once in 24,500-40,800 patients). Hemolytic anemia may result in patients with severe G-6-PD deficiency. Gray-baby syndrome of neonates results from their diminished ability to conjugate choramphenicol; if the drug must be used, the dosage should be decreased and levels monitored.

  C. **Drug interactions.** Chloramphenicol inhibits hepatic microsomal metabolism of the following drugs: tolbutamide, chlorpropamide, phenytoin, and warfarin. Increased serum levels and toxicity may result.

D. Dosage. Adults and Children, 50-100 mg/kg/d IV or PO divided q6h; Neonates, no more than 25 mg/kg/d IV divided q6h.

XVII. Tetracyclines inhibit protein synthesis by ribosomal binding. Tetracycline and doxycycline are therapeutically equivalent; doxycycline offers the advantage of twice-daily dosing. Tetracyclines have broad in vitro activity against aerobic and anaerobic bacteria, chlamydia, spirochetes, rickettsia, and mycoplasmas. However, for many bacterial strains, more consistently effective antibiotics are preferred.

A. Indications. Tetracyclines are the agents of choice to treat *C. trachomatis* genital infections, cholera, relapsing fever *(Borrelia recurrentis)*, psittacosis, and early Lyme disease. They are alternative agents to chloramphenicol for treatment of rickettsial illness, and to erythromycin for treatment of *M. pneumoniae* infections. Most pneumococci and *H. influenzae* are inhibited by tetracycline. Thus these agents are reasonable treatment for acute bronchitis. Tetracyclines are alternative agents to penicillin for treatment of syphilis in penicillin-allergic patients. Although many community-acquired *E. coli* are susceptible to tetracycline, there are other inexpensive and more effective antibiotics such as TMP/SMZ for treatment of uncomplicated urinary tract infection. Other indications include treatment of *Granuloma inguinale, Lymphogranuloma venereum,* melioidosis, *Mycobacterium marinum, Vibrio vulnificus,* acne, actinomycosis, anthrax, rat-bite fever *(Streptobacillus moniliformis),* tularemia, and *Yersinia enterocolitica.* Minocycline is used as alternative prophylaxis to rifampin for meningococcal disease.

B. Adverse reactions. Tetracycline can cause discoloration of teeth and depression of skeletal growth in children. Therefore, tetracycline should not be given to pregnant or nursing mothers or children up to the age of 8 years. Short courses can be given to children in unusual circumstances (e.g., Rocky Mountain spotted fever). Hypersensitivity reactions and especially photosensitivity rash and onycholysis are seen. Oral tetracycline frequently irritates the gastrointestinal tract. Food may decrease this effect for doxycycline; however, food significantly decreases absorption of tetracycline. Hepatotoxicity is seen with high doses, especially in pregnant women or in patients with high levels secondary to renal failure. Tetracycline may exacerbate azotemia by inhibiting protein synthesis and accelerating amino acid metabolism. Concurrent use of tetracycline may render oral contraceptives less effective. Tetracyclines have been associated with increased intracranial pressure. Minocyline has the unique side effect of reversible vertigo.

C. Drug interactions. Compounds containing divalent cations (e.g., Ca^{++}, Mg^{++}, Al^{++}, Fe^{++}) such as antacids may bind tetracycline and doxycycline and prevent gastrointestinal absorption. Tetracycline may potentiate azotemia associated with diuretics. Tetracyclines have been shown to depress plasma prothrombin activity. Therefore, patients on anticoagulants may need a decreased anticoagulant dosage.

D. Dosage: Adults and Children (>7 years), **Tetracycline (Achromycin, Sumycin, generic)** 250-500 mg PO or IV q6h; **Doxycycline (Doryx, Vibramycin, Vibra-Tabs, generic)** 50-100 mg PO or IV q12h.

XVIII. Metronidazole (Flagyl, Metric-21, Protostat, generic) is one of the most active antibiotics against obligate anaerobes. However, many facultative anaerobes such as anaerobic streptococci are resistant. It is active against *C.*

difficile. Metronidazole is also active against many protozoa including *Entamoeba histolytica, Giardia lamblia,* and *Trichomonas vaginalis.*

   A. Indications. Metronidazole is useful for anaerobic infections but must be combined with other antibiotics (e.g., ampicillin or penicillin) for treatment of anaerobic streptococci. Therefore it is used in combination therapy for abdominal and pelvic infections (e.g., metronidazole with ampicillin and gentamicin), brain abscess, anaerobic pneumonias and empyemas, head and neck infections, and mixed skin and soft tissue infections. Metronidazole is the drug of choice for *Trichomonas* and amoebic infections. Because of its low cost, metronidazole is preferred to oral vancomycin by many experts for treatment of pseudomembranous colitis caused by *C. difficile.* It is alternative therapy to quinacrine for *Giardia* infection.

   B. Adverse reactions. Metronidazole has been implicated in producing tumors in rodents and may also be mutagenic. Therefore it is contraindicated in the first trimester of pregnancy and should be avoided later in pregnancy and in nursing mothers. Gastrointestinal disturbances and metallic taste occur. Peripheral neuropathy has been reported rarely with intravenous metronidazole. It may cause darkening of the urine, transient leukopenia, and rashes.

   C. Drug interactions. Ingestion of alcohol while on metronidazole may cause an Antabuse reaction. Psychotic reactions have occurred in patients taking disulfiram. Metronidazole may potentiate the anticoagulant effect of warfarin. Drugs that induce the microsomal enzymes such as phenytoin and phenobarbital may accelerate elimination of metronidazole. Cimetidine may prolong the duration of action of metronidazole.

   D. Dosage: Adults, 500 mg PO or IV q6h. Patients with severe hepatic disease may metabolize metronidazole more slowly, and lower doses should be used in these patients.

XIX. Vancomycin inhibits cell wall synthesis and alters cell wall permeability and RNA synthesis. It is active against staphylococci (including MRSA and *Staphylococcus epidermidis*), streptococci (including enterococci), gram-positive anaerobes (including *C. difficile*), and *L. monocytogenes.* Vancomycin is not active against gram-negative bacilli.

   A. Indications. Vancomycin is an alternative to penicillins and cephalosporins for treating gram-positive infections in patients with a major allergy to these drugs. It is the drug of choice if methicillin-resistant staphylococci (e.g., infections of prosthetic devices, endocarditis in IV drug users in certain geographic areas) or penicillin-resistant pneumococci are suspected. Vancomycin does penetrate the CSF and can be used to treat meningitis. Oral vancomycin is not absorbed systemically; it is the drug of choice to treat pseudomembranous colitis due to *C. difficile.*

   B. Toxicity. Rapid intravenous infusion may cause flushing of the upper body ("red neck" syndrome) and muscle spasms, as well as anaphylactoid reactions. It is best to administer vancomycin at a rate of less than 10 mg/min. Vancomycin has been associated with nephrotoxicity, ototoxicity, and transient neutropenia.

   C. Drug interactions. Concomitant use of vancomycin and anesthetics has been associated with erythema and histamine-like flushing. Vancomycin may compound the nephrotoxicity of nephrotoxic drugs such as aminoglycosides.

D. Dosage
1. **Parenteral**—Adults, 2 gm/d IV divided q6h or q12h; Children, 10 mg/kg IV q6h; Neonates and infants, initial dose 15 mg/kg IV, followed by 10 mg/kg IV q12h for neonates in the first week of life and 10 mg/kg IV q8h in neonates after 1 week of age and up to 1 month of age.

In patients with renal dysfunction, 15 mg/kg initial dose IV can be given with subsequent dosing not required for over 24 hours.

2. **Oral preparation** (not systemically absorbed). Adults, 500 mg PO q6h; Children, 10 mg/kg/d PO divided q6-8h.

XX. **Rifampin (Rifadin, Rimactane)** inhibits bacterial DNA–dependent RNA polymerase. It has activity against *Mycobacterium tuberculosis, Mycobacterium leprae, N. meningitidis, H. influenzae, S. aureus,* and *S. epidermidis.*
  A. **Indications.** Rifampin is a primary treatment of tuberculosis (see p. 425). It is used for prophylaxis of persons exposed to *N. meningitidis* or invasive *H. influenzae,* and to treat the meningococcal carrier state.
  B. **Adverse reactions.** Occasionally dermatitis, "flu-like" syndrome, thrombocytopenia, hemolytic anemia, and renal failure have been associated with use of rifampin. Cholestatic hepatitis reactions may be seen more in the elderly and in patients on isoniazid. Rifampin will stain bodily secretions (also contact lenses) reddish orange.
  C. **Drug interactions.** Rifampin enhances the metabolism of warfarin, corticosteroids, cardiac glycosides, quinidine, oral contraceptives, oral hypoglycemics, narcotics, and analgesics. It has also been reported to diminish the effects of opiates, barbiturates, verapamil, beta-blockers, certain antiarrhythmics, theophylline, and anticonvulsants. Women on oral contraceptives should be advised as to the increased risk of pregnancy. Ketoconizole will diminish rifampin serum levels.
  D. Dosage
    1. **For prophylaxis of *N. meningitidis*:** Adults, 600 mg PO q12h for 2 days; Children, 10 mg/kg PO q12h for 2 days; Neonates, 5 mg/kg PO q12h for 2 days.
    2. ***H. influenzae*:** Adults, 600 mg PO qd for 4 days; Children, 20 mg/kg PO qd for 4 days; Neonates, 10 mg/kg PO qd for 4 days (also see Antituberculous Antibiotics).

Antifungal Therapy

I. **Amphotericin B (Fungizone)** disrupts the fungal cytoplasmic membrane by binding to sterols. Parenteral amphotericin B is useful for treatment of cryptococcosis, North American blastomycosis, disseminated candidiasis, coccidiomycosis, histoplasmosis, mucormycosis, sporotrichosis, and aspergillosis. Topical preparations are available for treatment of cutaneous or mucocutaneous candidiasis.
  A. **Indications.** Parenteral amphotericin B is rarely indicated in an emergency setting because either a fungal infection is not sufficiently suspected or confirmed, or because the infectious process is nonacute and does not demand immediate therapy. However, in certain circumstances (e.g., cryptococcal meningitis and rhinocerebral mucormycosis), rapid initiation of amphotericin B may be lifesaving.
  B. **Adverse reactions.** During administration, acute symptoms such as fever, chills, nausea, vomiting, headache, and thrombophlebitis often occur. These

may be lessened by premedication with acetaminophen and antihistamines, and the addition of 25-50 mg of hydrocortisone to each infusion. Chills often respond to meperidine. Long-term administration may result in anemia, hypokalemia, hypomagnesemia, renal tubular acidosis, and renal failure.
- **C. Drug interactions.** Amphotericin-induced hypokalemia must be monitored in patients on digitalis preparations. Carbenicillin and ticarcillin may exacerbate hypokalemia.
- **D.** Dosage (initial dose)
    1. **For critically ill patients:** Administer 1 mg test dose in 100 ml of D_5W IV over 1 hour. If tolerated then administer 25 mg/kg in 250 ml of D_5W IV over 4 hours.
    2. **For less ill patients:** Administer 1 mg test dose in 100 ml of D_5W IV over 1 hour. If tolerated administer 5 mg in 250 ml of D_5W IV over 4 hours.

II. Imidazoles and triazoles
- **A. Ketoconazole (Nizoral)** is an oral antifungal agent that interferes with fungal cytoplasmic membrane sterol metabolism.
    1. **Indications:** Ketoconazole is indicated in the treatment of chronic fungal infections such as nonmeningeal histoplasmosis, coccidiomycosis, blastomycosis in nonimmunocompromised hosts, treatment of chronic mucocutaneous candidiasis, and for oral and esophageal candidiasis in patients who do not respond to nystatin. Ketoconazole may rarely cause hepatitis, gynecomastia, decreased libido and spermatogenesis, and menstrual irregularities. Its absorption is inhibited by antacids and H_2-receptor blockers; occasional patients on phenytoin or warfarin may have elevated levels of these drugs.
    2. **Dosage:** Adults, 200-400 mg PO QD; Children older than 2 years, 3.3-6.6 mg/kg PO QD. A 2% cream is available for topical treatment of cutaneous candidiasis and for tinea corporis, cruris, and versicolor infections.
- **B. Fluconazole (Diflucan)** acts by a similar mechanism as ketoconazole and is available in tablets and as an intravenous preparation.
    1. **Indications:** Fluconazole is indicated in the treatment of oropharyngeal and esophageal candidiasis, and cryptococcal meningitis. Amphotericin B is preferred for initiation of therapy for acute cryptococcal meningitis; fluconazole is useful for subsequent treatment. Fluconazole is effective as single-dose oral therapy for vaginal candidiasis and may be useful for both meningeal and nonmeningeal coccidiomycosis infections. Rarely minor side effects such as gastrointestinal disturbance, headaches, and skin rash result. Concomitant use of fluconazole and warfarin, phenytoin, and oral hypoglycemics may increase the serum levels of these drugs.
    2. **Dosage:** Adults—for oropharyngeal or esophageal candidiasis, 200 mg PO on the first day and 100 mg PO QD thereafter; for systemic candidiasis or cryptococcal meningitis, 400 mg PO on the first day and 200 mg PO QD thereafter. For vaginal candidiasis, 150 mg PO once. The dosage must be reduced with renal dysfunction. The efficacy of fluconazole in children has not been established.

III. Griseofulvin (Fulvicin P/G, Fulvicin U/F, Grifulvin V, Grisactin, Gris-PEG) is an oral antifungal agent that is deposited in keratin precursor cells.
- **A. Indications:** treatment of dermatophyte (tinea) infections. It is most useful for infections of the scalp, hands, feet, and nails that are refractory to topical therapy. It is contraindicated in patients with porphyria, hepatic failure, and

in pregnancy. Skin rash is the most common side effect. Gastrointestinal disturbance is uncommon if the drug is taken after eating, and headaches, which are relatively common, usually subside in time. Peripheral neuropathy is rarely reported. Griseofulvin may decrease the anticoagulant effect of warfarin, and phenobarbital may increase metabolism of griseofulvin. Griseofulvin may increase the effects of alcohol and decrease the activity of oral contraceptives.

B. Dosage: Adults, 375 mg PO QD; Children, approximately 3.3 mg per pound of body weight PO QD.

IV. **Pentamidine (Pentam 300, NebuPent)** is a parenteral antiprotozoal agent that is now used mainly for treatment of *P. carinii,* which has been classified as a fungus.

   A. Indications: *P. carinii* pneumonia (PCP) in patients who cannot tolerate or who do not respond to TMP/SMZ. Monthly treatments of inhaled aerosolized pentamidine are used as prophylaxis for PCP. Rapid intravenous administration may be accompanied by hypotension; therefore, it should be administered over 1 hour. Other acute reactions include headache, tachycardia, dizziness, gastrointestinal disturbance, and hypoglycemia. With prolonged administration, diabetes, nephrotoxicity, hepatotoxicity, hypocalcemia, and blood cell abnormalities can occur.

   B. Dosage: Adults and Children, 4 mg/kg in 250 ml D_5W over 1 hour IV QD.

Antituberculous Therapy

In general, antituberculous therapy should not be initiated until an appropriate number of specimens from indicated sites have been obtained for culture and staining, and there is reasonable certainty of the diagnosis. However, if there is a significant likelihood of disease based on initial clinical evaluation and if the patient is severely ill (e.g., suspected TB meningitis), or if there is a public health concern of transmission, antituberculous therapy should not be delayed. Only first-line antituberculous medications, isoniazid, rifampin, pyrazinamide, ethambutol, and streptomycin will be discussed.

I. **Isoniazid (INH, Laniazid, generic)** is available in tablets and an injectable form, as well as in a fixed combination with rifampin (**Rifamate, Rimactazid**). It is the most active antituberculous drug and is the only agent known to be effective in chemoprophylaxis. For treatment of active disease, it is usually used in combination with one or more other antituberculous drugs; the standard adult regimen for all forms of tuberculosis, pulmonary and extrapulmonary, is isoniazid 300 mg and rifampin 600 mg PO QD for 9 months. Additional antituberculous drugs may be added initially while awaiting culture and susceptibility data if drug resistance is expected (e.g., previous treatment, contact with drug-resistant source, or acquisition in area with known high prevalence of INH resistance). Initial four-drug regimens are currently recommended because of concern for multi-drug-resistant strains. Isoniazid penetrates the CSF for treatment of meningitis. Overdose can result in mental status changes and seizures; peripheral neuropathy may also develop. These are prevented and treated with pyridoxine. The incidence of isoniazid-induced hepatitis increases with age and exceeds 1% in patients older than 35 years; hepatitis is four times more likely to occur in patients also taking rifampin. Hyperglycemia may be exacerbated in diabetes. Isoniazid may inhibit metabolism of phenytoin, thus increasing serum levels. Antacids may inhibit absorption. **Dosage:** Adults, 300 mg PO QD; Children, 10-20 mg/kg/d; Neonates and Infants, 5-10 mg/kg/d (as a single dose).

II. **Rifampin** is the standard therapy along with isoniazid for treatment of tuberculosis (see isoniazid above). It is also the drug of choice for chemoprophylaxis of invasive *H. influenzae* and *N. menigitidis* infections (see rifampin, p. 422). Rifampin penetrates the CSF for treatment of meningitis. **Dosage:** Adults, 600 mg PO QD; Children, 10 mg/kg/d (as a single dose).
III. **Pyrazinamide** is mycobactericidal and is used for intensive short-course antituberculous therapy (6 months) and initially if drug-resistance is suspected (see isoniazid above). Pyrazinamide penetrates the CSF for treatment of meningitis. It may increase serum uric acid levels and cause arthralgias, gastrointestinal disturbances, and in high dosages, hepatotoxicity. **Dosage:** Adults and Children, 20-30 mg/kg/d (as a single dose).
IV. **Streptomycin** is an aminoglycoside that is sometimes used as a third antituberculous drug in disseminated or resistant disease. It does not penetrate the CSF. It is also the agent of choice in combination with tetracycline for treatment of brucellosis, tularemia, and plague. Its primary toxicity is vestibular, especially in older patients, and its dosage must be reduced in patients with renal insufficiency. **Dosage:** Adults, 15 mg/kg/d IM (usually 1 gm) in one or two divided doses; Children, 20-40 mg/kg/d IM; Neonates, 20 mg/kg/d IM. Streptomycin may also be administered intravenously in a diluted form over 30-60 minutes.
V. **Ethambutol (Myambutol)** is a relatively weak first-line antituberculous drug and is occasionally used in initial regimens to decrease the chance of the development of drug resistance. Generally reversible optic neuritis with red-green blindness, decreased visual acuity, and central scotoma may occur with dosages of 25 mg/kg/d. **Dosage:** Adults and older Children, 15-25 mg/kg/d PO QD (in a single dose). It should not be given to children younger than 5 years because ocular toxicity cannot be monitored.

Antiviral Therapy

I. **Acyclovir (Zovirax)** is a guanosine analogue that inhibits viral DNA polymerase. It has significant antiviral activity against herpes viruses, including herpes simplex virus types 1 and 2 and varicella-zoster virus.
   A. **Indications:** Oral acyclovir is indicated for episodic therapy and long-term suppressive therapy of genital herpes. For localized zoster, high-dose oral acyclovir (600-800 mg five times daily for 7-10 days) has been shown to reduce acute pain, duration of viral shedding, and healing time of skin lesions; there is limited evidence to suggest that acyclovir decreases the incidence of postherpetic neuralgia. Intravenous acyclovir is indicated for localized herpes simplex (i.e., orofacial, esophageal, and genital infection) and varicella-zoster infections in immunocompromised hosts, and for herpes simplex encephalitis. It is also indicated for chickenpox in children and recommended by some for chickenpox in adults; for chickenpox it is most effective if administered within 24 hours of the onset of rash. Intravenous administration may be associated with precipitation of acyclovir crystals and acute renal dysfunction, and rarely mental status changes. Oral therapy may occasionally be associated with gastrointestinal disturbance and headache.
   B. **Dosage**
      1. **Oral:** Genital herpes—initial episode, 200 mg PO five times daily (or 400 mg TID) for 10 days; intermittent therapy, 200 mg PO five times daily for 5 days; chronic suppressive therapy, 400 mg PO BID for up to 12 months. Herpes zoster, 800 mg PO five times daily for 7-10 days. Chickenpox—

children, 20 mg/kg/d 4 times a day for 5 days; adults, 800 mg PO five times a day for 5 days. (For patients with renal dysfunction, the duration between doses should be increased: creatinine clearance <25 ml/min q12h-<12.5 ml/min q24h.)
   2. **Parenteral:** Disseminated herpes in immunocompromised host, herpes encephalitis, 12.4 mg/kg IV q8h for 7-10 days.
II. **Zidovudine (Retrovir)** is a thymidine analogue that inhibits viral RNA–dependent DNA polymerase. It has antiviral activity against HIV-1.
   A. **Indication:** Zidovudine is indicated for the treatment of patients with AIDS and for asymptomatic HIV-infected patients with CD4 lymphocyte counts <500/mm^3. In these patients zidovudine has been shown to significantly slow the progression to AIDS, decrease the incidence of opportunistic infections, and improve survival compared with placebo. Adverse effects occur more frequently in patients with advanced HIV disease. These frequently include anemia and granulocytopenia, which are dose related and usually reversible. Other side effects such as asthenia, gastrointestinal disturbance, CNS symptoms, and myalgia occur but have also been noted frequently in placebo-treated patients. For patients with significant baseline anemia (hemoglobin <7.5 gm/dl) or granulocytopenia (<750/mm^3), a reduction of daily dosage or interruption of continuous therapy is advised.
   B. **Dosage:** Adults, 200 mg PO q8h; Children (3 mo-12 years of age), 180 mg/m^2 PO q6h (not to exceed 200 mg q6h).
III. **Amantadine (Symmetrel)** inhibits replication of influenza A viruses. It has been demonstrated to have prophylactic and therapeutic efficacy for influenza A virus infections. Amantadine causes anticholinergic side effects and CNS complaints, particularly in high dosage. These side effects may be exacerbated by concomitant use of drugs with similar effects. **Dosage:** Adults, 200 mg PO QD (a split dose administered BID may reduce CNS side effects), Children (1-9 years of age), 4.4-8.8 mg/kg PO QD (not to exceed 150 mg/d). The dosage should be reduced in the elderly and those patients with renal impairment. Recently, a related anti-viral, rimantadine (Flumadine), has been approved; it appears to be as effective as amantadine with fewer CNS side effects.

Antiparasitic Therapy

I. **Metronidazole** (see p. 420) is the drug of choice for treatment of extraintestinal amoebic infections and vaginitis due to *Trichomonas vaginalis.* Although the cure rate is slightly less than quinacrine for giardiasis, it is generally preferred because it is better tolerated. **Dosage:** *T. vaginalis* vaginitis, 2 gm PO as one dose, or 250 mg PO TID for 7 days; Giardiasis, 250 mg PO TID for 5 days; Amebiasis, 750 mg PO TID for 10 days.
II. **Iodoquinol (Yodoxin)** is indicated for eradication of asymptomatic cysts; treatment of **intestinal** amebiasis is used for metronidazole.
   A. **Adverse effects** include gastrointestinal disturbance, acne, minimal thyroid enlargement, and optic atrophy with prolonged use.
   B. **Dosage:** Adults, 1 tablet (650 mg each) PO TID for 20 days; Children, 40 mg/kg PO QD divided into three doses, not to exceed 1.95 gm in 24 hours, for 20 days.
III. **Quinacrine HCl (Atabrine)** is an alternative drug to metronidazole for treatment of giardiasis (see comments on metronidazole above).

A. Adverse effects include bitter taste, gastrointestinal disturbance, and headaches. In high doses it may turn the skin and urine yellow. Less common side effects include skin rash and reversible acute toxic psychosis. It is contraindicated in patients with a history of psychosis. Quinacrine causes a disulfiram-like reaction to alcohol and may result in toxic serum levels of primaquine.

B. Dosage: Adults, 100 mg PO TID after meals for 5 days; Children, 2 mg/kg PO TID after meals for 5 days (maximum: 300 mg/d).

IV. Chloroquine HCl (Aralen HCl) is an antimalarial used for prophylaxis and therapy. It has activity against the erythrocytic phase of *Plasmodium vivax, P. ovale,* and *P. malariae;* however, *P. falciparum* strains are widely resistant.

A. Adverse effects of chloroquine include headache, fatigue, confusion, nausea, and vomiting. Rarely blood dyscrasias, rash, corneal opacities, retinal damage, and toxic psychosis may occur. It is contraindicated in patients with retinal disease, psoriasis, or porphyria and should be administered with caution in patients with G-6-PD deficiency. Chloroquine can be given by slow intravenous infusion; however, respiratory depression, circulatory collapse, and seizures can occur.

B. Dosage

1. Treatment of acute attack: Adults, 1 gm (600 mg base) initially, followed by 500 mg (300 mg base) in 6-8 hours, and 500 mg on each of the next 2 days PO; Children, 10 mg base/kg, followed by 5 mg base/kg in 6-8 hours, and 5 mg base/kg on each of the next 2 days PO.

2. Prophylaxis: Adults, 500 mg (300 mg base) PO same day of week, each week; Children, 5 mg base/kg weekly (suppression should begin 2 weeks before exposure and continue for 8 weeks after leaving the endemic area).

V. Mefloquine (Larium) is an antimalarial used for prophylaxis and treatment of chloroquine-resistant *P. falciparum* malaria. It is also active against the erythrocytic phase of *P. vivax.* Mefloquine is now the drug of choice for prophylaxis for travel to areas with chloroquine-resistant *P. falciparum* malaria. It can be used for oral treatment of *P. falciparum* malaria where quinine resistance is encountered (e.g., Thailand).

A. Adverse effects include nausea, dizziness, and transient sinus bradycardia.

B. Dosage

1. Treatment of acute attack. Adults, five tablets (1250 mg) PO as single dose with 8 oz of water. (The safety and effectiveness of mefloquine has not been established in children; however, when administered at a dose of 20-30 mg/kg as a single dose, it was found to be effective.)

2. Prophylaxis, one tablet (250 mg) PO as a single dose weekly for 4 weeks, then one tablet every other week. Suppression should begin 1 week before travel and should be continued 4 weeks after returning from the endemic area.

VI. Quinine and quinidine are dextrostereoisomers that are antimalarials active against the erythrocyte phase of *Plasmodium* species including chloroquine-resistant *P. falciparum* malaria. They are the drugs of choice to treat this condition.

A. Availability. Parenteral quinine is only available through the Centers for Disease Control and Prevention (CDC) (phone: 404-448-4046 or 404-638-2888), whereas parenteral quinidine is available in most hospitals but is considered an investigational agent for this condition. Quinine is relatively toxic and causes cinchonism (tinnitus, decreased hearing, headache, nausea, vomiting, and visual disturbance), rarely rashes, blood dyscrasias, massive hemolysis or hypoglycemia in patients with *P. falciparum* malaria, respiratory depression in patients with myasthenia gravis, and hemolysis in patients with G-6-PD deficiency. Quinine must be administered slowly when given intravenously to avoid shock secondary to cardiac depression and peripheral vasodilation. Quinidine gluconate is available for intravenous infusion. Prolongation of the QT interval, conduction disturbances, myocardial depression and hypotension, and cinchonism may occur. Quinidine may increase digoxin levels and potentiate warfarin.

B. Dosage
1. **Oral.** Quinine sulfate: Adults, 650 mg PO q8h for 3-7 days; Children, 25 mg/kg/d in three doses for 3 days.
2. **Parenteral.** Quinine sulfate or quinidine gluconate (same as above).

VII. Pyrimethamine (Daraprim) and a sulfonamide (sulfadiazine or **Fansidar** with sulfadoxine) is the therapy of choice for toxoplasmosis; pyrimethamine plus quinine (or mefloquine) is used for treatment of chloriquine-resistant *P. falciparum* malaria. The combination is no longer recommended for prophylaxis of chloroquine-resistant *P. falciparum* because of the risk of Stevens-Johnson syndrome and the advent of a safer agent, mefloquine.

A. Adverse effects of pyrimethamine (with a sulfonamide) include bone marrow suppression, which can be prevented with administration of folinic acid, and rarely, rash, gastrointestinal disturbance, and seizures. Pyrimethamine is contraindicated in the first trimester of pregnancy.

B. Dosage
1. **Malaria:** Adults, 25 mg PO q12h for 3 days; Children <10 kg, 6.25 mg/d; 10-20 kg, 12.5 mg/d; 20-40 kg, 25 mg/d, for 3 days.
2. **Toxoplasmosis (with sulfadiazine).** Adults, 100 mg, then 25 mg PO QD for 4-5 weeks; for patients with AIDS, 200 mg, then 75-100 mg PO QD (see sulfonamides pp. 415-416).

VIII. Primaquine phosphate (Aralen) is the only antimalarial drug available that is effective at eradicating the exoerythrocytic (liver) phase of *P. vivax* and *P. ovale*. It is used after a course of treatment or prophylaxis with chloroquine. Primaquine rarely causes gastrointestinal disturbance, anemia, methemoglobinemia, leukocytosis and other blood dyscrasias, hypertension, and arrhythmias.

A. The major concern with the use of primaquine is hemolysis in patients with G-6-PD deficiency. Groups at high risk for this deficiency (i.e., black, Asian, and Middle Eastern males) should be tested before primaquine administration.

B. Dosage: Adults, 26.3 mg (15 mg base) PO QD for 14 days; Children, 6.3 mg base/kg/d PO for 14 days.

IX. Suramin (Germainin) is used to treat non-CNS African trypanosomiasis (hemolymphatic).

A. Adverse effects include immediate effects of nausea, vomiting, shock, loss of consciousness, and urticaria. Later reactions up to 24 hours after administration include fever, rash, and paresthesias. Renal failure, prostration, jaundice, and chronic diarrhea may occur. The drug is available through the CDC (phone: 404-639-3670 or 404-639-2888).

B. Dosage: Adults, 100-200 mg (test dose) IV, then 1 gm IV on days 1, 2, 7, 14, and 21; Children, 20 mg/kg on days 1, 3, 7, 14, and 21.

X. Melarsoprol (Arsobal) is an arsenical used for treatment of CNS African trypanosomiasis. It is a highly toxic drug.

A. Adverse effects include fever, abdominal pain, vomiting, and arthralgia. The most serious side effect is reactive encephalopathy. Melarsoprol can cause severe hemolysis in patients with G-6-PD deficiency. The drug is available through the CDC (phone: 404-639-3670 or 404-639-2888).

B. Dosage: Adults, 2-3 mg/kg/d IV for 3 days, after 1 week 3-6 mg/kg/d IV for 3 days, repeat again in 10-21 days; Children, 18-25 mg/kg total over 1 month, initial dose 0.3 mg/kg IV, gradually increasing to 3.6 mg/kg (maximum) at intervals of 1-5 days for total of 9-10 doses.

XI. Nifurtimox (Lampit) is used for treatment of acute Chagas disease.

A. Adverse effects that are common and reversible include gastrointestinal disturbance, paresthesias, insomnia, disorientation, and rarely seizures. The drug is available through the CDC (phone: 404-639-3670 or 404-639-2888).

B. Dosage: Adult, 8-10 mg/kg/d PO q6h for 12 days; Children, 1-10 years, 15-20 mg/kg/d PO q6h for 90 days; 11-16 years, 12.5-15 mg/kg/d q6h for 90 days.

XII. Stibogluconate sodium (Pentostam) is an antimonial used for treatment of visceral and cutaneous leishmaniasis.

A. Adverse effects include abdominal pain, nausea, vomiting, headache, serum transaminase elevation, nephrotoxicity, fever, rash, and pneumonitis. There are dose-related ECG changes and arrhythmias, and sudden death has been associated with high doses. Antimonials are contraindicated in patients with myocarditis, hepatitis, and nephritis. The drug is available through the CDC (phone: 404-639-3670 or 404-639-2888).

B. Dosage: Adults and Children, 20 mg/kg/d (maximum 800 mg/d) IM/IV for 20 days.

XIII. Mebendazole (Vermox) is used for the treatment of intestinal roundworms, including *Ascaris lumbricoides* (common roundworm), *Necator americanus* and *Ancylostoma doudenale* (hookworm), *Trichuris trichiura* (whipworm), and *Enterobius vermicularis* (pinworm).

A. Adverse effects such as abdominal pain and diarrhea are uncommon. Occasionally the drug may provoke migration of ascaris worms from the nose or mouth. Mebendazole is contraindicated in pregnancy.

B. Dosage: Adults and children, Pinworm—one (100 mg) tablet PO once; Whipworms, hookworm, and common roundworm—one tablet PO BID for 3 days.

The use of mebendazole has not been extensively studied in children younger than 2 years.

XIV. Thiabendazole (Mintezol) is used for treatment of intestinal roundworms and larvae in tissues. It is indicated for treatment of strongyloidiasis, cutaneous larval migrans, visceral larval migrans, and for symptomatic relief in trichinosis. It may also be used if mebendazole is ineffective for hookworm, pinworm, and common roundworm.

A. Adverse effects commonly include nausea, vomiting, dizziness, malodorous urine, and, rarely, rash, abdominal pain, dysesthesias, diarrhea, bradycardia and hypotension, liver function test abnormalities, and biliary duct injury. Because of CNS side effects, activities requiring alertness should be avoided. Thiabendazole is relatively contraindicated in pregnancy.

B. Dosage: Adults and children, 0.1 gm/lb/dose. Strongyloidiasis, cutaneous larva migrans, and intestinal nematodes—two doses per day for 2 days; Visceral larva migrans—two doses per day for 7 days; Trichinosis—two doses per day for 2-4 days according to response of the patient.

XV. **Albendazole (Zentel)** is an antihelminth with broad activity against intestinal helminths including *A. lumbricoides, T. trichiura,* and hookworms. It is most useful for treatment of inoperable echinococcal cysts and for preventing postoperative recurrence of these cysts. Single-dose regimens for intestinal helminths are well tolerated; however, high-dose, prolonged therapy has been associated with hepatitis and obstructive jaundice. The drug is available through the CDC (phone: 404-639-3670 or 404-639-2888). **Dosage:** Adults, for intestinal helminths—400 mg PO as single dose; for echinococcal cysts—20 mg/kg PO QD for 28 days.

XVI. **Diethylcarbamazine (Hetrazan)** is active against lymphatic filariasis due to *Wuchereria bancrofti, Brugia malayi* and *B. timori, Mansonella ozzardi, Loa loa,* and the syndrome of pulmonary infiltrates with eosinophilia in the tropics. Ivermectin has replaced diethylcarbamazine as the treatment of choice for onchocerciasis.
  A. **Adverse reactions** are due both to the drug and the inflammatory reaction to released filarial antigens. Common reactions include headache, nausea, vomiting, arthralgia, and rarely acute psychosis. The drug is available through the CDC (phone: 404-639-3670 or 404-639-2888).
  B. **Dosage:** Adults, 50 mg PO after meal on day 1, 50 mg PO TID on day 2, 100 mg PO TID on day 3, 2 mg/kg TID days 4-21; Children, 1/2 the adult dose.
     (Note: for tropical pulmonary eosinophilia the dosage is 2 mg/kg PO TID for 7-10 days.)

XVII. **Ivermectin (Metizan)** is a recent advance for the treatment of onchocerciasis, with resultant local inflammatory reaction less severe than with diethylcarbamazine.
  A. **Adverse reactions** include fever, pruritus, headache, and cutaneous edema.
  B. **Dosage:** Adults and Children, 150 mg/kg PO as a single dose.

XVIII. **Praziquantel (Biltrizide)** is broadly active against flukes and tapeworms including schistosomiasis, liver flukes *(Clonorchis sinensis* and *Opisthorchis viverrini),* paragonimiasis (lung flukes), and intestinal flukes. It is highly active against adult and larval forms of tapeworms; however, niclosamide is preferred for tapeworm treatment. Praziquantel is indicated for treatment of neurocysticercosis under special circumstances; it is not effective against nonactive calcified cysts.
  A. **Adverse reactions** are common but mild including nausea, vomiting, abdominal pain, dizziness, and headache. Occasionally acute allergic reactions may follow treatment with release of worm antigens. Praziquantel may cause life-threatening reactions after treatment of neurocysticercosis, including increased intracranial pressure, cerebral edema, and seizures. Pretreatment with corticosteroids may help prevent these reactions.
  B. **Dosage:** Adults and children, 25 mg/kg PO TID for 1 day. (Note: paragonimiasis is treated for 2 days.)

XIX. **Niclosamide (Niclocide)** is the drug of choice for tapeworm infection due to *Taenia saginata* (beef tapeworm), *Diphyllobothrium latum* (fish tapeworm), and *Diphylidium caninum* (dog tapeworm).
  A. **Adverse effects** are rare and mild including gastrointestinal disturbance, drowsiness, dizziness, headache, and rash.

B. Dosage: *T. saginata* and *D. latum*—Adults, four tablets (2.0 gm) PO as single dose; Children >34 kg, three tablets (1.5 gm) PO as single dose; between 11 and 34 kg, two tablets (1.0 gm) PO as a single dose.

The safety of niclosamide has not been established in children younger than 2 years.

Suggested Readings

Center for Disease Control: 1993 sexually transmitted diseases treatment guidelines, *MMWR* 42:1-102, 1993.

The Medical Letter: *Handbook of antimicrobial therapy,* New Rochelle, NY, 1992, The Medical Letter.

Hessen MT, Kaye D: Principles of selection and use of antibacterial agents, *Infect Dis Clin North Am* 3:479-89, 1989.

Mustafa MM, McCracken GH: Antimicrobial agents in pediatric, *Infect Dis Clin North Am* 3:491-506, 1989.

Neu HC: General Concepts on chemotherapy of infectious diseases, *Med Clin North Am* 71:1051-64, 1987.

Physicians desk reference, ed 48, Montvale, NJ, 1994, Medical Economics Data.

The Medical Letter: Drugs for viral infections, *Med Lett Drugs Ther* 34:31-6, 1992.

The Medical Letter: The choice of antibacterial drugs, *Med Lett Drugs Ther* 34:49-56, 1992.

The Medical Letter: Drugs for tuberculosis, *Med Lett Drugs Ther* 35:99-102, 1993.

The Medical Letter: Drugs for parasitic infections, *Med Lett Drugs Ther* 35:111-22, 1993.

Sullivan TJ. Penicillin allergy. In Lichtenstein LM, Fauci A, editors: *Current therapy in allergy.* Philadelphia: BC Decker Inc., 1985.

Talan DA. The role of new antibiotics for the treatment of infections in the emergency department. *Ann Emerg Med* 24:473-489, 1994.

14

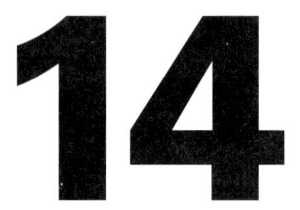

Treatment of Common Infections

Craig A. Wood, M.D.

Antibiotic therapy prescribed in the emergency department must be guided by an accurate clinical diagnosis and a thorough understanding of the microbiologic differential diagnosis. Neither the specific identification of the responsible organism nor the in vitro susceptibility results are generally available to the emergency practitioner to aid in guiding therapy.

Our understanding of the organisms responsible for a wide variety of infections has expanded tremendously. At the same time, the availability of antibiotics has also increased dramatically. The major goals of this chapter are to update the microbiologic causes of clinical infections and to recommend antibiotic therapy aimed at those organisms. The major emphasis will be on those illnesses amenable to treatment by the emergency physician. That will, in the majority of instances, dictate oral antimicrobial therapy. However, parenteral therapy does play a role, especially as single-dose therapy. The final decision to treat a patient in either an outpatient or inpatient setting requires sound clinical judgment. In addition to primary antibiotic therapy prescribed by emergency physicians, a variety of circumstances in which prophylactic or early empiric therapy is initiated within the emergency department will be discussed.

Each of the following sections will contain brief descriptions of clinical infections, a listing of the potential causative agents, and treatment recommendations. Additional antibiotic choices may also be effective in individual cases. The importance of knowing specific geographic and hospital microbiology cannot be overemphasized. An extensive differential diagnosis or discussion of the diagnostic work-up is beyond the scope of this chapter. Though it is not possible to cover the entire spectrum of infections encountered in the emergency department, the majority of the more commonly occurring infections will be discussed. For rapid reference, the recommended antibiotics will be found in tabular form at the end of most sections and will include first-line choices, as well as alternative agents. Individual choices are often dictated by antibiotic allergies or intolerances, drug availability, and cost. Recommendations of specific agents from a therapeutically equivalent class of antibiotics may allow substitution of other drugs of the same class. **Table 14-1** shows commonly used oral antibiotics, including available dosage forms and usual adult and pediatric dosages.

New antimicrobial agents are continually being introduced, and additional cephalosporins, β-lactam and β-lactamase combinations, fluoroquinolones, and others will become available. Our therapeutic armamenterium must necessarily evolve as the newer agents are carefully compared with our current choices.

Treatment of Common Infections 433

Table 14-1. Commonly Used Oral Antibiotics

Antibiotics	Dosage forms Tablets/capsules	Suspension	Usual dosage Adult	Children
Penicillins				
Natural penicillin				
Penicillin V	250, 500 mg	125, 250 mg/5 ml	250-500 mg qid	50 mg/kg divided tid-qid
Penicillinase-resistant penicillins				
Dicloxacillin	125, 250, 500 mg	62.5 mg/5 ml	250-500 mg qid	12.5-50 mg/kg divided qid
Cloxacillin	250, 500 mg	125 mg/5 ml	250-500 mg qid	50-100 mg/kg divided qid
Aminopenicillins				
Ampicillin	250, 500 mg	125, 250 mg/5 ml	250-500 mg qid	50-100 mg/kg divided tid
Amoxicillin	250, 500 mg	125, 250 mg/5 ml	250-500 mg tid	40 mg/kg divided tid
β-Lactam/β-Lactamase Combination				
Amoxicillin/clavulanic acid	250, 500 mg*	125, 250 mg*/5 ml	250-500 mg* tid	40 mg*/kg divided tid
Cephalosporins				
First generation				
Cephalexin	250, 500 mg	125, 250 mg/5 ml	250-500 mg qid	50-100 mg/kg divided qid
Cephradine	250, 500 mg	125, 250 mg/5 ml	250-500 mg qid	50-100 mg/kg divided qid
Cefadroxil	500 mg, 1 gm	125, 250 mg/5 ml	1 gm daily	30 mg/kg divided bid
Second generation				
Cefuroxime axetil	125, 250, 500 mg	Not available	250-500 mg bid	125-250 mg bid
Cefaclor	250, 500 mg	125, 187, 250, 375 mg/5 ml	250-500 mg tid	40 mg/kg divided tid
Cefprozil	250, 500 mg	125, 250 mg/5 ml	250-500 mg bid	15 mg/kg divided bid
Loracarbef	200 mg	100, 200 mg/5 ml	200-400 mg bid	15-30 mg/kg divided bid
Third generation				
Cefixime	200, 400 mg	100 mg/5 ml	400 mg daily	8 mg/kg daily
Cefpodoxime proxetil	100, 200 mg	50, 100 mg/5 ml	200-400 mg bid	10 mg/kg divided bid

Continued on next page

Table 14-1. Commonly Used Oral Antibiotics—cont'd

Antibiotics	Tablets/capsules	Suspension	Adult	Children
Macrolides				
Erythromycin	250, 500 mg	125, 250 mg/5 ml	250-500 mg qid	50 mg/kg divided tid-qid
Erythromycin ethyl succinate	400 mg	200, 400 mg/5 ml	400-800 mg qid	50 mg/kg divided tid-qid
Clarithromycin	250, 500 mg	Not available	250-500 mg bid	No recommendation
Azithromycin	250 mg	Not available	500 mg day 1, 250 mg daily days 2-5	No recommendation
Tetracyclines				
Doxycycline	50, 100 mg	25, 50 mg/5 ml	50-100 mg bid	5 mg/kg divided bid†
Tetracycline	250, 500 mg	125 mg/5 ml	250-500 mg qid	25-50 mg/kg divided qid†
Quinolones				
Ciprofloxacin	250, 500, 750 mg	Not available	250-750 mg bid	Not indicated
Norfloxacin	400 mg	Not available	400 mg bid	Not indicated
Ofloxacin	200, 300, 400 mg	Not available	200-400 mg bid	Not indicated
Lomefloxacin	400 mg	Not available	400 mg daily	Not indicated
Enoxacin	200, 400 mg	Not available	200-400 mg bid	Not indicated
Miscellaneous				
Trimethoprim-sulfamethoxazole	80/400, 160/800 mg (SS) (DS)	40/200 mg/5 ml	2 SS or 1 DS bid	10/50 mg/kg divided bid (or 8 mg/kg/d q12h based on trimethoprim component)
Metronidazole	250, 500 mg	Not available	250-500 mg tid	15 mg/kg divided bid
Clindamycin	150, 300 mg	75 mg/5 ml	150-450 mg qid	8-20 mg/kg divided tid
Erythromycin ethyl succinate/sulfisoxazole	Not available	200/600 mg/5 ml	Not used	50/150 mg/kg divided qid

SS, Single strength; DS, double strength.
*Amount of amoxicillin (clavulanate dose varies by preparation; two 250 mg tablets have twice the clavulanate as one 500 mg tablet).
†Tetracyclines not used in children younger than 8 years because they can cause primary tooth discoloration.

Skin and Soft Tissue Infections

Skin and soft tissue infections are among the most common infections seen in the outpatient or emergency department setting and occur in patients of all ages. Severity of illness varies from mild to life threatening. Therapy is often a combined medical and surgical approach **(Table 14-2)**.

I. Impetigo. Impetigo is a vesiculopustular infection that produces a characteristic golden yellow crust secondary to purulent drainage. The infection begins on exposed areas of the skin, such as the extremities, and quickly spreads to other parts of the body by self-inoculation. Preschool children are most often affected, but impetigo occurs in all age groups. Infection is caused by group A

Table 14-2. Antibiotic Therapy for Skin and Soft Tissue Infections

Clinical indication	Primary	Alternative
Impetigo	Penicillinase-resistant penicillins, first-generation cephalosporins, macrolides, clindamycin	Mupirocin topical
Cellulitis		
Including facial adult	Penicillinase-resistant penicillins, first-generation cephalosporins	Clindamycin
Facial in children	Amoxicillin/clavulanate	Second-generation cephalosporins
Abscess, acute furuncle, recurrent furunculosis, carbuncle	Drainage ±, clindamycin, penicillinase-resistant penicillins	First-generation cephalosporins, clindamycin, macrolides
Bites		
Human	Amoxicillin/clavulanate	Erythromycin or tetracycline, plus clindamycin
Dog/cat	Amoxicillin/clavulanate	Tetracycline ± clindamycin
Punctures	None, unless clinically infected; administer tetanus prophylaxis	—
Herpes zoster	High-dose oral acyclovir in selected patients; treat secondary infections with penicillinase-resistant penicillins or first-generation cephalosporins	—
Tinea corporis, cruris, pedis	Miconazole, clotrimazole, others	—
Tinea versicolor	Ketoconazole	—
Scabies	Permethrin, lindane 1%, 10% crotamiton	—
Lice	Permethrin, lindane	—

streptococci and *Staphylococcus aureus*. Though clinical differences are said to exist between streptococcal and staphylococcal infection (nonbullous versus bullous impetigo), differentiation is often impractical. Treatment consists of a penicillinase-resistant penicillin such as dicloxacillin, a first-generation cephalosporin such as cephalexin, or a macrolide antibiotic. Children often dislike the taste of dicloxacillin. Alternatives include amoxicillin/clavulanate or clindamycin. Topical mupirocin ointment provides a nonsystemic alternative but should be reserved for mild cases. Poststreptococcal glomerulonephritis is a potential sequela of impetigo that appears not to be influenced by antibiotic treatment.

II. **Cellulitis.** Cellulitis is an acute, superficial, spreading infection of the skin manifest by erythema and warmth. Infection is most commonly caused by group A streptococci (rarely other β-hemolytic streptococci) or occasionally, *S. aureus*. Erysipelas, an infection caused by group A streptococci, classically has a sharply demarcated, raised, advancing margin, whereas staphylococcal infection generally has a poorly defined, nonelevated border. Again, this distinction is often clinically impractical. Treatment consists of a penicillinase-resistant penicillin such as dicloxacillin or a first-generation cephalosporin. A macrolide (erythromycin, clarithromycin, or azithromycin) or clindamycin are alternatives, especially in the penicillin-allergic patient. Facial cellulitis in the adult has the same microbiologic cause and therapy as discussed above. Facial cellulitis in children may also be caused by *Haemophilus influenzae*, which characteristically causes a purple-blue skin discoloration. Treatment with amoxicillin/clavulanate or a second-generation cephalosporin would be appropriate. Trimethoprim/sulfamethoxazole is an additional alternative therapy for *H. influenzae*.

III. **Abscesses.** Furuncles (boils) are infections of obstructed hair follicles or sebaceous glands due to *S. aureus*. The treatment of choice is incision and drainage; antibiotic therapy is generally not indicated. If the patient is toxic or immunocompromised, if there is extensive cellulitis or involvement of any important structure (e.g., a hand), antibiotics are indicated. Antibiotic therapy should be directed primarily against *S. aureus* with an antistaphylococcal penicillin, first-generation cephalosporin, or macrolide. Recurrent furunculosis is a common and difficult problem. Traditional antistaphylococcal therapy is generally unsuccessful at interrupting recurrences. Recent data suggests that a 3-month course of low-dose clindamycin (150 mg once daily) may induce remission in a majority of those treated.

IV. **Bites.** Human and animal bites are all contaminated wounds and carry a substantial risk of infection, especially when involving the hand and distal arm. Cleaning, irrigation, and debridement are of primary importance, as is tetanus prophylaxis (discussed later in this section). Antibiotic therapy is often considered prophylaxis, if given within 12 hours of the injury, or empiric, if given later or for established infection. Improper management of bite injuries and subsequent infectious complications may have dramatic medicolegal implications. Thus a conservative approach with regard to hospitalization, parenteral antibiotics, and surgical therapy is generally advocated. Bite injuries of the hand, upper extremity, face, and neck are almost always treated with antibiotics. Though fresh, superficial bites of the hand may be managed as an outpatient with oral antibiotics, many injuries and most all established infections require hospitalization. The common clenched fist human bite injury carries a very high risk of infection, with potential involvement of bone, tendon sheath, and/or avascular spaces of the hand. Human bites are contaminated with normal oral and skin flora such as streptococci, *Eikenella corrodens, Bacteriodes* species, *Fusobacterium* species, *S. aureus,* coagulase-negative staphylococci, and group A streptococci. The majority of bite-related infections are polymicrobic. Therapy of hand bite wound infections consists of amoxicillin/clavulanate or, for the penicillin-allergic patient, a combination of erythromycin or tetracycline plus clindamycin (*E. corrodens* is resistant to clindamycin). Dog and cat bites are commonly contaminated with *S. aureus,* coagulase-negative staphylococci, streptococci, *Pasteurella multocida, Bacteroides* species, and *Fusobacterium* species. Dog bites may also be contaminated with *Capnocytophaga* (formerly DF-2). Therapy for either of these animal bites would be amoxicillin/clavulanate or alternatively, trimethoprim/sulfamethoxazole, a quinoline, or tetracycline with or without clindamycin. Cat bite infections of the finger that developed quickly in 24 to 48 hours are often due to *P. multocida* and may result in tenosynovitis or, occasionally, osteomyelitis.

V. Punctures. Puncture wounds are a common problem. Again, local measures and tetanus prophylaxis are of prime importance. Routine antibiotic therapy is generally not recommended unless soft tissue infection (as discussed elsewhere in this section) is manifest. Osteomyelitis of the small bones of the foot is a potential complication of this type of injury, with *Pseudomonas aeruginosa* the most common bacterial isolate. This complication requires a definitive combined medical and surgical approach. Ongoing pain after the initial injury is often a clue to the presence of this complication.

VI. Tetanus prophylaxis. The intensity of tetanus prophylaxis is dictated by the patient's previous history of vaccination with tetanus toxoid and the type of wound present. If three or more doses of tetanus toxoid have been given, a clean minor wound dictates no prophylaxis unless the last booster was given more than 10 years previously, in which case it is given as per the routine booster recommendation; all other wounds (contaminated wounds, punctures, avulsions, crush injuries, projectile injuries) dictate no prophylaxis unless the last tetanus booster was given more than 5 years previously, in which case it is given. Patients with an unknown history or a history of fewer than three doses of tetanus toxoid receive more aggressive prophylaxis. Clean minor wounds prompt a booster dose of tetanus toxoid, while all other wounds dictate both a booster dose and the administration of tetanus immune globulin, 500 units intramuscularly.

VII. Herpes zoster. Herpes zoster is the result of reactivation of latent varicella-zoster virus from the dorsal root ganglia. The cutaneous vesicles of zoster are indistinguishable from those caused by herpes simplex virus but tend to be dermatomal in distribution unless the disease is disseminated, as in the immunocompromised host. High-dose oral therapy using acyclovir, 800 mg five times per day, may make healing and acute pain reduction more rapid. Unfortunately, antiviral therapy with acyclovir is not effective in reducing the incidence or severity of postherpetic neuralgia. Herpes zoster may become secondarily infected with skin flora, dictating therapy with a penicillinase-resistant penicillin or a first-generation cephalosporin.

VIII. Dermatophytoses. The fungal skin infections most likely to be encountered in the emergency department include tinea corporis (ringworm), tinea cruris, and tinea pedis. These infections are due to a number of *Trichophyton* and *Epidermophyton* species. Topical therapy with a broad-spectrum antifungal agent such as miconazole, clotrimazole, or other "azole" agents is generally effective when used twice daily for 2 to 3 weeks. Tinea versicolor, a superficial skin infection caused by *Pityrosporum orbiculare,* is also common in young adults and results in hypopigmented macules on the upper trunk, neck, or shoulders. The diagnosis can be confirmed by a potassium hydroxide (KOH) preparation showing large, budding yeast and thick, tangled hyphae. Ketoconazole, 400 mg orally in a single dose, is very effective therapy with a minimal recurrence rate. Topical selenium sulfide therapy is also effective.

IX. **Infestations.** Scabies is a pruritic eczematous skin eruption caused by infestation with the mite *Sarcoptes scabiei*. The pruritic rash occurs most commonly in the finger webs, flexor surfaces of the wrist, extensor surfaces of the elbows, and intertriginous areas. A shaved biopsy specimen of a linear burrow examined under the microscope at high power will often demonstrate the organism or its products. Topical therapy is generally effective at curing infestation. Useful agents include permethrin 5% cream, lindane 1% (Kwell), and 10% crotamiton (Eurax). Lindane should be avoided in young children and pregnant women because of the potential neurotoxicity from absorbed drug.

Lice may infest the head (Pediculus humanus capitis), body (P. humanus corporis), or pubic area (Pthirus pubis). The louse bites produce an erythematous, maculopapular eruption that may be modified by excoriation. Lice may be difficult to see, but nits are usually present on hair shafts. Effective therapy includes permethrin and lindane.

The more serious, often life threatening, skin and soft tissue infections such as necrotizing fasciitis and clostridial myonecrosis will not be discussed in this section because aggressive inpatient medical and surgical care is dictated by the severity of these infections.

Ophthalmologic Infections

I. **Eyelid abscesses.** Infection of the glands adjacent to the eyelash follicles produces superficial pustules at the lid margin known as a style or hordeolum. Infection of the deeper glands of the tarsal plate results in a localized infection often appreciated from the conjunctival surface, known as a chalazion. *Staphylococcus aureus* is the implicated organism responsible for lid abscesses. Treatment generally consists of frequent warm compresses, with incision and drainage reserved for poor responses. If cellulitis is present, serious consideration should be given to the diagnosis of orbital cellulitis, and CT orbital imaging consultation may be indicated.

II. **Conjunctivitis.** Infectious conjunctivitis is most commonly caused by viruses, with adenovirus the most frequent etiologic agent. There are also a variety of bacterial causes of conjunctivitis such as *Streptococcus pneumoniae* and *Haemophilus* species. Marked conjunctival purulence is the hallmark of bacterial infections. Topical antibiotic therapy shortens the duration of illness and usually consists of neomycin and polymyxin, or sulfacetamide. Eye drops should be used frequently while awake, with ointment applied at bedtime. Topical ciprofloxacin or norfloxacin offer alternative therapy. More serious, vision-threatening eye infections such as keratitis and endophthalmitis should be referred to an ophthalmologist for rapid, accurate diagnosis and therapy.

III. **Orbital cellulitis.** In children this infection typically arises from the ethmoid sinus or maxillary sinus and is caused by *Haemophilus influenzae;* however, the etiology may be skin pathogens such as *Staphylococcus aureus*. Orbital cellulitis is an infectious disease emergency. Distinguishing orbital cellulitis and periorbital cellulitis may be possible if there is ophthalmoplegia or proptosis; however, orbital

CT scanning and consultation may be required. Therapy is surgical drainage of orbital abscesses and antibiotics with antistaphylococcal activity (e.g., nafcillin) with a third-generation cephalosporin (e.g., cefotaxime), or a β-lactamase inhibitor alone.

Upper Respiratory Tract Infections

I. **External otitis.** Superficial infection of the external auditory canal is caused by *S. aureus,* group A streptococcus, *Pseudomonas* species, or members of the Enterobacteriaceae family. Topical therapy with ear drops containing polymyxin B, neomycin, and hydrocortisone when used four times a day is generally effective **(Table 14-3)**. Malignant otitis externa, an invasive infection usually occurring in diabetics, involves the external canal, as well as deep soft tissues and bony structures. Often caused by *P. aeruginosa,* the seriousness of this infection often requires hospitalization and treatment with combination parenteral therapy. The excellent activity of ciprofloxacin may impact on the setting of this therapy when disease is less severe. Surgical drainage is occasionally required for this infection.

II. **Otitis media.** Though most common in young children, acute middle ear infection with an effusion may occur in patients of all ages, with similar microbiologic causes. The most commonly isolated organisms include *S. pneumoniae, H. influenzae,* and occasionally *Moraxella catarrhalis, S. aureus,* and group A streptococci. *Haemophilus influenzae* and even more frequently, *M. catarrhalis,* produce β-lactamase and thus influence antibiotic prescribing for refractory infections. Initial antibiotic therapy often consists of amoxicillin or trimethoprim/sulfamethoxazole; for refractory infections, amoxicillin/clavulanate, erythromycin plus sulfonamide (without sulfonamide for patients older than 4 years); or a sec-

Table 14-3. Antibiotic Therapy for Upper Respiratory Tract Infections

Clinical indication	Antibiotic therapy Primary	Alternative
External otitis	Polymyxin B/neomycin/hydrocortisone ear drops	—
Otitis media	Amoxicillin/clavulanate or erythromycin and sulfonamide (sulfonamide may be omitted if >4 years old)	Second- or third-generation cephalosporin, trimethoprim/sulfamethoxazole, clarithromycin
Sinusitis		
Acute	Amoxicillin/clavulanate	Second- or third-generation cephalosporin, trimethoprim/sulfamethoxazole, clarithromycin
Chronic	Amoxicillin/clavulanate	Clindamycin
Pharyngitis	Benzathine penicillin G	Penicillin V, macrolide, second- or third-generation cephalosporin
Odontogenic infection	Penicillin V and metronidazole	Clindamycin, amoxicillin/clavulanate

ond- or third-generation cephalosporin. Clarithromycin may also be considered for use. Therapy is generally given for 10 days.

III. **Sinusitis.** Patients with acute and chronic sinusitis are frequently seen in the outpatient setting, as well as in the emergency department. Maxillary sinuses are most frequently involved, though other sinuses are occasionally also infected. Facial pain and persistent purulent drainage are frequently present. Sinus radiographs or more sophisticated imaging may support the diagnosis. The most frequent pathogens recovered in acute sinusitis include pneumococci, *H. influenzae, M. catarrhalis,* group A streptococci, and occasionally oral anaerobes. *Staphylococcus aureus* is a very rare cause of acute sinusitis. Amoxicillin or trimethoprim/sulfamethoxazole or, for refractory or severe cases, amoxicillin/clavulanate, a second- or third-generation cephalosporin, or a new macrolide are rational antibiotic choices. Chronic sinusitis is caused by oral anaerobes such as *Bacteroides* species, peptostreptococci, and *Fusobacterium* species. Antibiotic therapy for chronic sinusitis consists of amoxicillin/clavulanate or clindamycin. However, medical therapy alone is often ineffective, and a definitive drainage procedure may be required. Consultation with an ear, nose, and throat (ENT) specialist is generally advised.

IV. **Pharyngitis.** Although a wide variety of viruses such as adenovirus, enteroviruses, and particularly Epstein-Barr virus cause the majority of cases of exudative pharyngitis, it is the bacterial causes that determine antibiotic therapy. In most cases of pharyngitis, the clinical findings do not indicate the specific etiologic agent. Group A streptococci and gonococci cause most cases of bacterial pharyngitis, while *Arcanobacterium hemolyticum* is also an etiologic agent. (*N. gonorrhaeae* is discussed separately in the chapter on sexually transmitted diseases [STDs].) Other β-hemolytic streptococci (group Co-G) may also cause pharyngitis. The major motivations for treating streptococcal pharyngitis are to eliminate streptococcal pharyngeal carriage in order to prevent acute rheumatic fever and to shorten the period to recovery. Effective therapy includes benzathine penicillin, 1.2 million units intramuscularly, or oral penicillin V, a macrolide, or cephalosporin. The oral agents other than azithromycin need to be continued for 10 days, a factor circumvented by the single intramuscular injection of benzathine penicillin.

V. **Odontogenic infections.** Dental abscesses and orofacial infection of odontogenic origin are caused by indigenous oral flora such as streptococci, fusobacteria, and *Bacteroides.* Penicillin V alone, or, for more severe infections, penicillin V plus metronidazole, clindamycin, or amoxicillin/clavulanate are effective therapies. Surgical drainage and debridement are often required in addition to medical therapy.

Lower Respiratory Tract Infections

I. **Acute bacterial exacerbation of chronic bronchitis (ABECB).** Exacerbations of bronchitis in patients with chronic obstructive lung disease are due to a variety of pathogenic organisms such as respiratory viruses (rhinovirus, influenza virus, parainfluenza virus, etc.) and bacteria (pneumococci, *H. influenzae, M. catarrhalis,* and others). Antibiotic therapy may contribute to improvement along with measures to improve pulmonary function (e.g., bronchodilators). Antibiotic therapy aimed at the usual bacterial isolates would include trimethoprim/sulfamethoxazole, or doxycycline, and, in more severe cases, second- or

third-generation cephalosporins, azithromycin or clarithromycin, or amoxicillin/clavulanate **(Table 14-4)**.
II. **Community-acquired pneumonia.** Selected patients with community-acquired pneumonia who have normal host defense mechanisms, little or no underlying disease, and relatively mild infection may be treated in the outpatient setting. Though "typical" and "atypical" pneumonias are often discussed separately, it is not possible on clinical grounds (history, physical examination, chest x-ray), to differentiate between the various typical bacterial pathogens and the atypical organisms. Therapy must, in most cases, be empirically based on the most frequently implicated pathogens. In patients younger than 60 years, respiratory viruses, *Mycoplasma pneumoniae, Chlamydia pneumoniae, S. pneumoniae, Legionella* species, and occasionally *H. influenzae* are the most commonly implicated organisms. Therapy for this group of patients generally consists of doxycycline, erythromycin, azithromycin, or clarithromycin. In patients older than 60 years, pneumococcus, *H. influenzae,* and group A streptococcus are most common; *M. pneumoniae* is rarely encountered. Therapy often consists of amoxicillin/clavulanate, a second- or third-generation cephalosporin, azithromycin or clarithromycin, or trimethoprim/sulfamethoxazole. For the older patient with underlying disease, the above organisms are still frequent, but *Legionella, C. pneumoniae,* and occasionally *Klebsiella pneumoniae* or other Enterobacteriaceae, and *S. aureus* must be added to the list. For mild disease in this patient group, amox-

Table 14-4. Antibiotic Therapy for Lower Respiratory Tract Infections

Clinical indication	Antibiotic therapy Primary	Alternative
Bronchitis	Amoxicillin/clavulanate	Second- or third-generation cephalosporin, trimethoprim/sulfamethoxazole, clarithromycin or azithromycin, ofloxacin
Community-acquired pneumonia*		
Age ≤40, without significant underlying disease	Azithromycin, clarithromycin	A tetracycline
Age ≥40, without significant underlying disease	Amoxicillin/clavulanate	Second- or third-generation cephalosporin, azithromycin or clarithromycin, trimethoprim/sulfamethoxazole
Age ≥40 with underlying disease	Amoxicillin/clavulanate OR second- or third-generation cephalosporin, OR trimethoprim/sulfamethoxazole PLUS a macrolide	—
Aspiration pneumonia/lung abscess*	Amoxicillin/clavulanate	Clindamycin, penicillin V plus metronidazole

*See text for outpatient candidates.

icillin/clavulanate, a second- or third-generation cephalosporin, or trimethoprim/sulfamethoxazole plus a macrolide antibiotic may provide effective oral therapy. Most patients with significant underlying diseases found to have pneumonia should generally be treated in the hospital, not only to deliver parenteral antimicrobial therapy, but to ensure adequate pulmonary toilet, hydration, and monitoring of overall pulmonary status, including the possible need for ventilatory support.

III. **Aspiration pneumonia and lung abscess.** Aspiration pneumonia and lung abscess occur in patients with poor dental and oral hygiene who are predisposed to aspiration. High-risk conditions associated with aspiration include drug or alcohol abuse, strokes, seizures, and esophageal dysmotility. These patients often have subacute or chronic complaints of cough, sputum production (often putrid), as well as systemic complaints. The usual bacteria responsible for aspiration pneumonia and lung abscess include *Bacteroides* species, *Prevotella* species, streptococci, and *Fusobacterium* species. Though most patients with lung abscess receive an initial period of parenteral therapy followed by oral therapy for a total duration of 6 to 8 weeks, occasional stable patients may be treated with entirely oral regimens. Effective therapy for aspiration pneumonia and lung abscess could include amoxicillin/clavulanate, clindamycin, or penicillin plus metronidazole.

Genitourinary Tract Infections

I. **Cystitis and Pyelonephritis.** Treatment of acute urinary tract infection is one of the most common indications for antibiotic use. These infections are an extremely common reason for seeking outpatient care, including visits to the emergency department **(Table 14-5)**. The largest group at risk are women between late adolescence and the mid 40s in their sexually active years. Other patients at risk include elderly patients. A small percentage of patients with acute urinary tract infection will need hospitalization for parenteral antibiotic therapy for acute pyelonephritis. These patients often have significant fever, costovertebral angle tenderness, and systemic toxicity including nausea and vomiting. For the majority of patients, it is more difficult to localize infection as cystitis, or occult or early renal infection. Until recently, the standard recommendation has been to treat cystitis

Table 14-5. Antibiotic Therapy for Genitourinary Tract Infections

	Antibiotic therapy	
Clinical indication	**Primary**	**Alternative**
Cystitis, pyelonephritis	Trimethoprim/ sulfamethoxazole	A quinolone, a cephalosporin, trimethoprim alone, nitrofurantoin (cystitis only)
Prostatitis and epididymo-orchitis		
<35 yr	(see STD section for treatment of gonococcus and *C. trachomatis*)	
>35 yr	Ofloxacin	Trimethoprim/sulfamethoxazole

Note: Ofloxacin could be used in all age groups and would be active against both STDs and uropathogens.

with single-dose therapy and to treat pyelonephritis for 2 weeks. Patients who have not responded to single-dose therapy have been retreated with an antibiotic regimen for pyelonephritis. Recent trials have shown that patients treated for cystitis with a single dose of trimethoprim/sulfamethoxazole had lower cure rates than patients treated for 3 days. The 3-day course has considerably fewer side effects than a longer course of therapy and is the preferred duration of therapy for cystitis.

Uncomplicated cystitis is caused by *Escherichia coli* and occasionally by other Enterobacteriaceae, *Staphylococcus saprophyticus,* or enterococci. The causes of uncomplicated pyelonephritis are the same as for cystitis, though *S. saprophyticus* is not implicated. Currently, patients with suspected acute uncomplicated cystitis should be treated with 3 days of antibiotic therapy. Patients with mild, uncomplicated pyelonephritis, amenable to outpatient therapy, should be treated for 2 weeks, as should patients with short-course treatment failures for acute cystitis. Uncomplicated cystitis may be treated with trimethoprim/sulfamethoxazole or a quinoline. Alternative antibiotics include a cephalosporin, trimethoprim alone, or nitrofurantoin. Uncomplicated pyelonephritis is treated identically, though nitrofurantoin is not utilized.

II. **Prostatitis and epididymo-orchitis.** Prostatitis in a sexually active man <35 years old is generally caused by either the gonococcus or *Chlamydia trachomatis*. Therapy for both organisms is continued for 14 days (see STD section for antimicrobial options). Acute bacterial prostatitis in older men with fever, perineal pain, and often symptoms of lower urinary tract infection is more often caused by members of the Enterobacteriaceae family and occasionally *Pseudomonas* species. Urine will contain leukocytes and the culture is generally positive, though not conclusive proof of a prostatic source. Examination will reveal an extremely tender prostate. Acute prostatitis is treated for 2 weeks with trimethoprim/sulfamethoxazole or ciprofloxacin, both of which penetrate the prostate well. Chronic prostatitis, often presenting as recurrent urinary tract infections, traditionally has been treated for 3 months with trimethoprim/sulfamethoxazole or a tetracycline, with improvement in the majority of patients but a cure in less than half. The availability of fluoroquinoles such as ciprofloxacin has allowed a shorter course of therapy (14 days) with equivalent or improved efficacy.

Epididymo-orchitis in men ≤35 years is generally caused by gonococcus or *C. trachomatis* (treatment recommendations as per STD section). In men older than 35 years, Enterobacteriaceae are causative in the majority of instances, and therapy consists of ciprofloxacin, ofloxacin, or trimethoprim/sulfamethoxazole for 10 to 14 days. Note that ofloxacin is active against gonorrhea, chlamydia, and *Enterobacteriaceae,* and this is reasonable empiric therapy in any age group.

Gynecologic Infections

I. **Vaginitis.** Vaginitis results in a variety of clinical presentations and is caused by a diverse group of organisms. Candida vaginitis often causes pruritis and a thick "cheesy" discharge. Hyphae are seen on KOH preparation. Miconazole, clotrimazole, or other topical azoles such as butoconazole, terconazole, ontioconazole used intravaginally for 5 to 7 days has a high cure rate. A single oral dose of fluconazole (150 mg) appears to be very effective. Vaginitis caused by the protozoan *Trichomonas vaginalis* often has an associated copious foamy discharge, and the organism can be seen on the saline preparation. The treatment of choice is metronidazole, 2 gm as a single dose (500 mg BID for 7 days is an alternative if the single dose is not tolerated). It is also necessary to treat sexual partners.

Women in the first trimester of pregnancy should be treated with clotrimazole intravaginal tablets for 2 weeks, or 20% saline douches. Bacterial vaginosis is caused by overgrowth of *Gardnerella vaginalis* along with nonfragilis *Bacteroides* species, peptococci, and *Mobiluncus*. This form of vaginitis produces a malodorous vaginal discharge. Wet preparations reveal "clue cells," which are cells covered with organisms, and KOH preparations often yield a "fishy" odor. Treatment options include metronidazole, 500 mg twice daily for 7 days; metronidazole vaginal gel for 5 days; clindamycin, 300 mg twice daily for 7 days; or clindamycin vaginal cream for 7 days.

II. **Cervicitis.** Mucopurulent cervicitis is caused by *Neisseria gonorrhoeae* and/or *C. trachomatis*. These infections generally result in the production of yellow or green pus, which on examination reveals greater than 10 leukocytes per oil field. Though Gram stain may reveal the gonococcus, in practice, therapy is prescribed that covers both isolates in case of coinfection. (Treatment as per VII.STD.)

III. **Salpingitis and pelvic inflammatory disease.** Infection of the fallopian tubes and/or the adnexal structures is a common reason for women to seek medical care in the outpatient clinic or emergency department. Risk factors for the development of acute salpingitis include sexual activity, use of an intrauterine device, and prior pelvic infection or surgery. The clinical criteria for a diagnosis of salpingitis include abdominal tenderness on motion of the cervix, adnexal tenderness, and at least one of the following: gram-negative intracellular diplococci in cervical exudate, temperature greater than 38° C, leukocytosis greater than 10,000, purulent material obtained by a culdocentesis or laparoscopy, or presence of a pelvic abscess. The microbiologic causes of salpingitis include *N. gonorrhoeae, C. trachomatis, Bacteriodes* species, Enterobacteriaceae, and streptococci. Patients able to take oral medications who have lower ranges of temperature and leukocytosis, as well as minimal peritonitis, may be candidates for outpatient therapy. Those not fulfilling these criteria and those with suspected abscess, the need for laparoscopy, failure to respond to outpatient therapy, as well as those who are pregnant, should be hospitalized for initial therapy. The outpatient treatment of acute salpingitis includes therapy for all usual organisms. Possible regimens include (1) ceftriaxone, 250 mg intramuscularly, or (2) cefoxitin, 2 gm intramuscularly plus probenecid, 1 gm orally; both are given with doxycycline 100 mg orally twice a day for 14 days. An alternative treatment consists of ofloxacin, with clindamycin or metronidazole for 14 days. In the treatment of pregnant patients, erythromycin should be substituted for tetracycline, and a quinolone should not be used.

   A. **Serious polymicrobic infections,** such as septic abortion and early postdelivery endomyometritis, warrant parenteral antimicrobial therapy and often require dilatation and curettage (D and C) in addition to medical therapy **(Table 14-6)**.

Sexually Transmitted Disease (STD)

I. **Syphilis.** Syphilis, caused by the spiral spirochete *Treponema pallidum,* is increasing in incidence. The duration and intensity of therapy for syphilis is dictated by the stage of disease. Penicillin remains the drug of choice for all stages of syphilis, and the physician should make all attempts to document penicillin allergy before choosing any alternative therapy **(Table 14-7)**. Primary syphilis is marked by the presence of the primary lesion of the infection, the chancre. Sec-

Table 14-6. Antibiotic Therapy for Gynecologic Infections

Clinical indication	Antibiotic therapy Primary	Alternative
Vaginitis		
Candidal	Miconazole, clotrimazole, other azoles	Oral fluconazole
Trichomoniasis	Metronidazole	Clotrimazole or 20% saline douche in pregnancy
Bacterial vaginosis	Metronidazole	Amoxicillin
Cervicitis	(see STD section for treatment of gonococcus and C. trachomatis)	
*Salpingitis/PID	Ceftriaxone or cefoxitin plus probenecid plus doxycycline or erythromycin	Ofloxacin plus clindamycin or metronidazole

*See text for outpatient candidates.

Table 14-7. Antibiotic Therapy for Sexually Transmitted Diseases

Clinical indication	Antibiotic therapy Primary	Alternative
Syphilis	Benzathine penicillin G	A tetracycline, erythromycin (see text)
Gonorrhea and	Ceftriaxone	—
	Ciprofloxacin, ofloxacin norfloxacin, or enoxacin	
	Cefuroxime axetil, cefixime	Doxycycline, erythromycin, ofloxacin
C. trachomatis	Azithromycin	
Genital herpes	Acyclovir	—
Chancroid	Ceftriaxone, azithromycin	Erythromycin
Lymphogranuloma venereum	Doxycycline	Erythromycin, sulfizoxaole

ondary syphilis occurs before or soon after healing of the chancre and consists of several skin manifestations such as the typical erythematous macular rash, condylomata lata, and mucous patches, as well as many other possible manifestations such as meningitis, hepatitis, arthritis, or uveitis. Latent syphilis is without clinical manifestations. Patients with tertiary or late syphilis develop gumma (granulomatous lesions of most any organ system), cardiovascular syphilis, or neurosyphilis. Patients with primary, secondary, or latent syphilis of less than 1-year duration (those patients most likely to be encountered in the emergency department) are all treated identically with benzathine penicillin G, 2.4 million units intramuscularly once. Alternative therapy may consist of either doxycycline, 100 mg twice a day for 14 days, or erythromycin, 500 mg four times a day for 14 days. Patients with latent syphilis of unknown or greater than 1-year duration, patients with cardiovascular syphilis, or patients with late, benign disease are treated with benzathine penicillin G, 2.4 million units intramuscularly weekly for 3 weeks (total dose of 7.2 million units). Alternative therapy, if neurosyphilis has been ruled out, consists of doxycycline, 100 mg twice a day for 28 days. The pregnant patient should be desensitized to penicillin and treated with benzathine penicillin G. The routine lumbar puncture during latent syphilis to rule out asymptomatic neurosyphilis has generally fallen into disfavor, and these patients are generally treated as above. Lumbar puncture is indicated for patients infected with human immunodeficiency virus (HIV) if the VDRL or RPR is greater than 1:32 or if nonpenicillin therapy is contemplated (unless the duration of infection is known to be less than one year). Patients with evidence of neurosyphilis should be treated with 10-20 million units of intravenous Penicillin G for 14 days. All patients treated for syphilis should have follow up arranged to obtain posttherapy serologic specimens and/or cerebrospinal fluid (CSF). Patients infected with HIV may be exceptions to the above outlined treatment guidelines due to increased recognition of treatment failures. It is generally recommended that HIV-infected patients receive more intense therapy than otherwise dictated by the stage of disease, and therefore many authorities recommend three weekly intramuscular injections of benzathine penicillin for early syphilis in these patients.

II. **Infections caused by *N. gonorrhoeae* and *C. trachomatis*.**
   A. **Urethritis and mucopurulent cervicitis** are both caused by *N. gonorrhoeae* and/or *C. trachomatis*. A definitive microbiologic diagnosis is rarely available in the emergency department, and therapy must be empiric and effectively treat both pathogens. Nongonococcal urethritis may also be caused by *Ureaplasma urealyticum*. Since a minority of *U. urealyticum* isolates are resistant to tetracycline, failures of tetracycline-based regimens should be retreated with a macrolide. In addition to urethritis and cervicitis, *N. gonorrhoeae* may cause pharyngitis and anorectal disease, as well as disseminated infection. Disseminated infection may include typical skin lesions, polyarthralgias, tenosynovitis, and later septic arthritis. Disseminated gonococcal infection requires 7 days of effective therapy directed at *N. gonorrhoeae*. Initial hospitalization is advised; after a good clinical response, therapy may be completed as an outpatient.
   B. **The treatment of urethritis or mucupurulent cervicitis** must effectively treat both the gonococcus and *C. trachomatis*. Regimens for *N. gonorrhoeae* include ceftriaxone, 125 mg intramuscularly once; ciprofloxacin, 500 mg once; ofloxacin, 400 mg once; norfloxacin, 800 mg once; enoxacin, 400 mg once; cefuroxime axetil, 1 gm once; cefpodoxime proxetil, 200 mg once; or cefixime, 400 mg once. Effective therapies for *C. trachomatis* include doxycycline, 100 mg twice daily for 7 days; erythromycin, 500 mg four times daily for 7 days; and azithromycin, 1 gm once. Ofloxacin, 300 mg twice daily for 7 days treats both gonococcal infection and *C. trachomatis*. The preferred single-dose oral regimen is cefixime, 400 mg, with azithromycin, 1 gm.

III. **Vesiculoulcerative diseases.** In the United States, the major cause of genital vesiculoulcerative lesions, other than syphilis, is herpes simplex virus. Chancroid, caused by *Haemophilus ducreyi,* is occasionally seen and is endemic in some areas of the United States. Chancroid may be clinically diagnosed when genital ulcers are present, especially with tender inguinal lymphadenopathy, and there is no evidence for herpes or syphilis. Lymphogranuloma vereum (LGV), caused by LGV strains of *C. trachomatis,* is rarely seen in the United States but may also occur in persons who have traveled in Asia or Africa. Diagnosis is based on inguinal lymphadenopathy and positive serologic tests. Primary genital herpes is often treated with acyclovir, 400 mg three times daily or 200 mg five times a day for 10 days, to increase the rate of healing. Unfortunately, treatment with acyclovir does not affect recurrent disease, which occurs at approximately 80% of patients infected with herpes simplex virus type 2 (HSV-2). Patients with frequent recurrent may be treated with acyclovir, 400 mg twice daily. Chancroid is effectively treated with azithromycin, 1 gm once; ceftriaxone, 250 mg intramuscularly once; erythromycin, 500 mg four times daily for 7 days; or ciprofloxacin, 500 mg twice daily for 3 days. Three weeks of doxycycline, erythromycin, or sulfisoxazole therapy is effective in the treatment of LGV.

Diarrhea

I. **Diarrhea and dysentery.** Patients with diarrheal syndromes and fever, bloody diarrhea, neutrophils in the stool, or travel history to a risk area may improve with empiric antimicrobial therapy. The microbiologic causes make up a diverse group of organisms, with individual likelihood dependent on the specific setting. These bacteria include *Campylobacter jejuni, E. coli* (enterotoxigenic, enteroinvasive, enterohemorrhagic [0157:H7]), *Shigella,* and *Salmonella.* Therapy consists of a quinolone or trimethoprim/sulfamethoxazole (does not cover *C. jejuni*).
   A. The protozoan parasite *Giardia lamblia* is also an etiologic agent responsible for either acute or chronic diarrhea, though blood and pus are generally absent from the stool. Treatment consists of either quinacrine (100 mg three times daily for adults or 6 mg/kg/day in three doses for children for 5 to 7 days) or metronidazole (250 mg times daily for adults or 15 mg/kg/day in three doses for children for 7 days). Treatment failure or relapse dictates an additional course of therapy with the same agent or an alternative.
II. **Antibiotic-associated diarrhea.** Antibiotic-associated diarrhea caused by a toxin produced by *Clostridium difficile* should be considered in all patients receiving, or having recently received, antibiotic therapy. Stool specimens often contain leukocytes, and the diagnosis is made by assaying for *C. difficile* toxin. Antibiotic therapy aimed at eradicating *C. difficile* includes metronidazole, 500 mg three times daily for 10 days, or vancomycin, 125 mg four times daily for 10 days. Relapses are not uncommon and require retreatment. No change in the antibiotic regimen chosen is indicated.

Antibiotic Prophylaxis

I. **Prophylaxis.** The emergency physician is rarely called on to prescribe true prophylactic antibiotic therapy but, more commonly, is responsible for the initial empiric therapy of the patient receiving care in the emergency department before being admitted to the hospital. The emergency practitioner may occasionally be in a position to prescribe prophylaxis, either for the prevention of bacterial endocarditis or for surgical prophylaxis of a clean or clean-contaminated case. These topics have been extensively reviewed and definitive recommendations have been made with regard to indications and the choice of antibiotic for prophylaxis. It would be prudent to refer to these recommendations as a guide to prescribing.
II. **Empiric therapy**
   A. **Open fractures.** Open fractures are contaminated wounds, with *S. aureus* the most commonly isolated pathogen. Early treatment should be initiated, generally with a first-generation cephalosporin such as cefazolin.

B. **Penetrating abdominal trauma.** The peritoneal contamination associated with penetrating abdominal trauma is polymicrobial bowel flora consisting predominately of members of the Enterobacteriaceae family and *B. fragilis.* A number of antibiotics and combinations of antibiotics having activity against these pathogens would be predicted to be, and have proven to be, effective in this setting. For the community-acquired disease seen in the emergency department, recommended empiric therapy consists of cefotetan, cefoxitin, or ampicillin/sulbactam. Any number of alternative regimens could be utilized, including the "gold standard" combination for abdominal sepsis, an aminoglycoside with either clindamycin or metronidazole.

Bacterial Meningitis

A. **Meningitis.** Acute bacterial meningitis is a life-threatening medical emergency requiring prompt diagnosis and initiation of bactericidal antimicrobial therapy. There should be no delay in performing a diagnostic lumbar puncture and starting antibiotic therapy in the patient with suspected pyogenic meningitis. Empiric therapy should be started before computed tomography (CT) imaging if an intracranial mass lesion needs to be ruled out before performing the lumbar puncture. A delay of several hours in obtaining CSF after initiating therapy will not affect culture results or other CSF parameters such as cell count, and protein or glucose concentrations. Antigen detection tests should still be utilized for rapid diagnosis.

1. The **choice of empiric therapy** is dictated by the patient's age and clinical setting, and is designed to have activity against the pathogens known to be predominant in that group. Meningitis in neonates (younger than 1 month) is caused by group B streptococci, Enterobacteriaceae, *Listeria monocytogenes,* and occasionally group D streptococci. Empiric therapy consists of ampicillin combined with cefotaxime. Infants (1 to 3 months old) are infected with *H. influenzae,* pneumococci, meningococci, group B streptococci, and occasionally the other neonatal pathogens. Empiric therapy with ampicillin and an extended-spectrum cephalosporin such as ceftriaxone is indicated. Infants and children (from 3 months to 10 years old) with meningitis have *H. influenzae,* pneumococci, and meningococci isolated most frequently. Note that invasive disease due to *H. influenzae* type B is becoming increasingly rare in vaccinated populations. These patients are treated with an extended-spectrum cephalosporin such as ceftriaxone. Neonates and infants should receive adjunctive corticosteroid therapy (dexamethasome, 0.15 mg/kg q6h for 4 days), which should be started before antibiotic therapy, if possible. Meningitis in children older than 7 years and in adults is caused by meningococcus, pneumococcus, or occasionally *L. monocytogenes.*

Recommended therapy in adults is high-dose penicillin, high-dose ampicillin, or the combination of ceftriaxone and ampicillin. Highly penicillin-allergic patients may be treated with chloramphenicol and trimethoprim/sulfamethoxazole. A growing problem with relative and high-level penicillin resistance in the pneumococcus may affect the therapy of meningitis. For geographic areas with a high prevalence of resistant isolates, empiric therapy should consist of vancomycin and ceftriaxone until susceptibility data is available. As with age, there are several patient groups whose expected microbiology dictates empiric therapy.

The elderly (older than 60 years) and the alcoholic patient may be infected with the same bacteria as listed for adults but may also be infected with Enterobacteriaceae or *H. influenzae.* Empiric therapy consists of penicillin or ampicillin with an extended-spectrum cephalosporin such as ceftriaxone. Chlorampenicol is an alternative choice. Patients with a CSF leak up to 3 days after trauma develop meningitis caused by pneumococci and should be treated with penicillin, ceftriaxone, or chloramphenicol. After neurosurgery, or more than 3 days after trauma, patients develop meningitis caused by *S. aureus,* Enterobacteriaceae, pneumococci, or *Pseudomonas.* These patients should be empirically treated with a combination of vancomycin, ceftazidime, and an aminoglycoside. Prophylactic therapy should be offered to selected contacts of patients with meningococcal or *H. influenzae* meningitis. Close household contacts of patients with meningococcal meningitis, as well as persons with unprotected intimate exposure (such as resuscitation), should be offered rifampin, 600 mg twice daily for 2 days (children receive a dose of 10 mg/kg. *Haemophilus influenzae* meningitis also dictates prophylaxis in all household contacts if there are children younger than 4 years present. Prophylaxis consists of rifampin, 20 mg/kg (maximum dose 600 mg) once daily for 4 days.

Protection of Health Personnel in the Emergency Department

Protection policies of the emergency department should attempt to minimize the risk of acquiring infectious diseases in the health care worker, as well as the risk of transmission of infectious diseases to patients. Immunization of the health care worker and precautions during health care delivery help to achieve these goals.

I. **Immunization.** Emergency personnel should receive immunization against both measles and rubella unless they are known to be immune. All health care workers should have received a complete primary series of both the polio vaccine and the tetanus–diphtheria toxoid vaccine. Td booster status should be up to date, administered every 10 years. Annual immunization with influenza vaccine is recommended. The risk of hepatitis B infection correlates directly with exposure to blood and blood products. Hepatitis B vaccine is recommended for health care workers with moderate or greater exposure, even if the risk of inoculation is low. However, the vaccine should be available to other personnel as well. An accidental or unavoidable exposure to infective material (stool) from a patient with hepatitis A dictates postexposure prophylaxis with gamma globulin (0.02 ml/kg intramuscularly). Prophylaxis for meningococcal disease was covered in the discussion of meningitis.

Selected Readings
Skin and Soft Tissue Infections
CDC: Tetanus—United States, 1985-1986, *MMWR* 36:477, 1987.
Feingold DS. What the infectious disease specialist should know about dermatophytes. In Remington JS, Swartz MN, editors: *Current topics in infectious diseases,* New York, 1987, McGraw-Hill.
Klempner MS, Styrt B: Prevention of recurrent staphylococcal skin infection with low dose oral clindamycin therapy, *JAMA* 260:2682-5, 1988.
McDonough JJ et al: Management of animal and human bites and resulting human infections. In Remington JS, Swartz MN, editors: *Current topics in infectious diseases,* New York, 1987, McGraw-Hill.
McLinn S. Topical mupirocin vs. systematic erythromycin treatment for pyoderma, *Pediatr Infect Dis J* 7:785-90, 1988.

Raush LJ, Jacobs PH: Tinea versicolor: treatment and prophylaxis with monthly administration of ketoconazole, *Cutis* 34:470-1, 1984.

Straus SE: The management of varicella and zoster infections, *Infect Dis Clin North Am* 1:367-82, 1987.

Ophthalmologic Infections

Barza M: Treatment of bacterial infection of the eye. In Remington JS, Swartz MN, editors: *Current topics in infectious diseases,* New York, 1980, McGraw-Hill.

Wilhelmus KR: The red eye: infectious conjunctivitis, keratitis, endophthalmitis, and periocular cellulitis, *Infect Dis Clin North Am* 2:99-116, 1988.

Upper Respiratory Tract Infections

Chow AW, editor: Infectious syndromes of the head and neck, *Infect Dis Clin North Am* 2:1-283, 1988.

Haydon GF et al: Management of the ambulatory patient with a sore throat. In Remington JS, Swartz MN, editors: *Current topics in infectious diseases,* New York, 1988, McGraw-Hill.

Klein JO: Management of acute and chronic otitis media. In Remington JS, Swartz MN, editors: *Current topics in infectious diseases,* New York, 1981, McGraw-Hill.

Medical Letter: Drugs for treatment of acute otitis media in children, *Med Lett Drugs Ther* 36:19-21, 1994.

Van Hare GF et al: Acute otitis media caused by *Branhamella catarrhalis:* biology and therapy, *Review of Infectious Diseases* 9:16-27, 1987.

Lower Respiratory Tract Infections

Anthonisen NR et al: Antibiotic therapy in exacerbation of chronic obstructive pulmonary disease, *Ann Intern Med* 106:196, 1987.

Cassell GH, Cole BC: Mycoplasmas as agents of human disease, *N Engl J Med* 304:80, 1981.

Marrie TJ et al: Pneumonia associated with TWAR strain of *Chlamydia, Ann Intern Med* 106:507-11, 1987.

Meyer RD: *Legionella* infection: a review of five years of research, *Review of Infectious Diseases* 147:362, 1983.

Genitourinary Tract Infections

Andriole VT, editor: Urinary tract infection, *Infect Dis Clin North Am* 1:713-977, 1987.

Fihn SO et al: Trimethoprim-sulfamethoxazole for acute dysuria in women, a single dose or 10-day course, *Ann Intern Med* 108:350-7, 1988.

Meanes EM JR: Prostatitis syndromes. In Remington JS, Swartz MN, editors: *Current topics in infectious diseases,* New York, 1984, McGraw-Hill.

Ronald AR, Conway B: An approach to urinary tract infection in ambulatory women. In Remington JS, Swartz MN, editors: *Current topics in infectious diseases,* New York, 1988, McGraw-Hill.

Stamm WE et al: Urinary tract infection from pathogenesis to treatment, *J Infect Dis* 159:400-6, 1989.

Gynecologic Infections

Burnakis TG, Hildebrandt NB: Pelvic inflammatory disease: a review with emphasis on antimicrobial therapy, *Review of Infectious Diseases* 8:86-116, 1986.

CDC: Pelvic inflammatory disease: guidelines for prevention and management, *MMWR* 40(RR-5):1-25, 1991.

Hager WD et al: Criteria for diagnosis and grading of salpingitis, *Obstet Gynecol* 61:113, 1983.

McCue JD: Evaluation and management of vaginitis, *Arch Intern Med* 149:565-8, 1989.

Rein MF, Holmes KK: "Non-specific vaginitis", vulvovaginal candidiasis and trichomoniasis: clinical features, diagnosis and management. In Remington JS, Swartz MN, editors: *Current topics in infectious diseases,* New York, 1983, McGraw-Hill.

Sexually Transmitted Diseases

CDC: 1993 STD treatment guidelines, *MMWR* 42(RR-14):1-102, 1993.

CDC: Antibiotic-resistant strains of *Neisseria gonorrhoeae:* policy guidelines for detection, management and control, *MMWR* 36(suppl 5):1S-18S, 1987.

Handsfield HH, editor: Sexually transmitted diseases, *Infect Dis Clin North Am* 1:341-82, 1987.

LeSaux N, Ronald AR: Role of ceftriaxone in sexually transmitted diseases, *Review of Infectious Diseases* 11:299-309, 1989.

Medical Letter: Treatment of sexually transmitted diseases, *Med Lett Drugs Ther* 36:1-6, 1994.

Mertz GJ: Diagnosis and treatment of genital herpes infections, *Infect Dis Clin North Am* 1:341-82, 1987.

Musher DM: Evaluation and management of an asymptomatic patient with a positive VDRL reaction. In Remington JS, Swartz MN, editors: *Current topics in infectious diseases,* New York, 1988, McGraw-Hill.

Diarrhea

Feckety R et al: Treatment of antibiotic-associated *Clostridium difficile* colitis with oral vancomycin: comparison of two dosage regimens, *Am J Med* 86:15-19, 1989.

Gorbach SL, editor: Infectious diarrhea, *Infect Dis Clin North Am* 2:557-778, 1988.

Teasley DG et al: Prospective randomized trial of metronidazole versus vancomycin for *Clostridium difficile*–associated diarrhea and colitis, *Lancet* 2:1043-6, 1983.

Antibiotic Prophylaxis and Empiric Therapy

Kaiser AB: Antimicrobial prophylaxis in surgery, *N Engl J Med* 315:1129-38, 1986.

Malangoni MA et al: Treatment of intraabdominal infections is appropriate with single agent or combination antibiotic therapy, *Surgery* 98:648-54, 1985.

Medical Letter: Antimicrobial prophylaxis in surgery, *Med Lett Drugs Ther* 35:91-4, 1993.

Medical Letter: Prevention of bacterial endocarditis, *Med Lett Drugs Ther* 31:112, 1989.

Patzakis MJ, Ivler D: Antibiotic and bacteriologic considerations in open fractures, *South Med J* 70:46, 1977.

Renkonen OV et al: Effect of ciprofloxacin on carrier rate of *Neisseria meningitidis* in army recruits in Finland, *Antimicrob Agents Chemother* 31:962-3, 1987.

Shulman ST et al: Prevention of bacterial endocarditis. A statement for health professionals by the Committee on Rheumatic Fever and Infective Endocarditis of the Council on Cardiovascular Disease in the Young, *Circulation* 70:1123A, 1984.

Swartz B et al: Comparative efficacy of ceftriaxone and rifampin in eradicating pharyngeal carriage of group A *Neisseria meningitidis, Lancet* 1:1239-42, 1988.

Talan DA et al: Role of empiric parenteral antibiotics prior to lumbar puncture in suspected bacterial meningitis: state of the art, *Review of Infectious Diseases* 10:365-76, 1988.

Tally FP, Ho JL: Management of patients with colonic perforation. In Remington JS, Swartz MN, editors: *Current topics in infectious diseases,* New York, 1987, McGraw-Hill.

Protection of Health Personnel in the Emergency Department

ACIP: General recommendations on immunization, *MMWR* 38:205-77, 1989.

CDC: Recommendations for prevention of HIV transmission in health care settings, *MMWR* 36(suppl 2):1S, 1987.

CDC: Update: acquired immunodeficiency syndrome and human immunodeficiency virus infection among health-care workers, *MMWR* 37:229,1988.

CDC: Update: universal precautions for prevention of transmission of human immunodeficiency virus, hepatitis B virus, and other blood borne pathogens in health-care settings, *MMWR* 37:377, 1988.

American College of Physicians and Infectious Disease Society of America: *Guide for adult immunization,* Philadelphia, 1990, American College of Physicians.

General Readings

Gorbach SL, Bartlett JB, Blacklow NR: *Infectious diseases,* Philadelphia, 1992, WB Saunders.

Holmes KK et al: *Sexually transmitted diseases,* ed 2, New York, 1990, McGraw-Hill.

Mandell GL, Douglas RG Jr, Bennett JE: *Principles and practice of infectious diseases,* ed 3, New York, 1990, Churchill Livingstone.

The Medical Letter, The choice of antibacterial drugs, *Med Lett Drugs Ther* 34:49-56, 1992.

Reese FE, Betts RF: *A practical approach to infectious diseases,* ed 3, Boston, 1991, Little Brown.

15

Management of Common Infectious Diseases: Rapid Access Guidelines

Jon Jui, M.D., M.P.H.

Pharyngitis

I. **Pharyngitis** is an inflammation of the posterior oral cavity involving the lymphoid tissues of the posterior pharynx and lateral pharyngeal bands.

II. **Etiology**
   A. **The most common** viral causes of pharyngitis include rhinovirus, coronavirus, adenovirus, influenza A and B viruses, parainfluenza viruses, and herpesviruses (Epstein-Barr virus [EBV], cytomegalovirus [CMV], herpes simplex virus types 1 and 2 [HSV-1, HSV-2]).
   B. **Bacterial causes** include group A β-hemolytic streptococci, non-group A (groups B, C, G) streptococci, *Corynebacterium* species *(C. diphtheriae, C. haemolyticum), Haemophilus influenzae, Moraxella catarrhalis, Bacteroides* species, *Neisseria gonorrhoeae, Mycoplasma pneumoniae,* and *Chlamydia pneumoniae.*
   C. **The incidence** of streptococcal pharyngitis is highest in children 5 to 15 years of age.
   D. **The method of transmission** is via airborne droplets.

III. **Clinical presentation**
   A. **History.** Sore throat, malaise, headache, chills, fever, myalgia, tachycardia, hoarseness, and drooling.
   B. **Physical examination.** Tender anterior cervical lymph nodes, pharyngeal exudates, and fever.

IV. **Clinical approach**
   A. **Detect** patients who may have life-threatening diseases: Patients with potential airway compromise.
      1. **Presence of stridor,** labored respirations, inability to swallow secretions (resulting in drooling), trismus, changes in voice are all warning signs of potential airway compromise.
      2. **The primary causes** that result in these warning signs are acute epiglottitis, peritonsillar or retropharyngeal abscess, severe tonsillar or uvular edema, and a foreign body in the airway.
      3. **Soft tissue radiologic examination** of the neck may be of use in the diagnosis of epiglottitis or retropharyngeal abscess. *The patient is always accompanied by a physician who is skilled in airway management.*
      4. **All patients** with these warning signs should have urgent nasopharyngoscopy performed in a controlled setting.
   B. **Potentially treatable infectious causes:** Is group A β-hemolytic streptococcal (GABHS) infection present?
      1. **It is extremely difficult** to distinguish between viral and bacterial pharyngitis; clinical scoring systems may be of assistance.

2. **The presence** of pharyngeal exudate, tender anterior cervical adenopathy, fever (>38° C), recent exposure, and the absence of cough all have been used to predict the presence of GABHS infection. The presence of two or three of these criteria support rapid antigen testing and/or culture, or, if follow-up is unlikely, the use of empiric antibiotic therapy (Wigton RS: *Arch Intern Med* 146:81-3, 1986).
   C. Noninfectious causes
   1. **In the pediatric population,** the presence of a foreign body should be considered.
   2. **In the geriatric population,** a malignancy of the vocal chords or esophagus must be considered. Burns from hot liquids, thermal inhalation, or exposure to caustic substances are among the remaining causes.

V. **Laboratory**
   A. Throat culture remains the "gold standard" for identification of GABHS infection in patients with sore throat. The false-negative rate for culture is estimated to be between 5% and 10%. Because the incidence of GABHS infection is markedly decreased in adults, the throat culture can be reserved for patients with a previous history of rheumatic fever, patients with multiple clinical risk factors, or failure to clear a pharyngeal infection despite therapy. Cultures for *N. gonorrhoeae* should be performed if the history suggests this cause.
   B. Rapid streptococcal antigen tests are highly specific (95% to 99%) and moderately sensitive (70% to 90%) compared with throat cultures. These tests permit early diagnosis and initiation of therapy if positive. However, if negative, this test does not exclude GABHS disease, and most clinicians then recommend obtaining a routine throat culture. Rapid antigen tests may be valuable in settings where routine throat cultures are not technically feasible, or access to health care providers is difficult and the outcome of the test will influence treatment.
   C. EBV infection (infectious mononucleosis) should be considered in patients with predominate signs and symptoms of fatigue, malaise, headache, adenopathy, and fever of 2 to 3 weeks or longer. These patients may benefit from a serologic test for infectious mononucleosis (Monospot test for heterophile agglutinin). This test is not usually positive until 1 to 2 weeks of illness. If a complete blood cell count is obtained, many of these patients will have >10% atypical lymphocytes present.
   D. The presence of a pharyngeal membrane should alert the clinician to consider *C. diphtheriae* or *C. haemolyticum* infection. Diphtheria can be identified by smears stained by Gram's method, methylene blue, or fluorescein-labeled antitoxin culture on Loeffler medium. The health department should be notified immediately in all cases of suspected diptheria.

VI. **Treatment**
   A. Viral: Symptomatic therapy for patients with viral pharyngitis consists of relieving pain and discomfort. Warm saline gargles, rest, antiinflammatory agents, and liquids are usually sufficient.
   B. Group A β-hemolytic streptococcus
   1. **Penicillin** remains the drug of choice for GABHS pharyngitis. Adults receive low-dose therapy (penicillin VK, 250 mg PO QID for 10 days), and children should receive 50,000 units/kg/day in three to four divided doses. Twice-daily regimens with double the standard dose also appear to be effective; however, durations shorter than 10 days are not as effective. A sin-

gle intramuscular dose of 1.2 million units of benzathine penicillin is also effective.
  2. **For penicillin-allergic patients,** erythromycin, 250 mg four times a day for 10 days or new macrolides (e.g., azithromycin for 5 days, clarithromycin for 10 days) are acceptable alternatives. Oral second- and third-generation cephalosporins are approved for the treatment of GABHS pharyngitis.
  3. **If the community has a reported high failure rate** with penicillins, the use of third-generation oral cephalosporins has been shown to be efficacious. Cefuroxime axetil, cefixime, cefprozil, loracarbef, and cefpodoxime proxetil are clinically efficacious, with bacteriologic and clinical cure in over 90% of cases. The recommended duration of treatment is 5 to 10 days.
  4. **Hospitalization** is indicated in patients unable to take oral fluids or who have the potential for airway obstruction.
 C. *Mycoplasma pneumoniae* or *C. pneumoniae:* **Pharyngitis secondary** to *M. pneumoniae* or *C. pneumoniae* responds to erythromycin, 250 mg QID for 14 days; tetracycline, 500 mg PO QID for 14 days; or doxycycline, 100 mg BID for 14 days, or new macrolides as mentioned above.

Acute Epiglottitis

I. **Definition.** Inflammation and edema of the supraglottic structure including the epiglottis, the arytenoids, and the false vocal cords.
II. **Pathophysiology.** The method of infection of the supraglottic region is currently unknown. Proposed mechanisms include mucosal surface trauma secondary to eating or viral infection, with subsequent direct invasion by bacteria (*H. influenzae* or other pathogens).
III. **Microbiology.** *H influenzae* type b is the predominate pathogen in both adults and children. Other organisms include *S. pneumoniae, S. aureus,* β-hemolytic streptococci, nontypeable *H. influenzae,* and *Pasteurella multocida.*
IV. **Clinical manifestations**
 A. Children
  1. **Symptoms.** Severe sore throat, fever, dysphagia, drooling, inspiratory stridor, and airway obstruction.
  2. **Signs.** Toxic appearance; frequently sitting upright in a "sniffing position," jaw protruding, drooling; inspiratory stridor; and tachycardia.
 B. Adults
  1. **Variable presentation.**
  2. **Symptoms.** "Severe unremitting sore throat," dysphagia, and fever.
  3. **Signs.** Toxicity and symptoms exceeding the physical findings.
V. **Diagnosis**
 A. **Visualization** of the epiglottis and supraglottic structures is the only reliable method of diagnosis. The epiglottis is erythematous and swollen. Occasionally, the supraglottic structures are the primary areas of involvement, with a normal appearing epiglottis.
 B. *In a child, visualization should be performed in the operating room with equipment and personnel ready to establish a surgical airway if necessary.*
 C. **Soft tissue lateral neck radiographs** may suggest the classic "thumb sign." The sensitivity of the radiograph is approximately 79%. The child should always be monitored by nursing and medical personnel during radiologic ex-

amination in the event airway obstruction occurs. Some investigators feel that this test is not helpful in the decision process.
- **D.** **A complete blood cell count** frequently reveal leukocytosis.
- **E.** **In children with acute epiglottitis,** the blood culture isolation rate is between 80% and 100%.

VI. Treatment
- **A.** **The primary and most immediate objective of treatment is to establish the airway.** Children with epiglottitis should routinely be intubated (via endotracheal tube or surgical tracheotomy). Endotracheal intubation is preferred to the surgical route.
- **B.** **Consensus on treatment of adults with epiglottitis is not available.** The airway should be assessed with direct visualization as soon as possible. If the findings are compatible with an impending airway obstruction, aggressive airway management with intubation would be recommended.
- **C.** **Antibiotics.** The choice of antibiotics must include coverage for *H. influenzae*. Because of the presence of β-lactamase–producing organisms, resistance to ampicillin is prevalent in many communities. A third-generation cephalosporin (ceftriaxone or cefotaxime) is recommended. Alternatively, ampicillin and chloramphenicol are acceptable.

VII. Prophylaxis.
Rifampin prophylaxis for *H. influenzae* type B is recommended (20 mg/kg/day not to exceed 600 mg/day) for all household contacts where there are susceptible members younger than 4 years, day-care and nursery school classroom contacts (including adults), and the patient (before discharge).

Septicemia

I. Introduction
- **A.** **Blood stream invasion** by bacteria and fungi remains common in the United States. In spite of newer and more potent antibiotics, death from septicemia has increased more than 10-fold in the last decade.
- **B.** **The microbiologic etiology** of septicemia varies with the patient population. In nosocomial- and community-acquired septicemia, gram-positive organisms, gram-negative organisms, anaerobes, and fungi account for 30% to 40%, 50% to 60%, 2% to 17%, and 2% to 12% of infections, respectively. Recent epidemiology suggests an increase in both polymicrobial sepsis and bacteremia by gram-positive cocci.
- **C.** **In the normal host,** the host defenses are usually capable of "containing" the invasion of microorganisms into the bloodstream. When underlying illness occurs or predisposing risk factors are present (malignancy, immunosuppression, burns, patients with indwelling prosthetic or other medical devices, renal or liver failure, alcoholism, diabetes, acquired immunodeficiency syndrome [AIDS], and the elderly), host defenses become overwhelmed and illness results. Endotoxin, exotoxins, and other products of bacterial cell walls cause a release of cytokines, which activate complement, intrinsic clotting, kinin, and fibrinolytic pathways. The most scrutinized of these cytokines has been tumor necrosis factor (TNF), interleukin-1, and γ-interferon.
- **D.** **Early recognition and initiation of treatment** is essential in the care of the patient with potential sepsis. Early appropriate therapy can reduce the mortality

rate in gram-negative sepsis and most likely in sepsis caused by other organisms as well.

- E. **Clinical approach.** The primary issues the emergency physician must address are as follows:
  1. **What is the hemodynamic and mental status of the patient?**
     a. **If the patient** has inadequate ventilation or oxygenation, and is unstable, airway and ventilatory support should be initiated.
     b. **If unstable hemodynamics** exist, fluid therapy, invasive monitoring (central venous pressure [CVP] or pulmonary capillary wedge pressure), and vasoactive drugs (dopamine, dobutamine) may be required.
  2. **Is sepsis present?** Early signs and symptoms of sepsis are nonspecific. Symptoms include malaise, lethargy, confusion, nausea, vomiting, hyperventilation, cough, and dysuria or increased urinary frequency. Abnormal signs include fever or hypothermia, wide or narrow pulse pressure, tachypnea, rash (petechiae, purpura, or diffuse erythema), and focal findings on pulmonary, cardiovascular, genitourinary, or abdominal examination.
  3. **If sepsis is possible, what is the most likely source of the sepsis?**
     a. **An assessment** of the presence of underlying medical conditions that would predispose a patient to sepsis is vital. Among these conditions are age (very old and young, recent medical intervention or instrumentation), a medical device implanted, evidence of drug abuse, and underlying medical disease.
     b. **After a careful history** and physical examination, the following laboratory and radiologic tests are useful in patients with sepsis:
        (1) Complete blood cell count with differential cell count and platelet count.
        (2) Serum electrolytes.
        (3) Renal and liver function tests.
        (4) Hemostasis studies (PT, PTT, fibrinogen, fibrin split products).
        (5) Arterial blood gases.
        (6) Chest radiograph.
        (7) Culture and Gram stain (along with tests for cells and chemistry) of blood and other body fluids suspected of being the site of infection (CSF, urine, ascites, pleural fluid, sputum).
        (8) Special studies if required (e.g., CT of the abdomen and sinuses, ultrasound of the biliary tract and kidneys).

II. Treatment

- A. **Therapy of sepsis** should be directed at supportive measures (oxygenation, fluid resuscitation, administration of pressor agents if needed and treatment of the underlying infectious cause.
- B. Airway and oxygenation
  1. **Significant hypoxia** and work of breathing occur in patients with sepsis.
  2. **Early correction** of hypoxia with aggressive measures such as endotracheal intubation and administration of positive end-expiratory pressure may be needed to maintain adequate oxygenation levels (PaO_2 >60 mm Hg).
- C. Fluids
  1. The initial fluid of choice for emergency resuscitation is **isotonic crystalloid solution** (normal saline, Ringer's lactate, or an equivalent). Close monitoring of fluid resuscitation with invasive monitoring (CVP or Swan-

Ganz measurements, cardiac output measurements, and arterial monitoring) is strongly recommended.

2. **Significant volume** may be required due to peripheral vasodilation and capillary leakage.
3. **Vasopressors (dopamine)** should be used if blood pressure cannot be maintained with fluids. Norepinephrine should be used if there is no response to dopamine.

D. Antibiotics
   1. **Prompt initiation** of appropriate empirical therapy can reduce the mortality rate in gram-negative sepsis, as well as sepsis of other etiologies. The objective of therapy is to control the bacteremia and prevent secondary sites of infection.
   2. **The choice of therapy** should cover all potential sites of infection, as well as the underlying infectious process suspected, based on host immunity factors.
   3. **Neonatal** (onset >5 days)
      a. **Coverage** should include group B streptococcus, gram-negative bacilli *(E. coli, Klebsiella)*, *S. aureus*, *Listeria* species (rare).
      b. **Ampicillin plus cefotaxime or ceftriaxone** is recommended.
   4. **Children nonimmunocompromised**
      a. **Coverage** of the following organisms must be included: *H. influenzae, Streptococcus pneumoniae, N. meningitidis,* and *S. aureus.*
      b. **Ceftriaxone, or cefotaxime, or cefuroxime** are suggested.
      c. **Acceptable alternatives** include antipseudomonal penicillins, ampicillin-sulbactam, or ticarcillin/clavulanate.
   5. **Adult nonimmunocompromised**
      a. **Organisms implicated** in these syndromes include gram-negative bacilli, gram-positive cocci, and anaerobes.
      b. **The combination** of a β-lactam antibiotic (third-generation cephalosporin, antipseudomonal penicillin, imipenem-cilastin, ticarcillin/clavulanate) plus an aminoglycoside is recommended for nonimmunocompromised adults with suspected sepsis.
      c. **If anaerobic infection** (primarily gastrointestinal, gynecologic, or soft tissue in origin), anaerobic coverage should be added (metronidazole, clindamycin, or β-lactamase inhibitor antibiotic).
      d. **For patients at high risk for aminoglycoside toxicity** (elderly), some authors recommend substitution of aminoglycoside with aztreonam.
   6. **Adult immunocompromised (neutropenic)**
      a. **Coverage** is the same as the nonimmunocompromised patients plus *Pseudomonas* species, coagulase-negative *Staphylococcus* species *(S. epidermidis),* and *Corynebacterium* species.
      b. **Standard regimens** have been a β-lactam antibiotic plus an aminoglycoside.
      c. **If the patient has an indwelling catheter** or other prosthetic device, or an obvious skin infection, vancomycin should be added to the regimen.
      d. **Imipenem** alone compared with ceftazidime and amikacin has had comparable results.

Pneumonia

I. **Introduction**
   A. **Pneumonia is the fifth leading cause of death** in the United States.
   B. Etiology
      1. **Community-acquired etiologic agents.** *S. pneumoniae, H. influenzae, S. aureus, Legionella pneumophila,* oral anaerobes (aspiration), *M. catarrhalis,* influenza virus, adenovirus, *C. pneumoniae, M. pneumoniae.*
      2. **Risk factors** include age and underlying cardiopulmonary disease (congestive heart failure, influenza viral infection, lung disease [asthma], immunosuppression, human immunodeficiency virus [HIV] infection, aspiration).

II. **Clinical presentation** of a patient with pneumonia consists of fever, cough, sputum production, hemoptysis, tachypnea (respiratory rate >18 in adults), hyperpnea (greater than normal minute ventilation), and tachycardia.

III. **Clinical approach**
   A. **An immediate determination of the adequacy of ventilation and oxygenation should be made.** Inability to speak, altered mental status, cyanosis, and preference for the upright position are clinical signs of inadequate ventilation or oxygenation. Pulse oximetry is very helpful if available.
   B. **A history of fever and cough** suggest the possibility of a respiratory tract infection. Key points in the physical examination include a complete evaluation of vital signs and general appearance (ability to speak, mental status, positioning, cyanosis), as well as a thorough examination of the ears, nose, and throat, lungs, heart, and extremities.

IV. **Diagnosis**
   A. **Chest x-rays** are essential in the evaluation of patients with suspected lower respiratory tract infections. Chest radiographic patterns may suggest an etiologic agent; however, there is significant overlap of radiographic presentations between most pathogens.
      1. **Lobar consolidation** is present in a minority of cases. The most frequent causes are *S. pneumoniae, Klebsiella/Enterobacter* group, *H. influenzae* type B, and *Legionella* species. *S. pneumoniae* is usually unilobar and located in the dependent portion of the upper and lower lobes. *Klebsiella/Enterobacter* species are frequently multilobar and have a predilection for the upper lobe.
      2. **Cavitation** is most frequently seen with *S. aureus,* gram-negative rods *(Klebsiella/Enterobacter, E. coli, Pseudomonas),* anaerobes, *Mycobacterium tuberculosis,* and fungi.
      3. **An interstitial pattern** is most frequently seen with *Mycoplasma,* viruses, and early *Pneumocystis* infections.
      4. **A wide variety of bacteria** are associated with bronchopneumonia including *Chlamydia, Mycoplasma, Legionella, S. pneumoniae,* and *H. influenzae.*
   B. **Pneumonias with significantly rapid onset** and toxicity are often due to *S. aureus, H. influenzae* type B, *Legionella, Klebsiella,* or *Pseudomonas.*
   C. **Leukocyte** and differential cell counts are useful tests in patients with suspected pneumonia. Patients with pneumonia usually are seen in the emer-

gency department with an elevation in their leukocyte count in the range of 15,000 to 20,000 with a shift to younger forms. The leukocyte count may be low in the elderly, in immunocompromised patients, and in patients with overwhelming infections.
- **D. A good sputum Gram stain** and culture may be useful in determining the causative organism in the patient with a chest x-ray consistent with pneumonia. Specimens containing greater than 10 epithelial cells per high-power field are unacceptable and represent oral flora.
- **E. Blood cultures and/or pleural fluid cultures** are valuable in select patients. The presence of toxicity, immunocompromised state, or difficulty in diagnosis are clinical settings where these cultures may be useful.
- **F. Invasive procedures.** Special techniques may be of value in select patient populations. Transtracheal aspiration, bronchoalveolar lavage, transbronchial lavage and/or bushings, and thoracentesis are among the most useful of these techniques.

V. Treatment

- **A. After adequate ventilation and oxygenation** have been assured and the diagnosis made, appropriate disposition of the patient is required. Commonly accepted indications for hospital admission are pulse rate >140, systolic blood pressure <90 mm Hg, respiratory rate >30, multilobe involvement, altered mental status, arterial hypoxemia (PaO_2 <60 mm Hg), and other concomitant suppurative complications. Other factors that affect morbidity and mortality include age >64 years, coexisting medical illness (diabetes, postsplenectomy, renal or cardiac insufficiency) or immunosuppression, and high temperature (>38.3° C).
- **B. Antibiotic selection for hospitalized patients.** It is usually necessary to begin empiric antimicrobial therapy for pneumonia before a definite microbiologic identification.
    1. **Infants younger than 3 weeks**
        a. **Group B streptococci, *K. pneumoniae*, *S. aureus*, *Pseudomonas* species, *E. coli*,** and occasionally *C. trachomatis* are the causes of pneumonia in this age group.
        b. **Treatment** should consist of a penicillinase-resistant penicillin and an aminoglycoside.
    2. **Infants 3 weeks to 4 months of age**
        a. ***C. trachomatis*** is an important consideration in this age group. The clinical course is frequently insidious with cough and diffuse infiltrates. Pertussis is also a frequent consideration in this age group.
        b. **Empiric treatment** with erythromycin is recommended with this presentation.
    3. **Infants and children <5 years of age**
        a. **Most pneumonia in children younger than 5 years** is caused by viruses. Most prominent of these viruses are respiratory syncytial virus (RSV), parainfluenza types 3 and 1, and influenza virus. Most children recover spontaneously from these pneumonias without specific treatment. Children with severe RSV can be treated with aerosolized ribavirin and those with severe influenza A may respond to oral amantadine or rimantadine.
        b. **Children with bacterial pneumonias** are most commonly infected with *S. pneumoniae*, *H. influenzae*, or *S. aureus*.

    (1) **If the child is moderately ill** and the chest x-ray shows diffuse or localized infiltrates without effusion, amoxicillin or ampicillin/clavulanate is recommended.
    (2) **If the child is severely ill** and the chest x-ray shows diffuse infiltrates, a third-generation cephalosporin is recommended (ceftriaxone or cefotaxime).
   c. **Alternatives** include a penicillinase-resistant penicillin and an aminoglycoside.
   4. **Adults.** Either a third-generation cephalosporin (ceftriaxone, cefotaxime), or ampicillin/sulbactam, or ticarcillin/clavulanate, or TMP/SMX plus erythromycin is recommended.
   5. **Immunocompromised neutropenic patients.** Aminoglycoside plus antipseudomonal penicillin or third-generation cephalosporin plus vancomycin. Imipenem is an acceptable substitute for the β-lactam/aminoglycoside combination.
   6. **Patients at high risk for aspiration.** Clindamycin, or cefoxitin, or ampicillin/sulbactam, ticarcillin/clavulanate, or piperacillin/tazobactam.
C. Antibiotic selection for outpatients
   1. **Appropriate candidates** for outpatient therapy include an otherwise young, healthy person with a nonproductive cough who has no "toxic (fever, chills)" manifestations, is not hypoxic, and usually has a diffuse infiltrate or a single lobar pneumonia (i.e., not meeting high-risk criteria delineated on p. 460). The organisms in this setting are more likely to be *S. pneumoniae, M. pneumoniae, C. pneumoniae, H. influenzae,* or viruses.
   2. **Azithromycin, clarithromycin, or erythromycin** are the preferred antibiotics. Clarithromycin should not be given to pregnant women. Doxycycline is an acceptable alternative.

Soft Tissue Infections Requiring a Surgical Approach

I. **Introduction**
   A. **Host Factors.** Presence of underlying diseases: peripheral vascular diseases, diabetes mellitus, malignancy, chronic renal failure, patients receiving immunosuppressive medications, chronic alcoholism.
   B. **Clues to early recognition**
      1. Extreme pain.
      2. Edema > erythema.
      3. Skin vesicles.
      4. Subcutaneous gas.
      5. Absent lymphangitis and lymphadenitis.
   C. **The three classic signs** are *late findings!*
      1. Fever.
      2. Crepitus.
      3. Shock.
   D. **The disease progresses** to result in skin anesthesia and local ecchymosis and necrosis. Systemic signs of fever, hypotension, and failure of antibiotics to arrest the infection will occur.
   E. **Operative findings**

1. Gray fascia.
2. Easy dissection and undermining of tissue planes.
3. Necrosis and thrombosis of tissue specimens will be visible.

II. Clostridial anaerobic cellulitis
A. Definition
1. **Necrotizing infection** of devitalized subcutaneous tissues.
2. **Deep fascia** and muscle are not usually involved.
3. **Gas formation** extensive.

B. Pathogenesis
1. **Clostridial species,** usually *Clostridium perfringens,* are usually introduced into the subcutaneous tissues through a dirty or inadequately debrided traumatic wound.

C. Clinical characteristics
1. **Incubation period** is several days.
2. **Frank crepitus** is present.
3. Thin, dark, sometimes foul-smelling **discharge.**
4. **Pain** is present but not to the degree it is present in gas gangrene.
5. Moderate amount of **swelling.**
6. Minimal **systemic toxicity.**

D. Diagnosis
1. **Made** on debridement and drainage.
2. **Gram stain** shows gram-positive bacilli.
3. **Radiologic films** show abundant gas, but none in muscles.

E. Treatment
1. **Appropriate drainage** and debridement is the foundation of treatment.
2. **If seen early,** does not require radical debridement or excision.
3. **Antibiotics**
   a. This is a polymicrobic infection. Appropriate selection of antibiotics should cover *Clostridia* species, group A and anaerobic streptococci, Enterobacteriaceae, and other anaerobes.
   b. Appropriate choices would be ampicillin/sulbactam, ticarcillin/clavulanate, piperacillin/tazobactam, or imipenem. Appropriate alternatives would be the combination of penicillin, an aminoglycoside, and anaerobic coverage (clindamycin or metronidazole).

III. Synergistic necrotizing cellulitis (nonclostridial anaerobic cellulitis)
A. Definition
1. Similar to above, but **etiology** is usually from non-spore-forming anaerobic bacteria (*Peptostreptococcus, Bacteroides,* coliforms).
2. Perineal form is responsible for most cases of gram-negative cellulitis described today as Fournier's gangrene.

B. Diagnosis and Treatment similar to clostridial anaerobic cellulitis.

IV. Necrotizing fasciitis
A. Definition
1. Term may be confusing.
2. Refers to all diffuse necrotizing soft tissue infections except clostridial myonecrosis.

B. Etiology
1. **Classification**
   a. **Type 1:** Anaerobic (*Bacteroides* or *Peptostreptococcus* species) plus facultative anaerobic species (non–group A streptococci, Enterobacteriaceae).

- **b. Type 2:** Hemolytic streptococcal gangrene—group A streptococcus plus a second organism (usually staphylococcus).
2. **Clinical characteristics**
   a. Usually an **acute process**.
   b. **Systemic toxicity** usually present (temperature of 102° F to 105° F usually present). This is usually the "clue" that should alert the physician to consider this diagnosis.
   c. Most commonly **affects the legs**.
   d. **Appearance**
      (1) **Early**
         Erythema.
         Swollen without sharp margins.
         Hot.
         Shiny.
         Exquisitely tender and painful.
         Lymphangitis and lymphadenitis are infrequent.
      (2) **Middle.** Color changes from red purple to blue gray.
      (3) **Late**
         Frank bullae.
         Cutaneous gangrene.
         Area has become anesthetic.
         Probing of the involved area reveals easy passage of the instrument along the plane just superficial to the deep fascia.
   e. **Diagnosis**
      (1) **Gram stains** are usually positive for leukocytes and the organisms.
      (2) **Blood cultures** are usually positive.
   f. **Therapy**
      (1) Immediate **surgical debridement** is indicated.
      (2) **Extensive debridement** usually required, extending beyond the area of involvement until normal fascia is found.
      (3) **Wound** should be left open.
      (4) **Antibiotics** recommended should cover anaerobic bacteria (metronidazole, clindamycin), streptococcal species (ampicillin or ampicillin/sulbactam), and Enterobacteriaceae (gentamicin).
      (5) **Prompt diagnosis** is critical.
      (6) **Mortality rate** 20% to 47%.
C. Special forms of necrotizing fasciitis
   1. **Fournier's gangrene**
      a. **Form of necrotizing fasciitis occurring about the male genitals.** May be confined to the scrotum or may extend up the perineum, penis, or abdominal wall.
      b. **Major role of anaerobic bacteria** in this disease; mixed cultures of facultative organisms (gram-negative enterococci) are often mixed with the anaerobic bacteria.
      c. **Clinical appearance**
         (1) **Area is usually swollen,** erythematous, and tender.
         (2) Patient is **toxic**.
         (3) **Pain** is prominent.
         (4) **Swelling** and crepitus are present.
         (5) **Eventually dark purple areas** and gangrene are present.

d. Diagnosis. Rapid diagnosis is critical to this presentation. The key is the presence of marked systemic toxicity out of proportion to local findings.
   e. Treatment
      (1) Immediate surgical debridement.
      (2) Antibiotics. Antibiotics should be directed at anaerobic bacteria, gram-negative rods. Appropriate choices would include ampicillin plus an aminoglycoside plus clindamycin or metronidazole. Imipenem would also be appropriate.
D. *Vibrio* infections
   1. Halophilic marine vibrios *(V. vulnificus)* are another cause of a form of necrotizing fasciitis
   2. Clinical presentation. Occasionally contaminates open wounds causing infection and necrosis.
      a. Ingestion of contaminated water or food may result in sepsis with cutaneous manifestations of hemorrhage, bullae, and necrotic lesions.
      b. More common in patients who are immunocompromised, especially those with hepatic cirrhosis.
   3. Treatment. Doxycycline plus ceftazidime are recommended. Acceptable alternative is chloramphenicol.
E. Clostridial Myonecrosis
   1. Definition
      a. Rapidly progressive, life-threatening, toxemic infection of the skeletal muscle due to clostridia.
      b. Usually follows muscle injury with secondary contamination.
   2. Clinical characteristics
      a. Intense wound pain.
      b. Marked swelling.
      c. Systemic toxicity.
         (1) Tachycardia.
         (2) Mental confusion.
   3. Etiology
      a. *C. perfringens*—70%.
      b. *C. novyi*—40%.
      c. C. septicum—10%.
   4. Clinical presentation
      a. Gas gangrene is a fulminant infection.
      b. Severe systemic toxicity is present.
         (1) Symptoms include diaphoresis, fever, tachycardia, and extreme anxiety of the patient.
         (2) Late complications include shock, renal failure, and hemolytic anemia.
      c. The wound is associated with extreme pain, tense edema, discoloration, hemorrhagic bullae, and evidence of gas in the soft tissues (crepitus). The wound has a characteristic sweetish offensive odor.
   5. Diagnosis
      a. Gram stain reveals the characteristic organisms (gram-positive rods—"box car") with few leukocytes.
      b. Radiographs will reveal gas.
      c. CT scan shows muscle involvement (not recommended as a way to diagnose this syndrome).

6. **Therapy**
   a. The most important and vital therapy is immediate surgical **debridement**. This should be extensive, with wide excision of the involved muscle.
   b. **Penicillin** still remains the drug of choice for patients with gas gangrene, although it should be accompanied by antibiotic providing staph and gram-negative coverage until the diagnosis is confirmed. Acceptable alternatives include imipenem, metronidazole, chloramphenicol, and clindamycin.
   c. **Adjuvant therapy** includes hyperbaric oxygen, but this therapeutic modality is less important than surgery and antibiotics.

Suggested Readings

Brown RB: Selecting the patients, *Hosp Pract* 28(suppl 1):11-15, 1993.

Dere WH: Acute bronchitis: results of US and European trials of antibiotic therapy, *Am J Med* 92:53S-57S, 1992.

Dipiro JT, Fortson NS: Combination antibiotic therapy in the management of intraabdominal infection, *Am J Surg* 165(suppl 2A):82S-88S, 1993.

Elder NC: Acute urinary tract infection in women. What kind of antibiotic therapy is optimal? *Postgrad Med* 92:159-62, 1992.

Hendrix WC et al: Aspergillus epidural abscess and cord compression in a patient with aspergilloma and empyema. Survival and response to high dose systemic amphotericin therapy, *Am Rev Respir Dis* 145:1483-6, 1992.

Hyslop DL: Efficacy and safety of loracarbef in the treatment of pneumonia, *Am J Med* 92:65S-69S, 1992.

Kane G, Wheeler NC, Cook S: Impact of the Los Angeles County Trauma System on the survival of seriously injured patients, *J Trauma* 32:576-83, 1992.

Katz PR: Antibiotics for nursing home residents. When are they appropriate? *Postgrad Med* 93:173-80, 1993.

Khan FA: Quinolones and macrolides: roles in respiratory infections, *Hosp Pract* 28:149-53, 1993.

Lancefield M, Conill AM: Antibiotic prophylaxis, *Hosp Pract (Off Ed)* 27:126-9, 1992.

Linn FV, Peppercorn MA: Drug therapy for inflammatory bowel disease: Part II, *Am J Surg* 164:178-85, 1992.

Morrow JD: The oral cephalosporins: a review, *Am J Med Sci* 303:35-9, 1992.

Nielsen RW: Acute bacterial maxillary sinusitis: results of US and European comparative therapy trials, *Am J Med* 92:70S-73S, 1992.

Nolan CM: Failure of therapy for tuberculosis in human immunodeficiency virus infection, *Am J Med Sci* 304:168-73, 1992.

Oishi CS, Carrion WV, Hoaglund FT: Use of parenteral prophylactic antibiotics in clean orthopaedic surgery. A review of the literature, *Clin Orthop* 296:249-55, 1993.

Orr PH et al: Randomized placebo-controlled trials of antibiotics for acute bronchitis: a critical review of literature, *J Fam Pract* 36:507-12, 1993.

Paluzzi RG: Antimicrobial prophylaxis for surgery, *Med Clin North Am* 77:427-41, 1993.

Rhodes KH, Henry NK: Antibiotic therapy for severe infections in infants and children, *Mayo Clin Proc* 67:59-68, 1992.

Robinson LA, Fleming WH, Galbraith TA: Intrapleural doxycycline control of malignant pleural effusions, *Ann Thorac Surg* 55:1115-21, 1993.

Seiter K, Kemeny N: Successful treatment of a desmoid tumor with doxorubicin, *Cancer* 71:2242-4, 1993.

Shands JW Jr: Empiric antibiotic therapy of abdominal sepsis and serious perioperative infections, *Surg Clin North Am* 73:291-306, 1993.

Stein GE, Havlichek DH: The new macrolide antibiotics. Azithromycin and clarithromycin, *Postgrad Med* 92:269-72, 1992.

Sweet RL: New approaches for the treatment of bacterial vaginosis, *Am J Obstet Gynecol* 169:479-82, 1993.

Tetteroo GW, Wagenvoort JH, Bruining HA: Role of selective decontamination in surgery, *Br J Surg* 79:300-4, 1992.

Therasse DG: The safety profile of loracarbef: clinical trials in respiratory, skin, and urinary tract infections, *Am J Med* 92:20S-25S, 1992.

Van Saene HK, Stoutenbeek CC, Stoller JK: Selective decontamination of the digestive tract in the intensive care unit: current status and future prospects, *Crit Care Med* 20:691-703, 1992.

Van Scoy RE, Wilkowske CJ: Prophylactic use of antimicrobial agents in adult patients, *Mayo Clin Proc* 67:288-92, 1992.

16 Selection of Antimicrobial Therapy for Sexually Transmitted Diseases

Charles A. Kennedy, M.D., F.A.C.P.
Gideon Bosker, M.D., F.A.C.E.P.

Overview of Therapeutic Principles for Sexually Transmitted Diseases (STDs)

Frequently managed in the emergency department, pelvic inflammatory disease (PID), also known as salpingitis, is a term that is most commonly used to describe infection of the uterus, fallopian tubes, and adjacent pelvic structures that is not associated with surgery or pregnancy. An estimated 1 million women per year are diagnosed with PID, and it is particularly common and problematic among lower socioeconomic groups in urban areas. In addition to the acute manifestations of the infection, long-term sequelae such as ectopic pregnancy and infertility occur in 25% of cases. In 1994, the direct and indirect costs of the disease and its complications are estimated to be greater than $4 billion. In view of the impact of this infection, a systematic approach to diagnosis and therapy is mandatory for all practitioners who encounter patients with this condition and its related complications.

In virtually all cases, PID results from ascending spread of organisms from the cervix and vagina to the upper genital tract. Sexual transmission of *Neisseria gonorrhoeae* and/or *Chlamydia trachomatis* account for more than half of all cases of PID. *Neisseria gonorrhoeae* is the major cause of PID in urban areas, where gonococcal infection is quite prevalent, whereas *C. trachomatis* is responsible for a greater proportion of cases among college students, in whom gonococcal infection is less common. Organisms such as *Escherichia coli* and other enteric organisms, including anaerobes, as well as organisms from the vaginal flora, also may cause PID, particularly when the normal vaginal flora (lactobacilli) are supplanted with other organisms. However, infection in the upper genital tract does not always result in clinically recognizable disease; indeed, many women with adverse sequelae associated with PID, such as infertility, have no known history of the disease. Risk factors for acquiring the disease include multiple sexual partners, young age, and use of intrauterine devices for contraception, with the greatest risk occurring during the first few months of use. More recently, vaginal douching and cigarette smoking have also been implicated. Barrier methods of contraception and oral contraceptives appear to protect against upper genital tract infection.

I. Manifestations and complications of PID

A. Abdominal pain. The most frequent presenting symptom of PID is lower abdominal pain that is usually bilateral and that may be associated with abnormal vaginal discharge or uterine bleeding, dysuria, fever, or other constitutional symptoms, such as nausea and vomiting. In general, infections with gonococci tend to have a more abrupt onset with more marked fever and signs of peritoneal irritation than nongonococcal disease. Infections are more likely to occur during the first half of the menstrual cycle, regardless of the pathogenic organism. Recurrent episodes of PID, ectopic pregnancy, chronic pelvic pain, and infertility may result from tubal damage and scarring that are caused by the initial episode of PID. In one prospective study, infertility caused by tubal occlusion occurred in 8% of women after one episode of PID, in 19.5% after two episodes, and in 40% after three or more episodes. Furthermore, many cases of PID are clinically silent, but as many as 70% of women who are infertile due to tubal obstruction have serum antibodies against *C. trachomatis* versus only about 25% of women who are infertile for other reasons.

B. **A high index of suspicion** and a low threshold for initiating treatment are important for facilitating detection and appropriate management. This approach should be applied to all women of childbearing age with pelvic pain. Although laparoscopic visualization of inflamed fallopian tubes and pelvic structures is possible and serves as a "gold standard" for the diagnosis, it is seldom practical. As a rule, the emergency physician must rely on clinical diagnosis, despite its limitations (one study found that only two thirds of patients with clinically diagnosed PID had this infection confirmed at laparoscopy). In addition to the clinical symptoms, lower abdominal tenderness, adnexal tenderness, and pain on manipulation of the cervix are present on physical examination in up to 90% of women with PID. Other manifestations such as elevated erythrocyte sedimentation rate or C-reactive protein, and abnormal vaginal discharge vary widely in frequency. At present, there are no effective ways to detect clinically silent disease.

II. Outpatient versus inpatient treatment

A. **Outpatient treatment is usually feasible** and is preferred for patients with mild cases of PID. There is limited data comparing the efficacy of inpatient versus outpatient therapy. Criteria for which hospitalization is generally recommended include (1) uncertain diagnosis; (2) when the possibility of appendicitis or ectopic pregnancy has not been excluded; (3) suspicion of a pelvic abscess; (4) the patient is pregnant or an adolescent; (5) the patient cannot follow outpatient treatment; (6) close follow-up within 48 to 72 hours cannot be ensured; or (7) previous outpatient treatment has been unsuccessful.

B. **Cervical cultures.** Although cervical cultures for *N. gonorrhoeae* and *C. trachomatis* should be performed, cultures for other organisms are not warranted.

C. **Therapy.** Antibiotic therapy directed at all potential organisms should be started empirically **(Table 16-1).** The Centers for Disease Control and Prevention (CDC) recommends a number of possible regimens, most of which are based on the use of a broad-spectrum cephalosporin administered parenterally, along with an oral agent effective against *Chlamydia* such as doxycycline.

D. **Follow-up and other considerations.** All women seen in the emergency department with suspected or confirmed PID require a pregnancy test to determine appropriate management. If present, intrauterine devices should be removed once antibiotic therapy is initiated. Close follow-up of outpatients within 24 to 48 hours after treatment is started is important. Failure to improve indicates the need for reassessment of the diagnosis (using laparoscopy, ultrasonography, or hospitalization) rather than a change in antibiotic therapy. Male sexual partners of patients with PID need to be examined; this should include examination for STDs other than chlamydial and gonococcal disease, although, as a minimum, they must be treated for these two infections. Women who have had PID should be advised against the use of in-

Overview of Therapeutic Principles for Sexually Transmitted Diseases (STDs)

Table 16-1. Rapid Access Management Guidelines for Treatment of PID and Other STDs in Women

Clinical condition	Drug of choice	Dosage	Alternative
C. trachomatis			
Cervicitis Urethritis	Azithromycin or Doxycycline	1 gm PO once 100 mg PO BID × 7 days	Erythromycin 500 mg PO QID × 7 days Ofloxacin 300 mg PO BID × 7 days (not in pregnancy)
Infection in pregnancy	Azithromycin or Erythromycin	1 gm PO once 500 mg PO QID × 7 days	Amoxicillin 500 mg PO TID × 7 days
Lymphogranuloma venereum	Doxycycline	100 mg PO BID × 21 days	Erythromycin 500 mg PO QID × 21 days
Gonorrhea			
Cervical Rectal	Cefixime	400 mg PO once	Ceftriaxone 125 mg IM once Ciprofloxacin 500 mg PO once Ofloxacin 400 mg PO once Spectinomycin 2 gm IM once
PID			
Outpatient therapy	Ceftriaxone or Cefoxitin plus probenicid plus Doxycycline or Ofloxacin plus clindamycin or metronidazole	250 mg IM once 2 gm IM once 100 mg PO BID × 14 days 400 mg PO BID × 14 days 450 mg PO QID × 14 days 500 mg PO BID × 14 days	—

Continued on next page

Table 16-1. Rapid Access Management Guidelines for Treatment of PID and Other STDs in Women—cont'd

Clinical condition	Drug of choice	Dosage	Alternative
PID—cont'd			
Hospitalized patients	Cefoxitin	2 gm IV q6h	—
	or Cefotetan	2 gm IV q12h	
	either regimen above plus		
	Doxycycline	100 mg IV q12h, until improved	
	followed by		
	Doxycycline	100 mg q12h to complete 14 days	
	or Clindamycin 900 mg IV q8h plus gentamicin 2 mg/kg IV once followed by gentamicin 1.5 mg/kg IV q8h until improved followed by doxycycline 100 mg PO BID to complete 14 days		
Vaginal Infection			
Vulvovaginal candidiasis	Fluconazole	150 mg PO once	Topical clotrimazole, miconazole, butoconazole, terconazole
Trichomoniasis	Metronidazole	2 gm PO once	Metronidazole 2 gm PO once
Bacterial vaginosis	Metronidazole	250 mg PO TID × 7 days	—

Table 16-1. Rapid Access Management Guidelines for Treatment of PID and Other STDs in Women—cont'd

Clinical condition	Drug of choice	Dosage	Alternative
Herpes Simplex			
Genital, first episode	Acyclovir	400 mg PO TID × 7-10 days	200 mg PO 5 times/day × 7-10 days
Proctitis, first episode	Acyclovir	800 mg PO TID × 7-10 days	Acyclovir 400 mg PO 5 times/day × 7-10 days
Prevention of recurrence	Acyclovir	400 mg PO BID	Acyclovir 200 mg PO 2-5 times a day
Chancroid	Azithromycin	1 gm PO once	Ciprofloxacin 500 mg PO BID × 3 days
	or Ceftriaxone	250 mg IM once	
Syphilis			
Early (primary, secondary, or latent less than 1 year)	Penicillin G benzathine	2.4 million U IM once	Doxycycline 100 mg PO BID × 14 days
Late (more than 1 year's duration)	Penicillin G benzathine	2.4 million U IM weekly × 3 weeks	Doxycycline 100 mg PO BID × 4 weeks

trauterine devices and to protect themselves as much as possible against subsequent STDs to reduce their likelihood of infertility and other long-term sequelae. In women with concomitant human immunodeficiency virus (HIV) infection, hospitalization and intravenous therapy are indicated.

Diagnosis and Management

The diagnosis and management of STDs has grown progressively complex over the last two decades. Previously unrecognized pathogens are reported with increasing frequency, and the emergence of antimicrobial resistance limits the utility of many antibiotics that were historically useful. Additionally, patients initially seen with signs and symptoms of an STD are at risk for coacquiring HIV infection.

I. General principles. Patients with STDs are usually examined in ambulatory care settings, and certain standards of practice should be followed. A careful history and physical examination should be obtained in all cases. The appearance of genital lesions in patients with STDs is often confusing; the microbiology laboratory should be used whenever feasible for cultures and pathologic confirmation.

  A. Partner notification should be attempted, appropriate cultures obtained, and empiric therapy offered, even when identified sexual contacts are asymptomatic.

  B. Reporting of an STD to county and state public health agencies is critical. Careful reporting of STD cases allows the identification of point-source outbreaks and the monitoring of antibiotic resistance patterns within communities.

  C. Serologic screening for syphilis and HIV should be considered in all patients with STDs; patients subsequently found to have a reactive Venereal Disease Research Laboratory (VDRL) test or rapid plasmin reagin (RPR) test, or those with a positive HIV enzyme-linked immunosorbent assay (ELISA), warrant referral to an infectious disease specialist for posttest counseling and clinical staging.

  D. Children with signs and symptoms of STDs must be assumed to be victims of sexual abuse. When the clinical suspicion of sexual abuse is present, children should be questioned in a sensitive and nonthreatening manner. Child protective services should evaluate these children and their parents/guardians before discharge from the emergency department (ED).

  E. Victims of sexual assault are frequently infected with one or more STD pathogens. Routine rape examinations should include cultures for *N. gonorrhoeae* and *C. trachomatis,* and serologic testing for syphilis and HIV infection.

II. Gonorrhea in males usually presents with dysuria and purulent urethral discharge; gonococcal cervicitis in females is often asymptomatic. Clinical symptoms begin within 2 to 7 days of sexual contact with an infected partner. Gram stain of the urethral exudate reveals numerous intracellular gram-negative diplococci. The presence of gram-negative diplococci in cervical secretions is not reliable for the diagnosis of GC in women as nonpathogenic *Neisseria* species are commensal flora in the female genital tract. Cultures should be obtained with calcium alginate swabs (cotton-tipped applicators inhibit the growth of *N. gonorrhoeae*) and plated rapidly on warmed chocolate or Thayer-Martin agar.

A. **Antibiotic-resistant isolates** of *N. gonorrhoeae* were first reported in 1976. Penicillinase-producing *N. gonorrhoeae* (PPNG) now account for >7% of all gonococcal isolates reported to the CDC. Chromosomally mediated penicillin resistance (CMRNG) occurs in <1% of *N. gonorrhoeae* isolates. Ceftriaxone, an injectable third-generation cephalosporin, is currently one of the drugs of choice for uncomplicated gonococcal urethritis and cervicitis; resistance to ceftriaxone has not been reported. Single-dose therapy with ceftriaxone or single-dose oral cephalosporins (e.g., cefixime) ensures compliance, is associated with minimal side effects, and provides some antimicrobial activity against incubating syphilis. Spectinomycin has been used for treatment of PPNG; however, plasmid-mediated resistance to this agent is now recognized. Tetracycline and doxycycline can no longer be relied on to eradicate GC from genital mucosal sites because of the emergence of resistant strains.

B. Treatment of gonococcal infections
   1. **Uncomplicated urethritis or cervicitis.** The recommended therapies for uncomplicated gonorrhea (urethritis and cervicitis, as well as pharyngitis and proctitis) are oral cefixime, 400 mg as a single dose, and ceftriaxone, 125 mg intramuscularly as a single dose. Single-dose fluoroquinolones (e.g., ciprofloxacin, 500 mg, and ofloxacin, 400 mg) are also effective; however, these are discouraged because of the need to rule out pregnancy, lack of activity against incubating syphilis, and contraindication for persons less than 18 years of age.
   2. **Pelvic inflammatory disease** is the leading cause of infertility, ectopic pregnancy, and chronic pelvic pain in women of reproductive age. It is a polymicrobial infection caused by *N. gonorrhoeae, C. trachomatis,* and pelvic anaerobes.
      a. **Hospitalization for intravenous antibiotic therapy** is indicated when (1) the diagnosis of PID is uncertain; (2) ectopic pregnancy, appendicitis, or ruptured ovarian cyst cannot be ruled out; (3) abscess cannot be excluded by pelvic ultrasonography or culdocentesis; (4) patients are unable to tolerate oral antibiotics or cannot return for follow-up evaluation within 48 hours; and (5) in adolescent females in an attempt to preserve fertility. Two intravenous antibiotic regimens are most frequently used for inpatient PID therapy: (1) doxycycline, 100 mg intravenously every 12 hours, plus cefoxitin, 2 gm intravenously every 6 hours; or (2) clindamycin, 600 to 900 mg intravenously every 8 hours, plus gentamicin, 1 mg/kg every 8 hours.
      b. **Outpatient therapy for PID** includes ceftriaxone, 250 mg intramuscularly once, and doxycycline, 100 mg orally twice a day for 14 days. An alternative oral regimen is ofloxacin, 400 mg plus either clindamycin, 450 mg four times daily or metronizadole, 500 mg twice daily for 14 days. All patients who receive outpatient therapy for PID must be reevaluated within 48 hours to document clinical improvement; if fever, pelvic pain, and nonmenstrual vaginal bleeding persist, hospitalization is indicated.
   3. **Disseminated gonococcal infection (DGI)** occurs in 1% to 3% of patients with untreated mucosal infection and presents clinically with a triad of pustular dermatitis, tenosynovitis, and monoarticular septic arthritis. Rarely, meningitis or fulminant endocarditis will be the initial manifestation of DGI. All patients with suspected DGI should be hos-

pitalized for parenteral antibiotic therapy. Ceftriaxone, 1 gm intravenously every 12 to 24 hours, is the preferred initial therapy. Amoxicillin, 500 mg orally three times daily, cefixime, 400 mg orally once daily, cefuroxime axetil, 500 mg orally twice daily, or ofloxacin, 400 mg orally once daily can be substituted when clinical improvement occurs and antibiotic susceptibilities are known. The diagnosis of DGI may be difficult to prove because cultures of blood, pustular skin lesions, and synovial fluid are positive in <50% of patients; culture specimens from the urethra, cervix, rectum, and pharynx may be helpful because extragenital gonococcal infection appears to enhance the risk of DGI.

III. **Nongonococcal urethritis (NGU)** is frequently difficult to distinguish from GC based on clinical presentation alone. The incubation period of NGU is longer than that of GC, and the urethral discharge is generally less purulent and of smaller volume. *Chlamydia trachomatis* accounts for most cases of NGU; *M. genitalium* and *U. urealyticum* are recently recognized pathogens capable of causing NGU. The diagnosis of NGU is made when gram-negative intracellular diplococci cannot be demonstrated on Gram stain of urethral discharge. Culturing *C. trachomatis* is not practical; however, immunofluorescent stains and rapid antigen detection kits are available in many emergency care settings.

   A. **Treatment of NGU** involves azithromycin, 1 g orally as a single dose, or doxycycline, 100 mg orally twice a day for 7 days; longer courses of therapy are not indicated. Some patients have symptomatic relapse of NGU after an appropriate course of antibiotic therapy; most relapses are due to tetracycline-resistant *Ureaplasma* and respond to a 7-day course of erythromycin, 500 mg orally four times daily.

   B. **The acute urethral syndrome** is characterized by the rapid onset of dysuria and urinary frequency in women. Despite lower urinary tract symptoms, urine cultures are sterile or have <100,000 bacteria per milliliter. *Chlamydia trachomatis* can be recovered from the urethra in two thirds of sexually active women with the acute urethral syndrome. Treatment is with tetracycline, doxycycline, 100 mg orally twice a day for 7 days, trimethoprim/sulfamethoxazole, double-strength orally twice a day for 7 days, or ofloxacin, 400 mg orally twice a day for 7 days.

IV. **Lymphogranuloma venereum (LGV)** is a systemic disease caused by a serovar of *C. trachomatis* that does not cause urethritis. Primary LGV is characterized by a painless genital papule or ulcer that spontaneously heals in 3 to 10 days. Secondary LGV occurs 2 to 6 weeks later with the development of suppurative lymphadenitis (bubos) and constitutional symptoms. Prominent lymphadenopathy above and below the inguinal ligament accounts for the characteristic "groove sign." Without treatment bubos eventually suppurate, and multiple fistulas and draining sinuses are seen; fluctuant inguinal lymph nodes should be aspirated before spontaneous rupture. *Chlamydia trachomatis* can be isolated from bubo aspirates, and complement-fixation antibody titers >1:64 are highly suggestive of LGV. Lymphogranuloma venereum is treated with either tetracycline, 500 mg orally four times a day, or doxycycline, 100 mg orally twice a day for 21 days; longer courses of therapy are sometimes required for complete healing of fistulous tracts.

V. **Syphilis** is a multisystem disease caused by *Treponema pallidum*. Primary chancres develop at the site of mucosal inoculation and are painless. Spontaneous resolution of the chancre occurs without antibiotic therapy in 1 to 2 weeks. Chancres are usually single, but multiple lesions may be seen. In addition to the characteristic genital location, chancres may be found in the mouth, perineum, and perianal areas. The secondary stage of syphilis occurs 2 to 6 weeks after resolution of the primary chancre and is characterized by a diffuse maculopapular eruption; papulosquamous plaques are present on the palms and soles. Mucous patches may be seen in the oropharynx, or condylomata lata in the perineum and perirectal area. Both the primary chancre and the cutaneous lesions of secondary syphilis have abundant spirochetes and are highly infectious. Uncommon manifestations of secondary syphilis include hepatitis, oligoarticular arthritis, patchy alopecia, and glomerulonephritis.

A. The diagnosis of syphilis is established by a reactive VDRL or RPR, and a confirmatory treponemal antibody test (microhemagglutination test for *T. pallidum* [MHA-TP] or the fluorescent treponemal antibody absorption test [FTA-ABS]) in patients with a compatible clinical syndrome. Darkfield microscopy can be performed on tissue scrapings from chancres, mucous patches, or condylomata lata.

B. Therapy. Parenteral penicillin remains the antimicrobial of choice for the treatment of all stages of syphilis.

1. **Primary and secondary syphilis** should be treated with benzathine penicillin, 2.4 million units intramuscularly. Penicillin-allergic patients should be given doxycycline, 100 mg orally twice a day for 2 weeks. Jarisch-Herxheimer reactions frequently accompany treatment of primary or secondary syphilis, and arthralgias, myalgias, fever, and orthostatic hypotension may occur. Most patients have symptomatic resolution with aspirin and volume replacement.

2. **Syphilis and HIV infection.** Controversy exists with regard to the appropriate amount and duration of penicillin therapy in patients with coexisting HIV infection. There are well-documented reports of meningovascular syphilis with catastrophic neurologic sequelae after a single benzathine penicillin injection for primary or secondary syphilis in HIV-infected patients. To date, the U.S. Public Health Service has not modified its treatment recommendations for HIV-infected patients with syphilis. It is the opinion of some authors that primary or secondary syphilis in HIV-seropositive patients be treated with a minimum of three benzathine penicillin injections (2.4 million units IM) at weekly intervals. All HIV-seropositive patients with primary or secondary syphilis should be referred to an infectious disease specialist so that serial quantitative VDRL tests can be performed; rising titers after initial therapy indicate relapse or reinfection and mandate lumbar puncture and retreatment.

VI. Chancroid is caused by *Haemophilus ducreyi,* a pleomorphic gram-negative coccobacillus. The ulcer of chancroid is typically painful, nonindurated, lined with granulation tissue, and associated with tender regional adenopathy; bubos may be seen with chancroid. *Haemophilus ducreyi* is fastidious but can be grown on chocolate agar. Appropriate treatment regimens include (1) azithromycin, 1 g orally as a single dose; (2) ceftriaxone, 250 mg intramuscularly once; (3) erythromycin, 500 mg orally four times a day for 7 days; (4) ciprofloxacin, 500 mg orally twice a day for 3 days; or (5) amoxicillin/clavulanate, 500 mg orally three times a day for 7 days. Recent outbreaks of chancroid have been reported in the United States and Canada and are associated with a high risk of HIV seroconversion.

VII. **Granuloma inguinale (donovanosis)** is caused by *Calymmatobacterium granulomatis*. Fewer than 100 cases of granuloma inguinale occur in the United States annually; however, *C. granulomatis* is a common cause of genital ulcer disease in certain tropical zones. The ulcer of donovanosis is usually painless and linked with exuberant granulation tissue. The diagnosis of granuloma inguinale is made by visualizing characteristic "donovan bodies" within macrophages from scrapings of the ulcer base. "Pseudobubos" are commonly seen. Unlike the suppurative lymphadenitis which accompanies LGV or chancroid, pseudobubos represent granulomatous infiltration of the subcutaneous tissue. Antimicrobial therapy for granuloma inguinale is suboptimal. Some patients respond to oral therapy with tetracycline, ampicillin, or cotrimoxazole. Patients with large ulcers or extensive involvement of the subcutaneous tissue should be hospitalized and treated with gentamicin, 1 mg/kg intravenously every 12 hours, or chloramphenicol, 500 mg intravenously every 8 hours for 2 to 3 weeks.

VIII. **Herpes simplex virus (HSV) type 2** is the most frequent cause of genital ulcer disease in the United States, and one of seven Americans are latently or actively infected. The typical lesions of HSV-2 are vesicular and clustered in groups of 5 to 10. Primary genital HSV-2 infection may be severe and is often associated with sacral radiculitis, perineal paresthesias, or urinary retention. Primary HSV-2 infection may be complicated by aseptic meningitis. Lumbar puncture reveals a lymphocytic pleocytosis. After primary infection, HSV-2 lies dormant in dorsal root ganglia, and reactivation of latent infection occurs during periods of physiologic or psychologic stress. Many patients have prodromal genital pruritus or burning paresthesias with recurrent episodes. Acute HSV-2 infection or recurrent episodes can be treated with acyclovir, 200 mg orally five times a day or 400 mg orally three times a day for 7 days. Suppressive therapy for patients with frequent or severe recurrences may be warranted (acyclovir 200 mg PO TID) and is more effective than intermittant courses of antiviral therapy. Currently there is no role for topical acyclovir in the treatment of genital HSV-2 infections.

IX. **Vaginitis**
   A. *Trichomonas vaginalis* is a protozoan that causes symptomatic vaginitis in women and urethritis in men. Vaginal discharge and vulvar pruritus are common; dysuria and urinary frequency occur rarely. The vaginal discharge is voluminous and usually gray in color. In men, the urethral discharge varies from clear to mucopurulent. Flagellate, motile trichomonads are easily seen in wet mount preparation of vaginal or urethral discharge. The pH of vaginal secretions is usually >5.0 and numerous polymorphonuclear neutrophils (PMNs) are present. Metronidazole, 250 mg orally three times a day for 7 days, is the drug of choice and reliably eradicates *Trichomonas* when sexual contacts are concomitantly treated. Single-dose therapy with metronidazole, 2.0 gm, is effective in females; however, single-dose therapy in men is associated with a substantial failure rate. Metronidazole is contraindicated during pregnancy in the first trimester. Clotrimazole vaginal suppositories and Betadine douches have been used with variable clinical success in pregnant patients with trichomoniasis.
   B. **Bacterial vaginosis,** formerly called nonspecific vaginitis, is due to the overgrowth of *Gardnerella vaginalis, Bacteroides* species, and anaerobic streptococci. Malodorous vaginal discharge, often described as "fishy," is charac-

teristic. Genital tract inflammation is absent, and dysuria and vulvar pruritis occur infrequently. The addition of 10% potassium hydroxide (KOH) solution to vaginal secretions produces a characteristic amine odor ("whiff test"). "Clue cells" represent denuded vaginal epithelial cells that are covered with adherant bacteria and are consistently found in bacterial vaginosis. Metronidazole, 250 mg orally three times a day for 7 days, is the preferred therapy. Metronidazole as a single 2 g oral dose is approximately 80% effective. Clindamycin-containing vaginal suppositories have recently been used with some success. At present, there is no indication for treatment of male sexual partners of women with bacterial vaginosis.

C. **Candida albicans** commonly causes vaginitis. The risk of *Candida* vaginitis is enhanced by a number of physiologic and disease states including pregnancy, diabetes mellitus, corticosteroid use, and broad-spectrum antibiotic therapy. Vulvar pruritis and dysuria are common. The vaginal discharge is typically white and "curd-like." Microscopic examination by wet mount or saline preparation readily demonstrates pseudohyphae. Topical antifungal creams and vaginal suppositories are the mainstays of therapy. Clotrimazole vaginal suppositories (100 mg) are effective when inserted daily for 1 week. Terconazole cream (5 gm) is also effective and can be administered for a shorter duration (3 days). Fluconazole, 150 mg PO, is effective as single-dose therapy for vaginal candidiasis; systemic side effects are infrequent with single-dose imidazole therapy. Refractory vaginal candidiasis may suggest defects in cell-mediated immunity, and HIV testing should be performed.

X. **Venereal warts** (condylomata accuminata) are caused by human papilloma virus (HPV) and are common in sexually active individuals. Venereal warts are papillary and usually found on the external genitalia or in the vaginal vault, ectocervix, or perianal area. Recognition and treatment of HPV infection is critical because of the association of venereal warts with cervical dysplasia and carcinoma. The application of vinegar or dilute acetic acid (acetowhite staining) to normal-appearing genital tissue often reveals HPV lesions that are not otherwise visible. All women with genital warts should be referred to a gynecologist for Pap smear and culposcopy. Similarly, homosexual males with perianal warts should undergo proctosigmoidoscopy because squamous carcinoma of the anus and rectum occurs with increased frequency in these patients. Podophyllin application and liquid nitrogen cryotherapy are the only treatment modalities that are widely available in emergency care settings. Patient-applied podophyllin preparations are available. Condylomata lata, a manifestation of secondary syphilis, may be confused with venereal warts, and syphilis serologic tests should be submitted on all patients with suspected genital HPV infection.

XI. **Hepatitis B** is frequently transmitted by sexual contact, and emergency physicians are frequently asked to provide guidance regarding postexposure immunoglobulin prophylaxis and vaccination. Sexual partners of patients with documented hepatitis B should receive hepatitis B immune globulin (HBIG), 0.06 ml/kg intramuscularly (maximum dose 5 ml), and the first of three vaccine injections (Recombivax 0.5 ml); follow-up should be arranged with additional vaccine injections administered 30 and 180 days later.

Suggested Readings

Katz BP, Zwickl BW: Compliance with antibiotic therapy for *Chlamydia trachomatis* and *Neisseria gonorrhoeae*, Sex Transm Dis 19(6):351-4, 1992.

Martens MG et al: Multicenter randomized trial of ofloxacin versus cefoxitin and doxycycline in outpatient treatment of pelvic inflammatory disease. Ambulatory PID Research Group, *South Med J* 86(6):604-10, 1993.

McCormack, WM: Pelvic inflammatory disease, *N Engl J Med* 330:115-119, 1994.

Med Lett Drugs Ther 36(913):1-4, 1994.

Soper DE, Brockwell NJ, Dalton HP: Microbial etiology of urban emergency department acute salpingitis: treatment with ofloxacin, *Am J Obstet Gynecol* 167(3):653-60, 1992.

Sweet RL: Pelvic inflammatory disease, *Hosp Pract* 28(suppl 2):25-30, July 1993.

Sweet RL et al: Evaluation of new anti-infective drugs for the treatment of acute pelvic inflammatory disease, *Clin Infect Dis* 15(suppl 1):S33-42, Nov. 1992.

Witkin SS, Ledger WJ: New directions in the diagnosis and treatment of pelvic inflammatory disease, *J Antimicrob Chemother* 31(2):197-9, 1990.

17

Human Immunodeficiency Virus (HIV) Infection

Jon Jui, M.D., M.P.H.

History

Over 250,000 people have acquired immunodeficiency syndrome (AIDS) in the United States, and over 1 million persons in the United States are believed to be infected with the causative agent, the human immunodeficiency virus (HIV-1, HIV-2). The major transmission routes of HIV-1 are sexual, parenteral blood and blood products, and perinatal exposure. The "1993 Revised Classification of HIV Disease" published by the Centers for Disease Control and Prevention (CDC) divides the clinical spectrum into three categories primarily based on clinical symptoms and CD4 counts **(Table 17-1)**.

The HIV virus is a member of the lentivirus subfamily of human retroviruses. The HIV virus infects peripheral blood nuclear cells (PMC), particularly T helper and B lymphocytes, and macrophages. The virus also has been recovered from promyelocytes, lymph nodes, bowel epithelium, brain, and epidermal Langerhans cells. HIV is also present in body fluids (serum, plasma, cerebrospinal fluid (CSF), tears, urine, semen, saliva, breast milk, and vaginal and ear secretions). The HIV virus is heterogenous with distinct biologic and morphologic features; different strains exist and even change in the same person with time. This heterogeneity is critical to the virus's pathogenicity and its resistance to antivirals. The major target for the anti-HIV attack has been its reverse transcriptase activity. Three antiviral agents have been licensed for use in HIV infections: zidovudine (AZT), didanosine (DDI), and zalcitabine (DDC). In addition, the importance of resistance to nucleosides has become a crucial area of intense investigation and interest.

Stages of HIV Infection

I. **Classification.** The two most widely utilized classification systems have been the CDC and Walter Reed Classification Systems. For the purposes of this chapter, the most recent 1993 revised CDC classification for adolescents and adults will be used (*MMWR* 41:RR-17, Dec 18, 1992).
II. **Acute primary infection**
   A. **Many HIV seroconversions are asymptomatic or subclinical.** The time from exposure to HIV-1 to onset of clinical symptoms is usually 2 to 4 weeks. The clinical presentation is usually similar to an infectious mononucleosis or influenza syndrome. This acute illness may consist of acute onset of fever, rigors, arthralgias, myalgias, lethargy, malaise, anorexia, weight loss, nausea, vomiting, diarrhea, sore throat, lymphadenopathy, and a maculopapular rash. Neurologic signs including headache, photophobia, retroorbital pain, stiff neck, peripheral neuropathy, or radiculopathy may be prominent features. Mucocutaneous ulceration is a distinctive feature and reported in 35% of patients in one series.

Table 17-1. 1993 Revised CDC HIV Classification System and Expanded AIDS Surveillance Definition for Adolescents and Adults

The revised system emphasizes the importance of CD4 lymphocyte testing in clinical management of HIV infected persons. The system is based on 3 ranges of CD4 counts and 3 clinical categories giving a matrix of 9 exclusive categories. The system replaces the 1986 classification.

CRITERIA FOR HIV INFECTION: Persons 13 years or older with repeatedly (2 or more) reactive screening tests (ELISA) + specific antibodies identified by a supplemental test, e.g., Western blot ["reactive" pattern = + vs any two of p24, gp41, or gp120/160 (*MMWR* 40:681, 1991)]. Other specific methods of diagnosis of HIV-1 include virus isolation, antigen detection, and detection of HIV genetic material by PCR.

Classification system

CD4 cells category	Clinical category*		
	A	B	C
(1) ≥500/mm³	A1	B1	C1
(2) 200-499/mm³	A2	B2	C2
(3) <200/mm³	A3	B3	B3

* See table for clinical definitions. Unshaded area indicates expansion of AIDS surveillance definition. Cat C currently "reportable." Cats A3 and B3 are "reportable" as AIDS effective January 1, 1993.
§ There is a diurnal variation in CD4 counts averaging 60/mm³ higher in the afternoon in HIV+ individuals and 500/mm³ in HIV-persons. Blood for sequential CD4 counts should be drawn at about the same time of day each time (*J*

Clinical category A

Asymptomatic HIV infection
Persistent generalized lymphadenopathy (PGL)¹
Acute (primary) HIV illness

Clinical category B

Symptomatic, not A or C conditions. Examples include but not limited to:
Bacillary angiomatosis
Candidiasis, vulvovaginal: persistent >1 month, poorly responsive to rx
Candidiasis, oropharyngeal
Cervical dysplasia, severe, or carcinoma in situ
Constitutional sx, e.g., fever (>38.5°) or diarrhea >1 month

Clinical category C*

Candidiasis: esophageal, trachea, bronchi
Coccidioidomycosis, extrapulmonary
Cryptococcosis, extrapulmonary
† Cercial cancer, invasive
Cryptosporidiosis, chronic intestinal (>1 month)
CMV retinitis, or other than liver, spleen, nodes
HIV encephalopathy
Herpes simplex with mucocutaneous uulcer >1 month, bronchitis pneumonia
Histoplasmosis: disseminated, extrapulmonary
Isosporiasis, chronic, >1 month
Kaposi's sarcoma
Lymphoma: Burkitt's, immunoblastic, primary in brain
M. avium or M. kansasii, extrapulmonary
M. tuberculosis, †pulmonary or extrapulmonary
Mycobacterium, other species disseminated or extra-pulmonary
Pneumocystis carinii pneumonia
†Pneumonia, recurrent (≥2 episodes in 1 year)

AIDS 3:144, 1990). The equivalence between CD4 counts and CD4 % of total lymphocytes is: ≥500 = ≥29%, 200-499 = 14-28%, <200 = <14%.			Progressive multifocal leukoencephalopathy Salmonella bacteremia, recurrent Toxoplasmosis, cerebral Wasting syndrome due to HIV
		The above must be attributed to HIV infection or have a clinical course or management complicated by HIV.	
	1 Nodes in 2 or more extrainguinal sites, at least 1 cm in diameter for ≥3 months		*These are the 1987 CDC case definitions (*MMWR* 36:15, 1987). The 1993 CDC *Expanded Surveillance Case Definition* includes all conditions contained in the 1987 definition *(above)* plus persons with documented HIV infection and any of the following: (1) CD4 T-lymphocyte count <200/mm^3 (or CD4 <14%), (2) pulmonary tuberculosis,† (3) recurrent pneumonia† (≥2 episodes within 1 year) or (4) invasive cervical carcinoma.†

From MMWR 41:RR = 17, Dec. 18, 1992.

B. Laboratory abnormalities include transient leukopenia, lymphopenia, elevated erythrocyte sedimentation rate, thrombocytopenia, relative monocytosis, and atypical lymphocytes on the peripheral smear. Seroconversion usually occurs 1 to 10 weeks after onset of acute illness.

C. Asymptomatic infection. Most patients enter a phase of asymptomatic infection after resolution of the acute primary infection. This period may last from months to years.

D. The role and benefit of "early antiretroviral therapy" is unclear. Some authorities start antiretroviral therapy in full dosage for 4 weeks to 6 months, while others advise no treatment.

E. Mother to child. A preliminary report by the Pediatric AIDS Clinical Treatment Group (ACTG) of the National Institute of Allergy and Infectious Diseases (NIAID) (Protocol 076) suggests that perinatal vertical transmission (mother to child) may be significantly reduced (67%) in mothers administered AZT (100 mg 5 times daily initiated at 14 to 34 weeks gestation and continued throughout pregnancy). Inclusion criteria were (1) any mothers who had not received antiretroviral therapy during the current pregnancy; (2) any mothers who had no clinical indications for antepartum antiretroviral therapy; and (3) any mothers with a CD4 count >200/mm^3 on initial assessment.

III. Early disease (CD4 count >500 cells/mm^3)

A. The natural history of progression of HIV infection is heterogenous. Differences may reflect variations in inoculum size, virulence of the strain of the virus, and the immunologic state of the patient. In the San Francisco City Clinic Cohort Study, 36% of the originally asymptomatic HIV carriers developed AIDS 88 months after infection; another 40% had other signs of infection. Other high-risk groups (transfusion recipients, hemophiliacs) indicate a 25% to 30% incidence of AIDS over a 5- to 6-year period.

B. The initial enzyme-linked immunosorbent assay (ELISA) test must have a confirmation test performed (Western blot or immunofluorescent antibody [IFA]). If the HIV confirmation test is positive, then the patient should have a comprehensive initial evaluation. This evaluation must include a comprehensive history with a specific focus on risks for opportunistic infections, immunization history, past medical illness, childhood infections, medications, and occupational and travel history. Particular attention in the physical examination should be focused on the ocular, pharyngeal, dermatologic, reticuloendothelial (lymph nodes, liver, and spleen), and urogenital systems.

C. Laboratory evaluation should include a complete blood cell count with differential, liver and renal function tests, syphilis, and toxoplasmosis serology, and when indicated, serology for hepatitis B and C. Additionally, an evaluation for tuberculosis (PPD with control) and a chest x-ray should be obtained. Finally, the percentage of total lymphocytes that are CD4 cells should be obtained.

IV. Middle stage disease (CD4 count between 200 and 500 cells/mm^3)

A. Asymptomatic. In this stage, the majority of persons will remain asymptomatic or have only mild disease manifestations. Patients with oral, skin, and constitutional symptoms will often have a worsening of symptoms.

B. Antiretroviral therapy is usually initiated during this stage of the disease.

C. Bacterial infections presenting as sinusitis, bronchitis, or pneumonia are commonly seen in this stage. The most common organisms are *Streptococcus pneumoniae, Haemophilus influenzae, Moraxella catarrhalis,* and *Mycoplasma pneumoniae.*

D. Disease progression. If left untreated, patients in this stage have a 20% to 30% chance of developing an AIDS-defining condition or dying within the next 18 to 24 months. With therapy, the risk of disease progression and mortality is reduced twofold to threefold.
 V. **Late disease (CD4 count between 50 and 200 cells/mm^3)**
   A. CD4 count below 200 cells/mm^3. The risk of developing AIDS-defining conditions rises substantially when the CD4 count falls below 200 cells/mm^3.
   B. Opportunistic infections. Patients in this stage of the disease are at high risk of developing opportunistic infections including esophageal candidiasis, *Pneumocystis carinii* pneumonia, *Toxoplasma* encephalitis, cryptosporidiosis, isosporiasis, tuberculosis, lymphoma, and Kaposi's sarcoma.
   C. Prophylaxis. As a rule, prophylactic therapy to prevent *P. carinii* pneumonia (PCP) is initiated when patients enter this stage of disease. Many clinicians will also expand the antiretroviral regimen to include two agents as opposed to monotherapy.
   D. With no treatment, patients in this stage of disease have a 50% to 70% likelihood of developing a new AIDS-related condition or dying within an 18- to 24-month period.
 VI. **Advanced HIV disease (CD4 count <50 cells/mm^3)**
   A. Certain opportunistic infections appear in this stage. Cytomegalovirus retinitis, disseminated *Mycobacterium avium,* cryptococcal meningitis, progressive multifocal leukoencephalopathy, and invasive fungal disease predominate the spectrum of infections. Patients who recover from these infections require lifelong maintenance therapy to prevent or diminish the possibility of relapse.
   B. Prophylaxis. Some clinicians initiate routine prophylaxis against cryptococcal meningitis, esophageal candidiasis, and *M. avium* complex disease.
   C. Neurologic disease and wasting syndrome are seen frequently in this stage of disease.

Antiretroviral Therapy

 I. **The initiation of antiretroviral therapy** is based primarily on the CD4 count.
   A. If the CD4 count is >500/mm^3, no antiviral therapy is indicated.
   B. If the CD4 count is between 200 and 500/mm^3, initiation of antiretroviral therapy is recommended. Monitoring for toxicity is recommended every 2 weeks × 2, then every 4 weeks × 6, then every 3 months. The question of monotherapy (AZT alone) versus combined therapy (AZT + DDI) is controversial.
   C. If the CD4 count is <200/mm^3, initiation of antiretroviral therapy and prophylaxis for PCP is recommended.
   D. If the patient is intolerant to the antiretroviral(s) or continues to clinically deteriorate (new constitutional symptoms, opportunistic infection, neoplasm or rapid decrease in CD4 count), then alternative antiretroviral regimens should be considered.
 II. **Zidovudine** is a thymidine analog that inhibits replication of HIV in vitro by inhibiting reverse transcriptase.
   A. The serum half-life of AZT is 1 hour, with the intracellular half-life of the triphosphate approaching 3 hours.
   B. The dosage for AZT in asymptomatic infection is 100 mg every 4 hours while awake (500 mg total daily dose). An alternative dosing regimen is 200

mg every morning, 100 mg at noon, and 200 mg at bedtime. In symptomatic infections the dosage is 100 mg every 4 hours (600 mg total daily dose). An alternative dosing regimen is 200 mg every 8 hours.

C. **The major toxicity of AZT** is bone marrow suppression. Anemia, neutropenia, and thrombocytopenia have been described. Constitutional adverse effects such as headache, nausea, and malaise usually subside with ongoing therapy.

III. Didanosine

A. **Didanosine is a nucleoside analog** that also inhibits the replication of HIV in vitro. It is approved for adults with advanced HIV infection who have received prolonged AZT therapy.

B. **The serum half-life** of DDI is 1.6 hours (after single oral dose).

C. **The dosage** for DDI is a 200 mg tablet twice a day or 250 mg powder twice a day for patients ≥60 kg; for patients <60 kg, a 125 mg tablet or 167 mg of powder is taken twice a day. The tablets must be crushed (or chewed before swallowing) and should be taken on an empty stomach.

D. **The major toxicities** of DDI include an increase in serum urate levels, diarrhea (28%), peripheral neuropathies (20%), hyperamylasemia (10%), and pancreatitis (6%). The diarrhea may be related to the citrate phosphate buffer that is used with current formulations. Mixing the tablet or powder with greater volumes of water may decrease the incidence of diarrhea.

E. **The major dose-limiting toxicity** is a painful sensorimotor peripheral neuropathy. Therapy should be interrupted if peripheral neuropathy develops; the symptoms gradually resolve over several weeks.

F. **Pancreatitis.** The major life-threatening complication is pancreatitis. Onset of abdominal pain with or without nausea should alert the physician to the possibility of pancreatitis. Didanosine therapy should be interrupted in any patient who has abdominal pain until the diagnosis of pancreatitis is excluded.

G. *P. carinii* **pneumonia.** Didanosine therapy should also be interrupted in patients who are receiving treatment for PCP with intravenous pentamidine because pentamidine can also precipitate pancreatitis.

IV. Dideoxycytidine (Zalcitabine, DDC)

A. **Dideoxycytidine in combination with zidovudine** is approved for the treatment of HIV-infected adults with CD4 counts <300/mm^3 who have demonstrated significant deterioration. The combination of DDC and AZT has synergistic inhibitory activity against HIV in vitro.

B. **In one trial**, HIV-infected patients who received DDC with little or no AZT had a greater mortality rate than patients who received AZT and DDC.

C. **Zalcitabine possesses a serum half-life** of approximately 1 hour.

D. **Dosage** of DDC is 0.75 mg every hour. Dosage is not decreased if weight is >30 kg.

E. **Toxicity.** Toxicity includes maculovesicular cutaneous eruptions, aphthous oral ulcerations, and fevers during the first 1 to 4 weeks of therapy.

1. **Painful sensorimotor peripheral neuropathy.** Approximately 10% of patients will have painful sensorimotor peripheral neuropathy. This side effect is the most common dose-limiting toxicity of DDC. If DDC is stopped at the first sign of peripheral neuropathy, the condition may resolve completely.

2. **Pancreatitis.** Zalcitabine on rare occasions may be associated with pancreatitis. As with DDI, onset of abdominal pain in a patient receiving DDC requires interruption of DDC therapy and evaluation for pancreatitis.

3. **Bone marrow suppression** (neutropenia, thrombocytopenia, and anemia) can also occur with the administration of DDC.

Cardiac Complications

I. **Myocarditis.** A number of investigators have noted a high incidence of myocarditis (nonspecific inflammation and interstitial edema) in autopsies of AIDS patients. The cause of the myocarditis is unclear in the majority of cases. Possible causes include opportunistic infections caused by *Cryptococcus, Toxoplasma,* mycobacteria, cytomegalovirus (CMV), coxsackievirus, and HIV. The work-up and treatment of AIDS-related myocarditis remains to be defined.

II. **Congestive cardiomyopathy.** Biventricular dilation is the hallmark of congestive cardiomyopathy in patients with AIDS. Suggested causes include viral infections, nutritional deficiency, cardiotoxins, and immunologic mechanisms. As a rule, drugs used to treat opportunistic infections in AIDS patients have been associated with significant cardiotoxicity. Case reports of reversible dilated cardiomyopathy in patients on interferon-α and phosphonoformate have been reported.

III. **Endocarditis.** Nonbacterial, thrombotic (marantic) endocarditis are frequently found in autopsies of AIDS patients. Although there has been no increase in the incidence of bacterial endocarditis in HIV patients, recent literature suggests a higher incidence of staphylococcal endocarditis in HIV-seropositive intravenous drug abusers.

IV. **Pericardial disease.** Pericardial effusion is a major cardiac manifestation of AIDS. A recent review reported that 23% of HIV-infected adult patients with cardiac disease have pericardial effusion. Most of these effusions are sterile. Symptomatic pericardial effusions and tamponade are usually infectious. Organisms causing pericardial effusions include *M. tuberculosis, M. avium* complex (MAC), and *Cryptococcus* species. Malignancies (disseminated lymphoma or Kaposi's sarcoma) have also been reported with pericardial or cardiac involvement.

Central Nervous System Disorders: *Cryptococcus neoformans*

Cryptococcal meningitis is the most common life-threatening opportunistic fungal infection encountered in patients with AIDS.

I. **Microbiology.** *C. neoformans* is a round, budding yeast-like fungus, 4 to 6 μm in diameter. It possesses a large polysaccharide capsule and has four serotypes (A through D).

II. **Epidemiology**
   A. *C. neoformans* **is ubiquitous in nature.** Its ecologic niche appears to be soil enriched by bird excrement, especially pigeon droppings.
   B. **Serotype A** is the most common isolate in the United States.
   C. **Incidence of infection** is 6% to 10% in AIDS patients, and in 2% to 4% of cases, it is the AIDS-defining opportunistic infection. *C. neoformans* is the fourth most common opportunistic infection after PCP, CMV and *M. avium–intracellulare* (MAI). In a recent study, over 90% of the HIV patients with cryptococcal infection had meningitis.

III. **Pathogenesis.** Infection is thought to be initiated by the inhalation of unencapsulated aerosolized yeast. In the absence of intact cell-mediated immunity

(CMI), the host is unable to contain the primary lung infection and *C. neoformans* disseminates widely, especially to the central nervous system (CNS).

IV. Clinical

- **A. Symptoms.** The most frequent presentation is in patients with CD4 counts <100/mm^3 and consists of symptoms suggestive of a subacute meningitis or meningoencephalitis. Symptoms include fever, headache (frontal or temporal), and malaise over a 2- to 4-week period. Stiff neck and photophobia, abnormal mental state, and fever were present in 20% to 30%, 20%, and 50% of cases, respectively. Focal deficits and seizures were uncommon (<10% of cases).
- **B. Other manifestations.** Approximately 30% of cases will also have evidence of pulmonary cryptococcosis, with cough, dyspnea, and pleuritic chest pain.
- **C. Painless skin lesions** may be the manifestation of dissemination in 5% to 10% of cases. Skin lesions can be ulcerative, pustular, or papular and may mimic molluscum contagiosum.

V. Diagnosis.
The "gold standard" for diagnosis remains a **positive fungal culture for** *C. neoformans* from body fluids or tissue.

- **A. Rapid diagnosis** can be made by a positive serum or CSF cryptococcal antigen (CRAG) assay. The sensitivity of this test for HIV patients with cryptococcal meningitis is 98% for serum and 91% for CSF specimens. A positive cryptococcal antigen titer >1:8 should be regarded as presumptive evidence of cryptococcal infection. CRAG should always be confirmed by a positive culture for *C. neoformans*.
- **B. The sensitivity of the India ink capsule stain** in detection of cryptococcal meningitis is approximately 70% to 80%.
- **C. The CSF can be deceptively normal** or demonstrate a mild lymphocytic pleocytosis with a cell count <20 leukocytes/ml. The concentrations of CSF glucose and protein may be normal in over 50% of cases. Opening pressures are elevated in 65% of cases and may have prognostic significance.
- **D. Abnormal findings** are seen on cranial computed tomography (CT) in 30% of cases. These findings include diffuse atrophy, mass lesions, hydrocephalus, and edema. All of these findings are neither sensitive nor specific for cryptococcal infection.
- **E. Chest radiographs** may show interstitial infiltrates, nodular patterns, pleural effusions, and/or hilar lymphadenopathy.

VI. Prognosis

- **A. The acute mortality rates** during initial therapy is 20%, and the 12-month mortality is 40% to 70%.
- **B. Factors associated with a poor prognosis** include altered mental status, CSF cryptococcal antigen titers >1:1024, and CSF cell counts <20/ml.

VII. Treatment

- **A.** Recommended initial therapy is amphotericin B (0.7 mg/kg/day) with or without flucytosine (5FC) for 2 to 3 weeks. The 5FC dosage is 100 mg/kg/day in four divided doses. A retrospective study showed no added benefit and increased toxicity when 5FC was added to an amphotericin regimen.
    - **1. Intravenous administration.** Amphotericin B is poorly absorbed and must be given intravenously. There is no advantage for dose escalation of amphotericin B in this setting; patients should receive the full therapeutic dose initially.

2. **Adverse reactions** associated with amphotericin B include reversible renal dysfunction (80%), fevers, arthralgias, headache, and thrombophlebitis.
3. **Serum monitoring.** If serum monitoring (60 to 120 minutes after dose is given) is available, 5FC doses should be adjusted to achieve levels of 50 µg/ml.
4. **Flucytosine** is associated with myelosuppression and gastrointestinal toxicity.
5. **A recent NIAID study** suggests that in mild cases, fluconazole alone (200 to 400 mg qd) may be adequate for induction therapy.
6. **Associated raised intracranial pressure** may be treated with shunts, daily lumbar punctures (remove 25 to 30 ml of CSF), or acetazolamide to inhibit CSF production. Corticosteroids are not recommended.

B. **Further therapy.** Once there is a clinical response, the initial induction therapy should be followed by consolidation, triazole therapy with fluconazole (400 mg PO daily) for a further 8 to 10 weeks. Side effects associated with fluconazole include skin rashes and liver function abnormalities.

C. **Maintenance therapy.** As with other opportunistic infections, maintenance therapy is necessary to prevent relapses. Fluconazole (100-200 mg PO daily) or amphotericin B (1 mg/kg/wk) are acceptable maintenance regimens.

VIII. **Prevention**
A. **Exposure to fungus.** Patients should avoid situations where exposure to fungus is likely (bird nests, heavily contaminated soils, etc.).
B. **Early initiation of triazole therapy** in association with falling CD4 counts (<100/mm^3) may be useful as a preventive adjunct in the future.

Central Nervous System Disorders: *Toxoplasma gondii*

Toxoplasmosis is the most common opportunistic infection to cause encephalitis and focal intracerebral lesions in patients with AIDS.

I. **Microbiology.** *Toxoplasma gondii* is an obligate intracellular protozoan parasite ubiquitous in nature, whose **definitive host is the cat.**
   A. Its **life cycle** consist of three stages: (1) **tachyzoite** (asexual invasive form); (2) **oocyst** (sexual form); and (3) **tissue cyst.**
   B. **Infection** in normal hosts results in parasite encystment and the development of humoral and cell-mediated immunity. Tissue cysts may be present in many organs but are most notable in the brain, heart, and skeletal muscle.
   C. **Common routes of infection** include exposure to cat feces containing oocysts or consumption of undercooked raw meat (beef, pork, lamb) containing viable tissue cysts.
   D. **The seroprevalence of *T. gondii* antibody** varies throughout the world depending on exposure and culinary habits.

II. **Epidemiology.** *Toxoplasma* encephalitis (TE) occurs almost exclusively in severely immunocompromised patients who are seropositive for *T. gondii*.
   1. It has a **reported incidence** of 10% to 40% in patients with AIDS, and it is the AIDS-defining illness in 5% of cases.
   2. **CD4 counts.** Ninety percent of AIDS patients with TE have CD4 counts less then 200 cells/mm^3.

III. Pathogenesis. TE in AIDS is secondary to reactivation of latent infection.
  A. **In the presence of impaired cell-mediated immunity,** tissue cysts in the brain are thought to rupture, resulting in the uncontrolled proliferation of tachyzoites and progressive encephalitis.
  B. **Extraneural toxoplasmosis** is also likely a result of the reactivation of a previously latent infection.
  C. **Pregnancy.** Primary or reactivated toxoplasmosis may be transferred transplacentally during pregnancy (congenital toxoplasmosis).

IV. Clinical presentation
  A. **Symptoms.** Most patients with TE present subacutely (5 to 28 days) with symptoms such as headache, confusion or altered mental status, and/or fever. Seizures are the initial symptom in one third of patients.
  B. **Focal neurologic deficits.** On physical examination, focal neurologic deficits (hemiparesis, ataxia, cranial nerve palsies) are present in 58% to 89% of patients. Fever, confusion, lethargy, delusional behavior, psychosis, and psychomotor retardation are also common.
  C. **Diffuse TE** is an uncommon presentation, characterized by generalized cerebral dysfunction and nonfocal findings.
  D. **Central involvement of areas critical to endocrine function** can result in panhypopituitarism, diabetes insipidus, and the syndrome of inappropriate secretion of antidiuretic hormone (SIADH).
  E. **Extraneural toxoplasmosis** is being recognized with increasing frequency. Pulmonary toxoplasmosis may mimic PCP and can be detected in bronchoalveolar lavage fluid. Ocular toxoplasmosis (retinochoroiditis) may present with pain and visual loss. The funduscopic lesions are usually fluffy and edematous, with ill-defined margins. The absence of hemorrhage helps differentiate toxoplasmosis from CMV-associated retinitis.

V. Diagnosis
  A. **Empiric therapy.** Although the definitive diagnosis of TE requires a **brain biopsy,** the accepted practice is to initiate empiric therapy in patients who have clinical and radiologic findings suggestive of toxoplasmosis and have positive serologic tests.
  B. **Serologic tests.** Since TE usually represents reactivation of latent disease, most patients (97% to 100%) have positive serologic tests for IgG *Toxoplasma* antibodies.
  C. **Cranial CT** has been the standard initial test for evaluation of AIDS patients with suspected toxoplasmosis. The magnetic resonance imaging (MRI) scan is more sensitive and frequently detects focal lesions missed by the CT scan. The CT scan shows bilateral, hypodense, ring-enhancing mass lesions in 70% to 80% of patients. Patients with a single lesion on CT should undergo MRI to attempt to determine if more than a single lesion is present. A single lesion on MRI is uncharacteristic of *Toxoplasma* infection; more than 50% of these lesions are lymphomas. *Toxoplasma* lesions have a predilection for the basal ganglia and corticomedullary junction.
  D. **The major differential diagnosis in TE is primary CNS lymphoma.** However, the presence of multiple lesions and positive serologic tests favors the diagnosis of TE.
  E. **The chest radiograph** in pulmonary toxoplasmosis frequently demonstrates bilateral interstitial infiltrates.

F. **Direct isolation or histopathology** may be helpful diagnostically in some patients. Antigen detection tests are still in their preliminary developmental stages.

VI. Prognosis
A. TE is uniformly fatal if untreated.
B. **Mean survival** in one series was 265 days.
C. **Factors** associated with a poor outcome included decreased level of consciousness at the time of presentation, history of Kaposi's sarcoma (KS) or PCP, fever, and a peripheral white blood cell lymphocyte percentage <24%.

VII. Treatment
A. **Empiric therapy.** HIV patients with a positive antibody (IgG) to *Toxoplasma* organisms are at risk for development of TE. Empiric therapy should be initiated in a patient with a compatible clinical presentation and characteristic radiographic findings on either MRI or CT consistent with toxoplasmosis. Brain biopsy is desirable in settings where the patient does not respond clinically or radiologically to therapy.
B. **Current recommendations for acute therapy** include pyrimethamine, 200 mg orally (loading dose), followed by 50 to 75 mg given orally every day, in conjunction with folinic acid (leucovorin), 10 to 50 mg given orally, intramuscularly, or intravenously every day, and sulfadiazine, 1 to 1.5 gm orally every 6 hours for at least 3 weeks. Side effects with this regimen are common and include nausea, vomiting, rash, and leukopenia.
C. **Sulfadiazine may be replaced by clindamycin,** 600 to 1200 mg given orally or intravenously every 6 hours, without loss of efficacy and with a reduction in the incidence of toxic side effects.
D. **Pyrimethamine/sulfadoxine** (Fansidar) administered intramuscularly has been reported to be efficacious in over 80% of patients, both clinically and radiographically. This combination is also effective in primary prophylaxis and maintenance therapy.
E. **Other agents** being investigated that have efficacy in animal models of toxoplasmosis include azithromycin (1200 to 1500 mg qd), clarithromycin (1 gm q12h), atovaquone (750 mg q6h), dapsone (100 mg qd), and minocycline. These agents must be used in combination with another agent (e.g., pyrimethamine with folinic acid) that has proven efficacy in the treatment of toxoplasmosis.
F. **Corticosteroids** may be helpful in the management of patients with intracranial hypertension secondary to a mass effect from *Toxoplasma* abscesses (midline shift present on CT), or in patients with a deteriorating level of consciousness. To date, no study has shown a superior outcome in patients with TE given corticosteroids. Corticosteroid therapy should be reduced rapidly once a clinical response is achieved. Most patients do not require more than 2 weeks of corticosteroid therapy. The use of corticosteroid therapy may complicate the interpretation of empiric *Toxoplasma* therapy because CNS lymphoma may also respond favorably to corticosteroid therapy.
G. **Patients with seizures** at presentation should receive anticonvulsive agents. These agents should be continued until the primary treatment is completed.
H. **Bone marrow suppression.** Because bone marrow suppression is associated with high-dose pyrimethamine, AZT is usually discontinued during therapy for active toxoplasmosis to avoid additive bone marrow suppression. Zidovudine may be reinstituted when maintenance therapy is started.

I. **Maintenance therapy** with pyrimethamine (25 to 50 mg PO qd), folinic acid (10 mg PO qd), and sulfadiazine (1 gm PO qd) or clindamycin (300 mg PO q6h) will be necessary in all cases to prevent relapse.
J. **Response.** An adequate clinical and radiologic response is normally seen within 14 days of starting therapy. Failure to respond during this period requires that the physician reconsider the differential diagnosis and proceed to brain biopsy for more definitive diagnosis.

VIII. **Prevention**
A. **Primary prophylaxis** has not been studied in controlled clinical trials but may be of value in patients with CD4 counts <200/mm^3 and positive serologic tests. Regimens may include TMP/SMX, pyrimethamine/dapsone, and pyrimethamine/sulfadoxine.
B. **Avoiding cat feces.** Patients should avoid contact with material potentially contaminated with cat feces.
C. **Hygiene.** Patients should wash their hands thoroughly after contact with raw meat and eat only well-cooked meat.

Dermatologic Manifestations: Infectious Cutaneous Disorders

I. **Bacterial infections**
A. **Soft tissue infections** are frequently seen in HIV-infected persons. *Staphylococcus aureus* is the most common cutaneous pathogen and can present as bacterial folliculitis, bullous impetigo, ecthyma, abscesses, and cellulitis.
B. **Bacterial folliculitis.** Folliculitis is the most common form of staphylococcal infection seen in HIV-infected persons. The primary presentation is the follicular pustule. These pustules usually involve the face, trunk, and groin, and may be associated with severe pruritus. Dicloxacillin, 500 mg orally four times a day, or other penicillinase-resistant antistaphylococcal agents are recommended for 7 to 21 days. In refractory cases, add rifampin 600 mg daily for the first 5 days.
C. **Bacillary angiomatosis**
  1. **Dermal bacillary angiomatosis** (BA) is an uncommon subacute or chronic bacterial infection occurring in the setting of immune suppression, especially late symptomatic HIV disease. In one study, patients with documented BA had an average CD4 count of 57/mm^3. The causative organisms are *Rochalimaea quintana* and *R. henselae*. Tissue biopsy is required to confirm the diagnosis.
  2. **Bacillary angiomatosis presents as an enlarging red papule that resembles a cranberry.** It often begins as a small red papule that enlarges to several centimeters in diameter and only rarely ulcerates. Lesions of BA may be single or multiple and may be associated with systemic dissemination of *R. henselae*. Patients with BA should be worked-up for osseous and parenchymal lesions. Differential diagnosis includes Kaposi's sarcoma, simple angioma, pyogenic granuloma, and angiokeratoma.
  3. **If untreated, BA can be fatal.** The treatment of choice is erythromycin, 500 mg orally or intravenously, four times a day for 7 to 10 days. Doxycycline, 100 mg orally or intravenously twice a day, and rifampin, 600 mg orally every day, have also been reported to be effective. The treatment may need to be extended for 4 to 6 weeks for complete resolution of the

lesions. Parenteral therapy may be required to treat relapses of cutaneous infection or disseminated infection.

II. Viral infections

A. **Herpes viruses** are frequently a cause of significant morbidity in patients with HIV disease.

1. **Herpes varicella-zoster (HVZ)** virus often reactivates during the asymptomatic and symptomatic period. Dermatomal presentations are the most common, although disseminated HVZ may also occur. In patients with more advanced HIV disease, herpes zoster may be very painful, severe, and prolonged. **Treatment** consists of acyclovir, 800 mg orally five times a day for 7 days for mild-to-moderate cases, and 10 to 12 mg/kg intravenously (infuse over 1 hour) every 8 hours for 7 to 14 days for severe cases.
2. **Both primary and reactivation herpes simplex** infection (HSV-1, HSV-2) are seen in HIV patients. Lesions usually occur in the genital, digital, and orofacial areas. Any persistent, nonhealing ulcer in an HIV-infected person must be suspected of being HSV related. Occasionally, *S. aureus* or other bacterial organisms may secondarily infect these ulcers.
3. **Treatment**
   a. **Acute attack:** Acyclovir, 5.0 mg/kg intravenously (infuse over 1 hr) every 8 hours for 7 days or 200 mg orally five times a day for 10 days is the treatment of choice. In patients known to have acyclovir-resistant HSV, foscarnet, 40 mg/kg intravenously (infuse over 2 hours) every 8 hours for 21 days is the treatment of choice. (Note that the patient must be well hydrated.)
   b. **Suppression therapy** should be initiated with the resolution of the acute attack. Acyclovir, 400 mg orally twice daily indefinitely, is the drug of choice. Foscarnet, in a dosage of 40 mg/day intravenously indefinitely, is indicated for suppression in patients with acyclovir-resistant HSV strains.

B. Hairy leukoplakia. Oral "hairy" leukoplakia has only been seen with HIV infection. The presentation is characterized by white verrucous or corrugated plaques along the lateral surface of the tongue or buccal mucosa. Although similar to oral candidiasis, the lesions are not easily scraped away. The implicated etiological organism is Epstein-Barr virus. Acyclovir, 800 mg orally five times a day (not FDA approved) is effective, but the condition tends to recur in most patients.

C. Human papillomavirus (HPV). HPV infection in HIV-infected patients can cause widespread warts (verrucae vulgares). Clinical presentations may include flat and filiform warts in the beard, anogenital warts (condylomata acuminata), plantar warts, and periungual cerrucae. Lesions caused by HPV are difficult to treat and respond poorly to local measures (topical caustic agent and/or electrocauterization). With condyloma acuminata, interferon-α-2b or interferon-α-n3, 1.0 million units (0.1 ml) intralesionally three times a week for 3 weeks, has been used with some success.

D. Molluscum contagiosum is a cutaneous poxvirus. The agent is transmitted by sexual or other close contact, and infection is extremely common in patients with symptomatic HIV disease.

1. **Molluscum lesions** are small, 2 to 5 mm in size, firm, umbilicated, painless papules with a pearly white surface. Lesions have a predilection for the eyelids, face, trunk, or genital areas and may number in the hundreds. Disseminated cryptococcosis has mimicked molluscum contagiosum.

2. Treatment with destructive therapies (cryotherapy with liquid nitrogen, light electrocautery, or curettage) is usually effective. α-Interferon is not effective. Retinoic acid (Retin A) applied once nightly to the face may decrease the rate of appearance of new lesions but does not affect established lesions. Retinoic acid must not be used on eyelid or genital lesions.

E. **Cutaneous CMV infection** is rare, and its presence suggests a poor prognosis. The most frequent presentation is that of persistent perianal ulcerations (similar to perianal herpes simplex infection) that fail to respond to acyclovir. Ganciclovir (5 mg/kg IV BID × 14 days) may result in clinical improvement. Recurrence is common after discontinuation of medication.

III. **Fungal infections: candidiasis**
   A. **Presentation.** The most common presentation of candidiasis in the HIV population is vaginal and oropharyngeal candidiasis. *Candida albicans* is the most commonly associated strain in these patients.
   B. **Female patients** with vaginal candidiasis complain of vulvar pruritus, burning pain, and dyspareunia. On examination, a creamy white abnormal discharge, pseudomembranous plaques, and mucosal erythema are present.
   C. **Most patients will respond to local therapies.** Clotrimazole troches, 10 mg (one troche) five times daily; miconazole 200 mg vaginal tablets, 1 tablet daily for 3 days; or nystatin oral suspension, 400,000 to 600,000 units (4 to 6 ml) four times daily for 3 days is effective.
   D. **Systemic therapy** is usually reserved for treatment failures or more severe disease. Oral fluconazole, 150 mg daily for 3 days, or itraconazole, 200 mg orally daily for 3 days, is effective. The cure rates between imidazoles are comparable. Relapse rates range from 20% to 60%.

IV. **Noninfectious disorders**
   A. **Seborrheic dermatitis.** Seborrheic dermatitis is extremely common in patients with symptomatic HIV disease. Erythematous scaling lesions are usually located in the hairy areas of the central face, scalp, chest, back, and groin. Facial and trunk lesions usually respond to topical imidazole cream (clotrimazole 1%, ketoconazole 2%) plus a medium-potency topical steroid (triamcinolone 0.1%) applied twice daily. Lesions on the scalp should be treated with dandruff shampoos containing selenium sulfide (Selsun Blue), zinc pyrithione (Head and Shoulders, Danex, Zincon), or sulfur and salicylic acid (Sebulex, Van Seb).
   B. **Psoriasis.** Psoriasis may flare or begin after HIV infection. Scaling psoriatic lesions of the axillae and groin are common, and lesions may also involve the elbows, knees, lumbosacral areas, palms, and soles. Mild-to-moderate psoriasis is managed with topical steroids and tar. Severe disease in the presence of HIV infection may improve with AZT therapy.
   C. **Eosinophilic pustular folliculitis.** This condition closely mimics bacterial folliculitis. The primary lesion is an edematous papule with a tiny central pustule. Numerous follicular papules may be present over the head, trunk, and extremities. Many of these lesions are excoriated due to the associated severe pruritus. Cultures are uniformly negative, and patients do not respond to antistaphylococcal antibiotics. Antihistamines, potent topical steroids, and phototherapy with ultraviolet B (UVB) are only partially effective.
   D. **Hypersensitivity. Drug reactions** are frequent in patients with HIV. Approximately 50% of patients being treated with TMP/SMX for *Pneumocystis pneumonia* will develop a widespread maculopapular reaction. Occasional cases of toxic epidermal necrolysis have also been reported.

Gastrointestinal Complications

Gastrointestinal complaints are commonly encountered in the management of patients with AIDS. In approximately 3% of cases in the United States, esophageal candidiasis is the AIDS-defining opportunistic infection.

I. **Esophagitis**
   A. **Etiology.** The most common etiologic agents of esophagitis are *C. albicans* (42% to 79%) and CMV (10% to 40%). Many will have both thrush and esophageal candidiasis. Other rare agents are *Torulopsis glabrata, Histoplasma capsulatum,* other herpes viruses (HSV and EBV), and HIV itself.
   B. **Presentation.** Esophagitis presents with dysphagia (difficulty swallowing), odynophagia (pain on swallowing), retrosternal chest pain (esophageal spasm), nausea, and weight loss.
      1. **The presence of thrush** in patients with odynophagia strongly suggests esophageal involvement.
      2. **Diagnosis.** The symptoms alone are not a reliable method of diagnosis. A classic "cobblestone" of the diffuse ulcerations and plaques will be present on barium contrast radiography. Definitive diagnosis requires endoscopy and biopsy.
      3. **Treatment.** In these patients, a course of antifungal therapy is recommended. Local agents are usually effective against oropharyngeal candidiasis, but esophageal disease usually requires systemic therapy. Most investigators favor fluconazole, 200 mg orally on the first day and 100 mg daily for the following 7 to 14 days. Some investigators are also placing these patients on suppressive therapy (fluconazole 100 mg PO every week). Alternatives include ketoconazole, 200 to 400 mg orally given daily until improvement. Endoscopy is not routinely performed unless the patient does not respond to therapy.
   C. **Herpes and CMV esophagitis** also present with dysphagia, odynophagia, and episodic retrosternal chest pain. Odynophagia and esophagospasm are more prominent in these patients than those with *Candida* esophagitis.
      1. **HSV ulceration.** Intense esophagitis, odynophagia, and dysphagia are present in patients with HSV-1 and HSV-2. These viruses cause deep clean-based ulcerations 1 to 2 cm in diameter and may be confused with those of CMV. However, HSV ulcerations tend to be fewer, deeper, and smaller. Biopsy and culture specimens are required to distinguish between these entities. These ulcers usually respond to acyclovir (5 mg/kg q8h × 7 days or 200 mg PO five times a day × 10 days). Suppression therapy with acyclovir (400 mg PO BID) is effective and must be continued indefinitely. If acyclovir therapy fails because of drug resistance, foscarnet is an effective alternative.
      2. **CMV ulceration.** CMV ulcers are extensive, extremely large (2 to 10 cm long), have sharp borders, and are frequently shallow and superficial. Extensive, circumferential involvement may be present. A biopsy specimen is required for definitive diagnosis. Ganciclovir (5 mg/kg IV BID × 14 days) has resulted in clinical improvement, but a significant portion of these patients relapse. Foscarnet (200 mg/kg daily × 21 days) is also reported to be effective. There is preliminary evidence that both drugs can be used together successfully for induction and maintenance treatment of CMV. The recommendations for maintenance therapy remain controversial.

D. Idiopathic esophagitis. A number of patients will have idiopathic esophagitis. Treatment of these patients is difficult and primarily supportive (antacids, low-acid diet, and sucralfate). Treatment of the underlying HIV disease may help as well. Primary lymphoma, Kaposi's sarcoma, histoplasmosis, and squamous cell carcinoma are other rare diseases that may involve the esophagus in HIV-infected patients.

II. Gastric disease

A. Gastric disease in the HIV patient is similar to that of the esophagus. *Candida* is less of a problem, most likely due to the presence of acid. In many HIV patients, hypochlorhydria may be present. Treatment of gastric pathogens is the same as esophageal pathogens. Because of the presence of hypochlorhydria, therapy with histamine (H_2) blockers is redundant and mucosal protective agents like sucralfate are the drugs of choice.

B. CMV may also cause gastritis with extensive ulcerations, intense inflammatory response, edema, and enlargement of rugal folds.

C. Gastric Kaposi's sarcoma is a common complication of cutaneous KS and is often asymptomatic. Gastric KS appears in radiographs as an ulcerative target lesion with underlying submucosal masses. Definitive diagnosis is made by endoscopy and biopsy.

D. B-cell non-Hodgkin's lymphoma involves the antrum and is associated with gastric outlet obstruction and occasionally hemorrhage.

III. Hepatobiliary disease

A. Signs. Right upper quadrant abdominal tenderness, hepatomegaly, and abnormal liver function tests have been noted with increased frequency in patients with AIDS.

B. An increased incidence of acalculous cholecystitis including gangrenous cholecystitis has also been reported. A number of these episodes follow infections such as *Campylobacter, Salmonella, Cryptosporidium,* or CMV enteritis. In patients with no clear cause, the pathophysiology is unknown but necrotizing vasculitis has been the proposed mechanism of injury. The patient typically has right hypochondrial pain and an elevated serum alkaline phosphatase level. Ultrasound examination often demonstrates a thickened gallbladder wall and/or gallbladder dilation. Cases associated with infection may respond to antibiotics. In severe cases, surgery may be required.

C. Significant hepatic parenchymal disease has been noted in patients with HIV infection. Steatosis, portal inflammation, congestion, and granuloma are the most common histologic abnormalities. AIDS-specific infections or malignancies have been detected in 40% of biopsy and autopsy specimens.

  1. **Hepatitis B virus (HBV).** HIV has been shown to increase HBV replication in established infection. The incidence of chronic HBV infection after exposure and the risk of reactivation of latent disease are also increased.
  2. **Other infectious causes include** hepatitis C virus, CMV, *M. avium–intracellulare, Cryptococcus, Histoplasma,* and *Coccidioides immitus* (coccidioidomycosis).
  3. **Neoplastic findings** have included KS and lymphoma.

IV. Small bowel disease

A. Large-volume diarrhea with abdominal pain and weight loss are common in AIDS patients. Many of these patients will have treatable infectious causes of diarrhea. Specific small bowel pathogens identified from stool cultures and ova and parasitic examination include *Salmonella* species, *Shigella* species,

Campylobacter species, *G. lamblia*, *Entamoeba histolytica*, *Cryptosporidium* species, and *I. belli*. In addition, HIV infection of enterocytes or the lamina propria has been described.
- B. **Treatment.** Some AIDS patients with severe dehydrating diarrhea may respond to octreotide (Somastatin). Responders were significantly more likely not to have enteric pathogens isolated from their stools. Dosages of octreotide range from 50 to 500 μg every 8 hours given subcutaneously.
- C. **Bacterial diarrhea.** Enteric infections caused by *Salmonella, Shigella,* or *Campylobacter* species can be treated with ciprofloxacin, 500 to 750 mg twice a day for 5 days. If relapse occurs, indefinite treatment may be indicated. Alternative therapy for *Campylobacter* enteritis is erythromycin, 250 mg four times a day for 10 days. Alternatives for *Salmonella* and *Shigella* enteritis are ampicillin, 500 mg four times a day for 10 to 14 days, or TMP/SMX, one double-strength tablet (160 mg TMP) twice a day for 10 to 14 days.
- D. Parasitic diarrhea
    1. ***Cryptosporidium* species.** No antimicrobial treatment has been shown to be effective with infection due to *Cryptosporidium* species. Paromomycin, 500 to 750 mg orally given three or four times a day for 10 days, has resulted in short-term improvement with a high relapse rate. Symptomatic treatment with imodium, diphenoxylate, tincture of opium, or octreotide may be beneficial.
    2. ***Giardia lamblia*** infections can be treated with metronidazole, 250 mg orally three times a day for 5 days, or quinacrine, 100 mg orally three times a day after meals for 5 days.
    3. ***Isospora belli*** infections can be treated with TMP/SMX, one double-strength tablet four times a day for 10 days, then twice daily for 3 weeks. Chronic suppression with TMP/SMX, one double-strength tablet given three times a week, is usually required in AIDS patients. Alternatives to this regimen are pyrimethamine, 75 mg orally daily for 14 days, with folinic acid, 10 mg orally for 14 days for acute treatment; and pyrimethamine, 25 mg orally daily, with folinic acid, 5 mg orally given daily, for chronic suppression.
    4. **Symptomatic *E. histolytica*** infection can be treated with metronidazole, 750 mg orally three times a day for 10 days, followed by iodoquinol, 650 mg orally three times a day for 20 days. Paromomycin, 500 mg orally given three times a day for 7 days, may be an acceptable substitute for iodoquinol. Asymptomatic carriers can be treated with paromomycin, 500 mg orally three times a day for 7 days, or iodoquinol, 650 mg orally three times a day for 20 days. An alternative to this regimen is dilanoxide furoate, 500 mg orally three times a day for 10 days.
- V. **Colorectal disease**
    - A. **Signs.** Left lower quadrant pain, suprapubic discomfort, rectal urgency, frequent small volume stools, proctalgia, and painful defecation are signs of colonic irritation or infection. The work-up parallels that of a patient with small bowel disease and includes stool for culture and examination for ova and parasites. In addition, stool for *Clostridium difficile* assay may be indicated for patients at risk for antibiotic-associated colitis. Patients with symptoms of proctitis should have a flexible sigmoidoscopy performed. Causes of proctitis in AIDS patients include CMV, HSV-1 and HSV-2, chlamydia, *N. gonorrhoeae*, syphilis, human papillomaviruses, and the enteric pathogens (see above).

- **B. Bacterial colonic infections.** Dosages and length of treatment are similar to the patients with small bowel disease.
- **C. The value of treatment of CMV** proctitis has not been established. Ganciclovir, 5 mg/kg given intravenously twice daily for 14 days, has resulted in clinical improvement (but with a high incidence of relapse). Foscarnet, 200 mg/kg intravenously daily for 21 days, is another alternative.
- **D. HSV proctitis** can be treated with acyclovir, 5 mg/kg intravenously every 8 hours for 7 days or 200 mg orally five times a day for 10 days, followed by 400 mg orally twice a day indefinitely. High-grade resistance to acyclovir has been reported with HSV in AIDS patients. These patients may respond to foscarnet, 40 mg/kg intravenously every 8 hours for 21 days, then 40 mg/kg every day indefinitely.

Hematologic Complications

Direct suppressive effects of HIV infection, ineffective hematopoiesis, infiltrative disease of the bone marrow, nutritional deficiencies, peripheral consumption, and drug effects can all contribute to the hematologic complications in the HIV-infected patient. Production of cytokines (colony stimulating factors and interleukin-α) is impaired in the HIV-infected patient, resulting in a suppressed bone marrow and ineffective hematopoiesis.

I. Anemia

- **A. Anemia is the most common hematologic abnormality** in patients with HIV disease. The approach to the diagnosis and management of anemia in the HIV-infected patient is based on the morphology of the peripheral blood smear.
- **B. Microcytosis.** Microcytosis is usually due to iron deficiency secondary to chronic blood loss from the GI tract. HIV-specific causes include KS, lymphoma, or infectious enteropathy.
- **C. Macrocytosis**
  1. **Hemolysis** with reticulocytosis secondary to autoimmunity, thrombotic thrombocytopenic purpura (TTP), hemolytic syndrome, disseminated intravascular coagulation, or drug reactions (most commonly sulfonamides) are the leading causes.
  2. **Vitamin B$_{12}$ or folate deficiency** may be encountered in patients with malabsorption as a result of severe enteropathy.
- **D. Normocytic**
  1. **If the hemoglobin level is >10 gm/dl** and the patient has no constitutional complaints or symptoms, the likely cause is anemia of chronic disease.
  2. **If the hemoglobin level is <10 gm/dl** and the patient has constitutional symptoms, bone marrow infiltration with infection or tumor is possible.
     a. **The most common infectious causes** are acid-fast bacilli and disseminated fungal disease.
     b. **Neoplastic causes include lymphomas.** The bone marrow is involved in up to one third of AIDS-related lymphomas. Kaposi's sarcoma is rarely found in the bone marrow.
- **E. Treatment.** If the patient is receiving AZT therapy, an erythropoietin level is advisable. If the level is less than 500 MU/dl, recombinant human erythropoietin therapy should be considered. The initial dose is 100 µg/kg/day ad-

ministered subcutaneously or intravenously three times a week. Pretreatment reticulocyte counts and ferritin levels should be obtained. The reticulocyte count should be used to monitor response to therapy. Patients may require iron supplementation if the reticulocyte count and ferritin level decrease.

II. **Granulocytopenia.** Granulocytopenia can be divided into two categories: (1) **drug induced**, and (2) **non–drug induced**.

   A. **Non-drug-induced** granulocytopenia is most frequently due to ineffective granulopoiesis. Other causes include direct destruction of lymphocytes by HIV and autoimmune disorders.

   B. **Granulocyte-macrophage colony-stimulating factor** (GM-CSF) has recently become available. Indications for GM-CSF include patients who are unable to sustain an absolute neutrophil count >500/mm^3. The initial dosage is 5 μg/kg/day subcutaneously for 1 week. In nonresponders, the dosage should be increased by 2.5 μg/kg weekly until 10 μg/kg is reached. If no response is noted at 10 μg/kg/day, GM-CSF should be discontinued.

III. **Thrombocytopenia**

   A. **HIV-related thrombocytopenia**

   1. **The most common platelet abnormality** in HIV-infected patients is HIV-related immune thrombocytopenia. Usually the clinical presentation is minor bleeding (petechiae, ecchymosis, epistaxis); rarely will patients initially be seen with GI bleeding. Laboratory examination reveals isolated thrombocytopenia (not accompanied by anemia or leukopenia). Peripheral smear shows rare large-form platelets, and the bone marrow will have an increased number of megakaryocytes.

   2. **The pathophysiology** is the presence of circulating immune complexes that precipitate on the platelet surface. These platelets are removed by the reticuloendothelial system (primarily the spleen). As the patient's disease process progresses, the circulating immune complexes and hypergammaglobulinemia block the spleen's ability to remove the platelets from the circulation and the platelet count rises.

   3. **Management** is similar to that used in the patient without HIV infection. In drug-induced thrombocytopenia, the medication causing the thrombocytopenia should be discontinued. Platelet transfusions should be administered when indicated. In general, HIV-infected patients with idiopathic thrombocytopenic purpura (ITP) are asymptomatic and healthy, and only close monitoring is required. Steroid therapy has been used with variable results. Prednisone, 1 mg/kg/day, has resulted in improvement; however, the improvement is not sustained when the steroid is tapered. In small series, splenectomy has been promising. Zidovudine administration has resulted in an improvement of the platelet count in two clinical trials. The role of high-dose intravenous gamma globulin therapy (400 mg/kg/day × 5 days), danazol, plasmapheresis, and vincristine in HIV-related ITP is currently being investigated.

   B. **Thrombotic thrombocytopenic purpura.** A number of reports have documented TTP in HIV-infected patients. The clinical syndrome in TTP includes fever, renal abnormalities, purpura, neurologic abnormalities, microangiopathic hemolysis, and thrombocytopenia. The cause is unclear but thought to be the result of circulating immune complexes or immunoglobulin dysregulation. The mortality rate is high. Therapy consists of platelet transfusions, high-dose steroids, and plasmapheresis.

Ocular Infections

Opportunistic ocular infections are common and important complications of AIDS. These have been traditionally divided into adnexal, and anterior and posterior segment infections. Molluscum contagiosum and KS have been reported in the ocular adnexa.

I. **Infection of ocular surface and adnexa**
   A. **Anterior segment infections** include recurrent conjunctivitis and/or keratitis. These are usually caused by viral (HSV, HVZ), fungal *(Candida),* or bacterial pathogens that cause similar infections in immunocompetent patients.
   B. **Herpes varicella-zoster.** The most common anterior segment infection is due to HVZ. The presentation and treatment are similar to that in the immunocompetent patient. Oral acyclovir (800 mg five times a day) has been shown to reduce the severity and incidence of ocular involvement. Some clinicians are treating newly diagnosed zoster ophthalmicus with intravenous acyclovir to reduce the risk of dissemination.
   C. **A previously rare disorder is corneal microsporidiosis.** This disorder is being recognized with increasing frequency in patients with AIDS. The infection presents with chronically red and irritated eyes with a decrease in visual acuity. Little corneal inflammation is present. Treatment has met with limited success; one reported case has responded to debridement and itraconazole.
   D. **Corneal infections** in the HIV patient are generally more severe and associated with a higher incidence of corneal perforation. Most anterior segment infections require prolonged and specific therapy with topical and/or systemic agents.

II. **Infection of the posterior segment.** Posterior segment infections that involve the retina and choroid, and result in visual loss are the most feared opportunistic ocular infections. Common retinal infections include CMV retinitis, ocular toxoplasmosis, and HVZ retinitis.
   A. **CMV retinitis** is the most common cause of visual loss in patients with AIDS. CMV is a member of the Herpesviridae (HSV, HVZ, EBV) family of viruses.
      1. **In immunocompetent patients,** CMV infection is often asymptomatic or results in a nonspecific viral syndrome. Like other herpesviruses, CMV enters a latent phase after infection in immunocompetent patients. The seroprevalence of CMV antibodies may be as high as 50% to 80% in the general population.
      2. Active CMV infection will develop in **90% of AIDS patients** at some point during their illness.
      3. **Histology.** Active CMV infection is histologically characterized by the presence of intranuclear and intracytoplasmic inclusions.
   B. Epidemiology
      1. **CMV retinitis is a late manifestation of AIDS,** with a reported incidence of 25% in clinical series and 30% in autopsy series.
      2. **CMV retinitis is associated with severe immunosuppression** and CD4 counts <50/mm^3 in the AIDS patient.
   C. Pathogenesis
      1. **CMV retinitis is secondary to the hematogenous spread of virus** to the retina after reactivation of a previously latent CMV infection.
      2. **The virus is thought to gain access to retinal tissue** as a result of HIV-mediated immune complex injury to retinal vessels. Direct retinal injury, optic nerve damage, or macular edema results in visual loss.

3. **CMV retinitis is often associated with infection** in other organ systems including the bone marrow, esophagus, colon, liver, and adrenal glands.
- **D.** Clinical presentation
    1. **Symptoms** will depend on location of the retinitis. Common complaints include blurred vision, floaters, and decreased visual acuity or loss of vision. CMV retinitis is *not* associated with photophobia, ocular pain, or a red eye. Peripheral retinal lesions may be asymptomatic or present as visual field defects (scotoma).
    2. **Classic funduscopic appearance** is that of perivascular yellow-white retinal infiltrates associated with central necrosis and retinal hemorrhage (cottage cheese and ketchup appearance). Vascular sheathing and retinal edema are common, and there is little overlapping vitreous inflammation.
    3. **As retinal lesions enlarge,** central areas atrophy and the resulting thinned retina is at an increased risk for detachment.
    4. **CMV retinitis begins insidiously and is initially unilateral.** If untreated, systemic viremia will eventually result in bilateral disease.
- **E.** Diagnosis
    1. **The diagnosis of CMV retinitis is based on immune status and classic funduscopic appearance.** Pupillary dilation and indirect ophthalmoscopy can assist in the early diagnosis of peripheral lesions.
    2. **Differential diagnosis** includes ocular toxoplasmosis and HVZ retinitis. Retinal hemorrhages are unusual and vitreous inflammation is prominent in ocular toxoplasmosis. HVZ retinitis is rare and causes a more rapid destruction of the retina.
- **F.** Treatment
    1. **Ganciclovir** (5 mg/kg IV q12h × 14 to 21 days) **or foscarnet** (60 mg/kg IV q8h × 14 to 21 days) are equally effective in the treatment of CMV retinitis. Induction therapy is followed by lifelong "maintenance" therapy of ganciclovir (5 mg/kg daily or 6 mg/kg out of 7 days) or foscarnet (90 to 120 mg/kg daily).
    2. **Both ganciclovir and foscarnet inhibit replication** by interfering with viral DNA polymerase. Since both agents are virostatic, maintenance therapy is necessary to prevent relapse. Maintenance regimens include ganciclovir, 5 mg/kg intravenously 5 days a week, or foscarnet, 90 mg/kg daily (adjusted for renal function) indefinitely.
    3. **Toxicity** is common and often a limiting factor in treatment with either agent. Dose-dependent, severe, reversible neutropenia (<1000 cells/mm^3) is seen in 40% of patients treated with ganciclovir. Zidovudine increases the incidence of severe neutropenia, and the two agents should not be used concurrently in the same patient. The use of granulocyte colony-stimulating factor (G-CSF) may help limit the neutropenia in some patients. Other common side effects include headache, confusion, nausea, vomiting, and abnormal liver function tests.
    4. **Toxic effects of foscarnet** include renal failure, hypocalcemia, hypophosphatemia, and anemia.
    5. **Patients that cannot tolerate systemic therapy** with either agent may benefit from repeated intravitreal injections of ganciclovir.
- **G.** Prognosis. If untreated, CMV retinitis will progressively enlarge and destroy the entire retina.
    1. **Visual acuity may improve** as a result of treatment and resolution of macular edema.

2. **Despite maintenance therapy, CMV retinopathy will eventually reactivate in most cases.** Reactivation may reflect worsening immunosuppression or drug resistance. Late reactivations may respond to alternating or combined therapy with ganciclovir and foscarnet.

Pulmonary Infections: *Pneumocystis carinii*

Pneumocystis carinii pneumonia is the most common AIDS-defining diagnosis in the United States and Europe.

I. **Microbiology**
   A. **Ascomycetes.** Although initially classified as a trypanosome, recent research suggests that the organism is related to Ascomycetes (yeasts).
   B. **The organism cannot be cultured,** and antibiotic sensitivities cannot be performed.
   C. **The life cycle** consists of three stages: (1) cysts; (2) sporozoites; and (3) trophozoites.

II. **Epidemiology**
   A. *P. carinii* **is believed to be ubiquitous** in nature, and infection is thought to be common early in life (ages 2 to 3 years).
   B. **Cell-mediated immunity** is thought to be the primary host defense mechanism.

III. **Pathogenesis.** The disease is thought to be reactivation of a "dormant" infection. The lack of cell-mediated immunity leads to the proliferation of organisms within the alveolar space, with subsequent attachment to type I alveolar cells. Injury to these cells results in increased permeability of the alveolar-capillary barrier with exudation of fluid into the alveolar space. Surfactant production is reduced, and there is intrapulmonary shunting of blood with associated decreased lung compliance.

IV. **Clinical presentation**
   A. The most common presentation of PCP is fever, nonproductive cough, and progressive shortness of breath in a patient with a CD4 count less than 200/mm^3. Atypical or subtle presentations including extrapulmonary PCP may occur in patients who are on prophylaxis. Physical findings are generally unremarkable. Arterial blood gases usually reveal significant hypoxia (PaO$_2$ <70 mm Hg) in 80% of the cases. The chest radiographs most often show diffuse interstitial infiltration involving all portions of the lung. Atypical radiographic presentations include spontaneous pneumothorax or upper lobe infiltrates.
   B. **Diagnosis** can be made by examination of sputum or bronchoalveolar lavage (BAL). The sensitivity of induced sputum was 77% in one report with the sensitivity of BAL ranging from 85% to 97% in patients with no previous treatment or prophylaxis for PCP.

V. **Treatment**
   A. TMP/SMX remains the treatment of choice for PCP. The dosage of TMP is 15 to 20 mg/kg daily for 21 days (normal adult: two double-strength tablets four times a day). With parenteral administration, TMP/SMX should be mixed in 250 ml of dextrose and water and given over 30 to 60 minutes at 6-hour intervals. Significant side effects occur at this dosage; over 60% of patients in one series were not able to complete a full course of therapy. The

most common side effects include skin rashes, fever, leukopenia, thrombocytopenia, hepatitis, nausea, and vomiting.
   1. **In acutely ill patients** (PaO_2 <70 mm Hg while breathing room air), the addition of prednisone has decreased the incidence of respiratory failure and death (*N Eng J Med* 323:1451, 1990). Prednisone dosage: 40 mg orally twice a day for 5 days, 40 mg daily for 5 days, and 20 mg daily for remainder of treatment (11 days). Give the first dose of prednisone 15 to 30 minutes before TMP/SMX, pentamidine, or clindamycin.
   2. **Measurement and concentration.** If possible, TMP or SMX concentration should be measured 90 to 120 minutes after administration of the oral or IV dose on day 2 or 3 of therapy. TMP concentration should range from 5 to 8 μg/ml and SMX concentration from 100 to 120 μg/ml.
   3. **Baseline laboratory tests.** Before initiation of therapy, the following baseline laboratory test results should be obtained: a complete blood cell count with differential, a platelet count, and liver, renal, and electrolyte chemistries.
   4. **Adverse reactions** requiring a change in therapy include a significant dermal reaction, neutropenia (<750 polymorphonuclear neutrophils (PMNs)/mm^3), thrombocytopenia (<40,000/mm^3), a serum creatinine level >3 mg/dl, and an increased serum alanine aminotransferase (ALT) level > five times the normal concentration.
B. **Dapsone/TMP** is equally efficacious as TMP/SMX in mild to moderate cases of PCP; it is an acceptable alternative in patients with significant side effects from TMP/SMX (*N Eng J Med* 323:776, 1990). The dosage regimen is dapsone, 100 mg/day, plus oral TMP, 20 mg/kg/day divided every 6 hours for 21 days.
C. **Pentamidine isethionate** (4 mg/kg/day IV × 21 days) is indicated in the acutely ill patient with PCP who cannot tolerate sulfonamides. This medication is only available in a parenteral form. The drug should be dissolved in 250 ml of 5% dextrose and water, and administered at a constant infusion rate over 1 hour. The most frequent adverse effect is neutropenia (<1000 PMNs/mm^3). Other adverse effects include abnormal liver and renal function, hyponatremia, hypoglycemia, pancreatitis, and a prolonged QT interval with torsades. The role of aerosolized pentamidine in the treatment of mild-to-moderate PCP remains undefined.
D. **Clindamycin,** 900 mg orally every 6 hours, plus **primaquine,** 30 mg base orally daily for 21 days, have been reported to be effective in patients with mild-to-moderate disease (*Clin Infect Dis* 14:183, 1992).
E. **Atovaquone** (750 mg PO TID × 21 days) is also reported to be efficacious in the treatment of PCP but with a higher failure rate than TMP/SMX. Lower toxicity is noticed with atovaquone compared with TMP/SMX.
F. **Lifelong maintenance therapy** will be required in all cases to prevent relapse. Treatment options and dosing are identical to the regimens used in primary preventive therapy (see below).

VI. Prevention
A. **Recommended prophylaxis.** TMP/SMX, one double-strength tablet daily or three times a week, is recommended for prophylaxis of PCP in patients with CD4 counts less than 200/mm^3. In one study, the mean survival time of patients given prophylactic TMP/SMX was 20 months compared with 11 months in control subjects.

B. Acceptable alternatives are dapsone, 100 mg orally daily (or 100 mg twice a week), or aerosolized pentamidine isethionate, 300 mg in 6 ml sterile water every 4 weeks. Two controlled studies have shown that TMP/SMX is a more effective regimen in preventing PCP than aerosolized pentamidine.
  1. **Pretreatment with a bronchodilator** is often needed with aerosolized pentamidine.
  2. Before beginning aerosolized pentamidine, tuberculosis (TB) should be ruled out with a chest x-ray and three sputum specimens examined for acid-fast bacilli (AFB).

Pulmonary Infections: Mycobacterial Disease

The presence of HIV infection has been identified as one of the most important risk factors for progression of latent *M. tuberculosis* infection to active TB in the United States. In contrast to historical data that suggest that 10% of persons infected with TB will progress to active TB, as many as 50% of persons infected with HIV and TB will develop active TB. Studies have also shown that TB preceded the diagnosis of AIDS in one half of patients and occurred concurrently or after the diagnosis of AIDS in the other half.

I. **The majority of TB in AIDS patients is thought to be secondary to reactivation TB.** The clinical presentation of TB is varied in patients with HIV. In patients with a relatively intact immune function (CD4 count > 500/mm^3), the clinical presentation is classic reactivation TB. In patients with AIDS, the clinical presentation resembles progressive primary TB. In patients with AIDS, the reported frequency of extrapulmonary TB ranges from 40% to 89% and increases with the severity of immunosuppression and extent of diagnostic evaluation. Disseminated disease and lymphadenitis are the most common forms of extrapulmonary TB. Cervical, supraclavicular, and axillary lymph nodes are the most common sites of peripheral TB lymphadenitis. The prevalence of bacteremia caused by *M. tuberculosis* has been reported to be as high as 26% to 42%. Central nervous system TB occurs in 5% to 10% of HIV-infected patients. Most have meningitis, but tuberculomas are also common. Pleural and pericardial disease are commonly recognized forms of extrapulmonary TB in HIV-infected African patients. Tuberculosis of the skin and soft tissues may occur in patients with *M. tuberculosis* bacteremia.

II. **The most frequent radiographic manifestations** of pulmonary TB in patients with AIDS are (1) hilar or mediastinal adenopathy (or both), (2) middle or lower lobe infiltrates, and (3) pleural effusions. Pulmonary cavitation is rarely seen. The classic radiographic picture of apical infiltrates in the absence of hilar or mediastinal adenopathy has been reported in less than 10% of AIDS-associated cases and occurs predominately in patients with relatively intact immune function (CD4 counts >500/mm^3).

III. **Diagnosis**
  A. PPD (tuberculin skin test—TST)
   1. **Patients with an earlier stage of HIV disease** and TB are more likely to have a positive PPD. Among these patients, 40% to 60% have TST reactions ≥10 mm.
   2. **In patients with AIDS,** anergy is frequent, with only 10% to 30% of patients reporting a positive PPD. Because of this increasing anergy, any patient with TST induration ≥5 mm should be considered to have presumptive evidence of TB infection.

3. **To improve the diagnosis of latent TB,** HIV-infected patients should undergo TSTs as early as possible in the course of their disease.
- B. **Culture and rapid diagnosis.** The diagnosis of TB in patients who are anergic depends on the recovery of *M. tuberculosis* from clinical specimens. Tuberculosis should be considered in any patient with unexplained fever, cough, pulmonary infiltrates, lymphadenopathy, meningitis, brain abscess, pericarditis, pleural effusions, or abscess formation. Appropriate specimens to culture include sputum, urine, blood, lymph node material, bone marrow, and liver tissue. Sputum specimens grow *M. tuberculosis* in 74% to 95% of HIV-infected patients. The sensitivity of the sputum examination is estimated to be between 40% and 67%. This is true even in patients with minimal radiographic changes.

IV. **Treatment.** The response rate of AIDS patients to antituberculosis treatment is generally as favorable as in non-AIDS patients, despite the fact that TB is more rapidly progressive and disseminated in patients with AIDS. Since it is difficult to distinguish tuberculosis from disseminated *M. avium* complex infection, anti-TB therapy should continue until culture results become final. Relapse after a proper course of therapy is uncommon.
- A. Drug-sensitive or unknown TB
    1. **The recommended initial regimen** for adults consists of four drugs daily.
        a. **Isoniazid (INH),** 300 mg/day.
        b. **Rifampin,** 600 mg/day (10 mg/kg/day or 450 mg/day in patients <50 kg).
        c. **Pyrazinamide (PZA),** 15 to 25 mg/kg/day (usually 2.0 gm) for the first 2 months.
        d. **Ethambutol,** 15 to 25 mg/kg/day orally (maximum daily dose 2.5 gm), or streptomycin, 15 mg/kg/day (maximum daily dose 1 gm) for first 2 months.
        e. **Isoniazid and rifampin** should be continued for either (whichever regimen is longer) a minimum of 9 months or at least 6 months after culture conversion (sputum culture is negative). After 2 months, the twice weekly regimen of INH, 900 mg, and rifampin, 600 mg, is efficacious. If INH or rifampin is not used in the regimen, the treatment should be continued for 18 months, or 12 months after sputum conversion.
    2. **Other regimens.** In areas where surveillance for drug-resistant TB has been carefully monitored and drug resistance rates <4% have been documented, three drugs (INH, rifampin, and PZA alone) may be used for initial therapy.
- B. Resistance of TB to INH and rifampin likely
    1. **Initial drug regimen.** If the possibility of resistance to both INH and rifampin is suspected, the initial drug regimen should include INH, rifampin, PZA and at least three drugs to which the local multidrug-resistant (MDR) TB organisms are susceptible. Improper use of drugs (selection of only one or two drugs that the strain is susceptible) for the treatment of MDR TB may result in the development of resistance. The selection and management of these cases should ideally be performed in conjunction with physicians experienced in treating MDR TB.
    2. **Multidrug-resistant (resistant to INH, rifampin, streptomycin, ethambutol, or PZA) TB**

a. **Satisfactory combinations have not been defined.** Most investigators recommend at least one injectable agent. One combination is ciprofloxacin, 750 mg twice a day; amikacin, 7.5 mg/kg intramuscularly every 12 hours; ethambutol, 15 mg/kg/day; and PZA, 15 to 25 mg/kg/day.
b. **Consider using rifabutin** as an alternative to rifampin if rifampin resistance is present (approximately 30% of rifampin-resistant organisms are sensitive to rifabutin).

V. **Prevention.** Antituberculous prophylactic therapy is effective in the HIV-infected population. The CDC recommends that all asymptomatic HIV-infected patients be administered a skin test (5 TU), and all symptomatic patients be given both a skin test and a screening chest x-ray examination. Any HIV-infected patients, whatever their age, with a tuberculin reaction ≥5 mm or a history of a positive skin test should receive preventive INH therapy (5 mg/kg/day, maximum dose 300 mg/day) for a minimum of 12 months. Some investigators recommend preventative therapy for any HIV-infected patients with anergy (negative TST and control skin test) if they belong to a group with a ≥10% prevalence of *M. tuberculosis* infection, or if they are a known contact of an infectious TB patient. Recent data suggest that 6 months of preventative therapy may also be effective. Sputum cultures should be obtained before therapy. Simultaneous administration of pyridoxine, 25 mg/day orally (50 mg/day if on DDC), is recommended.

VI. **Drug interactions and pharmacokinetics.** Significant changes in drug interactions and pharmacokinetics may occur in patients on INH or rifampin, and the antifungal azoles (ketoconazole, fluconazole, intraconazole), resulting in subtherapeutic levels of rifampin and the azoles.

Pulmonary Infections: Disseminated *Mycobacterium avium* Complex (MAC) Infection

Disseminated MAC is the most common opportunistic bacterial infection encountered in patients with AIDS.

I. **Microbiology**
A. *Mycobacterium avium* and *M. intracellulare* are two closely related nontuberculous atypical mycobacteria that are commonly grouped together as MAC.
B. **MAC organisms are ubiquitous** in the environment, with high concentrations present in water, soil, and aerosol droplets.
C. MAC has low pathogenicity in normal hosts.

II. **Epidemiology**
A. **The reported incidence** of MAC infection is 15% to 40%. Actual incidence may be higher since autopsy series have demonstrated evidence of disseminated MAC in over 50% of HIV-related deaths.
B. **MAC infection is rare** as an AIDS-defining opportunistic infection. It is normally a late manifestation after the occurrence of other opportunistic infections.
C. **Incidence.** There is a 20% incidence of infection per year after an AIDS-defining illness. MAC infection is seen almost exclusively in patients with advanced HIV disease and CD4 counts <100/mm^3.

III. Pathogenesis
  A. **Colonization** of the gastrointestinal tract and/or respiratory tract precedes dissemination.
  B. **Defective macrophage function** in patients with AIDS results in disseminated infection.

IV. Clinical presentation
  A. Asymptomatic. Colonized patients (positive sputum, stool, or urine cultures) may be asymptomatic.
  B. Common systemic findings include fever, night sweats, malaise, and weight loss. Symptoms may precede diagnosis by several months. Physical findings include lymphadenopathy and hepatosplenomegaly.
  C. Gastrointestinal manifestations include chronic diarrhea and abdominal pain (colonic invasion by MAC), chronic malabsorption (small intestine invasion by MAC), and jaundice (extrahepatic biliary obstruction from periportal lymphadenopathy).
  D. Associated multiple opportunistic infections are common and may delay diagnosis.
  E. Common laboratory abnormalities include anemia, neutropenia, and an elevated serum alkaline phosphatase level.

V. Diagnosis
  A. A **single positive blood culture** or positive culture from normally sterile sites (e.g., liver, bone marrow, or lymph node biopsy) is diagnostic for disseminated MAC.
   1. **The sensitivity** of the blood culture in diagnosing invasive MAC disease in a patient with AIDS approaches 100%.
   2. **The time for a culture to become positive** ranges from 5 to 51 days.
  B. The differential diagnosis of acid-fast bacilli on biopsy specimens includes *M. tuberculosis* and other atypical mycobacteria. In contrast to TB, the chest radiograph in MAC is frequently normal.

VI. Prognosis.
The mean survival after diagnosis is 3 to 4 months. In many patients it is difficult to separate the contribution of disseminated MAC infection from the effects of other opportunistic infections.

VII. Treatment.
Although once debated, recent therapeutic trials have correlated a reduction in MAC bacteremia with an improvement in systemic symptoms. No optimal treatment regimen has been identified. Therapy should include at least **two antimicrobial agents**.
  A. Suggested therapies include clarithromycin, 500 or 1000 mg orally twice a day, or azithromycin, 500 or 1000 mg orally daily, **plus** ethambutol, 15 to 25 mg/kg orally daily, or clofazimine, 100 to 200 mg orally daily. Ciprofloxacin, 750 mg orally daily, rifampin, 600 mg orally daily, rifabutin, 300 mg orally daily, or amikacin may be added as third and fourth agents.
  B. **Isoniazid and pyrazinamide have no role** in the treatment of disseminated MAC.

VIII. Prevention.
Prevention is important since disseminated MAC is common and appears to increase morbidity. Prevention is currently recommended in patients with CD4 counts <100/mm^3.
  A. **The recommended regimen is rifabutin, 300 mg orally daily.** Active infection with MAC should be ruled out (blood cultures and a chest radiograph) before initiating prophylaxis since rifabutin monotherapy is ineffective in an established infection.

B. **Rifabutin is generally well tolerated. Adverse effects** include uveitis, neutropenia, thrombocytopenia, rash, and gastrointestinal disturbances.

Renal Disorders

I. **Electrolyte and acid-base disorders**
   A. **Hyponatremia** has been observed in 36% to 56% of patients hospitalized with AIDS. The most frequent cause is gastrointestinal fluid loss. Other causes include renal salt wasting from tubulointerstitial disease or hormonal imbalances (hyporeninemic hypoaldosteronism, adrenal gland insufficiency, SIADH). Determination of urine and serum sodium concentration and osmolarity may clarify the cause of the hyponatremia. Hypernatremia in the HIV-infected patient is usually the result of drug-induced nephrogenic diabetic insipidus. The drugs most frequently implicated are amphotericin B and foscarnet.
   B. **Hypokalemia** occurs in up to 17% of hospitalized AIDS patients. Causes include gastrointestinal losses secondary to diarrhea and/or prolonged vomiting, and renal losses secondary to drug-induced tubular acidosis (amphotericin B, rifampin, cotrimoxazole). Hyperkalemia may be present in 16% to 24% of patients. Intrinsic renal nephropathy and insufficiency are the most common causes. Other causes are hypoaldosteronism, adrenal insufficiency, or pentamidine toxicity.
   C. **Hypocalcemia** is uncommon. The most frequent cause is hypomagnesemia due to renal losses of magnesium (pentamidine, amphotericin B) or drug-induced pancreatitis (pentamidine, DDI, foscarnet). Hypercalcemia is usually seen in granulomatous disorders, disseminated CMV infection, lymphoma, or with foscarnet administration.
   D. **Lactic acidosis** is expected with terminal AIDS and tissue hypoxia.

II. **Acute renal failure.** AIDS patients are at high risk of suffering renal complications including acute renal failure (ARF). ARF is seen in settings of sepsis, dehydration, hypoxia, and with administration of nephrotoxic drugs. Amphotericin B, pentamidine, TMP/SMX, foscarnet, aminoglycosides, and contrast agents have all been associated with nephrotoxicity. The approach and treatment of acute tubular necrosis (ATN) is similar to that in other clinical settings.

III. **Chronic glomerulopathies**
   A. **HVAN.** All types of glomerular lesions have been reported in HIV-seropositive patients. Investigators have described HIV-specific nephropathy (HVAN) presenting in HIV-infected patients with proteinuria and azotemia. Renal histology revealed focal and segmental glomerulosclerosis (FSGS) with intraglomerular deposition of IgM and C3. The role and interaction of HIV and heroin nephropathy with FSGS has not yet been elucidated.
   B. **Presentation.** The patients usually present with nephrotic syndrome or renal insufficiency. In contrast to other nephrotic syndromes, patients with AIDS frequently have minimal edema and a normal blood pressure. Dehydration and the high incidence of chronic diarrhea with intravascular volume depletion are the most common explanations for these findings. Findings supporting the diagnosis include large kidneys on ultrasound examination and severe proteinuria. Definitive diagnosis requires renal biopsy, although many physicians are diagnosing this condition clinically. The clinical course of AIDS

nephropathy is rapid progression to end-stage renal disease over weeks to months. Zidovudine in dosages of 300 to 800 mg/day has resulted in temporary remission of proteinuria and/or delayed occurrence of renal failure in anecdotal cases.

IV. **Diffuse glomerular mesangial hyperplasia.** Diffuse and global mesangial hyperplasia is identified histologically in approximately 25% of children with perinatal AIDS and nephrotic proteinuria, and in 13% of adults. The characteristics of HVAN are absent in these patients. These patients present with severe proteinuria with little or no decrease in renal function. Response to steroids is poor.

Suggested Readings

HIV and AIDS

Hirsch MS, D'Aquila RT: Therapy for human immunodeficiency virus infection, *N Engl J Med* 328(23):1686-95, 1993.

Niu MT, Stein DS, Schnittman SM: Primary human immunodeficiency virus type 1 infection: review of pathogenesis and early treatment intervention in humans and animal retrovirus infections, *J Infect Dis* 168(6):1490-501, 1993.

Pantaleo G, Graziosi C, Fauci AS: New concepts in the immunopathogenesis of human immunodeficiency virus infection, *N Engl J Med* 328(5):327-35, 1993.

Sande MA et al and the National Institute of Allergy and Infectious Diseases State-of-the-Art Panel on Anti-Retroviral Therapy for Adult HIV-Infected Patients: Antiretroviral therapy for adult HIV-infected patients. Recommendations from a state-of-the-art conference, *JAMA* 270(21):2583-9, 1993.

Sande MA, Volberding PA: *The medical management of AIDS,* ed 3, Philadelphia, 1992, WB Saunders.

Sperling RS, Stratton P, and the Obstetric-Gynecologic Working Group of the AIDS Clinical Trials Group of the National Institute of Allergy and Infectious Diseases: Treatment options for human immunodeficiency virus–infected pregnant women, *Obstet Gynecol* 79(3):443-8, 1992.

Talan DA, Kennedy CA: The management of HIV-related illness in the emergency department, *Ann Emerg Med* 20(12):1355-65, 1991.

Cardiac Complications

Acierno L: Cardiac complications in acquired immunodeficiency syndrome (AIDS): a review, *J Am Coll Cardiol* 13(5):1144-54, 1989.

Kaul S, Fishbein MC, Siegel RJ: Cardiac manifestations of acquired immune deficiency syndrome: a 1991 update, *Am Heart J* 122(2):535-44, 1991.

Central Nervous System Disorders

Porter SB, Sande MA: Toxoplasmosis in the central nervous system in the acquired immunodeficiency syndrome, *N Engl J Med* 327(23):1643-8, 1992.

Powderly WG: Cryptococcal meningitis and AIDS, *Clin Infect Dis* 837-42, 1993.

Dermatologic Manifestations

Dover JS, Johnson RA: Cutaneous manifestations of human immunodeficiency virus infection. Part I, *Arch Dermatol* 127(9):1383-91, 1991.

Dover JS, Johnson RA: Cutaneous manifestations of human immunodeficiency virus infection. Part II, *Arch Dermatol* 127(10):1549-58, 1991.

Zalla MJ, Su WP, Fransway AF: Dermatologic manifestations of human immunodeficiency virus infection, *Mayo Clin Proc* 67(11):1089-108, 1992.

Endocrine Disorders
Grinspoon SK, Bilezikian JP: HIV disease and the endocrine system, *N Engl J Med* 327(19):1360-5, 1992.

Gastrointestinal Complications
Bonacini M: Hepatobiliary complications in patients with human immunodeficiency virus infection, *Am J Med* 92(4):404-11, 1992.

Smith PD et al: NIH conference. Gastrointestinal infections in AIDS [see comments], *Ann Intern Med* 116(1):63-77, 1992.

Hematologic Complications
Groopman JE: Management of the hematologic complications of human immunodeficiency syndrome, *Rev Infect Dis* 12:931-7, 1990.

Scadden DT, Zon LI, Groopman JE: Pathophysiology and management of HIV-associated hematologic disorders, *Blood* 74:1455-63, 1989.

Ocular Infections
Bloom JN, Palestine AG: The diagnosis of cytomegalovirus retinitis, *Ann Intern Med* 109:963-9, 1988.

Holland GN: Acquired immunodeficiency syndrome and ophthalmology: the first decade, *Am J Ophthalmol* 114(1):86-95, 1992.

Pulmonary Infections: Pneumocystis
Bozette SA et al: A controlled trial of early adjunctive treatment with corticosteroids for *Pneumocystis carinii* pneumonia in the acquired immunodeficiency syndrome, *N Engl J Med* 323:1451, 1990.

Gagnon S et al: Corticosteroids as adjunctive therapy for severe *Pneumocystis carinii* pneumonia in the acquired immunodeficiency syndrome, *N Engl J Med* 323:1444, 1990.

Hardy WD et al: A controlled trial of trimethoprim-sulfamethoxazole or aerosolized pentamidine for secondary prophylaxis of *Pneumocystis carinii* pneumonia in patients with the acquired immunodeficiency syndrome. AIDS Clinical Trials Group Protocol 021, *N Engl J Med* 327(26):1842-8, 1992.

Masur H: Prevention and treatment of pneumocystis pneumonia, *N Engl J Med* 327(26):1853-60,

Pulmonary Infections: Tuberculosis
Barnes PF et al: Tuberculosis in patients with human immunodeficiency virus infection, *N Engl J Med* 324:1644-50, 1991.

Ellner JJ et al: Tuberculosis symposium: emerging problems and promise, *J Infect Dis* 168(3):537-51, 1993.

Hawkins CC et al: *Mycobacterium avium* complex infections in patients with the acquired immunodeficiency syndrome, *Ann Intern Med* 105(2):184-8, 1986.

Masur H, the Public Health Service Task Force on Prophylaxis and Therapy for *Mycobacterium avium* Complex: Recommendations on prophylaxis and therapy for disseminated *Mycobacterium avium* complex disease in patients infected with the human immunodeficiency virus, *N Engl J Med* 328:898-904, 1993.

Renal Disorders
Bourgoigine J, Meneses R, Pardo V: The nephropathy related to the acquired immune deficiency syndrome, *Adv Nephrol* 17:113-26, 1988.

18
Empiric Antibiotic Selection for Infectious Disease Emergencies in the Pediatric Age Group

Norman Christopher, M.D., F.A.A.P.

Variables

Appropriate emergency department management of a child who has an acute infectious process requires consideration of several important variables. Foremost among these is the determination of the child's general state of toxicity, extrapolated by carefully observing and examining the child, taking a careful history, and performing appropriate laboratory studies. Host-specific risk factors (see below) will further aid in the decision to initiate empiric antimicrobial therapy and, when indicated, will guide the choice of agents.

I. **Age** (clinical evaluation is particularly difficult in the newborn or young infant, complicating the assessment for disease presence and severity, even for the experienced practitioner).

II. **Perinatal risk factors** (i.e., active maternal infection or colonization at time of delivery with organisms such as herpesvirus, group B streptococcus, *Listeria monocytogenes,* and hepatitis B virus; prolonged rupture of amniotic membranes; and low Apgar scores).

III. **Prior infectious exposures** (differentiating primary from subsequent exposure may help define expected disease course in some situations).

IV. **Host immunocompetence** (affected by coexisting disease processes such as sickle cell disease or other hemoglobinopathies; human immunodeficiency virus [HIV] infection; or long-term immunosuppressive therapy for malignancy, reactive airways disease, or other chronic inflammatory conditions).

V. **Day-care attendance** (increases general exposure risk to gastrointestinal pathogens such as *Salmonella* species, *Giardia lamblia,* and *Shigella* species; and increases exposure to upper respiratory tract colonization or infection by pathogens such as respiratory syncytial virus, *Bordetella pertussis,* adenovirus, *Neisseria meningitidis,* and *Haemophilus influenzae*).

VI. **Immunization status**.

VII. **Presence of indwelling devices,** recent surgery, or other implementation.

VIII. **Underlying anatomic features** that predispose to infection (e.g., cardiac septal or valvular abnormalities, congenital abnormalities of the respiratory tract).

IX. **Modification of local respiratory tract immune defenses** by active or passive exposure to environmental toxins (including tobacco smoke).

Agents

The choice of antimicrobial agents in the emergency department is empiric and should be guided by a knowledge of the most likely pathogens for each clinical scenario and modified by local microbial resistance patterns **(Table 18-1)**. Cost and likelihood of patient compliance (affected by palatability of the antimicrobial agent, by dosing intervals, and by frequency of associated adverse effects) should be considered when choosing among several appropriate agents. Empiric coverage may be broadened but should not be limited by evidence gathered through laboratory studies and by microscopic examination of clinical specimens (cerebrospinal fluid, urine, wound exudate). Similarly, rapid antigen assays for common pathogens (group A β-hemolytic streptococcus, group B streptococcus, *H. influenzae, N. meningitidis*) are useful diagnostic supplements for use in the initial management of febrile or otherwise toxic children, but lack the sensitivity and specificity to replace cultures. Furthermore, antigen determinations reveal no information about specific antimicrobial sensitivity.

Suggested Readings

Baraff LJ: Management of the febrile child: a survey of pediatric and emergency medicine residency directors, *Pediatr Infect Dis J* 10:795-800, 1991.

Baraff LJ et al: Practice guideline for the management of infants and children 0 to 36 months of age with fever without source, *Ann Emerg Med* 22:1198-210, 1993.

Berman S et al: Acute respiratory infections during the first three months of life: clinical, radiologic, and physiologic predictors of, *Pediatr Emerg Care* 6:179-82, 1990.

Bonadio WA et al: Correlating infectious outcome with clinical parameters of 1130 consecutive febrile infants aged zero to eight weeks, *Pediatr Emerg Care* 9:84-6, 1993.

Committee on Infectious Diseases, American Academy of Pediatrics: *Report of the committee on infectious diseases,* ed 22, Elk Grove Village, Ill, 1991, American Academy of Pediatrics.

Dorfman DH, Craom EF, Bernstein LJ: Care of febrile children with HIV infection in the emergency department, *Pediatr Emerg Care* 6:305-10, 1990.

Downs SM, McNutt RA, Nargolis PA: Management of infants at risk for occult bacteremia: a decision analysis, *J Pediatr* 118:11-20, 1991.

Kravis E, Fleisher G, Ludwig S: Fever in children with sickle cell hemoglobinopathies, *Am J Dis Child* 136:1075-8, 1982.

Klassen TP, Rose PC: Selecting diagnostic tests to identify febrile infants less than 3 months of age as being at low risk for serious bacterial infection: a scientific overview, *J Pediatr* 121:671-6, 1992.

Krober MS et al: Bacterial and viral pathogens causing fever in infants less than 3 months old, *Am J Dis Child* 139:889-92, 1985.

Ledbetter EO: Antimicrobial therapy. In Hoekelman RA et al, editors: *Primary pediatric care,* St. Louis, 1987, Mosby–Year Book.

Lieu TA et al: Strategies for diagnosis and treatment of children at risk for occult bacteremia: clinical effectiveness and cost-effectiveness, *J Pediatr* 118:21-9, 1991.

McCarthy PL et al: Observation, history, and physical examination in diagnosis of serious illnesses in febrile children ≤24 months of age, *J Pediatr* 110:26-31, 1987.

Principi N et al: Occurrence of infections in children infected with human immunodeficiency virus, *Pediatr Infect Dis* J 10:190-3, 1991.

Rogers AR et al: Outpatient management of febrile illness in infants and young children with sickle cell anemia, *J Pediatr* 117:736-9, 1990.

Rosenberg NM et al: Sickle cell disease and fever, *Pediatr Emerg Care* 8:245-7, 1992.

Rothrock SG et al: Pediatric bacterial meningitis: is prior antibiotic therapy associated with an altered clinical presentation? *Ann Emerg Med* 21:146-52, 1992.

Talan DA, Zibulewsky J: Relationship of clinical presentation to time to antibiotics for the emergency department management of suspected bacterial meningitis, *Ann Emerg Med* 22:1733-8, 1993.

Williams JA et al: A randomized study of outpatient treatment with ceftriaxone for selected febrile children with sickle cell disease, *N Engl J Med* 329:472-6, 1993.

Table 18-1. Empiric Therapy for Infectious Disease Emergencies in the Pediatric Patient

Infectious disease	Antimicrobial and supportive therapy	Special considerations
Abscess, retropharyngeal and/or peritonsillar	Penicillin G 100,000-400,000 U/kg/day IV divided q4-6 hours (maximum 24 million U/day), or clindamycin 20-40 mg/kg/day IV divided q6-8 hours. Broad-spectrum cephalosporins (e.g., cefoxitin 80-160 mg/kg/d q4-6h) or β-lactamase inhibitor antibiotics (e.g., ticarcillin/clavulanate 200-300 mg/kg/d q4-6h) may be considered if either penicillin or clindamycin are not tolerated (cefuroxime 75-150 mg/kg/day IV divided q 8 hours × 10-14 days).	Consideration of airway patency and anticipation of impending obstruction is primary. Cellulitis and true abscess may be differentiated by plain radiography, sometimes supplemented by computed tomography or ultrasonography. Consideration for surgical drainage should be made when airway compromise is anticipated, or if the patient fails to improve after the administration of 24-48 hours of appropriate antibiotic therapy. Mild cases of peritonsillar abscess can be treated with needle aspiration and outpatient antibiotics.
Arthritis, suppurative	All patients should be admitted for parenteral therapy and possible surgical drainage. In the neonate, combination therapy with nafcillin (100-200 mg/kg/day IV divided q6 hours) and an aminoglycoside provide adequate initial coverage. (Cefotaxime may be used in place of the aminoglycoside if *Pseudomonas* infection is not a consideration.) In children older than 2 months, cefuroxime (100-150 mg/kg/day IV divided q8 hours) provides adequate coverage pending culture results. Single-agent therapy with nafcillin is adequate in children older than 10 years when disease due to *H. influenzae* is unlikely.	Definitive antimicrobial therapy must be guided by results of antibiotic sensitivity patterns of organisms isolated from the infected site. Gram stain results, while helpful in guiding therapy, should not *limit* initial therapeutic options.
Bacteremia	Empiric therapy of the nontoxic infant with presumed "occult bacteremia" with ceftriaxone (50-75 mg/kg IM single dose) pending culture results and next day fol-	Children with bacteremia due to *H. influenzae* or *N. meningitides* who remain febrile or ill should have a complete septic work-up and be admitted for parenter-

	low-up. Amoxicillin (60 mg/kg/day PO divided TID) may also be used, but is less effective at lowering risk of subsequent meningitis in children who later prove to have *H. influenzae* bacteremia. Successful vaccination programs against *H. influenzae* will change the epidemiology of occult bacteremia and may increase the utility of oral antimicrobial therapy when indicated.	al antimicrobial therapy. Some authorities feel that a child with *H. influenzae* bacteremia who is afebrile and well at follow-up can be treated with outpatient antimicrobial therapy with close follow-up. The well-appearing child with *S. pneumoniae* bacteremia may be treated as an outpatient without further laboratory evaluation pending results of follow-up blood cultures.
Bronchiolitis	Supportive care including oxygen administration, nebulized bronchodilator therapy, and maintenance of hydration are indicated in all children with bronchiolitis. If *Mycoplasma* infection is prevalent, erythromycin estolate (20-40 mg/kg/day PO divided QID × 10 days) should be administered. Aerosolized ribavirin therapy is indicated only in high-risk children with respiratory syncytial virus (RSV) infection (underlying heart disease or chronic lung disease with an oxygen requirement).	Oral bronchodilator therapy (albuterol 0.1 mg/kg/dose PO given TID-QID) should be initiated after discharge from the ED and continued until the child is reevaluated. Secondary bacterial infection may occur and, when present, will respond to standard antimicrobial therapy. Although inconsistently effective, corticosteroid therapy (prednisone 1-2 mg/kg/day PO × 5 days) is useful in some infants, making a therapeutic trial justifiable.
Buccal/periorbital cellulitis	*Preseptal/buccal cellulitis* may be treated empirically with ceftriaxone 100 mg/kg IV divided q12-24 hours, or cefuroxime 75-150 mg/kg/day IV divided q6-8 hours. If cellulitis is clearly related to a local infected wound or injury (and not related to bacteremic spread of *H. influenzae*), clindamycin (30-40 mg/kg/day IV divided q6 hours), nafcillin (150-200 mg/kg/day IV divided q4-6 hours), or a first- or second-generation cephalosporin may be used. *Orbital cellulitis* should be treated em-	Admission should be considered for all patients with facial cellulitis. Computed tomography should be considered if orbital involvement is suspected, and early surgical consultation should be sought if confirmed. Patients may be switched to oral antimicrobial therapy after defervescence and clinical improvement have occurred.

Continued on next page

Ch 18. Empiric Antibiotic Selection for the Pediatric Age Group

Table 18-1. Empiric Therapy for Infectious Disease Emergencies in the Pediatric Patient—cont'd

Infectious disease	Antimicrobial and supportive therapy	Special considerations
	pirically with nafcillin or vancomycin (40-60 mg/kg/day IV divided q6 hours), in combination with a third-generation cephalosporin (ceftriaxone 50-100 mg/kg/day IV given q12-24 hours, or cefotaxime 150-200 mg/kg/day IV divided q6-8 hours) or a β-lactamase inhibitor antibiotic (e.g., ticarcillin/clavulanate 200-300 mg/kg/d q4-6h).	
Chickenpox	Acyclovir (30 mg/kg/day IV divided q8 hours) is indicated in the immunocompromised host or in the toxic patient with widely disseminated disease. Localized varicella infection (pneumonia, meningitis) also require systemic antiviral therapy. Oral acyclovir (20 mg/kg/day divided q8 hours) may be indicated in the otherwise normal host who is at risk for severe disease after primary exposure (young infants, adolescents, and adults). To be effective, therapy must begin within 24 hours of the development of clinical disease. Although therapy may decrease the duration and magnitude of fever and lessen the number and duration of skin lesions, oral acyclovir should not be used indiscriminately for what is anticipated to be a routine disease course.	Salicylates should be avoided in children with varicella infection because of the increase in risk for development of Reyes syndrome. Varicella-Zoster Immune Globulin (VZIG) should be administered within 96 hours (for greatest effectiveness, within 48 hours) of exposure to all nonimmune persons at risk for severe and/or progressive disease. One vial (1.25 ml, 125 units) should be given for every 10 kg of body weight to a maximum of 5 vials. One vial is the minimum recommended dose. Immunocompromised patients and newborn infants whose mothers have had onset of varicella within 5 days before or 2 days after delivery should be treated with VZIG. An effective varicella vaccine has been developed but is not yet used routinely in otherwise normal or low-risk nonimmune patients.
Conjunctivitis (newborn)	*Neonatal chlamydial conjunctivitis* requires systemic therapy with oral erythromycin (either estolate or ethylsuccinate ester) 40 mg/kg/day divided QID for 14	Antibiotic therapy should be supplemented with frequent (q1-2 hour) ophthalmic irrigation with saline or other appropriate buffered solutions. The infant's

days. Topical therapy, when used alone, fails to eradicate systemic infection and nasopharyngeal colonization. Systemic erythromycin may be supplemented with topical therapy, but it is not required. Newer macrolide antibiotics have not been tested in infants and are not available in suspension. *Gonoccal conjunctivitis* requires parenteral therapy with ceftriaxone (50-75 mg/kg/day IV divided q12-24 hours × 7 days), or cefotaxime (25-50 mg/kg/day IV divided q8-12 hours × 7 days). Aqueous crystalline penicillin G (100,000 U/kg/day divided q6 hours × 7 days) may be used if sensitivity testing confirms its usefulness. Disease may be fulminant and ulcerations may develop early. Ophthalmologic consultation is urged. *Herpes simplex virus* may be localized to the conjunctiva or may simultaneously involve the skin and/or the central nervous system. Initial symptoms can occur shortly after birth or as late as 4-6 weeks postpartum. Disseminated disease usually occurs within the first 2 weeks of life. Corneal ulceration is common and may threaten vision. Systemic therapy (acyclovir 30 mg/kg/day IV divided q8 hours × 14 days) supplemented with topical vidarabine, 2% trifluridine, or 1% iododeoxyuridine is indicated. Ophthalmologic consultation is urged.

mother and partners should be treated if *Chlamydia*, herpes simplex, or *N. gonorrhoeae* are isolated. Gram stain may suggest the diagnosis of the latter and should be performed in all cases. Conjunctival scrapings should be obtained for *Chlamydia* culture; rapid antigen testing is available and approved for this indication but is less sensitive. Flourescein staining of the cornea should always be performed to evaluate for underlying ulceration or even perforation due to *N. gonorrhoeae* infection, as well as to identify typical dendritic ulceration secondary to herpes simplex infection.

| Croup (viral laryngotracheobronchitis) | Antimicrobial therapy is not indicated for routine presentations. Supportive care should include antipyretic therapy, ensuring adequate hydration, cool mist therapy, and oxygen administration when required. Racemic or L-epinephrine is indicated for severe croup | Foreign body aspiration and supra/epiglottitis must be considered and ruled out. A rapidly progressive course and a toxic appearance may suggest secondary bacterial infection, and should be managed as outlined for bacterial tracheitis. Corticosteroid therapy (dexametha- |

Continued on next page

Table 18-1. Empiric Therapy for Infectious Disease Emergencies in the Pediatric Patient—cont'd

Infectious disease	Antimicrobial and supportive therapy	Special considerations
		sone 0.6 mg/kg IM, given as a single dose) has proven beneficial when given to hospitalized patients and may be used as supplemental therapy for children discharged from the ED if close follow-up can be arranged.
Epiglottitis	Cefuroxime 75-150 mg/kg/day IV divided q8 hours, or ceftriaxone 50-100 mg/kg/day IV divided q12-24 hours, or cefotaxime 100-200 mg/kg/day IV divided q6-8 hours. The upper end of the dosage range should be used if meningitis is believed or shown to coexist.	Primary consideration is maintainence of airway patency. If the diagnosis is suspected, all interventions should be performed with surgical (airway) backup, preferably in the operating suite. All EDs should have in place a protocol for managing the child with suspected epiglotitits. Oral therapy with amoxicillin-clavulonate (40 mg/kg/day PO divided TID), or cefixime (8 mg/kg/day PO divided BID) may be used after observing clinical improvement on IV therapy. In cases due to *H. influenzae* type B, prophylaxis of household contacts is indicated (including the index case) if other children 4 years of age and younger live in the household (rifampin 20 mg/kg PO given once daily for 4 consecutive days, maximum dose 600 mg/day). Successful immunization programs against *H. influenzae* type B are changing the epidemiology of this disease.
Gastroenteritis (acute, of unknown etiology)	Acute therapy should be supportive and should focus on restoration and maintenance of adequate hydration. Mild or moderate dehydration may be safely and effectively corrected with oral rehydration therapy.	Most acute episodes of gastroenteritis in children have an infectious etiology and are accompanied by other related systemic signs. Lactose intolerance may develop even after a brief bout of infectious gastroenteritis,

	Evidence of inadequate organ perfusion is an indication for aggressive parenteral rehydration, but with continued oral supplementation. Vomiting alone is not a contraindication to oral rehydration. If addition of lactose-based formulas or of milk exacerbates diarrheal symptoms, they should be temporarily withheld. Early refeeding is desirable to prevent protein-calorie deprivation. Parenteral nutrition should be initiated if optimal nutrition is not attained in 5-7 days. Antidiarrheal preparations such as kaolin, pectin, paregoric, diphenoxylate, loperamide, and bismuth subsalicylate should not be prescribed. Empiric antibiotic therapy is unwarranted in the nontoxic infant with acute diarrhea. Stool cultures should be obtained in toxic-appearing infants or if there are public health concerns.	although most infants recover uneventfully. When indicated, empiric antimicrobial therapy should be initiated with trimethoprim-sulfamethoxazole (TMP-SMZ), with definitive therapy guided by local antimicrobial sensitivity patterns. When *Salmonella* species are isolated from a febrile patient at risk for disseminated disease (infants less than 6 months of age, patients with a known malignancy, patients with sickle cell hemoglobinopathy, or in an otherwise immunocompromised host), systemic therapy is indicated (TMP-SMZ or a third-generation cephalosporin).
Impetigo and pyoderma	Local cleansing and topical therapy have limited usefulness except for very localized infection. (Mupiricin applied TID for 5 days has shown to be particularly effective.) More extensive lesions require systemic antimicrobial therapy in conjunction with local care. Appropriate agents include erythromycin estolate (20-40 mg/kg/day divided TID-QID), or cephalexin (25-50 mg/kg/day divided q8-12 hours), or dicloxacillin (12.5-25 mg/kg/day divided q6 hours). Clindamycin (20-30 mg/kg/day divided q6 hours) is an acceptable alternative if other agents are poorly tolerated.	Acute poststreptococcal glomerulonephritis may follow skin infection with "nephritogenic" strains of streptococci.
Lymphadenitis, acute	When indicated, initial antimicrobial therapy should be directed against *S. aureus* and group A streptococci,	Cervical lymphadenopathy is extremely common in young children and frequently represents a response

Continued on next page

Table 18-1. Empiric Therapy for Infectious Disease Emergencies in the Pediatric Patient—cont'd

Infectious disease	Antimicrobial and supportive therapy	Special considerations
	and include dicloxacillin 12.5-25 mg/kg/day PO divided q6 hours, or cephalexin (or cephradine) 25-50 mg/kg/day PO divided q6-8 hours, or cefadroxil 30 mg/kg/day PO divided q6 hours. Clindamycin (20-30 mg/kg/day PO divided q6 hours) may be used in the patient allergic to penicillin.	to a nonspecific infection involving the upper respiratory tract. Systemic diseases associated with generalized involvement of the reticuloendothelial system should be considered, as should mycobacterial or other chronic infectious processes. Close follow-up is mandatory. Surgical drainage may be both therapeutic and diagnostic in certain situations and should be considered especially if there is no response to initial antibiotic therapy.
Mastoiditis, acute	Cefuroxime 75-100 mg/kg/day IV divided q8 hours, or nafcillin 100-200 mg/kg/day IV divided q4-6 hours. Ampicillin (150 mg/kg/day IV divided q4-6 hours) in combination with either an aminoglycoside or ceftazidime (100-150 mg/kg/day IV divided q8 hours) may be indicated for resistant cases.	Bacteriology is similar to that of acute otitis media. A trial of medical therapy is indicated prior to surgical drainage. Tympanocentesis of the ipsilateral infected middle ear may yield a specimen for culture and sensitivity testing. Patients with mastoid abscess will require partial or complete mastoidectomy.
Meningitis/Sepsis	*Newborn*—the usual pathogens include gram-negative enteric organisms, group B streptococcus, enterococcus, *L. monocytogenes*, and herpes simplex virus. Empiric therapy should include ampicillin 200-400 mg/kg/day IV divided q4-6 hours, and gentamicin (5 mg/kg/day IV divided q12 hours in the first week of life and 7.5 mg/kg/day IV divided q8 hours after the first week of life) or cefotaxime (100-200 mg/kg/day IV divided q12 hours in the first week of life and q8 hours thereafter). Acyclovir (30 mg/kg/day IV divided	Aggressive, supportive, and anticipatory therapy is indicated for all patients with meningitis. Antimicrobial therapy should be guided, but not limited, by preliminary results of the Gram stain of cerebrospinal fluid. Meningitis and sepsis often coexist in newborns and infants, and the clinical presentation of each may overlap the other. Ceftriaxone should be avoided in the newborn period because it may displace bilirubin bound to albumin.

	q8 hours) should be added if herpes simplex virus infection is suspected. *Infants 1-3 months old*—because of the broad variety of infectious pathogens in this age group, combination therapy with ampicillin and cefotaxime are indicated. (Cefotaxime alone is ineffective against *Listeria*, and ampicillin and an aminoglycoside together are ineffective against β-lactamase-producing *H. influenzae*). Third-generation cephalosporins provide adequate single-agent coverage in *older infants and children* (ceftriaxone 100 mg/kg/day IV divided q12-24 hours, or cefotaxime 200 mg/kg/day IV divided q6-8 hours).	Although still somewhat controversial, corticosteroid therapy (dexamethasone 0.15 mg/kg/dose IV q6 hours × 48-96 hours) should be administered before antibiotics to children >2 months of age with meningitis because postinfectious sequelae may be lessened (the greatest effect has been shown in children with *H. influenzae* infection).
Omphalitis	Ampicillin (100-200 mg/kg/day IV divided q4 hours) and gentamicin (5 mg/kg/day IV divided q12 hours in the first week of life and 7.5 mg/kg/day IV divided q8 hours thereafter) are appropriate empiric therapy for uncomplicated, community-acquired infection. Improved coverage against *Staphylococcus* species should be considered, such as with nafcillin (100-200 mg/kg/day IV divided q4-6h) or vancomycin (10 mg/kg/dose IV q8-18 hours, guided by serum levels), if there is inadequate response to initial antimicrobial therapy.	Coexisting bacteremia or sepsis should be assumed in the toxic infant with extensive disease. Abdominal wall cellulitis with fasciitis may require surgical debridement and aggressive supportive care. Omphalitis may be difficult to differentiate from uncomplicated umbilical granuloma, funisitis (inflammation of the umbilical stump without involvement of adjacent abdominal wall, patent urachus, and vitellointestinal fistula.
Osteomyelitis	Empiric therapy should be directed at *S. aureus*, the most likely pathogen. Nafcillin (100 mg/kg/day IV divided q6 hours) as a single agent is appropriate for empiric therapy for uncomplicated community-acquired	Early orthopedic referral should be obtained in all cases. Optimal therapy requires that the responsible pathogen be isolated and that antimicrobial sensitivity patterns be determined. Unlike suppurative arthritis,

Continued on next page

Table 18-1. Empiric Therapy for Infectious Disease Emergencies in the Pediatric Patient—cont'd

Infectious disease	Antimicrobial and supportive therapy	Special considerations
	infection. Vancomycin (10 mg/kg/dose IV divided q8 hours) should be administered if infection is hospital acquired and follows instrumentation or surgery. If gram-negative bacilli are present on Gram-stained specimens, an aminoglycoside should be added. *Salmonella* species and *Pseudomonas* species should be considered when osteomyelitis develops in a child with sickle cell disease or follows a puncture wound of the foot, respectively.	*H. influenzae* is not a common pathogen in the child with osteomyelitis.
Otitis Media	Initial therapy should be with amoxicillin 40 mg/kg/day PO divided TID × 10 days, or TMP-SMX 8-10 mg/kg/day (TMP component) PO divided BID × 10 days, or erythromycin ethylsuccinate and acetyl sulfisoxazole (Pediazole) 50 mg/kg/day PO (erythromycin component) divided q6h × 10 days. Intramuscular ceftriaxone may be useful in a child who will be treated as an outpatient but whose ability to tolerate PO antibiotics is temporarily limited.	Amoxicillin/clavulanate 40 mg/kg/day PO divided TID, cefixime (Suprax) 8 mg/kg/day PO in 1 or 2 doses, cefaclor (Ceclor) 40 mg/kg/day PO divided TID, or cefuroxime axetil (Ceftin) 40 mg/kg/day PO divided BID are acceptable alternatives in children who have failed first-line therapy or have recurrent/resistant disease. Tetracyclines, penicillin V or G, cephalexin, and erythromycin are not useful for therapy of acute otitis media. Cefuroxime axetil is not yet formulated in a suspension.
Pharyngitis, group A β-hemolytic streptococci	Benzathine penicillin G 1.2 million U IM (>60 lb) or 600,000 U IM (<60 lb). For oral therapy, penicillin VK 250 mg PO BID or TID <12 years of age) or 500 mg PO BID or TID (>12 years of age) may be given. Erythromycin estolate (20-40 mg/kg/day PO divided into 2-4 doses) or erythromycin ethylsuccinate (40-50	Other alternatives to penicillin or erythromycin may include a 10-day course of a first-generation cephalosporin (cephalexin or cephradine, each dosed at 25-50 mg/kg/day divided BID for children, and 500 mg BID for adolescents, or cefadroxil 30 mg/kg/day PO divided BID) or a second-generation cephalosporin

	(cefaclor or ceftin, 40 mg/kg/day PO divided TID). Because of its expanded spectrum, cefaclor is effective for use when middle ear infection coexists. TMP-SMX is inadequate treatment for streptococcal pharyngitis.
	mg/kg/day divided QID) are the best alternative for children with penicillin allergy. Ten days of therapy are required for all oral therapeutic regimens.
	Most authorities agree that, while the risk of postinfectious complications is small, symptomatic patients with either group C or group G streptococcal pharyngitis benefit from antimicrobial therapy.
Pharyngitis, non-group A β-hemolytic streptococci	Therapy is the same as for group A β-hemolytic streptococcal pharyngitis. See "comments."
Pneumonia, community acquired (presumed bacterial etiology)	Broad-spectrum empiric antimicrobial therapy should be directed toward the most likely age-dependent pathogens, with close follow-up arranged for all those treated as outpatients. In the acutely ill infant, broad-spectrum antibiotic therapy should be considered, as outlined in "Meningitis/Sepsis." If the infant is nontoxic, has no consolidation on CXR, has URI symptoms and wheezing, and presents during a local outbreak of similar illnesses, a viral pathogen is most likely, and therapy should commence as outlined under "Bronchiolitis." So-called "afebrile pneumonia," caused most often in young infants by *Chlamydia trachomatis*, *Ureaplasma urealyticum*, *Pneumocystis carinii*, and cytomegalovirus, should be treated with erythromycin after attempts are made to isolation of the suspected pathogen (nasopharyngeal swab for antigen testing and/or culture). Appropriate oral therapy for a child older than 3 months includes amoxicillin or amoxicillin/clavulanate (40 mg/kg/day PO divided	Pathogens are age-related. Viral pathogens are prevalent in all age groups, their presence suggested by local epidemiology and expected seasonal patterns of infection. In the immediate newborn period, the most commonly implicated agents include gram-negative enterics and group B streptococcus. In children between 2 weeks and 2 months of age, chlamydia, *S. pneumoniae*, *H. influenzae*, and *S. aureus* are the predominant bacterial etiologies. In older children, *S. pneumoniae*, *H. influenzae*, and *M. pneumoniae* are the dominant organisms causing pneumonia. RSV pneumonia should be considered in infants and young children in the winter and spring. Indications for admission include the presence of an oxygen requirement, respiratory compromise, lobar consolidation in a child less than 12 months of age, dehydration, and failure to improve or worsening after 24-48 hours of oral antimicrobial therapy.

Table 18-1. Empiric Therapy for Infectious Disease Emergencies in the Pediatric Patient—cont'd

Infectious disease	Antimicrobial and supportive therapy	Special considerations
	TID), or erythromycin/sulfisoxazole (50 mg/kg/day of erythromycin component PO divided TID-QID). Cefuroxime (150 mg/kg/day IV divided q8 hours) is appropriate therapy for children in this age group who require admission. In children older than 6-7 years, *M. pneumoniae*, *S. pneumoniae*, and viruses become the most frequently implicated pathogens, and the prevalence of disease caused by *H. influenzae* declines, making erythromycin or new macrolides appropriate choices for empiric antimicrobial therapy in this age group.	
Pyelonephritis	Newborn and younger infants are often toxic and bacteremic. Parenteral antibiotics are indicated and should include broad-spectrum coverage against the expected newborn pathogens. Ampicillin (200 mg/kg/day IV divided q4-6 hours), and gentamicin (2.5 mg/kg/dose IV given q12 hours in the first week of life, and q8 hours in older infants) or cefotaxime (100-200 mg/kg/day IV q8 hours) are appropriate empiric choices in this age group. For older children, single-agent therapy with a third-generation cephalosporin provides adequate coverage. Ampicillin and gentamicin are also appropriate in older children.	Because of the implications of the occurrence of pyelonephritis during infancy, careful documentation of infection by urine cultures obtained by catheterization must occur. Approximately 10-20% of infants with urinary tract infection will have a normal urinalysis, making microscopy and culture most important in this age group. Infants and young children with a first-time episode of pyelonephritis require radiographic evaluation to rule out the presence of underlying anatomic abnormalities of the genitourinary tract (most begin the evaluation with a voiding cystourethrogram followed by either an ultrasound or a nuclear imaging technique). The presence of vesicoureteral reflux

	Outpatient therapy in nontoxic, older children may be initiated with TMP-SMX (8 mg/kg/day of the TMP component PO divided BID) or a cephalosporin (e.g., cephalexin 50-100 mg/kg/d q6h or cefixime 8 mg/kg/d q24h). There is no urgency to begin therapy in the ED if the diagnosis is uncertain and the child otherwise appears well.	requires that prophylactic antibiotics be initiated and close follow-up ensured.
Sinusitis/Purulent Nasopharyngitis	Therapy is the same as for acute otitis media. Most authorities recommend at least 14 days of therapy. When parenteral therapy is indicated, cefuroxime (100 mg/kg/day IV divided q8 hours), or ceftriaxone (50-100 mg/kg/day IV divided q12-24 hours), or cefotaxime (100-200 mg/kg/day divided q6-8 hours) may be used, in conjunction with possible surgical drainage.	Parenteral antimicrobial therapy is indicated in the toxic-appearing child, in the presence of facial or periorbital cellulitis, or if there is evidence of intraorbital or intracranial extension of the infection. Surgical drainage is recommended in the immunocompromised host and in the presence of severe toxicity. Antihistamines, while often prescribed, have unknown value.
Tracheitis, presumed bacterial	Antimicrobial therapy as outlined for "Epiglottitis."	Primary consideration is maintenance of airway patency. Initially resembles viral laryngotracheobronchitis, but becomes progressive and severe with development of secondary bacterial infection.
Uvulitis	For uncomplicated disease, therapy is as outlined for group A β-hemolytic streptococcal (GABHS) pharyngitis. If the patient is febrile and toxic, treat as outlined for "Epiglottitis."	May coexist with supra/epiglottitis.

19

Empiric Antibiotic Selection for Infectious Disease Emergencies in the Elderly Patient

Gideon Bosker, M.D., F.A.C.E.P.

While bacterial infections in any age group are serious, in elderly patients they are more common and more frequently life threatening. In this regard, the most common cause of transfer from the nursing home to the short-stay, acute care hospital is infection which, in the frail elderly patient, may lead to what has been called the *geriatric cascade*. For example, a simple viral infection may lead to a bacterial pneumonia, which may cause death. The toxic delirium from even a mild infection may lead to a fall and a hip fracture, with the resulting immobility possibly leading to incontinence, pressure sores, or death.

Selection of Antibiotics

Given the wide range of organisms that infect elderly patients and the limited diagnostic database (i.e., lack of culture results) that is available in the ED, selection of an appropriate antibiotic can be extremely difficult. The enormous range and variety of antibiotics now available to the clinician can be confusing. As result, it is often times best to gain familiarity with the indications, spectrum, and side effects of the more commonly used, proven agents and learn how to use them well. When there is uncertainty regarding antibiotic selection, consultation with an infectious disease specialist is indicated.

Despite the broad spectrum of clinical infections encountered in the elderly patient, some sources of infection are more common than others. The most common sources of infection leading to septicemia are (1) the urinary tract; (2) the respiratory system; (3) gastrointestinal sources such as the biliary tree and gallbladder; (4) intraabdominal infection; (5) endocarditis; and (6) meningitis. Many of these infections will produce bacteremia, and in some cases, signs of sepsis will develop. Accordingly, in the emergency setting, rapid decisions must be made regarding antibiotic therapy, often without the benefit of culture material or even Gram stains of infected body fluids. In these cases, empiric antibiotic therapy must be initiated, based on the statistical likelihood of providing antimicrobial coverage against the most common offending organisms. A comprehensive guide to empiric antibiotic therapy in geriatric infectious disease emergencies is presented in **Table 19-1**. These recommendations for empiric therapy of common infections in the elderly take into account several modifying variables: clinical severity, the predominant organism(s) encountered in the specific infection, and the community or institutional microbiology.

Suggested Readings

American Thoracic Society, Medical Section of the American Lung Association: Treatment of community-acquired pneumonia. *Am Rev Respir Dis* 148:1418-26, 1993.

Bates, JH et al: Microbial etiology of acute pneumonia in hospitalized patients, *Chest* 101:1005-12, 1992.

Council of British Thoracic Society: The hospital management of community-acquired pneumonia, *J R Coll Physicians Lond* 21:267-9, 1987.

Fine MJ, Smith DN, Singer DE: Hospitalization decision in patients with community-acquired pneumonia: a prospective cohort study, *Am J Med* 89:713-21, 1990.

Woodhead MA et al: Aetiology and outcome of severe community-acquired pneumonia, *J Infect* 10:204-10, 1985.

Table 19-1. Empiric Therapy for Infectious Disease Emergencies in the Elderly Patient

Infectious disorder	Antibiotic regimen
Pneumonia	
Pneumonia (community acquired)	Cefuroxime, 1.5 mg IV q8h, **or** Ceftriaxone, 1-2 gm IV q12h, **plus** Erythromycin, 500-1000 mg IV or PO q6h, **or** Azithromycin, 500 mg PO day 1, followed by 250 mg PO × 4 days
Pneumonia (community-acquired, outpatient management, >60 years of age)	2nd-generation cephalosporin, 250-500 mg PO BID **plus** Erythromycin, 500-1000 mg IV or PO q6h
Pneumonia (community-acquired, outpatient management, otherwise healthy, <60 years of age)	Azithromycin, 500 mg PO day 1, followed by 250 mg PO BID × 4 days **or** Clarithromycin, 500 mg PO BID × 10 days
Pneumonia (with COPD)	Cefuroxime, 1.5 mg IV q8h, **plus** Azithromycin, 500 mg PO day 1, followed by 250 mg PO × 4 days
Pneumonia (frail, debilitated, underlying disease)	Cefuroxime, 1.5 mg IV q8h, **or** Ampicillin-sulbactam, 1.5-3 gm IV q6h, **plus** Erythromycin, 500-1000 mg IV or PO q6h
Pneumonia (nosocomial, hospital acquired)	Ceftriaxone, 1-2 gm IV q12h, **plus** Tobramycin, 80-100 mg IV q8h
Pneumonia (aspiration)	Ampicillin-sulbactam, 1.5-3.0 gm IV q6h, **or** Clindamycin, 600-900 mg IV q8h, **plus** Gentamicin, 100-120 mg (1.5-2 mg/kg) IV, followed by 80 mg IV q8h
Urinary Tract Infections	
Pyelonephritis	Ampicillin, 2 gm IV q4h, **plus** Gentamicin, 100-120 mg (1.5-2 mg/kg) IV, followed by 80 mg IV q8h **or** If gram-negative, Ceftriaxone, 1 gm IV q12h, **or** Ciprofloxacin, 250-500 mg PO BID
Lower urinary tract	Trimethoprim/Sulfamethoxazole, two double-strength tablets PO BID × 10 days, **or** Ciprofloxacin, 500 mg PO BID × 10 days (Note: quinolone is preferred in males with presumed prostatic source)

Selection of Antibiotics 527

Table 19-1. Empiric Therapy for Infectious Disease Emergencies in the Elderly Patient—cont'd

Infectious disorder	Antibiotic regimen
Complicated/catheter-associated UTI	Ampicillin, 2 gm IV q4h, **plus** Gentamicin, 100-120 mg (1.5-2 mg/kg) IV, followed by 80 mg IV q8h **or** If gram-negative, Ceftriaxone, 1 gm IV q12h, **or** Ciprofloxacin, 250-500 mg PO BID
Gastrointestinal Infections	
Cholecystitis	Mezloxillin, or Piperacillin, 3 gm IV q4-6h IV, **or** Gentamicin, 100-120 mg (1.5-2 mg/kg) IV, followed by 80 mg IV q8h
Bacterial cholangitis/biliary sepsis	Mezloxillin, or Piperacillin, 3 gm IV q4-6h IV, **plus** Metronidazole, 1.0 gm IV over 1 hour, then 500 mg IV q6h **or** Ampicillin-sulbactam, 3 gm IV q6h, **plus** Tobramycin, 80-100 mg IV q8h
Bacterial peritonitis	Ampicillin-sulbactam, 3 gm IV q6h, **plus** Gentamicin, 80-100 mg IV q8h, **or** Imipenem/cilastin, 0.5-1.0 gm IV q6-8h, **or** Ticarcillin/Clavulanate, 3.1 gm IV q4-6h **plus** Gentamicin, 80-100 mg IV q8h
Diverticulitis (moderate to severe)	Ampicillin-sulbactam, 1.5-3 gm IV q6h, **plus** Gentamicin (100-120 mg IV loading), then 80-100 mg IV q8h **or** Gentamicin (100-120 mg IV loading), then 80-100 mg IV q8h, **plus** Clindamycin, 600-900 mg IV q8h
Diverticulitis (mild)	Trimethoprim/Sulfamethoxazole, two double-strength tablets PO BID × 10 days **plus** Metronidazole, 500 mg PO BID × 10 days **or** Ciprofloxacin, 250-500 mg PO BID, **plus** Metronidazole, 250 mg PO TID × 10 days

Continued on next page

Table 19-1. Empiric Therapy for Infectious Disease Emergencies in the Elderly Patient—cont'd

Infectious disorder	Antibiotic regimen
Neurologic Infections	
Bacterial meningitis (empiric therapy for elderly, debilitated patients)	Ceftriaxone, 4 gm IV load, then 2 gm IV q12h, **plus** Ampicillin, 2 gm IV q4h
Cardiac Infections	
Acute bacterial endocarditis (empiric therapy)	Nafcillin, 2 gm IV q4h, **plus** Gentamicin, 120 mg load IV, followed by 80 mg IV q8h, **plus** Penicillin G, 18-24 million units/day q4h
Acute bacterial endocarditis (prosthetic valve)	Vancomycin, 500 mg IV q6h, **plus** Rifampin, 300 mg PO q8h × 6 weeks, **plus** Gentamicin, 1 mg/kg IV q8h × 2 weeks
Skin and Soft Tissue Infections	
Cellulitis (normal host, nondiabetic)	Cefazolin, 1-2 gm IV q8h
Cellulitis (diabetic, ulcerations, patient toxic)	Nafcillin, 1-2 gm IV q4-6h **plus** Gentamicin, 120 mg load IV, followed by 80 mg IV q8h **plus** Clindamycin, 600-1200 mg IV q6-8h, **or** Metronidazole, 1.0 gm IV over 1 hour, then 500 mg IV q6h **or** Ampicillin-sulbactam, 1.5-3 gm IV q6h, **plus** Gentamicin (100-120 mg IV loading), then 80-100 mg IV q8h
Sepsis—Unknown Source	
Nonimmunocompromised patient	Ceftriaxone, 1-2 gm IV q12h, **plus** Gentamicin (100-120 mg IV loading), followed by 80-100 mg IV q8h, **plus** Metronidazole, 1.0 gm IV over 1 hour, then 500 mg IV q6h (if anaerobes suspected, i.e., abdominal source)
Neutropenic patient	Ceftazidime, 2 gm IV q8h, **plus** Gentamicin (100-120 mg IV loading), followed by 80-100 mg IV q8h, **plus** Vancomycin, 500 mg IV q6h (if patient has indwelling catheter) **or** Imipenem alone, 500-1000 mg q6-8h (avoid if history of seizure or CVA)

20

Immunization

Jeffrey L. Arnold, M.D.
Joel M. Geiderman, M.D., F.A.C.E.P.

Immunization is the process by which a susceptible person acquires immunity to a disease through either active induction or passive administration of protective antibodies. Active immunization or vaccination stimulates the immune system to produce protective antibodies in 1 to 3 weeks if no prior exposure has occurred (in 4 days if previously exposed). Vaccines include live attenuated virus (measles, mumps, rubella, polio), killed virus (rabies), specific antigens (hepatitis B), and modified toxins or toxoids (tetanus, diphtheria). Passive immunization involves the administration of protective antibodies or immunoglobulin, providing immunity immediately but not permanently. Specific immune globulins include those against rabies, hepatitis B, varicella, and rhesus (Rh) factor.

Prevention of disease by immunization may take place before exposure occurs (preexposure immunization) or after exposure occurs (postexposure immunization). Because emergency physicians need to be able to identify patients at risk for infection, they should be familiar with the recommended preexposure immunizations for children and adults, and treat or refer these patients when appropriate **(Tables 20-1 and 20-2)**. Because patients commonly seek emergency medical care after possible exposure to disease, emergency physicians should be able to identify potentially significant exposures and to initiate appropriate immunoprophylaxis. Preventable diseases after exposure include tetanus, rabies, hepatitis A, hepatitis B, measles, varicella, and erythroblastosis fetalis (Rh isoimmunization).

Table 20-1. Recommended Immunization Schedule for Infants and Children

Age	Vaccine
2 months	DTP OPV Hib
4 months	DTP OPV Hib
6 months	DTP Hib
15 months	MMR DTP OPV Hib
4-6 years	DTP OPV MMR
14-16 years	Td

DTP, Diphtheria and tetanus toxoids with pertussis vaccine; *OPV*, oral trivalent live attenuated polio virus vaccine; *Hib*, Haemophilus influenza type b polysaccharide antigen vaccine; *MMR*, trivalent live attenuated measles, mumps, and rubella vaccine; *Td*, adult-type tetanus and diphtheria toxoids.

Table 20-2. Recommended Immunization Schedule for Adults

Vaccine	Recommendation
Tetanus-diphtheria	Td every 10 years if primary immunization complete (primary immunization: Td at 0, 1, and 6 months).
Measles	No vaccine if born before 1956. Measles vaccine or MMR if born after 1956 and no history of measles, or if not previously immunized with two live attenuated virus vaccines (after 1967).
Mumps	No vaccine if born before 1956. Mumps vaccine or MMR if born after 1956 and no history of mumps or if not previously immunized.
Rubella	Rubella vaccine if seronegative woman of childbearing age or health care worker.
Pneumococcal	Pneumovax if 65 years or older (booster in 5-10 years if immunocompromised) or if younger than 65 years and chronically ill (e.g., splenectomy).
Influenza	Influenza vaccine every year if 65 years or older or if younger than 65 years and chronically ill.

Tetanus

Tetanus is an acute neuroparalytic disease caused by a neurotoxin produced by *Clostridium tetani* in wounds. Although tetanus is uncommon in the United States (less than 100 cases per year), emergency physicians are routinely expected to evaluate patients for susceptibility to tetanus and to initiate immunoprophylaxis when appropriate **(Table 20-3)**.

I. **Pathophysiology.** *Clostridium tetani* spores are ubiquitous and are probably inoculated into wounds frequently. If anaerobic conditions occur (trauma, infection, foreign body), spores germinate and produce a neurotoxin that ascends peripheral motor neurons to the central nervous system (CNS) where it blocks γ-aminobutyric acid (GABA) release at inhibitory motor synapses, causing neuromuscular irritability; the toxin also stimulates the sympathetic nervous system.

II. **Clinical features.** Tetanus is characterized by progressive neuromuscular rigidity and spasm involving most muscle groups (trismus, risus sardonicus, opisthotonos, laryngospasm), and sympathetic hyperactivity (tachycardia, hypertension, diaphoresis); mental status is preserved.

III. **Evaluation of significant exposure.** Important factors to consider when evaluating susceptibility to tetanus include the following:

  A. **Immune status of patient.** Inadequately immunized patients who have had less than three previous tetanus toxoid doses or have unknown immunization status are at high risk for tetanus (elderly, immigrants, intravenous drug abusers [IVDA]). Patients older than 7 years who have received at least three previous tetanus toxoid doses are considered fully immunized if not more than 5 years have elapsed since their most recent immunization (tetanus-prone wounds) or 10 years (non-tetanus-prone wounds). Children younger than 7 years may or may not have completed their primary series and should have their immunization status evaluated according to **Table 20-1.** Previous tetanus disease does not confer immunity.

Table 20-3. Routine Diphtheria, Tetanus, and Pertussis Immunization Schedule for Persons Younger Than 7 Years

Dose	Age/interval	Vaccine
Primary 1	6 weeks or older	DTP
Primary 2	4 to 8 weeks after first dose	DTP
Primary 3	4 to 8 weeks after second dose	DTP
Primary 4	6 to 12 weeks after third dose	DTP
Booster*	4 to 6 years old	DPT

*Booster dose at 4 to 6 years of age not necessary if the fourth primary immunizing dose was administered after the fourth birthday.

    B. Type of wound. Tetanus-prone wounds are more than 6 hours old before treatment, contaminated with feces, soil, or saliva, infected, or surrounded by avascular or nonviable tissue (punctures, crush wounds, frostbite, burns, retained foreign body). Non-tetanus-prone wounds are less than 6 hours old; they are neither contaminated nor infected, and are surrounded by viable tissue (linear wounds). Tetanus may complicate any wound, no matter how trivial. No lesion is identified in 10% to 20% of cases; tetanus has been reported from skin tests, intramuscular injections, elective surgery, deliveries, abortions, electrical injuries, insect bites, corneal abrasions, dental infections, chronic skin ulcers, and abscesses.

IV. Postexposure prophylaxis. Management includes proper wound care and immunoprophylaxis. Immunoprophylaxis consists of active immunization with tetanus toxoid vaccine (Td or DTP) and, in select cases, passive immunization with tetanus immunoglobulin (TIG).

    A. Wound care includes washing with soap and water, debridement, irrigation with sterile normal saline solution, and suturing as indicated.

    B. Td is a combined diphtheria-tetanus toxoid prepared from diphtheria and tetanus toxins, and is recommended for persons 7 years of age or older. The diphtheria toxoid is added because adults often lack protective levels of antitoxin against diphtheria. Adverse reactions include local pain, erythema, edema, and rarely low-grade fever, headache, and malaise. Patients who have received tetanus toxoid boosters too frequently may develop an Arthus-type hypersensitivity reaction characterized by a severe local reaction 2 to 8 hours after immunization. Patients with a history of an Arthus-type hypersensitivity reaction should not receive Td more frequently than every 10 years. Systemic hypersensitivity reactions and neuropathy are rare but are contraindications to subsequent Td administration. The recommended dose of Td is 0.5 ml given intramuscularly; it should be administered as indicated in **Table 20-2.**

    C. DTP is a combined diphtheria-tetanus toxoid with pertussis vaccine and is recommended for children younger than 7 years (instead of Td). Contraindications to pertussis vaccine include a history of the following severe reactions to previous pertussis vaccine administration: encephalopathy, seizure, collapse, high fever, markedly abnormal crying, and anaphylaxis. If DTP is contraindicated because of a history of severe reaction to the pertussis component, then DT should be given (higher dose diphtheria toxoid). The recommended dose of DTP is 0.5 ml given intramuscularly and should be administered as indicated in **Table 20-3.**

Table 20-4. Tetanus Prophylaxis in Children Younger Than 7 Years

History of tetanus toxoid	Non-tetanus-prone wounds TIG*	Non-tetanus-prone wounds DTP†	Tetanus-prone wounds TIG*	Tetanus-prone wounds DTP†
Unknown or <3 doses	No	Yes	Yes	Yes
3 or more doses	No	No‡	No	No

*Dose of TIG is 250 ml IM.
†Dose of DTP is 0.5 ml IM; use DT if pertussis contraindicated.
‡Yes if routine immunization schedule has lapsed.

Table 20-5. Tetanus Prophylaxis in Persons 7 Years of Age and Older

History of tetanus toxoid	Non-tetanus-prone wounds TIG*	Non-tetanus-prone wounds Td†	Tetanus-prone wounds TIG*	Tetanus-prone wounds Td†
Unknown or <3 doses	No	Yes	Yes	Yes
3 or more doses	No	No‡	No	No**

*Dose of TIG is 250 ml IM.
†Dose of Td is 0.5 ml IM.
‡Yes if more than 10 years since last dose.
**Yes, if more than 5 years since last dose.

D. TIG is an antitetanus immunoglobulin prepared from human donors hyperimmunized with tetanus toxoid. It is indicated for inadequately immunized patients of all ages with tetanus-prone wounds **(Tables 20-4** and **20-5)**. Adverse reactions include local pain, erythema, edema, and low-grade fever. Peripheral neuropathy, urticaria, and systemic allergic reactions have been reported. The recommended dose of TIG is 250 ml given intramuscularly.

V. Disposition. A primary immunization series against tetanus consists of three doses of tetanus toxoid, with the first two doses administered at least 4 weeks apart and the third dose 6 months after the second. Patients remaining inadequately immunized after initial emergency department (ED) immunoprophylaxis should be referred to their primary care physician for completion of their primary series at the appropriate interval (usually 4 weeks).

Rabies

Rabies is an acute infectious viral disease of the CNS. Usually fatal, it is the most dreaded complication of an animal bite. Although human rabies is now rare in the United States (approximately one case per year), emergency physicians are commonly expected to evaluate patients for possible exposure to rabies and to initiate immunoprophylaxis when appropriate.

I. Pathophysiology. Rabies virus is transmitted by inoculation with infectious saliva from a rabid animal. Following bite or salivary contact through skin break or mucosa, the RNA-containing virus replicates in local myocytes, then ascends peripheral motor neurons to the CNS, where further replication occurs primarily in gray matter. The virus then disseminates via peripheral nerves to all organ systems and is shed in saliva, urine, and feces. The incubation period averages 1 to 2 months.

II. **Clinical features.** Rabies begins as a flu-like illness, then progresses to an encephalomyelitis with protean neurologic manifestations (altered mental status, delirium, hyperspasticity, paresis, paralysis, hypersensitivity to sensory stimuli, hydrophobia, cholinergic autonomic instability, seizures, coma). If untreated, death usually occurs in 4 to 7 days.

III. **Evaluation of significant exposure.** Critical factors to consider when evaluating a potential exposure to rabies include the following:
   A. **Species of biting animal.** High-risk wild species include skunk, bat, raccoon, fox, coyote, and bobcat; all should be considered rabid until proven otherwise. High-risk domestic species include dog, cat, and cow. Rodents (squirrels, chipmunks, rats, mice) and lagamorphs (rabbits) have never been reported as causing human rabies in the United States. The risk of rabies among various animal species varies greatly by region; therefore, it is best to consult with local public health authorities.
   B. **Type of exposure.** Any salivary exposure is potentially significant (e.g., a scratch that was then licked). A rare type of exposure is by inhalation (e.g., in bat-infested caves).
   C. **Presence of rabies in an area where bite has occurred.** Rabies is endemic worldwide, although it typically spares island nations (Australia, England, Japan). Dogs are the most important source of human infection in developing countries where animal immunizations are rare. In the United States, rabies is uncommon in New England, the Ohio Valley, and the Rocky Mountains. It is rare in most urban centers and has never been reported in Hawaii. One should consult local public health authorities or the Center for Disease Control and Prevention (404-639-1075 or 404-639-2888) regarding the current epidemiologic risk in a particular area.
   D. **Other important considerations** include behavior of the animal at the time of the bite (an unprovoked attack is more likely to be significant); immunization status of the animal (inactivated animal rabies vaccination confers immunity for at least 1 year); and immunization status of the patient (persons working in certain animal-related professions may have received preexposure immunoprophylaxis, which by standard regimens confers immunity for approximately 2 years). Wild animals, if captured, are sacrificed, and immunoprophylaxis should be initiated pending brain tissue analysis by public health authorities. Domestic animals, if captured, are quarantined for 10 days and observed for normal behavior. If an animal does not exhibit abnormal behavior, then immunoprophylaxis is not necessary **(Fig. 20-1).**

IV. **Postexposure prophylaxis.** Appropriate management of potential exposure to rabies consists of proper wound care and the initiation of immunoprophylaxis as early as possible. Immunoprophylaxis consists of both passive immunization with human rabies immune globulin (HRIG) and active immunization with the human diploid cell vaccine (HDCV).
   A. **Wound care** includes washing with soap and water, debridement, irrigation with sterile normal saline solution, and the avoidance of sutures if possible (suturing promotes viral replication).
   B. **HRIG is an antirabies immunoglobulin** prepared from hyperimmune human donors. It is indicated for any person with suspected exposure to rabies (except those previously immunized with documented adequate rabies anti-

Figure 20-1. Algorithm for Human Rabies Postexposure Immunoprophylaxis

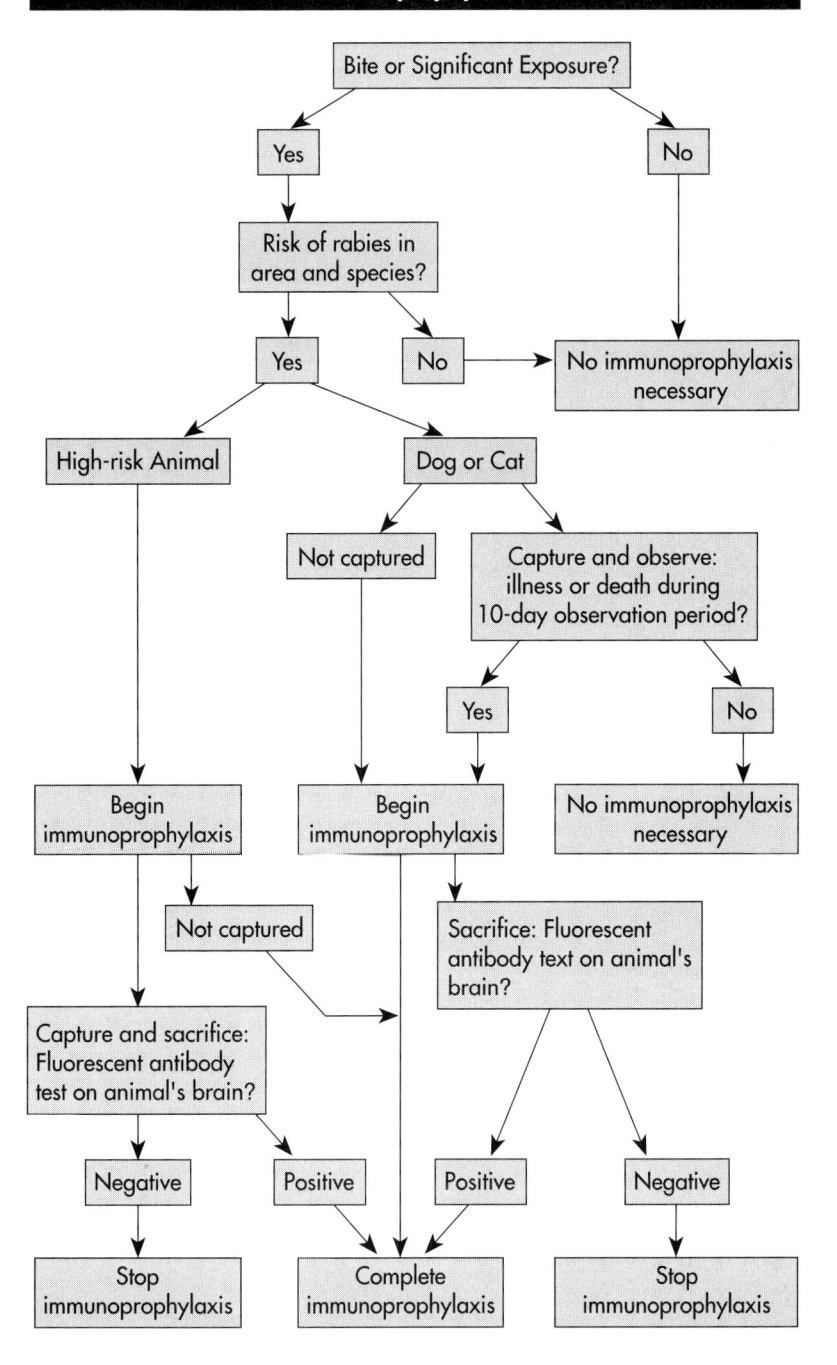

body titers). The most common adverse reactions include local soreness and low-grade fever. The recommended dose of HRIG is 20 IU/kg given intramuscularly. If possible, it is preferred that one half of the dose be infiltrated proximal to the wound and one half be given intramuscularly in the deltoid area. It is optimally given at the time of the first HDCV dose but may be given up to 8 days later (beyond this time, active immunity is established and sufficient).

C. **HDCV is an inactivated virus vaccine** that is also indicated for any person with suspected exposure to rabies as above. Adverse reactions include local pain, erythema, and edema (25%), as well as mild systemic symptoms such as headache, nausea, dizziness, and myalgias (20%). Anaphylaxis and Guillain-Barré syndrome have been reported but are rare. Active immunization should not be stopped because of local or mild systemic reactions. For more serious reactions, the risk of developing rabies should be weighed against the risk of continuing treatment. The recommended dose of HDCV is 1 ml administered intramuscularly on days 0, 3, 7, 14, and 28. It should be given as soon as possible after rabies exposure. The deltoid muscle is the preferred vaccination site.

Hepatitis A

Hepatitis A is an acute, self-limited febrile disease caused by hepatitis A virus (HAV), an RNA virus excreted in feces of persons with hepatitis A. Because hepatitis A is common, emergency physicians are frequently expected to evaluate a patient for exposure to hepatitis A and to initiate immunoprophylaxis when appropriate.

I. **Pathophysiology.** HAV is acquired by oral ingestion of fecally contaminated food or water or by person-to-person contact. Parenteral transmission does not occur. The incubation period ranges from 15 to 50 days (average 30 days). Viral shedding in feces is maximal during the 2 weeks before the onset of jaundice, becoming minimal by 1 week after the onset of jaundice; it is during these 3 weeks that a person is considered contagious to others. No carrier state or chronic infection occurs. The presence of IgM anti-HAV indicates recent infection, IgG anti-HAV indicates past infection, and the presence of either indicates lifelong immunity.

II. **Clinical features.** Hepatitis A is characterized clinically by four periods: incubation (asymptomatic), preicteric (malaise, anorexia, nausea), icteric (jaundice, dark urine), and convalescent. Fulminant hepatitis is rare. Hepatitis A cannot be distinguished from other causes of hepatitis on clinical grounds; serologic testing must be performed.

III. **Evaluation of significant exposure.** Important factors to consider when evaluating susceptibility to HAV include the following:
   A. **Source of exposure.** Persons with either clinical hepatitis (presumptive HAV infection) or serologically confirmed hepatitis A are considered at high risk for spreading HAV, for the purpose of administering immunoprophylaxis to others. In food- or water-borne outbreaks, the index case is rarely identified until it is too late for immunoprophylaxis to be effective.
   B. **Type of exposure.** Since hepatitis A is transmitted by the fecal-oral route, high-risk exposures include sexual and household contacts. Day-care facility contacts, especially with children less than 2 years old or children not yet toilet trained, are also at high risk since HAV is so readily spread in this age

group. School, institutional, hospital, and workplace contacts are not high risk unless an outbreak occurs.
- **C. Immune status of patient.** Serologic screening of the exposed patient is not recommended (expensive, delays immunoprophylaxis).
- **D. Timing of exposure.** Immunoprophylaxis is not indicated if more than 2 weeks has elapsed since last exposure to HAV.

IV. **Postexposure prophylaxis.** Immunoprophylaxis consists of passive immunization with immune globulin (IG).
- **A. IG contains anti-HAV** and is prepared from pooled human plasma. If given within 2 weeks of exposure, it is 80% to 90% effective in preventing clinical hepatitis A. Indications for administering IG include household or sexual contacts of persons with clinical or serologic hepatitis A; day-care facility contacts of persons with clinical or serologic hepatitis A (see *Red Book* published by the American Academy of Pediatrics); and persons exposed to HAV through contaminated food or water, or during epidemiologically defined outbreaks. Adverse effects are basically confined to a local reaction. Contraindications are a history of anaphylaxis or severe systemic reactions to IG. Dosage and administration of IG is 0.02 ml/kg given intramuscularly as soon as possible after exposure. IG should not be given later than 2 weeks after last exposure.

V. **Disposition.** Patients should be counseled that while IG usually prevents clinical hepatitis, it may not prevent asymptomatic infection and spread. Personal hygiene should be emphasized.

Hepatitis B

Hepatitis B infection is a potentially lethal viral disease acquired by percutaneous or permucosal exposure to infected blood or body fluids. Because it is also one of the most serious complications of needle-stick injuries to hospital personnel, emergency physicians are frequently expected to evaluate patients for significant exposure to hepatitis B virus (HBV) and to initiate immunoprophylaxis when appropriate.

I. **Pathophysiology.** HBV is a DNA virus whose outer protein shell contains the hepatitis B surface antigen (HBsAg) and whose inner core contains the hepatitis B core antigen (HBcAg). HBV is transmitted by percutaneous or permucosal exposure to infected blood, semen, or saliva. There is no fecal-oral transmission. The incubation period ranges from 30 to 180 days (average 75 days). After infection, a viremia occurs during which a person is infectious to others. This period of infectivity begins 2 to 7 weeks before symptoms occur and either continues until symptoms resolve (90% to 95%) or persists as a chronic infection (5% to 10%). The presence of HBsAg in serum indicates current infection; its persistence for 6 months indicates chronic infection (carrier state). The presence of the antibody to surface antigen (anti-HBs) indicates immunity by previous HBV infection or vaccination. Rarely, a window period occurs after the disappearance of HBsAg and before the appearance of anti-HBs during which acute infection is indicated solely by the presence of the antibody to core antigen (anti-HBc).

II. **Clinical features.** Acute hepatitis B is clinically similar to acute hepatitis A with incubation, preicteric, icteric, and convalescent periods. It cannot be distinguished from other causes of hepatitis on clinical grounds (serologic testing is required). Unlike HAV, HBV causes a range of infections from asymptomatic seroconversion to fulminant hepatitis with hepatic failure to chronic infection with

its dreaded sequelae (chronic active hepatitis, cirrhosis, hepatocellular carcinoma, extrahepatic disease).
- **III. Evaluation of significant exposure.** Important factors to consider when evaluating a potential exposure to HBV include the following:
  - **A. Type of exposure.** High-risk exposures include percutaneous (needle-stick, laceration, or bite) or permucosal exposure to HBsAg-positive blood; sexual or household contacts of persons with HBV infection; and perinatal exposure of infants to mothers who are HBsAg-positive.
  - **B. Source of exposure.** Persons at high risk for acquiring and transmitting HBV infection include homosexual males, heterosexuals with multiple partners, intravenous drug abusers, institutionalized persons, hemodialysis patients, household or sexual contacts of HBV carriers, members or populations in which HBV is highly endemic (native Alaskans, Pacific islanders, recent immigrants from Eastern Asia or Africa), and health care workers with frequent contact with the above persons. When the HBsAg status of the source is unknown, it is considered low risk, because an unknown source is 100 times less likely to transmit HBsAg than a known high-risk source (e.g., certain needle-stick exposures).
  - **C. Immune status of exposed person.** Persons *adequately vaccinated* against HBV have completed the recommended schedule of receiving a total of three doses of hepatitis B vaccine; the vaccine is given at 0, 1, and 6 months. Unvaccinated persons have not completed this series. Most adequately vaccinated persons develop a protective level of antibodies to HBsAg (anti-HBs ≥10 mIU) and are then called *vaccine responders* (82% to 97%). The remaining persons are partial or *nonresponders* to vaccine (anti-HBs <10 mIU). If a patient has been a documented responder within the past year, that person is considered protected and no further evaluation is required. Most often a person's response status is unknown at the time of ED evaluation.
- **IV. Postexposure prophylaxis.** Immunoprophylaxis consists of selective passive immunization with hepatitis B immunoglobulin (HBIG) and active immunization with hepatitis B vaccine. Percutaneous or permucosal exposures should be treated like other wounds, with consideration given to wound care and tetanus prophylaxis.
  - **A. HBIG is a pooled human immune globulin** prepared from donors with high titers of anti-HBs. It is indicated for persons not immunized against HBV infection who may be significantly exposed to HBsAg-positive blood or body fluid. It is most effective if given as soon as possible after exposure; it is ineffective if given more than 2 weeks after exposure. Adverse reactions include a local reaction at the site of infection. Urticaria and angioedema may occur; anaphylaxis is rare. Contraindications include a history of hypersensitivity to any component of HBIG. The recommended dose of HBIG is 0.06 ml/kg given intramuscularly in the deltoid area at a site distinct from hepatitis B vaccine if given **(Tables 20-6 and 20-7).**
  - **B. Three hepatitis B vaccines are currently licensed in the United States** for protection against hepatitis B: the plasma-derived Heptavax-B (pooled human plasma with high titers of HBsAg) and the recombinant Recombivax-HB and Engerix-B (genetically engineered in yeast culture). Hepatitis B vaccine is indicated for persons not immunized against HBV infection who may be significantly exposed to HBsAg-positive blood or body fluid. Heptavax-B is currently available in the United States only for hemodialysis and other immunocompromised patients, or persons with known allergy to yeast (consult

Table 20-6. Hepatitis B Immunoprophylaxis After Perinatal, Sexual, or Household Exposure

Exposure	Dose	HBIG timing	Vaccine* Dose	Vaccine* Timing
Perinatal	0.5 ml IM	Within 12 hours of birth	0.5 ml IM	Within 7 days
Sexual or household contact†	0.06 ml/kg	Within 14 days of last contact†	1.0 ml IM**	At time of HBIG

*Vaccine series should be completed at 1 and 6 months.
†Household contact immunoprophylaxis is indicated if person has had specific blood exposure to index patient (toothbrush or razor). Vaccination is indicated for all household contacts if index patient becomes hepatitis B carrier.
‡Prescreening contact for susceptibility to HBV recommended.
**For adults >19 years old; see package insert for other ages.

Table 20-7. Hepatitis B Immunoprophylaxis in ED After Percutaneous or Permucosal Exposure

Source	Unvaccinated HBIG*	Unvaccinated Vaccine†	Vaccinated Known nonresponder HBIG*	Vaccinated Known nonresponder Vaccine†	Vaccinated Known responder or unknown status HBIG*	Vaccinated Known responder or unknown status Vaccine†
HBsAg-positive or high-risk source	Yes	Yes	Yes	Yes	No‡	No‡
HbsAg-negative or low-risk or unknown source	No‡	Yes	No‡	No‡	No‡	No‡

*HBIG: dose is 0.06 ml/kg IM.
†Vaccine: Recombivax-HB or Engerix-B; dose is 1.0 ml IM for adults >19 years old. See package insert for other patients.
‡Yes, if indicated by serologic results on source and/or exposed person.

Heptavax-B package insert for further information). Adverse reactions to the recombinant vaccines include a local reaction at the injection site, transient systemic symptoms (fever, arthralgias, rash, nausea, malaise), and rarely neurologic sequelae. Contraindications include a history of hypersensitivity to any component of the vaccine or a history of neurologic sequelae. Dosage and administration of recombinant hepatitis B vaccine in an adult patient (>19 years old) is 1.0 ml intramuscularly in the deltoid area at a site distinct from HBIG. (Consult the package insert for dosages for persons 19 years old or less, or hemodialysis patients.) The vaccine should be administered within 7 days of exposure. The duration of protection and need for subsequent booster doses has not yet been defined **(Tables 20-6 and 20-7)**.

V. Disposition. In situations when immediate immunoprophylaxis is indicated, HBIG and hepatitis B vaccine may be administered in the emergency department. When the need for immediate immunoprophylaxis is unclear (e.g., certain "needle-stick" exposures of health care workers), the patient should be referred for serologic evaluation as soon as possible (e.g., to occupational health department of hospital). Since the hepatitis B vaccination series consists of three vaccinations, administered at 0, 1, and 6 months, patients initially vaccinated in the emergency department should be referred to their primary care physician for completion of the series at 1 and 6 months.

Hepatitis C

Hepatitis C, the most common cause of posttransfusion hepatitis (non-A, non-B hepatitis), is caused by hepatitis C virus (HCV), an RNA virus transmitted like hepatitis B. The incubation period is 7 to 9 weeks (range 2 to 12 weeks). About 15 weeks after the onset of clinical hepatitis, the antibody to HCV (anti-HCV) appears in serum, indicating infectivity. Clinically, the infection may be asymptomatic or mild, but frequently progresses to chronic hepatitis or cirrhosis (50% to 70%). Persons at high risk for acquiring and transmitting HCV include intravenous drug abusers, hemophiliacs, hemodialysis patients, health care workers exposed to such patients, and sexual or household contacts of infected persons. The efficacy of immunoprophylaxis with immunoglobulin (IG) is not yet established. Indications for administering IG include percutaneous or permucosal exposure to blood or body fluids from persons with non-A, non-B hepatitis (anti-HCV–positive or HBsAg-negative chronic hepatitis). Adverse reactions and contraindications to administering IG are discussed under "Hepatitis A." The dose and administration of IG is 0.06 ml/kg intramuscularly. It should not be administered to patients receiving HBIG.

Measles

Measles (rubeola) is an acute, highly contagious viral disease that can cause serious sequelae in the unimmunized or immunocompromised person. In particular, because the incidence of measles in the United States has increased recently, emergency physicians must be able to identify susceptible persons and initiate appropriate immunoprophylaxis.

I. **Pathophysiology.** Measles virus is an RNA paramyxovirus transmitted by direct or air-borne contact with infectious droplets. The incubation period to onset of characteristic rash is 14 days (range 7 to 18 days). Patients are contagious from 3 to 5 days before until 4 days after the onset of rash. Immunity is lifelong in healthy persons and is indicated serologically by the presence of antibodies to measles virus.

II. **Clinical features.** Measles is classically characterized by a prodrome of fever, cough, coryza, conjunctivitis, and a pathognomonic enanthem (Koplik's spots), followed by an erythematous maculopapular rash that begins on the face and descends distally. It is frequently complicated by otitis media and pneumonia and rarely by encephalitis. Adolescents and adults may present with atypical measles, characterized by fever, pneumonia, obtundation, and a variable rash that ranges from urticarial to maculopapular to petechial.

III. **Evaluation of significant exposure.** Important factors to consider when evaluating patients for immunoprophylaxis include the following:
  A. **Type of exposure.** High-risk exposures include household contacts of persons with measles and epidemiologically defined outbreaks of measles (schools, institutions, hospitals).

B. Immune status of patient. Patients considered immune to measles include those born before 1956 (when measles was universal), those with a history of measles, those with positive serology for measles antibody, and those with two prior live attenuated measles vaccinations (after 1967). Patients considered susceptible to measles include healthy persons not meeting the criteria above and immunocompromised patients, regardless of vaccination status.

C. Risk of serious complications. Patients at high risk for serious complications of measles include those with human immunodeficiency virus (HIV) infection, the severely immunocompromised (patients with leukemia, lymphoma, and generalized malignancy, as well as those undergoing therapy with alkylating agents, antimetabolites, radiation, or large doses of corticosteroids), and infants younger than 1 year.

IV. Postexposure prophylaxis. Immunoprophylaxis consists of passive immunization with human immune globulin (IG) or active immunization with measles vaccine.

A. IG is pooled human immune globulin. It is indicated for the following persons when significantly exposed to measles virus: infants younger than 1 year; healthy susceptible persons older than 1 year with a contraindication to measles vaccine or to whom measles vaccine cannot be given within 72 hours of exposure; pregnant women; and immunocompromised persons regardless of vaccination status. IG may prevent or attenuate the severity of measles. Adverse reactions include a local reaction at the site of injection, and it is contraindicated if there is a history of hypersensitivity to any component of IG. The dose of IG for healthy persons of any age is 0.25 ml/kg given intramuscularly. The dose and administration for immunocompromised persons is 0.5 ml/kg intramuscularly. The maximum dose is 15 ml. It should be administered within 6 days of exposure. If IG is administered, subsequent vaccination should be delayed for 3 months **(Table 20-8).**

B. Measles virus vaccine is a live attenuated virus vaccine prepared in chick embryo culture and is usually administered as trivalent measles-mumps-rubella vaccine (MMR); however it is also available as monovalent measles vaccine (M). The current U.S. *preexposure* immunization recommendation is for all children to first receive MMR at 15 months of age and again between 4 years and adolescence. In areas where measles is epidemic, local public health authorities may recommend that infants be given monovalent measles vaccine at age 6 months, in addition to subsequent routine preexposure immunization. As *postexposure* immunoprophylaxis, MMR is also recommended for healthy susceptible persons 1 year or older when significantly exposed to measles. Monovalent measles vaccine is recommended for infants from 6 months to 1 year of age. Adverse reactions include delayed febrile illness (approximately 6 days after vaccination), transient rash, and rarely neurologic sequelae. Because MMR is a live attenuated virus vaccine, it is contraindicated for pregnant women and the severely immunocompromised. HIV infection (in the absence of severe manifestation of disease) is not a contraindication to measles vaccine because these patients are at much higher risk for the deleterious effects of measles infection. It is also contraindicated for persons with a history of hypersensitivity to eggs or neomycin or any other component of vaccine, those with a history of neurologic sequelae after vaccine, those who have received a recent blood product transfusion, those who have received IG in the previous 3 months (IG blunts the immunogenicity of subsequent vaccine), and those with moderate or severe intercurrent febrile illness. The dose

Table 20-8. Measles Immunoprophylaxis

Exposure	IG* Dose	IG* Timing	Vaccine Dose	Vaccine Timing
Infants younger than 6 months	0.25 ml/kg IM	Within 6 days	—	—
Infants 6 months to 12 months old	—	—	0.5 ml SQ†	Within 72 hours
Healthy, susceptible‡ persons 1 year or older	—	—	0.5 ml SQ**	Within 72 hours
Healthy, susceptible persons with contraindication‡‡ to vaccine or in whom vaccine delayed more than 72 hours	0.25 ml/kg IM	Within 6 days	—	—
Pregnant women	0.25 ml/kg IM	Within 6 days	—	—
Immunocompromised#	0.5 ml/kg IM	Within 6 days	—	—

*IG, immune globulin.
†Monovalent measles virus vaccine (M) is preferred, but MMR may be given if M is not readily available.
‡Susceptible persons born 1957 or later, with no history of measles, no serologic evidence of measles, not previously immunized with two live attenuated virus vaccines (after 1967).
**Trivalent measles-mumps-rubella virus vaccine (MMR).
‡‡See text for contraindications to vaccine.
#Immunocompromised refers to patients with leukemia, lymphoma, generalized malignancy, or HIV infection, as well as those undergoing therapy with alkylating agents, antimetabolites, radiation, or large doses of corticosteroids.

of measles virus vaccine (MMR or M) is 0.5 ml given subcutaneously. It should be given no later than 72 hours after exposure **(Table 20-8)**.

V. **Disposition.** Patients passively immunized with IG who remain inadequately vaccinated should be referred to their primary care physician in 3 months for completion of their measles virus vaccine series.

Varicella

While primary varicella (chickenpox) is usually a benign, self-limited disease in the healthy child, it can cause serious life-threatening complications in normal adults and the immunocompromised. Because persons with varicella or zoster frequently expose other persons to disease at home and in the hospital, it is important for emergency physicians to be able to evaluate patients for susceptibility to varicella and to initiate immunoprophylaxis when appropriate.

I. **Pathophysiology.** Varicella-zoster virus (VZV) is a herpes virus transmitted person-to-person (by direct contact with contaminated hands) or by airborne droplets. The incubation period of primary varicella is 14 to 16 days (range 11 to 20 days). Patients are contagious 1 to 2 days before vesicular eruption until 5 days after its onset (usually until vesicles crust). Because reactivated vesicles are also infectious, persons with zoster (shingles) are also contagious. Airborne droplet transmission in zoster is rare. Once a person has varicella, immunity is lifelong and is indicated serologically by the presence of antibodies to VZV.

II. **Clinical features.** Primary infection with VZV produces chickenpox, characterized by its classic diffuse vesicular rash. In immunocompromised patients, vesicular eruption may be prolonged, continuing into the second week, and illness may be complicated by hepatitis, pancreatitis, pneumonia, and encephalitis. In healthy adults and pregnant women, chickenpox is often severe and may be complicated by pneumonia and subsequent hypoxemia.

III. **Evaluation of significant exposure.** Important factors to consider when evaluating patients for immunoprophylaxis include the following:
   A. **Type of exposure.** High-risk exposures include household contact, playmate contact for more than 1 hour indoors, certain hospital exposures (prolonged face-to-face contact or sharing same room with infected patient or health care worker), and perinatal exposure (neonates born to mothers with infection 5 days before or 2 days after delivery).
   B. **Immune status of patient.** Persons with a history of varicella are considered immune. Persons likely to be immune to VZV include those previously exposed to a person with varicella or zoster (persons with siblings who have had varicella, persons who attended urban schools, health care workers previously exposed to VZV at work). Serologic determination of immune status of patients with negative or uncertain histories may be performed if it does not delay the administration of immunoprophylaxis.
   C. **Risk of serious complication.** Persons at high risk for serious complications of VZV infection include the immunocompromised of any age, persons older than 15 years, pregnant women, and neonates.
   D. **Timing of exposure.** Immunoprophylaxis is not indicated later than 96 hours after exposure.

IV. **Postexposure prophylaxis.** Immunoprophylaxis consists of passive immunization with varicella-zoster immune globulin (VZIG). VZIG is an anti-varicella-zoster immune globulin prepared from hyperimmune human donors. It is indicated for susceptible persons at high risk for serious complications (e.g., immunocompromised patients) when significantly exposed to VZV. VZIG usually does not prevent infections but blunts the severity of disease and may prolong the incubation period and delay the onset of rash. The most common adverse reaction is a local reaction of the site of injection, and the only contraindication is a history of hypersensitivity to any component of VZIG. The dose and administration is one vial (125 units) per 10 kg of body weight given intramuscularly. The minimum dose is one vial, and the maximum dose is five vials. It should be administered within 48 hours of exposure and no later than 96 hours after exposure. The duration of protection is unknown. Reexposures occurring 2 weeks after initial immunoprophylaxis should be reevaluated for readministration of VZIG.

V. **Disposition.** Because VZIG may not prevent varicella infection, exposed susceptible persons are capable of transmitting VZV whether they receive VZIG or not. In particular, exposed susceptible health care workers with patient contact should be off work from day 8 to 28 after exposure if they receive VZIG, or day 8 to 21 if they do not receive VZIG (VZIG delays the onset of rash). Exposed, susceptible health care workers should be promptly referred to the occupational health department of the hospital for follow-up evaluation. Other patients should be referred to their primary care physician and cautioned that if a rash occurs and they require medical evaluation, they should wear a mask when returning to a health care facility.

Rh Isoimmunization

Rh isoimmunization is the most serious complication of fetomaternal hemorrhage (FMH) and occurs when Rh-negative mothers develop antibodies against the Rh antigen on the surface of Rh-positive fetal erythrocytes. Although the risk of Rh isoimmunization is low (0.1% in Rh-negative mothers receiving routine antepartum and postpartum Rh immunoprophylaxis), emergency physicians commonly evaluate bleeding during pregnancy and are expected to administer Rh immunoprophylaxis when appropriate.

I. **Pathophysiology.** When an Rh-negative mother is exposed to Rh-positive fetal erythrocytes, the Rh antigen efficiently induces her immune system to produce IG antibodies. These antibodies can then cross the placenta and attack Rh-positive erythrocytes in the fetal circulation, leading to hemolytic anemia, fetal hydrops, and death. Fetal prognosis ultimately depends on the maternal titer of these antibodies and the duration of fetal exposure.

II. **Clinical feature.** Maternal exposure to fetal erythrocytes may occur during any vaginal bleeding in pregnancy, including threatened abortion or ectopic pregnancy. Other causes of FMH include abortion (spontaneous or therapeutic), instrumentation (amniocentesis or chorionic villi sampling), blunt abdominal trauma, abruptio placentae, and delivery (vaginal or cesarean section). Trauma, placental abruptio, and traumatic delivery may be associated with large volumes of FMH that may be quantitated by using the Kleihauer-Betke test.

III. **Evaluation of significant exposure.** Important factors to consider when evaluating possible Rh isoimmunization include the following:

  A. **Whether fetomaternal hemorrhage has occurred.** Any event allowing fetal erythrocytes to enter the maternal circulation may lead to Rh isoimmunization.

  B. **Maternal Rh status.** Only Rh-negative mothers are at risk for Rh isoimmunization. Rh status can be obtained from historical sources (patient's physician, old chart, blood bank record) or by blood typing in the ED.

C. Maternal immune status. Previous Rh isoimmunization obviates the need for further evaluation. Blood banks routinely screen for anti–Rh antibodies (indirect Coomb's test) when an Rh-negative maternal blood type is determined.

D. Paternal Rh status. An Rh-negative father obviates the need for further evaluation.

IV. **Postexposure prophylaxis.** Immunoprophylaxis with Rh immunoglobulin (RhIG) is indicated when any Rh-negative nonimmunized mother is suspected of exposure to Rh-positive fetal erythrocytes. RhIG is an anti–Rh immune globulin prepared from immune human donors and acts by suppressing the immune response of Rh-negative persons to Rh-positive erythrocytes. The only contraindication is a history of anaphylaxis or severe allergic reaction to human immunoglobulin. The recommended dose of RhIG in first trimester bleeding is 50 µg given intramuscularly (MICRhoGAM). Later bleeding is treated with 300 µg intramuscularly (RhoGAM). Since 300 µg of RhIG only protects against 15 ml of fetal erythrocytes, if a larger volume of FMH is suspected (e.g., abdominal trauma), dosing should be guided by the Kleihauer-Betke test. RhIG, 300 µg intramuscularly, is also administered at the time of obstetric instrumentation, at 28 weeks gestation as routine antepartum prophylaxis, and at delivery if the newborn infant is Rh-positive. It is prudent to administer RhIG as soon as possible after potential FMH, with administration recommended no later than 72 hours. It is also recommended that the patient's physician and the blood bank be informed when RhIG is administered.

V. **Disposition.** Rh-negative mothers should be referred to their obstetrician for routine Rh immunoprophylaxis at 28 weeks gestation. When Rh testing is unavailable, women with first-trimester vaginal bleeding should be referred to their primary care physician for evaluation of the need for Rh immunoprophylaxis within 72 hours.

Suggested Readings

General

American College of Emergency Physicians: Immunization of the pediatric patient, *Ann Emerg Med* 22:627, 1993.

Zull D, Clark N: Vaccines and immunoprophylaxis. In *Principles and practices of emergency medicine,* ed 3.

Tetanus

American College of Emergency Physicians: Tetanus immunization recommendations for persons seven years of age and older, *Ann Emerg Med* 15:1111-2, 1986.

American College of Emergency Physicians: Tetanus immunization recommendations for persons less than seven years old, *Ann Emerg Med* 16:1181-3, 1987.

Center for Disease Control: Tetanus surveillance—United States, 1989-1990, *MMWR* 41:1-9, 1992.

Gareau A et al: Tetanus immunization status and immunologic response to a booster in an emergency department geriatric population, *Ann Emerg Med* 19:1377-82, 1990.

Grangrasso J, Smith RK: Misuse of tetanus immunoprophylaxis in wound care, *Ann Emerg Med* 14:573-9, 1985.

Grolean G: Tetanus, *Emerg Med Clin North Am* 10:351-60, 1992.

Rabies

Advisory Committee on Immunization Practice (ACIP): Rabies Prevention—United States, 1991, *MMWR* 40:1-19, 1991.

Dire D: Emergency management of dog and cat bite wounds, *Emerg Med Clin North Am* 10:719-36, 1992.
Fishbein D: *Rabies in current practice of emergency medicine,* ed 2, Philadelphia, 1991, BC Decker.
Grolean G: Rabies, *Emerg Med Clin North Am* 10:361-2, 1992.
Krebs J et al: Rabies surveillance in the United States during 1991, *JACMA* 201:1836-48, 1991.

Hepatitis A

Center for Disease Control: Recommendations for protection against viral hepatitis, *MMWR* 34:313-34, 1985.
Committee on Infectious Diseases, American Academy of Pediatrics: Hepatitis A. In Peter G, editor: *Report of the committee on infectious diseases,* ed 22, Elk Grove Village, Ill, 1991, American Academy of Pediatrics.
Kemon SM: Type A viral hepatitis: new development in an old disease, *N Engl J Med* 313:1059-67, 1985.
Robinson WS: Hepatitis A virus. *Principles and practices of infectious diseases,* ed 2, New York, 1985, Wiley and Sons.

Hepatitis B

Center for Disease Control: Recommendations for protection against viral hepatitis, *MMWR* 313-34, 1985.
Committee on Infectious Diseases, American Academy of Pediatrics: Hepatitis B. In Peter G, editor: *Report of the committee on infectious diseases,* ed 22, Elk Grove Village, Ill, 1991, American Academy of Pediatrics.
Go G, Baraff L, Schriger D: Management guidelines for health care workers exposed to blood and body fluids, *Ann Emerg Med* 20:1341-50, 1991.
Jaffe A, Kareta S: The prophylaxis of hepatitis B infection, *J Emerg Med* 4:487-95, 1986.
Romig D: Hepatitis B vaccination. In *Principles and practices of emergency medicine,* ed 3, 1992.

Hepatitis C

Center for Disease Control: Recommendations for protection against viral hepatitis, *MMWR* 34:333-4, 1985.
Committee on Infectious Diseases, American Academy of Pediatrics: Hepatitis C. In Peter G, editor: *Report of the committee on infectious diseases,* ed 22, Elk Grove Village, Ill, 1991, American Academy of Pediatrics.
Go G, Baraff L, Schriger D: Management guidelines for health care workers exposed to blood and body fluids, *Ann Emerg Med* 20:1341-50, 1991.

Measles

Aremillion D, Cranford G: Measles pneumonia in young adults, *Am J Med* 71:539-42, 1981.
Centers for Disease Control: Use of vaccines and immune globulins for persons with altered immunocompetence, *MMWR* 42:1-18, 1993.
Committee on Infectious Diseases, American Academy of Pediatrics: Measles. In Peter G, editor: *Report of the committee on infectious diseases,* ed 22, Elk Grove Village, Ill, 1991, American Academy of Pediatrics.

Varicella

Centers for Disease Control: Use of vaccines and immune globulins in persons with altered immunocompetence, *MMWR* 42:1-18, 1993.
Committee on Infectious Diseases, American Academy of Pediatrics: Varicella-zoster infections. In Peter G, editor: *Report of the committee on infectious diseases,* ed 22, Elk Grove Village, Ill, 1991, American Academy of Pediatrics.

Hockberger R, Rothstein R: Varicella pneumonia in adults: a spectrum of disease, *Ann Emerg Med* 15:931-4, 1986.

Sayre M, Lucid E: Management of varicella-zoster virus–exposed hospital employees, *Ann Emerg Med* 16:421-4, 1987.

Rh Isoimmunization

Bowman JM: Controversies in Rh prophylaxis. Who needs Rh immune globulin and when should it be given, *Am J Obstet Gynecol* 151:289-94, 1985.

Dayton VD et al: A case of Rh isoimmunization: should threatened first-trimester abortion be an indication for Rh immune globulin prophylaxis? *Am J Obstet Gynecol* 163:63-4, 1980.

Fisher M: Acute Rh isoimmunization following abdominal trauma associated with late abruptio placenta, *Acta Obstet Gynecol Scand* 68:657-9, 1989.

Grant J: Underutilization of Rh prophylaxis in the emergency department, *Ann Emerg Med* 22:868, 1993 (letter).

Grant J, Hyslop M: Underutilization of Rh prophylaxis in the emergency department: a retrospective survey. *Ann Emerg Med* 21:181-3, 1992.

Trauma

Ricardo Martinez, M.D., F.A.C.E.P.
Val Selivanov, M.D.

Trauma is the medical term for injury. Major trauma represents life- or limb-threatening severe injury. Energy transmission is the etiologic agent of trauma. Unlike other agents, such as bacteria or viruses, energy transmission occurs in an instant and the injuries are complete. From the time of injury, physiologic compensatory mechanisms attempt to maintain homeostasis.

In trauma care, time is at a premium. Care is directed at stabilizing identified injuries and returning the body to homeostasis. A multidisciplinary team approach is essential in the care of the major trauma victim. Each patient is considered to have multiple injuries until proven otherwise. Early surgical consultation and evaluation is essential for all major trauma patients with multisystem or abdominal trauma.

Pathophysiology

I. **Energy transmission** may cause disruption of bones, vessels, and organs producing fractures, lacerations, contusions, and disruption of organ systems. Hypovolemia is the major cause of shock in most major trauma victims, although spinal and septic shock may intervene.

II. **Specific compensatory mechanisms** are invoked in an attempt to maintain cardiac output and cellular perfusion.
   A. Activation of the sympathetic nervous system causes increased venous and arterial tone, bronchodilation, tachycardia, tachypnea, capillary shunting, and diaphoresis.
   B. Heart rate may increase. Cardiac output is equal to stroke volume times heart rate. As stroke volume falls, heart rate may increase.
   C. Respiratory rate increases. With inspiration, negative intrathoracic pressure is generated. This thoracic pumping action brings blood to the chest and preloads the right ventricle to maintain cardiac output.
   D. Urinary output decreases. Antidiuretic hormone and aldosterone are secreted to retain vascular fluid. A decreased glomerulofiltration rate contributes to this response.
   E. A decreased pulse pressure reflects a falling cardiac output (systolic) and increased vasoconstriction (diastolic). Normal pulse pressure is 35 to 40 mm Hg.
   F. Capillary shunting and transcapillary refill may cause cool, pale skin and dry mouth, respectively. Capillary refill may be delayed.
   G. Altered mental status and agitation may result from decreased perfusion to the brain or may be a direct result of head trauma.

Blunt versus Penetrating Trauma

I. **Penetrating trauma** results from a focal application of energy such that tissues are pierced or shattered. Gunshot wounds, knife wounds, and punctures are the most common examples of penetrating trauma. Single- or multiple-organ symptom injuries can occur depending on the path and depth of penetration. Low-velocity wounds from knives, and punctures from falls and assaults differ from high-velocity impacts such as gunshot wounds. The latter transmits shock waves that cause stretching and tearing of body tissue. Bullets may also fragment and ricochet, creating multiple paths.

II. **Blunt trauma** results when kinetic energy is absorbed either focally or diffusely. Falls from a height, motor vehicle impacts, and beatings are the most common mechanisms of blunt injury. Multisystem injury is common. Thorough repetitive evaluations are often necessary to identify all the injuries sustained.

Approach to the Trauma Patient

A systematic approach is necessary to identify and prioritize injuries and rapidly stabilize the patient. The American College of Surgeons advocates a four-phased approach to evaluating the trauma patient. This approach to trauma care is divided into a primary survey in which a quick assessment is done to check priority systems, and a secondary head-to-toe examination to identify all injuries. Occurring between the surveys is a resuscitative phase that initiates stabilization procedures. A final definitive care phase is directed toward providing definitive treatment for identified injuries.

I. **Primary survey.** The primary survey follows the mnemonic "ABCDE."

   A. *A*irway patency has the highest priority. In trauma patients, the most common cause of airway obstruction is an altered level of consciousness, allowing the tongue or other matter to block the posterior pharynx. Other causes of airway obstruction are massive swelling, foreign bodies, blood and secretions, and loss of bony support for soft tissue.

   1. **Clearing the airway** may be as simple as suctioning blood and debris or inserting a nasopharyngeal or oropharyngeal airway to lift the tongue out of the posterior pharynx. However, since cervical injury may be of concern in these patients, extension of the neck is contraindicated unless the cervical spine has been cleared of injury. Cervical spine immobilization is mandatory until clearance occurs.

   2. **A nasopharyngeal tube** may be inserted in the nares of patients who are conscious or have a gag reflex. An oropharyngeal airway may be placed in patients without a gag reflex. In either instance the appropriate-sized airway may be approximated by determining the distance from the aperture to the angle of the jaw.

   3. **If facial trauma,** massive bleeding, or swelling precludes establishing a secure airway, intubation is indicated. Orotracheal intubation is preferred in almost all situations. Patients with major facial or laryngeal trauma require surgical airways. Patients with laryngeal trauma may initially be seen with cough, dysphonia, hoarseness, stridor, hematemesis, hemoptysis, and dysphagia.

B. *Breathing* is the mechanics of ventilation. Consider breathing as dependent on anatomical structures below the larynx. Breathing is contingent on the integrity of three factors:
  1. **Neural supply**—phrenic nerve and brain stem. Consider head injury, neck trauma, and spinal injury.
  2. **The bony chest.** Consider the ribs, chest wall, costochondral junctions, and diaphragm. Flail segments and open wounds in the chest wall negate efforts to generate negative intrathoracic pressures. As wound size increases, air will preferentially flow through an opening in the chest wall rather than through the trachea. The diaphragm acts as a movable floor of the chest cavity. Disruption of the diaphragm can severely affect ventilation.
  3. **Chest contents.** Consider pulmonary injury and loss of integrity of the pleural sac. Air or blood in the pleural sac causes pneumothorax and hemothorax, respectively. Evacuation of the pleural sac with a chest tube is necessary to stabilize patients with respiratory compromise. Patients with pulmonary contusions require oxygenation and often need positive pressure ventilation. Herniation of abdominal contents into the thoracic cavity requires surgical intervention.

C. To access *Circulation* in the primary survey, palpation of pulses provides immediate information about the patient's circulatory status. Radial and carotid pulses should be palpated. Pulses are palpable at the following approximate systolic blood pressures: carotid artery, 60 mm Hg; artery, 70 mm Hg; brachial artery, 80 mm Hg; and radial artery, 90 mm Hg. Consider systolic blood pressures less than 90 mm Hg as evidence of shock.
  1. **Pulse** rate should be noted. Pulse rates greater than 120 beats/min represent approximately a 30% hemorrhage, and rates greater than 140 beats/min represent a loss of approximately 40% or more of blood volume. In these cases, the capillary refill time generally exceeds 2 seconds.
  2. **Obvious bleeding** should be controlled with direct pressure. Avoid ligatures in the uncontrolled setting because nerves frequently run alongside arteries and may be injured.

D. Assessing *Disability* requires continuous assessment of the neurologic status and is essential to identifying central nervous system injury. Prehospital care provider assessments can help in determining the patient's neurologic trend. The Glasgow Coma Scale **(Table 21-1)** is often used to score a patient's neurologic response.

A simple, readily repeatable scoring system describes the patient's level of consciousness as follows:

A - Alert
V - Verbal; responsive to verbal stimulus
P - Pain; responsive to painful stimuli
U - Unresponsive to painful stimuli
Note pupils for equality and reactivity to light.

E. *Expose* the patient completely to evaluate him/her for injury. The only way to diagnose the injury is to look for it. Do not forget the patient's back.

II. Resuscitative phase. After the primary survey, direct efforts toward resuscitation of the patient. If adequate personnel are available, this phase may be ongoing during the primary survey. The mnemonic for the resuscitative phase is "AEIOU."

Table 21-1. Glasgow Coma Scale

Criteria	Response	Score
Eyes opening	Opens eyes spontaneously	4
	Opens eyes to command	3
	Opens eyes to pain	2
	None	1
Best verbal response	Spontaneous and appropriate	5
	Confused	4
	Inappropriate words	3
	Incomprehensible sounds	2
	None	1
Best motor response	Obeys commands	6
	Localizes pain	5
	Withdraws from pain	4
	Abnormal flexion (decorticate posturing)	3
	Abnormal extension (decerebrate posturing)	2
	No response	1

A. *A*irway. The airway should be reevaluated. Definitive care with intubation will be necessary if conditions warrant. Patients with head trauma requiring hyperventilation and protection of the airway from aspiration may need intubation at this point.

B. *E*lectrocardiographic (ECG) monitoring identifies changes in heart rate, as well as signs of cardiac irritability and perfusion. These changes may occur despite normalization of blood pressure.

C. *I*ntravenous access is accomplished by the use of two large-bore peripheral intravenous lines. Resistance to flow is a function of length and is inversely proportional to the radius by the fourth power. Large-bore tubing is necessary to overcome this resistance and provide high flow. Peripheral catheters are short and over the needle. Central lines are usually longer and may have smaller internal diameters. For these reasons, central lines are usually reserved for monitoring purposes and should be placed on an elective basis to avoid complications. When peripheral access is unobtainable, large-bore cutdowns and femoral lines with large-bore catheters are preferable to subclavian or internal jugular lines. Crystalloid solution is usually given as Ringer's lactate. A 2 L bolus is given during the resuscitative phase. Patients who are only temporarily stabilized may have ongoing bleeding that needs operative intervention. Patients in whom no response is noted may need immediate operative intervention and blood replacement.

D. *O*xygen is given to all trauma patients to maintain hemoglobin saturation. Oxygen content is a function of saturation and the hemoglobin concentration. Hemoglobin levels are assumed to be falling in trauma patients until proven otherwise.

E. *U*rinary and nasogastric tubes are placed as both therapeutic and diagnostic adjuncts. A urinary catheter should be passed only after examination of the perineum for signs of injury (scrotal or labial hematoma, meatal blood), and a rectal examination is done in males to ensure that the prostate is in proper position. Urine flow should be at least 40 ml/hr. A drop in urine output may signify inadequate perfusion. Urine should be evaluated for the presence of hemoglobin and erythrocytes. Nasogastric tubes will decompress the stomach and decrease the risk of aspiration. Check the aspirate for blood and monitor for ongoing bleeding. Placing a nasogastric tube before performing a chest x-ray enhances the interpretation of the film (see Chest Injury, below).

III. **Secondary survey and definitive treatment.** The secondary survey evaluation of the patient proceeds in a head-to-toe manner to identify all possible injuries. The definitive treatment plan is formulated based on the injuries identified and their relative priorities. As a rule, injuries identified as needing rapid surgical intervention take priority over prolonged, detailed evaluation unless failure to diagnose a suspected injury would jeopardize a patient during the period of anesthesia.

   A. Head injury is the leading cause of trauma deaths. Intracranial injury may cause increased intracranial pressure (ICP), resulting in decreased cerebral perfusion, herniation, and death. The injured brain is extremely sensitive to hypoxia, hypercarbia, hypoglycemia, and hypotension. Early neurosurgical involvement in operative lesions is essential. The cervical spine must be assumed to be injured until proven otherwise, and cervical immobilization should be maintained until cervical spine injury is ruled out.

   1. **Evaluation.** Altered mental status may be the result of intoxication (drugs, alcohol), insufficient perfusion, or intracranial injury. Disability should be continually evaluated with the Glasgow Coma Scale or "AVPU" method. Signs of trauma to the head are usually present with intracranial injury because direct impact to the head is required. Battle's sign (hematoma at the mastoid area), hemotympanum, raccoon's eyes (bilateral black eyes), and cerebrospinal fluid (CSF) leak from the nose or auditory meatus are synonymous with basilar skull fracture. Focal neurologic deficits indicate surgical lesions. Posturing may occur from diffuse axonal injury or increased ICP. Bradycardia and hypertension (Cushing's sign) can occur in response to elevated ICP.

   2. **Radiographic evaluation** is best accomplished with computed tomography (CT) or magnetic resonance imaging (MRI). Noncontrast CT studies in trauma patients will identify most acute bleeding sites and are excellent for evaluating bone and sinuses. Performing an MRI is technically more difficult in many trauma patients. An MRI can evaluate blood flow but is less valuable for bone evaluation. Plain skull films are of little value since they do not demonstrate intracranial architecture.

   3. **Treatment** is directed to minimizing ICP and evacuating focal surgical lesions. Subdural, epidural, and intracerebral hematomas require immediate neurosurgical evaluation. The approach to reducing ICP should be discussed with the admitting physician when possible to ensure continuity of care. Treatment of intracranial pressure includes the following:

      a. **Intubation and hyperventilation** should occur only after a complete baseline neurologic examination is done. Hypocarbia decreases cerebral blood flow and decreases brain edema. Arterial carbon dioxide pressure ($PaCO_2$) should be maintained at 26 to 28 mm Hg. Too low a $PaCO_2$ can cause ischemia.

      b. **Mannitol,** 1 gm/kg, can be administered to cause diuresis and decrease brain edema. Care must be taken not to cause hypovolemia in the traumatized patient.

      c. **Monitor fluid administration.** Overhydration contributes to brain edema. Once hypotension is treated, reduce intravenous fluids to maintenance levels.

- **d. An ICP monitor** may be placed by a neurosurgeon directly through the dura. Cerebral perfusion pressure (CPP) can be calculated as follows: CPP = Mean arterial pressure (MAP) − ICP. Optimal ICP is below 15 mm Hg.
- **e. New therapies** such as high molecular weight dextromorphan and other N-methyl-D-aspartate (NMDA) inhibitors are under study and may soon be given in the early treatment of the head-injured patient to minimize ongoing cellular brain damage caused by propagation of glutaminergic acids.

B. Vertebral and spinal cord injuries can lead to lifelong disability. Early detection and evaluation are mandatory to minimize additional injury. Blunt trauma patients and patients with penetrating wounds that track near the spinal column are at risk for vertebral and spinal injury. In these patients, spinal column injury should be suspected and **immobilization maintained until physical or radiographic examination dictates otherwise.** Prehospital history regarding the mechanism of injury and the patient's condition may give clues to the underlying injury. Computed tomography scanning is useful in evaluating the relationship between vertebral injury and injury to the spinal cord. Obtain neurosurgical or orthopedic consultation as soon as vertebral injury, spinal cord injury, or both are suspected.

1. **Physical findings** suggestive of vertebral fracture are pain, swelling, crepitance, or deformity found on palpation of the vertebral column. Ecchymosis or deformity may be visible. Physical findings vary by dermatomal distribution of injury location. Sensation, motor, and propioception must all be tested. Diaphragmatic breathing, priapism, flaccid areflexia, loss of sensation, and paresis are indicative of spinal injury.

2. **Cervical spine injury** usually is associated with falls, motor vehicle impacts, and diving. Immobilization consists of an appropriately sized cervical collar, lateral supports, a spinal backboard, and stabilization of the head and chest. Awake, alert patients with no physical findings or cervical pain to palpation are candidates for clinical clearance. In all cases, a complete neurologic examination should be done and documented. Patients with an altered level of consciousness, severe multiple trauma, an abnormal neurologic examination, and those with other vertebral fractures require radiographic evaluation of all seven cervical vertebrae. At a minimum, lateral, odontoid, and anteroposterior (AP) radiographs are required. Additional views or CT scanning may be required for evaluation of suspicious lesions. Patients with real or suspected injury should be maintained in cervical immobilization until cleared. Other injuries may take priority over radiographic clearance.

3. **Thoracic spine injuries** are often associated with motorcycle and bicycle impacts in which the patient has been thrown forward and has landed on the base of the neck. Interscapular pain is common. Compression fractures are likely, but burst fractures may cause complete disruption and complete spinal injuries. Radiographic examination should be done on suspected injuries with the patient on a spinal backboard.

4. **Lumbar fractures** are also associated with motor vehicle impacts and falls. A vertebral body distraction fracture (Chance fracture) is associated with seat belt marks across the soft abdomen. Lumbar fractures can cause impingement on the cauda equina, with resultant neurologic findings. Small, stable anterior compression fractures heal with bed rest.

5. **Spinal cord injury** demands special attention. Neurosurgical consultation should be sought immediately. Care should be taken to minimize movement of unstable injuries and further damage the spinal cord. High cervical injuries demand attention to the patient's ventilatory status. Examination of the patient can determine whether a spinal injury is complete or incomplete. Incomplete injuries have sparing of some sensory or motor function and are associated with improved recovery. Therefore, a thorough neurologic examination is essential. Sacral sparing, anal wink, and bulbocavernosus reflexes should be noted. Once a spinal injury is identified, high-dose methylprednisolone therapy (30 mg/kg bolus, followed by an infusion of 5.4 mg/kg/hr for the next 24 hours) is associated with improved prognosis, but only if initiated within 8 hours of injury. Tirilozad is under investigation for use in spinal injuries but is not yet approved by the Food and Drug Administration (FDA).
6. **Spinal shock** can occur with spinal injuries above the T-6 cord segment. Spinal shock represents a loss of sympathetic tone. Physical findings include bradycardia, warm and dry skin from vasodilation, and hypotension. Systolic blood pressure of 80 to 90 mm Hg is acceptable, and the impulse to increase the heart rate or give massive amounts of fluid should be resisted. A lower blood pressure in the face of bradycardia can be treated with atropine, 0.5 to 1 mg given intravenously, with a maximum dose of 2 mg.

C. Chest injury can cause respiratory distress or massive hemorrhage. Approximately 90% of chest injuries can be managed without thoracotomy. Nonoperative management or simple placement of a chest tube is definitive treatment in 95% of chest injuries. Patients with blunt chest injury usually have associated extrathoracic injuries. The major initial working diagnostic and treatment categories of chest trauma are as follows:

1. **Chest wall crepitance** suggests a **rib fracture** and the potential for a pneumothorax. Tenderness may be elicited by direct or remote palpation. If no pneumothorax is noted on an initial chest radiograph, observation with a second radiograph in 4 to 6 hours is appropriate. Simple rib fractures can be treated with analgesia or intercostal nerve block in difficult cases. Older patients with rib fractures may require hospitalization and attention to pulmonary status until ventilation is unrestricted by pain. Patients requiring positive pressure ventilation must have a tube thoracostomy to prevent development of a tension pneumothorax.
2. **Pneumothorax, hemothorax, and hemopneumothorax** are secondary to entry of air, blood, or both into the pleural sac. Collapse of the lung is related to the loss of pleural space. Physical findings include decreased movement of the involved hemithorax, decreased breath sounds, and decreased tactile fremitus. Percussion elicits resonant sounds for pneumothorax and dull sounds for hemothorax. A small pneumothorax, hemothorax, or hemopneumothorax can be managed with serial observations. Most require large-bore chest tube insertion in the midaxillary line. If more than a liter of blood is returned or the subsequent output is more than 200 ml/hr, thoracotomy is indicated. Massive hemothorax may tamponade itself, and sudden vascular collapse will occur with insertion of a chest tube. These patients need aggressive volume resuscitation and urgent thoracotomy. Particulate matter aspirated by a chest tube and large air leaks are suggestive of esophageal rupture and may need radiographic imaging and surgical exploration.

3. **Tension pneumothorax** occurs when positive pressure builds up within the pleural space, causing a shift of the mediastinum, decreasing venous return, and resulting in hemodynamic compromise. Physical findings include tracheal shifting to the opposite side, jugular venous distention, respiratory distress, absence of breath sounds on the affected side, and a tympanic percussion note. Positive pressure ventilation from a bag-valve mask or from endotracheal ventilation is a common cause, though tension pneumothorax may occur in patients with pulmonary injury. Immediate needle decompression of the affected side of the chest is mandatory. A chest tube must be placed to prevent reoccurrence.
4. **Widened mediastinum** occurs with high-energy deceleration injury and is suggestive of **central great vessel and traumatic aortic dissection.** Physical findings and symptoms suggestive of traumatic aortic disruption are swelling at the base of the neck, bruits, pulse and blood pressure differentials between arms, dysphagia, and chest pain, especially radiating to the back or shoulder blades. Blood from thoracic spine injuries may cause a widened mediastinum on AP chest films. Blood distribution changes in the supine position; therefore an erect film is preferred. A mediastinal shadow greater than 6 cm at the T-4 level is considered wide. **Table 21-2** shows the six common radiographic findings of aortic arch disruption. If three or more findings are present, arch study is indicated. Angiography is the diagnostic modality of choice because CT findings are less sensitive and give less anatomic information. Coronary arteries can be visualized at the same time. Angiography should be used liberally with a ratio of nine negative per one positive arch study deemed appropriate utilization. Transesophageal Doppler ultrasound can be used to evaluate aortic arch integrity and anatomy, but is operator dependent.

    Treatment is surgical, but free bleeding in the peritoneum and pleural cavities, as well as neurosurgical evaluation and interventions, take precedence over performance of arch studies.
5. **Multiple rib fractures and flail chest segment** may compromise ventilation (see **Breathing II., B**). Diagnosis of free-floating flail segment is clinical, demonstrating a paradoxical movement to the rest of the chest. Initial treatment is supportive. Intubation (internal splinting) is required for proven hypoxia. Associated pulmonary injury often mandates intubation and tube thoracostomy placement.
6. **Pulmonary contusion** is identified as a hazy opacity or infiltrate on chest radiograph, usually segmental or lobar in distribution. This represents alveoli containing blood and is usually self-limited correcting with time. Hemoptysis may occur. Patients showing respiratory distress or hypoxia require intubation and positive pressure ventilation. Extrapleural hemor-

---

Table 21-2. Radiographic Signs of Potential Aortic Arch Disruption

Loss of aortic knob
Left pleural cap
Trachial deviation to right
Depressed left main stem bronchus
Loss of aorta pulmonary window
Deviation of nasogastric tube to right (2 mm to right of spinous process of T-4)

rhage from central, rib, or supraclavicular vessels may mimic these radiographic findings. Chest CT scan and angiography can distinguish extrapleural hemorrhage from pulmonary contusion. Chest CT scan often shows pleural laceration associated with pulmonary contusion.

7. **Cardiac contusion** is an overused diagnosis in patients with chest wall pain and is clinically important only in those patients with dysrhythmias, ectopy, or cardiac dysfunction during the initial phases of their evaluation. Serum levels of creatine phosphokinase **(CPK) and CPK-MB fraction, nuclear scans, and echocardiography do not correlate with autopsy studies.** Multisystem trauma and head injuries cause cardiac dysrhythmias, ectopy, and serum enzyme elevations unrelated to direct cardiac trauma. Patients with dysrhythmias should be treated accordingly. A Swan-Ganz catheter may be useful in optimizing fluid and inotropic support for true cardiac contusions.

8. **Cardiac tamponade** may be due to blunt or penetrating trauma. The prognosis is much better for penetrating trauma since the site of bleeding is usually focal. Cardiac tamponade depresses preload and causes hemodynamic compromise secondary to inadequate cardiac filling. Physical findings are hypotension, tachycardia, pulsus paradoxus, distended jugular veins, and muffled heart sounds. A rise in central venous pressures may aid in diagnosis and rule out hypovolemia. Intravenous infusion of crystalloid may improve cardiac output while preparing the patient for pericardiocentesis. Subxiphoid pericardiocentesis may be lifesaving but is a temporizing measure, and emergent thoracotomy is indicated. Large hemorrhage into the pericardial sac will overwhelm its thrombolytic system, resulting in clotted blood that cannot be aspirated.

9. **Gun shot wounds to chest.** Except for mediastinal traverse, most lateral gunshot wounds to the chest may be managed by chest tube placement and monitoring the rate of blood loss from the tube. The majority will not require thoracotomy. Ceftriaxone, 500 mg, or ampicillin-sulbactam, 3 gm, should be given intravenously in the emergency department.

10. **Mediastinal traverse with penetrating foreign body.** If a gunshot wound entry is on one side of the chest and the exit or foreign body is on the other side of the chest, a presumption of mediastinal crossing or penetration is made. This mandates adjunctive diagnostic studies such as subxiphoid pericardial window to rule in hemopericardium, an arch study, an esophogram, a lateral cross-table chest film, or occasionally a CT scan of the chest.

D. **Abdominal injuries.** Death from abdominal hemorrhage is a common cause of preventable death in trauma patients. In the emergency department, initial evaluation and treatment is not geared toward identification of a specific abdominal injury but rather toward determining whether a surgical intraabdominal injury exists. Patients who are unstable need rapid resuscitation and a chest and pelvic radiograph. If these are negative the active bleeding is assumed to be in the abdomen, and rapid surgical exploration is warranted. Patients that stabilize with initial resuscitation are candidates for further evaluation and possible nonoperative management. In the multiply injured patient, the ability to assess the abdomen by manual and visual examination is often limited. A CT scan and peritoneal lavage offer adjuncts to this evaluation.

1. **A CT scan** is preferred because of the gain in accuracy and specificity, allowing selective nonoperative management of stable patients with solid organ injuries. An abdominal CT scan can be done sequentially to CT of the

head if nonoperative cranial lesions are present. Indications for abdominal and pelvic CT scans are listed in **Table 21-3.** Oral contrast enhances identification of bowel integrity and is given before CT scanning, either orally or by nasogastric tube. Intravenous contrast should be given to visualize renal function. Presence of free fluid on CT scan with evidence of solid organ injury suggests perforation of a hollow viscus and is an indication for laparotomy. **Peritoneal lavage** is used when a patient needs other urgent surgical interventions (open fracture, emergency craniotomy or thoracotomy), and the presence of hemoperitoneum or intraperitoneal bacteria will alter the algorithm sequencing of operative procedures. After 1 L of normal saline or Ringer's lactate solution is infused into the peritoneum, the lavage fluid is siphoned back by gravity. The presence of $\geq 100,000$ erythrocytes/cm^3 (50,000 for penetrating injury), 500 leukocytes/cm^3, or bacteria on Gram stain of lavage fluid mandates simultaneous exploratory laparotomy in the case of craniotomy or thoracotomy, and delay of orthopedic procedures until intraabdominal injuries are controlled at laparotomy. Peritoneal lavage is useful in evaluating blunt trauma patients with abdominal pain and patients with penetrating injury but negative abdominal CT scans. Tears and lacerations of viscus organs will leak stool, sucus entericus, and bile and pancreatic fluids into the peritoneum. Gram stain can identify bacteria and fecal material, and should be done on all peritoneal lavage fluid.

2. **Plain films of the abdomen** add little information but may be used to determine the presence of free air or gastric distention.
3. **Physical findings** associated with intraabdominal injury include guarding, peritoneal signs, diffuse and focal tenderness, and nausea. Abdominal wall contusion and fractures of the lower ribs often make it difficult to examine the abdomen by palpation. Bowel sounds are unreliable. Lower rib fractures are associated with a spleen or liver injury 10% to 20% of the time. Seat belt marks across the soft abdomen are associated with intestinal injury, especially at the proximal jejunum, terminal ileum, and mesentery. Direct blunt trauma usually causes ruptures or tears of the solid organs. Rectal examination should be done, and stool checked for blood.
4. **Retroperitoneal bleeding** may come from bleeding of the aorta, vena cava, kidneys and ureters, pancreas, pelvic fractures, and retroperitoneal portions of the large and small intestine. Physical findings may be minimal, and peritoneal lavage may be negative. A CT scan will identify sig-

Table 21-3. Indications for Abdominal and Pelvic CT Scans*

Equivocal abdominal examination
Blunt trauma patient with closed head injury
Blunt trauma patient with spinal cord injury
Gross hematuria
Pelvic fractures, with or without suspected bleeding
Patient requiring serial examinations, but will be unavailable for physical examination for a prolonged period (i.e., orthopedic procedures, general anesthesia, etc.)
Patient with dulled or altered sensorium caused by toxic, metabolic, or psychiatric event

*CT scans are contraindicated in unstable patients.

nificant retroperitoneal bleeding. Flank pain and contusions are often late findings.
5. **Penetrating wounds.** Stab wounds differ from gunshot wounds in that stab wounds usually are low velocity and can be managed selectively. The evaluation is geared to early identification of either systemic symptoms of hemorrhage or the potential for peritonitis. Stab wounds are stratified by location.
    a. **Anterior abdominal wounds** are anterior to the anterior axillary line, below the costal margin, and above the inguinal ligament. In the absence of hypotension, peritonitis, or obvious evisceration, these wounds are explored locally under sterile technique. Liberal enlargement of the initial wound may be necessary to clearly visualize the wound depth to fascia. If fascia is penetrated (most often the rectus muscle anterior fascial sheath), the patient undergoes peritoneal lavage. If fascia is not penetrated, the wound is irrigated and closed, and the patient is a candidate for discharge. Local exploration is used only to determine anterior fascial penetration, not peritoneal penetration. *Under local anesthesia, it is cruel and difficult to determine peritoneal penetration with accuracy.*
    b. **Flank stabs** are between the anterior and posterior axillary lines, and the lower ribs to the iliac crests. These wounds are treated the same as anterior abdominal wounds; however, because of the retroperitoneal attachments of the ascending and descending colon, there is an added need for evaluation with a contrast enema and with an abdominal and/or pelvic CT scan.
    c. **Back stabs** are posterior to the posterior axillary lines. If there is no anterior abdominal tenderness and bowel sounds are present, back stabs are managed selectively, with nonoperative management initially. It is difficult to explore the deep muscles of the back locally. In the absence of peritonitis or external bleeding, patients with back stabs should be admitted for observation, unless the stabs are clearly seen to be superficial slashes. High-lumbar and low-thoracic right paravertebral stabs have the potential for causing posterior duodenal or hepatic injury. A CT scan can reveal these injuries, but they are easily missed. Admission for observation is advised.
    d. **Lower chest stabs** below the nipples in any locus—anterior, lateral, or posterior—carry potential for intrathoracic and intraabdominal injury. Because of the potential for transdiaphragmatic traverse, this area remains a diagnostic dilemma. Small diaphragm wounds may not bleed significantly and may not have caused significant subdiaphragmatic injury. However, the pressure gradient between the intraabdominal and pleural space may cause diaphragmatic wound enlargement and herniation of the stomach, omentum, or spleen. Interpreting peritoneal lavage results by using a low threshold for the erythrocyte count (e.g., 10,000/ml) may determine the need for laparotomy. Thoracoscopy may be useful to visualize the diaphragm.
    e. **Peristernal potential mediastinal wounds** are in the vicinity of the cardiac silhouette and the base of the neck in the suprasternal notch. Examine the patient for clinical signs of cardiac tamponade. Liberal use of central venous pressure monitoring and echocardiography is encouraged to diagnose cardiac tamponade early. Patients

with chest and parasternal stabs without initial evidence of hemopneumothorax or tamponade should be observed a minimum of 6 hours, and a chest radiograph should be repeated to detect occult or developing pneumothorax.

   6. **Gunshot wounds to the abdomen** are associated with high-energy transmission and have a very high incidence of serious injury. Compared with stab wounds, there is less room for selectivity and stratification in these higher energy injuries. Grazing wounds occur, but most gunshot wounds have a high potential to cause hemorrhage and perforation. Most gunshot wounds to the abdomen should be explored with laparotomy. Antibiotics providing coverage for gram-negative enteric organisms and anaerobes (ampicillin-sulbactam, 3 gm IV; or cefotetan, 2 gm IV) should be initiated in the emergency department.

E. **Peripheral vascular injury** usually occurs from a penetrating mechanism, but fractures and dislocations of the tibia and fibula, distal femur, or midshaft of the humerus not infrequently causes concomitant arterial vascular injury to the popliteal trifurcation, superficial common femoral artery, and radial artery, respectively. A distal pulse is present in up to 10% of transected major arteries due to collateral flow or transmission of the pulse across a clot. Pallor, pulselessness, paresthesias, paralysis, pain (ischemic), and poikilothermia are the six classic "P's" of peripheral vascular arterial injury. Except for paresthesias these are all considered "hard signs." If the extremity is cadaveric, exploration of the most likely injured vascular structure is indicated without benefit of arteriography. Another indication for immediate surgical exploration is a continued brisk external hemorrhage with a rapidly expanding hematoma. A machinery bruit is also an indication for surgery, with or without arteriography depending on the location of the bruit.

Without signs of rapid hemorrhage, a cadaveric extremity, or the presence of any of the above-mentioned "hard signs," arteriography is useful to identify the site of the lesion. Selective management of "minimal angiographic findings" is now practiced, and a vascular surgery consultation is indicated. If there are no "hard signs" and the injury is only in proximity to a major vascular structure, an angiogram is not needed emergently, but the patient's injury requires serial observation.

F. **Extremity injuries** are rarely life threatening but are a leading cause of long-term surgical intervention and disability for these patients. Initial treatment should consist of control of hemorrhage, evaluation of function and neurovascular status, and splinting. Direct pressure may decrease or stop obvious hemorrhage.

   1. **Physical findings** include obvious deformity, crepitance, loss of normal contours, shortening, rotation, angulation, and loss or decreased function beyond a wound. Injury to tendons can cause inability to extend or flex specific anatomical parts of the body. Neurovascular status can be evaluated by palpation of pulses, noting perfusion, color, and temperature, and testing for motor function and sensation.

   2. **Wounds** may be an obvious source of bleeding or cause an expanding hematoma. Distal neurovascular status and tendon function should be assessed. Wounds should be cleaned with copious irrigation and explored for foreign bodies before repair. Wounds in the vicinity of a fracture suggest an open fracture. Administer tetanus prophylaxis as indicated.

3. **Radiographic evaluation** of potential fractures should be used liberally. Failure to locate a fracture results in delayed treatment and the potential for the injury to worsen. Radiographs should include the joint above and below the fracture site.
4. **Fractures** should be aligned as best as possible and splinted to minimize further injury to neurovascular structures, as well as to decrease pain. Neurovascular status should be reassessed after splinting. In many instances, simply realigning the extremity will improve vascular status. Open fractures should be cultured and antibiotics given. Orthopedic consultation is mandatory.
5. **Dislocations and fracture-dislocations** should be relocated as soon as possible. Radiographs are essential to determine dislocation from fracture-dislocation. Both are associated with malalignment and may cause neurovascular injury and ischemic necrosis to overlying skin.
6. **Femur fractures** are associated with neurovascular compromise and may cause severe bleeding. Physical findings include external rotation and shortening of the lower leg, a firm expanding hematoma of the thigh, and thigh or hip pain. These fractures should be placed in a traction device and pulled out to length. Doing so may relieve thigh spasm, decrease bleeding at the fracture site, and improve neurovascular status.

G. **Renal and genitourinary injury.** Gross hematuria and blood at the urethral meatus are the two hallmarks of significant renal and genitourinary injury. Microscopic hematuria is ubiquitous in blunt trauma and has little clinical significance in the absence of flank pain.
1. **A urethral tear** is suspected if there is blood at the urethral meatus. Urethral tears are much more common in males and quite rare in females. A urethrogram must be performed before insertion of a urinary catheter is attempted. If the urethrogram is normal, then a urinary catheter is passed, and 400 ml of contrast media is instilled into the urinary bladder. The catheter is clamped and a cystogram is performed to determine **bladder extravasation**. At times it is difficult to distinguish free intraperitoneal bladder perforation from extraperitoneal extravasation of contrast media. A CT scan of the abdomen and pelvis with the catheter clamped is useful in this circumstance.
2. **Gross hematuria** on insertion of a urinary catheter, when no urethral meatal blood had been present, mandates an abdominal and pelvic CT scan with a clamped catheter. Intravenous contrast media will help evaluate kidney perfusion, ureteral integrity, and urinary bladder integrity (no extravasation from urinary bladder if intact). Renal arteriography, complete intravenous pyelogram (IVP), and single-image IVP to evaluate gross hematuria resulting from genitourinary trauma have been supplanted by abdominal and pelvic CT scan with intravenous and oral contrast media. Occasionally, to accommodate urgent laparotomy, a single-image IVP (50 ml renal contrast media given intravenously, followed by a plain film of the kidneys, ureters, and bladder (KUB) done at 2 minutes) done in the emergency department may give assurance that two perfused kidneys are present before laparotomy is begun.

H. **Pelvic injury** may be the source of major hemorrhage from vascular and bony structures into the retroperitoneal space. **Physical findings** include scrotal or labial hematoma, displaced prostate in males, and pain and instability on palpation of the iliac crests or pubis, or from inward compression of both iliac wings. Of major pelvic fractures, 5% are associated with urethral injury. In unconscious patients, a plain AP pelvis radiograph is advised. If fractures are noted and the patient is stable, an abdominal and pelvic CT scan will define the extent of fracture involvement and any retroperitoneal and extraperitoneal hemorrhage. Generally, crush injuries, symphysis diastasis, and iliac wing fractures are greater sources of bleeding than pubic rami fractures. Peritoneal lavage is often falsely positive but may be necessary in unstable patients to determine therapeutic options. Patients with **open pelvic fractures** or deep perineal lacerations may need a diverting colostomy performed. Therefore an exploratory laparotomy will be performed, obviating the need for peritoneal lavage. In females with severely displaced pubic rami fractures, a speculum examination of the vagina is essential to detect bony protrusion and lacerations, both of which constitute an "open pelvic fracture." Rectal contrast can augment CT evaluation of suspected left-sided colon injuries.

If **pelvic fractures** are suspected of causing significant ongoing extraperitoneal hemorrhage, early external fixator placement by an orthopedic surgeon may stop or slow the hemorrhage. If fixator placement is not effective, angiographic embolization is indicated for diagnosis and therapy.

I. **Perineal wounds and suspected rectal traverse wounds.** The extraperitoneal rectum is encased in the deep pelvis and pelvic floor musculature and is not easily evaluated for penetrating or blunt injury. The potential for devastating deep perineal muscle infections, both abscess and synergistic fasciitis, warrants a liberal use of diverting colostomy. In stable patients, anoscopy and sigmoidoscopy may determine the presence of a rectal injury, but they may be equivocal or impractical to perform in the face of proximity bleeding, an unstable pelvis, or long bone fractures. If anoscopy and sigmoidoscopy reveal blood or clots, the presumption of a rectal tear is made and diverting colostomy with presacral drainage is indicated. If rectal penetration is highly suspected but not definitively proven, a high index of suspicion is an indication for fecal diversion and presacral drainage.

J. **Blood component therapy** in the emergency department is based on patient requirements. For initial resuscitation of the trauma patient, type O ("universal donor") packed erythrocytes are used for patients who remain hypotensive, with signs of poor perfusion (i.e., decreased mental status, oliguria, cool skin with >3 seconds capillary refill) despite receiving at least 2 L of warm crystalloid infusion. In general, packed erythrocytes are given with the supposition that definitive operative therapy is available within the hour. It is counterproductive to aggressively transfuse packed erythrocytes with crystalloid simply to transiently increase intravascular volume and systolic blood pressure, which may increase the rate of hemorrhage and precipitate rapid vascular collapse with lethal arrhythmias. Considerable judgment must be exercised in balancing the need for transfusion with the need and availability of immediate operative therapy. When universal donor blood is unavailable, type O-positive blood may be given, but females should be given rhesus (Rh) prophylaxis. Type-specific and, when possible, cross-matched erythrocytes should be given to augment hemoglobin content of stable patients. Platelets and fresh frozen plasma are not indicated prophylactically, and platelets are rarely necessary. Infusion of fresh frozen plasma for the treatment of disseminated intravascular coagulation should be dictated by the results of coagulation studies.

K. Medications
  1. **Pain control** is contraindicated in patients with severe shock and significant closed head injuries. Lucid patients with milder injuries who have been examined and resuscitated need adequate analgesia. Small doses of intravenous morphine sulfate, 2 to 4 mg, may be used in monitored patients. Agitation is often due to hypoxia, pain, or both, and should be treated by ensuring adequate oxygenation and providing compassionate analgesia. Chemical restraint with muscle paralysis, though often needed to accomplish intubation, should not be used as first-line treatment of agitation. There should be a primary need for intubation, and muscle relaxants should only be used to facilitate intubation. Pain control for fractures and soft tissue injury may be accomplished with morphine sulfate, administered orally, intramuscularly, or intravenously; codeine, administered orally; or ketorolac (Toradol), 60 mg given intramuscularly. Elevation of extremity injuries minimizes the throbbing associated with vascular congestion and swelling. There is no indication for epidural analgesia in the emergency department, though temporary peripheral nerve blocks may be helpful to facilitate procedures and wound repair.
  2. **Antibiotics** are used in the emergency department for penetrating abdominal or chest trauma. A number of options should be considered for initial treatment **(Table 21-4)**. For blunt abdominal trauma with a sus-

Table 21-4. Empiric Antibiotic Therapy for Traumatic Emergencies

Penetrating Abdominal Trauma
Regimen 1   or   Regimen 2
  Ampicillin-sulbactam, 3 gm IV   Clindamycin, 600 mg IV q6h
  or   plus
  Cefoxitin, 1 gm IV   Gentamicin, 1.5 mg/kg IV q8h
  or
  Cefotetan, 1 gm IV
  +/−
  Gentamicin, 1.5 mg/kg IV q8h

Penetrating Chest Trauma
Cefoxitin, 1 gm IV
  or
Cefotetan, 1 gm IV

Penetrating Head and Neck Trauma
Ampicillin-sulbactam, 3 gm IV
  or
Cefazolin, 1 gm IV
  or
Clindamycin, 600 mg IV

Orthopedic Trauma
Cefazolin, 1 gm IV
  or
Vancomycin, 1 gm IV

Penetrating Soft Tissue Trauma
Cefazolin, 1 gm IV
  plus (in case of human, cat, or dog bites)
Amoxicillin-clavulanic acid, 500 mg PO TID × 14 days

pected perforated viscus, the same regimen (ampicillin/sulbactam, 3 gm IV; or cefotetan, 2 gm IV) is used. For large soft tissue destructive injuries, initial use of cefazolin, 1 to 2 gm given intravenously, is a safe initial regimen and should be followed by copious irrigation in the operating room with the jet lavage device with bacitracin, 50,000 units in 2 to 3 L of saline solution. Subsequent choices of antibiotics should await Gram stain and culture results. Tetanus prophylaxis is indicated for open fractures and tetanus-prone wounds.

Suggested Readings

Flancbaum L, Choban PS: Newer aspects of trauma care, *Surg Annu* 25:19-42, 1993.

Lacqua MJ, Sahdev P: Effective management of penetrating abdominal trauma, *Hosp Pract (Off Ed)* 28:31-32, 1993.

Maslanka AM: Scoring systems and triage from the field, *Emerg Med Clin North Am* 11:15-27, 1993.

Moran GJ, Talan DA: Hand infections, *Emerg Med Clin North Am* 11:601-619, 1993.

Mulder DS, Marelli D: The 1991 Fraser Gurd lecture: evolution of airway control in the management of injured patients, *J Trauma* 33:856-862, 1992.

Nichols RL et al: Prospective alterations in therapy for penetrating abdominal trauma, *Arch Surg* 128:55-63, 1993.

Pollack CV Jr: Prehospital fluid resuscitation of the trauma patient. An update on the controversies, *Emerg Med Clin North Am* 11:61-70, 1993.

Raimonde AJ, Rodriguez A: Priorities and diagnostic studies in the management of the injured patient, *Compr Ther* 18:27-32, 1992.

Schmidt J, Moore GP: Management of multiple trauma, *Emerg Med Clin North Am* 11:29-51, 1993.

Trunkey DD: Decision making in management of critically injured patients, *Surgery* 111:481-483, 1992.

22

Ear, Nose, and Throat Emergencies

H. Brian Goldman, M.D., A.B.E.M., M.C.F.P. (EM)
Patricia L. Johnson, B.Sc., M.D., C.C.F.P. (EM)

Emergencies of the ear, nose, and throat (ENT) are among the most commonly seen in the emergency department. Emergencies in this region run the gamut from life-threatening conditions such as upper airway obstruction and malignant otitis externa to less urgent disorders such as otitis media and allergic rhinitis. Emergency physicians must be well prepared to deal with both. Frequently they must act without the aid of consultants. Life-threatening emergencies often require intervention before the consultant can arrive; less urgent conditions may not warrant immediate consultation at all.

Otitis Externa

Otitis externa is also known as "swimmer's ear" because it often follows aquatic activities such as swimming and scuba diving. It is an infection of the external auditory canal that occurs if the integrity of the external auditory canal is breached. Common causes include immersion in water, high humidity, excessive dryness, preexisting eczema or psoriasis, benign and malignant growths, and foreign bodies such as cotton swabs and insects. The key symptom is intense and unremitting auricular pain of sudden onset. A rare variant of otitis media, known as malignant otitis externa, is often fatal if not treated aggressively. Malignant otitis generally occurs in elderly patients with suppressed immune function.

I. **Causative organisms.** The most common causative bacterial organisms are *Pseudomonas aeruginosa, Streptococcus pyogenes,* and *Staphylococcus aureus* (see **Table 22-1**). Fungal organisms that cause otitis externa include *Aspergillus* and *Candida albicans.* Herpes zoster oticus (Ramsay Hunt syndrome) is a rare cause of otitis externa.

II. **Clinical presentation**
   A. History
      1. **Otitis externa.** Patients usually complain of a mild itch or dull ache that often progresses to severe pain over hours to days. There may be muffled hearing because of swelling of the external auditory canal, as well as a watery discharge.
      2. **Malignant otitis externa.** The course may be insidious, beginning with dermatitis of the external canal, and progressing to cellulitis, chondritis, osteitis, and osteomyelitis of the temporal bone and skull base. Complications include meningitis, multiple cranial nerve palsies, and sphenoidal sinusitis. Elderly patients initially seen with a history of auricular pain and fever should be asked about a history of insulin-dependent diabetes mellitus and other causes of a suppressed immune state.

Table 22-1. Causative Organisms in ENT Infections

Disease	Bacterial	Viral	Fungal
Otitis externa	P. aeruginosa P. mirabilis S. aureus S. pneumoniae	Herpes zoster	Aspergillus Candida
Otitis media	S. pneumoniae (30%-60%) H. influenzae (20%-30%) Moraxella (Branhamella) catarrhalis (8%-18%) S. pyogenes—group A (4%-8%) S. aureus (1%-2%) S. epidermidis (1%-2%)		

- **B. Physical examination.** Unlike otitis media, otitis externa does not usually begin with an upper respiratory tract infection. The external auditory canal is swollen, erythematous, and tender. There is often debris present in the canal that can be removed with gentle suction. Movement of the auricle causes exquisite pain. This is a key finding that distinguishes otitis externa from otitis media. Unlike otitis media, the tympanic membrane is not erythematous. The preauricular lymph nodes may also be swollen and tender. Low-grade fever occasionally occurs in otitis externa. Patients with malignant otitis externa initially have high fevers and a toxic appearance.
- **C. Laboratory aids.** Laboratory tests are not usually necessary to make the diagnosis of otitis externa. Auricular discharge can be Gram-stained and cultured to determine the causative organism. Patients with suspected malignant otitis externa should have blood drawn for glucose levels, complete blood cell counts (CBCs), and blood cultures.

III. **Management.** Because the condition is both difficult to eradicate and often recurrent, all patients with otitis externa should be treated with aggressive topical therapy. Oral antibiotics are reserved for patients with systemic signs and symptoms. The specific therapy for malignant otitis externa is discussed below.
- **A. Patient instructions.** Patients should be encouraged to keep the external canal dry and to avoid inserting any objects such as cotton swabs into the canal. Patients should be advised to keep water out of the ear for 2 to 3 weeks and not to swim for 4 to 6 weeks.
- **B. Clean the external auditory canal** under direct vision with gentle suction and a small cotton swab.
- **C. Antibiotic therapy**
    1. **First-line therapy.** Topical antibiotic therapy is the treatment of choice. Since the causative organisms are *P. aeruginosa, S. pyogenes,* and *S. aureus,* specific topical antibiotics of choice include a combination of polymixin B and either neomycin or colistin. Combining a mild corticosteroid such as hydrocortisone treats the inflammation, as well as the infection. A combination antibiotic-corticosteroid drop is usually effective if used three or four times a day for 10 days. Initial agents of choice include Cortisporin Otic Solution, Cortisporin Otic Suspension, and VoSol HC Otic Solution.
    2. **Second-line therapy.** Patients who do not respond to first-line therapy may have a concomitant fungal infection; this is often the case with patients who have recurrent otitis externa.

a. **Ear wick.** In some patients the canal is so swollen that the introduction of a strip of gauze or a hydroxycellulose wick soaked in the antibiotic solution of choice is necessary. These facilitate distribution of the solution and can usually be removed in 3 or 4 days.
  b. Patients who do not respond to first-line antibiotic therapy should be switched to a more potent antibiotic and corticosteroid combination. A good second-line agent is the combination of clioquinol (which is both antifungal and antibacterial) and flumethasone, a fluorinated corticosteroid. The combination is contained in Locacorten Vioform, and the dosage is 2 to 3 drops twice a day.
D. **Analgesics.** It is all too common for emergency physicians to underestimate the degree of pain caused by otitis externa. This disorder should be regarded as causing moderate to severe pain. Thus pain should be managed with a potent oral analgesic such as acetaminophen with codeine 30 mg, oxycodone, naproxen, ketorolac, or floctafenine.
E. **Oral antibiotics.** Oral antibiotics are not usually required for otitis externa. However, they are indicated in two particular circumstances. First, oral antibiotics should be started if the patient has a fever or is systemically ill. Second, it should be appreciated that otitis media and otitis externa can sometimes coexist. Moreover, the external canal may be so occluded that the external auditory canal cannot be visualized. If there is a possibility that the patient has a coincident otitis media, then oral antibiotics should be started. The antibiotic of choice depends on the organism involved. The treatment of otitis media is described elsewhere in this chapter. If the diagnosis is otitis externa and antibiotics are prescribed because the patient is somewhat febrile, then the choice of antibiotics depends on the suspected organism. The antibiotics of choice for staphylococcus and streptococcus are a first-generation cephalosporin such as cephalexin or cloxacillin with or without penicillin. If the suspected organism is *Pseudomonas,* then the oral antibiotic of choice is ciprofloxacin, 250 to 750 mg PO BID. A Gram stain of the exudate from the ear may help determine the causative organism.
F. Malignant otitis externa
  1. **Patients with fever** and toxic appearance should be admitted to the hospital. The primary causative agent in malignant otitis media is *P. aeruginosa.* Initiate intravenous antibiotic therapy with either of the following four choices.
  2. **Therapy.** Therapy must be continued for several weeks and surgical debridement may be necessary.
     a. ticarcillin or carbenicillin plus an aminoglycoside.
     b. ceftazidime 1 to 2 gm IV q8h
     c. aztreonam 1 to 2 gm IV q8 to 12h
     d. ciprofloxacin 1 gm PO q12h (can be used in lieu of IV medication)

Herpes Zoster Oticus (Ramsay Hunt Syndrome)

This condition is uncommon but can mimic severe otitis externa. It is due to recurrence of varicella zoster infection along the distribution of cranial nerve VIII. Associated symptoms may include facial paralysis, hearing loss, or balance problems. Tiny vesicles may appear on the concha, face, or ear canal. Mild cases require observation only. In severe cases, such as those patients with underlying immunosuppression or facial nerve paralysis, treatment with acyclovir should be instituted. The dosage is 800 mg five times daily for 10 days. For intravenous use, 5 mg/kg is infused over 1 hour every 8 hours; this dosage should be adjusted for abnormal renal function.

Otomycosis

Otomycosis is a fungal infection of the external auditory canal that usually occurs in patients with chronic or recurrent bacterial otitis externa. High humidity is another predisposing factor.

I. **Causative organisms.** Otomycosis is usually caused by *Aspergillus* or *Candida*.
II. **Clinical presentation.** Most patients have auricular pain, as well as scaling in the external auditory canal. The diagnosis is confirmed by obtaining scrapings from the external canal, which are then dissolved in potassium hydroxide (KOH) solution and examined for fungal filaments under a microscope.
III. **Management.** Remove all debris from the external canal. Then administer a 2% acetic acid otic solution (five drops four times a day) or a solution containing equal parts vinegar and isopropyl alcohol three or four times a day for 14 days. Gentian violet and tolnaftate solutions are also acceptable alternatives, as are antibiotic preparations mentioned above.

Furunculosis

I. **Definition.** Furunculosis is an infection of the pilosebaceous follicles that sometimes occurs in the ear and may be mistaken for otitis externa. It causes intermittent sharp pain in the ear. It can sometimes progress to occlusion of the canal, causing muffled hearing and postaural swelling. *Staphylococcus aureus* is the most common cause.
II. **Management.** Warm compresses help promote spontaneous drainage. Incision and drainage may be necessary. Topical antibiotics are not useful. However, systemic antibiotics such as cloxacillin or cephalexin should be employed if the patient has systemic signs or if cellulitis appears to be present.

Impacted Cerumen

I. Patients with impacted cerumen complain of a conductive **hearing loss.** The problem is compounded by the use of cotton swabs that push the wax deeper, causing further irritation. There may be secondary infection.
II. **Management.** The wax must be removed. This is made easier by prior softening, which can be accomplished by instilling either mineral oil or a commercially available cerumenolytic such as Cerumenex. The wax is then removed by irrigating the canal with a syringe filled with tepid water. Alternatively, suction or gentle curettage under direct vision may be used. After removing the cerumen, the tympanic membrane is examined for perforations.

Barotitis

I. **Pathogenesis and clinical presentation.** Barotitis arises when the tympanic membrane is stretched due to a change in air pressure without a change in middle ear pressure. This can occur during air travel, scuba diving, and high-altitude activities. Water skiers may also have barotrauma if they fall into the water at high speeds, resulting in pressure being applied to the eardrum. Patients have mild to excruciating auralgia. Hearing loss, tinnitus, and vertigo may also be present. On examination, the tympanic membrane is usually red but may change to a deep blue or yellow color.

II. Management. Resolution is often spontaneous, within hours. If symptoms persist, a systemic decongestant such as pseudoephedrine may be prescribed.

Otitis Media

Otitis media is an acute suppurative infection of the middle ear. It is the most common diagnosis in childhood, accounting for one third of all office visits in children younger than 5 years. The peak incidence of otitis media is between 6 months and 3 years of age; a second peak occurs in children aged 4 to 7 years.

I. Etiology and pathogenesis. Acute otitis media is characterized by inflammation and accumulation of infected exudate in the middle ear. It usually occurs because of a dysfunctional eustachian tube, due either to abnormal patency or frank obstruction. It is usually preceded by a viral infection of the nasopharynx. The viruses associated with acute otitis media include adenovirus, influenza, and respiratory syncytial virus.

   A. Acute suppurative otitis media is most commonly caused by bacteria; it is rarely caused by viral infection. *Streptococcus pneumoniae* continues to be the most common pathogen, followed by *H. influenzae* and *B. catarrhalis.*

   B. Recurrences of otitis media are common. Risk factors for recurrence include a family history of otitis media, parental smoking, large family size, attendance at day-care centers, and low socioeconomic status.

II. Clinical presentation

   A. History. The presentation of otitis media varies with the age of the patient. Preverbal children may have nonspecific symptoms such as fever, irritability, anorexia, vomiting, and diarrhea. Older children and adults usually complain of pain or pressure sensation in the ear, temporomandibular joint, or throat. Other symptoms in this age group include nausea, heaviness in the head, and discharge from the ear. A preceding upper respiratory tract infection is common.

   B. Physical examination. On physical examination, fever is a common finding; the temperature can be as high as 40.5° C. The tympanic membrane appears dull, bulging, and erythematous. The ossicles may be obscured by the swelling. Mobility of the tympanic membrane is reduced when examined by pneumatic otoscopy; note that this finding is seldom present in adults. Fluid may be visible through the membrane.

   C. Laboratory. Tympanometry may show a flat tracing indicating effusion. Audiometry may disclose a conductive hearing loss. If the tympanic membrane is perforated, then an exudate may be present in the external auditory canal, which can be Gram-stained and cultured to determine the causative organism.

III. Management. The mainstay of treatment in acute otitis media is antibiotic therapy. Supportive therapy, including effective management of pain, is another important priority.

   A. Antibiotic therapy. Acute otitis media requires systemic antibiotic therapy; unless otitis externa is present, topical antibiotics have no role in this condition. The choice of antibiotic is a function of the causative organism. Because the bacteria is seldom identified, the choice of antibiotic is usually empiric.

The most common causative organisms are *S. pneumoniae, H. influenzae,* and *B. catarrhalis.* The in vitro sensitivities are shown in **Table 22-2.**

1. **Antibiotics of choice.** The selection of an appropriate antibiotic depends on the patient's history of past infections, a history of allergy to antibiotics, and the incidence of β-lactamase–producing strains of *H. influenzae* and *B. catarrhalis* that are found in the community where the patient lives. Until recently, amoxicillin or ampicillin has been the drug of choice for patients not allergic to penicillin; trimethoprim/sulfamethoxazole has been the drug of choice for patients allergic to penicillin. However, the emergence of β-lactamase–producing strains of both *H. influenzae* and *B. catarrhalis* has meant that such organisms are resistant to amoxicillin and ampicillin. Resistance levels depend on the community; some areas now report an incidence of β-lactamase–producing *H. influenzae* of more than 30%.

   a. **A consensus** is now emerging on the choice of antibiotics. If the incidence of β-lactamase resistance is 20% or less, amoxicillin (40 mg/kg/day divided TID) remains the antibiotic of choice for patients with acute otitis media. If the incidence of resistance is greater than 30%, then the drugs of choice are cefaclor (20 to 40 mg/kg/d divided TID) or amoxicillin/clavulanate (40 mg/kg/d and 10 mg/kg/d respectively, divided TID).

   b. Patients with a suspected **β-lactamase–producing strain** who are allergic to penicillin may receive either the combination of erythromycin and sulfisoxazole (50 and 150 mg/kg/day divided QID) or trimethoprim/sulfamethoxazole (see above).

   c. **New antibiotics** such as cefuroxime and cefixime are also available for the treatment of otitis media. However, they are more expensive without providing substantial benefits over conventional agents. At present, these agents should be reserved for patients who do not respond to standard therapy.

2. **Duration of therapy.** The duration of therapy is still controversial. Although most authors recommend a 10-day course of antibiotics, up to 90% of patients respond to 5 days of therapy. Overall, 90% of patients with acute otitis media respond to initial therapy.

Table 22-2. In Vitro Sensitivities of Organisms Causing Acute Otitis Media

Antibiotic	*S. pneumoniae*	*H. influenzae* β-*lactamase* +	*H. influenzae* β-*lactamase* −	*B. catarrhalis* β-*lactamase* +	*B. catarrhalis* β-*lactamase* −	Group A streptococci
Ampicillin	+	−	+	−	+	+
Penicillin V	+	−	+	−	+	+
Cefaclor	+	+	+	+/−	+	+
Erythromycin	+	−	−	+	+	+
Trimethoprim/ sulfamethoxazole	+	+	+	+	+	−
Amoxicillin/ clavulanate	+	+	+	+	+	+

3. **Close follow-up.** Infants and children with acute otitis media should be seen by their physicians within 48 hours of beginning antibiotics. Patients who do not respond to antibiotics after 48 hours of therapy (decreased fever and pain) should be switched to another antibiotic. If such patients were initially given amoxicillin, then switching to cefaclor would be appropriate. Newer antibiotics such as cefuroxime and cefixime appear promising and are indicated for treatment failures or documented resistance.
    a. Patients who have deteriorated are at risk for developing the complications of **otitis media** such as meningitis, mastoiditis, brain abscess, cavernous sinus thrombosis, and facial nerve paralysis.
    b. Such patients may be suffering from less common causes of otitis media such as *P. aeruginosa* or *S. aureus*. In such cases, patients should be admitted to the hospital and given intravenous antibiotics, pending the outcome of blood cultures and other studies.
4. **Recurrent otitis media.** This condition is present in any child who has six or more episodes of otitis media by 6 years of age, as well as any child who has three or more episodes within a 6-month period. Studies have shown that such patients should be given chemoprophylaxis with one of the following three regimens for 3 to 4 months each:
    a. Amoxicillin 20 mg/kg qd.
    b. Sulfisoxazole 50 mg/kg qd.
    c. Trimethoprim/sulfamethoxazole 4 mg/kg qd.
5. **Chronic otitis media with effusion (COME).** This entity can bedevil emergency physicians. By definition, COME consists of an effusion after an attack of acute otitis media that lasts more than 3 months. In most children, the effusion associated with acute otitis media disappears within 1 month of onset. In 10% of cases, the effusion persists for more than 3 months. There is growing concern that children with COME are prone to develop hearing loss.

    Antihistamines and decongestants are commonly prescribed but appear to be of no value. Treatment with amoxicillin is marginally effective. Although steroids alone have not been shown to be effective, it appears that the combination of prednisone (0.5 to 1.0 mg/kg/day) along with trimethoprim/sulfamethoxazole (5 mg/kg/dose BID) for 30 days is 70% effective in resolving COME.

B. **Supportive care.** Pain is a common complaint in otitis media. Pain control is described elsewhere in the Manual. Until antibiotic therapy begins to work, severe pain should be expected. Patients with severe auralgia who do not respond to acetaminophen often require oral narcotics such as codeine. In addition, the instillation of two to five drops of a 5% solution of topical cocaine onto the affected tympanic membrane is often quite efficacious. Patients with acute otitis media may require acetaminophen for the control of fever.

Vertigo

Vertigo is defined as the sensation of motion without actual movement. Vertigo often has a spinning or hurtling quality. Patients perceive that either they or the environment is moving. Many patients complain of dizziness, and it is important to differentiate between this and true vertigo.

I. Etiology and classification

A. Causes. Approximately 85% of patients with vertigo have peripheral vestibular disorders, while the rest have a central nervous system (CNS) disorder. The causes of peripheral vertigo include Meniere's disease, trauma, infection, drugs, otosclerosis, paroxysmal positional vertigo, and syphilitic vestibular dysfunction.

B. Clinical features. The critical determination to make is whether the vertigo is peripheral or central in origin. In general, peripheral vertigo tends to have a benign cause; most patients with peripheral vertigo may be investigated as outpatients. Central vertigo points toward severe CNS pathology such as brain stem tumors, vertebrobasilar insufficiency, and cerebellar disorders. Such patients require urgent diagnostic imaging of the CNS, as well as referral to a neurologist or neurosurgeon. The features that distinguish peripheral from central vertigo are described in **Table 22-3**.

II. Peripheral vertigo

A. Meniere's disease. This disorder primarily affects adults and may be bilateral in 50% of cases. The cause appears to be multifactorial inheritance and results in endolymphatic hydrops. It consists of a triad of vertigo, tinnitus, and hearing loss. The vertigo usually persists for 3 to 6 hours and may be accompanied by nausea and vomiting. The tinnitus is described as a low-pitched roaring that reaches a peak just before an attack. The hearing loss is unilateral and is worse just before an attack. Although hearing typically returns to normal after an attack, some patients with long-standing disease may have permanent deafness of varying severity. During an acute attack there may be a transient spontaneous nystagmus. Gait is unsteady, and the patients veer toward the affected ear.

1. Diagnosis. Meniere's disease is usually diagnosed clinically. Audiometry usually demonstrates a low-frequency hearing loss. Other tests include the glycerol test, caloric stimulation test, and the short increment sensitivity index (SISI) test. Magnetic resonance imaging may be considered to rule out an acoustic neuroma. Patients with frequent attacks or disabling symptoms should be referred to an otolaryngologist for definitive management.

2. Treatment

a. Diazepam 2 to 10 mg IV by slow push, followed by 2 to 10 mg PO q8h p.r.n.

Table 22-3. Peripheral versus Central Vertigo

	Peripheral	Central
Onset	Sudden, explosive	Slow
Pattern	Paroxysmal, intermittent	Constant
Fatigues with provocative testing	Yes	No
Duration	Hours	Days-months
Nystagmus	Horizontal; fatigues; fast	Vertical; doesn't fatigue; slow
Hearing loss	Yes	No
Tinnitus	Yes	No
Abnormal tympanic membrane	Often	No
CNS abnormalities	No	Yes

b. Diphenhydramine 25 to 50 mg PO or IM q6-8h p.r.n. (Benadryl is an effective antinausea drug.)
   c. Meclizine hydrochloride 25 mg PO q8-12h is also effective. However, the nicotinic acid contained in meclizine may provoke facial flushing.
B. **Trauma.** Trauma may occur to the labyrinth because of a temporal bone fracture, a blow to the head, or a flexion-extension (whiplash) injury. After treatment of associated injuries, the dizziness will respond to symptomatic treatment and gradually improve over 1 year. A fistula may develop between the inner and middle ear because of a direct blow, secondary to coughing or straining, or from an idiopathic cause. Hearing loss may accompany the vertigo. Spontaneous resolution may occur, but surgery is indicated if this does not occur.
C. **Viral infections.** Viral infections may cause vertigo either through involvement of the ganglion of the vestibular nerve or the labyrinth. The presentation of vestibular neuronitis and labyrinthitis is similar and consists of intermittent vertigo without hearing loss. Spontaneous resolution within weeks or months is the rule. In some cases of otitis media a toxic labyrinthitis may develop, resulting in vertigo. This will clear with the infection. The same may occur in chronic otitis media, or a fistula between the middle ear and labyrinth can occur; the latter should be suspected in patients with a cholesteatoma and vertigo.
D. **Drugs.** Drugs may be a cause of vertigo. The offending agents include aminoglycoside antibiotics, acetylsalicylic acid (ASA), nitrogen mustard, or cisplatin. These drugs should be discontinued if possible; resolution of vertigo is often complete.
E. **Paroxysmal positional vertigo.** This is thought to occur when otoliths impinge on the posterior canal cristae. With positioning of the head, nystagmus will usually occur toward the ear placed down. Resolution is usually spontaneous within 6 to 12 months.

III. **Central vertigo.** Central nervous system causes of vertigo are less common but more serious. They include multiple sclerosis, cerebellopontine-angle tumors, epilepsy, vascular accidents, migraine headache, and basilar artery insufficiency. After a complete history and physical examination is completed, paying special attention to the otologic and neurologic systems, a referral to an otolaryngologist may be necessary for a definitive diagnosis. For the majority of patients treatment is supportive and multifactorial. Admission need only be considered in those with severe symptoms. For mild symptoms dimenhydrinate, 50 to 100 mg IM or PO every 4 hours, or meclizine hydrochloride (HCL), 25 to 50 mg twice a day may be used. For more severe symptoms promethazine HCL, 25 to 50 mg PO every 6 to 8 hours, or diazepam, 5 to 10 mg every 6 hours is effective. In Meniere's disease salt restriction to 1 g/day, along with a diuretic such as hydrochlorothiazide-triamterene may be effective.

Sinusitis

I. **Clinical presentation.** This common disorder typically presents with headache, facial pain, nasal obstruction, and rhinorrhea. Children may simply have generalized irritability. The pain is exacerbated by changes in position, straining, or barometric pressure changes. Fever and chills are uncommon. Mucopurulent nasal discharge may be present, but their absence does not preclude the diagnosis because inspissation can prevent drainage. On examination there may be tenderness over the involved sinus, eyelid and medial canthus edema, inability to transilluminate the sinus, erythema of the mucosa of the turbinates, and conjunctivitis. In immunosuppressed patients, fungal infections may cause a fulminant infection with fever, altered mental status, a black discoloration of the nasal mucosa and nasal discharge and metabolic derangement.

II. **Etiology.** The most common organisms are *S. pneumoniae, H. influenzae, B. catarrhalis,* and *Bacteroides.* Anaerobic organisms are found commonly in chronic infections, and gram-negative organisms are normally found in hospital-acquired sinusitis. *Aspergillus* may be invasive or noninvasive.

III. **Diagnostic studies.** Radiographs show involvement of the maxillary and frontal sinuses but may not identify cases despite symptoms and signs. Computerized tomography (CT) or magnetic resonance imaging (MRI) is better at delineating the mucosa and soft tissue masses within the sinuses.

IV. **Treatment.** Initial treatment aims to restore normal aeration of the sinuses. Antibiotics are efficacious. First-line treatment includes amoxicillin, 500 mg TID; amoxicillin/clavulanic acid, 500 mg/125 mg TID; azithromycin; clarithromycin; trimethoprim/sulfamethoxazole, 160 mg/800 mg BID; cefaclor, 500 mg TID; and erythromycin, 250 mg QID. These should be continued for 10 days in acute cases and longer for recurrent or chronic sinusitis. Saline nasal sprays help to liquefy secretions. Phenylpropanolamine orally can increase the diameter of the maxillary opening and therefore aid in promoting drainage.

Mastoiditis

Mastoiditis as a clinical entity has declined since the advent of antibiotics for the treatment of suppurative otitis media. The symptoms include otalgia, retroauricular swelling or erythema, protrusion of the auricle, and otorrhea. Mastoiditis is often complicated by a subperiosteal abscess. Although mastoiditis is recognized as a complication of otitis media, the organisms responsible differ in that *H. influenzae* is rarely isolated. Recommended treatment includes intravenous antibiotics for 48 hours if a subperiosteal abscess of the CNS is not present. The combination of amoxicillin and clavulanic acid is a good choice after initial IV therapy. If clinical improvement is not apparent in 2 days or if a subperiosteal abscess is present, then surgery is indicated. In addition, myringotomy and insertion of ventilation tubes in children with otitis media with effusion should be considered.

Parotitis

Parotitis is an inflammation of the parotid gland that can result from a number of causes. Infectious parotitis can be caused by viruses, of which mumps is the prototype. Other viruses that cause parotitis include parainfluenza type 3A, coxsackievirus, and influenza type B. The swelling may be unilateral or bilateral, and there are usually associated findings of fever, chills, and malaise. The gland is tender to palpation, and there is clear saliva expressed from Stensen's duct. Bacterial parotitis is usually caused by *S. aureus* and is most often unilateral, occurring after surgery in debilitated patients or premature newborns. The gland is warm, hard, and very tender with erythema of the overlying skin. Purulent material may be expressed from Stensen's duct. Some drugs such as iodine, phenylguatazone, athiouracil, and guanethidine can also cause a bilateral enlargement without associated symptoms. Tumors, cysts, and obstruction caused by stones or strictures usually result in swelling that progresses more slowly than with infectious causes. Treatment of mumps is symptomatic, consisting of analgesics and hot or cold packs to help ease the discomfort. Bacterial parotitis should be treated with hydration, attention to oral hygiene, and antibiotics active against penicillinase-producing staphylococci, such as cloxacillin, 500 mg four times a day orally, or methicillin or cephalexin parenterally. Vancomycin may be used in penicillin-allergic patients. Surgical drainage is rarely necessary.

Foreign Bodies in the Ear

This is a common presenting complaint, especially in children who are naturally curious. Most adults can give a history of the type of foreign body and the duration it has been present; however, this is not always true in children. Sudden pain, ear fullness, and altered hearing are all symptoms of a foreign body. The removal usually employs one of three methods: irrigation, suction, or instrumentation. The former can use water, saline solution, or alcohol. Some advocate a solution of isopropyl alcohol and water when trying to remove organic foreign bodies, since this may cause less swelling. Devices include a standard 20 ml syringe with an 18-gauge Silastic catheter, a commercially available ear syringe, or a Water Pik. The stream should be directed around the edge of the foreign body to force it out with back pressure. Wall suction may be attached to an instrument that is smaller than the diameter of the canal. These include Frazier suction tubes or sections of intravenous tubing. For foreign bodies that are impacted or associated with edema, removal with instrumentation under direct visualization is usually the best method. For irregular objects, fine tissue forceps or alligator forceps can be used. For smooth or spherical objects, an instrument that can be passed behind it and used to pull it out is more useful. These include right angle hooks, ear curettes, and shin hooks. Insects need to be killed first by using 2% lidocaine solution or mineral oil. The former may have an advantage in that retrieval is easier from an aqueous solution. The canal should be inspected after removal of the foreign body for tympanic membrane perforation, canal abrasion, or bleeding. Otitis externa should be treated appropriately. Perforation warrants referral, as does failure to remove the foreign body.

Oral Candidiasis

I. **Clinical presentation.** This disorder can present as an acute or chronic infection. Acute pseudomembranous candidiasis is more common, and patients initially have diminished taste and a burning sensation and sensitivity to foods that are spicy or acidic. On examination there are white, curd-like lesions that are easily scraped off, leaving an erythematous base that bleeds. In the chronic form, generalized burning is often the only complaint. There is diffuse redness of the oral cavity, and the lips and commissures may also be affected. There is usually a history of chronic irritation such as dentures.

II. **Etiology.** *Candida albicans,* the most common causative organism, exists as a commensal in the mouth that becomes an opportunistic infection when there is a local or systemic change that causes decreased resistance. These range from extremes of age to antibiotic or immunosuppressive therapy, hematologic dyscrasias, endocrine disorders, and malignancy. At present, acquired immune deficiency syndrome is also an important cause.

III. **Treatment.** Management consists of controlling predisposing causes and antifungal therapy. This can be local, such as Nystatin suspension, 100,000 units four times a day, held in the mouth as long as possible, or using the vaginal tablets as a lozenge. Nystatin ointment may be applied directly to small areas after they have been allowed to dry. If the disease is resistant to local therapy or more extensive, oral ketoconazole, 200 mg once daily for 14 days, may be used. Liver toxicity may occur, and liver enzyme levels should be measured if used for more than 14 days.

Aphthous Stomatitis

In this disorder oral mucosal ulcers appear and remain for days or weeks with periods of remission. The cause is likely multifactorial. The prevalence rate is 10% to 20% in the general population.

I. **Clinical presentation.** The clinical course has four stages. In stage one premonitory symptoms appear with tingling or burning at the site. Approximately 24 hours later, the preulceration stage appears, which can last 18 to 72 hours. This is manifested by macules, papules, and a membrane with a reddened halo. The pain may be severe. During the ulcerative stage the pain gradually begins to decline. The membrane sloughs and a depressed ulcer with an erythematous border and a fibrinous base is left. This may last 1 day to 2 weeks. In the fourth stage healing occurs.

II. **Treatment.** Management includes topical anesthetics, such as 2% viscous xylocaine or a mixture of 50% diphenhydramine elixir and 50% Maalox with or without viscous xylocaine added. The Maalox coats the base of the ulcers; sucralfate suspension accomplishes the same end. These may be painted directly on for children or gargled and expectorated for adults. Topical corticosteroids may treat the immunologic mechanisms. Triamcinolone acetonide dental paste applied four times a day or betamethasone valerate ointment 0.1% four times daily can be used. Tetracycline suspension in a dose of 250 mg rinsed in the mouth for 2 minutes four times a day for 7 days probably acts locally. A mouthwash containing chlorhexidine gluconate may be used for recurrences; it is usually used three times daily for 5 weeks followed by 2 weeks of abstinence before restarting again.

Acute Necrotizing Ulcerative Gingivitis

I. **Clinical presentation and etiology.** Also called Vincent's angina or trench mouth, this disease causes sudden onset of tender bleeding gums, halitosis, and bad taste. Systemic symptoms such as fever, anorexia, malaise, tachycardia, cervical lymphadenopathy, and leukocytosis may be present. The lesions are characteristically punched out depressions of the interdental papilla and margin. A gray pseudomembrane covers them, and there is bleeding when it is removed. The disease is caused by a combination of *Treponema vincentii, Fusobacterium,* anaerobic organisms, and underlying tissue changes that facilitate destruction by the bacteria. It is not contagious.

II. **Treatment.** The mouth may be rinsed with one-half strength hydrogen peroxide and the necrotic tissue removed by swabbing with it. Penicillin V in a dosage of 500 mg four times a day is the drug of choice. Tetracycline or erythromycin in dosages of 500 mg four times a day is a good alternative.

Herpetic Gingivostomatitis

I. **Clinical presentation and etiology.** This is caused by the herpes simplex virus (HSV). Primary HSV infection includes systemic and local symptoms. Fever, malaise, headache, dysphagia, and regional lymphadenopathy accompany painful, red gingival inflammation that proceeds to clusters of small vesicles. These coalesce and rupture to form ragged, shallow, painful ulcers with a red border and yellow-gray center. They may occur throughout the oral cavity and lips. These will heal in 1 to 2 weeks without scarring. Self-inoculation may occur to areas such as the eyes, genitalia, and hands. Recurrent infections are mild and occur at mucocutaneous junctions, with a prodrome of tingling, burning, pain, and swelling before the vesicles appear.

II. **Treatment.** Symptomatic treatment consists of hydration and nutrition with cool fluids and pureed foods. Other measures include application of ice, rubbing alcohol, Betadine, and ether. Local anesthetics as outlined in the section on aphthous stomatitis may also be used. Lysine, 2 or 3 g daily for recurrences and 1 g daily for recurrences has also been advocated. Vidarabine ophthalmic ointment applied every 2 hours from the onset and used for 4 days has been suggested, as well as topical acyclovir applied in the same manner. For severe symptoms or recurrences, oral acyclovir, 200 mg five times daily for 5 days may decrease viral shedding and reduce healing time.

Epistaxis

I. **Etiology.** Epistaxis is commonly seen in the emergency department and can result from local factors or reflect systemic platelet or clotting system dysfunction. It is uncommon for epistaxis to be the first manifestation of the latter. Most bleeding from the nose arises anteriorly from the anterior, inferior septal region. This is known as Little's area and contains Kiesselbach's plexus. Posterior epistaxis, which is less common and usually more severe, can be concluded to be the cause if the source of bleeding cannot be located after adequate anterior examination, persists despite anterior packing, or occurs primarily down the pharynx. This type of bleeding usually arises from larger nasal branches of the internal maxillary or ethmoid arteries.

II. **Treatment.** Management of bleeding consists of identification of the source, control of bleeding, and appropriate investigations determined by the clinical situation. The source should be identified by suctioning the nose free of clots. Vasoconstriction and anesthesia can be achieved simultaneously by using cotton pledgets soaked in a 4% to 10% solution of cocaine. These should be applied for 5 minutes to the bleeding area. Alternatively, 1% phenylephrine followed by xylocaine spray may be used.

   A. **Anterior epistaxis.** Cautery of an anterior bleeding source with silver nitrate sticks pressed firmly over the bleeding site will usually suffice. Smearing it over a wide area should be avoided because this causes mucosal trauma. After cautery, topical antibiotic ointment should be applied and the patient instructed to continue the application three times daily for 1 week. The patient should also be asked not to blow the nose for 24 hours. If the bleeding site cannot be identified because it is under a turbinate or cannot be cauterized, then packing is required. Use ½ inch petroleum jelly iodoform gauze that has been coated with antibiotic ointment. This is packed in layers along the floor of the nose, with the loose ends at the nostril; this prevents them from slipping posteriorly and choking the patient. Each layer should be compressed firmly, making sure that the bony nose is adequately packed; if this is not done, hemorrhage can continue. The nostrils should be pinched together and taped to maintain the packing. It should be left in place for 2 or 3 days during which time physical exercise, hot showers, and hot beverages should be avoided. A humidifier may help counteract the dryness that occurs in the mouth.

B. **Posterior epistaxis.** Posterior bleeding may be managed with a number of methods including commercially available nasal balloons that have both a posterior and anterior balloon. A Foley catheter can also be placed through the nostril until the tip is seen below the soft palate and then filled with 10 ml of saline solution. This can gently be pulled until resistance is met. If excessive pain occurs, 1 to 2 ml of saline solution should be withdrawn. The catheter is held on the nasal floor while the anterior nose is packed. The catheter is secured by wrapping it with gauze to protect the alar rim, and a small hemostat is used to maintain tension. Alternatively, a 3 × 3 inch piece of gauze is folded and tied in the middle with number 2 silk, leaving the ends long. A second piece of silk is tied to the loop and attached to a straight catheter that has been placed through the nose and brought out through the mouth. The catheter is used to pull the pack into the nasopharynx, with the opposite index finger guiding it into place. The ends of the first silk tie are allowed to hang down the pharynx to facilitate removal later. The anterior pack is inserted and the ends of the silk protruding from the nose are tied to a roll of gauze at the nostril. Patients with a posterior pack require hospitalization, oxygen administration, and antibiotic therapy. The antibiotic chosen should be effective against organisms comprising the nasal flora, as well as *S. aureus.* Cephalexin, 500 mg three times daily, or amoxicillin/clavulanic acid, 500 mg/125 mg with clavulanic acid three times daily, are good oral and/or intravenous choices. The posterior pack is left in place for 48 to 72 hours and then removed; at this time the antibiotics can be stopped. If a Foley catheter was used, it is deflated after 48 hours and removed after another 24 hours if the bleeding does not recur. The patient is examined in 1 or 2 weeks to look for underlying causes and to make certain that septal perforation has not occurred.

Peritonsillar Abscess

This can occur in all age groups and treatment of tonsillitis with antibiotics does not preclude its formation. It can occur in patients who have had a previous tonsillectomy.

I. **Etiology and clinical presentation.** The most common causative organism is group A β-hemolytic streptococcus. Pharyngitis may have been present for a variable period and may have been treated with antibiotics. The patient describes a severe sore throat (often unilateral), accompanied by difficulty swallowing and referred ear pain. A fever may be present, as well as drooling and a muffled voice. Trismus is almost always present, with an inability to open the mouth more than 2.5 cm as measured between the tips of the upper and lower incisors. Halitosis is also common. Examination shows generalized erythema, with swelling of the anterior tonsillar pillar and palate. The tonsil is displaced forward, inferiorly, and medially. The uvula may be shifted to the opposite side. The differential diagnosis includes peritonsillar cellulitis, lateral pharyngeal space abscess, tonsillar abscess, retromolar abscess, and prevertebral and retropharyngeal abscess.

II. **Treatment.** Outpatient management is successful in most cases, with needle aspiration, Penicillin V, 300 mg orally four times a day, salt water gargles, and pain medication. Erythromycin, 500 mg orally four times a day, is an alternative in patients with penicillin allergy. Needle aspiration is successful in 80% to 85% of patients and can be done with a 10 ml syringe and an 18- or 20-gauge needle, 2.5 cm long, or a spinal needle. Anesthesia is obtained with xylocaine spray, and the most fluctuant part of the affected side is entered and aspiration is attempted. The needle may be redirected until successful. The carotid artery is lateral to the tonsillar bed and may be entered with deep penetration, especially in the inferior part of the tonsil. If blood is obtained, the procedure should be stopped and pressure applied. Removal of pus brings resolution of trismus and odynophagia; if this does not occur or no pus is obtained, then hospitalization with incision and drainage or tonsillectomy may be required.

Pharyngitis

Patients with pharyngitis are commonly seen in the physician's office or in the emergency department.

I. **Etiology and clinical presentation.** The most common organisms are viral, accounting for approximately 40% of cases, and group A β-hemolytic streptococcus, accounting for 30%. Other organisms such as those causing diphtheria or gonorrhea should be considered in patients at risk. In the remainder of cases, no pathogen is isolated. Differentiating viral from bacterial pharyngitis is not always easy, even in experienced hands. This is especially true in children, although the presence of a sore throat without a fever is unlikely to be due to group A β-hemolytic streptococcus. Common symptoms include dysphagia, fever, and a red throat, while classic signs include tonsillar exudate and cervical adenopathy. Cough, coryza, conjunctivitis, and posterior node involvement suggest a viral cause.

II. **Treatment.** Treatment is instituted to prevent acute rheumatic fever, to reduce the contagious period, and to reduce the incidence of suppurative complications. Recent studies indicate that early treatment may reduce the duration of symptoms but may increase recurrences by not allowing formation of beneficial antistreptococcal antibodies. Antibiotic treatment does not protect against acute glomerulonephritis. The rapid tests that are available have a sensitivity approaching 80% and a specificity of more than 90%. If the rapid test is positive, then treatment can be instituted with Penicillin V, 15 mg/kg/day for children or 300 mg for adults, given by mouth four times daily. Erythromycin estolate is a good substitute in penicillin-allergic patients; the dosage is 20 mg/kg/day for children or 250 mg for adults, given four times daily by mouth. Therapy should be continued for 10 days. Patients with fever, especially children or those with a high probability of having streptococcal pharyngitis, should be treated if the rapid test is not available or negative. In these cases a throat culture should be obtained. Ampicillin should not be used because of the possibility of a rash occurring in those patients who are infected with the Epstein-Barr virus; in addition to the discomfort, those patients will be erroneously labelled as allergic to penicillin. Recently it has been reported that failure of penicillin therapy may occur as the result of copathogens present in the pharynx. These may include *S. aureus, M. catarrhalis,* and *H. influenzae.* Therefore, in patients who have been compliant with an adequate dose of penicillin but fail to respond, then a β-lactamase–resistant antibiotic should be used. These include cephalexin, 30 mg/kg/day in children and 250 mg in adults, given orally three times daily, or cefadroxil, 30 mg/kg/day in children or 1 g in adults, given orally once daily. These are both first-generation cephalosporins, and although they have limited activity against β-lactamase–producing strains of *H. influenzae* and *M. catarrhalis,* they are very effective against group A streptococcus and *S. aureus.* There are two useful second-generation cephalosporins, cefaclor and cefuroxime axetil. The dosage for cefaclor is 30 mg/kg/day in children, divided every 8 hours, and 250 mg every 8 hours for adults. Cefuroxime axetil is given twice daily at a dosage of 8 mg/kg/day for children and 125 mg per dose in adults. Cefaclor is inactive against about 25% of β-lactamase–producing strains of *H. influenzae* and the majority of *M. catarrhalis* strains producing this enzyme. Cefixime is a third-generation cephalosporin that has excellent activity against the β-lactamase producers, but poor activity against *S. aureus.* It has convenient once daily dosing at 8 mg/kg for children and 200 mg for adults; however, it is expensive.

Epiglottitis

I. **Etiology and clinical presentation.** This disorder most frequently affects children between the ages of 3 and 7, although it can affect adults as well. It is caused by *H. influenzae* type B. The typical case is rapid in onset with high fever, difficulty swallowing, a muffled voice, and drooling. Respiratory distress may follow with tachycardia, tachypnea, retractions, stridor, cyanosis, and fatigue. If epiglottitis is suspected, steps must be taken to ensure that an artificial airway can be secured. Lateral soft tissue views of the neck will aid in making the diagnosis, with the classic "thumb sign" indicating a swollen epiglottis. These patients should be accompanied to the radiology department.

II. **Treatment.** Once the diagnosis is made, an artificial airway should be secured under controlled conditions, with experienced personnel attempting intubation but prepared to insert a surgical airway should this fail. The antibiotics of choice are cefotaxime, 150 mg/kg/day given every 8 hours for children and 1 g every 6 hours for adults, or ceftriaxone, 50 mg/kg once daily for children or 1 to 2 g once daily for adults. These should all be given intravenously. An alternative would be to use ampicillin and chloramphenicol initially and to stop the chloramphenicol if cultures showed the organism to be susceptible to ampicillin. The dosages are 75 mg/kg/day for children and adults, given every 8 hours, for ampicillin, and 50 to 75 mg/kg/day given every 6 hours for children and adults, for chloramphenicol.

Suggested Readings

Bluestone CD: Modern management of otitis media, *Pediatr Clin North Am* 36:1371-87, 1989.

Fairbanks DN: Inflammatory diseases of the sinuses: bacteriology and antibiotics, *Otolaryngol Clin North Am* 26:549-59, 1993.

Hedges JR, Lowe RA: Approach to acute pharyngitis, *Emerg Med Clin North Am* 5:335-51, 1987.

Karma P et al: Otoscopic diagnosis of middle ear effusion in acute and non-acute otitis media. I. The value of different otoscopic findings, *Int J Pediatr Otorhinolaryngol* 17:37-49, 1989.

Mabry RL: Corticosteroids in rhinology, *Otolaryngol Head Neck Surg* 108:768-70, 1993.

Medoff G: Antimicrobial use in otolaryngeal infections: general considerations, *Ann Otol Rhinol Laryngol Suppl* 155:5-8,1992.

Reich JJ: Ear infections, *Emerg Med Clin North Am* 5:227-42, 1987.

23

Ophthalmologic Disorders

James Dougherty, M.D., F.A.C.E.P.

Patients frequently present to the emergency department with such acute ophthalmologic disturbances as ocular pain, visual loss, red eye, or other visual aberrations (i.e., peripheral field cuts, haloes, tunnel vision, etc.). Unfortunately, deciphering the causes and selecting therapy for these conditions are frequently difficult for the nonophthalmologist. Nevertheless, because of the potential for loss of sight particularly in the elderly, many of whom already have compromised vision, such symptoms are usually cause for great concern on the part of most patients. Consequently, acute ophthalmologic disturbances require diagnostic acumen so that therapy is implemented promptly and consultation, when indicated, is obtained as early as possible. Finally, ophthalmologic emergencies not only can be the first manifestation of underlying systemic disease, but many pharmacotherapeutic agents used to treat ophthalmologic conditions can produce systemic toxicity that is easily overlooked.

Evaluation

I. **History.** As with other acute medical disorders, a thorough symptom-oriented history is invaluable for sorting out precipitating factors and identifying the most likely diagnosis in acute disorders of the eye. Not surprisingly, there are certain "red flags" that the examining physician should recognize when evaluating patients with ophthalmologic complaints. For example, glaucoma should be suspected in any elderly patient who complains of seeing haloes, even in the absence of ocular pain or other symptoms. On the other hand, a history of significant blunt ocular trauma should lead to a diligent examination of the entire retina for signs of retinal detachment, which may be preceded by such symptoms as flashing lights or drifting shadows across the visual field. In the majority of cases, monocular diplopia is hysterical in origin; it can be caused be retinal detachment, macular edema, subluxation of the lens, or cataracts. Binocular diplopia most often results from dysfunction of the extraocular muscles, ischemic insult to the vertebrobasilar system, or disruption of the orbit as can be seen in retroorbital abscess. Momentary loss of vision (amaurosis fugax) may be the first sign of an impending cerebrovascular accident, spasm of the central retinal artery, or partial occlusion of the internal carotid artery. Quivering or scintillating blind spots (scotomas) may occur transiently as a result of localized constriction of cerebral or retinal arteries.

II. **Visual acuity** is to the ophthalmologic exam what routine vital signs are to the general physical exam. In order to be considered complete, the ophthalmologic exam must include a description of visual acuity, whether it is a formal Snellen chart recording or documentation of the patient's ability to count fingers. In general, baseline measurements of central acuity at a distance (20 feet) and at close range (comfortable reading distance) must be augmented by the increased physiologic need for additional light. Note that remarkable tol-

erance especially by the elderly to spectacle misalignment is common, so it is important that lenses are clean and properly centered.
III. **The lids and the adnexa** should be examined closely, noting symmetry, swelling, abnormal discharge, secretions, edema, erythema, or ecchymosis. In addition, if there is suspicion of a foreign body, eversion of the upper and lower lids is mandatory. The tear points (lacrimal puncta) must also be examined. Normally these are directed slightly backward so that the opening is in contact with the bulbar conjunctiva or "lacrimal lake." If lid relaxation has allowed them to rotate forward and open into the air, there will be poor tear siphoning and epiphora. Impairment of lid closure is suggestive of senile or relaxation ectropion of the lower lid. Pupillary light responses should be checked with a flashlight, including the "swinging flashlight test" for a Marcus Gunn afferent pupillary defect.
IV. **Peripheral vision.** A number of important conditions, such as glaucoma, are associated with loss of peripheral vision. A simple confrontation test should be performed as a rough test for such gross defects. The physician and patient face each other at arm's length. The patient is then told to hold one hand lightly over the left eye and look with the right eye at the examiner's left eye. The examiner can then use his or her fingers to enter the peripheral fields and ask the patient to recognize when they appear and how many are present. The fullness of the reported field is compared to that of the physician's perception. The test is then repeated for the other eye.
V. **Next, the intraocular pressure** of each eye should be estimated by one of several available methods. Finger palpation is useful only when a large difference exists between the intraocular pressure of the two eyes, as in unilateral angle-closure glaucoma. The Schiotz tonometer, although not as accurate as the air puff tonometer or the Goldmann applanation tonometer (used with a slit lamp), is much less expensive than either of these. It relies upon a known quantity of weight to indent the corneal surface after instillation of topical anesthesia. The intraocular pressure (IOP) is generally between 10 and 20 mm Hg.
   A. **A slit lamp examination,** which should be a routine part of any emergency ophthalmologic exam, is particularly useful for accurate assessment of corneal integrity as well as anterior chamber anatomy. The use of a light source directed horizontally across the cornea is helpful in estimating the depth of the anterior chamber. If there is dangerous shallowing, a shadow will be seen on the opposite side of the anterior chamber. Conversely, broad illumination of the entire chamber signifies adequate depth **(Figure 23-1).** The presence of a shallow anterior chamber should elicit a thorough evaluation for glaucoma by tonometry and is a contraindication to pupillary dilation.
   B. **Ophthalmoscopy** can be performed safely using a 2.5% phenylephrine for topical mydriasis. Contraindications to pupillary dilation include: recent head injury, history of angle-closure glaucoma, or the presence of an iris-fixated intraocular lens. The optic disk and iris will appear paler with age. Funduscopic exam ordinarily reveals a cup/disk ratio not exceeding 0.3 or 0.4 when measured across the 3 to 9 o'clock diameter of the optic nerve head. If it exceeds this or if there is a difference of 0.2 or greater between the two eyes, the patient should be evaluated for glaucoma. Aging retinal arterioles normally show some physiologic sclerosis with slight yellowing of the arteriolar reflections of light and diffuse narrowing and straightening of arterioles, which tend to obscure venules at crossing points.

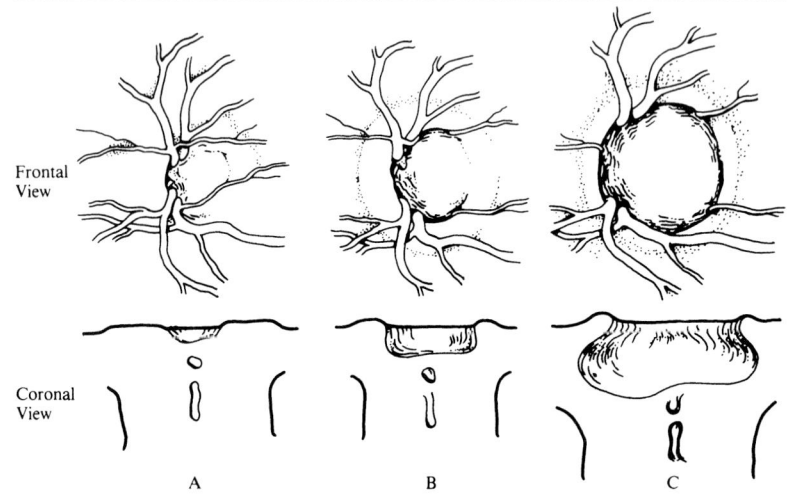

Figure 23-1. Changes in the optic disk with increasing intraocular pressure showing on both the frontal and coronal views: A, normal; B, early change; C, late change. (Reproduced with permission from Kidwell EDR: Glaucoma. In Barker LR, Burton JR, and Zieve PD, editors: Principles of ambulatory medicine, Baltimore, 1986, Williams & Wilkins, p 1376.)

C. **Red-free light** (a white light with a green filter) allows details of hemorrhages, focal irregularity of blood vessels, and nerve fibers to be seen more clearly.

The Red Eye (Table 23-1)

I. **Conjunctivitis**
   A. Allergic conjunctivitis
      1. **The conjunctivae** are exposed to many environmental allergens, microorganisms, and noxious agents, some of which can cause edema, inflammation, hypertrophy, cell death, and exfoliation. Allergic or contact conjunctivitis can produce edema of the stromal layer (chemosis) or hypertrophy of the lymphoid layer of the stroma (follicle formation). Not infrequently, a conjunctival exudate forms on the lid margins.
      2. **Itching and tearing.** Patients with allergic conjunctivitis complain of ocular itching and tearing, which is usually accompanied by sneezing and nasal congestion. Conjunctival injection is usually mild, but there may be dramatic chemosis. Oral antihistamines (diphendyramine, 25 mg PO QID) may provide relief. Many patients find substantial relief from the eye symptoms with the use of antihistamine-decongestant over-the-counter preparations (e.g., Visine AC, containing a decongestant tetrahydrozoline hydrochloride, and an analgesic astringent, zinc sulfate; or a prescription combination such as Vasocon-A, containing naphazoline hydrochloride 0.05% and antazoline phosphate 0.5%). Cool compresses can also be soothing.
   B. Bacterial conjunctivitis
      1. ***Staphylococcus aureus*** is the most common cause of bacterial conjunctivitis in adults, whereas *Streptococcus pneumoniae* and *Haemophilus influenzae* are prominent pathogens in children. Patients complain of irrita-

Table 23-1. Conditions Causing Red Eye

Eyelid
Blepharitis
Hordeolum (sty)
Chalazion
Lacrimal
Dacryoadenitis
Dacryocystitis
Orbit
Periorbital cellulitis
Orbital cellulitis
Conjunctiva
Ophthalmia neonatorum
Bacterial
Viral
Allergic
Sclera
Episcleritis
Scleritis
Cornea
Corneal abrasions
Keratitis
Iris
Uveitis
Glaucoma—acute narrow angle
Trauma
Burns (chemical and thermal)
Corneal abrasions
Intraorbital foreign body
Ruptured globe
Penetrating ocular injury
Neurologic
Cavernous sinus thrombosis

tion, a gritty sensation, and tearing in one or both eyes. A mucopurulent discharge is common. Visual acuity is seldom affected. The conjunctiva is diffusely injected without involvement of the perilimbic area. There may also be subconjunctival petechial hemorrhages, which are most characteristic of *H. influenzae* infection. Examination of the superior tarsal conjunctiva may reveal follicles, which suggest infection with *Chlamydia trachomatis*.

2. **Treatment (Table 23-2).** Although many bacterial infections of the conjunctiva are self-limited, standard practice includes treatment with topical 10% sulfacetimide (Sodium Sulamyd Ophthalmologic Solution, available in 10% to 30% preparations) or sulfisoxazole (Gantrisin). If drops are chosen, two drops should be instilled every 2 to 4 hours while the patient is awake and every 4 hours at night. Ointment preparations can be applied four times daily. Alternative antimicrobial agents include gentamicin, chloramphenicol, or a combination antibiotic. One commonly used formulation combines neomycin, polymyxin, and bacitracin. Although this combination is not contraindicated, the physician should recognize that neomycin may produce a hypersensitivity reaction in as many as 15% of patients.

Table 23-2. Topical Antibiotic Preparations

Drug	Preparation	Indications	Comments
Bacitracin	500-1000 µg ointment	Gram-positive organisms	Limited ophthalmic use
Chloramphenicol	0.5% solution, 1% ointment	Gram-positive and some gram-negative and anaerobic organisms	Bacteriostatic; aplastic anemia reported from topical use
Erythromycin	0.5% ointment	*Chlamydia* and *staphylococcus*	Chlamydial infection requires topical and oral therapy
Gentamicin	3 mg/ml solution	Gram-negative organisms	Used for serious ocular infections and corneal ulcers
Neomycin	2.5 mg/ml solution, 5 mg/gm ointment	Limited coverage of gram-negative and gram-positive organisms	Usually combined with polymyxin and bacitracin as Neosporin
Sulfacetamide	10-30% solution, 10% ointment	Broad coverage of gram-negative and gram-positive organisms	Initial therapy for conjunctivitis, reasonable cost, low risk of allergic reaction; stinging on instillation
Sulfisoxazole	4% solution, 4% ointment	Same as sulfacetamide sodium	Same as sulfacetamide
Tetracycline	1% solution and ointment	*Chlamydia*	Ophthalmologic *Chlamydia* should be treated topically and systemically

3. **Purulent, hyperacute bacterial conjunctivitis** is most often caused by *Neisseria gonorrhoeae*. There is an intense, inflammatory response resulting in copious purulent discharge, as well as edema of the eyelids and conjunctiva. The exudate contains gram-negative intracellular diplococci. *Neisseria* conjunctivitis is a reportable disease; sexual partners should be evaluated.
4. **Penicillin** (10 million units/day in divided doses, for at least 5 days) remains the treatment of choice, although many experts recommend therapy with intravenous cefoxitin (1 gm four times daily) or a single injection of ceftriaxone, 1 gm intramuscularly daily for 5 days, if penicillinase-producing strains of *N. gonorrhoeae* are suspected. Ophthalmologists recommend irrigation of the conjunctiva on a regular basis, as well as topical therapy with erythromycin. Sexual partners should also be treated.

C. Viral conjunctivitis
 1. **Viral conjunctivitis ranges** from a mild, self-limited infection to a severe, disabling disease. Follicular conjunctivitis caused by adenovirus is the most common form. There may be bilateral involvement with a profuse serous discharge and photosensitivity. The clinical picture is characterized by conjunctival injection, chemosis, lid edema, and a marked follicular response that is best seen on the inner surface of the inferior eyelid. There

may be punctate fluorescein staining of the cornea. Adenovirus is the most common cause. Because this condition is difficult to distinguish clinically from bacterial conjunctivitis, most experts recommend a 5-day course of 10% sulfacetimide to prevent secondary bacterial infection.
   2. **Infection with herpes simplex virus** (HSV) is reported to cause up to 500,000 cases of HSV conjunctivitis in the United States annually. Herpes simplex virus produces discrete epithelial lesions on the cornea that usually form branching (dendritic) ulcers. Herpetic vesicles are often present on the face or eyelids. In the newborn infant, HSV infection must be treated with intravenous acyclovir. The physician should attempt to exclude concurrent encephalitis, chorioretinitis, and hepatitis in the newborn infant with HSV conjunctivitis.
   3. **Patients with herpes simplex keratitis,** herpes simplex conjunctivitis, or both should be referred to an ophthalmologist. Topical antiviral treatment includes idoxuridine 0.1% solution every 1 to 4 hours or idoxuridine 0.5% ointment every 4 to 6 hours. Adverse reactions include lacrimation, irritation, and a foreign body sensation.
   4. **Acute hemorrhagic conjunctivitis** is endemic to most countries and is commonly seen in Florida. Its onset is abrupt with conjunctivitis, edema, serous drainage, and conjunctival hemorrhage. Acute hemorrhagic conjunctivitis usually resolves spontaneously within 5 to 7 days.
D. Neonatal conjunctivitis (**ophthalmia neonatorum**)
   1. **Microbial inoculation** of the newborn conjunctiva from the maternal genital tract occurs during birth. Bacterial conjunctivitis in the immunologically immature or premature infant has the potential to produce meningitis or sepsis. Bacterial causes of neonatal conjunctivitis include *Escherichia coli, S. aureus,* and *H. influenzae.* However, *N. gonorrhoeae* and *C. trachomatis* are the most virulent pathogens causing neonatal conjunctivitis and usually require hospitalization of the newborn infant. Conjunctival smears for Gram stain, culture, and chlamydial assay are required.
   2. **Chemical conjunctivitis** is the most common form of conjunctivitis in the newborn infant due to the inflammation caused by silver nitrate prophylaxis. It is usually mild and resolves within 3 days.
E. Treatment of conjunctivitis
   1. **Topical antibiotic therapy.** Most conjunctival infections resolve spontaneously, but topical antibiotic therapy may hasten the resolution. Since conjunctivitis is quite contagious, antibiotics are applied to both eyes, even when unilateral disease is present; this prevents the spread of infection from one eye to the other. Sodium sulfacetamide is widely used and is available in a 10% or 30% concentration. *Staphylococcus aureus* is increasingly resistant to sodium sulfacetamide. Gentamicin and tobramycin are aminoglycosides that are effective against *Pseudomonas aeruginosa* and gram-negative bacilli; they have less activity against *Neisseria* and *Haemophilus.*
   2. **Bacitracin** is effective against gram-positive organisms (e.g., *Staphylococcus, Streptococcus*). Erythromycin is effective against *N. gonorrhoeae, Neisseria meningitidis,* and *H. influenzae,* but less so against *S. aureus, S. pneumoniae,* and *Streptococcus pyogenes.* Fluoroquinolones are highly effective against a broad spectrum of organisms including *P. aeruginosa.* Specifically, ciprofloxacin is effective in almost 90% of patients without causing serious side effects.

3. **Fluoroquinolones** are contraindicated in children and pregnant patients, and are expensive.

II. Eyelid disorders

A. **Blepharitis.** Blepharitis is an inflammatory disorder of the eyelid margins. Anterior blepharitis involves the lid margins and may be associated with conjunctivitis. There are two types of anterior blepharitis: staphylococcal (ulcerative) and seborrheic (nonulcerative). The seborrheic form is identified by hyperemia of the lid margins and greasy scales surrounding the eyelashes. The seborrheic type is treated by lid hygiene and scale removal with gentle washing, using baby shampoo in a shower. Neonates may have seborrheic blepharitis associated with seborrheic dermatitis of the scalp (cradle cap).

1. **The ulcerative (staphylococcal) form** causes inflammation of the follicles and lashes, which may lead to abscess formation. The eyelid margins are red and inflamed with multiple, crusting, suppurative lesions. This crust is extracted with difficulty often resulting in the removal of eyelashes. Staphylococcal blepharitis may be further complicated by formation of a hordeolum (sty), chalazion, or keratitis (inflammation of the cornea). Anterior staphylococcal blepharitis is treated with a topical antistaphylococcal agent (bacitracin, erythromycin, or sulfacetimide) for mild infections; oral antibiotics (dicloxacillin, 500 mg PO QID for 7 days) are added for severe cases.

2. **Posterior blepharitis** occurs when the meibomian gland becomes plugged, producing a caseous secretion. The lids may eventually roll inward, causing injury to the tarsal conjunctiva and cornea. Treatment usually consists of oral antistaphylococcal antibiotics.

B. **Hordeolum.** A hordeolum or sty is an abscess of the meibomian glands of the eyelids. The patient has an acutely tender, reddened, inflamed swelling of the lid margin often pointing at the eyelash follicle. A hordeolum may point to the conjunctival surface or to the skin. Treatment consists of warm compresses three or four times a day. If there is no resolution of symptoms in 48 hours, surgical drainage may be necessary. Antistaphylococcal antibiotic ointment should be applied to the conjunctival sac every 3 hours.

C. **Chalazion.** A chalazion is a granuloma that develops around a sebaceous gland in the eyelid. It may evolve from a hordeolum. The acute process may produce marked lid edema. It may spontaneously drain through the skin or through the subconjunctival surface. Treatment in the early stages consists of warm compresses to achieve localization and spontaneous drainage. Topical antibiotics do not directly affect the inflammation but are sometimes empirically used as adjunctive therapy to decrease local bacterial flora. Surgical drainage may be necessary in the chronic stage.

III. Lacrimal disorders

A. **Dacryoadenitis.** Dacryoadenitis is an acute inflammation of the lacrimal gland and is seen most often in children. The lacrimal gland is in the superior temporal quadrant of the orbit. In children, it is usually associated with a viral infection; in adults, it is associated with gonorrhea. Dacryoadenitis may also result from extension of bacterial conjunctivitis or lid infection. The patient will have pain, swelling, and redness of the temporal aspect of the upper lid. Treatment consists of warm compresses and oral antibiotics effective against both streptococcal and staphylococcal organisms (e.g., dicloxicillin, 500 mg PO QID for 10 days; or cephalexin, 500 mg PO QID for 10 days).

B. Dacryocystitis. Dacryocystitis is a suppurative infection of the lacrimal sac that is precipitated by obstruction of the nasolacrimal duct. The lacrimal sac is in the inferonasal quadrant of the orbit. Dacryocystitis is most common in infants and postmenopausal women; it is rare in others unless caused by trauma or a dacryolith. Acute dacryocystitis in children is usually caused by *H. influenzae*.
   1. **Prompt antimicrobial treatment** will minimize the risk of orbital cellulitis. *Staphylococcus aureus* and β-hemolytic streptococcus are the most common pathogens in adults. The patient has swelling, redness, and tenderness surrounding the medial canthus. Mucoid material may be expressed from the lacrimal sac.
   2. **Treatment in children** that are afebrile consists of amoxicillin-clavulanate. Severely ill children should be hospitalized and treated with intravenous cefuroxime. Adults with mild cases should be treated with oral dicloxacillin or oral cephalexin. Febrile or acutely ill adults require hospitalization and treatment with nafcillin or cefazolin. Acute dacryocystitis usually responds to antibiotics, warm compresses, and relief of the obstruction, which may require surgery.

IV. Periorbital cellulitis. Periorbital cellulitis is an infection that is anterior to the orbital septum. Periorbital cellulitis is associated with an elevated temperature, erythema and edema of the eyelids, chemosis, orbital pain, and conjunctivitis. Extraocular muscle use is unrestricted with periorbital cellulitis but restricted with orbital cellulitis. A violaceous discoloration of the eyelids is characteristic of *H. influenzae* infection. Common predisposing factors include a recent history of respiratory tract infection, sinusitis, acute or chronic otitis media, eyelid or facial trauma, and infection of adjacent structures.

   A. Children. Periorbital cellulitis is most common in children, with an increased frequency in children younger than 5 years (with a peak between 6 months and 2 years). It occurs with greater frequency than orbital infections. The most common pathogens are *H. influenzae* and *S. pneumoniae*. In adults, *S. aureus* and β-hemolytic streptococcus most commonly cause periorbital cellulitis. Human bites increase the risk of infection by anaerobic organisms.

   B. Laboratory evaluation should include a complete blood cell count. The leukocyte count is frequently elevated to between 10,000 and 15,000 cells/mm^3, with counts over 20,000 cells/mm^3 in some cases. Blood cultures should be obtained, although most will not yield the pathogen.

   C. Oral penicillinase-resistant penicillins or a cephalosporin (cefaclor) are indicated for outpatient therapy in mild or equivocal cases. Intravenous nafcillin for gram-positive organisms and chloramphenicol for anaerobic organisms should be used for infections requiring hospitalization. A computed tomography (CT) scan or magnetic resonance imaging (MRI) scan is indicated if orbital cellulitis is suspected. Because of the severity of central nervous system (CNS) complications, hospitalization is strongly recommended. Intravenous cefuroxime is frequently used, due to its efficacy against *H. influenzae* and *S. pneumoniae*.

V. Orbital cellulitis. Orbital cellulitis is a serious infection that may lead to CNS infection, visual loss, cavernous sinus thrombosis, osteomyelitis, and even death. The patient has proptosis, orbital discomfort, and ophthalmoplegia from edema of the orbital adipose and soft tissues.

A. Signs. Patients are usually older than 6 years, febrile, and appear ill. Most cases result from a sinus infection. Pain, redness, edema of the eyelids, chemosis, and conjunctival injection is found in both periorbital and orbital cellulitis. However, with orbital cellulitis, diffuse orbital soft tissue inflammation may cause axial displacement of the eye. Nonaxial displacement of the eye occurs with a focal subperiosteal or orbital abscess.

B. The most common organisms are *S. aureus, S. pyogenes, S. pneumoniae,* and *H. influenzae.* When orbital cellulitis results from trauma, infections caused by *S. aureus, Clostridium* species, anaerobes, and polymicrobial infections are more common. Orbital cellulitis is rare in infancy but when present is usually caused by *H. influenzae.* The assessment of visual acuity may be difficult in infants. Nevertheless, the presence of an ipsilateral afferent pupillary defect (Marcus Gunn pupil) is considered a sign of significant visual impairment.

C. Intravenous antibiotics. All patients with orbital cellulitis should be hospitalized for intravenous antibiotics. In patients younger than 6 years, cefuroxime is recommended. Older patients are treated with cloxacillin or nafcillin in combination with chloramphenicol. Vancomycin is substituted for a penicillinase-resistant penicillin in allergic patients. Patients should be reassessed frequently while in the emergency department, specifically noting the clinical condition, changes in temperature, mental status, visual acuity, proptosis, ophthalmoplegia, pupillary findings, and funduscopy.

VI. Uveitis (iritis). Uveitis is an inflammation of the uveal tract that is usually confined to the iris and the anterior chamber. The uveal tract is composed of the iris, the ciliary body, and the choroid (the middle layer of the globe). Acute uveitis usually causes blurred vision, ocular pain, conjunctival injection, a watery discharge, and photophobia. Inflammation of the anterior uvea and spasm of the ciliary body produce photophobia. A simple bedside test to assess for uveitis is the consensual light reflex. The affected (red) eye is covered, and a bright light is shined into the uncovered, unaffected eye. If the red eye hurts, uveitis is strongly suspected. Blurred vision usually results from clouding of the aqueous humor, cornea, or lens. Uveitis is associated with minor trauma, systemic diseases (e.g., ulcerative colitis), and systemic infections (e.g., Lyme disease). Uveitis can be difficult to diagnose in the absence of ocular redness; patients may have isolated pain that is relieved by ibuprofen.

A. Circumcorneal flush. Conjunctival vascular congestion produces a circumcorneal (ciliary) "flush." The inflamed anterior uveal tract causes protein and cells to extravasate into the aqueous humor, which can be detected by slit-lamp examination. Increased protein circulating within the aqueous is called *flare.* Fine white deposits (keratic precipitates) on the surface of the cornea may occur. Accumulation of fibrin in the anterior chamber can result in *synechiae,* which are adhesions between the pupillary margin of the iris and the lens. Synechiae may produce miosis and pupillary irregularities.

B. The intraocular pressure (IOP) may elevate from decreased flow of aqueous humor out of the anterior chamber. Anticholinergic preparations (e.g., homatropine 1% to 5%, Isoptoatropine 1%) dilate the pupil to help prevent synechiae formation. However, atropine is contraindicated if acute narrow-angle glaucoma is suspected. Topical steroids (prednisolone acetate 1% solution [Econopred Plus, Pred Forte]) that decrease the inflammatory response are used cautiously because they can result in secondary glaucoma and cataract formation, as well as exacerbate herpes simplex keratitis. Oral non-

steroidal antiinflammatory agents are also used. Patients with uveitis should be referred for ophthalmologic evaluation.
- C. **Corneal abrasion.** Corneal abrasions produce immediate intense pain, lacrimation, a foreign body sensation, photophobia, and blepharospasm. A topical anesthetic agent may be required to relieve blepharospasm. There is ciliary injection and an area of epithelial loss that stains with fluorescein and is easily seen with a cobalt blue filter. Careful inspection of the bulbar and tarsal conjunctiva by everting the eyelids will reveal a retained foreign body or contact lens. Multiple corneal abrasions caused by the retained foreign body repeatedly grating across the cornea is referred to as the *ice rink* sign. Some patients with a corneal abrasion will suffer from recurrent corneal erosion. Recurrent corneal erosion can occur weeks to months after the initial injury. Pain is frequently present during the night or on awakening.
  1. **Treatment** includes using a topical broad-spectrum antibiotic (sulfacetimide) for infection prophylaxis. A cycloplegic agent (e.g., Cyclogyl 1%) may increase comfort. A pressure patch (using two eye pads together) can be applied to provide comfort and to shield the epithelium as it heals. The patch should be left on for at least 36 hours. A follow-up examination is essential in contact lens–related abrasions due to the increased incidence of gram-negative bacterial infection especially from *Pseudomonas.*
  2. **With lens abrasions,** an antibiotic with gram-negative coverage (gentamicin, tobramycin) is used and an eye patch is avoided. Oral analgesics may be given. Topical anesthetics are contraindicated; they delay healing and can promote further injury as a result of a loss of the protective reflexes. Contact lens wearers should abstain from lens wear for at least 1 week.
- D. **Chemical injuries.** The most serious chemical burns are caused by strong alkalis such as ammonia, lye, potassium hydroxide, magnesium hydroxide (found in sparklers), and lime (plaster, cement). Alkalis rapidly penetrate the cornea and may damage the entire anterior segment. The hydroxyl ion in alkali compounds causes liquefaction necrosis. Opacification of the cornea or an extensive avascular segment of the sclera suggests considerable ocular damage.
  1. **Acid burns,** although severe, are often limited to the ocular surface because most acids coagulate epithelial and stromal proteins, forming a barrier to deep penetration. Of the many acids that can cause injury, sulfuric acid (found in automobile batteries) is the most common.
  2. **For serious chemical burns,** treatment must begin at the scene, with copious water irrigation by using the nearest available source (hose, shower). Irrigation should be continued during transport to the emergency department. On arrival, treatment should continue and the examination should be started without any interruption of therapy. Topical anesthetic agents are given. Eyelid retractors are inserted to allow the greatest amount of visualization. Irrigation should be continued for up to 40 minutes with a physiologic solution (Dacriose, 0.9% normal saline solution). Morgan lens can be used to facilitate irrigation. The eyelids must be everted to find any retained particles. A litmus paper test should be performed after irrigation to make certain that the pH of the tears is 7.3 to 7.7. Alkali material can continue to leach out of the anterior chamber for several hours, requiring repeated litmus testing and continued irrigation. A severely injured patient must be examined by an ophthalmologist.

E. Traumatic hyphema
1. **Blunt trauma.** Hyphema (blood in the anterior chamber) is a common manifestation of blunt trauma. The extent of hyphema should be described by the volume of blood filling the anterior chamber (e.g., one third, one half, all of the anterior chamber). Blunt impact to the eye distorts the normal architecture, producing a rapid increase in IOP, equatorial stretching of the globe, and posterior displacement of the lens and iris. Hemorrhage originates from the blood vessels of the iris and ciliary body.
2. **Complete eye examination.** In all patients with blunt trauma, a complete eye examination is required to exclude a ruptured globe. The visual acuity, the IOP, and an illustration of the hyphema must be documented. Rebleeding is suggested by bright red blood layering over darker, clotted blood and an increase in the hyphema size. Traumatic iritis and traumatic mydriasis may accompany a hyphema. The patient should have the head of the bed elevated to 30 degrees, receive analgesics or sedatives, and be referred to an ophthalmologist for follow-up evaluation.

Ophthalmologic Manifestations of Systemic Disease

Although a complete listing of systemic diseases that can cause ocular abnormalities is beyond the scope of this review, some of the more common ocular manifestations of systemic diseases are shown in **Table 23-3**.

I. **Diabetic changes.** Diabetes, for example, should be considered in all patients with cataracts, unexplained retinopathy, optic neuropathy, extraocular muscle palsy, or sudden changes in refractive error. The onset of retinopathy frequently cannot be dated by the elderly diabetic. In most cases, hypertensive or arteriosclerotic vasculopathy is already present and, when combined with diabetes, leads to a maculopathy that is uniquely resistant to therapy. Intraretinal microvascular anomalies occur and result in loss of vascular integrity and leakage of intravascular fluids into the retinal space, especially the macula. Once present, macular edema causes structural distortion that can reduce vision to the level of legal blindness (20/200 or less).

II. **Hypertension.** Hypertensive retinopathy may be categorized into four groups initially described by Wagner and Keith in 1939. Stages I and II are characterized by mild arteriolar changes with attenuation and an increased light reflex ("copper" or "silver" wiring). Stages III and IV include cotton wool spots, hemorrhages, extensive microvascular changes, and hard exudates. Stage IV is differentiated by the additional features of optic disk edema. The appearance of the fundus in hypertensive retinopathy is determined by the degree of elevation of the blood pressure and the state of the retinal arterioles. Note that elderly patients with fixed arteriosclerotic vessels are partially protected from the vascular damage associated with accelerated hypertension. Thus, older individuals seldom exhibit signs of florid hypertensive retinopathy.

III. **Arteriosclerosis.** Arteriosclerosis is characterized by diffuse fibrosis and hyalinization of the retinal vessels beyond the disk. As the walls of the arterioles become infiltrated with fatty acids and cholesterol, the vessels become sclerotic, and the vessel wall gradually loses its transparency. The blood column appears wider than normal, and the thin light reflex becomes broader. A typical "copper wire" appearance is seen as grayish-yellow, fat products in the vessel wall that

Table 23-3. Ocular Manifestations of Systemic Disease

Sign/symptom	Systemic diseases
Retinal hemorrhages	Hypertension, diabetes mellitus, leukemia, polycythemia, acute blood loss, subacute bacterial endocarditis
Uveitis	Toxoplasmosis, sarcoid, rheumatoid arthritis, Behcet's disease, sinusitis, dental disease
Amaurosis fugax	Carotid disease, valvular heart disease, dysrhythmia, anemia, polycythemia, hypotensive or hypertensive episodes, arteritis
Occulusive disease of retinal vessels	Hypertension, atheromatous disease (carotid/vertebral) systems, abnormal blood viscosity syndromes, glaucoma, temporal arteritis
Papilledema	Tumors, benign increased intracranial pressure, hydrocephalus, drugs, trauma, middle ear disease, endocrine abnormalities, blood dyscrasias
Cataracts	Steroid use, diabetes mellitus, uveal disease, retinal detachment, trauma
Optic neuritis	Multiple sclerosis, diabetes mellitus, Graves' disease, toxins (methanol), temporal arteritis
Conjunctivitis	Infections, allergy, chemical exposure
Scleral discoloration	Jaundice, Atabrine (yellow), osteogenesis imperfecta (blue), blacks, alkaptonuria (brown)
Macular degeneration	Senile degeneration, hereditary, traumatic, cystic, histoplasmosis
Dry eye syndrome	Sjögren's syndrome, tranquilizers, other collagen disorders
Angioid streaks	Pseudoxanthoma elasticum, sickle cell disease, Paget's disease, high myopia
Proptosis	Graves' disease, ocular tumors, hemorrhage, orbital cellulitis, carotid-cavernous sinus fistula, leukemia, lymphoma, aneurysms
Oculomotor paralysis	Diabetes mellitus, multiple sclerosis, botulism, Wernicke's encephalopathy, posterior communicating aneurysm, Graves' disease, polyarteritis nodosa
Optic atrophy	Tertiary syphilis, diabetes mellitus, pernicious and other anemias, brain tumor
Diplopia	Myasthenia gravis (worse in the evening), Graves' disease, ptosis, oculomotor palsies
Central retinal vein occlusion	Diabetes mellitus, hypertension, collagen vascular disease, hyperviscosity syndromes

blend with the red of the blood column. As sclerosis proceeds from moderate to severe, the vessel wall light reflection resembles a "silver wire," and, at times, even complete occlusion of an arteriolar branch may occur.

IV. Neoplasms. Neoplastic disease may involve the eye and optic pathways by direct spread or by metastatic infiltration. The most frequent tumor metastasizing to the eye is bronchial carcinoma in men and carcinoma of the breast in women, followed by neoplasms of the genitourinary and intestinal tract. Orbital involvement with Hodgkin's disease or lymphosarcoma is not uncommon and usually presents beneath the conjunctiva of the upper cul-de-sac; it may be the only sign of lymphoma.

Ocular Pain

Precise evaluation of the painful eye is an especially difficult and challenging problem. Potential diagnoses range from minor ocular problems to catastrophic events that may not directly involve the eye, such as a leaking or ruptured internal carotid aneurysm. Emergency physicians should be particularly aware of those conditions which are most likely to cause ocular pain **(Table 23-4).**

Ocular pain can be defined as gritty irritation or discomfort in the eye and can be especially severe when the trigeminal nerve is involved. The patient complaining of acute pain of the eye or orbit will generally fall into one of two groups: those with signs of external inflammation (i.e., a red eye) and those without such signs. As a rule, pain that occurs in an eye free of inflammation is unlikely to be ocular in origin and is usually of referred origin. Contrary to popular belief, refractive errors are an infrequent source of ocular pain or eye strain.

I. Dry eye syndrome. Dry eye syndrome is quite common particularly in the elderly and results from deficient tear secretion. Patients with dry eyes complain of a burning sensation or sandy feeling. Other common symptoms include itching, excessive mucous secretion, blurred vision, photosensitivity, redness, and difficulty in moving the lids. The eye is usually minimally inflamed with an absent tear meniscus at the lower lid margin. Diagnosis of a dry eye is confirmed most easily by assessing the extent of wetting of a thin strip of litmus paper after 5 minutes (Schirmer's test). In severe cases, there may be signs of keratoconjunctivitis sicca, which is manifested by punctate staining with 1% rose bengal of the cornea and interpalpebral areas of the conjunctiva. Treatment consists of replacement with artificial tears as often as necessary and lubricating ointment at bedtime. For more severe cases, a sustained-release tear insert (Lacrisert, one insert in each eye daily) may be employed.

    A. Exposure keratopathy occurs whenever the cornea is not properly moistened and covered by the eyelids. This can be seen in patients with exophthalmos, ectropion, facial nerve palsies, loss of consciousness, and anesthetic corneas.

Table 23-4. Causes of Ocular Pain

Condition	Diagnostic signs
Keratoconjunctivitis sicca	Check tear secretion with Schirmer's tear test, strip and stain for corneal ulceration with rose bengal
Exposure keratopathy	Facial palsy (imperfect lid closure), ulcer in lower third of cornea
Corneal ulcer	Grayish ulcer with crescentic margin; pus in floor of anterior chamber may be seen
Herpetic keratitis	Branching dendritic figures on fluorescein staining
Herpes zoster ophthalmicus	Keratitis or iridocyclitis likely if vesicles on side of nose
Acute iritis	Pupil small, possible irregular; keratic precipitates may be present
Intraocular tumor	Painful blind eye may mask malignancy; eye congested and hard due to secondary glaucoma, does not transilluminate
Angle-closure glaucoma	Pupil semidilated, oval; fixed eye hard to palpate through upper lid

The two factors at work are the drying of the cornea and its exposure to minor trauma. In addition to conjunctival swelling and hyperemia, the cornea will usually stain abnormally with fluorescein, indicating an epithelial defect or deeper corneal ulceration. The therapeutic objective is to provide protection and moisture for the entire corneal surface. Artificial tears or ointment may be of benefit; treatment requires that the eyelids be taped to maintain closure.

B. Entropion and ectropion of the lower eyelid cause inflammation of the conjunctiva that is predominantly inferior in location. Loss of posterior support from shrinkage of orbital fat, combined with atony of the tarsoorbital fascia and relaxation of the palpebral skin, are important contributing factors. Trichiasis (turning inward of the lashes so they rub on the cornea) results from senile entropion. It causes corneal irritation and may encourage corneal ulceration. Temporary relief of entropion may be obtained by taping the lower lid to the cheek with tension temporally and inferiorly. Ectropion (sagging and eversion of the lower lid) may precipitate desiccation and hypertrophy of the tarsal conjunctiva of the lid. When this occurs, the eye becomes irritable, watery, and prone to conjunctival infection and exposure keratitis. Marked ectropion is treated by surgical shortening of the lower lid in a horizontal direction.

II. Corneal ulcer. A corneal ulcer is a true medical emergency necessitating immediate intervention. Opacification of the cornea with fluorescein staining should alert the physician to this potentially dangerous condition. Hypopyon keratitis is an infective corneal ulcer accompanied by pus in the floor of the anterior chamber. The pus is usually sterile, and the ulcer is grayish with a crescentic advancing edge. Corneal ulcers may result from foreign body injury, but can occur spontaneously in debilitated patients with a degenerate cornea or poor hygiene. Swabbing the cornea with the cotton swab supplied in the culture tube and sending it to the laboratory is insufficient to make a bacteriologic diagnosis, with the yield approaching only 10% or less. The ulcer must be scraped with a scalpel blade or platinum spatula and plated directly from the blade onto culture media. The usual bacterial offender is *Staphylococcus aureus,* pneumococcus, or a more virulent organism such as *Pseudomonas.* Any of these can cause corneal perforation and loss of the eye in 12 hours, so any delay in hospitalization or treatment may turn a potentially treatable disease into a blind eye.

III. Herpes simplex keratitis

A. Dendritic keratitis, or necrotizing herpes simplex keratitis, is the most common cause of corneal ulceration in the United States. It is often painful as a result of concomitant corneal epithelial edema, uveitis, and secondary glaucoma due to trabecular dysfunction. A branching dendritic figure that stains with fluorescein is characteristic and is composed of small erosions united by branching fissures. Left untreated, the dendrites coalesce to form a shallow geographic ulcer with scalloped margins. Bacterial or fungal keratitis can mimic herpetic keratitis or can occur concomitantly. Appropriate cultures are, therefore, always necessary. Treatment is by topical antiviral agents, such as idoxuridine, every 2 hours or vidarabine ointment under the supervision of an ophthalmologist. Topical steroids are contraindicated in the presence of epithelial loss.

B. Herpes zoster ophthalmicus, a viral infection of the trigeminal ganglion, is usually heralded by pain in the trigeminal nerve distribution. After 3 or 4 days, a vesicular eruption appears in the supra- or infraorbital area, depending on which division of the nerve is involved. Vesicles on the tip of the nose indicating nasociliary involvement should have an ophthalmic evaluation. Ocular complications may involve the cornea, uveal tract, and optic nerve. Topical steroids are indicated, provided there is no coincidental herpes simplex infection; atropine drops are required once or twice a day.

IV. Iritis. Acute iritis and iridocyclitis may produce trigeminal-type pain and ciliary congestion. In contrast to acute angle-closure glaucoma, vision is less severely depressed, the intraocular pressure may be low, and the pupil is small and irregular. Deposits of cells (keratic precipitates) are found on the back of the cornea. Posterior synechiae or adhesions of the iris to the lens occur in untreated cases. In the elderly, phacoanaphylactic iridocyclitis may result from hypersensitivity to lens protein after extracapsular cataract extraction. More often, however, iridocyclitis in this group is secondary to ankylosing spondylitis, diabetes, herpes simplex, herpes zoster, and a focal infection, such as dental root abscesses. Although tuberculosis may occasionally be an etiologic factor in iritis or iridocyclitis, as many as 50% of the cases have no known cause.

V. Pain without Inflammation. Patients who present with a painful eye or orbit, but with no external signs of inflammation, are at high risk for having a number of conditions. Sudden onset of pain combined with an oculomotor palsy (i.e., dilated pupil with or without ophthalmoplegia) should suggest an expanding or leaking internal carotid aneurysm. An aneurysm above the clinoid process may impinge on the optic nerve or chiasm and cause visual field deficits. Temporal arteritis may cause acute pain that is referred to the orbit. Visual loss due to ischemic optic neuropathy is frequent, and a few cases have a central retinal artery occlusion. A painful eye associated with an afferent pupillary deficit (Marcus Gunn pupil) and diminished visual acuity suggests optic neuritis—particularly if associated with painful ocular motion or a tender globe. There may or may not be signs of inflammation of the optic disk depending on whether the process is intraocular or retrobulbar. Finally, migraines and cluster headaches may present as an acutely painful eye or orbit.

Glaucoma

I. Open-angle glaucoma. In glaucoma, the intraocular pressure is sufficiently elevated to cause characteristic optic disk changes and visual field defects, eventually leading to blindness in some patients. A pressure greater than 22 mm Hg is considered abnormal but not necessarily an absolute indication for treatment. Glaucoma can be primary or secondary to other disease processes (e.g., trauma or following cataract extraction). Primary glaucoma is further subdivided into open-angle and angle-closure types. The vast majority of affected individuals have chronic open-angle (or "simple") glaucoma. The prevalence of this condition increases with age, rising from a very low level in young adults to as high as 5 to 10% in the eighth decade.

A. The term "chronic open-angle glaucoma" is used when optic nerve damage and visual field loss result from elevated intraocular pressure in an eye with an open angle (as determined by gonioscopy), and no etiology is found. In the trabecular meshwork there is a poorly understood block to the outflow of the aqueous humor. With continued production of aqueous humor, the intraocular pressure gradually increases. The peripheral field is usually lost first. As the visual fields become progressively constricted later, only a small central island of vision remains and then disappears, causing loss of central visual acuity. Patients are often unaware that there is a problem until the disease is far advanced. A family history, complaints of blurred vision not correctable with lenses, or a halo effect around lights should raise the examiner's level of suspicion. The pupil may be slightly dilated and react sluggishly to light, but otherwise the eye appears perfectly normal externally. Ophthalmoscopic exam may reveal glaucomatous cupping of the disk and atrophy of the optic nerve (see **Figure 23-1**). In glaucomatous cupping, there is a true loss of the substance of the optic nerve head so that it becomes carved out and excavated. A pale, chalk-white nerve head with a large cup/disk ratio (0.5 or greater) is indicative of late open-angle glaucoma.

B. Treatment. Goals of therapy are to preserve visual function and prevent visual damage in the safest way possible. Because only 5 to 10% of patients with ocular hypertension (pressure greater than 22 mm Hg) develop open-angle glaucoma, most patients with ocular hypertension should be observed without treatment to avoid therapeutic complications. Medications available for open-angled glaucoma are shown in **Table 23-5**. Medical treatment can lower the intraocular pressure by increasing aqueous outflow with miotics (pilocarpine) or by decreasing aqueous formation with carbonic anhydrase inhibitors (Diamox). Epinephrine may be added to the miotics or used as the primary drug to decrease aqueous production and increase aqueous outflow. Timolol maleate, a beta-adrenergic blocking agent with few side effects, also decreases aqueous production and may increase outflow by an as-yet-unknown mechanism. This drug is used only twice daily and may be extremely effective in responsive patients. When medical therapy has failed to control the intraocular pressure adequately, laser trabeculoplasty or surgical intervention becomes necessary. The operation for open-angle glaucoma creates a fistula between the anterior chamber and the subconjunctival space, allowing an exit for the aqueous humor.

II. Angle-closure glaucoma.
Angle-closure glaucoma results from forward displacement of the iris against the cornea and obstruction of flow of the aqueous humor into the chamber angle and the spaces of Fontana **(Figure 23-2)**. The aging eye is more susceptible to this disease as the anterior chamber becomes shallower and the lens increases in size. An attack may be precipitated by the use of mydriatics, sitting in a darkened room, or a sudden increase in the volume of the posterior chamber (e.g., hemorrhage or congestion).

In contrast to chronic open-angle glaucoma, acute angle-closure glaucoma is marked by striking and prominent symptoms:

1. Abrupt onset of blurred vision
2. Rainbow-colored haloes around lights
3. Moderate to severe unilateral pain
4. Dramatic loss of vision
5. Nausea, vomiting, and abdominal pain

A. There may be a family history of angle-closure glaucoma, and the patient may also have a history of previous, less severe attacks. Often, patients find relief in well-lighted rooms or out of doors where daylight causes constriction of the pupil and opening of the angle of the anterior chamber. Examination during an acute attack usually reveals a markedly increased intraocular pressure (50 mm Hg or more), a shallow anterior chamber, an edematous cornea, decreased visual acuity, ciliary injection, and a fixed, semidilated pupil.

B. Emergency treatment. Emergency treatment consists of frequent instillation of miotics, parenteral administration of carbonic anhydrase inhibitors, and

Table 23-5. Antiglaucoma Medications

Class and name	Dosage	Route	Side effects	Contraindications
I. Miotics (Cholinergic)				
Pilocarpine 0.25-10%	1 to 2 drops 4 times/day	Topical	Ciliary muscle spasm, ↓ visual acuity, ↓ dark adaptation, follicular conjunctivitis, headache, nausea, bronchial constriction, ↑ salivation	Hypersensitivity, iritis, asthma hypertension
Carbachol 0.75-3%	2 drops up to 4 times/day	Topical	As per pilocarpine, transient ciliary, and conjunctival injection	As per pilocarpine
II. Hyperosmotics				
Glycerol 50%	1.0-1.5 g/kg	Oral	Nausea, vomiting, headache, confusion, dehydration, cardiac arrhythmias, blood sugar, hyperosmotic coma	Hypersensitivity, hypervolemia, congestive heart failure (CHF), confusional states
Mannitol 20%	1.5-2.0 g/kg	Intravenous	Headache, chills, chest pain, diuresis	Hypersensitivity, anuria, pulmonary edema, severe dehydration, intracranial hemorrhage
III. Carbonic Anhydrase Inhibitors (Used with Miotics)				
Acetazolamide (Diamox)	250 mg tablets 4 times/day	Oral	Paresthesias, anorexia, nausea	Na^+, K^+, abnormalities, marked renal and hepatic disease
	500 mg sequels 2 times/day	Oral	Polyuria, occasional drowsiness, and confusion	Chronic noncongestive angle-closure glaucoma, hypersensitivity, Addison's disease, severe COPD
	250-500 mg 2 times/day	Intravenous	Acidosis (long-term usage), all adverse reactions to sulfonamides	

Table 23-5. Antiglaucoma Medications—cont'd

Class and name	Dosage	Route	Side effects	Contraindications
III. Carbonic Anhydrase Inhibitors (Used with Miotics)—cont'd				
Dichlorphenamide (Daranide)	100 mg 2 times/ 2day until desired response obtained. Then 25-50 mg 1-3 times/day	Oral	As above	As above
Ethoxzolamide (Ethamide)	125 mg 1-2 times/day	Oral	As above	As above
Methazolamide (Neptazane)	50-100 mg 2-3 times/day	Oral	Anorexia, nausea, vomiting, malaise, fatigue, drowsiness, headache, paresthesias, confusion, vertigo	As above
IV. Adrenergics				
Epinephrine 0.25-2%	1 drop 1-2 times/day	Topical	May cause reversible cystoid macula edema (CME) in aphakics, blurred vision, conjunctival hyperemia, HTN, allergy, pigment deposition in conjunctiva	Narrow-angle glaucoma, use with caution in patients with hypertension, coronary artery disease
Dipivefrin HCl (Propine) 0.1%	1 drop 2 times/day	Topical	Aphakic CME, tachycardia, arrhythmias, hypertension, adenochrome deposits, burning, stinging	Narrow-angle glaucoma, hypersensitivity
Timolol (Timoptic) 0.5%	1 drop 2 times/day	Topical	Conjunctivitis, blepharitis, keratitis, visual disturbance, bradyarrhythmia, syncope, hypertension, bronchospasm, rarely confusion, depression, palpitations	Hypersensitivity, bronchospastic disease, bradycardia, first-degree block, CHF, cardiogenic shock, concomitant usage of adrenergic-augmenting psychotropic drugs

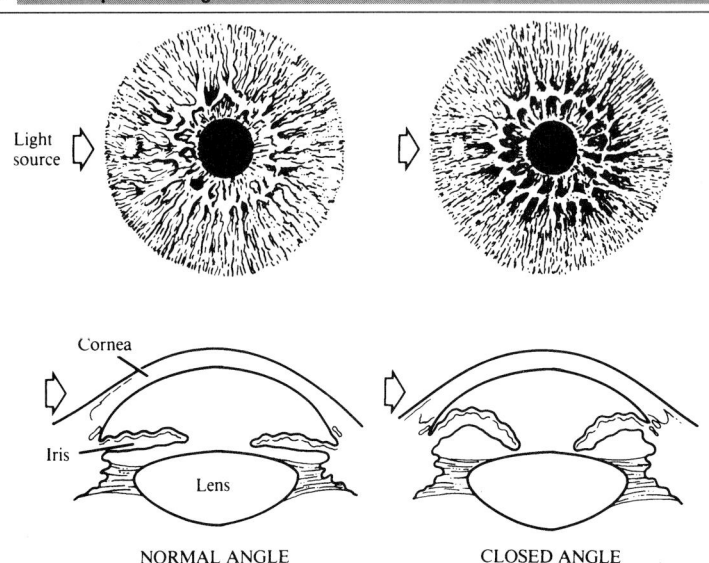

Figure 23-2. Illustration shows a shadow cast on the iris resulting from the bowed iris in angle-closure glaucoma. (Reproduced with permission from Kidwell EDR: Glaucoma. In Barker LR, Burton JR, and Zieve PD, editors: Principles of ambulatory medicine, Baltimore, 1986, Williams & Wilkins, p 1375.)

oral administration of hyperosmotic agents (such as glycerol). If treatment with glycerin is not successful or if the patient is nauseated, intravenous hypertonic mannitol (20%) may be effective. Miotics should be instilled in the other eye, which is also susceptible to acute angle closure. Definitive treatment is surgical. A peripheral iridectomy is performed when the symptoms have diminished and later on the unaffected eye as a prophylactic measure. (See **Table 23-5.**)

Cataracts

A cataract is an opacification of the crystalline lens. Cataracts vary markedly in degree of density and may be due to a variety of causes but are usually associated with aging. The crystalline lens is a unique structure: New lens fibers are constantly being formed throughout life, and old lens fibers are not lost but come to lie progressively deeper and more distant from the capsule of the lens. As the lens ages, its nucleus becomes increasingly dark, dense, and relatively opaque with a high refractive index (nuclear sclerosis). Cataracts diminish vision by decreasing the transparency of the lens and by altering the refractive power of the lens. Some degree of cataract formation is to be expected in all persons over the age of 70. Most are bilateral, although the rate of progression in each eye is seldom equal. Traumatic cataract, steroid-induced cataract, and other types are less common.

  I. **Visual loss is usually gradual,** although occasionally a patient first notices a monocular cataract when the better eye is covered and may interpret this as visual loss of sudden onset. Visual loss is always painless, and the patient may describe a constant fog over the eye. Occasionally, there is annoying diplopia or polyopia due to irregular refraction of the lens. Cataracts that affect the posterior surface of the lens may cause the vision to be much worse for close objects in bright light, because, when the pupil is small, all the light must pass through the area of the cataract.

II. **Slit-lamp.** Cataracts are easily identified by illuminating the lens with a slit lamp, but most emergency practitioners will find that they can see a cataract easily through the plus 4-10 lens of their direct ophthalmoscope. With pupillary dilation, the cataract may be manifested by a general dullness in the red reflex (nuclear sclerosis), peripheral "spokes" (cortical), or a central discrete opacity (posterior subcapsular). The depth of the anterior chamber should be checked, since in some cataracts the lens may swell and reduce the anterior chamber. Likewise, checking the intraocular pressures may identify glaucoma as a complication or cause of the cataract. The clinical degree of cataract formation, assuming that no other eye disease is present, is judged primarily by visual acuity.

III. **There are no medications** that have any direct beneficial effect upon cataract formation or progression. Occasionally, dilation of the pupil with mydriatic or cycloplegic drops may enlarge the pupil sufficiently to improve vision by allowing light to enter the eye around the cataract. These drops may improve vision sufficiently to enable elderly patients to function for years without surgery. The decision to remove a cataract is determined by the visual needs of the patient, as well as by the degree of capsular involvement and of any other ocular abnormalities. Surgical intervention, which has a 90 to 95% success rate, is the only definitive treatment.

Acute Vascular Occlusions

A number of entities can cause painless monocular visual loss: 1) central retinal artery or vein occlusion, 2) temporal arteritis, 3) retinal detachment, 4) macular degeneration, and 5) vitreous hemorrhage resulting from diabetic retinopathy or retinal hole formation. It is imperative that the patient suspected of having retinal artery or venous occlusion be evaluated by an ophthalmologist early in the course of the disease in order to increase the possibility of returning the eye to normal vision.

I. **Emboli or thrombi** from the carotid system or cardiac valves may occlude the central retinal artery or one of its branches. When the central retinal artery is affected, the result is sudden, complete or almost complete loss of vision. Total occlusion may be preceded by transient episodes of decreased vision, blindness in the affected eye (amaurosis fugax), or flickering vision. Ophthalmologic examination usually reveals the etiology of the visual loss. The direct pupillary reaction is absent but consensual light reaction is normal. The posterior retina is usually pale and opaque because of ischemic changes in the axons of the nerve fiber layer. Because the fovea lacks this layer, the choroid can be seen as a cherry-red spot. The veins appear dark, and the arteries may be narrowed, with segmentation of the blood column ("boxcar" appearance). Later, the vessel may appear normal, but emboli or plaque is often visible in the arterial tree.

A. **Treatment.** Unfortunately, in most cases, treatment is ineffective. If the patient is seen within 2 hours of the onset of symptoms, one should attempt to restore the blood flow. Treatment is directed toward relief of vasospasm (breathing a mixture of CO_2 and O_2, using a paper bag if necessary) or an attempt to dislodge the embolus by digital massage. The globe is massaged by pressing firmly through the closed lids for 5 seconds and then released for 5

seconds. Acetazolamide, 500 mg given orally, may lower the intraocular pressure to decrease resistance to arterial blood flow.
  B. **Other methods** that may be used by the ophthalmologist are a retrobulbar lidocaine block or anterior chamber paracentesis. The use of thrombolytic agents is recommended by some clinicians, but clinical evidence for effectiveness is lacking.
II. **Retinal vein occlusion** is encountered with some frequency and also has a poor prognosis for visual recovery. It may occur secondary to diabetes mellitus, hypertension, glaucoma, leukemia, and other conditions that impede venous flow. Arteriosclerosis is the most important systemic condition. External compression of the retinal vein by the rigid arterial wall may severely restrict blood flow, leading to venous stasis and eventual occlusion. Painless loss of vision ensues, although some degree of visual acuity may be preserved in up to 20% of patients. Venous occlusion is often preceded by episodes of transient decrease in vision lasting several hours, in contrast to the brief prodromal episodes associated with central retinal artery occlusion. Ophthalmoscopic examination reveals vascular dilation and tortuosity accompanied by retinal hemorrhage and occasionally retinal edema. When present in its classical form, this hemorrhagic retinopathy is described as "blood and thunder." Emergency medical therapy includes steroids, anticoagulants, vasodilators, and hemodilution, but treatment is even less effective than in central retinal artery occlusion. The natural history of this condition is variable, with spontaneous resolution not uncommon. Patients with branch retinal vein occlusion have a much better prognosis for useful vision, but many will require photocoagulation.

Temporal Arteritis

I. **Age.** One cause of retinal and ophthalmic artery occlusion that merits separate consideration is temporal or giant cell arteritis. This condition is clearly a disease of the elderly, with a median age of 75 years at diagnosis. It is characterized by giant cell infiltration of the media, progressing to panarteritis and intimal fibrosis. The superficial temporal, ophthalmic, vertebral, and internal carotid arteries are most commonly involved. Patients feel ill and have excruciating pain over the temporal or occipital arteries. Systemic symptoms include fever, malaise, weakness, and altered mentation. The scalp is often tender. Jaw claudication may occur and is sometimes worsened with chewing. The temporal arteries may be pulseless and are usually indurated with overlying erythema. Visual symptoms, such as blurring, diplopia, and transient or permanent visual loss, result when arteritis compromises blood supply to the retina or optic nerve. Approximately 40% of patients with temporal arteritis eventually suffer visual loss secondary to the ischemic optic neuropathy. Ischemic optic neuritis may also result from arteriosclerotic involvement of the small vessels supplying the optic nerve.
II. **Ophthalmoscopy** may initially produce unremarkable findings. Commonly, however, there are signs of iritis, extraocular muscle palsies, or manifestations of retinal artery occlusion, including pallor, hemorrhage, or exudates. The sedimentation rate is almost always over 50 mm/hr and frequently over 100 mm/hr. Many patients with active temporal arteritis have a low-grade anemia, leukocytosis, and elevated liver function tests. The definitive diagnosis is accomplished by temporal artery biopsy. Prompt treatment is recommended in suspected cases to prevent further vision loss. Patients with visual symptoms should be hospitalized and treated with high-dose intravenous steroids. Temporal artery biopsy should be

Retinal Detachment

It is essential that the emergency physician suspect retinal detachment in all cases of visual loss. There are 25,000 new cases of retinal detachment annually. Surgical repair is often effective if undertaken soon after onset. A complaint of "lightning flashes," cloudy or smoky vision, shower or floaters, or a curtain-like sensation falling over the visual field is an indication for an emergent ophthalmoscopic examination through a dilated pupil to detect the presence of retinal detachment. This is particularly true if the patient has undergone cataract surgery, is myopic, or has sustained recent trauma.

I. **Definition.** Retinal detachment does not represent true dislocation of the retina from the choroid but, rather, a separation of two retinal layers—the rod and cone layer—from the pigment epithelium. Accumulation of the fluid between these layers causes the detachment. The fluid usually originates in the vitreous, having passed through a hole in the retina. Physical examination will usually demonstrate a relative loss of visual field in the area of the detachment. When the detachment spreads very slowly, the patient may be unaware of any problem until the macula is affected. There may a disturbance of the red reflex, and, on funduscopic examination, one can observe a grayish mound that appears out of focus or a folding of the retina. The other eye must be examined, since it often has retinal holes or vitreoretinal adhesions that can lead to tears.

II. **Diagnosis.** It is difficult to make the diagnosis of retinal detachment without indirect ophthalmoscopy and scleral depression to visualize the peripheral retina—the area that is most commonly detached. Thus, the diagnosis should be suspected primarily on the basis of symptoms, confrontation field, and visual acuity, and, if these are abnormal, the patient should be referred immediately for a complete ophthalmologic evaluation. Treatment of retinal detachment requires urgent surgical intervention. Reattachment can be achieved in 95% of cases, and, even with macular involvement, visual restoration to a 20/40 or better acuity level can be accomplished in over half of patients. However, the longer the retina remains detached, the poorer the visual prognosis.

Macular Degeneration

Macular degeneration affects nearly one third of the geriatric population and is the leading cause of registered blindness in the United States. The risk of senile macular degeneration increases dramatically with age. Unlike cataracts or retinal detachment, macular degeneration is not amenable to surgery and, therefore, constitutes one of the most serious ocular diseases encountered in the geriatric patient. The exact etiology is unknown, although macular degeneration probably results from a decrease in the vascular supply to the macula from the lamina choriocapillaris. The overlying pigment epithelium is disturbed, especially in the macula and at the disk margin. Drusen—discrete hyaline deposits beneath the pigment epithelium—may be present as further evidence of degeneration. Retinal neovascularization may follow formation of the drusen. Disciform scars, macular cysts, and retinal detachment also may develop.

I. **Clinically, senile macular degeneration** is marked by a painless, progressive loss of central vision (e.g., close reading) over many months or years. Because retinal involvement is generally limited to the macular region, peripheral vision remains essentially intact. Ophthalmologic examination shows a relative central scotoma and loss of the foveal light reflex. In most patients, a disturbance in the smooth retinal pigment epithelial layer causes a fine stippling or clumping of black pigment associated with varying degrees of depigmentation in the macular region. The neovascularization may hemorrhage, and the patient presents with blood in the vitreous or beneath the retina. A grayish membrane appearing below the retina suggests the existence of neovascularization.

II. **Laser photocoagulation** may be useful in some patients who have focal areas of neovascularization identified with fluorescein angiography. However, the vast majority of patients are either never amenable to laser therapy (generalized atrophy) or are diagnosed too late (large disciform scar). Therapy is then confined to prescribing corrective lenses and assuring the patient that total blindness will not result from this disease.

Ophthalmologic Drugs

I. **Systemic reactions.** It is important to recognize that certain topical ocular medications may result in significant systemic reactions, such as cardiac failure (timolol), respiratory distress, myocardial infarction, depression, or suicidal ideation. Systemic side effects of these topical drugs are a result of three basic factors:
   A. First-order pass effect
   B. Typically high concentrations of the drug
   C. Higher concentration of drug retained by the conjunctival sac

   With the rapid absorption of medications particularly through the aging conjunctiva, merely one drop of a potent medication may have a marked systemic effect. This occurs because the drug reaches various target organs without first passing through the liver or kidney to be detoxified (first-order pass effect). Because of the variation in dosage forms, the clinician must carefully prescribe the topically applied preparation with the least potential systemic side effects.

II. **Eye medications are often concentrated** because their ocular exposure is short. This phenomenon is especially important in the elderly in whom the conjunctival sac retains a greater volume of medication because the eyelids are more lax. When drugs are given in eyedrop form, an estimated 80% of the dose drains rapidly through the nasolacrimal system and is absorbed by the nasal mucosa. Instructing the elderly patients to occlude the punctum by pressing the inner aspect of the lower lid with a finger for several minutes can markedly decrease the amount of systemic dissemination of an eyedrop, enhancing the safe topical use of medication. (See **Table 23-6**.)

III. **Topical ocular medications.** Outlined below are common topical ocular medications and their potential systemic side effects.
   A. **Corticosteroids.** Their use may reduce the facility of aqueous outflow, thereby increasing intraocular pressure. Approximately one third of patients will develop intraocular pressure elevation within 6 weeks of topical steroid therapy. This may induce or aggravate preexisting open-angle glaucoma. Corticosteroid drops may also potentiate herpes simplex or fungal keratitis. In addition, patients with tissue antigen HLA A1 are likely to develop posterior subcapsular cataracts, whether the steroid is given topically or systemically.
   B. **Antibiotics.** Any of the topical antibiotic drops can cause a local allergic reaction and are capable of causing anaphylaxis in patients with prior histories of hypersensitivity. A skin sensitivity to neomycin—manifested by an erythematous, pruritic scaling dermatitis—may appear in as many as 10 to 15% of

Table 23-6. Safe Use of Ocular Drugs in the Elderly

- Prescribe the topically applied preparation with the least potential systemic side effects.
- Instruct the patient to occlude the nasolacrimal punctum for a few minutes after drug application, thereby decreasing systemic absorption.
- Because of the marked variation in "generic equivalents," brand name medications are preferred.
- Use small amounts of ointment rather than drops when possible.
- Use a more dilute concentration.
- Wipe excess solution or ointment from the eye immediately after application.
- Because an informed patient is a better patient, actions as well as undesirable side effects should be discussed with elderly patients.

patients. Chloramphenicol and Sodium Sulamyd 10% rarely cause local sensitization.

C. Phenylephrine. Systemic reactions to topical ocular instillation of phenylephrine for dilation of pupils are uncommon but can be serious and even lethal when they occur. Only the 2.5% concentration is recommended for use in the elderly. Blood pressure should be carefully monitored in patients with cardiac disease, hypertension, arteriosclerosis, and aneurysms. Other rare reactions are ventricular arrhythmias, tachycardia, myocardial infarction, and subarachnoid hemorrhage. Tropicamide 0.5% (Mydriacyl) is probably the safest mydriatic, with weak cycloplegic action, for dilation of eyes in the elderly.

D. Cycloplegics. These sympathomimetic drugs (e.g., atropine, homatropine, scopolamine, and cyclopentolate) blur near vision by interfering with accommodation and are inferior for routine pupil dilation. They should be used with caution in patients with diabetes, hypertension, hyperthyroidism, heart disease, and bronchial asthma. In addition, the pressor response from these drugs may be markedly exaggerated in patients who have received tricyclic antidepressants, MAO inhibitors, propranolol, and anticholinergic drugs.

E. Epinephrine. The amount of epinephrine absorbed from topical ocular glaucoma therapy is comparable with the amount used systemically for various conditions. Adverse systemic effects include direct cardiovascular toxicity (e.g., hypertension, arrhythmias) and indirect central nervous system (CNS) toxicity (e.g., delusions, psychosis). Local ocular side effects of long-term epinephrine treatment for glaucoma are common. They range from corneal edema to conjunctival scarring, blepharitis, and deposition of pigment in the conjunctiva.

F. Parasympathomimetic drugs. The miotics are used almost exclusively for the treatment of glaucoma. Pilocarpine is one of the most commonly used and has the lowest reported incidence of systemic side effects. It does produce blurring of vision because of the accommodative spasm, as well as decreased vision due to miosis. This may severely reduce vision in an eye with a cataract. Adverse parasympathetic effects may include nausea, vomiting, diarrhea, headache, bradycardia, muscle cramps, perspiration, and respiratory distress. The anticholinesterase drugs may also be responsible for the development of cataracts, blurred vision, conjunctivitis, and retinal detachment.

G. Beta-blockers. The adverse effects associated with timolol maleate are more frequent and more severe than those associated with epinephrine and pilocarpine. Systemic side effects of topical ocular timolol are the same as those observed with oral beta-blockers. Cardiovascular, respiratory, CNS, gastrointestinal, and dermatologic reactions can occur. Timolol has been implicated as a causative agent in pulmonary edema, myocardial infarction, respiratory failure, and death and should be used with caution especially in elderly patients with peripheral vascular disease, asthma, ventricular failure, or bradycardia.

H. **Carbonic anhydrase inhibitor.** Diamox, a carbonic anhydrase inhibitor, markedly reduces the output of aqueous humor by the ciliary body. Its principal use is in the management of acute angle-closure glaucoma not responding to combinations of eyedrops. Diamox is chemically similar to the sulfonamides and may cause potassium depletion, gastric distress, diarrhea, exfoliative dermatitis, renal stone formation, shortness of breath, acidosis, and fatigue. These side effects, although not entirely absent, are less frequent with methazolamide (Neptazane).

Suggested Readings

Abrahamson IA: Eye changes after forty, *Am Fam Physician* 29:171-181, 1984.

Berson FG: The eye in old age. In Rossman I, editor: *Clinical geriatrics,* Philadelphia, 1986, JB Lippincott.

Davidorf FH: Retinal breakdown in the aging eye: what are the consequences? *Geriatrics* 36:103-107, 1981.

Eifrig DE, Simons KB: An overview of common geriatric ophthalmologic disorders, *Geriatrics* 38:55-57, 1983.

Ferris FL: Senile macular degeneration: review of epidemiologic features, *Am J Epidemiol* 118:132-151, 1983.

Fraunfelder FT, Meyer SM: Safe use of ocular drugs in the elderly, *Geriatrics* 39:97-102, 1984.

Hayreth SS, Hayreth MS: Hemicentral retinal vein occlusion: pathogenesis, clinical features and natural history, *Arch Ophthalmol* 98:1600-1609, 1980.

Kasper RL: Eye problems of the aged. In Reichel W, editor: *Clinical aspects of aging,* Baltimore, 1978, Williams & Wilkins.

Keeney AH, Keeney VT: A guide to examining the aging eye, *Geriatrics* 35:81-91, 1980.

Keltner JL: Giant-cell arteritis: signs and symptoms, *Ophthalmology* 89:1101-1109, 1982.

Kollarits CR: The aging eye. In Calkins E, Davis PJ, Ford AB, editors: *The practice of geriatrics,* Philadelphia, 1986, WB Saunders.

Leighton DA: Special senses: aging of the eye. In Brocklehurst JC, editor: *Textbook of geriatric medicine and gerontology,* New York, 1985, Churchill Livingstone.

Rosenfield SJ: Treatment of temporal arteritis with ocular involvement, *Am J Med* 80:143-146, 1986.

Sakamoto DK: Retinal detachment: where an early diagnosis is important, *Geriatrics* 36:87-90, 1981.

Schlichtemeier WR: Corneal disease: an approach to primary care, *Geriatrics* 39:56-66, 1984.

Stokoe NL: Ocular pain in the elderly: simple symptom or hidden danger? *Geriatrics* 35:41-50, 1980.

Vaughan D, Taylor A: *General ophthalmology,* Los Altos, Calif, 1983, Lange Medical Publishers.

Suggested Readings

Walshe TM, editor: *Manual of clinical problems in geriatric medicine,* Boston, 1985, Little, Brown.

Weale R: The eye of the elderly. What is normal aging? *Geriatr Med Today* 4:29-37, 1985.

Weinstock FJ: Ophthalmic disorders. In Covington TR, Walker JI, editors: *Current geriatric therapy,* Philadelphia, 1984, WB Saunders.

Yanofsky NN: The acute painful eye, *Emerg Med Clin North Am* 6:21-42, 1988.

Zun LS: Acute vision loss, *Emerg Med Clin North Am* 6:21-42, 1988.

This chapter is modified from Dougherty J: A systematic approach to acute ophthalmologic disorders in the geriatric patient. In Bosker et al, editors: *Geriatric emergency medicine,* St. Louis, 1990, Mosby–Year Book.

24

Dermatologic Disorders

Stephan A. Billstein, M.D., M.P.H.

Papulosquamous Eruptions

A. Papules and scaling. Papulosquamous eruptions are characterized by papules and scaling. Papules are raised lesions. The surface of a papule may be smooth, irregular, and occasionally vesiculated or scaly. When papules merge together, they can produce lesions termed macules. Squamous implies that a lesion is characterized by a scale or is scaling. The epidermis usually consists of four layers (a fifth layer is present in the skin of the palms and soles). From outward in, the layers are the stratum corneum, stratum lucidum (palms and soles), stratum granulosum, stratum malpighii (spinous cell layer), and stratum basale. Hyperkeratosis and parakeratosis are evidenced by increased thickening of the stratum corneum, which clinically is represented by scaling.

B. Questions to ask. When an emergency physician sees a patient with a papulosquamous eruption, there are several questions that should come to mind. They include the following: Is itching present? Are excoriations apparent? What is the distribution of the eruption? What is the history of progression of lesions of the eruption? Do systemic symptoms such as fever accompany the eruption? Is there a history of recent trauma such as an insect bite or penetrating wound? Is there a family history of a similar eruption? Does anyone who has had intimate exposure to the patient have a similar eruption at present or within the past few weeks? What medications or food has the patient recently taken or is regularly taking?

Eczema

Eczema and dermatitis (inflammation of the skin) are interchangeably used as synonyms for one another. The characteristics of eczema on physical examination are papules accompanied by scaling, redness, and often excoriations. In order to treat this disease effectively, the physician must understand the basic pathophysiologic process. The physician then will be able to explain to the patient with eczema how and why the skin eruption occurs.

I. Itching. The initial physiologic event in eczema is itching. The patient begins to itch and then to scratch. The eruption then occurs because of the scratching, as the skin tries to protect itself. The rash causes the patient to scratch more, eventually leading to an itch-scratch-itch cycle. On examination of the skin during an acute exacerbation, the physician will see papules, erythema, and scaling, with occasional evidence of actual excoriations. On close examination along with taking a comprehensive history, the physician can determine that the lesions seen are not "true" skin lesions but rather a response of the skin trying to protect itself from the patient's constant scratching.

When a comprehensive history is taken in the emergency department, it is important to ask the patient which came first, the rash or the itching. The physician can accurately assess the patient by taking a careful history and by performing a complete physical examination. This assessment gives the emergency physician the necessary information to formulate a good differential diagnosis in many skin eruptions that present with papules, erythema, and scaling.

II. Definition. Eczema is a chronic, recurrent eruption seen in an atopic person. It is associated with allergy and characterized by exacerbations and remissions. The dermatologic definition of eczema is dermatitis (inflammation) of the skin characterized by erythema, itching, vesiculation, and scaling. On histopathologic examination, the vesiculation is intraepidermal. Intercellular edema of the malpighian layer of the epidermis (microscopic spongiosis) occurs, eventually leading to the vesiculation. Also present is hyperkeratosis of the stratum corneum, the outer layer of the epidermis, which is the cause of scaling seen on physical examination.

   A. Early definitions. In 1923, **Coca defined atopy** as hypersensitivity based on hereditary influence. Originally, the definition included just asthma, hay fever, and then eczema. Now it also includes urticaria and dermatographism. In 1933, Sulzberger first defined atopic dermatitis. He implied that the patient with atopic dermatitis had a predisposition to asthma and/or hay fever.

   B. Current thought is that atopic persons can have any one or more of the five manifestations of the allergic diathesis: asthma, hay fever, dermatitis, urticaria, and dermatographism. The patient that sees an emergency physician can have evidence of acute, subacute, or chronic signs and symptoms of eczema. The subacute and chronic forms of this disease will have less inflammation and will be characterized by greater thickening and even a leathery appearance, especially in areas that have been chronically scratched. Often, hypopigmentation and hyperpigmentation of the skin in areas of predilection are present.

III. Age. The infantile form of eczema is most often seen on the cheeks, the trunk, and the extremities. In the childhood form, the eruption is seen most often in antecubital areas, the popliteal fossae, and over the extensor surfaces of the body. Older children, adolescents, and adults will show high activity on the flexural surfaces of the skin, the face, and the neck. Presentation of atopic dermatitis can take many shapes or forms depending on the underlying pruritus and the ability of the patient to reach and scratch particular areas of the skin. One form of presentation is nummular eczema. This type is usually coin-like or circular in appearance, with scaling, erythema, and occasionally vesiculation. One place on the body where it is especially important to recognize nummular eczema is on the scalp. Often patients will have an insect bite or some other antecedent event that produces itching. They will get into an itch-scratch-itch cycle and eventually come to the physician with a large area of hair loss dominated by a nummular thickened, scaled, erythematous, vesiculated patch of dermatitis. A thorough history is very important in this case to determine the true etiologic nature of the dermatitis. Prescribing medication may not be enough to improve the dermatitis, since behavioral modification is often necessary.

IV. Patients with atopic dermatitis often have certain stigmata. They seem to have an abnormal physiologic response to epinephrine and/or norepinephrine. Their skin tends to be pale. They demonstrate dermatographism, which is localized edema and urtication of the skin in response to pressure, such as streaking with the blunt end of a pencil. They may show a hyperactive cold pressure response, as well as a tendency toward hypotension. A number of atopic patients demonstrate a flat glucose tolerance curve. Over time, if a large number of atopic patients are examined, they seem to get cataracts earlier than those persons in the general population that do not have the atopic diathesis. Sweat retention is common. The skin of the atopic person tends to be so dry that it may demonstrate keratosis pilaris (chicken-like skin), pleats under the eyes, and sometimes prominent palmar creases. Dry skin alone (xerosis) is not enough to state that a patient has eczema. The other characteristics previously described, both clinically and histopathologically, also have to be present.

  A. **Psychologic characteristics. Atopic persons** often have psychologic behavioral characteristics that tend to precipitate the exacerbation of the dermatitis. They are usually active and aggressive people. Often they are precocious and very bright. Evaluating the psychologic profile is important when taking a thorough history on the patient with eczema. Management of this patient may require behavioral modification, and this knowledge will be helpful.

  B. **In summary,** the actual cause of the pathogenesis of atopic dermatitis is unknown. Atopic patients have abnormal itching associated with dry skin. The itch tends to spread, and atopic persons scratch. The body responds by building up a thickness or hyperkeratosis of the epidermis, and eventually an itch-scratch-itch cycle results. An imbalance of the autonomic nervous system in atopic persons seems to be present, caused by adrenergic blockade. In hot or cold weather, atopic persons tend to overreact at the site of the peripheral nerves. In cold weather, their feet and/or the tips of their fingers will become very cold, simulating a Raynaud's phenomenon. When they enter a warm area or warm themselves, they have an abnormal throbbing of the body parts that were previously cold. Increased levels of serum IgE have also been associated with patients with the atopic diathesis.

V. **Therapy and management.** The first principle in managing the patient with atopic dermatitis patient is to know thy patient. A thorough history needs to be taken from the patient by the physician. Once the pathophysiology of atopic dermatitis in a particular patient is understood, the physician will be able to give that patient an understanding of, and insight into, his or her own disease. This transferral to the patient of how the rash occurs following the itching is vitally important for therapy to succeed.

  A. **Intervention.** To successfully manage the atopic patient, intervention must be directed at the patient's scratching and the hypersensitivity of the skin that causes itching. If the itching can successfully be stopped, then the scratching will stop and the eruption will resolve. Systemic medications may serve as an adjunct, but by themselves will not be successful in the management of this disease. Medications that are characterized as "antiitch" pills usually gain their antipruritic effects by virtue of other pharmacologic actions. These pills are usually hypnotics, antihistamines, sedatives, or tranquilizers. By inducing a sedative or tranquilizing effect, they make the patients so relaxed that they are unable to lift their hand to scratch. Systemic and/or topical antibiotics may be necessary if the eczematous dermatitis becomes superinfected.

  B. **Hydration of the skin** is often helpful as an adjunct to primary intervention therapy because the skin of most atopic patients is usually dry. Tepid or lukewarm water should be used by patients for general hydration, such as in baths or showers. Emollient oils, gels, or other preparations designed to make the baths more soothing and pleasant to the skin are often useful in helping to debride scales and crusts and minimize pruritus. Patients must be instructed when using these emollients to be careful getting in and out of the bathtub because they could slip and fracture a hip. The frequency and duration of bathing and showering should be kept to a minimum. When itching or pruritus is prolonged, it is more apt to occur shortly after bathing is over.

C. Creams and ointments. The hallmark of therapy for atopic dermatitis is an antiinflammatory cream or ointment. Five percent crude cold tar preparations are available over-the-counter and often are effective therapy in a number of cases providing the patient is willing to apply them three or four times daily. The major objections to crude cold tar preparations are that they have an offensive odor and stain all clothing and other apparel black. Corticosteroid creams have essentially become the norm for managing atopic dermatitis **(Table 24-1)**. Systemic corticosteroid therapy is not usually prescribed. Topical therapy will work as long as enough dosage is given. Because other measures are available that provide effective treatment, the adverse effects associated with continuous systemic corticosteroid therapy outweigh the benefits. In addition, tolerance and habituation may occur. On withdrawal, a rebound exacerbation of the dermatitis may occur that is often worse than the initial bout.

    1. Acute phase. There are many corticosteroid creams and ointments available by prescription, and most will be effective when used properly. In the acute phase or after the first visit to the physician, patients should be instructed to follow a regular application schedule, as well as applying the preparation additionally anytime that they want to scratch. Within a few days of a regularly scheduled and an as-needed regimen, the dermatitis will come under control. Oftentimes patients will state that they cannot apply the topical preparation on a regular basis. When this occurs, the physician has to be creative and make the schedule fit the patients' daily routine. An example of this would be a four-time-a-day regimen such as before work, after work, at dinner time, and at bedtime.

    2. Vanishing creams and ointments are usually the corticosteroid preparations that are available. The vanishing cream has the advantage of being able to be rubbed in until it disappears, whereas the ointment with a petrolatum base can be rubbed in but will leave a petrolatum ointment coating on the skin. Patients should be consulted as to which preparation they would prefer from a cosmetic standpoint, since either will effectively treat the dermatitis providing it is used. If a vanishing-cream base is prescribed, it is important to instruct patients that a minimal amount of cream is necessary and that it must be rubbed into the skin thoroughly. If any cream remains on the skin that looks like icing on a pie or cake, it can be wiped away and really has no effect, since it has not been rubbed into the skin. Often there are areas of the skin that are markedly raw and inflamed. The patient, especially a child (or parent), needs to know that the initial application of a corticosteroid cream or ointment may burn. If the physician does not inform the patient of this side effect, often the patient will stop using the preparation after the first application. Corticosteroid creams and ointments have been divided into low-potency, medium-potency and high-potency preparations. Also, they can be categorized as nonfluorinated and fluorinated. High potency and/or fluorinated preparations, when used for long periods, can induce skin atrophy and/or telangiectasis. However,

Table 24-1. Topical Corticosteroid Preparations

Corticosteroid	Brand name (vehicle)	Cost[a]
Lowest Potency		
Dexamethasone 0.1%	Decadron[c]	++++
	Decaderm[d]	++++
Hydrocortisone 1.0%	Cort-Dome[c]	++++
	Cortef[e]	++++
	Penecort[c]	+
Hydrocortisone 2.5%	Penecort[c]	+++
	Synacort[c]	+++
	Hytone[f]	+++
Methylprednisolone acetate 0.25%	Medrol[e]	++++
Methylprednisolone acetate 1.0%	Medrol[e]	++++
Low Potency		
Betamethasone valerate 0.01%	Valisone, decreased strength[c]	+++
Clocortolone 0.1%	Cloderm[c]	++++
Desonide 0.05%	Desowen[c]	+++
	Tridesilon[c,e]	+++
Fluocinolone acetonide 0.01%	Generic[c]	+
	Synalar[c]	+++
Flurandrenolide 0.025%	Cordran, Cordran SP[c,e]	+++
Hydrocortisone valerate 0.2%	Westcort[c,e]	+++
Triamcinolone acetonide 0.025%	Generic[c,e]	+
	Aristocort[c]	+++
	Aristocort A[c]	+++
	Kenalog[c,e,f]	++++
Intermediate Potency		
Betamethasone benzoate 0.025%	Benisone[c,d,e,f]	+++
	Uticort[c,d,e,f]	+++
Betamethasone valerate 0.1%	Generic[c,e,f]	+++
	Valisone[c,e]	++++
Desoximetasone 0.05%	Topicort LP[c]	+++
	Topicort Gel[d]	+++
Fluocinolone acetonide 0.025%	Generic[c,e]	+
	Fluonid[c,e]	+++
Flurandrenolide	Generic[f]	+
	Cordran, Cordran SP	++++
Halcinonide 0.025%	Halog[c]	++++
Triamcinolone acetonide 0.1%	Generic[c,e,f]	+
	Aristocort[c,e]	+++
	Aristocort A[c,e]	++++
	Kenalog[c,e,f]	+++,++++
High Potency		
Amcinonide 0.1%	Cyclocort[c,e]	++++
Betamethasone dipropionate 0.05%	Generic[c,e]	+++
	Alphatrex[c,e,f]	+++
	Diprosone[c,e]	++++
Desoximetasone 0.25%	Topicort[c,e]	+++
Diflorasone diacetate 0.05%	Florone[c,e]	++++
	Maxiflor[c,e]	++++
Fluocinolone 0.2%	Synalar HP[c]	++++

Continued on next page

Table 24-1. Topical Corticosteroid Preparations—cont'd

Corticosteroid	Brand name (vehicle)	Cost[a]
Fluocinonide 0.05%	Lidex, Lidex-E[c,d,e]	++++
Halcinonide 0.1%	Halog, Halog-E[c,e,g]	++++
Triamcinolone acetonide 0.5%	Generic[c,e]	+++
	Aristocort A[c]	++++
	Aristocort[c,e]	++++
	Kenalog[c,e]	++++
Highest Potency		
Betamethasone dipropionate 0.05%	Diprolene[c,e]	++++
Clobetasol propionate 0.05%	Temovate[c,e]	++++

From Koda-Kimble A, Young LY: *Applied therapeutics: the clinical use of drugs*, ed 5, Vancouver, 1992, Applied Therapeutics.
[a] + = <$2; ++ = $2-$5; +++ = $5-$10; ++++ = >$10.
[b] May be ineffective for some indications.
[c] Cream.
[d] Gel.
[e] Ointment.
[f] Lotion.
[g] Solution.

once use of the preparation has stopped, the skin will usually regain its normal appearance, unless over time it has been permanently scarred by the chronic nature of the dermatitis.

3. **In chronic recurrent eczema** where use of topical corticosteroids is the norm, tolerance to a particular preparation will often develop. The physician needs to be aware of this phenomenon and when it occurs, prescribe a different corticosteroid formulation. The use of the new topical cream or ointment will usually work. Tolerance to a preparation usually lasts about 10 days. Hence, the patient should be instructed not to discard the old prescription. In fact, a good method of management in patients with atopic dermatitis is to have them rotate several topical medications.

4. **Initial management** of patients who are seen with acute atopic dermatitis should include a topical corticosteroid, equivalent to 0.1% triamcinolone cream or ointment. Patients should be instructed to apply this preparation thoroughly at least four times a day and any time they wish to scratch. In addition, if the lesions are markedly vesicular, edematous, or macerated, local astringent solutions may be applied such as Burow's solution. This solution is usually applied as an open, wet dressing; it is soothing, cooling, antipruritic, and helps to remove debris and crusts. It also helps to hydrate the skin, dry up the vesicular component of the crust, and has some mild antibacterial action. The technique in applying Burow's solution is to use a handkerchief or strips of bed sheeting soaked with the solution, which is kept at room temperature. The compresses should be moderately wet, not dripping, and moistened at intervals. Burow's is available commercially as a solution, tablets, and a powder. Adding a single tablet or packet of powder to a pint of water produces a 1:40 solution. The usual regimen is that the patient apply the Burow's solution for 15 to 20 minutes four times daily. Patients with eczema should also use soaps that

have a minimal amount of perfume and are not excessively drying. Various companies market soaps of a hypoallergenic nature. During the summertime, air conditioning is often helpful because excessive sweating by the eczematous patient is not handled well. Harsh detergents, bubble baths, feather pillows, stuffed animals, wool, fuzzy toys, and some types of cats and dogs should be avoided.

D. The differential diagnosis of atopic dermatitis include seborrheic dermatitis, lichen planus, psoriasis, parapsoriasis, secondary syphilis, tinea or ringworm infections, pityriasis rosea, contact dermatitis, insect bites, miliaria, lice and scabies infestations, and moniliasis. These diseases will be discussed in the forthcoming pages.

Seborrheic Dermatitis

Seborrheic dermatitis is a papulosquamous eruption that presents with minimal pruritus. This eruption is most prevalent when sebaceous glands are active. Therefore, it will be seen in patients where estrogen and/or testosterone levels are present, since these hormones are necessary for sebaceous gland activity. The newborn infant can have seborrheic dermatitis until the sebaceous glands atrophy when maternal estrogen disappears. The sebaceous glands again become active as the sex hormones are secreted at the time that puberty begins.

I. The initial papular lesions begin around the pilosebaceous unit. They are characterized by erythema and a yellowish, crusty, sometimes vesicular scaling. They may appear in areas of the skin anywhere sebaceous glands are present. Involvement of the body may be minimal, that is localized to one or two areas, or it can be extensive, sometimes involving greater than 50% of the body surface. Papules can merge and form macules, and even get larger, with macules merging to form plaques. Occasionally, it may be difficult to differentiate seborrheic dermatitis from psoriasis. Differentiation from eczema can be made because itching is not the initial symptom.

II. Age. In the infant, the eruption is most characteristically seen on the scalp where it is called cradle cap. It also frequently involves the central areas of the face and chest, and occasionally the diaper area. In the adult, the most frequent sites are the central areas of the face and chest, the groin, and the scalp, where the disease is termed dandruff. Seborrheic dermatitis is a chronic inflammatory skin eruption that is characterized by exacerbations and remissions. Environmental conditions and overt and subconscious tension can precipitate exacerbations of this disease.

III. Pathophysiology. In treating seborrheic dermatitis, both the physician and the patient need to understand the pathophysiology of the disease. If the physician perceives that environmental factors or tension are precipitating factors in exacerbations of the dermatitis, then the physician must make the patient aware of this. Therefore, part of the implementation of a therapeutic course may involve behavioral modification. The emergency physician usually does not see the patient except for the acute diagnosis and treatment. However, the emergency physician still can discuss behavioral changes with the patient and give the patient insight into the precipitating factors of the eruption. If the patient works as a short-order cook in a diner and the heat of the stove seems to precipitate the dermatitis, it may be necessary for the patient to enter into a new occupation. If there is a problem in the patient's interpersonal relationships that is producing either overt or subconscious tension, that issue may need to be addressed.

IV. **Creams and ointments.** Specific medications to treat seborrheic dermatitis include topical antiinflammatory creams and ointments. Five percent crude cold tar preparations, available over-the-counter, are effective but have a tar odor and can stain clothing black. Topical corticosteroid creams, ointments, and lotions (for the scalp) are currently the mainstay of therapy. A preparation approximating the potency of 0.1% triamcinolone cream or ointment should be the initial treatment and prescribed a minimum of three or four times daily. For seborrhea of the scalp, various shampoos are effective when used daily. They include those that contain tar, salicylic acid, and selenium sulfide. In addition, Burow's solution may be useful to help debride crusts. If the area of seborrheic dermatitis is extensive, antibiotics, whether given systemically or applied topically either in combination or alternating with the corticosteroid preparation, are helpful. Erythromycin and tetracycline have been used systemically, as well as topically, in addition to topical neomycin or topical chloramphenicol. It is important to let the patient know that the management and/or treatment of seborrheic dermatitis will not usually effect a cure. This eruption is chronic and characterized by exacerbations and remissions.

Lichen Planus

Lichen planus is a papulosquamous eruption that is intensely pruritic. The cause of this dermatitis is unknown. Overt and subconscious tension are thought to play a role in precipitating this disease.

I. **The lesions of lichen planus** are characterized by violaceous papules present most often on the volar surfaces of the wrists, on both sides of the ankle, and on the penis. More often than not, when lesions are present on the skin, the buccal mucosa of the mouth has a lacy-white pattern. The eruption on the buccal mucosa if untreated can progress to ulceration. Lichen planus is also characterized by the "Koebner phenomenon," in which new lesions appear on parts of the skin that are traumatized or irritated. This phenomenon is also seen in psoriasis; however, the lesions of psoriasis usually do not itch. The lesions of lichen planus will start as papules but can become confluent to the point of being macular, and can form plaques if treatment is not instituted.

II. **The histopathology** of lichen planus is diagnostic. Most prominent is a band-like infiltrate of monocytic cells in the upper dermis adjacent to the epidermis. The epidermis shows hyperkeratosis and sometimes parakeratosis along with vesiculation, depending on how much excoriation has occurred. Also at times, the vesiculation may be at the dermal-epidermal junction, as well as being intraepidermal.

III. **Management** of the patient with lichen planus is often helped by behavioral modification if psychologic factors are deemed to be precipitating events. When the physician gives this type of insight to the patient, the patient can often relate some psychologic trauma that was close to or preceded the onset of the eruption. Specific therapy for lichen planus that works 100% of the time does not exist. Both systemic and topical corticosteroids have been used, either as single therapy or in combination. Triamcinolone, 40 mg/ml by intralesional injection, is often given in the dosage of 1 ml/wk. This is accompanied by a topical regimen of a medium- to high-potency corticosteroid cream rubbed into the skin lesions a minimum of four times a day and anytime the patient wants to scratch. As the itching of the eruption comes under control, the systemic corticosteroids can be tapered off and the patient can be maintained on topical preparations. Tranquilizers such as diazepam, 5 mg three times a day, are often useful in helping patients cope with their psychologic precipitating problems, as well as providing sedation and relieving, to a degree, the itching. They should be prescribed sparingly. To avoid tolerance and physical dependence, tranquilizers should not be prescribed beyond 1 month's duration.

Psoriasis Vulgaris

Psoriasis vulgaris is a chronic papulosquamous eruption characterized by exacerbations and remissions. The disease is rarely associated with itching. The eruption starts as a raised erythematous papule with scaling, gradually enlarging so that many papules will often merge or coalesce and eventually form macular and plaque-like lesions. Scaling that occurs with this eruption is probably the most intense compared with all the other papulosquamous eruptions.

I. **The cause** of psoriasis is unknown. In up to 80% or more of the cases, there is a hereditary predisposition that seems to be precipitated by environmental and psychologic factors. The underlying pathophysiology of psoriasis is that the metabolism of the epidermis is speeded up from 28 days to 3 days. This means that the cells from the stratum basale, the deepest layer of the epidermis, take 3 days to migrate up to the skin surface and become the stratum corneum. Because the transit time is so rapid, often the nuclei of the cells have not disappeared. Therefore, the histopathology of psoriasis vulgaris is characteristic; hyperkeratosis and parakeratosis with thickening of the epidermis are seen. There may be a mild perivascular infiltrate in the dermis. It is unclear whether psoriasis vulgaris begins first in the epidermis, first in the dermis, or in both layers of the skin at the same time.

II. **The distribution of psoriatic papules, macules, plaques, or patches** can occur anywhere on the body. New lesions arise often resulting from Koebner phenomenon (see Lichen Planus). Most often, the lesions of psoriasis are on the dorsal surface of the body, especially prominent in areas of constant friction, such as the elbows, the knees, and the glans penis. Psoriasis can also appear on apposed surfaces of the body where it is more likely to see erythematous papules and macules with minimal scaling. This is termed inverse psoriasis. Psoriasis may also occur on the scalp and simulate the dandruff appearance of seborrheic dermatitis. One characteristic unique to psoriasis is pitting of the nails. If a patient has had the eruption for a period of time, the emergency physician can often confirm that the papulosquamous eruption is psoriasis by examining the fingernails.

III. **Management and treatment** of psoriasis will have its greatest chance of success when the physician is able to explain to the patient what the precipitating factors of each exacerbation might be. By taking a thorough history from the patient and by showing interest and empathy for the patient's plight, the physician can gain the confidence of the patient so that together they can decide on the course of treatment. The treatment for each psoriatic patient needs to be individualized so that the patient feels confident that the physician cares. The use of topical antiinflammatory preparations such as 5% crude cold tar, liquor carbonis detergent (cold tar solution), salicylic acid, lactic acid, corticosteroids, nonsteroidal antiinflammatory agents such as ibuprofen, imidazoles, and vitamin D_3

have all been tried in some patients. The *power of positive sell,* regardless of what is prescribed for the patient, is important. The physician must convince the patient that the topical preparation has a chance of working. The physician must prescribe a specific regimen and explain exactly how to apply the topical medication so there is no confusion in the patient's mind on how to use the medication. All the topical medications that were previously mentioned when applied three or four times a day or more, will usually work initially until either a tolerance develops and/or compliance fails. It is important that the attending physician follow the patient closely to maintain the rapport gained at the first visit. The emergency physician, in this case, should refer the psoriatic patient to a *caring* dermatologist. A psoriatic patient that has been previously treated with a number of different medications often is hostile and switches doctors often.

IV. **Systemic drugs.** When topical medications no longer are effective in managing the psoriatic patient, a number of systemic drugs are available. Corticosteroids have been used for short-term treatment, although they are not usually recommended because their side effects outweigh their therapeutic benefit. Also, the eruption recurs via a rebound phenomenon when corticosteroids are discontinued. Methotrexate, hydroxyurea, PUVA (photochemotherapy combined with the use of psoralens), etretinate, and cyclosporine have all been prescribed for the psoriatic patient who no longer responds to topical therapy alone. Often these drugs are used in combination with each other and with topical therapy. The systemic medications all have pronounced side effects, and the physician who prescribes them must weigh the risks of these drugs with their benefits. Systemic medications and PUVA should be prescribed only by experienced dermatologists because of the greater risk of toxicity.

Parapsoriasis

I. **Parapsoriasis is a catch-all term** for eruptions that accompany various types of vasculitis. Parapsoriasis is a papulosquamous eruption, and itching may or may not occur depending on the stage and the degree of the vasculitis. The cause of most types of vasculitis that cause parapsoriatic-type eruptions is unknown. The diseases are often tagged with eponyms and characterized by histopathologic and clinical descriptions. Many times the course is typified by erythematous scaling papules erupting, becoming larger, possibly coalescing or merging with other similar lesions, vesiculating, crusting, and resolving, often with scarring of the skin, especially if the underlying dermis is involved.

II. **Recurrence.** Many patients with a vasculitis have recurrent parapsoriatic eruptions. Therefore it is imperative that the emergency physician take a good history when examining a patient with a papulosquamous eruption. Knowing the past history of similar eruptions and the possibility of hereditary influence are vitally important in helping to diagnose this disease on the initial visit. Biopsy of a new lesion is necessary to confirm the diagnosis of parapsoriasis. Management and treatment of parapsoriasis will be dependent on the type of vasculitis identified. Systemic and/or topical corticosteroids are the most common medications used. Parapsoriasis would not normally be treated by the emergency physician; however, it is important for the emergency physician to recognize this disease from other papulosquamous eruptions.

Syphilis

Syphilis is an infectious disease caused by a spirochete, *Treponema pallidum*. Syphilis can affect all the organs of the body, including the skin. It is classified by stages. The primary stage is characterized by an incubation period of approximately 2 to 6 weeks. The lesion seen in the primary stage is a chancre. The chancre usually occurs at the point of contact. Occasionally there are multiple chancres. Without treatment, the chancre remains for up to 4 weeks and then will disappear. However, the disease will usually continue subclinically and systemically. On physical examination, the chancre is firm and nontender. A rubbery feeling, shoddy lymphadenopathy may be present in the lymphatic area that drains the site of the chancre.

I. **Diagnosis.** The most consistent method used to correctly diagnose the chancre of syphilis is darkfield examination. The emergency physician should scrape the base of the chancre and place a wet mount preparation on a slide for darkfield examination. The *T. pallidum* spirochete usually has three coils and is motile on darkfield examination. If the ability to examine the wet mount is not readily available, then the wet mount needs to have a cover glass applied, with Vaseline put around the periphery of the cover glass. The slide then can be sent to a laboratory for fluorescent darkfield examination. Nonspecific serologic tests, such as the VDRL or RPR, as well as specific tests such as the FTA, are rarely positive when the chancre first appears. However, a specimen of blood should be drawn for a baseline examination.

II. **Secondary syphilis.** In order to make the diagnosis of secondary syphilis, the patient must have a rash and a positive nonspecific serologic test for syphilis. Eruptions of secondary syphilis can mimic any other dermatologic disease. Because of this, syphilis has been called *the great imitator*. Hence, papulosquamous eruptions can be present that simulate eczema, seborrheic dermatitis, psoriasis, parapsoriasis, and other dermatologic entities. The emergency physician should always have a high index of suspicion of this disease in sexually active patients, especially those from ages 15 to 35 years who are seen with a recent onset of dermatitis. Papulosquamous eruptions can also occur as part of the congenital syphilis syndrome. Therefore it is imperative that the emergency physician take a thorough history and do a comprehensive physical examination before arriving at a tentative diagnosis of the papulosquamous eruption. As stated before, to make a diagnosis of secondary syphilis or even congenital syphilis, the VDRL or RPR must be positive.

   A. **Characteristically the papulosquamous eruption of secondary syphilis** is often bilateral, symmetrical, and involves the palms and soles. Evidence of the eruption is often present at the corners of the mouth and about the ala nasi. Bilateral symmetrical loss of the outer edges of the eyebrows is common. Mucous patches of the genitals, perianal area, and buccal mucosa are often seen, appearing as denuded papules or ulcerations. If the patient is seen during the first few days of this eruption, the mucous patch–type lesions are often darkfield positive, and a rapid diagnosis can be made as opposed to waiting for serologic test results. Wart-like lesions, termed condyloma lata, appear in apposed areas, such as about the anus, in the axillae, or between the toes.

   B. **The incubation period for secondary syphilis** is roughly 3 to 6 months after contact with the infection. The chancre stage will usually have occurred. Patients will often not know that they had a chancre because it is a painless, firm ulceration. When the chancre occurs internally, patients may not have ever seen, or had symptoms from, the chancre. In the case of congenital syphilis, depending on when the infant acquired the disease in utero, the eruption may be present at birth or take several months to appear.

III. The use of penicillin remains the standard treatment for syphilis. Tetracycline and erythromycin are used as alternatives when the patient is allergic to penicillin. This section will not include a discussion of latent and late syphilis because the management is not usually handled by an emergency physician. See the chapter on sexually transmitted diseases for current drug choice and dosage.

Tinea Infections

Tinea infections are known by the lay public as ringworm and by the medical public as dermatophytoses. These are superficial mycotic infections of the dead cornified layers of the skin and its appendages (hair and nails). These infections are not usually severe and rarely become systemic.

I. Etiology. Three genera and a multitude of species, known collectively as the dermatophytes, are the etiologic agents of ringworm. Most human infections are caused by the following fungi: *Microsporum canis, Microsporum audouinii, Trichophyton rubrum, Trichophyton mentagrophytes, Trichophyton tonsurans, Trichophyton schoenleinii,* and *Epidermophyton floccosum.* A variety of papulosquamous eruptions can be caused by a singular dermatophyte species, and in different parts of the body, the same clinical picture may be due to dermatophytes of different species and different genera.

II. Classification. Clinically, ringworm is classified according to the body area involved. The Latin word *tinea,* meaning gnawing worm, is used with the designated site of infection to describe ringworm of the scalp (tinea capitis), body (tinea corporis), feet (tinea pedis), and so on. Dermatophytes seek the area of newly forming keratin deep in the skin or hair follicles for maximum development.

III. Symptoms. Infection with dermatophytes most often appears on the skin as red, scaly patches. The lesions usually begin as red papules and become progressively larger if untreated; the border extends while the center area clears, and this process gives rise to a ring-like, wormy-appearing lesion. The presenting eruption may include erythema, scaling, and vesiculation—more than normally would be expected from a superficial infection. A large part of the skin response is a result of the host's reaction to the fungus. Itching is rare. Most lesions are relatively asymptomatic. Poor hygiene, hyperhidrosis, inadequate drying of apposed areas such as the feet and groin, and immunoincompetence are factors that may contribute to infection. Once this infection has been acquired, it may remain throughout life and exhibit periods of exacerbation and remission.

IV. Diagnosis. The existence of these fungal infections is often suspected by the morphology of the individual lesions and their anatomic distribution. A presumptive diagnosis can be made by treating scrapings from skin lesions with a 10% potassium hydroxide solution and examining this preparation under a microscope for the presence of arthrospores or for segmented, branched filaments known as hyphae. Confirmation of the diagnosis is made by culture on Sabouraud's agar medium, a procedure requiring 1 to 4 weeks. This is reserved for patients for whom identification is not made on Kolt solution.

A. To obtain a specimen for either method, the emergency physician can rub a sterile, moist cotton swab over the surface of a suspected ringworm lesion, especially the outer periphery and then on to the culture medium, or use a scalpel and scrape the same area. Both techniques have been equally successful in producing positive cultures. However, the scalpel method for potassium hydroxide examinations is preferred because the scales would have to be removed from the fibers of the cotton swab, a difficult procedure.

B. Suspected scalp infections with *M. canis* or *M. audouinii* can be diagnosed by using a Wood's light (3600 Å ultraviolet light). When the hair is involved, this ultraviolet light will produce a yellow-green fluorescence that is presumptive of a diagnosis of infection with a *Microsporum* species. The other genera do not fluoresce. Tinea infections are common in patients with human immunodeficiency virus disease. Despite being immunocompromised, an inflammatory response to the fungus is often quite pronounced. Therefore, in patients who are seen with marked inflammatory lesions that are diagnosed as dermatophyte infections, it is prudent to evaluate for the possibility that this patient may have AIDS or another immunocompromising disease such as diabetes mellitus.

V. Transmission. The source of human infections can be infected persons, infected animals, or soil. When animals are implicated, it is important to identify and treat them at the same time that the patient is treated. Otherwise, the person who continues to consort with these animals will be reinfected. Dermatophyte infections can be spread by personal contact, as well as by fomites such as combs, towels, blankets, and barber shears. However, infection transmission is not always 100% on exposure. The person must be susceptible to become infected.

VI. Tinea pedis (athlete's foot) may be precipitated by poor hygiene coupled with hot, humid conditions. Efforts to control this disease are primarily directed toward education of the affected patient about the need to maintain good personal hygiene. Careful drying of the toes after bathing and an application of dusting powder containing an effective fungicide will prevent many infections. Topical dyes and imidazole derivatives applied to overt lesions will often clear up local areas of dermatophytosis and prevent spread from treated lesions.

VII. Tinea capitis and tinea corporis. In contrast to the treatment of athlete's foot, treatment of tinea capitis or tinea corporis by topical medications is usually ineffective. Topical medications often miss incubating lesions that are not easily visible but are still contagious. Therefore, griseofulvin is the treatment of choice for these infections, together with a topical agent. Griseofulvin given orally reaches the epidermal skin within 24 hours and probably renders a patient with contagious ringworm noninfective within 24 to 48 hours. To get the best results when prescribing griseofulvin, it should be administered or taken with the largest meal of the day. Griseofulvin is best absorbed with a meal containing fat. Also, when taken in this manner, it is least likely to cause gastrointestinal upset, a common side effect. Ketoconazole, an orally administered imidazole, has also been used systemically as an alternative to griseofulvin. One other aspect of treatment is to identify the human or animal source. To prevent reinfection, the source must also be treated.

Pityriasis Rosea

Pityriasis rosea is a papulosquamous eruption that has been called the *Christmas tree rash*. The term pityriasis means bran-like. Therefore, the clinical presentation of the typical lesion is bran-like scaling on a red base. This eruption most often occurs between the ages of 10 and 30 years. The cause is unknown.

I. **The eruption** begins with the characteristic *herald patch*. This lesion is larger than all of the rest that will appear. It most often precedes the general eruption by 3 or more days. It is most often seen over the anterior aspect of the shoulder joint but may occur anywhere. Most commonly the heaviest concentration of lesions is between the neck and the thighs. Rarely it may extend to the face and below the inguinal ligaments; occasionally it will extend distal to the elbows. Within 3 to 5 days after the herald patch appears, the rest of the eruption will occur in a descending manner from neck to inguinal ligaments in a bilateral symmetrical presentation that resembles the appearance of a *Christmas tree*. The eruption will last approximately 12 weeks before it disappears with or without treatment. The eruption usually does not itch if not treated.

II. **Bathing.** Taking hot baths or showers may produce postbathing itching. Therefore, lukewarm water should be used. Current topical medications that are available either over-the-counter or by prescription have no effect on this eruption. Systemic corticosteroids can cause the rash to temporarily disappear; however, once the course of systemic corticosteroids has ended, the eruption will reappear and last for the average of 12 weeks.

III. **Diagnosis.** The most important aspect of pityriasis rosea, from the standpoint of emergency physicians, is that they must make the correct diagnosis by performing a complete physical examination and taking a complete history. Differentiating this papulosquamous eruption from others, such as secondary syphilis, is very important as far as institution of proper management. By reviewing the age of onset of the other papulosquamous eruptions discussed in this chapter, it can be seen that the age range of 10 to 30 years is common for all. Just evaluating the herald patch without waiting a couple of days before the eruption appears can cause confusion with tinea infections, contact dermatitis, and other skin eruptions. Once the total eruption is apparent, secondary syphilis, psoriasis, and eczema should be considered in the differential diagnosis. Treatment in general for pityriasis rosea is judicious neglect and reassurance to the patient that the disease is benign.

Contact Dermatitis

I. **Symptoms.** Contact dermatitis in its acute phase has a similar appearance to allergic eczema. It is characterized by redness, edema, papules, vesiculations, weeping, and crusting and is accompanied by itching. When it becomes chronic, similar to allergic eczema, the involved skin can become thickened, lichenified, fissured, and pigmented. The difference between allergic contact dermatitis and allergic eczema is that with the former, an identified cause can be determined. The emergency physician, by taking a comprehensive history and doing a thorough physical examination, can usually make the diagnosis. When the patient is questioned regarding possible causes of the eruption, the emergency physician should have a high index of suspicion that the rash may be due to allergic contact dermatitis.

II. **Sensitization.** It is important that the emergency physician realize that the patient who is seen with a true contact dermatitis has undergone a period of sensitization. The incubation period after an initial sensitizing exposure to a contactant is usually 5 to 21 days. During this time changes develop in the skin that lead to clinical dermatitis on either continual exposure or reexposure to the specific allergen. If the dermatitis occurs on reexposure, the time between exposure of the previously sensitized subject to the specific sensitizing allergen and the development of the clinical reaction is termed the reaction time. This can vary from 8 to 120 hours but usually takes place in 12 to 48 hours, and even may occur as early as an hour after reexposure.

The emergency physician must realize that the extent of dermatitis that develops on exposure to a contactant in a sensitized person will depend on many of the following factors:

A. **The intensity,** duration, and frequency of exposure to the allergen.
B. **The degree** of allergic sensitivity.
C. **The presence** of infected, inflamed, burned, or eczematoid skin.
D. **The area exposed** to the contactant.
E. **Mechanical factors,** such as pressure and friction, which may increase the intimacy of contact of the sensitizer with the skin.
F. **Perspiration** could either dilute a contactant or in some persons enhance the development of the dermatitis.
G. **Alkalinity of the skin,** because a shift of normal acid skin pH toward alkalinity seems to enhance allergic eczematous contact dermatitis.
H. **Cachexia, lymphomas and sarcoidosis,** since these conditions appear to decrease reactivity to developing an allergic eczematous contact dermatitis.
I. **Genetic factors,** because children whose parents have previously been sensitized to certain contact allergens seem to have a higher rate of also becoming sensitized than children whose parents have not previously had contact dermatitis.

III. **Topical applications.** When a patient is seen with an acute, pruritic, seemingly localized eczematous dermatitis, it is important for the emergency physician to be aware of, and have a high index of suspicion of, topical medications, cosmetics, and articles of clothing that may have been in contact with the affected areas involved in the dermatitis. An example would be a dermatitis of the eyelids. The eyelids are one of the most sensitive areas to contact allergens. Any substance used on the scalp, face, or hands can produce an allergic eczematous dermatitis of the eyelids, while the primary sites remain unaltered. An example of this would be a new nail polish applied to the fingernails. Another area of the body that reacts to sensitizers conveyed to it by the hands is the penis and scrotum. Poison ivy may occur in this area because the hands have brought the Rhus antigen to it.

IV. **The management** of acute allergic contact dermatitis is primarily to eliminate the allergen. In addition, the emergency physician should prescribe medication that will eliminate the signs and symptoms already present. Most often, a topical corticosteroid preparation applied to the affected area at least three times daily and every time the patient wishes to scratch will be effective. This preparation should be at least equivalent to 0.1% triamcinolone cream or ointment. If the area is exudative, then Burow's solution may also be helpful in drying the area before cream or ointment application. If excessive excoriations have occurred before the patient sees the emergency physician, then the physician must make sure that a superimposed infection is not present. If infection is present, then appropriate antibiotics should be prescribed.

Insect Bites

I. **Symptoms.** Insect bites may appear as localized papulosquamous lesions. They can also appear as papules without scales, vesiculated papules, or even bullae. Depending on when the first lesions appeared on the patient and when that patient first sees the emergency physician, the appearance of the insect bites may mimic any of the other eruptions discussed.

II. **Questions.** The emergency physician must have a high index of suspicion when discrete papules are seen that are localized to one or two specific areas. The physician should also be aware of the patient's activities, both indoors and outdoors, before the appearance of the lesions. The physician should know that if the patient hasn't been rolling on the floor or out in the grass, that flea bites rarely occur above the knees. Fleas do not jump very high. The physician also should be aware of other insect activity in the geographic area in which the patient resides. Are mosquitos currently active in the community. Has a dog or cat previously lived in the home of the patient? Does the dog and/or cat still live in the residence of the patient? Is the patient an avid outdoors person? What clothing does the patient wear when outdoors? Taking a good history from the patient regarding the first appearance of the lesions, what happened before the appearance of the lesions, and asking the patient what he or she thinks may be the antecedent cause is often very helpful in identifying that insect bites are the cause of the dermatitis.

III. **Treatment.** Once the diagnosis is made, management of the acute dermatitis caused by insect bites is easily handled by applying a topical corticosteroid preparation equivalent to 0.1% triamcinolone cream or ointment at least three times a day and any other time the patient wishes to scratch. Also, if the insect source is identified as being within the home, then proper methods of eradication should be suggested and hopefully implemented by the patient.

Miliaria

I. **Definition.** Miliaria is a general designation for those eruptions that occur when the free flow of sweat to the surface is impeded. Miliaria is a three-stage process. The initial stage is a change in the distal portion of the sweat duct that impedes the egress of sweat in some manner. The second stage is an accumulation of material that stains Schiff-positive and is diastase resistant in the distal sweat pore. This material is excreted by small dark cells of the eccrine secretory coil, and the accumulation of it produces a plug so that the flow of sweat to the surface of the skin is blocked. With further sweating, there is rupture of the sweat duct. In miliaria crystallina, the rupture occurs within or just beneath the stratum corneum. In miliaria rubra, the rupture takes place more deeply within the epidermis. The third stage of miliaria is when the injured epidermal sweat duct unit degenerates and forms a hyperkeratotic or parakeratotic "keratin plug." This plug will then obstruct the pore of the newly regenerated epidermal sweat duct unit. With sweating, a new lesion of miliaria rubra is then produced and the sequence is repeated. The keratin plug will slough within 5 to 7 days, so that episodes of sweating must occur at least every few days to continue the process.

   A. **Varieties.** The old terminology for miliaria was *prickly heat*. Clinically, there are four varieties of miliaria. Miliaria crystallina lesions are superficial, noninflammatory, crystal-clear vesicles that resemble dew drops on the skin. These lesions are usually asymptomatic and transient. Miliaria rubra appears as small, discrete erythematous papules, vesicles, or papulovesicles at the sweat pores. These lesions are never associated with hair follicles. There is a predilection for the covered parts of the skin, especially where there is friction from clothing. Palms and soles are not involved, and the face is rarely affected. These lesions can burn, sting, or itch. If sweating stops, the eruption will fade within a few days, but if sweating continues or recurs, the lesions begin all over again. With each additional episode of sweating, more sweat glands become involved and the area of the eruption becomes wider. Miliaria pustulosa is a variant of miliaria rubra, consisting of discrete, distinct, superficial sterile pustules not associated with hair follicles. These lesions tend to appear in areas of the skin that have been previously inflamed. Miliaria pustulosa and miliaria rubra can coexist. In miliaria profunda, the infected skin has discrete, flesh-colored noninflammatory papules resembling goose flesh, and these lesions are localized to the sweat pores. They are asymptomatic. If the person exercises or is exposed to a hot environment, the lesions will increase in size.

    B. Miliaria rubra can resemble eczema, insect bites, viral exanthems, and drug eruptions. The emergency physician must distinguish miliaria pustulosa from true pyodermas. Secondary bacterial infection can, on occasion, complicate miliaria rubra and miliaria pustulosa.

II. Treatment. It is important for the emergency physician to recognize and differentiate miliaria from other papulosquamous eruptions. Once having done so, he or she can implement effective therapy, which is the elimination of the need to sweat. Therefore, the treatment regimen consists of adequate ventilation, lightweight clothing, and if needed, cool compresses or swimming in a lake or a pool. Also important is the elimination of the hot environment that induced the miliaria eruption. If available, air conditioning is invaluable since only 4 or more hours daily in that environment can completely prevent miliaria.

Ectoparasitic Infestations

I. Lice

    A. Species. The emergency physician should be able to recognize lice infestations. Lesions caused by these insects itch. Three species of lice infest human beings: *Phthirus pubis,* the crab louse; *Pediculus humanus corporis,* the body louse; and *Pediculus humanus capitis,* the head louse. These sucking lice are dorsoventrally compressed, wingless, and small, with retractable, piercing, sucking mouthparts. They are most often transmitted from one person to another or via fomites that another person has used. Lice are host specific. Therefore, lice that infest human beings will usually bite only human beings unless the normal host is not around. This is true also of lice that infest dogs, cats, and other animals.

    B. Common types. Patients who are seen in the emergency department with a lice infestation will usually complain of marked itching. They may or may not be aware that they have lice or their eggs (nits) present on their body. The two most prevalent lice infestations that the emergency physician should be able to recognize are those caused by the head louse and the pubic louse. The difference between these two lice is their grasping ability. The grasp of the pubic louse's claw matches the diameter of pubic and axillary hairs; hence, it is not only found in the pubic area but also has been recovered from the axillae, beard areas, eyelashes, and eyebrows. The grasp of the head louse's claw seems uniquely adapted to the diameter of the scalp hair. Therefore, it is very difficult to transplant head lice to other areas of the body. Another difference between these two lice is in their rate of movement. Pubic lice seem to be the most sedentary. Pubic lice can move a maximum of 10 centimeters in a day, whereas body lice can wander as much as 35 mm in a 2-hour period.

    C. Sensitivity to louse bites varies with the person. When previously unexposed persons are bitten, there may either be no signs or symptoms, or a slight sting with little or no itching or redness. At least 5 days must pass before allergic sensitization can occur. At that point the main symptom is itching, which then leads to scratching, causing erythema, irritation, and inflammation. A person who has been bitten by a large number of lice during a short period may even have a mild fever, malaise, and increased irritability. Lesions on the body either induced by the body louse or pubic louse may present as a papulosquamous eruption. It is important for the emergency physician, on careful examination of the lesions on the body, to look for both adult lice and their eggs. Both can be seen by the naked eye. Head lice characteristically are found on the scalp surface with the nits attached to the hair. Because scalp hair grows at a rate of about 0.4 mm/day, and the nits of the head louse usually hatch within 9 days, most of the unhatched nits are within 5 mm of the scalp surface. Nits on scalp hair are usually cemented at an oblique angle, which helps to distinguish them from foreign material that slides up and down and frequently surrounds the hair. On examination of the groin or pudendal area, pubic lice may be perceived as scabs or crust over what first were thought to be *scratch* papules. When the emergency physician takes a closer look and sees nits on the hairs, then the correct diagnosis is obvious. If the crust is removed and placed on a glass slide for microscopic examination, the crust often walks away before the cover glass is in place. When no adult lice are available, the demonstration of nits under the microscope will also confirm the diagnosis.

D. **The treatment regimen** in this infection should be individualized. The ideal pediculicide should effectively kill both the adult lice and the eggs. Examination of partners and other household contacts of the patient is mandatory so that both source and spread cases can be treated. There are effective nonprescription and prescription medications available. For these medications to be ovicidal, the pediculicide should remain in contact with the eggs for 1 hour or longer. In my experience, the most effective nonprescription products contain pyrethrins and piperonyl butoxide. Two products, RID (Pfizer Inc., New York, N.Y.) (liquid and shampoo) and Triple X (Youngs Drug Product, Weatherfield, Conn.) (liquid and shampoo), contain 0.3% pyrethrins and 3.0% piperonyl butoxide. One application of either of these preparations will usually eradicate adult lice and nits. Results of two studies suggest that a small percentage of patients will require another application 7 to 10 days after the first treatment. RID packaging has a fine-toothed comb that helps the patient dislodge the dead nits at the end of treatment. A-200 Pyrinate shampoo (Beecham Products, Bristol, Tenn.) also contains pyrethrins and piperonyl butoxide but in concentrations of 0.165% and 2.0%, respectively. Two applications, 1 week apart, are required for this preparation because the first application is often not lethal to the nits. BARC (Commerce Drug Company, Farmingdale, N.Y.) is another over-the counter pediculicide containing pyrethrins and piperonyl butoxide, but it is less effective than the other drugs already mentioned.

   1. **Kwell** (lotion, cream, or shampoo) (Reed and Carnrick, Jersey City, N.J.) is the most commonly used prescription medication for the treatment of louse infestations in the United States. It contains the insecticide lindane, which is 1% gamma benzene hexachloride. Lindane is also available without prescription as a commercial insecticide. I instruct patients using prescription 1% lindane preparations to divide the day into three 8-hour segments, showering before each of two applications. During the first two 8-hour segments, the application of 1% lindane should remain on the af-

fected area for the entire 8-hour period. An additional shower or bath should be taken after completion of the two 1% lindane applications.

2. **The use of 1% lindane** has several disadvantages. It may be absorbed percutaneously, and case reports have described mild signs and symptoms of neurotoxicity when it has been applied too frequently, not washed off as directed, or applied to massively excoriated skin. In one study, 9% of a single dose was found in the urine of a patient with badly excoriated skin 5 days after treatment. Other studies, however, have not found evidence of the drug in blood, tissue, or urine. Use of lindane should be avoided in small children, pregnant women, and patients with massive excoriations or multiple lesions over the scrotum.

3. **Nix** (Burroughs Wellcome, Research Triangle Park, N.C.), now available without prescription, is a 1% creme rinse. It is marketed for the treatment of head lice. The manufacturer suggests that it be used after the hair has been washed with regular shampoo, rinsed with water, and towel dried. A sufficient amount should then be applied to saturate the hair and scalp (especially behind the ears and on the nape of the neck). The creme rinse should be left on the hair for 10 minutes but no longer. Then the scalp should again be rinsed with water. A single application has been shown to kill both adult lice and eggs. Retreatment is required in less than 1% of patients. This occurs when live lice are still observed 7 days or more after the first application. Nix packaging also provides a fine-toothed comb. If neither RID or Kwell were available, then Nix would be a treatment option for pubic lice infestations.

4. **Other prescription medications** available for the treatment of lice infestations include emulsions of 20% or greater benzyl benzoate, 10% sulfur ointment, and Eurax (crotamiton 10%). All three preparations are effective but have disadvantages in that they require several days of application and impart an unpleasant odor to the patient. Six percent sulfur in petrolatum may be useful in treating infants who cannot tolerate other therapy. Malathion 0.5% lotion (Ovide) was remarketed in the United States in 1989. This lotion requires one application of 8 to 12 hours. It is both ovicidal and pediculicidal.

5. **Application of petrolatum** (petroleum jelly) is the treatment of choice for pubic lice attached to the eyelids or eyelashes. Petrolatum acts by mechanically obstructing the respiratory apparatus of the louse. Insecticides are not used near the eyes because they can cause severe irritation. Itching is the prominent feature in all louse infestations. Although initial treatment with the pediculicide will usually eradicate both adult lice and nits, itching may continue because of an allergic reaction or irritation. The possibility that pruritus may continue after treatment should be discussed with each patient; a mild topical antiinflammatory cream or ointment may be prescribed. Each case should be reevaluated 4 to 7 days after treatment. Attention to all these details is important so that the emergency physician can prevent excessive pediculicide use. Patients who continue to itch after treatment and who have not been informed about this reaction may suffer from parasitophobia and the feeling of "being unclean."

6. **Clearing the patient's clothing** and fomites of adult lice and nits is an important part of the treatment for louse infestation. Laundering these items in hot water (125° F) or dry cleaning kills the adult lice, nymphs, and nits. Articles that cannot be washed may be treated with any of several insecti-

cides that are intended for home use and contain pyrethrin and piperonyl butoxide. R&C spray, Li-ban spray, Black Flag, and Raid are examples of these. It is important that patients understand that these preparations must only be used on inanimate or nonwashable items.

E. Outbreaks. The emergency physician must realize that when seeing a child or adult with lice that this patient could well be the index case of a much larger outbreak. Therefore, it is important to take a history from these patients on their social interactions, and if the history warrants, then appropriate authorities or medical personnel at work or school should be notified.

II. Scabies. Scabies is an infestation caused by the human itch mite, *Sarcoptes scabiei*. Clinically it can present as a papulosquamous eruption. The eruption of scabies is usually very pruritic. Scabies can exist with other skin diseases, and the symptoms can be altered by drug therapy and by secondary infection with pyogenic bacteria. The drying effects of aging and the use, abuse, or overuse of topical medications can affect the clinical presentation. It is important for the emergency physician evaluating a patient's pruritic dermatitis to *think scabies*. The chronology of the signs and symptoms of the dermatitis can assist the emergency physician in making the diagnosis.

A. The clinical course of a scabietic infestation, other than Norwegian scabies, is usually associated with a 4- to 6-week latent period without itching from the time of initial infestation. After initial contact with the mite, the female mite burrows into the skin, resulting in its presentation to the immune system of the patient. The symptoms that appear 4 to 6 weeks later reflect the earliest development of the primary immune response. In contrast, because the immune system is already primed, persons who have been previously infested may develop symptoms as quickly as 24 hours after reinfestation. **During the initial reproductive phase** of the scabietic mite in a healthy person, there are usually fewer than 100 mites on the body. When the allergic reaction begins to occur and itching begins, an itch-scratch-itch cycle evolves. This allergic response paradoxically kills the mites and leaves fewer mites than there were originally. The greatest concentration of scabietic mites are seen at the finger webs, wrist folds, axillae, naval, under the breasts, between the buttocks, around the nipples, and on the genitalia. Both the rash and the burrows are rare above the neck and on the palms and soles.

B. Scratching. When the emergency physician enters the examining room, it is not unusual to notice that the patient with a pruritic eruption caused by scabies is continually scratching and is often not aware that this has become a habit. This activity alone should immediately put scabies at the top of the clinician's list of possible diagnoses for that patient.

C. Norwegian scabies is most often seen in immunosuppressed patients who may or may not itch. An especially high index of suspicion by the physician is needed to diagnose scabies in these patients because the disease is often mistaken for eczema, seborrheic dermatitis, or contact dermatitis caused by the use of topical preparations (scabies and contact dermatitis may coexist). This type of scabies is most often characterized by thickened, yellow, scaly skin and, in several cases, a thick crust with moisture often oozing from deep cracks. The number of mites on the body of patients with Norwegian scabies can exceed 10,000, compared with that on the body of nonimmunosuppressed patients who may have one to three dozen mites at the height of their infestation. This variant of scabies is very contagious. Besides burrows and the crusted impetiginized lesions, cutaneous manifestations also include papules, nodules, and eczematoid plaques. All these lesions can occur simultaneously on the same person.

D. Transference. The mites of a scabies infestation are transferred directly between persons by skin-to-skin contact or, rarely, by dislodged mites found in fomites. Both in Norwegian scabies (crusted scabies) and in reinfestations, fomites probably play a more important role than they do in primary infestations. Transmission seems to require prolonged intimate contact, as suggested by the high incidence in sexual partners of an index case and the infrequent transmission that seems to occur among roommates or nonintimate family members. Younger children who are continually hugged are also more likely to have the disease than older children.

E. Diagnosis. A definitive diagnosis of *S. scabiei* infestation requires identification of the mite, its eggs, or fecal pellets. The fecal pellets, or scybala, appear as brown, irregularly shaped clumps that are smaller than the eggs. The presence of burrows alone supports only a presumptive diagnosis. One method of examining the burrow is to shave off the top with a scalpel and examine the contents with a microscope. However, a virgin burrow is often difficult to find on patients who have been itching (and scratching) for some time or who have used a number of over-the-counter topical preparations to treat their pruritus. Therefore, it is important to look carefully over the entire skin and consider the use of a magnifying lens with good illumination to identify a burrow that has yet to be excoriated. These appear as raised, round, or elongated papules with little or no erythema, often surrounding a dot that represents the mite within. The best places to find a virgin burrow are in the apposed areas of the body, such as the axillae, the webs of the fingers, the webs of the toes, under the breasts, and on the penile shaft and scrotum. Areas that are difficult to reach with the fingernail are especially promising.

F. Treatment. Once the scalpel blade has removed the burrow, the mite will be found at the blind end. The mite can be removed by using a sewing needle or pin, swabbing the skin with ether, or applying clear cellophane adhesive tape and quickly removing the tape. Visualization of the mite can be accomplished by the application of a drop of mineral oil, ink from a pen, or topical tetracycline. A positive biopsy specimen may show the entire organism, or parts of it, existing within the epidermis. Most of the mite will be seen in the stratum corneum, with the mouth parts occasionally seen penetrating the lower strata of the epidermis and occasionally reaching the dermal-epidermal interface. The organism does not invade dermal structures. A clinician's selection of the method to view the scabies mite within the lesion will depend on the one that feels most comfortable to use on the basis of trial and error, and experience. The treatment of a scabies infestation should comprise three parts: the use of an insecticide, the use of a topical corticosteroid after the insecticide application, and psychologic support for the patient. The most commonly used insecticide for the treatment of a scabies infestation is 1% lindane (gamma benzene hexachloride) lotion or cream (Kwell) (Reed and Carnrick, Jersey City, N.J.). I instruct patients to divide a 24-hour day into three 8-hour segments. Upon showering at the beginning of the first two 8-hour segments, the lotion should be applied to the affected areas of the body, usually from the neck down for each of two 8-hour applications separated by a shower. At the end of the second application, a shower should again be taken and the patient should begin to apply a corticosteroid preparation similar in strength to 0.1% triamcinolone cream or ointment. The patient is instructed to apply this cream three or four times a day after the Kwell applications are completed and at any other time there is a need to scratch. It is also important for the emergency physician to help patients understand that they are not unclean, that the insecticide will kill the parasite, and that they may continue to itch for as long as 4 weeks. In the case of nodular scabies, itching may continue for as long as 2 months because the skin eruption is an allergic response to the mite. The use of Kwell has been associated with adverse reactions, especially central nervous system toxicity. In reviewing the literature regarding adverse events, the number of reports are few, compared with the enormous amount of this preparation that is used to treat both lice and scabies. The toxicity from this preparation has usually occurred when it has been misused, overused, or ingested. It is also possible that when the skin is excessively inflamed and the patient is small, such as in the case of an infant, excessive transdermal absorption of this compound could occur. Resistance of the scabies mite to the use of Kwell has not been reported in the United States. Other treatments for scabies have included crotamiton (Eurax; Westwood Pharmaceuticals, Buffalo, N.Y.), 5% or 10% sulfur ointment (sulfur petrolatum), 25% benzyl benzoate (ascabiol), Nix (Burroughs-Wellcome, Research Triangle Park, N.C.), malathion (Ovide lotion; Genderm Corp., Northbrook, Ill.), and NBIN (WHO treatment for large populations). A recent addition to the prescription products is a 5% permethrin cream (Elimite; Herbert Labs, Irvine, Calif.). One 8- to 14-hour application is recommended followed by bathing.

G. **Further steps in treatment.** Two other aspects of the management of a scabies infestation include the treatment of the patient's intimate contacts and decontamination of fomites. Clothing, bedding, and other intimate articles should be machine washed. Insecticide sprays (see *Lice*) are also effective for killing mites on furniture or on objects that cannot be cleaned in a washing machine. These measures provide patients with psychologic reassurance that they will not be reinfested after wearing or using these articles or pieces of furniture. Treatment failures may be due to the following:
  1. **Inadequate patient education** about infestation, treatment, and itching after treatment.
  2. **Inadequate or improper application** of medication.
  3. **Overmedication.**
  4. **Excessive bathing** or cleansing.
  5. **Reinfestation** from untreated fomites.

Moniliasis

Topical yeast infections, termed moniliasis, can present as papulosquamous eruptions that may or may not itch. They are most often caused by the yeast, *Candida albicans*. The eruption in infants is often seen not only in the groin and termed diaper rash, but also is seen on the face, especially on the cheeks, and commonly on the torso.

I. **Age.** In the infant, other than in the groin, the eruption often appears as dry scaling on a moderately inflamed base. These lesions do not appear to be overly pruritic because the infant is not usually scratching them. They are easily misdiagnosed as infantile eczema, and corticosteroid topical preparations are prescribed. Within a few days to a week when it is noted that treatment with corticosteroid creams has been unsuccessful, the diagnosis of moniliasis should be considered. The diaper area may or may not be involved with an eruption at the time of presentation on other parts of the body. If the emergency physician does a thorough physical examination of the infant, then the diagnosis of monilia should be considered, especially when pruritus and excoriations are lacking. In older patients, both children and adults, moniliasis of the skin is typified by inflamed papules and macules accompanied by satellite lesions. A fine scale may be present. These lesions may be asymptomatic, itch, or even burn, depending on how raw the erythematous base is. The lesions in the older child and adult most often appear in apposed areas of the body such as the groin on the medial thighs, in the axillae, under pendulous breasts, and in paronychial swellings. Another clue to making the diagnosis of a monilial rash is to examine the mucous membranes of the buccal mucosa, as well as those of the vaginal and perianal areas. Lesions in the mouth are termed oral thrush. They are most commonly seen in the newborn infant and appear about the seventh day of life. From 4% to 6% of infants will have oral thrush. The lesions are characteristically white, raised papules that have erupted on the buccal mucosa, gingivae, and tongue. They can proceed to ulceration. They may also coalesce to form extensive cheesy deposits that may spread to the hard and soft palate, tonsils, and fauces. Thrush patches adhere closely to the mucosa and on removal leave an eroded, bleeding site, thus distinguishing them from milk curds. Similar lesions may be seen along the vaginal mucosa and may be accompanied by leukorrhea, a profuse, cheesy white discharge. The vaginal wall becomes edematous and erythematous. The discharge is often intense and accompanied by painful itching and burning, along with painful urination.

II. **Use of antibiotics or hormonal preparations.** In older children and adults, use of antibiotics and/or hormonal preparations such as birth control pills, can often upset the ecologic balance along the mucous membranes and cause *C. albicans* to overgrow, producing the eruptions described above. A patient who has an intense disseminated *Candida* infection that does not easily respond to topical and/or systemic therapy should be evaluated for a possible underlying immunodeficiency state such as AIDS.

III. **Diagnosis.** In order for emergency physicians to make a rapid diagnosis of a *Candida* skin infection, they should take a scraping from one of the lesions and make a wet mount preparation. The material should be emulsified in a drop of sterile diluted water and examined microscopically with a reduced light source under a cover glass. If a yeast is present, the physician should be able to see budding and the method of bud attachment, as well as the presence or absence of pseudohyphae, true hyphae, or arthroconidia. The size and shape of the yeast present should also be noted. Any round or slightly oval budding yeast with rare or no pseudohyphae should be examined further for the presence of a capsule. The same wet preparation used for the initial microscopic examination can be used for an India ink examination. A small drop of India ink is added close to the edge of the cover slip and allowed to diffuse underneath. The preparation can then be examined for the presence of encapsulated yeast. The outline of the yeast cell, surrounded by a clear area that is a mucopolysaccharide capsule, will be obvious against the dark India ink background. False-positive preparations usually result from contaminated ink or artifacts that can exhibit ragged edges. The presence of a capsule does not automatically ensure that the yeast is *Cryptococcus neoformans*.

IV. **Treatment** of skin infections caused by yeasts can be accomplished with topical antiyeast preparations and/or systemic ketoconazole and fluconazole administration. Topical preparations include Mycostatin and imidazoles such as clotrimazole, econazole, ketoconazole, and miconazole, available in cream, ointment, and liquid preparations. These are usually applied to the affected areas at least three or four times a day. They may be used alone for the treatment of these infections or can be combined with oral ketoconazole, 200 mg daily. Other options include fluconazole, 100 mg orally every day. The other aspect of management of the yeast-infected patient is for the emergency physician to take a thorough history and define, if possible, an underlying problem that would make the patient more susceptible to yeast infections. If an underlying problem is present and not identified, the topical and/or oral therapy will not be effective.

Dermatologic Disorders: Brian Goldman, M.D.

I. **Erythema multiforme (EM).** This is a disorder of the epidermal and dermal layers of the skin. It has a spectrum of presentations, varying from a relatively insignificant skin eruption to a multisystem disease causing severe morbidity.
   A. **Incidence.** Erythema multiforme can occur at any age. Males are more likely to be affected than females.
   B. **Etiology.** Although the precise cause of EM is unknown, the disorder is generally regarded as being caused by the presence of circulating immune complexes. Common conditions associated with the disorder include infectious diseases, malignancies, and concomitant use of drugs **(Table 24-2)**. In half the cases of EM, a cause is not identified.
   C. **Clinical presentation.** As mentioned above, the skin manifestations of EM are protean. Erythema multiforme can present as erythematous macules or as nonpruritic urticaria-like eruptions. Unlike hives, however, the urticaria-like lesions of EM are not evanescent. Once lesions arrive, they tend to remain for 7 to 10 days, often coalescing. The classic lesion of EM is known as a "target lesion." Targets consist of a ring-like erythematous plaque with a dusky (sometimes petechial) center. Vesicobullous lesions can also develop. Lesions tend to develop on the dorsa of the hands, palms, and soles of the feet. Vesicobullous eruptions may appear on the mucous membranes.
   D. **Stevens-Johnson syndrome.** This is an extremely severe variant of EM. It is preceded by a prodrome of malaise, fever, myalgias, and arthralgias. These quickly give rise to a severe illness characterized by widespread vesicobullous eruptions on the skin and most mucous membranes, as well as constitutional symptoms. Stomatitis can lead to difficulty feeding. Corneal ulceration can develop, leading to blindness. Multiorgan failure (*especially* renal failure) helps contribute to an overall mortality rate of 10%.
   E. **Differential diagnosis.** The differential diagnosis should include other erythematous maculopapular and papulosquamous disorders. Examples include erythema nodosum and nonspecific drug eruptions. When vesicles are promi-

Table 24-2. Conditions Associated with Erythema Multiforme

Condition	Examples
Drug induced	Oral hypoglycemics, anticonvulsants, sulfonamides
Malignancies	Lymphomas
Infections	*Mycoplasma pneumoniae,* influenza, cat-scratch fever, herpes simplex infection

nent, diagnoses such as pemphigus vulgaris and bullous pemphigoid should be entertained.
- **F. Diagnosis.** The diagnosis is usually made by the appearance of the typical features, including target lesions. A skin biopsy specimen showing lymphocytic infiltration in the upper dermis can be helpful in equivocal cases. Patients with constitutional symptoms or extensive skin and mucous membrane involvement should have serum electrolytes, urea, and creatinine levels determined, as well as a urinalysis. Once the diagnosis is made, an appropriate history, physical examination, and laboratory investigations should be done to search for associated conditions such as infections and underlying malignancies. This can often be carried out by the patient's primary care physician.
- **G. Treatment.** The treatment depends on the severity of the illness.
  1. **Mild to moderate skin involvement only.** Patients in this category may be treated with a topical corticosteroid. A mild corticosteroid such as 1% hydrocortisone cream applied three times a day as needed may be prescribed as the initial agent. Often, more potent steroids such as betamethasone 0.05% are required. An alternative approach is to use systemic corticosteroids. An acceptable choice is prednisone. Begin with a dosage of 40 to 60 mg/day for 4 days, and then slowly taper the dose over the next 10 to 14 days. If the patient has urticaria, an antihistamine such as diphenhydramine, 25 to 50 mg every 6 to 8 hours, may be prescribed. Follow-up with the primary care physician should be arranged. Patients not responding to the above therapy after 4 or 5 days should be referred to a dermatologist.
  2. **Stevens-Johnson syndrome.** Patients with this disorder should be admitted to the hospital for intravenous fluid hydration and monitoring of electrolyte levels and renal function. An ophthalmology consultation should be obtained to rule out eye involvement. Typically, the equivalent of 80 to 120 mg/day of prednisone is required for these patients.

II. Toxic epidermal necrolysis (TEN). This disorder, also known as the scalded skin syndrome, is a rapidly progressive disorder characterized by widespread denuding of skin.
- **A. Etiology.** There are two etiologic agents. In children, this condition is usually caused by a toxin produced by a staphylococcal infection. The toxin cleaves the epidermis beneath the stratum granulosum. In adults, the disorder is usually drug induced (e.g., sulfonamides, griseofulvin, sulindac, and phenytoin). The key difference between the adult and child variants is that in the adult variant, the cleavage point is at the dermal-epidermal junction.
- **B. Clinical presentation**
  1. **Scalded skin syndrome.** This childhood variant begins as extremely tender areas of erythema, typically located on the face and intertriginous areas. The lesions quickly develop into large bullae, after which the overlying epidermis sloughs off in sheets, leaving exfoliated areas with a glistening erythematous base. The mucous membranes are not involved.
  2. **Adult variant.** As in the childhood variant, the disorder affecting adults is widespread. However, in this case, the mucous membranes are commonly involved. Extensive fluid loss and secondary infection are common, contributing to the 5% to 50% mortality rate associated with the adult variant.
- **C. Diagnosis.** The diagnosis is usually made by the clinical appearance of the patient. The diagnosis is confirmed by a skin biopsy of the affected areas. An infectious cause is determined by obtaining cultures growing *Staphylococcus au-*

reus from skin lesions. Serum electrolyte levels should be monitored. Blood cultures will confirm a diagnosis of sepsis.
  D. **Treatment.** The condition is not unlike that of a burn patient. Adults with this condition may lose up to 4 L/day. Thus, the key to successful early management is the repletion of previous and ongoing fluid losses. Standard formulas for calculating fluid losses and appropriate repletion should be used. Because sulfonamides can cause TEN, silver sulfadiazine creams should not be used on scalded areas of skin. Systemic antibiotics such as cloxacillin should be reserved for situations in which *S. aureus* is the causative agent. In adults, parenteral antibiotics should only be used if secondary sepsis is strongly suspected.
  E. **Disposition.** Patients with involvement of more than 10% of the surface of their skin should be admitted to a burn unit. Patients with less than 10% skin involvement may be discharged provided they are given dressings soaked in silver nitrate (0.5%) and are followed by a dermatologist or a plastic surgeon every 1 or 2 days.

Suggested Readings

Fegan D, Glennon J: Use of steroids in dermatological emergencies, *Trop Doct* 23:15-17, 1993.

Heng MC: Drug-induced toxic epidermal necrolysis, *Br J Dermatol* 113:597-600, 1985.

Heng MC, Allen SG: Efficacy of cyclophosphamide in toxic epidermal necrolysis. Clinical and pathophysiologic aspects, *J Am Acad Dermatol* 25:778-86, 1991.

Levy M, Shear NH: *Mycoplasma pneumoniae* infections and Stevens-Johnson syndrome. Report of eight cases and review of the literature, *Clin Pediatr* 30:42-9, 1991.

Patterson R et al: Erythema multiforme and Stevens-Johnson syndrome. Descriptive and therapeutic controversy, *Chest* 98:331-6, 1990.

Renfro L et al: Drug-induced toxic epidermal necrolysis treated with cyclosporine, *Int J Dermatol* 28:441-4, 1989.

Renfro L et al: Controversy: are systemic steroids indicated in the treatment of erythema multiforme? *Pediatr Dermatol* 6:43-50, 1989.

Williams RE, MacKie RM: The staphylococci. Importance of their control in the management of skin disease, *Dermatol Clin* 11:201-6, 1993.

25 Rheumatoid Emergencies

Ernest A. Kopecky, B.Sc., Ph.D.
(Candidate)

Modern medicine has elucidated the etiology and pathophysiology of numerous rheumatologic disorders commonly seen in the patient population. However, there are certain conditions that are seen at a higher frequency in the emergency department. This chapter is presented in a quick reference format providing the essential information needed for rapid recognition and treatment of common rheumatoid emergencies. The primary goal of the emergency physician is to treat the pain and inflammation associated with rheumatoid emergencies and increase the patient's debilitated range of motion.

Rheumatoid Arthritis (RA)

I. **Definition.** Chronic systemic inflammatory disorder, of unknown cause, characterized as a symmetric inflammation of synovial tissues, deforming polyarthritis, and numerous extraarticular manifestations.

II. **Salient features**

Female/male dominance ratio of 3:1.

Prevalence is age dependent where disease manifestations increase with age.

Slow onset.

Early symptoms include malaise, fatigue, morning stiffness, and diffuse musculoskeletal pain affecting the joints bilaterally, with hands, wrists, and feet affected first.

Hand metacarpophalangeal (MCP) and proximal interphalangeal (PIP) joints affected, with distal interphalangeal (DIP) joints spared.

Eventually elbows, knees, shoulders, ankles, hips, temporomandibular joints (TMJs), sternoclavicular joints, and glenohumeral joints become involved.

A. Characteristics
1. Soft tissue swelling, heat sensation, decreased range of motion, and muscle atrophy in some cases.
2. Advanced disease exhibits irreversible joint disease encompassing ulnar deviation of fingers and PIP flexion or DIP hyperextension deformities.

B. Extraarticular characteristics
1. Evidence of spontaneous rheumatoid nodules on the extensor surface of the olecranon process, proximal ulna, and also on the hands, sacral areas, eyes, lungs, heart, plantar aspect of the foot, and the Achilles tendon.
2. Pleuropulmonary and cardiac manifestations, fibrosis, serositis, vasculitis in any organ, and presentation of syndromes (e.g., Sjogren's syndrome: keratoconjunctivitis sicca, xerostomia, and connective tissue disease; or Felty's syndrome: chronic arthritis, splenomegaly, neutropenia, thrombocytopenia, anemia, and lymphadenopathy).

C. Differential diagnosis
   1. Sjogren's syndrome.
   2. Felty's syndrome.
   3. Rheumatoid vasculitis.
III. **Management**
   A. Rest, heat, physiotherapy, occupational therapy consultation, and emotional support.
   B. **Laboratory** erythrocyte sedimentation rate (ESR), hemoglobin (Hgb) level, serum albumin level, and rheumatoid factor (RF)—tests and results are not diagnostic alone.
   C. Pharmacologic treatment
   1. **First-line treatment**
      a. **Nonsteroidal antiinflammatory drugs (NSAIDs)—salicylates. Aspirin,** 600 to 1200 mg every 4 to 6 hours, or 3.6 to 7.5 gm/day; antiinflammatory dose to be taken with meals.
      b. **Nonaspirin NSAIDs**
         Naproxen, 750 to 1000 mg/day to maximum 1500 mg/day.
         Piroxicam, 20 mg/day PO or 10 mg PO BID to maximum 20 mg/day.
         Sulindac, 150 to 200 mg PO BID to maximum 400 mg/day.
         Indomethacin, 25 mg TID to QID or slow-release (SR) preparation at a dose of 75 mg = 25 mg TID.
         Ibuprofen, 1600 to 2400 mg/day to maximum 3200 gm/day.
   2 **Second-line treatment: disease-modifying antirheumatic drugs (DMARDs)**
      a. **Gold salts,** 300 to 1000 mg, with 10 mg IM initially and after 1 week, 25 to 50 mg/wk.
      b. **Antimalarials. Hydroxychloroquine,** 6.0 to 6.5 mg/kg/day.
      c. **Penicillamine,** 10 to 12 mg/kg/day; 125 mg/day in a single dose for 3 months, then 500 mg for 3 months, then 750 mg/day in two doses to 500 mg BID for 3 months.
      d. **Glucocorticoids. Prednisone,** 5.0 to 7.5 mg in a single dose; acute dosing in hospital, 20 to 30 mg/day for 3 to 5 days with tapering; 40 to 60 mg/day for rheumatoid vasculitis if manifested by mesenteric and other internal organ ischemia.
      e. **Cytotoxics. Azathioprine,** start at 1.5 mg/kg/day orally and increase to 2.5 to 3.0 mg/kg maintenance by 50 mg increments; **Cyclophosphamide,** 1.0 to 1.5 mg/kg orally initially, then 2.5 to 3.0 mg/kg to maximum 3 mg/kg; **Methotrexate,** 7.5 to 15 mg/wk range; initially, 2.5 mg orally every 12 hours for three doses given once a week.
   D. **Surgery.** Joint fusion, synovectomy, total joint arthroplasty, and reconstruction procedures are among the prominent surgical interventions.

Juvenile Rheumatoid Arthritis (JRA)

I. **Definition**
   A. Chronic idiopathic synovitis is defined as a pediatric form of arthritis commencing before the age of 16 years.
   B. Most common pediatric connective tissue disease.

II. **Salient features.** Morning stiffness and joint pain manifested in children as increased irritability, guarding of involved joints, or refusal to walk; fatigue, low-grade fever, anorexia, and weight loss often associated.
   A. Disease classifications
      1. **Polyarthritis/polyarticular.** JRA commencing in more than five joints with few if any systemic manifestations:
         - Affects the knees, wrists, elbows, ankles, and hands and feet.
         - A TMJ problem is common causing limited bite and micrognathia.
         - Subcutaneous nodules are evident but may also exhibit low-grade fever, slight hepatosplenomegaly, lymphadenopathy, pericarditis, and chronic uveitis.
      2. **Oligoarthritis/pauciarticular.** Initial involvement in four or less joints encompassing the knees, ankles, or wrists. Extraarticular facets are rare, but young girls exhibit iridocyclitis.
      3. **Systemic.** Characteristic features include a high spiking fever and rheumatoid rash, increased body temperature, and a small, discrete, erythematous, morbilliform macular rash on the trunk and extremities. Hepatosplenomegaly, lymphadenopathy, pericarditis, anemia, serositis, and leukocytosis are commonly present.
   B. **Differential diagnosis.** Bone and joint infection, rheumatic fever, bacterial infections, viral infections, systemic lupus erythematosus (SLE), vasculitis syndromes, hemoglobinopathies, malignancies, serum sickness–like syndromes, inflammatory bowel disease, traumatic synovitis, hemophilia (may present with acute arthritis in infancy), normocytic hypochromic anemia, elevated ESR, thrombocytosis, and leukocytosis.

III. **Management**
   A. Rest initially in acute episode, heat, nutrition and social work consultations, physiotherapy, occupational therapy consultation, exercise, splint to prevent deformity, ophthalmology consultation to examine for uveitis, and an orthopedic surgery consultation.
   B. **Laboratory.** ESR, RF, antinuclear antibody (ANA), human leukocyte antigen (HLA) B27 (if ankylosing spondylitis, psoriatic arthritis, or arthritis associated with inflammatory bowel disease [IBD]), levels of serum immunoglobulins and liver function tests (LFTs), urinalysis, C3 and C4 (if SLE suspected), CBC and differential, X-rays, blood cultures (BCs), bone scan (if osteomyelitis suspected), and arthrocentesis (if septic arthritis suspected).
   C. **Diagnosis based on** (1) arthritis in one or more joints for 6 weeks; (2) onset in children younger than 16 years; (3) other rheumatic diseases have been ruled out; and (4) the classification of JRA (polyarticular, pauciarticular, or systemic) has been established.
   D. Pharmacologic treatment
      1. **First-line treatment**
         a. **NSAIDs—salicylates.** Aspirin, 60 to 80 mg/kg/day to 130 mg/kg/day for antiinflammatory effect.
         b. **Nonaspirin NSAIDs**
            Tolmetin Sodium, 30 to 40 mg/kg/day given orally in divided doses three or four times a day to maximum 1.6 gm/day.
            Naproxen, 10 to 20 mg/kg/day orally in divided doses twice a day to 1000 mg maximum.
            Indomethacin, 1.5 to 3.0 mg/kg/day orally in divided doses three times a day with meals to maximum 200 mg/day.

2. Second-line treatment

a. **Antimalarial.** Hydroxychloroquine, 60 mg/kg/day orally in a single dose with food/milk to maximum 300 mg/day.
b. **Gold salts,** initially 5 mg parenterally with food/milk to 0.75 mg/kg/wk to maximum 50 mg/wk.
c. **D-Penicillamine,** 5 mg/kg/day PO in a single dose daily, then increase in increments of 5 mg/kg/day at intervals of 2 to 3 months to 15 mg/kg/day PO in divided doses two to four times daily; maximum initial dose is 250 mg and final maximum dose 1.5 gm/day; dose on empty stomach—either 1 hour before meals or 2 hours after meals.
d. **Sulfasalazine,** 40 to 60 mg/kg/day PO in divided doses two to four times a day with food/milk; begin with one third recommended dose and increase every 2 days to maximum dosage—maintain fluid intake.
e. **Corticosteroids,** intraarticular or systemically administered with life-threatening systemic JRA, fever unresponsive to NSAIDs, chronic uveitis, or severe polyarticular JRA. **Prednisone,** 1 mg/kg/day PO in single or divided doses initially to maximum 60 mg/day; to discontinue after ≥ 10 days, decrease dosage by 50% every 48 hours until 2.5 ± 0.8 mg/m^2/day, then reduce by 50% every 10 to 14 days.
f. **Cytotoxics/immunosuppressives. Methotrexate,** 5 mg/m^2/dose PO once a week, then may double dose prn after 6 to 8 weeks; dose on empty stomach either 1 hour before or 2 hours after meals and monitor liver function.

E. **Surgery.** Synovectomy, total joint replacement, reconstructive jaw surgery.

Osteoarthritis (OA)

I. **Definition.** Degenerative joint disease marked by focal deterioration of articular cartilage and concomitant generation of new bone at the articular surface (subchondral bone) and at the joint margins (osteophytes).

II. **Salient features.** Symptomatology is limited to involved joints exhibiting synovial joint inflammation. Morning stiffness and stiffness after rest during the day are characteristic and limited to < 30 minutes duration of the involved joints. Crepitus is associated with passive and active motion in the involved joints.

A. **Effected areas.** DIP And PIP joints of the hands, first carpometacarpal joint, hips, knees, cervical and lumbar spine leading to spinal stenosis (neurogenic claudication), and first metatarsophalangeal joints.

B. **Prevalence.** Increases with age, congenital malformations, chronic inflammatory arthritis, and joint trauma.

C. **Primary symptoms.** Localized, deep, aching pain in the affected joint.

D. **Pathologic processes**
1. Fissuring, focal and diffuse erosion of the cartilagenous surface, and thinning and complete denudation of the articular cartilage contribute to the structural breakdown of that cartilage.
2. Sclerosis, cyst formation, bone thickening, and proliferation of new bone and cartilage-producing osteophytes contribute to changes in the subchondral bone.
3. Occasional occurrence of synovitis.

E. **Radiographic criteria.** Joint space narrowing, periarticular ossicles, subchondral bone cysts, and altered shape of the articular surface.

F. Differential diagnosis. Inflammatory monoarticular and polyarticular RA, infectious arthritis, neoplastic synovitis, tendinitis and bursitis, psoriasis, Reiter syndrome, IBD, ankylosing spondylitis, gout, and pseudogout.

III. Management

A. Therapy is aimed at pain relief, correcting the causative factors, and minimizing or preventing disability.

B. Laboratory. X-rays, CBC, blood chemistry profile, ESR, RF, and urinalysis are not diagnostic but contribute to ruling out differential diagnoses.

C. Rest, physiotherapy and occupational therapy, and a social work consultation concurrently aid in the patient's recovery and rehabilitation. This disease is painful and debilitating, often resulting in an agitated and difficult patient, strained employer-employee relations, family stress, and eventually, in the patient's withdrawal from social interaction. Arranging social work follow-up, after medical intervention, can help the individual resume employment and a healthy, active lifestyle with family and friends.

D. Pharmacological treatment

  1. **NSAIDs—salicylates.** Enteric-coated aspirin, 500 mg QID after meals to maintenance of 20 to 30 mg/dl; 15 to 20 mg/dl in elderly patients.
  Salsalate, 750 to 1000 mg two or three times a day.
  Sulindac, 150 to 200 mg BID with meals.
  Piroxicam, 20 mg/day in a single dose.
  Naproxen, 250 to 1000 mg/day BID.
  Ibuprofen, 1200 to 1400 mg/day in divided doses three or four times a day.
  Phenylbutazone, 300 to 600 mg/day in divided doses three or four times a day to maximum of 400 mg/day in long-term therapy.

  2. **Glucocorticoids. Prednisone,** 1 mg/kg/day PO in single or divided doses initially to maximum of 60 mg/day; to discontinue after $\geq$ 10 days, decrease dose by 50% every 48 hours until 2.5 $\pm$ 0.8 mg/m^2/day, then reduce by 50% every 10 to 14 days.

  3. **Acetaminophen,** 325 to 650 mg QID for analgesia.

E. Surgery. Osteotomy, arthrodesis, total knee prosthesis, total hip replacement, and arthroscopic debridement.

Reiter Syndrome

I. Definition.
Syndrome consisting of asymmetric oligoarthritis, urethritis, conjunctivitis, and skin and mucous membrane lesions.

II. Salient features
Male/female ratio of 15:1 with young adult predominance.
Possible genetic predisposition (HLA-B27 lymphocyte antigen).
Generally manifests after epidemic dysentery or sexual intercourse.

A. Causative bacterial organisms. *Mycoplasma, Chlamydia, Shigella, Salmonella, and Yersinia.*

B. Symptomatology. Low-grade fever, fatigue, arthritis, mucopurulent/mucoid urethral discharge in males and urethral ulcers in females, prostatitis and hemorrhagic cystitis, pericarditis, conjunctivitis, iritis, diarrhea, balanitis circinata, and keratoderma blennorrhagicum.

C. Laboratory. Elevated WBC (10,000 to 18,000 cells/mm^3), hematocrit normal acutely but rises if chronic, increased ESR (>100 mm/hr), pyuria and hematuria, PMN leukocytes in sterile urethral discharge, stool negative for

enteric pathogens, joint fluid turbid and grossly purulent (2000 to 50,000 cells/mL)—neutrophils seen early followed by lymphocytes in chronic joint effusion, synovial fluid glucose usually normal but decreases if leukocytosis is present, complement may be increased (this is nondiagnostic: serum complement frequently is increased).
- D. **Diagnostic features.** Arthritis, urethritis, conjunctivitis with/without mucocutaneous manifestations.
- E. **Differential diagnosis.** Gonorrhea, Behcet syndrome, RA, and psoriasis.

III. **Management**
- A. **Laboratory.** CBC and differential, urinalysis, stool cultures, joint aspiration, and X-rays.
- B. **Control pain and inflammation. Aspirin,** 600 to 900 mg PO QID, and **Indomethacin,** 25 to 50 mg TID **OR Naproxen,** 250 mg BID **OR Sulfasalazine,** 40 to 60 mg/kg/day PO in divided doses two to four times a day with food/milk; begin with one third recommended dosage and increase every 2 days to maximum dosage—maintain fluid intake. For severe cases, **Methotrexate** 5 mg/m^2/dose PO once a week, then may double dose prn after 6 to 8 weeks; dose on empty stomach either 1 hour before or 2 hours after meals and monitor liver function.

Septic/Infectious Arthritis

I. **Definition.** A hematogenously acquired sepsis of the articular joint through the higher vascular synovium, which allows unimpeded passage of bacteria from the blood into the synovial space.

II. **Salient features.** At 15 to 40 years of age, the clinician should suspect gonococcal arthritis. At < 1 year of age, the diagnosis is problematic because the capillaries perforate the epiphyseal growth plate. *S. aureus* is the predominant cause of nongonococcal arthritis with predisposing factors encompassing chronic illness (cancer, diabetes mellitus, cirrhosis), prior arthritis, prior arthrocentesis, joint prosthesis, and immunosuppression, trauma, osteoarthritis, and chronic granulomatous disease.

Symptoms include fever and chills, multiple joint migratory polyarthralgias, flu-like symptomatology, malaise, and diffuse aching. Septic arthritis is associated with menstruation, urethral and vaginal discharge, and IV drug use. The joints appear swollen, warm, erythematous, painful, and manifest a decreased range of motion. Tenosynovitis involving the fingers, wrists, ankles, and feet may represent gonococcal arthritis.
- A. **Causative organisms.** *N. gonorrhoeae, S. aureus, S. pneumoniae, S. hemolyticus,* and gram-negative bacilli *(E. coli, Salmonella, Pseudomonas)* are associated with the primary joint infection.
- B. **Portals of infection.** Skin, sinuses, middle ear, oropharynx, pelvis, urethra, rectum, lungs, and conditions such as pyelonephritis, prostatitis, vaginitis, proctitis, and endocarditis.
- C. **Diagnostic features.** Aspirated fluid findings and organism isolation.
- D. **Differential diagnosis.** Viral arthritis, osteoarthritis, trauma, gout, pseudogout, and RA.

III. **Management**
- A. **Laboratory.** CBC and differential, culture all possible portals of infection, X-rays, radioisotope bone scan, arthrocentesis (aspirate synovial fluid for CBC

and differential, synovial fluid glucose, countercurrent immunoelectrophoresis to detect bacterial antigens, lactic acid level, cultures, and Gram stain).
- **B. Initial treatment.** Antibiotic therapy based on Gram stain results:
    1. ***Staphylococcus.*** **Nafcillin,** 100 to 150 mg/kg/day in divided doses four times a day, **OR Cephalothin,** 100 mg/kg/day, **OR Methicillin,** 2 gm IV q6h.
    2. ***N. gonorrhoeae.*** **Penicillin** G 15 to 20 million U/day in divided doses four times a day, **OR Erythromycin,** 2 gm/day, **OR Procaine penicillin,** 600,000 U IM q12h.
    3. **Gram-negative bacilli. Gentamicin,** 5 mg/kg/day in divided doses three times a day, **OR Amikacin,** 15 mg/kg/day.
    4. ***H. influenzae.*** **Ampicillin,** 50 mg/kg/day in divided doses four times a day, **OR Chloramphenicol,** 50 mg/kg/day.
    5. ***Streptococcus.*** **Penicillin G,** 15 to 20 million U/day in divided doses four times a day, **OR Cephalothin,** 100 mg/kg/day.
    6. ***Pseudomonas.*** **Tobramycin,** 5 mg/kg/day in divided doses three times a day, **OR Amikacin,** 15 mg/kg/day.
    7. **Unknown organism. Gentamycin or Tobramycin,** 5 mg/kg/day IV q8h, plus **Cefazolin,** 2 to 6 gm/day IV.
- **C.** **Analgesics** with no effect on fever. **Codeine,** 30 mg q4h.
- **D.** **Antiinflammatory medications** are not used initially until antibiotic therapy is assessed.
- **E.** Temporary **splinting** to reduce discomfort, pain, and flexion deformities.
- **F. Exercise,** serial joint aspirations, and open surgical drainage as clinically indicated.
- **G. Gonococcal arthritis** is exemplified by positive cultures, monoarthritis and polyarthritis, tenosynovitis, and pustulovesicular lesions that are treated with the following antibiotics:
    1. **Erythromycin,** 0.5 gm PO QID for 7 days, **OR**
    2. **Ampicillin,** 3.5 gm, or **Amoxicillin,** 3.0 gm PO, with **Probenecid,** 1.0 gm, followed by 0.5 gm **Ampicillin** or 0.5 gm **Amoxicillin** PO QID for 7 days, **OR**
    3. **Tetracycline,** 0.5 gm PO QID for 7 days (not for gravid women), **OR**
    4. **Aqueous Crystalline Penicilline G,** 10 million U IV daily until improvement, followed by **Ampicillin,** 0.5 gm QID to complete 7 days of treatment, **OR**
    5. **Spectinomycin,** 2.0 gm IM BID for 3 days for penicillinase-producing *N. gonorrhoeae.*
- **H. Fungal arthritis** exhibits typically as chronic monoarticular disease; however, an acute polyarthritis with/without erythema nodosum may be seen. Causative organisms include sporotichosis, candidiasis, blastomycosis, cryptococcosis, coccidioidomycosis, and histoplasmosis that are **treated** as follows:
    - a. **Amphotericin B,** 1.0 mg/kg/day IV for total dose of 2 to 3 gm over 10 weeks, and **occasionally,**
    - b. **5-Fluorocytosine** 150 mg/kg/day PO for 6 weeks.
    - c. **Surgical debridement** may be required.
- **I. Viral arthritis** is caused by hepatitis B and rubella, although it may be due to mumps, Epstein-Barr virus (EBV), or arbovirus infections. Patients can present with polyarthritis or hepatitis B infection for which there is no specific available therapy. However, the physician can control symptoms with **Aspirin,** 600 mg PO q6h.

J. Tuberculous arthritis exhibits a chronic monoarthritis or spondylitis, with a PPD skin test that is always positive. **Treatment** is with **Isoniazid,** 300 mg/day, and **Ethambutol,** 15 to 20 mg/kg/day for a minimum of 24 months.

Acute Gout

I. **Definition**
   A. **Primary gout** is a metabolic disorder of purine metabolism characterized by hyperuricemia, acute and chronic recurrent arthritis, and deposits of monosodium urates.
   B. **Secondary gout** is a hyperuricemia caused by a number of disorders (e.g., lymphoma, psoriasis, hemolytic anemia, chronic renal failure, lead neuropathy, lactic acidosis, or glycogen storage disease) as a result of excessive production or impaired excretion of uric acid.

II. **Salient features**
   Male predisposition.
   Nocturnal occurrence.
   Low-grade fever may be evident.
   Shoulder, hip, and vertebrae involvement are extremely rare.
   A. Joint involvement
      1. **Acutely affects a single joint** and predominates in the lower extremities (e.g., podagra, foot dorsum, ankle, knee, and rarely the upper extremity joints).
      2. **Joints are quite tender** and painful, with periarticular swelling and erythema mimicking cellulitis or thrombophlebitis.
      3. Pain is due to **microcrystal deposition** in the joints and periarticular tissues.
   B. Frequency
      1. **First attack** is usually monoarticular, while recurrent attacks are longer in duration, polyarticular, and occur in an ascending and asymmetrical profile.
      2. **Older patients** have an increased frequency of attacks after surgery and medical illnesses such as myocardial infarction (MI), urinary tract infection (UTI), cerebrovascular accident (CVA), or pneumonia.
   C. Podagra
      1. An acute attack of the great toe is the **most frequent manifestation** of acute gouty arthritis.
      2. **Acute podagra attacks** have no obvious precipitating event; however, trauma, excessive alcohol consumption, initiation of hypouricemia therapy, diuretic use, rapid weight reduction, or stress may contribute to exacerbating an acute attack.
   D. Diagnostic features. Identification of polymorphonuclear leukocytes containing phagocytosed monosodium urate crystals in the joint aspirate, presence of pain involving the joint, tophi, hyperuricemia, oligoarthritis, erythema over the joints, asymmetric swelling within a joint on radiologic examination, more than one arthritic attack, unilateral podagra, and joint inflammation that reaches a maximum within 1 day.
   E. **Differential diagnosis.** Septic arthritis, trauma, atypical RA, pseudogout; if no aspirate available, consider calcium oxalate deposition disease, calcium pyrophosphate dihydrate deposition disease, or calcium hydroxyapatite deposition disease.

III. Management

A. Laboratory
CBC, electrolytes, blood urea nitrogen (BUN), serum creatinine, serum uric acid, ESR, synovial fluid examination with crystal identification, arthrocentesis, and X-rays.

B. Pharmacologic treatment
1. **Drug of choice. Indomethacin,** 150 to 200 mg PO; 50 mg TID for 2 days, then 50 mg BID for 1 day, and ending with 50 mg/day for 1 day, **OR Phenylbutazone or Oxyphenbutazone,** 800 mg PO in divided doses four times a day for initial 24 hours, then taper over 3 to 5 days.
2. **NSAIDs. Sulindac,** 400 mg initially, then 200 mg BID with gradual tapering over 3 to 5 days; **OR Naproxen,** 500 mg initially, then 250 mg q8h with gradual tapering over 5 days; **OR Ibuprofen,** 800 mg initially, then 400 mg q6h with gradual tapering over 5 days.
3. **Colchicine,** 1 to 2 mg IV in 15 to 20 ml normal saline solution slowly over 3 to 5 minutes, then 0.5 mg q6-12h to a maximum of 4 mg/day **OR** 1 to 2 tablets (0.5 mg or 0.6 mg), which equals 0.5 to 1.2 mg PO, followed by 0.5 to 1.2 mg PO q1-2h until therapeutic effect or GI side effects to a maximum of 8 mg/day.

Pseudogout

I. Definition
Inflammatory arthropathy caused by calcium pyrophosphate dihydrate crystal deposition in the synovial tissues.

II. Salient features
Signs and symptoms are similar to gout without tophi, and an abrupt onset with severe joint inflammation is characteristic.

A. Pathogenesis
Abnormalities in the cartilage structure caused by age, metabolic disorders, genetic defects, and osteoarthritis.

B. Associated diseases
Hyperparathyroidism, hypothyroidism, gout, neuropathic arthropathy, hemochromatosis, hypophosphatasia, and hypomagnesemia.

C. Diagnostic features
Identification of rod-shaped or rhomboid birefringent crystals of calcium pyrophosphate—use a red lens to distinguish from urate crystals.

D. Differential diagnosis
Gout, septic arthritis, hydroxyapatite crystal deposition disease, metabolic disorders (e.g., hyperthyroidism, hypothyroidism, Wilson disease, ochronosis, hypomagnesemia, diabetes mellitus, hemochromatosis, hypophosphatasia), and other associations such as postseptic arthritis, trauma, neuropathic joints, and osteoarthritis.

III. Management

A. Laboratory
1. No specific biochemical abnormalities for pseudogout.
2. Obtain serum levels of thyroxin, magnesium, calcium, iron, uric acid, and phosphate, which may be abnormal and indicative of the associated diseases. X-rays, arthrocentesis, and synovial fluid aspiration should be performed.

B. Combine joint aspiration and pharmacologic treatment
1. **Joint aspiration and intraarticular steroids. Depo-Medrol,** 40 to 60 mg with a maximum of three treatments per year; **Phenylbutazone,** 400 to 600 mg PO in divided doses for several days, **OR Indomethacin,** 50 mg q6h with tapering over 5 days.
2. **Naproxen and Sulindac** are also effective.
3. **Hospitalized patients. Colchicine,** 2 mg IV in 15 ml of normal saline solution if NSAIDs are not tolerated.

4. **Chronic pseudogout. Aspirin,** 900 mg QID or equivalent dosage of NSAIDs.

C. Bed rest

Systemic Lupus Erythematosus (SLE)

I. **Definition.** SLE is a chronic, inflammatory, multisystem systemic disease of autoimmune origin, exhibiting a course of alternating exacerbations and remissions.

II. **Salient features**

Female/male predominance of 9:1.

Onset usually before 40 years of age; however, any person may be affected, and presentation in elderly may differ.

Higher prevalence in the U.S. black population, indicating a genetic predisposition.

A. **Presenting manifestations.** Fatigue, arthritis or arthralgias, malaise, weight loss, fever, nephritis, photosensitivity, serositis, cerebritis, cerebral vasculitis, pneumonitis, inflammatory myositis, myocarditis, thrombocytopenia, anemia, leukopenia, facial erythema, pericarditis, endocarditis, vasculitis, aortic insufficiency, pleuritis, as well as conjunctivitis, episcleritis, and retinal exudates.

B. **Clinical manifestations.** Musculoarticular, abnormal hematology, cutaneous disease, fever of unknown cause, fatigue, neuropsychiatric, pulmonary, renal, and cardiac diseases, and GI complaints.

C. **Inducing agents.** Chlorpromazine, hydralazine, isoniazid, lithium, methyldopa, penicillamine, phenytoin, procainamide, propylthiouracil, quinidine, and sulfasalazine.

D. **Diagnostic features.** Patient must have more than four of the following features: malar rash, discoid rash, photosensitivity, oral ulcers, arthritis, serositis, renal disorder, neurologic disorder, hematologic disorder, immunologic disorder, and ANA.

E. **Differential diagnosis.** Discoid lupus, drug-induced LE, sicca syndrome, scleroderma, RA, membranoproliferative glomerulonephritis, cryoglobulinemia, hereditary complement deficiency, and angioedema.

III. **Management**

A. **Laboratory.** CBC, PT/PTT, RF, ANA, anti–smooth muscle antibody, ESR, and Coombs' test.

B. Adequate sleep, rest, and for skin eruptions, *para*-**aminobenzoic acid skin protection factor (SPF)** 40 (if sun sensitive) lotions applied liberally every 1 to 2 hours, especially before sun exposure or after sweating or swimming; topical corticosteroids—**Triamcinolone OR Fluocinonide,** two or three times a day, **OR Hydroxychloroquine,** 200 mg PO BID plus topical agents for systemic therapy.

C. **Fever and arthritic pain.** Aspirin, 600 to 900 mg QID for fever, **OR Indomethacin,** 25 to 50 mg TID if aspirin sensitive, **OR Prednisone,** 10 to 20 mg PO daily.

D. **Serositis.** NSAIDs as for arthritis and **Prednisone,** 20 mg PO TID.

E. **Pneumonitis. Prednisone,** 20 mg PO TID, plus **Azathioprine,** 2 to 3 mg/kg/day, **OR Cyclophosphamide,** 2 to 3 mg/kg/day.

F. **Hemolytic anemia. Prednisone,** 40 to 60 mg/day orally in divided doses two or three times a day and taper quickly.

- **G. Immune thrombocytopenia. Prednisone,** 60 mg/day PO plus **gamma globulin** IV to increase platelet count.
- **H. Vasculitis. Prednisone,** 20 to 60 mg/day PO depending on size of vessel.
- **I.** Seizures. **Phenytoin,** 300 to 400 mg/day initially, and add Phenobarbital, 20 to 60 mg TID for seizure control.
- **J.** Steroid-induced psychosis. **Haloperidol,** 1 mg BID.
- **K. Renal failure, active CNS disease, or severe thrombocytopenia. Methylprednisolone,** 500 mg IV infusion over 30 minutes q12h for 3 to 5 days, then **Prednisone,** 50 mg PO BID and taper.
- **L. Side effects.** Changes in physical appearance and mental status, immunosuppression, adrenal suppression, fluid and electrolyte abnormalities, hyperglycemia, hypertension, osteopenia, steroid-induced myopathy, ischemic bone necrosis, and ocular effects.

Temporal Arteritis (TA)

I. Definition. Giant cell arteritis is a vascular inflammatory syndrome affecting medium- and large-sized arteries, with predominant effects on the temporal and other cranial arteries; hence, the term "temporal arteritis."

II. Salient features

Peak incidence at 60 to 80 years of age; rarely if younger than 50 years.

Temporal headaches, blindness, scalp necrosis, tongue gangrene, as well as jaw claudication, ear canal, pinna, or parotid gland pain, and TMJ pain.

Internal carotid artery association causing ocular damage encompasses amaurosis fugax, unilateral or complete blindness, bilateral blindness, and diplopia secondary to ischemic paresis.

- **A. Presenting manifestations.** Fatigue, malaise, fever, myalgia, arthralgia, weight loss, depression, temporal artery tenderness, tortuosity, and visual field altitudinal defects.
- **B. Diagnostic features.** Elevated ESR (50 to greater than 100 mm/hr), along with a biopsy indicating an inflammatory mononuclear infiltrate, fragmentation of the internal elastic lamina, intimal proliferation, and the presence of giant cells.
- **C. Differential diagnosis.** Systemic necrotizing vasculitis, arteriosclerotic vascular disease, and Takayasu arteritis.

III. Management
- **A. Laboratory.** ESR and temporal artery tissue biopsy.
- **B. Pharmacologic treatment**
    1. **Prednisone,** 40 mg/day PO in divided doses; with acute TA-associated visual changes.
    2. **Methylprednisolone,** 80 to 100 mg/day IV STAT and taper to oral **prednisone** dose after 7 to 10 days.
- **C. Maintenance therapy. Prednisone,** 5 to 10 mg/day for 2 to 5 years.

Vasculitis

I. Definition. A general term for describing a number of inflammatory and necrotic blood vessel diseases, with multiple clinical manifestations, encompassing primary disorders involving only the blood vessels, and secondary disorders involving blood vessels as a component of a more serious systemic disease.

II. Salient features. Headache, fever, weight loss, rash, arthritis, myositis, renal disease, hypertension, cardiac failure, arrhythmias, CNS disturbances, neu-

ropathies, arthralgias, episcleritis, abdominal pain, and gastrointestinal dysfunction; elevated ESR, anemia, leukocytosis.
   A. Diagnostic features. Diagnosis confirmation via biopsy of specific lesion, "blind" muscle biopsy, sural nerve biopsy, and arteriography.
III. **Management**
   A. Laboratory. ESR.
   B. Pharmacologic treatment
      1. Glucocorticoids. Prednisone, 60 to 100 mg/day PO; if life-threatening manifestations occur, use **Methylprednisolone,** 500 mg IV q12h for 3 to 5 days.
      2. Immunosuppressives. Cyclophosphamide, 1.5 to 2.0 mg/kg/day PO, or 0.5 to 1.0 gm/m^2 IV per month added to steroid treatment if major organ system involvement occurs.
   C. Short-term plasmapheresis for life-threatening vasculitis—DO NOT use with immunosuppressive drugs.

Suggested Readings

Alercon GS et al: Lack of association between HLA-DR2 and clinical response to methotrexate in patients with rheumatoid arthritis, *Arthritis Rheum* 30:218, 1987.

Aweeka FT: Bone and skin infections. In Koda-Kimble MA, Young LY, editors: *Applied therapeutics: the clinical use of drugs,* ed 5, Vancouver, 1992, Applied Therapeutics.

Beary JF III: Osteoarthritis. In Beary JF III, Christian CL, Johanson NA, editors: *Manual of rheumatology and outpatient orthopedic disorders: diagnosis and therapy,* ed 2, Boston, 1987, Little, Brown.

Boss GR, Seegmiller JE: Hyperuricemia and gout: classification, complications, management, *N Engl J Med* 300:1459, 1979.

Cardenosa G, Deluca SA: Radiographic features of gout, *Am Fam Physician* 4:539, 1990.

Cassidy JT: Juvenile rheumatoid arthritis. In Kelly WN et al, editors: *Textbook of rheumatology,* ed 3, Philadelphia, 1989, WB Saunders.

Copass MK, Eisenberg MS, editors: *Emergency medical therapy,* ed 3, Philadelphia, 1988, WB Saunders.

Dahl SL: Rheumatic disorders. In Koda-Kimble MA, Young LY, editors: *Applied therapeutics: the clinical use of drugs,* ed 5, Vancouver, 1992, Applied Therapeutics.

Fauci AS, Haynes BF, Katz P: The spectrum of vasculitis: clinical, pathologic, immunologic, and therapeutic considerations, *Ann Intern Med* 89:660, 1978.

Fink CW: Treatment of juvenile rheumatoid arthritis, *Bull Rheum Dis* 32:21, 1982.

Freed JF et al: Acute monoarticular arthritis: A diagnostic approach, *JAMA* 342:2314, 1980.

Fries JF, Holman HR: *Systemic lupus erythematosus: a clinical analysis,* Philadelphia, 1975, WB Saunders.

Gibofsky A: Reiter syndrome. In Beary JF III, Christian CL, Johanson NA, editors: *Manual of rheumatology and outpatient orthopedic disorders: diagnosis and therapy,* ed 2, Boston, 1987, Little, Brown.

Goldenberg DL, Reed JI: Bacterial arthritis, *N Engl J Med* 312:764, 1985.

Hahn BH: SLE. In Parker CW, editor: *Clinical immunology,* Philadelphia, 1980, WB Saunders.

Harris ED Jr: The clinical features of rheumatoid arthritis. In Kelly WW et al, editors: *Textbook of rheumatology,* ed 3, Philadelphia, 1989, WB Saunders.

Healy LA, Wilske K: *The systemic manifestations of temporal arteritis,* New York, 1979, Grune & Stratton.

Hughes GRV: Systemic lupus erythematosus, *Clinics in Rheumatic Diseases* 8:(1):1-323, 1982.

Huskisson EC, Balme HW: Pseudopodagra: differential diagnosis of gout, *Lancet* 2:269, 1972.

Inman RD: Infectious arthritis. In Beary JF III, Christian CL, Johanson NA, editors: *Manual of rheumatology and outpatient orthopedic disorders: diagnosis and therapy,* ed 2, Boston, 1987, Little, Brown.

Kahl LE: Arthritis and rheumatologic disease. In Woodley M, Whelan WH, editors: *Manual of medical therapeutics: the Washington manual,* ed 27, St. Louis, 1992, Little, Brown.

Kelly PJ et al: Bacterial (suppurative) arthritis in the adult, *J Bone Joint Surg [Am]* 52(8):1595-1602, 1970.

Kimberly RP: Lupus erythematosus. In Paget S, Pellicci P, Beary JF III, editors: *Manual of rheumatology and outpatient orthopedic disorders: diagnosis and therapy,* ed 3, Boston, 1993, Little, Brown.

Klearman M, Pereira M: Arthritis and rheumatologic diseases. In Dunagan C, Ridner ML, editors: *Manual of medical therapeutics,* ed 26, Boston, 1989, Little, Brown.

Lo B: Hyperuricemia and gout, *West J Med* 142:104, 1985.

Mankin HJ: Clinical features of osteoarthritis. In Kelly WN et al, editors: *Textbook of rheumatology,* ed 3, Philadelphia, 1989, WB Saunders.

Morris R et al: HLA-A W27: a clue to the diagnosis and pathogenesis of Reiter's syndrome, *N Engl J Med* 289:554, 1987.

Nelson JD, Koontz WC: Septic arthritis in infants and children: a review of 117 cases, *Pediatrics* 38:966, 1966.

Paget S, Bryan W: Rheumatoid arthritis. In Paget S, Pellicci P, Beary JF III, editors: *Manual of rheumatology and outpatient orthopedic disorders: diagnosis and therapy,* ed 3, Boston, 1993, Little, Brown.

Paulus HE et al: Azathioprine vs d-penicillamine in rheumatic arthritis patients who have been treated unsuccessfully with gold, *Arthritis Rheum* 27:721, 1984.

Resnick D: Crystal induced arthropathy: gout and pseudogout, *JAMA* 242(22):2440-2, 1979.

Scarpa NP: Gout. In Beary JF III, Christian CL, Johanson NA, editors: *Manual of rheumatology and outpatient orthopedic disorders: diagnosis and therapy,* ed 2, Boston, 1987, Little, Brown.

Scarpa NP: Pseudogout (calcium dihydrate crystal arthropathy). In Beary JF III, Christian CL, Johanson NA, editors: *Manual of rheumatology and outpatient orthopedic disorders: diagnosis and therapy,* ed 2, Boston, 1987, Little, Brown.

Sergent JS: Vasculitis. In Paget S, Pellicci P, Beary JF III, editors: *Manual of rheumatology and outpatient orthopedic disorders: diagnosis and therapy,* ed 3, Boston, 1993, Little, Brown.

Shefler AG, editor: *The HSC handbook of pediatrics,* ed 8, St. Louis, 1992, Mosby–Year Book.

Simkin PA: Management of gout, *Ann Intern Med* 90:812, 1979.

Simkin PA et al: The pathogenesis of podagra, *Ann Intern Med* 86:230, 1977.

Singser BH: Pediatric rheumatic disease. In Schumacher HR Jr, editor: *Primer on the rheumatic diseases,* ed 9, Atlanta, 1988, Arthritis Foundation.

Spruill WJ, Wade WE: Other connective tissue disorders and the use of glucocorticoids. In Koda-Kimble MA, Young LY editors: *Applied therapeutics: the clinical use of drugs,* ed 5, Vancouver, 1992, Applied Therapeutics.

Stern R: Polymyalgia rheumatica and temporal arteritis. In Beary JF III, Christian CL, Johanson NA, editors: *Manual of rheumatology and outpatient orthopedic disorders: diagnosis and therapy,* ed 2, Boston, 1987, Little, Brown.

Tabatabai MR, Cummings MA: Intravenous colchicine in the treatment of acute pseudogout, *Arthritis Rheum* 23:370, 1980.

Wagener HP, Hollenhorst RW: Ocular lesions of temporal arteritis, *Am J Ophthalmol* 45:617, 1958.

Wedgwood JF, Larouche SJ: Juvenile rheumatoid arthritis. In Beary JF III, Christian CL, Johanson NA, editors: *Manual of rheumatology and outpatient orthopedic disorders: diagnosis and therapy,* ed 2, Boston, 1987, Little, Brown.

Young LY: Gout and hyperuricemia. In Koda-Kimble MA, Young LY, editors: *Applied therapeutics: the clinical use of drugs,* ed 5, Vancouver, 1992, Applied Therapeutics.

Zvaifler NJ et al: Rheumatoid arthritis. In Schumacher HR Jr, editor: *Primer on the rheumatic diseases,* ed 9, Atlanta, 1988, Arthritis Foundation.

26

Psychiatric Emergencies

H. Brian Goldman, M.D., A.B.E.M., M.C.F.P. (EM)

Few patients invoke anxiety in emergency physicians more than those with psychiatric complaints. There are several obvious reasons for this. First, psychiatric illness tends to be unpredictable in its presentation and course. Not surprisingly, it often takes more time to assess the psychiatric well-being of a patient than it does to assess the well-being of a patient with complaints related to other systems. Second, assessment and management tend to be both time-consuming and labor-intensive, as anyone who has had to deal with a dangerously violent patient will attest. Third, the origins of psychiatric symptoms are not always apparent. The emergency physician must always be aware that organic illness may masquerade as a primary psychiatric disorder. Finally, no other type of emergencies demands a greater awareness of consent and other medicolegal issues than psychiatric emergencies.

This chapter deals with the rapid assessment and management of patients presenting with depression, suicidal ideation, acute psychosis, schizophrenia, violent behavior, and panic agoraphobia. It details critical issues such as assessment for risk of suicide or violent behavior, criteria for involuntary admission, as well as effective techniques for chemical and physical restraint of patients.

Presenting Illnesses

The most common psychiatric disorders include personality disorders, acute psychoses, schizophrenia, unipolar depression, bipolar affective disorder, anxiety disorder, and panic attacks. While the above disorders usually arise from a primary psychiatric condition, organic pathology is frequently involved. For example, the elderly patient with violent behavior may have a subdural hematoma or an anticholinergic syndrome. Likewise, the patient with acute psychosis may have taken an overdose of cocaine. Ethanol intoxication is a frequent concomitant to psychiatric emergencies. In a study of patients requiring restraints to control violent behavior, half the patients had abused ethanol, while another 25% had taken a drug overdose. **Therefore it is imperative to consider organic pathology in all psychiatric patients (Table 26-1 and 26-2).**

Initial Assessment

The purposes of the initial assessment are to arrive at a provisional diagnosis, to evaluate the risk of suicide or violent behavior (and to neutralize such risks by using verbal, physical, or chemical techniques), to rule out significant organic factors, and to arrange for appropriate referral and disposition. Such evaluation begins as soon as the patient arrives at the registration desk. It continues with an appropriate history and physical examination, and usually requires the search for confirmatory information by contacting the attending physician or psychiatrist, and by judicious use of laboratory testing.

Table 26-1. Clues to Organic Etiology

Alterations in vital signs
Respiratory distress
Facial flushing
Constricted or dilated pupils
Nystagmus
Stiff neck
Focal central nervous system (CNS) abnormalities
Tremors, ataxia, abnormal gait
Focus of infection

Table 26-2. Causes of Delirium in the Elderly

Intoxications: anticholinergic drugs, benzodiazepines, antihypertensives, cimetidine
Alcoholism
Electrolyte disturbances/hypovolemia
Sepsis
End-organ failure, myocardial infarction
Postoperative/anesthetic-related disorders

I. **Triage: recognition of risk factors.** Both the registration clerk and triage personnel must be able to assess the risk of impending suicide, as well as violent behavior. High-risk patients should be brought into an examining room immediately; prolonged waiting in the reception area intensifies agitation and places other patients and their families at risk.
   A. **Risk factors for suicide** include alcoholism, male sex, major depression, a history of suicidal attempts and threats, increasing age, unemployment, lack of social supports, and chronic illness. Many such patients do not recognize their own risk but are accompanied by concerned relatives. It is important to take the concerns of relatives and friends seriously.
   B. **The risk factors for violent behavior** include loud or pressured speech, pacing, lunging hand movements, clenched fists, standing close to others, verbal threats of violent behavior, delusions (especially command delusions), abnormal vital signs, and evidence of drug or alcohol intoxication.
II. **Security procedures** should be implemented in all high-risk situations, before the psychiatric interview takes place. Security guards should be contacted by using an innocuous command, such as requesting that "Dr. Armstrong" be contacted. Only flagrantly violent patients have to be subdued at this point. In most cases, a "show of force" actually calms patients down by demonstrating that they need not fear losing control.
III. **The psychiatric assessment room** should consist of heavy furniture that is difficult to lift or throw, soft objects to shield attacks, two doors, an emergency call button, pink walls, stimulus regression music, closed circuit television, and room for a restraining stretcher. All sharp objects must be removed in advance.
IV. **The psychiatric interview** should take place in the psychiatric assessment room. At least one door to the room should remain open. If the security team has been summoned but is not required to intervene, they should remain out-

side the room but within site of the entrance. Both the physician and the patient should stand an equal distance from the door; neither should be permitted to block the exit from the other. The essential parts of the psychiatric history include the following:

- **A. Presenting complaint.** As the patient gives a history of the present illness, assess the patient for tangential thought processes, delusions, general appearance and grooming, nutritional status, and evidence of agitation or depression.
- **B. Past history of psychiatric illness.** Obtain the name of the attending psychiatrist and family physician, as well as the names of all hospitals where the patient was previously admitted. Examine the patient's old chart; look specifically for a past history of violent behavior or suicide attempts.
- **C. Psychiatric medications.** Obtain the names and dosages of all psychoactive medications. Attempt to assess patient compliance, since noncompliance is a common etiologic factor in exacerbations of schizophrenia.
- **D.** Ask about **alcohol** and **drug abuse**.
- **E. Review of systems** and a past history of medical complaints should also be obtained.
- **F. Social history.** An interruption in the patient's usual social circumstances can trigger an acute psychiatric presentation. Ask about recent changes in accommodation, social welfare assistance, family conflicts, as well as a change of attending psychiatrists.
- **G. Obtain corroborating history** from outside sources such as the patient's family, friends, and psychiatrist.

V. Mental status examination. Perform a mental status examination on all patients with psychiatric complaints. The key parts of the examination include the following:

- **A. Level of consciousness.** Use the Glasgow Coma Scale for patients with a decreased level of consciousness. Patients who are alert should be assessed for orientation to person, time, date, and place.
- **B. Appearance and behavior** should be assessed, including nutritional status, grooming, motor activity (psychomotor agitation or retardation), and eye contact.
- **C. Mood and affect.** These should be described (examples include anger, anxiety, depression), with specific examples taken from the conversation. Blunted affect, suggestive of schizophrenia, should be noted.
- **D. Form and content of thought.** Tangential thoughts suggest schizophrenia, while flight of ideas and grandiose thoughts suggest hypomania. Incoherent thinking suggests dementia or toxic delirium. Abnormalities of thought content include delusions (fixed firm beliefs that are held despite evidence to the contrary) and ideas of reference (the idea that neutral objects or events hold special significance to the patient). Delusions and ideas of reference suggest schizophrenia. Suicidal ideation or ideas of worthlessness and hopelessness usually suggest depression, although they may occur with psychoses. The most worrisome kind of delusions are command delusions, which are usually manifested as a verbal command to harm oneself or others. **Command delusions are a cardinal sign of an acute psychiatric emergency.**

VI. Physical examination. The purpose of a physical examination is to look for evidence of organicity and for evidence of drug intoxication or withdrawal. Important clues to organicity include alterations in vital signs, respiratory distress, facial flushing, constricted or dilated pupils, nystagmus, stiff neck, abnormal CNS examination, tremors, ataxia, abnormal gait, or a focus of infection.

VII. **Laboratory investigations** depend on the past history and the findings on physical examination. Patients with a well-established history of primary psychiatric illness do not require extensive investigations. If the history or physical examination warrant it, potentially relevant tests include arterial blood gases, serum electrolytes, serum osmolality, serum calcium, serum magnesium, a complete blood cell count, serum liver enzymes, serum and urine drug screens, cultures (blood, urine, and cerebrospinal fluid), as well as diagnostic imaging studies such as computed tomography and magnetic resonance imaging.

Referral and Disposition

I. **Psychiatric consultation.** In general, it is best to obtain a psychiatric consultation of all patients with psychiatric disorders, especially if the emergency physician intends to discharge the patient. Note that many psychiatric services ask that all psychiatric patients be "cleared" of any potential medical or organic problems before referring them. Emergency physicians should not be coerced into providing such blanket assurances and should not write notifications such as "medically clear" on the patient chart.

II. **Criteria for discharge from hospital.** Patients may be discharged provided there is a high degree of certainty that neither the patients nor their intended victims are in danger. The patient's psychiatrist (if he has one) should be contacted before discharge. If the patient does not have a psychiatrist, a consultation should be obtained, and the patient should be provided with the name and telephone number of the psychiatrist providing follow-up care. If in doubt about the decision to discharge, it is best to arrange an immediate consultation or admission.

III. **Involuntary admission to hospital.** In general, emergency physicians should admit patients to a psychiatric service with their consent. However, it is permissible to admit such patients and to restrain them (physically and/or chemically) without their consent, provided there is evidence that patients are at risk of harming themselves or others. Such evidence may include stated intentions to harm themselves or others, psychosis or hypomania, violent behavior, intoxication, organic brain syndrome, as well as patients with life-threatening conditions who wish to leave against medical advice. It is important to **judge each case on its own merits**. It is always prudent to attempt to obtain consent before proceeding to involuntary commitment. The physician should document the reasons for involuntary commitment, using verbatim quotations from the patient and from witnesses. In addition, since circumstances change, the decision to involuntarily commit a patient should be reevaluated frequently. Note that terms and conditions for involuntary admission vary from state to state. In all cases, the hospital attorney should be consulted, although restraint should not be delayed by this step in emergency circumstances.

Legal Issues

I. **Consent to treatment.** All patients have an a priori right to refuse treatment. A refusal of consent should be honored without fear of legal reprisal provided the consent is voluntary, competent, and informed. It is legally permissible to treat without consent in four cases. The first case occurs if the patient is incompetent to give consent. Conditions possibly leading to a finding of incompetence include a head injury, ethanol or drug intoxication, and toxic delirium. In these cases, it is necessary to obtain consent from a next of kin or a legal guardian appointed by the courts. Issues such as the definition of incompetence and determination of substitute consent vary from state to state. A second exception to the rule of consent is in the case of an emergency; treatment may be given without consent if time is of the essence. The third and fourth exceptions have to do with the danger criteria; patients may be treated without consent if they are a danger to themselves or others. Physicians may only use chemical or physical means to restrain patients until a proper examination is completed.

II. **Use of force to detain and restrain patients.** It is prudent to use the minimum force necessary to restrain the patient, to document reasons for the use of force, and to examine the patient for injuries resulting from the use of restraints. Court cases have obliged the physician to demonstrate that professional judgement was exercised in making the decision to use restraints.

III. **Physician's duty to warn.** Court cases have established that physicians have a duty to warn intended victims of violence. If a patient escapes or cannot be held, the physician should notify the intended victims and notify the police to provide protection for the intended victims.

The Violent Patient

Violent patients are the most difficult of all patients seen with psychiatric emergencies, both from a diagnostic and a management point of view.

I. **Etiologic factors associated with violent behavior.** Contrary to popular belief, the majority of violent people do not suffer from a definable psychiatric illness.

   A. **Psychiatric disorders associated with violent behavior** include schizophrenia and other paranoid states, bipolar affective disorder (hypomania and mania), and personality disorders such as antisocial and borderline personalities.

   B. **Drug intoxications** of ethanol, cocaine (crack), amphetamines, hallucinogens such as phencyclidine (PCP), lysergic acid diethylamide (LSD), benzodiazepines (especially triazolam), short-acting barbiturates and anticholinergic drugs are associated with violent behavior.

   C. **Drug withdrawal** from ethanol, barbiturates, and benzodiazepines can precipitate violent behavior.

   D. **Organic conditions** may be associated with violence. Common examples include hypoglycemia, hypoxemia, hyponatremia, CNS infections, hepatic encephalopathy, and endocrinopathies such as Cushing's syndrome and thyrotoxicosis. Uncommon organic causes of violence include carbon dioxide (CO_2) retention, temporal lobe epilepsy, and vitamin deficiencies.

   E. **Situational crisis.** The most common precipitant of violent behavior is an acute situational crisis. Examples include family conflict, recent unemployment, loss of a significant relationship, loss of accommodation, and perceived personal or racial insults.

   F. **Episodic nonpsychotic violence** is typified by spousal and child abuse.

II. **Characteristic profile.** Violent persons tend to be males between the ages of 15 and 40 years. They frequently have a history of alcohol abuse and come from disadvantaged social and educational backgrounds. They lack friends and social supports, tend to blame others for their problems, and are conditioned to violence. The most important etiologic factor in predicting violent behavior is a past history of violence.

III. **Predicting violent behavior.** The overt clues of impending violence include pacing in the waiting room, motor restlessness, loud, forceful, or pressured speech, threats to injure or kill others, as well as the presence of weapons. Subtle clues include evidence of intoxication, hypomania or history of bipolar affective disorder, psychosis with command delusions, delirium, and acute onset of confusion in the elderly. The best clue is often a "gut feeling" of impending violence that is held by the staff.

IV. Protection of staff and other patients. Since violence may erupt quickly and without warning, appropriate precautions should preceed the psychiatric interview of potentially violent patients. Assemble a uniformed security team. Two security officers may present a show of force, but a minimum of five persons are required to physically restrain a patient. They should be available on a prearranged signal. If the patient is known to be carrying a weapon, the security team should carry out the search and seizure.

V. Personal protection. When interviewing potentially violent patients, take special precautions. Remove dangerous clothing that could be used as a weapon, such as neckties, stethoscopes, belts, glasses, pens, and jewelry. It is not advisable to see a potentially dangerous person alone or without nearby assistance. When interviewing potentially violent patients, remain at least 3 to 4 feet from the patient. Sit facing the patient, and do not sit behind a desk. Both patient and physician should have equal access to the door, which remains open during the interview.

VI. Assessment. The dual purposes of taking a history, as well as defusing the potential for violence, occur simultaneously.

A. Essential history. Try to determine the potential for violence by direct questioning. Ask whether the patient is afraid of harming someone. Obtain the names of intended victims, as well as the method of intended harm. Ask whether the patient is afraid of losing control, and whether the patient is able to control his or her violent intentions. Other details to obtain include a past psychiatric history, prescribed psychoactive medications and compliance, ethanol and drug abuse, as well as complicating medical problems such as a recent head injury.

B. Techniques to deescalate tension. Techniques such as offering food and verbal techniques can greatly diffuse the risk of violent behavior. The physician should speak slowly and quietly. The first technique is to identify oneself by using a formal title. It is important to always by overtly respectful of the patient and to empathize with the patient early and often. An offer of food or a cold drink can be helpful; never offer a hot drink. Explain the purpose of the interview and any anticipated procedures in advance. Build the patient's confidence by focusing on what the patient is doing well. Focus on the patient's feelings, not the situation precipitating the feelings. Summarize frequently what has been said by the patient.

Verbal techniques should be used in all cases of incipient violence but are unlikely to suffice when the patient is suffering from florrid psychosis, toxic delirium, intoxication, organic brain syndrome, hypomanic episode, and extreme agitation.

VII. Restraint techniques. Both physical and chemical restraints are available and are often used simultaneously. They are indicated when verbal techniques are unlikely to be effective (see VI), and when verbal techniques have failed to stop or prevent violence.

A. Physical restraints are indicated when patients are imminently at risk of harming themselves or others (including staff), when patients are allergic to anxiolytics and/or neuroleptics, and when the cause of agitation mandates

ongoing neurologic assessment. Restraints should not be used as a long-term strategy unless sedation is either ineffective or contraindicated.
- **B. Technique.** The team should wear disposable gloves and should be assembled in advance. A minimum of five persons is required to restrain a patient; if the patient is female, at least one member of the team must be female. Assign the most experienced member of the team as leader. Remove all persons from the room except the five people who will restrain the patient. Each person should have a preassigned limb (or head) to grasp. Each person should begin by standing 20 ft from patient. The leader should inform the patient why physical restraints are being used, and may briefly offer the patient one chance to voluntarily lie face down on the stretcher. If the patient refuses to cooperate, divide the team into two and have them approach the patient from opposite sides. Use a light mattress or cushion if the patient is holding a sharp object or is flailing about. Sandwich the patient on the floor between the two teams. The head, elbows, and knees are individually grasped, and the patient is taken to the stretcher. Each limb is secured to the stretcher with a leather restraint. Do not used rolled sheets or adhesive tape to restrain a patient because these are easily removed by the patient.
- **C. Positioning.** Young adult patients should be placed in a supine, head-up position. Extremely violent patients should be placed in the prone position. Elderly patients should be placed on their side.
- **D. Weapons search.** Once restraints are applied, search the patient and remove all weapons and drugs.
- **E. Postrestraint observation.** Examine the patient for injuries caused by using restraints, such as lacerations, contusions, and abrasions. Examine the limbs for pulses and capillary refill every few minutes to ensure that circulation is adequate. Reposition the patient every hour to prevent pressure sores. Observe the patient constantly while restrained.
- **F. Disposition.** It is important to document why restraints are being implemented. Obtain a psychiatric consultation. Do not remove restraints until the patient is seen by a psychiatrist, unless the patient has been sedated.

VIII. Chemical restraints are extremely effective and rapidly acting in controlling violent behavior. Alone and in combination, both benzodiazepines and neuroleptic agents are used in the emergency setting.
- **A. Benzodiazepines.** These agents cause rapid and effective sedation, anxiolysis, muscle relaxation, and anterograde amnesia. The use of benzodiazepines can result in a significant reduction in the dosage of neuroleptic agents required to control violent behavior. The agents of choice in the emergency sedation of violent patients include lorazepam, diazepam, and alprazolam. Midazolam, with its relatively brief duration of action, is not indicated for the effective control of violent behavior. Because of their differing pharmacokinetics, each agent has its advantages and disadvantages.
  - **1. Lorazepam.** This agent is the benzodiazepine of choice for the sedation of violent patients. It has an elimination half-life intermediate to that of midazolam and diazepam. It has the most effective and predictable intramuscular absorption of all the benzodiazepines, and has a rapid onset of action when administered sublingually. The intramuscular and sublingual routes have virtually identical absorption profiles, so there is no particular advantage to the intramuscular route. Lorazepam may also be administered intravenously, although it should be administered

slowly to minimize the risk of respiratory depression. In addition, the drug should be administered cautiously, since lorazepam can sometimes cause severe irritation to surrounding tissues when given intravenously. The dosage and route of administration for patients with mild agitation is 1 to 2 mg sublingually, while the dosage and route of administration for severe agitation is 2 mg sublingually, intramuscularly, or intravenously every 1 to 2 hours as needed until sedated, or up to a maximum of 5 to 6 mg.
2. **Diazepam**. Since diazepam initially binds with high affinity to the CNS (particularly the limbic system and the cerebral cortex), it has the most rapid onset of action of the benzodiazepines used in the sedation of violent patients. Redistribution throughout the body occurs within 30 to 60 minutes, after which the CNS effects usually wear off rapidly. However, this is not always the case. Because the elimination half-life is 24 to 48 hours, prolonged sedation and an associated inability to complete a psychiatric assessment are a possibility when diazepam is given. The half-life is prolonged in the elderly and in patients with liver disease.
   a. **Dosage and routes of administration.** In cases of mild agitation, diazepam may be given orally, but the intravenous route is preferred in cases of extreme agitation. Although the intramuscular route is often used, the absorption of diazepam is erratic and unpredictable. The dose of diazepam is 5 to 10 mg orally or intravenously. Use half the recommended dose in patients who are elderly, have liver disease, or who are receiving concomitant narcotics. Because of the risk of severe respiratory depression, equipment for endotracheal intubation and bag ventilation must be kept near the patient's bedside. Continuous monitoring of oxygen (O_2) saturation is optional. Since circulatory impairment has been observed after an intravenous bolus injection, it is advisable to use a cardiac monitor and to maintain a secure intravenous drip during and after the procedure.
   b. **Adverse effects and contraindications.** The most common adverse effects are drowsiness and ataxia. Less frequent adverse effects include headache, vertigo, tremors, euphoria, dysarthria, hypotension, and paradoxical excitement. Contraindications to the use of intravenous diazepam include myasthenia gravis, acute angle-closure glaucoma, coma of unknown cause, shock, severe chronic obstructive pulmonary disease (COPD), advanced liver disease, and hypersensitivity reactions.
3. **Alprazolam.** Although there is less clinical experience with this agent than with lorazepam and diazepam, alprazolam is emerging as an effective adjunct to neuroleptic agents. The dosage of alprazolam is 1 mg orally as needed every 2 hours, to a maximum dose of 4 mg. Alprazolam has not been studied alone as a sedating agent for violent patients; its use has been documented in combination with haloperidol administered as an oral concentrate.

B. Neuroleptic agents
   1. **Haloperidol: high-dose intravenous administration.** Haloperidol has been used for decades in small intramuscular boluses in the management of acute schizophrenia and other psychoses. Concern over hemodynamic and extrapyramidal adverse effects has resulted in a reluctance to use larger dosages. However, recent studies have shown that

haloperidol may be administered intravenously in much larger doses than previously believed.
2. **Intravenous haloperidol** has emerged as a first-line drug in the treatment of agitation of virtually any cause. In particular, it has been used to sedate agitated patients requiring diagnostic procedures such as magnetic resonance imaging and computed tomography.
3. **The use of intravenous haloperidol as described below** is currently the focus of intensive research. The results of preliminary studies are extremely encouraging. However, until definitive studies are completed, the use of intravenous haloperidol as recommended below must be considered experimental.
    a. **Pharmacokinetics.** Haloperidol produces peak sedation effects 5 to 10 minutes after an intravenous bolus, compared with 20 minutes after intramuscular administration.
    b. **Dosage and route of administration.** Haloperidol is titrated for optimal effect. The starting dose is 5 to 10 mg by slow intravenous push. If the patient tolerates this dose, increments of 5 to 10 mg may be given every 10 minutes until the patient is calm. In elderly patients, administer 1 to 2 mg intravenously every 5 to 10 minutes for three doses, and increase the incremental dosages to 5 mg every 10 minutes if tolerated. There is no maximum dose of intravenous haloperidol. Severely agitated patients in critical care settings have required boluses as large as 50 to 75 mg intravenously every 30 to 60 minutes.
    c. **Adverse effects and contraindications.** Intravenously administered haloperidol does not cause adverse hemodynamic, respiratory, or neurologic effects. Extrapyramidal effects are rarely observed and tend to be milder than those occurring after intramuscular administration; they respond well to diphenhydramine.
    d. **Indications.** Intravenous haloperidol is indicated for the rapid relief of agitation of any cause, such as psychosis, organic brain disease, CNS pathology, metabolic or endocrine abnormalities, major organ failure, and drug-induced deliria. Haloperidol is also indicated for the sedation of patients requiring diagnostic imaging or painful procedures when benzodiazepines are contraindicated.
  C. **Combined haloperidol and lorazepam.** The above combination provides both rapid and long-lasting sedation across the spectrum of causes of acute delirium. The combination is administered intravenously in a dosage of haloperidol, 5 mg intramuscularly, with lorazepam, 2 mg intramuscularly or sublingually, every 2 to 3 hours as needed until the patient is sedated.
IX. **Evaluation.** Because of the high association of organic factors in patients with violent behavior, a thorough evaluation guided by the history and physical examination must be done to exclude an organic cause.
  A. **Physical examination.** Once sedated, all violent patients must have a complete general physical examination, a complete neurologic examination, and a complete set of vital signs. Particular findings to look for include alterations in vital signs (especially elevations in temperature and blood pressure), diaphoresis, focal signs of infection (especially stiff neck), and focal neurologic signs such as pupillary abnormalities and nystagmus.
  B. **Laboratory investigations.** Determine serum levels of electrolytes, glucose, urea, and creatinine in all violent patients. Because of the high correlation

between alcohol and drug intoxication and violent behavior, determine a serum osmolality, a serum ethanol level, and perform a drug screen in violent patients. When warranted, a septic work-up should be performed, including blood and urine cultures and a lumbar puncture. If CNS abnormalities are found, a computed tomography or magnetic resonance imaging scan of the head should be done.

X. Treatment. The principles of treatment include rapid control of violent behavior, followed by specific therapy for the cause of the violent behavior.

Acute Psychosis

Acute psychosis is a clinical syndrome characterized by thought disturbances, agitation, and affective derangements.

I. Etiology. The cause of acute psychosis is multifactorial. Common causes include mania, depression, drug abuse (amphetamines, cocaine, PCP, and hallucinogens), schizophrenia, and withdrawal from psychoactive medications, chiefly benzodiazepines. Less common causes include medical disorders such as Cushing's syndrome, hypernatremia and hyponatremia, thiamine deficiency, and hypoglycemia.

II. Clinical presentation. Patients with acute psychosis typically present with delusions, ideas of reference, hallucinations, flight of ideas, insomnia, psychomotor agitation, and anxiety. Patients with hypomania may initially be seen with pressure of speech, insomnia and elation, and evidence of grandiose actions. Patients with depression may present with suicidal ideation and dysphoria. In general, patients with acute psychosis exhibit poor judgement. Patients with psychosis of organic etiology may have abnormal vital signs such as fever and tachycardia.

III. Diagnosis. A patient with acute psychosis is investigated in the same manner as a violent patient. Since most patients have a significant thought disorder, it is essential to obtain corroborative history from friends, family, attending physicians and psychiatrists, and other witnesses.

  A. Premorbid state and course of illness. It is important to determine the patient's premorbid state. Normal premorbid mentation and behavior suggests drug abuse as the cause, while a preexisting abnormal mental status suggests a primary psychiatric cause. Patients with bipolar affective disorder, as well as schizophrenia, usually have a history of repeated psychotic episodes.

  B. Medical history. Determine whether the patient has a history of organic illness.

  C. Medications. Obtain a list of prescription and over-the-counter drugs, as well as illicit drugs, used by the patient.

  D. Physical examination. Perform a detailed mental status examination (see mental status examination p. 648). Signs associated with organic delirium include disorientation to time and place, visual hallucinations (auditory hallucinations are more common in primary psychiatric disorders), and fluctuating levels of consciousness. Specific criteria for schizophrenia include delusions, incoherent thinking or loose associations, flat affect, auditory hallucinations, and catatonic behavior.

  E. Laboratory testing should be individualized. Patients initially seen with their first episode of acute psychosis and those with suspected organic delirium should have the following laboratory tests done: serum levels of electrolytes, urea, creatinine, glucose, liver transaminases, bilirubin, alkaline phosphatase, thyroid indices, calcium, and magnesium, as well as complete blood cell count, serum and urine drug screens, and a urinalysis.

IV. Management. The principles of appropriate management were detailed in the management of "The Violent Patient" (VII through X).

A. Admission. Most patients with acute psychosis should be admitted to the hospital for management of their symptoms and treatment of the underlying cause. Although most patients will voluntarily consent to admission, involuntary admission should be considered for patients who meet the previously mentioned criteria (Referral and Disposition, III).

B. Management of psychotic behavior. Violent patients should be managed as described previously. Patients not requiring physical or chemical restraint should have all weapons, sharp objects, cigarette lighters, and other dangerous objects confiscated. Patients should be kept under close observation in a psychiatric examining room. A security team should be rapidly available on a prearranged signal.

C. Pharmacologic management

  1. Sedating violent patients: see The Violent Patient, VIII A through C.

  2. Management of the compliant patient is not as urgent as management of the violent patient. Generally, lower doses are required to control psychotic symptoms in nonviolent patients than to control symptoms in patients exhibiting violent behavior. Although neuroleptic agents are specific therapy for schizophrenia and mania, they are not specific therapy for the control of psychotic symptoms in drug-abusing patients. Therefore, many clinicians prefer to sedate compliant psychotic patients with short-acting benzodiazepines until the cause of the psychosis is clear.

  a. Benzodiazepines. Lorazepam is the benzodiazepine of choice for controlling symptoms of mild psychosis. The dosage is 2 to 5 mg by mouth or sublingually.

  b. Neuroleptic agents. Haloperidol is the agent of choice for emergency tranquillization. Chlorpromazine is not recommended because it causes profound sedation and anticholinergic symptoms. The dosage of haloperidol is 5 mg of a liquid concentrate administered orally twice a day. Since haloperidol can cause acute dystonias (torticollis, oculogyric crises, etc.), many clinicians prophylactically administer benztropine, 2 mg intramuscularly or orally twice a day. It is acceptable to wait for dystonia to appear before administering antiparkinsonian medication.

The Suicidal Patient

I. Incidence and demographic factors. The annual suicide rate in the United States is 12 per 100,000 persons. Although males commit suicide three to four times more often than females, females attempt suicide three to four times more often than males. The peak incidence for males is 75 years of age; for females the peak incidence is 60 years of age.

II. Etiology. The vast majority of suicidal patients have a significant underlying psychiatric disorder. Half of all psychiatric patients are suffering from depression (including postpartum depression in females), while a quarter suffer from alcoholism. A smaller proportion have an underlying psychosis such as schizophrenia. Command delusions urging the patient to commit suicide is a dangerous symptom.

III. **Risk factors.** Factors associated with an increased risk of suicide include male sex, major depression, alcoholism, tenuous economic status, chronic pain, chronic illness and disability, and lack of social supports.
IV. **Clinical presentation.** The key to a successful work-up is a history from the patient, as well as a corroborating history from family, friends, and the attending psychiatrist.
   A. **The purposes of the history** are to determine the likelihood of further suicide attempts and to establish a trusting relationship with the patient. It is essential to obtain a detailed account of the present suicide attempt and any other past suicide attempts.
   B. **Symptoms to illicit** include recent depressed affect (depression) and hypomania (bipolar affective disorder). Delusions, thought blocking, and ideas of reference suggest schizophrenia. In addition, look for indications of risk factors for a successful suicide attempt, such as evidence of alcoholism and other chronic illnesses (see III).
   C. **Evaluation of suicidal intent.** The seriousness of intent varies with patients and their circumstances. Indicators of serious intent include detailed preparations for suicide, a dangerous method of suicide (e.g., handgun or potentially lethal overdose), anger or sorrow at being discovered, strong intent to repeat the act, recent recovery from a bout of depression, and the presence of psychotic delusions, especially command delusions urging the patient to commit suicide.
   D. Some patients with a **history of borderline and other personality disorders** frequently are seen with the latest in a long series of nonlethal suicide gestures. They are not usually at high risk for immediate suicide. However, the long-term prognosis for these patients is such that a significant percentage will ultimately succeed in committing suicide.
V. **Management and disposition**
   A. **Obtain a psychiatric consultation** in all cases in which a suicide attempt has taken place and in all cases in which the suicidal intent is judged to be high. In addition, it is prudent to obtain a consultation in low-risk situations when doubt exists as to the seriousness of suicidal ideation.
   B. **Involuntary admission.** Patients who are judged to have a high risk of committing suicide should be involuntarily held for psychiatric referral if the patient refuses admission to the hospital. The reasons for involuntarily holding the patient should be thoroughly documented.
   C. **Voluntary admission.** The decision to admit the patient on a voluntary basis should be made by the attending or consultant psychiatrist, and should be made on the basis of a prompt evaluation (Referral and Disposition, III).
   D. **Discharge from hospital.** The decision to discharge a patient who has attempted or contemplated suicide should be made by the consultant psychiatrist after a thorough and timely evaluation.
   E. **Remove objects** that could harm the patient, such as knives, handguns, and pills.
VI. **Treatment.** Management includes antidepressant medication, as well as a combination of individualized and group psychotherapy.
   A. **Antidepressants.** These include heterocyclic antidepressants, monoamine oxidase inhibitors (MAOIs), and second-generation antidepressants (such as fluoxetine and sertraline). As a rule, antidepressant medication takes several days to begin to treat symptoms of depression and reduce suicidal ideation. In addition, agents such as MAOIs and heterocyclic antidepressants cause sig-

nificant toxicity when taken in overdose. **For these reasons, it is inappropriate for the emergency physician to initiate antidepressant therapy.** Such therapeutic decisions are best left to the consultant psychiatrist.
- **B. Anxiolytics.** Patients manifesting symptoms of agitation and suicidal ideation may be given lorazepam, 1 to 2 mg sublingually or intramuscularly. The dose may be repeated once.
- **C. Antipsychotic medication.** Patients with severe agitation (often associated with psychotic features) may alternatively be treated with haloperidol administered orally or parenterally, depending on the severity of symptoms and the urgency of the need to restrain the patient (see The Violent Patient, VIII, B).

Panic Disorder

- **I. Panic disorder** is part of the general psychiatric category of anxiety disorders. It is characterized by brief intermittent episodes of extreme anxiety associated with a feeling of impending doom. It is often accompanied by symptoms of cardiorespiratory distress, as well as symptoms caused by catecholamine excess.
- **II. Epidemiology.** Panic disorder occurs three times more often in women than in men. It usually begins early in adult life, frequently after a major life stress such as loss of a loved one or a change in employment. Often there is a family history of panic disorder.
- **III. Pathophysiology.** Abnormalities in the noradrenergic and seritonergic systems have been implicated in panic disorder. The disorder also involves Y-aminobutyric acid (GABA) and benzodiazepine receptors. Administration of lactic acid precipitates panic attacks, but the reason is unknown.
- **IV. Clinical presentation**
  - **A. Primary symptoms.** Patients with panic disorder typically have recurrent episodes of paralyzing anxiety. These may occur spontaneously or in response to stereotypic situations. The first attack, called a herald attack, is often associated with a premonition of future episodes. Symptoms of a panic attack include overwhelming anxiety, tachypnea with hyperventilation syndrome, tachycardia, chest pain or tightness, dyspnea, weakness, and nonspecific dizziness.
  - **B. Precipitants.** Patients with panic disorder may have panic attacks in response to situational precipitants, caffeine, alcohol, cocaine, and pseudoephedrine.
  - **C. Secondary symptoms.** Patients with recurrent panic attacks often develop agoraphobia. Other secondary symptoms include depression, substance abuse, and generalized anxiety disorder.
- **V. Diagnosis of panic attack.** According to the Diagnostic and Statistical Manual of Mental Disorders (DSM-III-R), patients must have a minimum of four of the following symptoms that develop suddenly and increase in intensity within the first 10 minutes of the attack:
  - **A.** Shortness of breath or smothering sensations
  - **B.** Dizziness, unsteady feelings, or faintness
  - **C.** Palpitations or tachycardia
  - **D.** Trembling or shaking
  - **E.** Sweating
  - **F.** Choking
  - **G.** Nausea or abdominal distress
  - **H.** Depersonalization or derealization
  - **I.** Numbness or tingling sensations (paresthesias)

- **J.** Flushes (hot flashes) or chills
- **K.** Chest pain or discomfort
- **L.** Fear of dying
- **M.** Fear of going crazy or doing something uncontrolled

VI. Differential diagnosis. Patients with panic disorder frequently visit several physicians before obtaining the correct diagnosis. Medical disorders that mimic panic disorder include myocardial infarction, mitral valve prolapse, hyperthyroidism, pheochromocytoma, hypoglycemia, benign positional vertigo, as well as alcohol and drug withdrawal syndromes. Psychiatric disorders that are part of the differential diagnosis include generalized anxiety disorder, depression and hypomania, somatoform disorders, phobic disorders, and posttraumatic stress disorder.

VII. Treatment. Successful therapy usually involves a combination of medication and behavioral modification.

- **A. Nonpharmacologic therapy.** One of the most important initial interventions is to reassure patients that they do not suffer from disorders listed in the differential diagnosis. Behavioral modification is used to eliminate secondary phobias. In some cases of herald attacks, rapid reexposure to the precipitating situation prevents further attacks. Nonpharmacologic interventions are carried out by a consultant psychiatrist or psychologist on an outpatient basis. Specialized clinics are usually available in most communities.

- **B. Pharmacotherapy of panic disorder.** Tricyclic antidepressants, MAOIs, and benzodiazepines are effective in the management of panic disorder.

- **C. Antidepressants are the mainstay of therapy.** They produce fairly rapid control of symptoms and have a negligible risk of psychologic dependence. The most efficacious agents are imipramine and fluoxetine.
    1. **Imipramine.** The usual starting dosage is 10 to 25 mg orally at bedtime. If the patient tolerates it, the dose may be titrated to a maximum of 150 to 200 mg. Most patients respond to less than antidepressant doses of imipramine. Patients should be warned that it takes 2 weeks of continuous therapy for a clinical response. Antidepressants may cause an initial period of psychomotor stimulation; this can be lessened by briefly reducing the dose. Contraindications include prostatism, glaucoma, and coexistent suicidal ideation. The duration of therapy is individualized.
    2. **Fluoxetine.** The usual starting dosage of fluoxetine is 5 mg orally in the morning. The dose may be titrated in units of 5 to 10 mg every 2 or 3 days to a maximum of 30 mg. Fluoxetine does not produce anticholinergic symptoms. However, it can cause psychomotor stimulation in the initial phase of treatment. Patients started on fluoxetine in the emergency department should have close follow-up with the treating psychiatrist.

- **D. MAOIs.** Because of significant drug and food interactions, MAOIs should not be prescribed as a drug of choice by emergency physicians.

- **E. Benzodiazepines** can produce rapid control of symptoms associated with panic attacks. However, their potential for psychologic abuse merits judicious prescribing of these agents.
    1. **Alprazolam** is the benzodiazepine of choice for relieving panic symptoms. The starting dose is 0.25 to 0.50 mg four times a day. Although 1 to 2 mg/day will control the symptoms of most patients, the dose may be titrated to a maximum of 4 mg if the initial response is unsatisfactory. Because of the risk of addiction, the drug should be prescribed at the mini-

mum dose necessary to control symptoms. Nonpharmacologic therapy should be arranged, and the duration of therapy should be limited to several weeks or months. Slow withdrawal of medication is usually required.
2. **Clonazepam** may be prescribed instead of alprazolam. The starting dosage is 0.25 to 0.50 mg once or twice a day, and the usual daily dosage is between 2 and 6 mg/day.

F. **Other agents.** β-Blockers and buspirone have been prescribed for patients with panic disorder; however, neither are considered drugs of choice at present.

Suggested Readings

Barbee JG et al: Alprazolam as a neuroleptic adjunct in the emergency treatment of schizophrenia, *Am J Psychiatry* 149:506-10, 1992.

Blummenreich P et al: Violent patients. Are you prepared to deal with them? *Postgrad Med* 90:201-6, 1991.

Clinton JE et al: Haloperidol for sedation of disruptive emergency patients, *Ann Emerg Med* 16:319-22, 1987.

Cross-National Collaborative Panic Study, Second Phase Investigators: Drug treatment of panic disorder: the comparative efficacy of alprazolam, imipramine, and placebo, *Br J Psychiatry* 160:191-202, 1992.

Lavoie F. Consent, involuntary treatment, and the use of force in an urban emergency department, *Ann Emerg Med* 21:25-32, 1992.

Lipowski ZJ. Delirium in the elderly patient, *N Engl J Med* 320:578-82, 1989.

Schweizer E et al. Double-blind, placebo-controlled study of a once-a-day, sustained-release preparation of alprazolam for the treatment of panic disorder, *Am J Psychiatry* 150:1210-15, 1993.

Sheline Y, Beattie M. Effects of the right to refuse medication in an emergency psychiatric service, *Hosp Community Psychiatry* 43:640-42, 1992.

Silverstein S et al: Parenteral haloperidol in combative patients: a prospective study, *Ann Emerg Med* 15:636, 1986.

Tardiff K. The current state of psychiatry in the treatment of violent patients, *Arch Gen Psychiatry* 49:493-9, 1992.

Tesar GE et al: Use of high-dose intravenous haloperidol in the treatment of agitated cardiac patients, *J Clin Psychopharmacol* 5:344-7, 1985.

27 Drugs in Pregnancy

Matthew G. Fahey, M.D.

Risk to Fetus

Though few medications have been proven to be teratogenic, all medications are a potential risk to the fetus. Almost all drugs and environmental toxins pass through the placenta and thus expose the fetus. Since nearly all expectant mothers use some form of medication during pregnancy, it is important to know which medications (prescribed or otherwise) are considered safe and which are potentially harmful.

I. Birth defects. It is estimated that 1% to 4% of all birth defects are caused by drugs, chemicals, or radiation exposure. The types of drug effects on the fetus are teratogenic, direct toxicity, and neurobehavioral effects. The first trimester usually is the most dangerous for the fetus.

II. Timing of toxic exposures. Toxic exposures during the first 1 to 3 weeks of gestation can cause spontaneous abortions. Major organ damage tends to occur with exposure from 3 to 10 weeks, especially in the neurologic and vascular systems. Toxic exposure after 10 weeks is more likely to cause neuropsychiatric and growth retardation. Exposure to anticoagulants and psychotropic drugs near term can have direct adverse effects on the newborn infant.

III. Prescribing medications. General principles in prescribing medications to best limit adverse effects on the fetus are as follows:
  A. Use the best drug for a particular class of medications.
  B. Use the lowest dose for the shortest period possible to treat effectively.
  C. Avoid using drugs altogether if possible.

Table 27-1 lists medications commonly prescribed or taken over-the-counter; Food and Drug Administration (FDA) pregnancy categories are provided in parentheses.

Suggested Readings

Briggs et al: *Drugs in pregnancy and lactation,* Baltimore, 1983, Williams and Wilkins.
Drug facts and comparisons, 1993 edition. St. Louis, 1993, Facts and Comparisons.
Drug therapy in obstetrics and gynecology, 1987, Appleton Century Crofts, Prentice-Hall.
Med Lett Drugs Ther 29(743), 1987.

Table 27-1. Medications Commonly Prescribed or Taken Over-the-counter

Type of medication	Safe (A and B)	Potential risks (C)	Known risks (D)	Contraindicated (X)
Analgesics		All narcotics Codeine Hydrocodone Oxycodone Morphine Meperidine Fentanyl		
Antibiotics Aminoglycosides		Amikacin Gentamicin Neomycin	Kanamycin Streptomycin Tobramycin	
Antifungals	Amphotericin B Clotrimazcle Nystatin	Miconazole	Griseofulvin	
Antituberculosis	Ethambutol	Isoniazid Pyrazinamide Rifampin		
Antiviral		Acyclovir Amantadine Vidarabine		Ribavirin
Cephalosporins Erythromycins Fluoroquinones	All All except estolate		Erythromycin estolate Ciprofloxacin Norfloxacin	

Risk to Fetus

Penicillins		All	
Antimalarials			Chloroquine Primaquine Pyrimethamine Quinacrine	Quinine
Scabicide		Lindane Permethrin	
Sulfonamides				All
Tetracyclines				All
Others		Clindamycin Polymixin B Nitrofurantoin Metronidazole	Bacitracin Chloramphenicol Trimethoprim Vancomycin	Ofloxacin Lomefloxacin

Anticoagulants/coagulants

			Heparin Protamine	Coumarin Warfarin
Antidiarrheals		Loperamide	Diphenoxylate	
Antiemetics		Cyclizine Meclizine Metoclopramide Dimenhydrinate	Droperidol Prochlorperazine Trimethobenzamide Ondansetron	
Antiflatulents			Simethicone	
Antihistamines (H_1 and H_2)		Cimetidine Ranitidine Meclizine Chlorpheniramine Diphenhydramine	Brompheniramine Clemastine Diphenhydramine Hydroxyzine Promethazine	

Table 27-1. Medications Commonly Prescribed or Taken Over-the-counter—cont'd

Type of medication	Safe (A and B)	Potential risks (C)	Known risks (D)	Contraindicated (X)
Antineoplastics			All	
Antitussive/expectorants			All iodine compounds	
Anticholinergics	Dicyclomine Glycopyrrolate	Guaifenesin Atropine Benztropine Homatropine Isopropamide Methixene Scopolamine		
Bronchodilators	Fenoterol Terbutaline	Albuterol Isoetharine Isoproterenol Metaproterenol Theophylline		
Cardiovascular				
Angiotensin converting enzyme inhibitors (ACEI)			Captopril Enalapril Lisinopril Ramapril	
β-Blockers	Acebutolol Metoprolol Pindolol	Atenolol Esmolol Labetolol Nadolol Propranolol Timolol		
Calcium channel blockers		Verapamil Nifedipine		

Risk to Fetus 665

Other antihypertensives	Clonidine	Diltiazem
Nimodipine
Reserpine
Diazoxide
Hydralazine
Sodium nitroprusside
Trimethaphan
Methyldopa
Cholestyramine
Dextrothyroxine
Antilipemics		Amiodarone
Amrinone
Bretylium
Digoxin compounds
Procainamide
Lidocaine
Quinidine
Adenosine
Antiarrhythmics		
Central Nervous System		
Analgesics	Acetaminophen	Aspirin
(low dose, 1st and 2nd trimester only)
Propoxyphene
Antipyretics	Phenacetin	
Anticonvulsants	Magnesium sulfate
Metharbital	Carbamazepine
Clonazepam
Ethosuximide
Mephenytoin
Methsuximide
Aminoglutethimide
Paramethadione
Phenobarbital
Phenytoin
Primidone
Trimethadione

Continued on next page

Table 27-1. Medications Commonly Prescribed or Taken Over-the-counter—cont'd

Type of medication	Safe (A and B)	Potential risks (C)	Known risks (D)	Contraindicated (X)
Anticonvulsants—cont'd			Valproic acid	
Antidepressants	Maprotiline	Desipramine	Amitriptyline	
		Doxepin	Imipramine	
			Nortriptyline	
Cholinergics		Neostigmine		
		Physostigmine		
Diuretics	Amilor de	Furosemide	Spironolactone	
	Triamterene	Hydrochlorothiazide		
	Ethacrynic acid	Mannitol		
	Metalazone			
	Indapamide			
Hormones				
Adrenal	Prednisolone	Beclomethasone	Cortisone	
	Prednisone	Betamethasone		
		Dexamethasone		
Antidiabetic	Insulin		All oral hypoglycemics	
Antithyroid			I^{131}	
Estrogens			All	
Pituitary	Desmopressin	Corticotropin		
	Somatostatin	Lypressin		
	Vasopressin			
Progestogens			All	
Thyroid	Levothyroxine (T_4)	Thyrotropin	Propylthiouracil	
	Liothyronine (T_3)		Methimazole	
Other	Calcitonin			
Narcotic antagonists	Naloxone			

Nonsteroidal antiinflammatory drugs (1st and 2nd trimester only) (NSAIDs)	Ibuprophen Indomethacin Ketoprophen Naproxen	Tolmetin Ketorolac	Oxyphenbutazone Phenylbutazone
Sedative/hypnotics		Chloral hydrate	Chlordiazepoxide Diazepam Ethanol Lorazepam Meprobamate Oxazepam Phenobarbital Yellow fever
Serums, toxoids, vaccines	Immune globulins Tetanus Rabies Hepatitis	Diphtheria/tetanus BCG Cholera Hepatitis B Influenza Meningococcus Pneumococcal Polio inactivated Polio live Rabies Tularemia Typhoid	Measles Mumps Rubella Smallpox
Skeletal muscle relaxants	Cyclobenzaprine	Chlorzoxazone Decamethonium	
Spermicides		All	
Stimulants		Phentermine	

Table 27-1. Medications Commonly Prescribed or Taken Over-the-counter—cont'd

Type of medication	Safe (A and B)	Potential risks (C)	Known risks (D)	Contraindicated (X)
Sympathomimetics		Dobutamine Dopamine Epinephrine Ephedrine Phenylpropanolamine Pseudoephedrine	Levarterenol Metaraminol	
Tranquilizers		Butaperazine Chlorpromazine Chlorprothixene Droperidol Fluphenazine Haloperidol Hydroxyzine Loxapine Perphenazine Piperacetazine Prochlorperazine Thioridazine Thiothixene Trifluoperazine All neuroleptics	Lithium	
Thrombolytics	Urokinase	Streptokinase t-PA		
Vitamins		Folic acid Thiamine		Etretinate Isotretinoin

28

Drugs in Lactation

Judith R. Logan, M.D., F.A.C.E.P.

This list of drugs in breast milk is of necessity limited by a lack of primary literature on the topic. Many recommendations are made based on single case reports, and many on data on drug excretion into milk without study of the effects in infants. Many other recommendations are based on theoretical considerations alone, and for some drugs only the data can be reported without specific recommendations to the practicing physician. In addition, different reviewers may make different recommendations on the same agents. Avoidance of drugs may be required for one of two reasons: either the drug has a detrimental effect on lactation, primarily through a decrease in maternal prolactin levels; or there are adverse effects in the infant. A classification system such as with drugs in pregnancy (A, B, C, D, X) might be useful, but none is in wide use. Fortunately for the emergency physician, there are few agents where caution has been advised that cannot be used with monitoring or for which a substitution cannot be found. For example, oral contraceptives are commonly used after establishment of the milk supply, especially the progestin-only pills. Antiepileptic levels can be monitored in infants. Irritability from theophylline can be monitored by the mother, with a decreased likelihood of side effects with dosing recommendations below. A dosing alternative that should be acceptable to most nursing mothers is available for metronidazole. Short-term use of many drugs is probably acceptable, such as corticosteroids, the psychotropic agents, and most analgesics.

What's missing: good data for phenazopyridine (Pyridium), antianginal agents, antispasmodics other than atropine and belladonna, and most muscle relaxants; antinausea agents, antacids, and antifungal agents, including the topical or vaginal preparations; and a number of agents within many classes such as oral hypoglycemic agents. While it is tempting to use drugs on theoretical grounds and because no adverse effects have been reported, the physician must be cautious about use of drugs for which no toxicity data exist, and as always, to weigh the risks and benefits.

Analgesics

I. **Preferred**
   A. Acetaminophen
   B. Ibuprofen (Motrin), flubiprofen (Ansaid)
II. **Safe**
   A. **Codeine, oxycodone, propoxyphene (Darvon), meperidine (Demerol), morphine, butorphanol (Stadol).** In limited doses, all narcotics appear safe, although it might be prudent to minimize use in neonatal period, especially if infant has had episode of bradycardia, apnea, or cyanosis; meperidine may cause more depression in the infant than morphine.
   B. **Tolmetin (Tolectin), piroxicam (Feldene), naproxen (Naprosyn, Anaprox), fenoprofen (Nalfon), ketorolac (Toradol) PO.** Amounts of

most NSAIDs in milk is low. Shorter-acting agents are preferred, especially in the newborn period.

III. Caution
  A. **Aspirin (salicylates).** Case report of metabolic acidosis (dose related); potential antiplatelet effect; rash; risk of Reye's syndrome due to salicylates in milk is unknown but must be a concern.
  B. **Methadone.** Signs of opiate withdrawal if rapidly withdrawn; probably compatible with breast-feeding if maternal dosage 20 mg/day or less.
  C. **Indomethacin (Indocin), phenylbutazone (Azolid, Butazolidin), mefenamic acid (Ponstel).** These inherently more toxic NSAIDs should be avoided if possible although all are felt to be compatible with breast-feeding by the American Academy of Pediatrics (AAP).
  D. **Ketorolac (Toradol) IM or IV.** Has not been studied.

Antibiotics, Antiinfective Agents

All antibiotics transfer into breast milk in limited amounts; any antibiotic has the potential for disruption of the GI flora (diarrhea, thrush), for allergic sensitization (rash), and can interfere with culture results if a fever work-up becomes necessary.

I. Safe
  A. **Aminoglycosides.** Systemic effects unlikely because of small amounts in milk and poor oral absorption by the infant; eliminated more slowly by neonates than older infants.
  B. **Antihelmintic: mebendazole (Vermox).** Case report of inhibition of lactation, questionably related to drug; unlikely to cause adverse effects.
  C. Antimalarials
   1. **Hydroxychloroquine (Plaquenil).** Concentrated in human milk; caution during daily therapy; weekly doses probably safe.
   2. **Chloroquine (Aralen).** Extensive use with no adverse effects.
   3. **Quinine.** Allergic reactions may occasionally occur.
   4. **Pyrimethamine.** Extensive use without adverse effects.
  D. **Aztreonam (Azactam).** Active against normal GI flora, so watch for disruption of normal flora (thrush, diarrhea).
  E. **Cephalosporins.** All appear in milk in low amounts; watch for disruption of the GI flora (thrush, diarrhea) especially with third-generation agents (ceftriaxone), which are more active against normal GI flora.
  F. **Erythromycin.** Concentrated in human milk but probably safe anyway; no information on other macrolides (azithromycin, clarithromycin).
  G. Penicillins
   1. **Sulbactam (with amoxicillin: Unasyn)**
  H. **Tetracyclines.** Minimal GI absorption by the infant occurs; because of theoretical risk of effect on bone growth and teeth discoloration, limit maternal therapy to 10 days for this and related antibiotics.
  I. Urinary germicides
   1. **Methenamine hippurate (Hiprex, Urex)**
   2. **Methenamine mandelate (Mandelamine, UroqidAcid)**
   3. **Nitrofurantoin (Macrodantin, Macrobid).** Case report of hemolysis in infant with glucose-6-phosphate dehydrogenase (G6PD) deficiency.

4. **Nalidixic acid (NegGram).** Case report of hemolytic anemia; hemolysis may occur with G6PD-deficient infants.
  J. **Vancomycin.** Little data; since drug poorly absorbed orally, its use in nursing is probably safe.
II. **Caution**
  A. **Acyclovir.** Concentrated in human milk; topical application to small areas should pose no risk but uncertain risk with oral or IV therapy, although it is used to treat neonates and therefore should be safe.
  B. **Antituberculous agents: cycloserine (Seromycin), rifampin (Rifadin, others), ethambutol (Myambutol), streptomycin, isoniazid (INH).** Caution advised because many of these drugs can cause hepatotoxicity, although risk to infant may be greater if the mother is not treated adequately than the risk from the drug exposure; minimize exposure by a single bedtime dose, with bottle feeding during the night.
  C. **Metronidazole (Flagyl).** Theoretical risk of carcinogenicity, infant plasma concentrations relatively high; for trichomoniasis, use single 2 gm dose, restrict breast-feeding for 12-24 hours.
  D. **Dapsone (DDC, a sulfone).** May produce hemolytic anemia; newborns and G6PD-deficient infants especially susceptible; felt to be usually compatible with breast-feeding by the AAP.
  E. **Sulfonamides.** Use with caution in infants with G6PD deficiency or jaundice, or who are ill, stressed, or premature; can be used safely by nursing mothers of older, healthy, term infants.
  F. **Dapsone (DDC, a sulfone).** May produce hemolytic anemia; newborns and G6PD-deficient infants especially susceptible; felt to be usually compatible with breast-feeding by the AAP.
  G. **Lindane (Kwell).** Excreted in milk with persistent elevation of levels; alternative drugs such as permethrin (Nix) and pyrethrins (multiple, in combinations) are preferred.
III. **Avoid**
  A. **Fluoroquinolones: ciprofloxacin (Cipro), norfloxacin (Noroxin), ofloxacin (Floxin).** Slightly concentrated in milk; avoid until more safety data obtained.
  B. **Chloramphenicol.** Safety unknown, possible risk of idiosyncratic bone marrow suppression, although doses not sufficient to induce "gray baby" syndrome; case report of refusal to feed, intestinal gas, heavy vomiting.
  C. **Clindamycin.** Not certain of effect on infants' GI flora (e.g., induction of pseudomembranous colitis); one case of bloody stools in an infant with normal stool flora reported, infant also on gentamicin; best avoided if possible.
  D. **Iodine (povidone-iodine vaginal douche).** Case report: elevated iodine levels in breast milk, odor of iodine on infant's skin; theoretical risk of effect on thyroid function.

Anticoagulants

I. **Preferred**
  A. Heparin
  B. Warfarin (Coumadin)
II. **Avoid: anisindione (Miradon).** A related inandione, phenindione, is contraindicated.

Antiepileptics

I. **Caution.** Generally all agents can be used, and if needed, drug levels in the infant can be monitored; withdrawal symptoms after abrupt weaning have been reported, and breast-feeding can prevent withdrawal symptoms in infants whose mothers took anticonvulsants during pregnancy; mild drowsiness is common, especially in the neonatal period. Long-term effects have not been studied well and are of concern.
   - A. **Carbamazepine (Tegretol).** Case report probable idiosyncratic reaction (cholestatic hepatitis).
   - B. **Clonazepam (Klonopin).** Limited studies, monitor for CNS depression, apnea.
   - C. **Ethosuximide (Zarontin).** Infants may attain significant plasma levels; drowsiness, fussiness reported; keep maternal levels in low therapeutic range or use an alternative.
   - D. **Phenobarbital.** Case report: methemoglobinemia, drowsiness leading to feeding difficulties; monitor infant behavior, weight gain, and drug plasma concentration.
   - E. **Phenytoin (Dilantin).** Case report: drowsiness, decreased sucking activity, and methemoglobinemia (when ingested with phenobarbital).
   - F. **Primidone (Mysoline).** Case reports of sedation, feeding problems; use in low to moderate doses, and monitor infant behavior, weight gain, and drug plasma concentrations.
   - G. **Valproic acid (Depakene, Depakote).** Observe for rare idiosyncratic effects such as hepatotoxicity.

Antihypertensives and Cardiovascular Drugs

I. **Cardiac glycosides: digoxin (lanoxin).** Safe: Infants receive trivial doses.
II. **Antiarrhythmic agents**
   - A. Safe
     1. **Quinidine**
     2. **Lidocaine (Xylocaine)**
     3. **Mexiletine (Mexitil)**
     4. **Flecainide (Tambocor)**
   - B. Caution
     1. **Disopyramide (Norpace).** Infants may attain levels below but near therapeutic levels; watch for anticholinergic effects; felt to be usually compatible with breast-feeding by the AAP.
     2. **Procainamide (Pronestyl, Procan).** More concentrated in milk than in plasma, but absolute amount small; felt to be usually compatible with breast-feeding by the AAP.
     3. **Tocainide (Tonocard).** Possibly concentrated in breast milk.
   - C. Avoid: **amiodarone (Cordarone).** Infant can get significant dose, although no adverse effects reported; long elimination half-life with long-term therapy and high levels of iodine; breast-feeding not recommended if the mother is currently taking the drug or has taken it chronically within the past several months.
III. **Calcium channel blockers**
   - A. Preferred: **verapamil (Calan, Isoptin)**

 B. Safe
  1. Diltiazem (Cardizem)
  2. Nifedipine (Procardia)
IV. Beta-adrenergic blockers. With all agents, observe infants for signs of β-blockade including hypotension and bradycardia.
 A. Preferred, especially in the neonatal period
  1. Labetolol (Normodyne, Trandate)
  2. Metoprolol (Lopressor)
  3. Propranolol (Inderal)
 B. Safe in older infants and low doses
  1. Acebutolol (Sectral)
  2. Atenolol (Tenormin)
  3. Betaxolol (Kerlone)
  4. Nadolol (Corgard)
  5. Sotalol (Betapace)
  6. Timolol (Blocadren)
V. Antihypertensive agents
 A. Safe
  1. Methyldopa (Aldomet and others)
  2. Hydralazine (Apresoline)
  3. Minoxidil (Loniten)
 B. Caution
  1. **Reserpine.** May cause nasal stuffiness and increased tracheobronchial secretions.
  2. **Clonidine (Catapres).** Milk levels high, may decrease maternal prolactin secretion.
  3. **Guanfacine (Tenex).** May decrease maternal prolactin secretion.
VI. ACE inhibitors
 A. Safe
  1. Captopril (Capoten)
  2. Enalapril (Vasotec)

Antineoplastic Agents

All agents are CONTRAINDICATED because of the theoretical risk of immune suppression and unknown effect on growth or association with carcinogenesis.

Bronchodilators

I. Preferred: β₂ agonists, inhaled. Not studied, but should transfer less drug to the infant.
II. Safe
 A. Epinephrine (Adrenaline). Degraded in the infant gut.
 B. Terbutyline (Brethine, Bricanyl)
III. Caution
 A. Diphylline (Dilor and others). Concentrated in breast milk.
 B. Theophylline (many). Irritability, fretful sleep reported; newborns most likely to be affected; theobromines and caffeine should not be taken with theophylline to avoid a cumulative effect; keep maternal plasma levels in lower part of therapeutic range, may check infant plasma concentrations.

Cold Preparations

I. **Preferred: nasal decongestant sprays**
II. **Safe: antihistamines and/or decongestants (many combinations).**
    Lactation inhibition seems to occur occasionally with oral decongestants.
III. **Caution**
    A. Clemastine (Tavist). Case report of drowsiness, irritability, refusal to feed, high-pitched cry, neck stiffness.
    B. Expectorants: KI, SSKI. Iodine is concentrated in breast milk, inorganic salts especially have potential for thyroid suppression and rashes; felt to be usually compatible with breast-feeding by the AAP.

Diuretic Agents

I. **Safe**
    A. Chlorothiazide (Diuril, others), hydrochlorothiazide (Esidrix, Hydrodiuril, others). Lactation suppression reported from thiazide diuretics, especially long-acting agents; may be considered safe in usual doses.
    B. Furosemide (Lasix)
    C. Spironolactone (Aldactone)
II. **Caution**
    A. Bendroflumethiazide (Naturetin). Reports of suppression of lactation.
    B. Chlorthalidone (Hygroton, others). Excreted slowly.

Endocrine Drugs

I. **Estrogenic hormones**
    A. High doses. In high doses, estrogens are used to suppress postpartum breast engorgement; in lower doses, problems are unlikely except for questionable decrease in milk production, and nitrogen and protein content as noted with oral contraceptives.
    B. Safe in low doses
        1. **Estrogens, conjugated (Premarin)**
        2. **Mestranol**
        3. **Ethinyl estradiol (Estinyl, Feminone)**
        4. **Dienestrol (as vaginal preparation)**
        5. **Estradiol (Estrace, Estraderm, and others, IM)**
II. **Progestogenic hormones: safe in low doses**
    A. Medroxyprogesterone (Provera and others)
    B. Progesterone
    C. Norethynodrel (from 19-nortestosterone, with mestranol in Enovid, also in OCs)
    D. Norethindrone (from 19-nortestosterone, Norlutin, Norlutate, Aygestin, also in OCs)
III. **Oral contraceptives (OCs)**
    A. Preferred
        1. **Progestin-only pills**
        2. **Levonorgestrel implants**

B. Safe: combination pills. Rare reports of breast enlargement and proliferation of vaginal epithelium reported; questionable decrease in milk production and protein and nitrogen content may occur; this may be of nutritional import with malnourished mothers.

IV. Antidiabetic agents
A. Preferred: insulin. Does not cross into breast milk due to its high molecular weight.

B. Safe: tolbutamide (Orinase). Potential for jaundice, hypoglycemia, although excreted in small amounts that should produce no harm; no information available on other oral sulfonylurea agents.

V. Corticosteroids.
Potential risk with high doses of growth and adrenal suppression.

A. Preferred: prednisolone. Excretion in milk minimal with daily doses <20 mg or with single large doses.

B. Safe
1. **Prednisone.** Excretion in milk minimal with daily doses <20 mg or with single large doses.
2. **Methylprednisolone (Medrol)**
3. **Depot injections, inhaled beclomethosone, topical corticosteroids.** Little data but should present little to no risk; case report of infant with symptoms of corticosteroid excess in mother who used topical steroids on her nipples.

VI. Thyroid preparations: safe
A. Levothyroxine (T_4, Synthroid). Levels are too low to effect neonatal screening tests but may offer a little protection against neonatal hypothyroidism.

B. Liothyronine (T_3, Cytomel). Replacement therapy may pass larger amounts to infant than with 1-thyroxine.

VII. Antithyroid agents
A. Safe: propylthiouracil (PTU). Measure infant hormones periodically.

B. Caution: methimazole (Tapazole). Potential for decreased thyroid function; passes more freely into milk more than PTU; may be used in low doses ≤10 mg/day.

Gastrointestinal Drugs

I. Anticholinergic antispasmodics
A. Caution: atropine and other belladonna alkaloids. Conflicting reports: infants may be sensitive to anticholinergic effects (drying of secretions, temperature elevation, CNS disturbances); may suppress lactation; felt to be usually compatible with breast-feeding by the AAP.

II. Antidiarrheal agents
A. Preferred: kaolin, attapulgite, and pectin (in many combinations). Not known to be absorbed from the GI tract.

B. Safe: preparations containing opium powder (paregoric). See morphine.

C. Caution
1. **Diphenoxylate (with atropine: Lomotil).** Use caution because of the atropine; a few small doses probably acceptable.

2. **Loperamide (Imodium).** Less central action that diphenoxylate, but excretion into milk has not been studied.
   D. **Avoid: bismuth subsalicylate (Pepto-Bismol).** Should probably be avoided because of systemic salicylate absorption.
III. **Mesalamine derivatives: caution**
   A. **Sulfasalazine (Azulfidine).** Case report: bloody diarrhea in one infant; sulfapyridine has risk of jaundice; use with caution at high doses, avoid in first month of life.
   B. **Mesalamine (Asacol, Rowasa).** Case report of diarrhea.
   C. **Olsalazine (Dipentum).** Recent report found low level of metabolite in milk; no effects noted in the infant after 3 weeks of therapy; more study needed.
IV. **Antiulcer agents**
   A. Safe: sucralfate (Carafate). Should be safe because virtually nonabsorbable.
   B. Caution
      1. **Cimetidine (Tagamet).** Concentrated in human milk with potential for suppression of gastric acidity, inhibition of drug metabolism, and CNS stimulation; felt to be usually compatible with breast-feeding by the AAP, although other authors suggest it be avoided.
      2. **Ranitidine (Zantac).** Concentrated in milk but to lesser extent than cimetidine; no data available on effect in infants.
      3. **Famotidine (Pepcid), nizatidine (Axid).** Less concentrated, so may be preferable, although no data available.
V. **Laxative agents**
   A. Preferred
      1. **Methylcellulose (Citrucel, others), psyllium (Metamucil, Konsyl, others), polycarbophil (FiberCon, others)**
      2. **Docusate sodium (DSS, Colace, and others)**
   B. Safe
      1. **Milk of magnesia (magnesium hydroxide), magnesium sulfate (Epsom salts), magnesium citrate.** Absorption of Mg occurs but effects unknown; if in significant quantities, might be associated with diarrhea, drowsiness, reduced muscle tone, and respiratory difficulties in the neonate.
      2. **Sodium phosphate/biphosphate (Fleet Phospho-soda)**
      3. **Mineral oil.** Little if any absorbed; theoretically would not appear in breast milk.
      4. **Bisacodyl (Dulcolax, others).** Virtually unabsorbed, so should be safe; not listed by AAP.
   C. Caution
      1. **Cascara.** Increased bowel activity in infants reported; felt to be usually compatible with breast-feeding by the AAP; other authors disagree.
      2. **Senna (Senokot, others).** Risk of inducing diarrhea in the infant present but probably low at normal doses.
      3. **Phenolphthalein (Ex-Lax, Feen-a-Mint, others).** 40% incidence of increased bowel activity reported, although little found in breast milk.
VI. **Motility agents**
   A. **Caution: metoclopramide (Reglan).** Concentrated in human milk; no case reports of effects on infants but potent central nervous system drug; augments milk production.

Psychotropic Drugs

Little data on effects of long-term use; the benefits to the mother and to the maternal-infant bond may outweigh the risks.

I. **Caution**
   A. Antidepressants (tricyclics and related)
      1. **Amitriptyline (Elavil, Endep)**
      2. **Amoxapine (Asendin)**
      3. **Desipramine (Norpramin)**
      4. **Doxepin (Sinequan, Adapin).** Case report: respiratory depression.
      5. **Imipramine (Tofranil).** Found in high concentrations in milk.
      6. **Trazadone (Desyrel)**
      7. **Nortriptyline (Aventyl, Pamelor)**
      8. **Maprotiline (Ludiomil).** Appears in milk; effect on infants not studied.
   B. Antipsychotics. Reports of drowsiness with some agents; extrapyramidal reactions possible but not reported.
      1. **Chlorpromazine (Thorazine).** Drowsiness and lethargy reported.
      2. **Chlorprothixene (Taractan)**
      3. **Haloperidol (Haldol)**
      4. **Mesoridazan (Serentil)**

II. **Avoid**
   A. **Lithium.** One-half to one-third therapeutic blood concentration attained in infants.
   B. **Phenelzine (Nardil).** Contraindicated because of potential toxicity; may suppress lactation.

Sedatives and Hypnotics

Caution should be used with all benzodiazepines because of concern about effects of long-term exposure on the infant's neurobehavioral development.

I. **Preferred.** Short-acting agents of any class preferred.
   A. Oxazepam (Serax)
   B. Lorazepam (Ativan)
   C. Secobarbital (Seconal)
   D. Pentobarbital (Nembutal)

II. **Safe**
   A. Prazepam (Centrax)
   B. Quazepam (Doral)
   C. Alprazolam (Xanax). Infant withdrawal symptoms noted after abrupt weaning or cessation of long-term therapy.
   D. Midazolam (Versed). IV use not studied.
   E. Butabarbital (Butisol)
   F. Methyprylon (Noludar). Case report of drowsiness.

III. **Caution**
   A. **Chloral hydrate.** Case report of sleepiness; appears in milk in significant amounts; felt to be usually compatible with breast-feeding by the AAP.
   B. **Diazepam (Valium).** Can accumulate in infants, especially neonates because of decreased metabolism, and has caused adverse effects (sedation); withhold feeding 6-8 hours when used for procedures.

C. Phenobarbital. Long-acting; case report of sedation in infant with hypnotic doses.

Vaccines

Breast-feeding not a contraindication to use of any vaccine.
 I. **Polio.** Concern over prevention of active immunization in infants because of maternal antibodies; by recommended immunization age of 6 weeks, breast-feeding does not appear to have an effect; for earlier immunization, withhold breast-feeding for 6 hours before and after administration of the vaccine.
 II. **Rubella.** Vaccine transferred to milk and produces an immune response in half of cases; appears to be of little consequence; recommended in postpartum period.

Vitamins

Maternal supplementation to RDA amounts recommended for those patients with inadequate nutritional intake.
 I. **Vitamin A.** Not known if high maternal doses present a danger.
 II. **B-vitamins, C, K.** Safe even in high doses.
 III. **Vitamin D.** Follow infant's serum Ca^{+2} levels if mother receives it in pharmacologic doses.
 IV. **Vitamin E.** Case report: when applied to nipples, infant serum levels rose; long-term effects on infants not known; maternal supplementation recommended only if the diet does not provide RDA levels.

Miscellaneous

 I. **Acetazolamide (Diamox).** Safe: appears in milk in very small amounts, may accumulate if exposure prolonged.
 II. **Colchicine.** Avoid: no studies in humans but decreases milk production and alters composition in animals.
 III. **Magnesium sulfate.** Safe: potential for infant drowsiness and difficulty establishing milk supply and nursing when given IV for preeclampsia or eclampsia.
 IV. **Anesthetics.** Anesthetic agents felt to be safe, especially if nursing stopped for 12-24 hours postoperatively.
   A. Halothane
   B. Thiopental (Pentothal)
 V. **Amantidine (Symmetrel).** Probably safe: poorly documented risk of adverse effects (urinary retention, vomiting, skin rash).
 VI. **Diagnostic agents**
   A. Fluorescein (topical). Safe: case report of phototoxic effects in newborn undergoing phototherapy.
   B. Iodinated compounds (contrast materials)
     1. **Safe: Diatrizoate (Hypaque), gadopentetate (Magnevist), iodamide (Renovue), iohexol (Omnipaque), iopanoic acid (Telepaque), metrizoate, metrimazide (Amipaque).** A number of ionic and nonionic agents are found in breast milk after IV administration; no adverse effects reported; concern over suppression of thyroid functions; except for ethiodized oil probably safe to use but may wish to withhold breast-feeding 24-36 hours.

2. **Avoid: ethiodized oil (Ethiodol)**. Large amounts of iodine are excreted for weeks after lymphangiography; discontinue nursing after this procedure.

VII. **Retinoids**
   A. **Caution: tretinoin (Retin-A)**. Minimal absorption from topical administration, but avoid contact of the infant's skin with treated areas.
   B. **Avoid**
      1. **Etretinate (Tegison)**. Metabolized to acetretin, which passes into breast milk in significant quantities; effects in infants uncertain but contraindicated in pregnancy due to teratogenicity.
      2. **Isotretinoin (Accutane)**. Potential for adverse effects (teratogenicity, premature closure of epiphyses, tumorigenicity).

VIII. **Ergot alkaloids**
   A. **Ergotamine (Ergostat and others, DHE45, combination drugs including Cafergot, Wigraine, Midrin)**. Avoid: case reports of ergotism; vomiting, diarrhea, and convulsions with crude ergot extracts; excessive dosing or prolonged use may inhibit lactation.
   B. Oxytocics
      1. **Ergonovine (Ergotrate)**. Caution: can lower maternal prolactin levels.
      2. **Methylergonovine (Methergine)**. Safe: does not lower maternal prolactin levels; preferred over ergonovine.
   C. **Bromocriptine (Parlodel)**. Avoid: suppresses lactation.

IX. **Local anesthetics: safe**
   A. **Lidocaine (Xylocaine)**
   B. **Bupivicaine (Marcaine)**. Not detected in milk when administered by intrapleural or epidural route.

X. **Parasympathomimetic/cholinergic agents**
   A. Safe
      1. **Neostigmine (Prostigmin)**. Not found in milk although cannot be totally excluded because of the analytical technique; no adverse effects reported.
      2. **Pyridostigmine (Mestinon)**. Has been used safely in patients with myasthenia gravis.
   B. **Caution: bethanechol (Urecholine)**. Case report: abdominal pain, diarrhea.

XI. **Muscle relaxants: safe**
   A. Baclofen (Lioresal)
   B. Methocarbamol (Robaxin and others)

XII. **Radiopharmaceutical agents**. Temporary cessation of breast-feeding required.

Nonmedical Drugs

I. **Drugs of abuse**. All drugs of abuse should be CONTRAINDICATED based on their hazard to the nursing infant, as well as their potential detrimental effects on the physical and emotional health of the mother.
   A. **Amphetamines**. Case reports of irritability, poor sleep patterns; inhibits prolactin release.
   B. **Cocaine**. Case report of cocaine intoxication (vomiting, diarrhea, irritability, dilated pupils).
   C. Heroin
   D. Marijuana

E. Phencyclidine. Potent hallucinogen; concentrated in milk and remains detectable for weeks after heavy use.
II. **Nicotine (smoking).** AVOID: reports of shock, vomiting, diarrhea, rapid heart rate, restlessness; prolactin levels are decreased; smokers wean their infants earlier; increase in infantile colic reported; risk of increased respiratory irritation and infection from secondary smoke.
III. **Caffeine.** Safe in usual doses; reports of irritability, poor sleep pattern; excreted slowly especially in newborns; no effect with usual amount of caffeine beverages; watch for cumulative effects; may be ingesting caffeine from many sources such as soft drinks, teas, chocolate, and coffee.
IV. **Alcohol.** Caution: reports of drowsiness, diaphoresis, deep sleep, weakness, decrease in linear growth, abnormal weight gain; pseudo-Cushings syndrome; rapidly equilibrates between blood and milk; maternal ingestion of 1 gm/day may decrease the milk ejection reflex; a recent report indicates that chronic exposure may have an adverse effect on psychomotor development; use in moderation is acceptable; heavy use is contraindicated.

How to Minimize Drug Transfer to the Infant

I. **Whenever possible, nursing mothers should avoid drugs.** Breast milk is the ideal food for infants. Rather than interrupting breast-feeding for drug treatment, the question should be whether the nursing mother can do without drug treatment.
II. **Temporary cessation of breast-feeding** has been recommended on occasion; for example, with single-dose metronidazole therapy and with radiopharmaceutical agents. Caution should be exercised in recommending temporary cessation of breast-feeding, however, because manual or machine pumping can be difficult and uncomfortable for the inexperienced mother, the equipment can be expensive to buy or rent, and this may lead to decreased milk production and discouragement on the mother's part. Temporary cessation for more than a few hours may jeopardize continued breast-feeding. In addition, exclusively breast-fed babies often reject bottle-feeding.
III. **Keep the maternal plasma drug level to a minimum** to minimize the infant's exposure. First, use the lowest dose of drug necessary to treat the maternal condition. Second, use a drug or route of administration that will lead to a lower risk of maternal systemic drug exposure. For example, use an inhaled bronchodilator or steroid rather than an oral agent for treatment of asthma; a nasal decongestant spray rather than an oral decongestant agent; and a poorly absorbed bulk-forming laxative agent instead of a stimulant cathartic agent.
IV. **Schedule drug dosing** to minimize the amount passed on to the infant. Transportation of most drugs into milk is generally rapid, such that the half-lives in milk and plasma are the same. Plasma and milk concentrations are lowest just before taking a medication, at least with drugs with a short half-life relative to dosing; recommending breast-feeding at this time can help minimize drug exposure to the infant. In addition, drugs may be given just before the infant's longest sleep periods. Bedtime dosing is especially useful with drugs that can be given once daily; if further caution is warranted, the infant can be given a bottle during the night.
V. **Educate the mother** to observe for untoward signs in the infant.

Suggested Readings

Anderson PO: Drug use during breast-feeding, *Clin Pharm* 10:594-624, 1991.

Bennett PN, editor, and the WHO Working Group: *Drugs and human lactation: a guide to the content and consequences of drugs, micronutrients, radiopharmaceuticals, and environmental and occupational chemicals in human milk,* 1988.

Briggs GG, Freeman RK, Yaffe SJ, editors: *Drugs in pregnancy and lactation: a reference guide to fetal and neonatal risk,* ed 3, 1990.

Committee on Drugs, American Academy of Pediatrics: Transfer of drugs and other chemicals into human milk, *Pediatrics* 84(5):924-36, 1989.

29 Thermoregulatory Disorders

Louis J. Perretta, M.D., F.A.C.E.P.

Pathophysiology of Hypothermia

Hypothermia is defined as a core temperature less than 35° C. A number of disorders can predispose an individual to hypothermia by decreasing heat production, increasing heat loss, or interfering with the central or peripheral control of thermoregulation. Environmental exposure to cold, probably the most common cause of hypothermia, lowers core temperature by increasing heat loss.

I. **Body temperature** is closely regulated through a balance between heat production and heat dissipation. Metabolic activity in the heart and liver is responsible for the majority of endogenous heat production. Heat is subsequently dissipated at the body surface, with the skin accounting for 90% of heat loss and the lung contributing the rest. The thermal load is dissipated primarily through radiation cooling (70%) with a smaller amount given off by the evaporation of insensible perspiration. The preoptic nucleus of the anterior hypothalamus is the thermal control center, maintaining body temperature at a given set value.

II. **Elevation.** When the core body temperature is elevated, the hypothalamus stimulates the autonomic nervous system to produce sweating and cutaneous vasodilation, both of which decrease core body temperature. Conversely, when core body temperature or skin temperature decreases, the hypothalamus conserves heat by producing cutaneous vasoconstriction. In addition, the hypothalamus can increase heat production by stimulating muscular activity in the form of shivering. The appreciation of cold at a conscious level induces the individual to exercise, wear more clothing, and move to a warmer environment. Exposure to heat influences the decision to remove clothing and move to a cooler environment. In addition, nonthermal stimuli, such as the consumption of alcohol or drugs, produce vasomotor changes that affect temperature regulation.

Medical Causes

Medical conditions associated with heat loss include dermal disorders, such as psoriasis and exfoliative dermatitis, which cause excessive heat loss through two possible mechanisms: increased peripheral blood flow and transepidermal water loss with evaporation. Paget's disease and malnutrition with lack of subcutaneous fat are also associated with increased heat loss and hypothermia.

I. **Central nervous system (CNS) disease** can produce or contribute to hypothermia in the elderly by impairing central thermoregulation. Stroke, subarachnoid hemorrhage, subdural hematoma, tumor, head trauma, and Wernicke's encephalopathy have all been associated with hypothermia. Low cardiac output, secondary to acute myocardial infarction, has been shown to cause thermoregulatory disturbances resulting in hypothermia. Hypothermia has also been reported with severe infections, bacteremia, and sepsis. These patients have a significantly higher mortality than those with hypothermia associated with other conditions. It has been shown that hypothermic patients with severe infection and bacteremia have an increased cardiac index and decreased systemic vascular resistance. Cardiac index is decreased, and systemic vascular resistance is increased in hypothermic patients without severe infection. Infection may also cause central thermoregulatory or hypothalamic dysfunction, leading to hypothermia.

II. **Hypothermia is a well-known complication of diabetic ketoacidosis and hypoglycemia.** Other systemic diseases that cause hypothermia via their effect on the hypothalamus include uremia, hepatic failure, and carbon monoxide poisoning.

III. **Hypothermia can be induced with drugs** (see the box below). Ethanol causes hypothermia by inducing vasodilation, reducing shivering, and depressing central thermoregulation. Hypothermia may be seen as a complication of acute Wernicke's encephalopathy, while phenothiazines and cyclic antidepressants such as imipramine act on the hypothalamus to inhibit shivering. Benzodiazepines, barbiturates, and reserpine may lead to hypothermia by impairing centrally mediated vasoconstrictor response to the cold. Other causes of hypothermia are shown in **Table 29-1**.

Presentation

Initial symptoms include diminished mental status, extremity stiffness, weakness, shivering, increased muscle tone, and hypertension. If core temperatures drop below 35° C, many patients no longer complain that they are cold. Consciousness becomes further impaired as the central temperature falls, eventually leading to coma. Other earlier and more subtle neurologic signs include slurred speech, ataxia, and extensor plantar responses. Unfortunately, most signs and symptoms of hypothermia are nonspecific, and the only reliable way to make the diagnosis is by measuring core body temperature. This is difficult because most standard thermometers measure temperature in the range of 35° C to 42° C (95° F to 104° F). More accurate measurement of core body temperature can be made by a rectal, rather than oral, temperature, taken with a low-reading thermometer capable of measuring temperatures from 25° C to 40° C.

I. **Other signs** of hypothermia include gastric dilatation, impaired hepatic function, decreased renal blood flow, and renal tubular dysfunction. The clinician may have difficulty distinguishing hypothermia from primary hypothyroidism. Obtaining TSH levels, which are raised in hypothyroid hypothermia and normal in primary hypothermia, will help distinguish between these two conditions. Hy-

---

Pharmacologic Agents Causing Hypothermia

Phenothiazines	Ethanol
Antidepressants	Reserpine
Benzodiazepines	Barbiturates

Table 29-1. Causes of Hypothermia*

	In-hospital (%) (n = 26)	Out-of-hospital (%) (n = 28)
Infection		
Urinary tract	38	32
Pneumonia	31	21
Skin infection	4	7
Peritonitis	8	0
Gastroenteritis	0	7
Cholecystitis	4	0
Unknown source	0	4
Cerebrovascular accident	8	11
Terminal heart failure	8	7
Myxedema coma	0	4
Barbiturate overdose	0	4
Intestinal obstruction	0	4

Reproduced with permission from Kramer MR et al: Arch Intern Med 149:1521, 1989. Copyright 1989, American Medical Association.
*None of the differences between in-hospital and out-of-hospital cases are significant.

pothermia will also tend to alter the oxygen dissociation curve so that less oxygen is given up to the tissues, thus leading to tissue anoxia.

II. **Dysrhythmias.** As temperature falls, cardiac dysrhythmias become common. These dysrhythmias include supraventricular tachycardias, atrial fibrillation, ventricular tachycardia, and ventricular fibrillation. In addition, heart block and asystole can occur, leading to cardiac arrest at temperatures below 32.2° C. Ventricular fibrillation is the principal cause of death at core temperatures below 28° C. A characteristic Osborn, or J, wave, which is a positive deflection in the left ventricular leads at the junction of the QRS and ST segments, occurs in one fourth to one third of all hypothermic patients. The presence of a J wave is neither pathognomonic nor prognostic. As the body temperature reaches 30° C, patients become hypopneic and hypotensive.

Treatment

Two methods are commonly used to treat hypothermia: slow, spontaneous rewarming and rapid, active rewarming. The treatment regimen selected depends upon whether or not there is a life-threatening complication of hypothermia. If such a complication exists, rapid, active rewarming should be utilized. It should be noted that rewarming alone is adequate treatment for environmental causes of hypothermia. However, when hypothermia is caused by an associated medical disease, rewarming may be inadequate unless the underlying disease is aggressively treated as well.

I. **Slow, spontaneous rewarming.** Slow, spontaneous rewarming is done without the use of external heat and is best accomplished by wrapping the patients in warm blankets in order to gradually raise the core temperature at a rate of 1° F per hour (0.5° C). The ambient temperature should exceed 21° C, and the air should contain a high amount of humidity. If the temperature fails to rise more than 0.5° F per hour, other causes of hypothermia such as myxedema crisis, hypoglycemia, and gram-negative sepsis may be present. This rewarming technique presupposes that the patient is able to metabolically generate a sufficient amount of heat in order to spontaneously rewarm. When there is no shivering, metabolic heat production may be insufficient to raise core temperature. Shivering could be absent because of core temperatures below 30° C, associated medical conditions, drug ingestions, or uncorrected hypoglycemia.

II. **Rapid, active rewarming.** Rapid, active rewarming, which involves a transfer of exogenous heat to the patient, can be accomplished by internal or external methods. Active rewarming is mandatory when there is cardiac instability and decompensation since defibrillation is rarely successful at temperatures below 28° to 30° C. Active rewarming is also indicated for patients with impaired CNS control of thermoregulation or when endogenous thermogenesis is insufficient. Examples of diseases that cause insufficient thermogenesis are hypopituitarism, adrenal insufficiency, hypothyroidism, and cerebral infarction.

   A. **Active external rewarming** (AER) can be achieved by placing the patient in a warm bath or water. This method presents several problems: difficulty in monitoring patients, performing cardiopulmonary resuscitation (CPR), and forcing them to remain in a hemodynamically disadvantageous head-up position. Other methods of external rewarming include plumbed garments that circulate warm fluids, water bottles, heating pads, and blankets.

   B. **Elderly.** In the elderly, AER has been shown to be dangerous for a majority of patients, since the extensive vasodilatation that usually accompanies AER can result in hypotension and inadequate coronary perfusion. In addition, dilation of peripheral and core vessels can result in sudden cooling of the core as well as a sudden exposure of the core to lactic acid. This "after drop" can cause fatal arrhythmias. The reported mortality rate with AER is 60.3% as compared with a mortality rate of 44% when using slow, spontaneous rewarming in all age groups.

   C. **Active internal rewarming** (AIR) allows for active rewarming, while minimizing the possibility of rewarming collapse (after drop) in patients with core temperatures below 30° C. Techniques for AIR include mediastinal irrigation, peritoneal dialysis, hemodialysis, gastric irrigation, and extracorporeal blood warming. Rewarming through the airway with heated gases may prove to be a very effective means of core rewarming in the elderly. In fact, airway rewarming, by inducing selective warming of the endocardium via pulmonary venous blood, may reduce the risk of ventricular fibrillation.

   D. **Ventricular fibrillation.** Lastly, the association of ventricular fibrillation with orotracheal intubation in the hypothermic patient is worth mentioning. Although ventricular fibrillation has been described as a complication of intubation, there is no evidence showing this relationship in the setting of a normal arterial blood gas (ABG). It has been demonstrated that correction of hypoxia and acidosis prior to intubation will decrease the incidence of ventricular fibrillation in hypothermic individuals undergoing intubation.

Hyperthermia

Hyperthermia is a serious problem with a high mortality rate. Hyperthermia can also be a manifestation of systemic illness. The raised body temperature is usually caused by exposure to excessive heat, impaired thermoregulatory reflexes, or the effect of circulating pyrogens. Hyperthermia is defined as the presence of a temperature of at least 40.5° C for at least 1 hour. Heat stroke is characterized by hyperthermia, along with severe CNS disturbances such as delirium, seizures, or coma. Hyperthermia and heat stroke are usually thought to be problems encountered in younger individuals undergoing physical exertion in the warm weather; however, the elderly often acquire heat illnesses during heat waves without exercise.

Etiology

Heat illness or hyperthermia is a disease that encompasses a comprehensive spectrum from minor heat syndromes such as heat edema, heat cramps, and heat syncope to the most serious syndrome—heat stroke. Heat exhaustion, which can be viewed as a precursor to heat stroke, is between the two poles of this spectrum. In addition to the usual heat syndromes, severe and prolonged fever may be difficult or impossible to distinguish from hyperthermia.

I. **Infectious causes.** As already mentioned, circulating endogenous pyrogens can cause fever by raising the hypothalamic set point. Infection usually causes release of pyrogens, but several other medical conditions have been associated with the release of endogenous pyrogens and subsequent temperature elevations **(see the box below).** Fever is often encountered with malignant disease, such as malignancy of the reticuloendothelial system, lung, liver, pancreas, kidney, and colon.

II. **Pharmacologic causes.** There are many pharmacologic agents that can cause hyperthermia by 1) increasing muscular activity and heat production, 2) increasing metabolic rate, or 3) impairing heat dissipation **(see the box on page 690).** Drugs that cause muscular hyperactivity include cyclic antidepressants and monoamine oxidase inhibitors. Drugs such as salicylates and thyroid hormones lead to hypermetabolism. Ethanol and phenothiazines impair thermoregulation, while anticholinergics, tricyclic antidepressants, and phenothiazines impair the body's ability to dissipate heat. Diuretics, beta-blockers, and sympatholytic antihypertensive agents all impair cardiovascular compensation, which is necessary to prevent hyperthermia.

III. **Environmental causes.** The majority of hyperthermia is usually environmental in etiology. Heat illnesses are often seen during heat waves, especially when coupled with strenuous activity, a lack of air conditioning, or poor ventilation. These instances will be the major focus because they are the most common, often preventable, and usually readily treatable.

Presentation

There are several different types of heat illness that can present. These can be divided into minor heat emergencies, which include heat edema, heat cramps, and heat syncope. The more serious heat emergencies include heat exhaustion and heat stroke.

I. **Heat edema** presents as swelling of the hands and feet. Many patients may present simply with pitting edema, which usually occurs in the first few days after exposure to a hot environment and is self-limiting, usually resolving after acclimatization occurs. It is important to distinguish heat edema from other (i.e.,

Medical Conditions Causing Fever/Hyperthermia	
Infectious disorders	Neoplastic disease
Mechanical trauma	Vascular accidents
Crush injury	Immune disorders
	Collagen vascular disease

Pharmacologic Agents Causing Hyperthermia

Increased Muscular Activity
Amphetamines
PCP
Monoamine oxidase inhibitors
Cocaine
Tricyclic antidepressants
Halothane, succinylcholine ("malignant hyperthermia")
Antipsychotics, lithium ("neuroleptic malignant syndrome")
Increased Metabolic Rate
Salicylates
Thyroid hormone
Impaired Thermoregulation
Phenothiazines
Ethanol
Impaired Heat Dissipation
Anticholinergics
Antihistamines
Tricyclic antidepressants
Phenothiazines

cardiac) causes of edema that are treated with diuretics, since administration of diuretics to patients with heat edema will make them more likely to develop heat stroke.

II. **Heat cramps** are caused by salt depletion. The hyponatremia that results may interfere with calcium-dependent relaxation. Patients with heat cramps usually develop painful but benign involuntary skeletal muscle spasms that occur in muscles after cessation of exercise. This condition is more likely to occur in physically active individuals. Treatment of heat cramps includes oral fluid replacement with a solution such as Gatorade or intravenous saline if the patient is unable to tolerate oral fluids.

III. **Heat syncope.** A variation of vasovagal syncope, heat syncope, is seen primarily in those who stand or work in the heat for a prolonged period of time. It is caused by arteriolar vasodilatation without compensatory tachycardia, resulting in a pooling of the blood in the lower extremities. This condition is easily treated by postural changes, which involve elevating the feet or lowering the head. The use of support hose on the lower extremities to promote venous return may prevent heat syncope.

IV. **Heat exhaustion** is characterized by weakness, dizziness, nausea, or syncope due to excessive loss of both water and salt. This condition is classified as either hypernatremic (primary water loss) or hyponatremic (primary sodium loss). Vague symptoms and signs complicate the diagnosis of heat exhaustion. The diagnosis is usually made after ruling out other underlying illnesses and identifying a precipitating factor, such as a broken air conditioner, poorly ventilated apartment, or the presence of a heat wave. Heat exhaustion and heat stroke should be considered in patients who present with confusion and elevated temperature, especially during heat waves in which environmental temperatures exceed 95° F for more than 3 days.

V. **Heat exhaustion vs. heat stroke.** Obtaining a rectal temperature is the only way of accurately measuring core temperature and subsequently being able to differentiate heat exhaustion from heat stroke. Studies have demonstrated that the presence of tachypnea alone can raise the average temperature difference (rectal versus oral) significantly. In heat exhaustion, most patients will have temperatures of less than 39° C; they may even be normal. In addition, mental function is basically intact in these individuals with only slight confusion or irritability present.

VI. Heat stroke occurs when the body's ability to dissipate heat becomes unable to compensate for the heat burden imposed by the environment, endogenous sources, or exertion. Heat stroke should always be suspected in patients with a history of heat exposure, temperatures greater than 41° C, and CNS manifestations such as delirium, psychosis, violent behavior, loss of consciousness, focal findings, and seizures. Two types of heat stroke are usually described: classical and exertional. Both types are true medical emergencies associated with a mortality rate ranging from 10 to 80%.

   A. Classic heat stroke typically affects patients during a heat wave. Most of these patients are older than 70 years and may have underlying medical problems such as congestive heart failure, diabetes mellitus, alcoholism, or diuretic and anticholinergic use. Classic heat stroke develops over a period of several days during a heat wave in persons who are unable to take adequate fluids or move to a cooler environment. CNS manifestations are usually the first to appear and include confusion, bizarre behavior, seizures, and coma. Other neurologic abnormalities—such as dystonia, muscle rigidity, decerebrate posturing, and transient hemiplegia—may also be present, requiring careful differentiation from meningitis. Sweating may be present or absent. Patients with heat stroke have elevated rectal temperatures, sometimes greater than 41° C.

   B. Other manifestations. In addition to hyperthermia and CNS dysfunction, there are several other clinical manifestations of hyperthermia that may be life threatening. Shock and acidosis can result from the inability to maintain cardiac output in the presence of peripheral vasodilatation and dehydration. Hyperthermia may also impair cardiac output by causing myocardial necrosis, pulmonary hypertension, or both.

   C. Hyperventilation. Patients with heat stroke will also hyperventilate, at rates up to 60 per minute, in order to lose heat. The respiratory alkalosis that results can produce paresthesias, carpal spasm, tetany, and hypokalemia. Abnormal bleeding, which results from thrombocytopenia or impaired synthesis of clotting factors, is frequently seen in patients with hyperthermia. Disseminated intravascular coagulation can result from activation of the coagulation system by direct thermal injury to vascular endothelium. Muscle breakdown may also occur as a result of direct thermal injury, muscle hyperactivity, or tissue ischemia. Renal failure can occur secondary to the shock state and dehydration as well as the aforementioned rhabdomyolysis. Cardiac arrhythmias may also occur in acute hyperthermia because of myocardial injury, acidosis, hyperkalemia, or hypokalemia. Hypokalemia is more common in elderly patients with classic heat stroke.

Differential Diagnosis

Recognition of heat illness can be difficult in situations when there is no heat wave and the presentation is subtle. A high index of suspicion should always be maintained, and a rectal temperature should always be obtained. It is also essential that the physician consider other medical conditions that can present with significant temperature elevations.

A lumbar puncture can usually distinguish meningitis and encephalitis from heat stroke. Malaria, although rare in nonendemic areas, can be distinguished with a peripheral blood smear. Other diseases such as epilepsy, head trauma, cerebrovascular accidents, thyroid storm, diabetic ketoacidosis, and infection-sepsis can also mimic heat stroke. A careful history and laboratory findings help make the distinction, with initial SGOT, LDH, and CPK levels being high in heat stroke and normal or slightly elevated in the infectious or other diseases.

Treatment

Cooling should be started immediately in patients with temperatures above 41° C, and this should take precedence over all other diagnostic measures. The two methods of cooling involve the use of ice water baths and evaporative cooling.

I. **Evaporative cooling** can be performed by moving air over a wet, disrobed patient. Patients should be suspended and warm water should be used in order to prevent shivering. This method is similar to the methods developed in Saudi Arabia, which have been shown to be very successful. The use of ice water baths is impractical, is often dangerous, causes shivering, and makes monitoring and airway management more difficult. A specific tank for cooling has been developed but is not in widespread use.

II. **The airway** may require protection, since coma, convulsions, and vomiting put patients at risk for aspiration. Patients with hyperthermia have high tissue-oxygen needs and require supplemental oxygen administration.

III. **An intravenous (IV)** line should be started, and fluid administration should be initiated. Fluid requirements are usually low in patients with environmental heat illness, and fluids should be administered cautiously. Elderly people should have Swan-Ganz catheterization prior to large amounts of fluid administration in order to avoid pulmonary edema. The fluid of choice is normal saline.

IV. **Monitoring.** All patients with hyperthermia should be monitored for dysrhythmias and carefully evaluated for gastrointestinal (GI) bleeding. Shivering is best treated with diazepam or chlorpromazine, although chlorpromazine may cause hypotension and lower the seizure threshold.

Prevention involves avoiding heat, reducing activity, and maintaining adequate hydration.

Suggested Readings

Beezer CB: Heat stress and the young athlete: recognizing and reducing the risks, *Postgrad Med* 76(1):109, 1984.

Billen JP et al: Ventricular fibrillation during orotracheal intubation of hypothermic dogs, *Ann Emerg Med* 15:412-416, 1986.

Clowes GH and O'Donnell TF: Heat stroke, *N Engl J Med* 291:564, 1974.

Collins KJ: *Hypothermia: the facts,* New York, 1983, Oxford University Press.

Collins KJ, Easton JC, and Exton-Smith AN: Shivering thermogenesis and vasomotor responses with convective cooling in the elderly, *J Physiol* 320:76, 1981.

Collins KJ, Exton-Smith AN, and Dore C: Urban hypothermia: preferred temperature and thermal perception in old age, *Br Med J* 282:175, 1981.

Cooper KE: *Temperature regulation and its disorders: hypothermia in recent advances in medicine,* ed 15, London, 1986, Churchill Livingstone.

DeMonchaux C: *Psychological factors in hypothermia,* Social Science Research Council Report, 1975.

Doherty NE et al: Hypothermia with acute myocardial infarction, *Ann Intern Med* 101(6):797-798, 1984.

Ellis FP: Heat illness, *Trans R Soc Trop Med Hyg* 70:402, 1976.

Gabow PA, Kaehny WD, and Kelleher SP: The spectrum of rhabdomyolysis, *Medicine* 61:141, 1982.

Gale EAM and Tattersal RB: Hypothermia: a complication of diabetic ketoacidosis, *Br Med J* 4:1387, 1978.

Hart GR et al: Epidemic classical heat stroke: clinical characteristics and course of 28 patients, *Medicine* 61:189, 1982.

Kallman H: Protecting your elderly patients from winter's cold, *Geriatrics* 40(12):69, 1985.

Kelleher JP and Sales JEL: Pyrexia of unknown origin and colorectal carcinoma, *Br Med J* 293(6):1475, 1986.

Khogali M, Mustafa MK, and Gumaa K: Management of heatstroke, *Lancet* 2(8309):1225, 1982.

Knochal JP: Dog days and siriasis: how to kill a football player, *JAMA* 233(6):513, 1975.

Knochel JP: Environmental heat illness: an eclectic review, *Arch Intern Med* 133:841, 1974.

Kramer MR, Vandijk J, and Rosin AJ: Mortality in elderly patients with thermoregulatory failure, *Arch Intern Med* 149:1521, 1989.

Leads from the MMWR: Hypothermia associated deaths—United States 1968-70, *JAMA* 255(3):307, 1986.

Lewin S, Brettman LR, and Holzman RS: Infection in hypothermic patients, *Arch Intern Med* 141:920, 1981.

Lloyd E: Accidental hypothermia treated by central rewarming through the airway, *Br J Anaesth* 45:41, 1973.

Lloyd E and Mitchell B: Factors affecting the onset of ventricular fibrillation in hypothermia, *Lancet* 2:1294, 1974.

Maclean D and Emslie-Smith D: *Accidental hypothermia,* 1977, Philadelphia, J.B. Lippincott Co.

MacNichol MW: Respiratory failure and acid base status in hypothermia, *Postgrad Med J* 43:674, 1967.

Matz R: Hypothermia: mechanisms and countermeasures, *Hosp Pract* 21(1A):45, 1986.

Molnar GW and Read RC: Hypoglycemia and body temperature, *JAMA* 227:916, 1974.

Morris DL et al: Hemodynamic characteristics of patients with hypothermia due to occult infection and other causes, *Ann Intern Med* 102(2):153, 1985.

Murray HW et al: Fever and pulmonary thromboembolism, *Am J Med* 67:232-235, 1979.

Neil HA, Dawson JA, and Baker JE: Risk of hypothermia in elderly patients with diabetes, *Br Med J* 293:416, 1986.

O'Donnell TF: Acute heat stroke: epidemiologic, biochemical, renal and coagulation studies, *JAMA* 234:824, 1975.

Olson KR and Benowitz NL: Environmental and drug induced hyperthermia, recognition and management, *Emerg Med Clin North Am* 2:459, 1984.

Pizelonski MM et al: Fever in the wake of a stroke, *Neurology* 36:427, 1986.

Petersdorf RG and Beeson PB: Fever of unexplained origin: report on 100 cases, *Medicine* 40:1, 1961.

Rango N: Exposure related hypothermia mortality in the United States, 1970-79, *Am J Public Health* 74:1159, 1984.

Restivo KM et al: Accumulation of polyamines and their weak association with lower body temperature in elderly convalescent patients, *J Lab Clin Med* 110(2):217-220, 1987.

Reuler JB: Hypothermia: pathophysiology, clinical settings and management, *Ann Intern Med* 89:519, 1978.

Rew MC, Bershas I, and Sefteh H: The diagnostic and prognostic significance of serum enzyme changes in heat stroke, *Trans R Soc Trop Med Hyg* 63:325, 1971.

Rosenberg J et al: Hyperthermia associated with drug intoxication, *Crit Care Med* 14(11):964, 1986.

Rousseaux P et al: Fever and cerebral vasospasm in ruptured intracranial aneurysms, *Surg Neurol* 14:459, 1980.

Schoenfeld Y and Odassin R: Age and sex difference in response to short exposure to extreme dry heat, *J Appl Physiol* 44:1, 1978.

Stewart CE: Preventing progression of heat injury, *Emerg Med Rep* 8(16):121, 1987.

Tandberg D and Sklar D: Effect of tachypnea on the estimation of body temperature by an oral thermometer, *N Engl J Med* 308(16):945, 1983.

Treatment of myxedic coma, *Lancet* 2:768, 1956 (editorial).

Watts AJ: Hypothermia in the aged: a study of the role of cold sensitivity, *Environ Res* 5:119, 1971.

Weiner JS and Kohgali M: A physiologic body cooling unit for treatment of heatstroke, *Lancet* 1(8167):507, 1980.

Wilson GM: Hypothermia in clinical medicine, *Med Sci Law* 9:231, 1969.

Wollner L and Spalding JMK: The autonomic nervous system. In Brocklehurst JC, editor: *Textbook of geriatric medicine and gerontology,* ed 3, London, 1978, Churchill Livingstone.

Woolf PD et al: Accidental hypothermia: endocrine function during recovery, *J Clin Endocrinol Metab* 34:460, 1972.

Zell SC and Kurtz KJ: Severe exposure hypothermia: a resuscitation protocol, *Ann Emerg Med* 4:339, 1985.

This chapter appeared in part in Bosker G et al: *Geriatric Emergency Medicine.* St. Louis: Mosby–Year Book, 1990.

Index

A

A-200 pyrinate shampoo, 626
Abdominal hernias, 311, 312
Abdominal injuries
  diagnosis and treatment of, 599, 560t, 560-562, 565, 565t
  penetrating, treatment of, 450, 451
Abdominal pain, 121, 122t, 124
Abortions, 447
Abscesses
  carbuncles, 439
  dental, treatment of, 443
  diagnosis and treatment of, 438t, 439
  eyelid, diagnosis and treatment of, 441
  furuncles, 439
  furunculosis, 439
  lung, treatment of, 444, 444t, 445
  peritonsillar, antimicrobial therapy for in pediatrics, 516t
  retropharyngeal, antimicrobial therapy for in pediatrics, 516t
  treatment of, 438t
Accutane (isotretinoin), 682
ACE inhibitors
  in antihypertensive treatment, 36t
  effects on metabolic disorders, 32t
  FDA pregnancy safety classification of, 667t
  in lactation, 676
  in treatment of myocardial infarction, 153
Acebutolol
  FDA pregnancy safety classification of, 667t
  in lactation, 676
Acetaminophen
  antidote for, 182t, 195, 196
  with codeine
    street price of, 133t
    in treatment of
      dental pain, 95t
      dysmenorrhea, 95t
      otitis externa, 569
      pain, 94t
      pain for fractures, 95t
  FDA pregnancy safety classification of, 668t
  in lactation, 672
  with oxycodone, in treatment of pain, 94t
  in treatment of
    osteoarthritis, 639
    otitis media, 573
    pain, 84, 95t
      for cancer, 95t

Acetazolamide
  in lactation, 681
  in treatment of
    emboli/thrombi, 603
    glaucoma, 598, 599t
      adverse reactions to, 607
      contraindications to, 599t
    metabolic alkalosis, 369
Acetic acid otic solutions, 570
Acetohexamide, 44t
Acetyl sulfisoxazole (Pediazole) with erythromycin ethylsuccinate, in treatment of
  otitis media in pediatrics, 524t
  sinusitis/purulent nasopharyngitis in pediatrics, 527t
Acetylsalicylic acid (ASA)
  as cause of peripheral vertigo, 575
  with codeine and butalbital, drug seekers of, 132
  in treatment of
    myocardial infarction, 153
    pain, 80, 81t, 82-84
      with codeine, 76
      with oxycodone, 94t
Acid and alkaline ingestions, 296, 297, 297t
Acid burns, 592
Acid-base disorders
  case presentations of, 354-358
  diagnosis and treatment of, 346, 347t, 348, 349t, 350, 351t, 352t, 353– 356, 357, 358, 359t, 360, 361t
ACLS drugs; *see* Advanced cardiac life support drugs
ACTH cosyntropin (Cortosyn), 393
Active external rewarming (AER), 688
Active internal rewarming (AIR), 688
Acute gout; *see* Gout, acute
Acyclovir
  FDA pregnancy safety classification of, 665t
  in lactation, 674
  precautions for use, in pregnancy, 405
  recommendations and adverse reactions to, 427, 428
  in treatment of
    bacterial pneumonia, in pediatrics, 525t
    chickenpox, 518t
    hairy leukoplakia, 495
    herpes simplex virus
      genital herpes, 448t, 449, 473t, 480
      proctitis, 473t, 480
    herpes simplex virus (HSV), 588
    herpes zoster oticus, 91, 438t, 440, 569, 570

Page numbers in *italics* indicate illustrations; *t* indicates tables.

Index   693

HIV related
  herpes esophagitis, 497
  herpes simplex virus, 495
  herpes varicella zoster, 495
  HSV proctitis, 500
  ocular herpes varicella zoster, 502
  meningitis/sepsis, in pediatrics, 522t, 523t
  neonatal gonococcal conjunctivitis, 519t
  pain, 95t
Adapin (doxepin),680
Adenosine
  FDA pregnancy safety classification of, 668t
  in treatment of
    arrhythmias, 217, 218
    paroxysmal supraventricular tachycardia (PSVT), 238
    supraventricular tachycardia (SVT), pediatric, 249
    tachycardias, 233
    Wolff-Parkinson-White syndrome (WPW), 225, pediatric, 248
Adnexa, 584
Adrenal hormones, 669t
Adrenaline (epinephrine), 676
β-Adrenergic antagonists, 193
β-Adrenergic blockers, 676
Adrenergics, 600t
β-Adrenoceptor Antagonists; see β-blockers
Adrenocortical hypofunction (Addison's disease), 393
Advanced cardiac life support (ACLS) drugs
  atropine, 219, 220
  digitalis, 222
  dopamine, 221
  epinephrine, 219
  isoproterenol, 221
  morphine, 220, 221
  oxygen, 218, 219
  sodium bicarbonate, 220
Adverse drug interactions, over-the-counter-drugs, 6, 7
Adverse drug reactions; see also Specific drug names
  causes and risks among the elderly, 1–3, 2t, 3t
  pathophysiology and pharmacokinetics, 7, 8
  patient risk factors, 6, 7
  physician-related risk factors, 3t–5t, 3–6
  drug management
    anticoagulants, 54, 56t, 57–60
    antidepressants, 51, 52t, 53, 54
    antihistamines, 65–67, 66t
    antihypertensive agents, 39–41, 41t
    antipsychotics, 54, 55T
    anxiolytic and sedative hypnotic drugs, 47, 48t, 49, 50
    bronchodilators, 61–65
    cholesterol-reducing agents, 46, 47
    H_2 antagonists, 60, 61, 61t
    nitrate therapy, 41
    NSAIDs, 41–43
    oral hypoglycemic agents, 43, 44t, 45, 46
    salicylates, 65
  emergency/ambulatory situations
    with ACE inhibitors, 16–18
    with antihypertensive agents, 27–29, 29t, 30t, 31, 31t–33t, 34–35, 36t, 37, 38
    with calcium channel blockers, 14–16
    with cardiovascular medication, 12–14, 24–27
    with digitalis, 22–24
  preventive care and the elderly, 67, 68
  types of, 8t–10t, 8–10
AER; see Active external rewarming
Aerobic gram-negative bacilli, 406
Agitation, acute
  causes of, 273t
  differential diagnosis of, 272
  treatment of, 272
β₂-agonists
  inhaled, in lactation, 676
  precautions/contraindications for the elderly, 280
  in treatment of
    asthma, 277t–279t, 279–282
    chronic obstructive pulmonary disease (COPD), 283, 284
AIR; see Active internal rewarming
Air puff tonometers, 584
Ajmaline, 217
Albendazole, 432
Albumin, 399
Albuterol
  FDA pregnancy safety classification of, 667t
  in treatment of
    asthma, 277t, 278t, 280
      compared to salmeterol, 280
    bronchiolitis, in pediatrics, 517t
    hyperkalemia, 380
Alcohol
  adverse drug interactions of, with anticoagulants, 56t
  as cause of vertigo, 270
  in lactation, 683
  withdrawal seizures
    emergency room procedures for, 257
    with status epilepticus, 257
Alcohol, rubbing, 579
Alcoholic ketoacidosis (AKA); see Ketoacidosis, alcoholic
Alcoholic patients, 451
Aldactone (spironolactone), 677
Aldomet (methyldopa), 676
Alfentanil, 109
Alkali therapy, 363
Alkaline ingestions; see Acid and alkaline ingestions
Alkaloids
  belladonna, in lactation, 678
  ergot, in lactation, 682
Alkaptonuria, scleral discoloration (brown) as symptom of, 594t
Alkylating agents, 56t
Allergies, 594t
Allopurinol, 56t
Alpha-blockers; see α-blockers
Alprazolam
  anxiolytic effects on the elderly, 48t
  drug seekers of, 132
  in lactation, 680
  in treatment of

694　Index

Alprazolam—*Continued*
　　panic disorders, 662, 663
　　violent behavior, 656
Amanita phalloides, 182*t*, 198, 199
Amantadine
　　breast feeding and, 681
　　contraindications of, in pregnancy, 404
　　FDA pregnancy safety classification of, 665*t*
　　in lactation, 681
　　recommendations and adverse reactions to, 428
　　in treatment of pediatric pneumonia, 463
Amaurosis fugax
　　as symptom of
　　　anemia, 594*t*
　　　arteritis, 594*t*
　　　carotid disease, 594*t*
　　　dysrhythmia, 594*t*
　　　hypotension/hypertension, 594*t*
　　　polycythemia, 594*t*
　　　valvular heart disease, 594*t*
Amcinonide, 613*t*
Amebiasis, *324,* 328
AMI; *see* Myocardial infarction, acute
Amikacin
　　FDA pregnancy safety classification of, 665*t*
　　recommendations and adverse reactions to, 417
　　in treatment of, HIV related
　　　Mycobacterium avium, 509
　　　tuberculosis, 508
　　　septic arthritis, 641
Amiloride, 669*t*
Aminoglutethimide, 668*t*
Aminoglycosides
　　with ampicillin, in treatment of acute mastoiditis in pediatrics, 522*t*
　　with ampicillin and clindamycin, in treatment of
　　　Fournier's Gangrene, 466
　　　gram-negative synergistic necrotizing cellulitis, 466
　　with ampicillin and metronidazole, in treatment of
　　　Fournier's Gangrene, 466
　　　gram-negative synergistic necrotizing cellulitis, 466
　　with antipseudomonal penicillin, in treatment of septicemia in nonimmunocompromised adults, 461
　　with β-lactam antibiotic, in treatment of septicemia in immunocompromised adults, 461
　　with carbenicillin, in treatment of malignant otitis externa, 569
　　as cause of peripheral vertigo, 575
　　with cephalosporins, in treatment of septicemia in nonimmunocompromised adults, 461
　　with clindamycin, in treatment of penetrating abdominal traumas, 450, 451
　　FDA pregnancy safety classification of, 665*t*
　　with imipenem-cilastin, in treatment of septicemia in nonimmunocompromised adults, 461
　　in lactation, 673
　　with metronidazole, in treatment of penetrating abdominal traumas, 450, 451
　　with nafcillin, in treatment of suppurative arthritis in pediatrics, 516*t*
　　with penicillin, in treatment of
　　　clostridial anaerobic cellulitis, 465
　　　gram-negative synergistic necrotizing cellulitis, 465
　　　pediatric pneumonia, 463
　　precautions for use in pregnancy, 404
　　recommendations and adverse reactions to, 416, 417
　　with ticarcillin, in treatment of malignant otitis externa, 569
　　with ticarcillin/clavulanate, in treatment of septicemia in nonimmunocompromised adults, 461
　　with tipseudomonal penicillin, in treatment of pneumonia in immunocompromised adults, 463
　　in treatment of
　　　conjunctivitis, 588
　　　meningitis in neurosurgery/trauma patients, 451
Aminopenicillins, 436*t*
Aminophylline, 277*t*, 278*t*, 281
Amiodarone
　　FDA pregnancy safety classification of, 668*t*
　　in lactation, 675
　　in treatment of
　　　arrhythmias, 214
　　　atrial fibrillation, 235
　　　　pediatric, *251*
　　　atrial flutter, 235
　　　　pediatric, *251*
　　　Wolff-Parkinson-White syndrome (WPW), pediatric, *248*
Amipaque (metrizamide), 681
Amitriptyline
　　FDA pregnancy safety classification of, 669*t*
　　with fluphenazine, in treatment of pain, 96*t*
　　in lactation, 680
　　in treatment of pain, 86, 88
　　　for fibromyalgia, 95*t*
　　　for neuropathic disorders, 95*t*
Amoxapine, 680
Amoxicillin, with clavulanic acid, in treatment of mastoiditis, 576
　　dosing frequencies for, 403*t*
　　with probenecid, in treatment of
　　　gonococcal cervicitis and urethritis, 476, 477
　　recommendations and adverse reactions to, 407
　　in treatment of
　　　COPD, 285
　　　disseminated gonococcal infections, 478
　　　gonococcal cervicitis during pregnancy, 471*t*
　　　infectious diseases, 436*t*
　　　otitis media, 572
　　　　in pediatrics, 524*t*
　　　　recurrences of, 573
　　　pediatric bacteremia, 516*t*, 517*t*
　　　pediatric pyelonephritis, 526*t*
　　　pediatric sinusitis/purulent nasopharyngitis, 527*t*
　　　septic arthritis, 641
　　　sinusitis, 576
Amoxicillin-clavulanic acid
　　dosing frequencies for, 403*t*
　　with penicillin, in treatment of
　　　dental abscesses, 443
　　　orofacial infections, 443
　　recommendations and adverse reactions to, 414
　　in treatment of
　　　acute sinusitis, 442*t*, 443
　　　animal bites, 438*t*, 439, 440
　　　aspiration pneumonia, 444, 444*t,* 445
　　　chronic bronchitis, 443, 444*t*
　　　chronic sinusitis, 443
　　　community-acquired pneumonia, 443, 444, 444*t*

cystitis, 445, 445t, 446
dacryocystitis, 590
human bites, 439, 440
impetigo, 438, 439
infectious diseases, 436t
lung abscesses, 444, 444t, 445
odontogenic infections, 443
otitis media, 442, 442t, 572
pediatric bacterial pneumonia, 525t
pediatric epiglottitis, 520t
pediatric facial cellulitis, 438t, 439
pediatric otitis media, 524t
penetrating soft tissue trauma, 566t
posterior epistaxis, 580
pyelonephritis, 445, 445t, 446
sinusitis, 576
Amoxicillin-sulbactam, 673
Amphetamine-like drugs, 132
Amphetamines
acute psychosis and, 658
agents causing hyperthermia, 690t
in lactation, 682
violent behavior in psychiatric emergencies and, 653
Amphotericin B
FDA pregnancy safety classification of, 665t
recommendations and adverse reactions to, 424, 425
in treatment of, HIV related
cryptococcal meningitis, 490, 491
hyponatremia, 510
septic arthritis, 641
Ampicillin
with aminoglycosides, in treatment of pediatric acute mastoiditis, 522t
with aminoglycosides and clindamycin, in treatment of
Fournier's Gangrene, 466
gram-negative synergistic necrotizing cellulitis, 466
with aminoglycosides and metronidazole, in treatment of
Fournier's Gangrene, 466
gram-negative synergistic necrotizing cellulitis, 466
with cefotaxime, in treatment of
meningitis in neonates, 451
pediatric meningitis/sepsis, 522t, 523t
septicemia in neonates, 461
with ceftazidime, in treatment of pediatric acute mastoiditis, 522t
with ceftriaxone, in treatment of bacterial meningitis in elderly, 531t
meningitis in neonates, 451
septicemia in neonates, 461
with chloramphenicol, in treatment of epiglottitis, 582
contraindications for, in treatment of, pharyngitis, 581
dosing frequencies for, 403t
with gentamicin, in treatment of pediatric
bacterial pneumonia, 525t
meningitis/sepsis, 522t, 523t
omphalitis, 523t
pyelonephritis, 526t
with probenecid, in treatment of
gonococcal cervicitis and urethritis, 476, 477
recommendations and adverse reactions to, 407
in treatment of
acute epiglottitis, 459

granuloma inguinale (donovanosis), 480
HIV related bacterial diarrhea, 499
infectious diseases, 436t
listeriosis, 330
meningitis
in alcoholic patients, 451
in elderly, 451
pediatric, 451
necrotizing fasciitis, 466
pediatric pneumonia, 463
salmonellosis, 324, 327
septic arthritis, 641
shigellosis, 322, 324t
Ampicillin-clavulanate, 463
Ampicillin-sulbactam, with gentamicin in treatment of pneumonia in elderly, 530t
with metronidazole, in treatment of pneumonia in high-risk aspiration adults, 464
recommendations and adverse reactions to, 414
with tobramycin, in treatment of elderly
with bacterial cholangitis/biliary sepsis, 531t
with bacterial peritonitis, 531t
with cellulitis, 532t
with diverticulitis, 531t
with pyelonephritis, 530t
with urinary tract infections, 531t
in treatment of
abdominal trauma, 566t
cholecystitis in elderly, 531t
clostridial anaerobic cellulitis, 465
gram-negative synergistic necrotizing cellulitis, 465
gun shot wounds, 559, 562
necrotizing fasciitis, 466
penetrating abdominal traumas, 450, 451
pneumonia in elderly, 530t
pneumonia in adults, 463
septicemia in nonimmunocompromised children, 461
Amrinone, 668t
Amyl nitrite
antidotal action of, 182t, 189, 197, 198
in treatment of
cyanide poisoning, 343t
ergotism, 343t
Anabolic steroids, 56t
Analgesics
breast feeding and, 672, 673
in emergency medicine, 72–96
FDA pregnancy safety classification of, 665t, 668t
ideal properties of, 100t
in lactation, 672, 673
parenteral, in treatment of perirectal abscesses, 311
in treatment of corneal abrasions in uveitis, 592
hemorrhoids, 310
Anaprox (naproxen), 672, 673
Anemias
amaurosis fugax as symptom of, 594t
HIV related, diagnosis and treatment of, 500, 501
optic atrophy as symptom of, 594t
pernicious, optic atrophy as symptom of, 594t
Anesthesia, general, 259
Anesthetics
contraindications to, in treatment of corneal abrasions in uveitis, 592
in lactation, 681
local, in lactation, 682
topical
lidocaine gel, 91
in treatment of hemorrhoids, 310

Anesthetics—*Continued*
    in treatment of chemical injuries in uveitis, 592
Aneurysms
    internal carotid, 597
    posterior communicating, oculomotor paralysis as symptom of, 594*t*
    proptosis as symptom of, 594*t*
Angina, 122*t*, 125
Angioconverting enzyme inhibitors (ACE inhibitors); *see* ACE inhibitors
Angiography
    in diagnosis of subarachnoid hemorrhages (SAH), 265
    in treatment of gastrointestinal bleeding, 300
Angioid streaks, as symptom of
    high myopia, 594*t*
    Paget's disease, 594*t*
    pseudoxanthoma elasticum, 594*t*
    sickle cell disease, 594*t*
Angiokeratoma, 494
Angioma, 494
Angiomatosis, 494
Anion gap, 350, 352*t*, 353, 355, 356, 357, 358
Anisindione (Miradon), 674
Anoscopy, 309
Ansaid (flubiprofen), 672
Antazoline phosphate, 585
Antiacids, 498
Antiarrhythmic drugs
    classification of, 205*t*, 206*t*, 207*t*, 208–222
        ACLS drugs, 218–222
        class I, 206*t*, 207*t*, 208–212
        class II, 207*t*, 212, 213
        class III, 207*t*, 213–215
        class IV, 207*t*, 215, 216
        new agents, 216–218
    FDA pregnancy safety classification of, 668*t*
    in lactation, 675
Antibacterials, 403*t*
Antibiotic ointments, 579
Antibiotics
    aminoglycosides, 575
    breast feeding and, 673, 674
    combination, in treatment of bacterial conjunctivitis, 586, 587
    cost of, 404
    FDA pregnancy safety classification of, 665*t*
    β-lactamase-inhibitors, 414
        piperacillin/tazobactam, 414
    ophthalmologic uses of, adverse effects of, 606
    oral
        in treatment of
            otitis externa, 569
            posterior blepharitis, 589
            ulcerative (staphylococcal) blepharitis, 589
    prophylactic, in treatment of first onset seizures in children, 257
    recommendations and adverse reactions, in pregnancy, 404, 405
    topical
        in treatment of
            conjunctivitis, 588
            corneal abrasions in uveitis, 592
    in treatment of
        abdominal hernias, 312
        blunt abdominal injuries, 565, 566*t*
        elderly, 528, 529, 530*t*–532*t*
        mastoiditis, 576
        midgut volvulus and malrotation, 303
        posterior epistaxis, 580
        trauma, 565
Anticholinergic drugs, 66*t*
Anticholinergics
    antidote for, 182*t*, 199
    as cause of hyperthermia, 689, 690*t*
    FDA pregnancy safety classification of, 667*t*
    in lactation, 678
    in treatment of
        asthma, 279, 281
        COPD, 284
        dystonic drug reactions, 272, 273
        uveitis, 591
Anticholinesterase drugs, 272, 273
Anticoagulants
    adverse drug interactions, 56*t*
    adverse drug reactions, 56*t*
    breast feeding and, 674
    in lactation, 674
    in treatment of retinal vein occlusions, 603
Anticoagulants/coagulants, 666*t*
Anticoagulation, 262
Anticonvulsants
    FDA pregnancy safety classification of, 668*t*
    in treatment of
        discarism, 343*t*
        new onset seizures, 256, 257*t*
        pain, 88, 89
        recurrent seizures, 257, 258, 258*t*
        subarachnoid hemorrhages (SAH), 264, 265
Antidepressants
    as cause of hypothermia, 686, 690*t*
    cyclic, antidote for, 182*t*, 202, 203
    FDA pregnancy safety classification of, 669*t*
    in lactation, 680
    in treatment of
        pain, 86, 88
        panic disorders, 662
        suicidal patients, 660, 661
    tricyclic, as cause of hyperthermia, 689, 690*t*
Antidiabetic agents, 678
Antidiabetic hormones, 669*t*
Antidiarrheals
    drug seekers feigning colitis for, 135*t*
    FDA pregnancy safety classification of, 666*t*
    in lactation, 678, 679
    in treatment of shigellosis, 322
Antiemetics
    as cause of dystonic reactions, 272
    FDA pregnancy safety classification of, 666*t*
    in treatment of
        hepatitis, 308
        migraines, 268
Antiepileptics, 675
Antiflatulents, 666*t*
Antifungals, 424–426
    FDA pregnancy safety classification of, 665*t*
    recommendations and adverse reactions to, 424–426
Antihelminthics
    in lactation, 673
    precautions for use, in pregnancy, 405
Antihistamine-decongestants, 585
Antihistamines
    as cause of hyperthermia, 690*t*
    FDA pregnancy safety classification of, 666*t*, 667*t*
    in lactation, 677
    in treatment of
        allergic conjunctivitis, 585
        dystonic drug reactions, 273
        fish poisonings, 344*t*

Index 697

HIV related eosinophilic pustular folliculitis, 494
Antihypertensives
  breast feeding and, 675, 676
  effects on coexisting disease of, 32*t*
  effects on metabolic disorders of, 32*t*
  FDA pregnancy safety classification of, 668*t*
  in lactation, 676
  in parenteral treatment of pain in thoracic aortic aneurysm, 126
Antiinfectives, 673, 674
Antiinflammatory agents, 284
Antiinflammatory creams, in treatment of
  eczema, 612
  psoriasis vulgaris, 617, 618
  seborrheic dermatitis, 615, 616
Antilipemics, 668*t*
Antimalarials, 636, 638
  FDA pregnancy safety classification of, 666*t*
  in lactation, 673
  precautions for use, in pregnancy, 405
  in treatment of rheumatoid arthritis, 636
Antimetabolites, 56*t*
Antimicrobial agents, 405–424
  in pediatrics
    choice of, 513, 514
    variables in, 513
  precautions for use, in pregnancy, 404, 405
  recommendations and adverse reactions to, 402, 403*t*, 404-433
Antimotility agents, 324, 326
Antineoplastic agents, 676
Antiparasitics, 428–432
Antipseudomonal penicillin, 461
Antipsychotics
  in lactation, 680
  lithium, as cause of hyperthermia, 690*t*
  precautions/contraindications for the elderly, 55*t*
  in treatment of suicidal patients, 661
Antipyretics
  FDA pregnancy safety classification of, 668*t*
  for pediatric croup, 519*t*
Antistaphylococcal drugs, in treatment of
  HIV related bacterial folliculitis, 494
  hordeolum, 589
  posterior blepharitis, 589
  ulcerative blepharitis, 589
Antithyroid agents
  FDA pregnancy safety classification of, 669*t*
  in lactation, 678
Antituberculous drugs
  FDA pregnancy safety classification of, 665*t*
  in lactation, 674
  precautions for use, in pregnancy, 404
  recommendations and adverse reactions, 426, 427
Antitussives/expectorants, 667*t*
Antiulcer agents, 679
Antivenins, 181, 183*t*, 184*t*
Antivert (meclizine), 270*t*
Antivirals
  FDA pregnancy classification of, 665*t*
  precautions for use, in pregnancy, 405
  recommendations and adverse reactions, 427, 428
  in treatment of necrotizing herpes simplex keratitis, 596
Anxiolytics, in treatment of
  abdominal hernias, 312
  suicidal patients, 661
Aphthous stomatitis, 578
Appendicitis, 308, 309

Appetite suppressants 132
Apresoline (hydralazine), in lactation, 676
Aqueous crystalline penicillin G, 641
Aralen; *see* Primaquine phosphate
Aralen HCl; *see* Chloroquine HCl
Arosabal; *see* Melarsoprol
Arrhythmias
  life-threatening
    asystole, *223, 224, 228, 229*
    atrial fibrillation, *234,* 235, 236
    atrial flutter, *234,* 235, 236
    atrioventricular blocks, *237, 240, 241*
    diagnosis and treatment of, *223–234,* 235, *236–241*
    multifocal atrial tachycardia (MAT), *231,* 232
    paroxysmal supraventricular tachycardia (PSVT), *236, 238, 239*
    pulseless electrical activity (PEA), *223, 224, 228, 229*
    pulseless ventricular tachycardia (VT), *223, 224, 226, 227*
    sinus bradycardia, *237, 240, 241*
    sinus tachycardia, *231*
    tachycardias, 232, *233*
    torsades de pointes (TDP), 232
    ventricular ectopy, *225, 230,* 231
    ventricular fibrillation (VF), *223, 224, 226, 227*
    ventricular tachycardia, 236, 237
    Wolff-Parkinson-White syndrome (WPW), *225*
  pediatric
    asystole, 241, *246, 247*
    atrial fibrillation, 245, *251*
    atrial flutter, 245, *251*
    paroxysmal supraventricular tachycardia (PSVT), 245, *250*
    pulseless electrical activity (PEA), 241, *246, 247*
    pulseless ventricular tachycardia (VT), 241, *246, 247*
    sinus bradycardia, 245, *252*
    supraventricular tachycardia (SVT), 245, *249*
    ventricular fibrillation (VF), 241, *246, 247*
    ventricular tachycardia with pulse, 241, *244*
    Wolff-Parkinson-White syndrome (WPW), 241, *248*
  ventricular fibrillation/pulseless ventricular tachycardia (VF/VT), 166, 167
Arsenic, 182*t,* 189
Arterial blood gases, 348
Arteriosclerosis, 593, 594, 594*t*
Arteritis
  amaurosis fugax as symptom of, 594*t*
  temporal
    age and, 603
    diagnosis and treatment of, 269, 603, 604
    biopsies in, 604
    occlusive disease of retinal vessels as symptom of, 594*t*
    ocular pain as symptom of, 597
    optic neuritis as symptom of, 594*t*
Arthritis; *see also* Osteoarthritis; Rheumatoid arthritis
  septic, diagnosis and treatment of, 640–642
  suppurative, antimicrobial therapy for, in pediatrics, 516*t*
ASA; *see* Acetylsalicylic acid
Asacol (mesalamine), 679
Ascabiol, 630
Ascorbic Acid, 314*t*
Asendin (amoxapine), 680
Aspergillus, as cause of
  otitis externa, 567, 568*t*

Aspergillus, as cause of—*Continued*
  otomycosis, 570
  sinusitis, 576
Aspirin
  FDA pregnancy safety classification of, 668*t*
  in lactation, 673
  in treatment of
    myocardial infarction, 152, 154
    osteoarthritis, 639
    pseudogout, 643
    Reiter's syndrome, 640
    rheumatoid arthritis, 636
    septic arthritis, 641
    systemic lupus erythematosus, 644
Asthma
  acute
    diagnosis and treatment of, 276, 277, 277*t*, 278*t*, 278–285, 279*t*
  precautions in parenteral treatment of, 107, 108
Asystole, 167, *223*, *224*, *228*, *229*
Atabrine, 594*t*
Atenolol
  FDA pregnancy safety classification of, 667*t*
  in lactation, 676
  in treatment of
    atrial fibrillation, 235
    atrial flutter, 235
    myocardial infarction, 153
Atheromatous disease, 594*t*
Ativan (lorazepam), 680
Atovaquone, in treatment of, HIV related encephalitis, 493
  focal intracerebral lesions, 493
  pneumocystis pneumonia, 505
  toxoplasmosis, 493
Atrial fibrillation, *234*, 235, 236
Atrial flutter, *234*, 235, 236
Atrioventricular blocks, *237*, *240*, *241*
Atropine
  antidotal action of, 182*t*, 185, 186, 199, 200
  contraindications to, in treatment of uveitis, 591
  with diphenoxylate, in lactation, 678
  FDA pregnancy safety classification of, 667*t*
  in lactation, 678
  in treatment of
    asystole, *229*
    atrioventricular blocks, *242*, *243*
    bradycardia, 168
    cardiac arrest, recommendations and adverse reactions to, 219, 220
    pulseless electrical activity (PEA), *229*
    sinus bradycardia, *242*, *243*
      pediatric, *252*
    supraventricular tachycardia (SVT), pediatric, *249*
Attapulgite, 678
Attention deficit syndrome, 135*t*
Aventyl (nortriptyline), 680
Axactam; *see* Aztreonam
Axid, 679
Azactam (aztreonam), 673
Azathioprine, in treatment of
  rheumatoid arthritis, 636
  systemic lupus erythematosus, 644
Azithromycin
  with cefoxitin and probenecid, in outpatient treatment of PID, 471*t*
  with cefuroxime, in treatment of pneumonia in elderly, 530*t*
  dosing frequencies for, 403*t*
  with gentamicin, in treatment of pneumonia in elderly, 530*t*
  recommendations and adverse reactions to, 421
  with TMP/SMX, in treatment of pneumonia in adults, 463
  in treatment of
    cellulitis, 439
    chancroid, 448*t*, 449, 473*t*
    chronic bronchitis, 443, 444*t*
    community-acquired pneumonia, 443, 444, 444*t*
    erysipelas, 439
    gonococcal cervicitis, 471*t*
      during pregnancy, 471*t*
    gonococcal urethritis, 471*t*
    HIV related
      encephalitis, 493
      focal intracerebral lesions, 493
      Mycobacterium avium, 509
      toxoplasmosis, 493
    infectious diseases, 43/*t*
    nongonococcal urethritis, 478
    pneumonia, 464
      in elderly, 530*t*
Azlocillin
  recommendations and adverse reactions to, 408
  with tobramycin and vancomycin, in treatment of neutropenic elderly patients, 532*t*
  in treatment of cholecystitis in elderly, 531*t*
Azoles, 446, 447*t*
Azolid (phenylbutazone), 673
Aztreonam
  with antipseudomonal penicillin, in treatment of septicemia in elderly, 461
  with cephalosporins, in treatment of septicemia in elderly, 461
  with imipenem-cilastin, in treatment of septicemia in elderly, 461
  in lactation, 673
  recommendations and adverse reactions to, 413
  with ticarcillin/clavulanate, in treatment of septicemia in elderly, 461
  in treatment of malignant otitis externa, 569
Azulfidine (sulfasalazine), 679

B

B. cereus; *see Bacillus cereus*
Bacampicillin
  dosing frequencies for, 403*t*
  recommendations and adverse reactions to, 407
Bacillus cereus, 328, 329
Bacitracin
  FDA pregnancy safety classification of, 666*t*
  in treatment of
    conjunctivitis, 588
    ulcerative blepharitis, 589
Back pain, low
  floctafenine as alternative for drug seekers, 141, 142*t*
  NSAIDs as alternative for drug seekers, 141, 142*t*
Baclofen
  in lactation, 682
  in treatment of
    muscle spasms, 89
      recommendations and adverse reactions to, 89
    trigeminal, 96*t*
Bacteremia
  antimicrobial therapy for, in pediatrics, 516*t*, 517*t*

Index 699

Haemophilus influenzae, antimicrobials in treatment of, precautions for use in pediatrics, 516*t*
Streptococcus pneumoniae, antimicrobials in treatment of, in pediatrics, 516*t,* 517*t*
Bacteria, 406
Bacterial endocarditis, 594*t*
Bacteroides, 576
Bacteroides fragilis, 406
Barbiturates
  acute psychosis and, 658
  adverse drug interactions
    with anticoagulants, 56*t*
  as cause of hyperthermia, 686
  drug seekers of, 132
  violent behavior in psychiatric emergencies and, 653
Barium enemas
  in diagnosis of appendicitis, 309
  in treatment of
    intussusception, 301
    sigmoid volvulus, 302
Barotitis, 570, 571
Basal artery insufficiency, 575
BCG vaccines, 670*t*
Beclomethasone
  FDA pregnancy safety classification of, 669*t*
  in lactation, 678
Behcet's disease, 594*t*
Belladonna alkaloids, 678
Benadryl (diphenhydramine), in treatment of
  acute labyrinthitis, 269, 270*t*
  drug side effects with hepatitis, 308
Bendroflumethiazide (Naturetin), 677
Benzathine penicillin, 407
Benzathine penicillin G, in treatment of
  cardiovascular syphilis, 448
  latent syphilis, 448
  pharyngitis, 443, 457
  syphilis, 448, 448*t,* 473*t, 479*
    in HIV patients, 448, 449
    during pregnancy,, 448
Benzodiazepines
  adverse drug interactions with warfarin, 61*t*
  antidote for, 182*t,* 192, 193
  as cause of hyperthermia, 686
  drug seekers of, 132, 135*t*
  in parenteral treatment of pain, recommendations and adverse reactions of, 104*t,* 117, 119
  in treatment of
    acute agitation, 272
    acute psychosis, 659
    panic disorders, 662, 663
    rectal foreign bodies, 310
    violent behavior, 655, 656
Benzothiadiazides, 33*t*
Benztropine
  antidotal action of, 182*t,* 191
  FDA pregnancy safety classification of, 667*t*
  in treatment of dystonic drug reactions, 272, 273
Beta-adrenergic antagonists; *see* β-Adrenergic antagonists
Beta-blockers; *see* β-Blockers
Betadine, in treatment of
  herpetic gingivostomatitis, 579
  perirectal abscesses, 311
Betadine douches, 480
Betamethasone
  benzoate, in treatment of dermatologic disorders, 613*t*

dipropionate, in treatment of dermatologic disorders, 613, 614*t*
FDA pregnancy safety classification of, 669*t*
valerate
  ointment, in treatment of aphthous stomatitis, 578
  in treatment of dermatologic disorders, 613*t*
Betapace (sotalol), 676
Betaxolol (Kerlone), 676
Bethanechol
  in lactation, 682
  in treatment of GERD, 298, 298*t*
Biaxin; *see* Clarithromycin
Bicarbonate, 247
Bicillin L-A; *see* Benzathine penicillin
Biliary colic
  definition of, 305
  diagnosis of, 305, 306
  parenteral treatment of, 122*t,* 125
Bipolar affective disorder, 649, 653
Bisacodyl (Dulcolax), 679
Bismuth subsalicylate (Pepto-Bismol), 679
Bites
  animal, diagnosis and treatment of, 438*t,* 439, 440
  human, diagnosis and treatment of, 438*t,* 439, 440
Bitrizide; *see* Praziquantel
Blepharitis, anterior
  seborrheic (nonulcerative), diagnosis and treatment of, 589
  staphylococcal (ulcerative), diagnosis and treatment of, 589
  posterior, diagnosis and treatment of, 589
Blocadren (timolol), 676
α-blockers
  in antihypertensive treatment, 32*t*
  in treatment of pheochromocytoma, 395
β-Blockers
  adverse drug interactions with cimetidine, 61*t*
  in antihypertensive treatment, 36*t*
    effects on coexisting disease, 32*t*
    effects on metabolic disorders, 32*t*
  ophthalmologic use of, adverse effects of, 607
  in treatment of myocardial infarction, 153
β-blockers
  drug seekers of, 132
  FDA pregnancy safety classification of, 667*t*
  in treatment of
    arrhythmias, 212, 213
    hyperthyroidism, 391
    paroxysmal supraventricular tachycardia (PSVT), 239
    sinus tachycardia, 231
Blood component therapy, 564, 565
Blood dyscrasias, 594*t*
Blood level measurement, 257, 258, 258*t*
Blood viscosity, 594*t*
Boils; *see* furuncles
Botulinum antitoxin (ABE Trivalent), 182*t,* 186
Botulism
  antidote for, 182*t,* 186
  diagnosis and treatment of, 317–321
  oculomotor paralysis as symptom of, 594*t*
  reporting requirements for, 317
Bowel disease, 498
Bradycardias, 167, 168
Brain edema, 555
Brain tumors; *see also* Tumors
  as cause of increased intracranial pressure, treatment of, 271
  new onset seizures with, treatment of, 256, 271

700 Index

Brain tumors—*Continued*
optic atrophy as symptom of, 594*t*
treatment of, 271, 272
Branhamella catarrhalis
as cause of sinusitis, 576
β-lactamase-producing, as cause of otitis media, 568*t*, 571, 572*t*
Brethine (terbutaline), 676
Bretylium
FDA pregnancy safety classification of, 668*t*
orthostatic hypotension cause of, 33*t*
in treatment of
asystole, pediatric, *247*
pulseless electrical activity (PEA), pediatric, *247*
pulseless ventricular tachycardia (VT), *227*
pediatric, *247*
tachycardias, *233*
ventricular arrhythmias, 167
ventricular fibrillation (VF), *227*
pediatric, *247*
ventricular tachycardia, *237*
ventricular tachycardia with pulse, pediatric, *244*
Bretylium tosylate, in treatment of
arrhythmias, 213, 214
ventricular ectopy, *230*
ventricular tachycardia, 237
Bricanyl (terbutaline), 676
Bromocriptine (Parlodel), 682
Brompheniramine, 666*t*
Bronchiolitis, 517*t*
Bronchitis
chronic, diagnosis and treatment of, 443, 444*t*
drug seekers feigning, 136, 136*t*
for cough syrups with dihydrocodone, 135*t*
Bronchodilators
breast feeding and, 676, 677
FDA pregnancy safety classification of, 667*t*
in lactation, 676, 677
in treatment of
asthma, 277*t*, 278*t*, 279t, 279–282
COPD, 283, 284
pediatric bacterial pneumonia, 525*t*
pediatric bronchiolitis, 517*t*
sulfite food poisoning, 344*t*
Buccal/preseptal cellulitis, 517*t*
Bumetanide, in treatment of
acute renal failure, 399
hyponatremia, 373
BUN/Cr ratio, 348
Bupivacaine
in lactation, 682
in parenteral treatment of
pain in costochondritis spasm, 126
pain in rib fractures, 126
Bupivacaine hydrochloride, 141, 142*t*
Buprenorphine, 110
Burow's solution, in treatment of
contact dermatitis, 623
eczema, 614
Buspirone, 663
Butabarbital (Butisol), 680
Butalbital, 132
Butaperazine, 671*t*
Butazolidin (phenylbutazone), 673
Butisol (butabarbital), 680
Butoconazole, 446, 472*t*
Butorphanol
in lactation, 672
in parenteral treatment of pain, 99*t*

Butyrophenones
antidote for, 182*t*, 191
as cause of dystonic reactions, 272

C

C. perfringens; see Clostridium perfringens
C. pneumonia, 458
Cafergot (ergotamine), 267*t*
Caffeine, 683
Calan (verapamil), 676
Calcitonin
FDA pregnancy safety classification of, 669*t*
in treatment of
hypercalcemia, 383
vitamin D intoxication, 316*t*
Calcium
contraindications in treatment of hyperkalemia, 379, 380
disorders
diagnosis and treatment of, 381–383
hypercalcemia, 382, 383
hypocalcemia, 381, 382
Calcium antagonists
in antihypertensive treatment, 36*t*
effects on coexisting disease of, 32*t*
effects on metabolic disorders of, 32*t*
Calcium channel blockers
antidote for, 182*t*, 186, 187
FDA pregnancy safety classification of, 667*t*, 668*t*
in lactation, 675, 676
Calcium chloride, 182*t*, 186, 187
Calcium gluconate
antidotal action of, 182*t*, 186
in treatment of
atrial fibrillation, 235
atrial flutter, 235
hyperkalemia, 379, 380
hypermagnesemia, 385
hypocalcemia, 381
paroxysmal supraventricular tachycardia (PSVT), *239*
Campylobacter enteritis, *324,* 330
CaNa2EDTA, 182*t*, 187, 188, 189
Cancer, 95*t*
Candida albicans, as cause of
oral candidiasis, 577
otitis externa, 567, 568*t*
Candidiasis
oral, diagnosis and treatment of, 577
oropharyngeal, HIV related, diagnosis and treatment of, 496
vaginal, HIV related, diagnosis and treatment of, 496
Capoten (captopril), 676
Captopril
as cause of orthostatic hypotension, 33*t*
FDA pregnancy safety classification of, 667*t*
in lactation, 676
Carafate (sucralfate), 679
Carbachol, in treatment of glaucoma, 599*t*
contraindications to, 599*t*
Carbamates, 182*t*, 199, 200
Carbamazepine
adverse drug interactions of
with anticoagulants, 56*t*
with cimetidine, 61*t*
FDA pregnancy safety classification of, 668*t*
in lactation, 675
for treatment of new onset seizures, 257*t*
in treatment of

pain, 88
petit mal status epilepticus, 259
Carbenicillin
  with aminoglycosides, in treatment of malignant otitis externa, 569
  dosing frequencies for, 403t
  recommendations and adverse reactions to, 408
Carbonic anhydrase inhibitors
  with miotics, in treatment of glaucoma, 598, 599t, 601
  ophthalmologic use of, adverse effects of, 607
Carboxypenicillins, 408
Carbuncles, 438t, 439
Cardiac arrest, 170–177
Cardiac arrhythmias; *see* Arrhythmias
Cardiac glycosides
  antidote for, 182t, 190, 191
  in lactation, 675, 676
Cardiogenic shock (CS), 164, 164t, 165, 166
Cardiovascular drugs
  breast feeding and, 675, 676
  in lactation, 675, 676
Cardizem (diltiazem), 676
Carisoprodol, 86, 87t
Carotid disease, 594t
Carotid-cavernous sinus fistula, 594t
Cascara, 679
CAT scans, in treatment of
  new onset seizures, 255
  severe head injuries, 259
Catapres (clonidine), 676
Cataracts
  definition of, 601
  diagnosis and treatment of, 602
  as symptom of
    diabetes mellitus, 594t
    retinal detachment, 594t
    steroid use, 594t
    trauma, 594t
    uveal disease, 594t
Catheters, Foley, in treatment of
  esophageal foreign bodies, 295
  gastrointestinal bleeding, 300
  midgut volvulus and malrotation, 302
  posterior epistaxis, 580
  rectal foreign bodies, 310
CDC classification system, 484, 485t
Cecal volvulus, 302
Cefaclor
  dosing frequencies for, 403t
  recommendations and adverse reactions to, 410, 411
  in treatment of
    infectious diseases, 436t
    otitis media, 572
      in pediatrics, 524t
    periorbital cellulitis, 590
    pharyngitis, 581
      in pediatrics, 524t
    sinusitis, 576
Cefadroxil
  dosing frequencies for, 403t
  recommendations and adverse reactions to, 410
  in treatment of
    acute lymphadenitis in pediatrics, 521t
    infectious diseases, 436t
    pharyngitis, 581
      in pediatrics, 524t
Cefamandole, 411
Cefazidime, 467

Cefazolin, in treatment of
  cellulitis in elderly, 532t
  dacryocystitis, 590
  open fractures, 450
  septic arthritis, 641
  traumas
    head and neck, 566t
    orthopedic, 566t
    penetrating soft tissue, 566t
Cefixime
  recommendations and adverse reactions to, 413
  in treatment of
    cervical gonorrhea, 471t
    epiglottitis in pediatrics, 520t
    gonorrhea, 448t, 449
    infectious diseases, 436t
    otitis media, 442, 572
      in pediatrics, 524t
    pharyngitis, 581, 582
      group A β-hemolytic streptococcus, 458
    rectal gonorrhea, 471t
Cefizox; *see* Ceftizoxime
Cefmetazole
  recommendations and adverse reactions, 411
  in treatment of penetrating abdominal traumas, 450, 451
Cefobid; *see* Cefoperazone
Cefocime, 403t
Cefonicid, 411
Cefoperazone, 412, 413
Cefotan; *see* Cefotetan
Cefotaxime
  with ampicillin, in treatment of
    pediatric meningitis, 451
    pediatric meningitis/sepsis, 522t, 523t
    septicemia in neonates, 461
  with nafcillin, in treatment of pediatric suppurative arthritis, 516t
  recommendations and adverse reactions to, 412
  in treatment of
    epiglottitis, 582
      in pediatrics, 520t
    gonococcal cervicitis, 476, 477
    gonococcal urethritis, 476, 477
    neonatal gonococcal conjunctivitis, 519t
    pediatric bacterial pneumonia, 525t
    pediatric bacterial tracheitis, 527t
    pediatric meningitis/sepsis, 522t, 523t
    pediatric pneumonia, 463
    pediatric purulent nasopharyngitis/sinusitis, 527t
    pediatric pyelonephritis, 526t
    pediatric uvulitis, 527t
    pneumonia in adults, 463
    septicemia in nonimmunocompromised children, 461
Cefotetan
  with doxycycline, in treatment of PID, 472t, 477
  recommendations and adverse reactions to, 411
  in treatment of
    abdominal traumas, 566t
    penetrating, 450, 451
    chest trauma, 566t
Cefoxitin
  with doxycycline, in treatment of
    PID, 447, 447t, 472t, 477
    salpingitis, 447, 447t
  with erythromycin, in treatment of
    PID, 447, 447t
    salpingitis, 447, 447t

Cefoxitin—*Continued*
  with probenecid and azithromycin, in treatment of PID, 471*t*
  recommendations and adverse reactions to, 411
  in treatment of
    abdominal traumas, penetrating, 450, 451
    bacterial conjunctivitis, 587
    chest traumas, 566*t*
    pneumonia in high risk aspiration adults, 464
Cefpodoxime
  dosing frequencies for, 403*t*
  proxetil in treatment of
    gonorrhea, 448*t*, 449
    infectious diseases, 436*t*
  recommendations and adverse reactions to, 413
  in treatment of pharyngitis, group A β-hemolytic streptococcus, 458
Cefprozil
  dosing frequencies for, 403*t*
  recommendations and adverse reactions to, 411, 412
  in treatment of
    infectious diseases, 436*t*
    pharyngitis, group A β-hemolytic streptococcus, 458
Ceftazidime
  with ampicillin, in treatment of, pediatric acute mastoiditis, 522t
  recommendations and adverse reactions to, 412, 413
  in treatment of malignant otitis externa, 569
  in treatment of meningitis in neurosurgery/trauma patients, 451
Ceftin (cefuroxime axetil), 524*t*
Ceftizoxime
  recommendations and adverse reactions to, 412
  in treatment of
    gonococcal cervicitis, 476, 477
    gonococcal urethritis, 476, 477
Ceftriaxone
  with ampicillin, in treatment of
    bacterial meningitis
      in elderly, 531*t*
      meningitis in neonates, 451
      septicemia in neonates, 461
  with erythromycin, in treatment of pneumonia in elderly, 530*t*
  with probenecid, in treatment of, gonococcal pharyngitis, 477
  recommendations and adverse reactions to, 412
  with tobramycin, in treatment of pneumonia in elderly, 530*t*
  with tobramycin and metronidazole, in treatment of nonimmunocompromised elderly patients, 532*t*
  in treatment of
    acute epiglottitis, 459
    anorectal gonorrhea, 477
    antibiotic-resistant gonorrhea, 476
    bacteremia in pediatrics, 516*t*, 517*t*
    bacterial conjunctivitis, 587
    bacterial pneumonia in pediatrics, 525*t*
    bacterial tracheitis in pediatrics, 527*t*
    cervical gonorrhea, 471*t*
    chancroid, 479, 480
    disseminated gonococcal infections, 478
    epiglottitis, 582
      in pediatrics, 520*t*
    gonococcal cervicitis, 476, 477
    gonococcal urethritis, 476, 477
    gonorrhea, 448*t*, 449
    gun shot wounds, 559
    meningitis, 451
      in alcoholic patients, 451
      in elderly, 451
      in patients with CSF leak, 451
      pediatric, 451
    meningitis/sepsis in pediatrics, 522*t*, 523*t*
    neonatal gonococcal conjunctivitis, 518*t*, 519*t*
    PID, 471*t*, 477, 478
    pneumonia in adults, 463
    pneumonia in children, 463
    preseptal/buccal cellulitis in pediatrics, 517*t*
    purulent nasopharyngitis/sinusitis in pediatrics, 527*t*
    pyelonephritis in elderly, 530*t*
    rectal gonorrhea, 471*t*
    salmonellosis, *324,* 327
    septicemia in nonimmunocompromised children, 461
    urinary tract infections in elderly, 531*t*
    uvulitis in pediatrics, 527*t*
  in treatment of chancroid, 448*t*, 449
Cefuroxime
  with azithromycin, in treatment of pneumonia in elderly, 530*t*
  with erythromycin, in treatment of pneumonia in elderly, 530*t*
  recommendations and adverse reactions to, 411
  in treatment of
    acute epiglottitis, 459
    dacryocystitis, 590
    orbital cellulitis, 591
    otitis media, 572
    pediatric acute mastoiditis, 522*t*
    pediatric bacterial pneumonia, 525*t*
    pediatric bacterial tracheitis, 527*t*
    pediatric epiglottitis, 520*t*
    pediatric preseptal/buccal cellulitis, 517*t*
    pediatric purulent nasopharyngitis/sinusitis, 527*t*
    pediatric retropharyngeal and peritonsillar abscesses, 516*t*
    pediatric suppurative arthritis, 516*t*
    pediatric uvulitis, 527*t*
    periorbital cellulitis, 590
    pharyngitis, group A β-hemolytic streptococcus, 458
    pneumonia in elderly, 530*t*
    pneumonia in children, 463
    septicemia in nonimmunocompromised children, 461
Cefuroxime axetil
  dosing frequencies for, 403*t*
  recommendations and adverse reactions to, 411, 412
  in treatment of
    disseminated gonococcal infections, 478
    gonorrhea, 448*t*, 449
    infectious diseases, 436*t*
    otitis media in pediatrics, 524*t*
    pharyngitis, 581
      in pediatrics, 524*t*
Cefzil; *see* Cefprozil
Cellulitis
  antimicrobial therapy for, in pediatrics, 517*t*
  clostridial anaerobic, diagnosis and treatment of, 464, 465

Index 703

diagnosis and treatment of, 438–441
gram-negative synergistic necrotizing, diagnosis and treatment of, 465, 466, 467
periorbital
  definition of, 590
  diagnosis and treatment of, 590
treatment of, 438t, 439
Centers for Disease Control (CDC), 317, 319
Centrax (prazepam), 680
Cephalexin
  dosing frequencies for, 403t
  recommendations and adverse reactions to, 410
  in treatment
    of parotitis, 576, 577
  in treatment of
    acute lymphadenitis in pediatrics, 521t
    dacryoadenitis, 590
    dacryocystitis, 590
    furunculosis, 570
    impetigo and pyoderma in pediatrics, 521t
    infectious diseases, 436t
    otitis externa, 569
    pharyngitis, 581
      in pediatrics, 524t
    posterior epistaxis, 580
Cephalosporins
  with aminoglycosides, in treatment of septicemia in nonimmunocompromised adults, 461
  with aztreonam, in treatment of septicemia in elderly, 461
  FDA pregnancy safety classification of, 665t
  in lactation, 673
  recommendations and adverse reactions to, 409–413
  in treatment of
    abscesses, 438t
    acute epiglottitis, 459
    acute sinusitis, 442t, 443
    antibiotic-resistant gonorrhea, 476
    bacterial pneumonia in pediatrics, 525t
    carbuncles, 438t, 439
    cellulitis, 438t, 439
    chronic bronchitis, 443, 444t
    community-acquired pneumonia, 443, 444, 444t
    cystitis, 445, 445t, 446
    erysipelas, 439
    eyelid abscesses, 441
    facial cellulitis in pediatrics, 438t, 439
    furunculosis, 438t
    gonococcal cervicitis, 476, 477
    gonococcal urethritis, 476, 477
    herpes zoster, 438t, 440
    impetigo, 438, 438t, 439
    infectious diseases, 436t
    meningitis
      in alcoholic patients, 451
      in elderly, 451
      in pediatrics, 451
    meningitis/sepsis in pediatrics, 522t, 523t
    open fractures, 450
    otitis externa, 569
    otitis media, 442, 442t
    periorbital cellulitis, 590
    pharyngitis, 443, 581, 582
      group A β-hemolytic streptococcus, 458
      in pediatrics, 524t
    pneumonia in pediatrics, 463
    pneumonia in adults, 463

preseptal/buccal cellulitis in pediatrics, 517t
pyelonephritis, 445, 445t, 446
  in pediatrics, 526t
retropharyngeal and peritonsillar abscesses in pediatrics, 516t
with vancomycin, in treatment of pneumonia in immunocompromised adults, 463
Cephalothin, 641
Cephradine
  dosing frequencies for, 403t
  recommendations and adverse reactions to, 410
  in treatment of, acute lymphadenitis in pediatrics, 521t
  infectious diseases, 436t
  pharyngitis, in pediatrics, 524t
Cerebellar hemorrhages, 270
Cerebellopontine-angle tumors, 575
Cerebral edema, 260
Cerebrovascular disease
  intracranial hemorrhages, treatment of, 262–265, 264
  thromboembolic strokes, treatment of, 261
  transient ischemic attacks (TIAs), treatment of, 260
Cerumen, 570
Cerumenex, 570
Cerumenolytics, 570
Cervicitis
  diagnosis and treatment of, 446
  gonococcal
    diagnosis and treatment of, 471t, 476, 477
    during pregnancy, treatment of, 471t, 476, 477
Chalazion
  definition of, 589
  diagnosis and treatment of, 441, 589
Chancroid, 448t, 449, 473t, 479, 480
Charcoal, in treatment of
  botulism, 320
  fish poisonings, 343t
  salicylates ingestions, 365
Chemical conjunctivitis, 588
Chemical exposure, 594t
Chemoprophylaxis, 573
Chenodiol, 306
Chest injuries, 557, 558, 558t, 559, 565t
Chest pain, 122t, 125
Chest wall injuries, 95t
CHF; *see* Congestive heart failure
Chickenpox
  antimicrobial therapy for, in pediatrics, 518t
  diagnosis and treatment of, 546, 547
Chlamydia trachomatis
  as cause of
    neonatal conjunctivitis, 518t, 519t, 588
    pediatric pneumonia, 525t
  treatment of, 448t, 449
Chloral hydrate
  FDA pregnancy safety classification of, 670t
  in lactation, 680
Chloramphenicol
  adverse drug interactions, with anticoagulants, 56t
  with ampicillin, in treatment of epiglottitis, 582
  FDA pregnancy safety classification of, 666t
  in lactation, 674
  with nafcillin, in treatment of orbital cellulitis, 591
  ophthalmologic uses of, 606
  precautions for use, in pregnancy, 404
  recommendations and adverse reactions to, 421
  in treatment of

Chloramphenicol—*Continued*
  acute epiglottitis, 459
  bacterial conjunctivitis, 586, 587*t*
  clostridial myonecrosis, 468
  granuloma inguinale (donovanosis), 480
  meningitis
    in adults, 451
    in alcoholic patients, 451
    in elderly, 451
    in patients with CSF leak, 451
    in pediatrics, 451
  mushroom poisoning, 335
  periorbital cellulitis, 590
  salmonellosis, *324,* 327
  seborrheic dermatitis, 616
  septic arthritis, 641
  vibrio infections, 467
Chlordiazepoxide, 670*t*
Chlorhexidine gluconate, 578
Chlorinated insecticides, 56*t*
Chlorine gas, 182*t*
Chlorisondamine, 33*t*
Chloroquine
  FDA pregnancy safety classification of, 666*t*
  in lactation, 673
  precautions for use, in pregnancy, 405
Chloroquine HCl, 429
Chlorothiazide (Diuril), 677
Chlorpheniramine, 667*t*
Chlorpromazine
  as alternative for drug seekers with migraines, 142, 142*t*
  FDA pregnancy safety classification of, 671*t*
  in lactation, 680
  in parenteral treatment of
    acute migraine headaches, 98
    migraine, cluster, and tension headaches, 106*t*, 117
    pain in migraine headaches, 123*t*, 127, 128
  precautions/contraindications for the elderly, 55*t*
Chlorpropamide
  dosage, duration, and effects of, 44*t*
  indicators of possible toxicity, 13*t*
Chlorprothixene
  FDA pregnancy safety classification of, 671*t*
  in lactation, 680
Chlorthalidone (Hygroton), 677
Chlorzoxazone
  FDA pregnancy safety classification of, 671*t*
  in treatment of pain, 86, 87*t*
Cholecystitis, 305–307
  definition of, 305
  diagnosis and treatment of, 305, 306
Cholecystograms, in diagnosis
  of biliary colic, 306
  of cholelithiasis, 306
Cholelithiasis, 306
Cholera, 329, 330
Cholera vaccines, 670*t*
Cholestyramine
  adverse drug interactions, with anticoagulants, 56*t*
  FDA pregnancy safety classification of, 668*t*
Choline magnesium trisalicylate, 81*t*
Cholinergic crisis, 274
Cholinergics, 669*t*
Chondrocalcinosis, 643
Christmas tree rash; *see* Pityriasis rosea
Chronic obstructive pulmonary disease (COPD), 283–285

Cibenzoline, 216
Cimetidine
  adverse drug interactions, 56*t*
  FDA pregnancy safety classification of, 666*t*
  in lactation, 679
  in treatment of
    asthma, 281
    fish poisonings, 344*t*
    food poisonings, staphylococcal, 331
    gastrointestinal bleeding, 300
    GERD, 298, 298*t*
Ciprofloxacin
  contraindications of
    in pregnancy, 404
  dosing frequencies for, 403*t*
  FDA pregnancy safety classification of, 665*t*
  in lactation, 674
  with metronidazole, in treatment of diverticulitis in elderly, 531*t*
  recommendations and adverse reactions to, 415
  in treatment of
    acute prostatitis, 446
    asthma, 281
    campylobacter enteritis, *324,* 330
    cervical gonorrhea, 471*t*
    chancroid, 448*t*, 449, 479, 480
    cholera, *324,* 330
    conjunctivitis, 441, 589
    epididymo-orchitis, 445*t*, 446
    Escherichia coli, enteropathic (traveler's diarrhea), *324,* 328
    gonococcal cervicitis, 476, 477
    gonococcal urethritis, 476, 477
    gonorrhea, 448*t*, 449
    HIV related
      bacterial diarrhea, 499
      Mycobacterium avium, 509
      tuberculosis, 508
    infectious diseases, 437*t*
    lower urinary tract infections in elderly, 530*t*
    malignant otitis externa, 569
    otitis externa, 569
    otitis malignant externa, 442
    rectal gonorrhea, 471*t*
    salmonellosis, *324,* 327
    shigellosis, 322, 324*t*
Circumcorneal flush, 591
Cisapride, 298, 298*t*
Cisplatin, 575
Citrucel (methylcellulose), 679
Claforan; *see* Cefotaxime
Clanthromycin, 403*t*
Clarithromycin
  recommendations and adverse reactions to, 421
  with TMP/SMX, in treatment of pneumonia in adults, 463
  in treatment of
    acute sinusitis, 442*t*, 443
    cellulitis, 439
    chronic bronchitis, 443, 444*t*
    community-acquired pneumonia, 443, 444, 444*t*
    erysipelas, 439
    HIV related
      encephalitis, 493
      focal intracerebral lesions, 493
      Mycobacterium avium, 509
      toxoplasmosis, 493
    infectious diseases, 437*t*

otitis media, 442, 442*t*
pneumonia, 464
Clemastine
FDA pregnancy safety classification of, 666*t*
in lactation, 677
Clindamycin
with aminoglycosides, in treatment of penetrating abdominal traumas, 450, 451
ampicillin and aminoglycosides, in treatment of Fournier's Gangrene, 466
gram-negative synergistic necrotizing cellulitis, 466
FDA pregnancy safety classification of, 666*t*
with gentamicin, in treatment of PID, 472*t*, 477
in lactation, 674
with ofloxacin, in treatment of
PID, 447, 447*t*, 471*t*
salpingitis, 447, 447*t*
with penicillin, in treatment of
dental abscesses, 443
orofacial infections, 443
precautions for use, in pregnancy, 404
recommendations and adverse reactions to, 419
with tetracycline, in treatment of
animal bites, 438*t*, 439, 440
human bites, 439, 440
with tobramycin, in treatment of diverticulitis in elderly, 531*t*
in treatment of
abdominal trauma, 566*t*
abscesses, 438*t*
acute lymphadenitis in pediatrics, 521*t*
animal bites, 439, 440
aspiration pneumonia, 444, 444*t*, 445
carbuncles, 438*t*, 439
cellulitis, 438*t*, 439
chronic sinusitis, 443
clostridial anaerobic cellulitis, 465
clostridial myonecrosis, 468
erysipelas, 439
furunculosis, 438*t*, 439
gram-negative synergistic necrotizing cellulitis, 465
HIV related
encephalitis, 493
focal intracerebral lesions, 493
toxoplasmosis, 493
HIV related pneumocystis pneumonia, 505
human bites, 438*t*
impetigo, 438, 438*t*, 439
impetigo and pyoderma in pediatrics, 521*t*
infectious diseases, 437*t*
lung abscesses, 444, 444*t*, 445
necrotizing fasciitis, 466
odontogenic infections, 443
pneumonia in high risk aspiration adults, 464
preseptal/buccal cellulitis in pediatrics, 517*t*
retropharyngeal and peritonsillar abscesses in pediatrics, 516*t*
vaginitis, 446
vaginal suppositories, in treatment of bacterial vaginitis, 481
Clioquinol, 569
Clitocybe/inocybe, 182*t*, 185, 186
Clobetasol propionate, 614*t*
Clocortolone, 613*t*
Clofazimine, 509
Clonazepam
FDA pregnancy safety classification of, 668*t*
in lactation, 675
in treatment of
acute labyrinthitis, 270*t*
panic disorders, 663
positional vertigo, 269, 270*t*
Clonidine
as cause of orthostatic hypotension, 33*t*
drug seekers of, 133
FDA pregnancy safety classification of, 668*t*
in lactation, 676
side effects of, 31*t*
Clorazepate dipotassium, 132
Clostridial myonecrosis, 467, 468
Clostridium, 591
Clostridium botulinum, 317, 318
Clostridium perfringens, 328
Clotrimazole
FDA pregnancy safety classification of, 665*t*
in treatment of
candidal vaginitis, 446, 447*t*, 472*t*, 481
moniliasis, 631, 632
tinea corporis, 438*t*, 440, 441
tinea cruris, 440, 441
tinea pedis, 440, 441
vaginitis during pregnancy, 446, 447*t*
troche, in treatment of HIV related candidiasis, 496
vaginal suppositories, in treatment of trichomoniasis vaginitis, 480
Clotting disorders, 263
Cloxacillin, in treatment of
furunculosis, 570
infectious diseases, 436*t*
orbital cellulitis, 591
otitis externa, 569
parotitis, 576
toxic epidermal necrolysis (TEN), 634
Cluster headaches
definition of, 265
diagnosis and treatment of, 265, 266, 267t, 269
CNS infections, 257
Cocaine
acute psychosis and, 658
as cause of hyperthermia, 690*t*
in lactation, 682
in treatment of
epistaxis, 579
vascular headaches, 90
violent behavior in psychiatric emergencies and, 649, 653
Codeine, 76
with acetaminophen
street price of, 133*t*
in treatment of otitis externa, 569
with butalbital and acetylsalicylic acid (ASA), drug seekers of, 132
drug seekers of, 132
FDA pregnancy safety classification of, 665*t*
with fiorinal
drug seekers feigning migraines for, 135*t*
street price of, 133*t*
in lactation, 672
oral narcotic equivalency table, 74*t*
in parenteral treatment of pain, adverse drug reactions and, 102
parenteral/oral narcotic equivalency index, 101*t*
plasma half lives of, 75*t*
precautions/contraindications for the elderly, 76
in treatment of

Codeine—*Continued*
  otitis media, 573
  septic arthritis, 641
Colace (docusate sodium), 679
Colchicine
  breast feeding and, 681
  in lactation, 681
  in treatment of
    acute gout, 643
    pseudogout, 643
Cold preparations
  breast feeding and, 677
  in lactation, 677
Colistin, 568
Colitis, 135*t*
Collagen disorders, 594*t*
Collagen vascular disease, 594*t*
Colonoscopy, 300
Colorectal disease, 499, 500
Comas
  Glasgow coma scale, use in psychiatric emergencies of, 651
  in hyperthermia, 692
  trauma and, 554
COME (chronic otitis media with effusion), 573
Compazine (prochlorperazine)
  as alternative for drug seekers with migraines, 142, 142*t*
  in treatment of
    acute labyrinthitis, 269, 270*t*
    hepatitis, 308
Congestive cardiomyopathy, 489
Congestive heart failure (CHF)
  diagnosis and treatment of, 164–166
  stroke and, 261
Conjunctivitis
  acute hemorrhagic, diagnosis of, 588
  allergic
    causes of, 585
    diagnosis and treatment of, 585
  bacterial
    causes of, 586, 587
    diagnosis and treatment of, 586, 587, 587*t*
  diagnosis and treatment of, 441, 588, 589
  HIV related, diagnosis and treatment of, 502
  neonatal
    antimicrobial therapy for, 518*t*, 519*t*
    chemical, 588
    microbial, 588
  as symptom of
    allergies, 594*t*
    chemical exposure, 594t
    infections, 594*t*
  viral
    acute hemorrhagic conjunctivitis, 588
    diagnosis of, 587, 588
    herpes simplex virus (HSV), 588
Contact dermatitis, 622, 623
Controlled Substances Act, 143
COPD; *see* Chronic obstructive pulmonary disease
Copper, 182*t*, 188
Cordarone (amiodarone), 675
Corgard (nadolol), 676
Corneal abrasions, 592
Corneal microsporidiosis, 502
Corneal ulceration, 519*t*
Corneal ulcers, 595*t*, 596
Corticosteroids, 613, 614*t*
  in lactation, 678
  ophthalmologic uses of, adverse effects of, 605
  in treatment of
    aphthous stomatitis, 578
    asthma, 277*t*–279*t*, 279–282
    bronchiolitis, in pediatrics, 517*t*
    contact dermatitis, 623
    COPD, 284
    eczema, 612, 613, 614*t*
    HIV related
      encephalitis, 493
      focal intracerebral lesions, 493
      toxoplasmosis, 493
    insect bites, 624
    lichen planus, 616
    meningitis/sepsis, in pediatrics, 522*t*, 523*t*
    myasthenia gravis, 273
    otitis externa, 568
    parapsoriasis, 618
    pericarditis, 96*t*
    psoriasis vulgaris, 617, 618
    rheumatoid arthritis, in pediatrics, 638
    scabies, 629
    seborrheic dermatitis, 616
Corticotropin, 669*t*
Cortisone, 669*t*
Cortisporin Otic Solution, 568
Cortisporin Otic Suspension, 568
Costochondritis (Tietze syndrome), 122*t*, 126
Cotrimoxazole, 480
Cough syrups
  analgesic, drug seekers of, 132
  with dihydrocodone, drug seekers feigning bronchitis for, 135*t*
  with hydromorphone, street price of, 133*t*
Coumadin (warfarin) 83, 674
Coumarin
  derivatives of, antidote for, 182*t*, 200, 201
  FDA pregnancy safety classification of, 666*t*
Cramps, night; *see* Night cramps
Cricopharyngeus muscle, 294
Cromolyn sodium, 282, 283
Crotamiton, 438*t*, 441, 630
Croup (viral laryngotracheobronchitis), 519*t*
Cryotherapy, 495, 496
Cryptococcal meningitis, 489–491
CS; *see* Cardiogenic shock (CS)
CT scans, in diagnosis of
  appendicitis, 309
  pancreatitis, 304
Curettage, 495, 496
Cushing's syndrome, 658
Cutaneous CMV, 496
Cyanide poisoning
  antidote for, 182*t*, 189, 197, 198
  diagnosis and treatment of, 343*t*
Cycad poisoning, 343*t*
Cyclic antidepressants, 33*t*
Cyclizine, 666*t*
Cyclobenzamine, in treatment of pain, 88
  in fibromyalgia, 95*t*
Cyclobenzaprine
  FDA pregnancy safety classification of, 671*t*
  in treatment of
    chronic neuralgias, 96*t*
    muscle contraction headaches, 267*t*
    pain, 85, 86, 87*t*
Cyclogyl, 592
Cyclophosphamide, in treatment of
  rheumatoid arthritis, 636

Index 707

vasculitis, 646
Cycloplegics
  ophthalmologic uses of, adverse effects of, 606
  in treatment of corneal abrasions in uveitis, 592
Cycloserine (Seromycin), 674
Cyclosporin, 618
Cystitis, 445, 445t, 446
Cysts, 594t
Cytomegalovirus, 525t
Cytomel (liothyronine), 678
Cytotoxins, 636, 640
  in treatment of rheumatoid arthritis, 636
    pediatric, 638
Cytriaxone
  with doxycycline, in treatment of
    PID, 447, 447t
    salpingitis, 447, 447t
  with erythromycin, in treatment of
    PID, 447, 447t
    salpingitis, 447, 447t

D

Dacriose, 592
Dacryoadenitis
  causes of, 589, 590
  definition of, 589
  diagnosis and treatment of, 589, 590
Dacryocystitis, 590
Dandruff shampoos, 496
Dapsone
  in lactation, 674
  in treatment of, HIV related
    encephalitis, 493
    focal intracerebral lesions, 493
    toxoplasmosis, 493
Dapsone/TMP, 505
Daranide (dichlorphenamide), 600t
Daraprim; see Pyrimethamine
Darvon (propoxyphene), 672
Decamethonium, 671t
Decongestants
  in lactation, 677
  in treatment of barotitis, 571
Deferoxamine
  antidotal action of, 182t, 188
  in treatment of favism, 343t
Dehydroemetine/emetine, 404
Delirium
  causes in the elderly patient of, 650t, 651
  diagnosis of, 651
Demerol (meperidine)
  in lactation, 672
  in treatment of migraines, 267t
Dendritic keratitis; see Herpes simplex keratitis, necrotizing
Dental abscesses, 443
Dental caries, drug seekers feigning, 136, 136t
  diagnosis of, 139
Dental disease, 594t
Dental pain, 95t
Depakene (valproic acid)
  in lactation, 675
  in treatment of
    new onset seizures, 257t
    petit mal status epilepticus, 259
    recurrent seizures, 258t
Depakote (valproic acid)
  in lactation, 675
  in treatment of
    new onset seizures, 257t
    petit mal status epilepticus, 259
    recurrent seizures, 258t
Depo-Medrol, 643
Dermal bacillary angiomatosis, 494
Dermatologic disorders
  contact dermatitis, 622, 623
  diagnosis and treatment of, 609–612, 613, 614t, 615–631, 632t, 633, 634
  ectoparasitic infestations, 625–630
  eczema, 609–612, 613, 614t, 615
  erythema multiforme (EM), 632t, 633
  insect bites, 623, 624
  lichen planus, 616, 617
  miliaria, 624, 625
  moniliasis, 630, 632
  parapsoriasis, 618
  pityriasis rosea, 621, 622
  psoriasis vulgaris, 617, 618
  seborrheic dermatitis, 615, 616
  Stevens-Johnson syndrome, 632
  syphilis, 618, 619
  tinea infections, 620, 621
  toxic epidermal necrolysis (TEN), 633, 634
Dermatophytoses
  diagnosis and treatment of, 440, 441, 620, 621
  tinea corporis, 440
  tinea cruris, 440
  tinea pedis, 440
  tinea versicolor, 440, 441
Desipramine
  FDA pregnancy safety classification of, 669t
  in lactation, 680
Desmopressin, 669t
Desonide, 613t
Desoximetasone, 613t
Desyrel (trazodone), 680
Dexamethasone
  FDA pregnancy safety classification of, 669t
  in treatment of
    bacterial pneumonia in pediatrics, 525t
    croup in pediatrics, 519t
    dermatologic disorders, 613t
    hyperthyroidism, 392
    increased intracranial pressure from brain tumors, 271
    meningitis, 451
    meningitis/sepsis in pediatrics, 522t, 523t
    spinal cord compression, 272
Dextrose
  antidotal action of, 182t, 190
  with saline solution in treatment of migraines, 268
  in treatment of
    grand mal status epilepticus, 258
    hepatitis, 308
Dextrose solutions, 393
Dextrothyroxine, 668t
DGI; see disseminated gonococcal infections
DHE; see Dihydroergotamine
Diabetes mellitus, 593, 594t
Diagnostic agents, 681
Diagnostic imaging, 122t
Dialysis, in treatment of
  hypercalcemia, 383
  hyperkalemia, 380
Diamox (acetazolamide)
  in lactation, 681
  in treatment of glaucoma, 598, 599t
    adverse reactions to, 607

Diamox (acetazolamide)—*Continued*
  contraindications to, 599*t*
Diarrhea
  antibiotic-associated, diagnosis and treatment of, 450
  bacterial, HIV related, diagnosis and treatment of, 498, 499
  diagnosis and treatment of, 450
  HIV related, diagnosis and treatment of, 498, 499
  parasitic, HIV related, diagnosis and treatment of, 498, 499
  symptomatic, HIV related, diagnosis and treatment of, 499
Diascorism, 343*t*
Diatrizoate (Hypaque), 681
Diazepam
  anxiolytic effects on the elderly, 48*t*
  drug seekers of, 132
  FDA pregnancy safety classification of, 670*t*
  in lactation, 680
  in parenteral treatment of pain, 104*t*, 117, 118
    in cardioversion, 122*t*
    in diagnostic imaging, 122*t*
    painful procedures, 123*t*, 127, 128
  street price of, 133*t*
  in treatment of
    acute agitation, 272
    acute labyrinthitis, 270*t*
    central vertigo, 575
    grand mal status epilepticus, 258, 259
    side effects of, 258, 259
    lichen planus, 616
    muscle contraction headaches, 267*t*, 268
    pain, 87*t*
    petit mal status epilepticus, 259
    positional vertigo, 269, 270*t*
    violent behavior, 656
Diazoxide
  adverse drug interactions with anticoagulants, 56*t*
  antidotal action of, 182*t*, 190
  FDA pregnancy safety classification of, 668*t*
Dichlorphenamide (Daranide), 600*t*
Diclofenac, 81*t*, 83
Dicloxacillin
  recommendations and adverse reactions to, 409
  in treatment of
    acute lymphadenitis in pediatrics, 521*t*
    carbuncles, 439
    cellulitis, 439
    dacryoadenitis, 590
    dacryocystitis, 590
    erysipelas, 439
    HIV related bacterial folliculitis, 494
    impetigo, 438, 439
    impetigo and pyoderma in pediatrics, 521*t*
    infectious diseases, 436*t*
    ulcerative blepharitis, 589
Dicyclomine 667*t*
Didanosine (DDI), 488
Dideoxycytidine (Zalcitabine DDC), 488, 489
Dienestrol, 677
Diethylcarbamazine, 432
Diffuse esophageal, 122*t*, 126
Diflorasone diacetate, 613*t*
Diflucan; *see* Fluconazole
Digoxin
  compounds of, FDA pregnancy safety classification of, 668*t*

immune FAB (Digibind), antidotal action of, 182*t*, 190, 191
  indicators of possible toxicity, 13*t*
  in lactation, 675
  in treatment of
    atrial fibrillation, pediatric, *251*
    atrial flutter, pediatric, *251*
    cardiac arrest, 222
    paroxysmal supraventricular tachycardia (PSVT), *239*
    Wolff-Parkinson-White syndrome (WPW), pediatric, *248*
Dihydrocodone, in cough syrups
  drug seekers feigning bronchitis for, 135*t*
  drug seekers of, 132
Dihydroergotamine (DHE) in parenteral treatment of
  migraine, cluster and tension headaches, recommendations and adverse reactions of, 105*t*, 116
  migraine headaches, 123*t*, 127, 128
Dihydroergotamine (DHE-45), 267*t*, 268
Dihydromorphone, 135*t*
Diiodohydroxyquin, 322
Dilanoxide furoate, 499
Dilantin (phenytoin)
  in lactation, 675
  in treatment of
    new onset seizures, 256, 257*t*
      side effects of, 256
    recurrent seizures, 258*t*
    seizures with brain tumors, 271
Dilor (dyphylline), 676
Diltiazem
  FDA pregnancy safety classification of, 668*t*
  in lactation, 676
  in treatment of
    atrial fibrillation, 235
    atrial flutter, 235
    paroxysmal supraventricular tachycardia (PSVT), 239
Dimenhydrinate
  FDA pregnancy safety classification of, 666*t*
  in treatment of
    acute labyrinthitis, 270*t*
    central vertigo, 575
Dimercaprol (BAL), 182*t*, 188
Dimercaptosuccinic acid (DMSA), 182*t*, 188, 189
Dipentum (olsalazine), 679
Diphenhydramine
  antidotal action of, 182*t*, 191
  FDA pregnancy safety classification of, 666*t*, 667*t*
  with Maalox, in treatment of aphthous stomatitis, 578
  in treatment of
    acute labyrinthitis, 269, 270*t*
    allergic conjunctivitis, 585
    dystonic drug reactions, 273
Diphenhydramine (Benadryl), 308
Diphenoxylate
  with atropine, in lactation, 678
  FDA pregnancy safety classification of, 666*t*
  in treatment of HIV related parasitic diarrhea, 499
Diphtheria
  tetanus vaccines, FDA pregnancy safety classification of, 670*t*
  tetanus/diphtheria/and pertussis, immunization schedule for, 534*t*, 535*t*

Dipivefrin HCI (Propine), 600t
Diplopia, 594t
Dipyridamole, 56t
Disease-modifying antirheumatic drugs (DMARDs), 636
Disopyramide, 208, 209
Disopyramide (Norpace), 675
Disseminated gonococcal infections, 478
Disulfiram, 56t
Diuretics
  in antihypertensive treatment, 36t
  effects on coexisting disease of, 32t
  effects on metabolic disorders of, 32t
  breast feeding and, 677
  as cause of hyperthermia, 689
  FDA pregnancy safety classification of, 669t
  in lactation, 677
Diuril (chlorothiazide), in lactation, 677
DMSA; see Dimercaptosuccinic acid (DMSA)
DNA vaccines, recombinant, 307
Dobutamine
  FDA pregnancy safety classification of, 671t
  in treatment of
    acute renal failure, 399
    congestive heart failure/cardiogenic shock, precautions with, 165
    hyponatremia, 373
    lactic acidosis, 363
Docusate sodium (DSS, Colace), 679
Dopamine
  FDA pregnancy safety classification of, 671t
  in treatment of
    acute renal failure, 399
    atrioventricular blocks, *242, 243*
    bradycardias, 168
    cardiac arrest, 221
    congestive heart failure/cardiogenic shock, precautions with, 165
    lactic acidosis, contraindications of, 363
    sinus bradycardia, *242, 243*
Doral (quazepam), 680
Doxazosin
  adverse side effects of, 31t
  in treatment of pheochromocytoma, 395
Doxepin
  FDA pregnancy safety classification of, 669t
  in lactation, 680
Doxycycline
  with cefotetan, in treatment of PID, 472t, 477
  with cefoxitin, in treatment of
    PID, 447, 447t, 472t, 477
    salpingitis, 447, 447t
  with ceftazidime, in treatment of vibrio infections, 467
  with cytriaxone, in treatment of
    PID, 447, 447t
    salpingitis, 447, 447t
  dosing frequencies for, 403t
  in treatment of
    acute nongonococcal urethritis, 478
    angiokeratoma, 494
    Chlamydia trachomatis, 448t, 449
    chronic bronchitis, 443
    cystitis, 445, 445t, 446
    Escherichia coli, enteropathic, *324,* 327
    gonococcal cervicitis, 471t, 476, 477
    gonococcal urethritis, 471t, 476, 477
    HIV related dermal bacillary angiomatosis, 494
    infectious diseases, 437t
    Kaposi's Sarcoma, 494
    latent syphilis, 448
    lymphogranuloma venereum, 448t, 449, 471t, 478, 479
    nongonococcal urethritis, 478
    pharyngitis
      secondary to c. pneumonia, 458
      secondary to mycoplasma pneumonia, 458
    PID, 471t, 477, 478
    pneumonia during pregnancy, 464
    pyogenic granuloma, 494
    simple angioma, 494
    syphilis, 448, 473t, 479
D-Penicillamine
  antidotal action of, 182t, 187, 188, 189
  in treatment of rheumatoid arthritis, pediatric, 638
Dramamine (dimenhydrinate), 270t
Droperidol
  FDA pregnancy safety classification of, 666t, 671t
  in treatment of hepatitis, 308
Drug addicts
  confrontation of, 142, 143
  definition of, 133, 134t
Drug combinations, in treatment of
  atrial fibrillation, 235
  atrial flutter, 235
Drug seekers, 131–143
  confrontation of, 142, 143
  definition of, 131
  detection of, in emergency rooms, 131
    methods of, 131
    of prescription drugs, 131, 132, 133, 134, 134t
      controlled
        amphetamine-like drugs, 132
        barbiturates, 132
        benzodiazepines, 132
        narcotics, 132
    diagnosis of, 138–141
      through history, 138, 138t, 139, 140
      through laboratory tests, 139, 140
      through physical examination, 139
    diseases feigned by, ςt, 135, 136, 136t
      with flawed objective tests, 136, 136t
    drug addiction confession of, in emergency rooms, 138
    emergency room policies for, 141–143
    noncontrolled
      β-blockers, 132
      clonidine, 133
      NSAIDs, 133
    parent and child scams of, in emergency rooms, 137
    prescription forgeries of, 138
    psychologic tactics of, in emergency rooms, 136, 137
    techniques of, 134–138
    types of, 133, 134, 134t
      drug addicts, 133, 134t
      entrepreneurial, 133, 134, 134t
      professional patients, 133, 134, 134t
  withdrawal symptoms of, 143
Dry eye syndrome
  diagnosis and treatment of, 595, 595t, 596
  exposure keratopathy, 595t, 596
  eyelid entropion/ectropion, 596
  as symptom of
    collagen disorders, 594t

Dry eye syndrome—*Continued*
   Sjögren's syndrome, 594*t*
   from tranquilizers, 594*t*
DSS (docusate sodium), 679
Dulcolax (bisacodyl), 679
D$_5$W
   in treatment of
      hypernatremia, 375
      methanol ingestions, 364
      nonanion gap metabolic acidosis, 368
D$_5$W1/2NS, 375
D$_5$W1/4NS, 375
Dyphylline (Dilor), 676
Dyscrasias, 594*t*
Dysentery, 450
Dysmenorrhea, 95*t*
Dysrhythmias
   amaurosis fugax as symptom of, 594*t*
   occurring with hypothermia, 687
Dystonic drug reactions
   causes of, 272
   diagnosis and treatment of, 272, 273

E

E. histolytica; see Entamoeba histolytica
Ear, nose, and throat (ENT) emergencies
   treatment of, 567–582
      acute necrotizing ulcerative gingivitis, 578
      aphthous stomatitis, 578
      barotitis, 570, 571
      epiglottis, 582
      epistaxis, 579, 580
      foreign bodies in ear, 577
      furunculosis, 570
      herpes zoster oticus, 569, 570
      herpetic gingivostomatitis, 578, 579
      impacted cerumen, 570
      mastoiditis, 576
      oral candidiasis, 577
      otitis externa, 567–569
      otitis media, 571–573
      otomycosis, 570
      parotitis, 576, 577
      peritonsillar abscess, 580, 581
      pharyngitis, 581, 582
      sinusitis, 575, 576
      vertigo, 573–575
Ear disease, 594*t*
Ear drops, 441, 442, 442*t*
Ear infections, 270; *see also* Otitis media
Ear wicks, 569
Econazole, 631, 632
Econopred Plus, 591, 592
Ectoparasitic infestations
   diagnosis and treatment of, 625–630
   lice, 625–628
   scabies, 628–630
Ectropion, 596
Eczema, 609–612, 613, 614*t*, 615
EDB; *see* Emergency department battery (EDB)
Edrophonium, 249
Edrophonium chloride test, 273
Elavil (amitriptyline), 680
Electrocardiograms (ECG), in diagnosis of
   myasthenia gravis, 273
   new onset seizures, 255
   trauma, 554
Electrocardiography

   hemorrhagic stroke, 147*t*
   myocardial infarction, 146, 147, 147*t*
   pericarditis, 147*t*
   ventricular aneurysm, 147*t*
Electrocautery, 495, 496
Electroencephalograms (EEGs), 255
Elimite, 630
EM; *see* Erythema multiforme (EM)
Emboli, 602, 603
Emergency department battery (EDB), 347, 348
Enalapril
   FDA pregnancy safety classification of, 667*t*
   in lactation, 676
Encainide, 212
Encephalitis
   HIV related, diagnosis and treatment of, 493
   toxoplasma, HIV related
      diagnosis and treatment of, 491–494
      maintenance therapy, 494
      preventative medicine, 494
Encephalopathy, 308 *see also* Wernicke's encephalopathy
Endep (amitriptyline), 680
Endocarditis
   bacterial, HIV related, diagnosis and treatment of, 489
   nonbacterial, HIV related, diagnosis and treatment of, 489
   subacute bacterial, retinal hemorrhages as symptom of, 594*t*
Endocrine abnormalities, 594*t*
Endocrine drugs
   breast feeding and, 677
   in lactation, 677, 678
Endocrine emergencies, 385–400
Endophalmitis, 441
Endorphins, 98
Endoscopy, in treatment of
   acid and alkaline ingestions, 297
   gastrointestinal bleeding, 300
Enemas
   barium
      in diagnosis of appendicitis, 309
      in treatment of
         intussusception, 301
         sigmoid volvulus, 302
   lactulose, in treatment of hepatic encephalopathy, 308
   radiographic contrast, in diagnosis of rectal foreign bodies, 309
Enoxacin
   recommendations and adverse reactions, 416
   in treatment of
      gonorrhea, 448*t*, 449
      infectious diseases, 437*t*
ENT emergencies; *see* Ear, nose, and throat emergencies
Entamoeba histolytica, 324, 328
Enterococcus, 522*t*
Entrepreneurial drug seekers, 133, 134, 134*t*
   techniques of, 134–138
Entropion, 596
Ephedrine, 671*t*
Epididymo-orchitis, 445*t*, 446
Epidural analgesia, 565
Epiglottitis
   acute, diagnosis and treatment of, 458, 459
   antimicrobial therapy for, in pediatrics, 520*t*
   causes of, 582

diagnosis and treatment of, 582
Epilepsy, 575
Epinephrine
  FDA pregnancy safety classification of, 671t
  in lactation, 676
  in treatment of
    asthma, 277t, 278t, 280
    asystole, 167, 229
      pediatric, 247
    atrioventricular blocks, 242, 243
    bradycardias, 168
    cardiac arrest, 219
    croup, in pediatrics, 519t
    glaucoma, 598, 600t
      contraindications to, 600t
    perirectal abscesses, 311
    pulseless electrical activity (PEA), 167, 229
      pediatric, 247
    pulseless ventricular tachycardia (VT), 226
      pediatric, 247
    sinus bradycardia, 242, 243
      pediatric, 252
    ventricular fibrillation (VF), 226
      pediatric, 246
Epistaxis
  anterior, diagnosis and treatment of, 579
  causes of, 579
  diagnosis and treatment of, 579, 580
  posterior, diagnosis and treatment of, 579, 580
Epsom salts (magnesium sulfate), 679
Equine antiserum, 320, 321
Ergomar (ergotamine), 267t, 269
Ergonovine (Ergotrate), 682
Ergostat (ergotamine), 682
Ergot alkaloids, 682
Ergotamine
  in lactation, 682
  tartrate
    in parenteral treatment of acute migraine headaches, 98
    in treatment of
      cluster headaches, 95t
      vascular headaches, 95t
    in treatment of
      cluster headaches, 267t, 269
      migraines, 267t
Ergotism, 343t
Ergotrate (ergonovine), 682
Erysipelas, 438t, 439
Erythema multiforme (EM), 632t, 633
Erythromycin
  with cefoxitin, in treatment of
    PID, 447, 447t
    salpingitis, 447, 447t
  with ceftriaxone, in treatment of pneumonia in elderly, 530t
  with cefuroxime, in treatment of pneumonia in elderly, 530t
  with cytriaxone, in treatment of
    PID, 447, 447t
    salpingitis, 447, 447t
  dosing frequencies for, 403t
  erythromycin ethylsuccinate, 420, 421
  FDA pregnancy safety classification of, 665t
  in lactation, 673
  with quinolone, in treatment of
    diarrhea, 450
    dysentery, 450

recommendations and adverse reactions to, 420, 421
sulfisoxazole, 420, 421
  in treatment of otitis media, 572
with sulfonamides, in treatment of otitis media, 442, 442t
with TMP/SMX, in treatment of pneumonia in adults, 463
in treatment of
  acute necrotizing ulcerative gingivitis, 578
  angiokeratoma, 494
  asthma, 281
  bacterial conjunctivitis, 587
  campylobacter enteritis, 324, 330
  cellulitis, 439
  chancroid, 448t, 449, 479, 480
  Chlamydia trachomatis, 448t, 449
  conjunctivitis, 588, 589
  erysipelas, 439
  gonococcal cervicitis, 471t
    during pregnancy, 471t, 476, 477
  gonococcal urethritis, 471t
  HIV related bacterial diarrhea, 499
  HIV related dermal bacillary angiomatosis, 494
  human bites, 438t, 439, 440
  impetigo, 438, 439
  infectious diseases, 437t
  Kaposi's Sarcoma, 494
  lymphogranuloma venereum, 448t, 449, 471t
  nongonococcal urethritis, 478
  peritonsillar abscesses, 580
  pharyngitis
    group A β-hemolytic streptococcus, 458
    secondary to c. pneumonia, 458
    secondary to mycoplasma pneumonia, 458
  pneumonia, 464
    in elderly, 530t
  pneumonia in infants, 463
  pyogenic granuloma, 494
  salpingitis during pregnancy, 447, 447t
  seborrheic dermatitis, 616
  septic arthritis, 641
  simple angioma, 494
  sinusitis, 576
  syphilis, 448, 448t
  ulcerative (staphylococcal) blepharitis, 589
with trimethoprim/sulfamethoxazole, in treatment of
  diarrhea, 450
  dysentery, 450
Erythromycin estolate
  contraindications of, in pregnancy, 404
  FDA pregnancy safety classification of, 665t
  in treatment of
    bacterial pneumonia, in pediatrics, 525t
    impetigo and pyoderma, in pediatrics, 521t
    mycoplasma infection, in pediatrics, 517t
    neonatal chlamydial conjunctivitis, 518t
    pharyngitis, 581
      in pediatrics, 524t
    uvulitis, in pediatrics, 527t
Erythromycin ethylsuccinate
  with acetyl sulfisoxazole, in treatment of
    otitis media, in pediatrics, 524t
    sinusitis/purulent nasopharyngitis, in pediatrics, 527t
  recommendations and adverse reactions to, 420, 421

Erythromycin ethylsuccinate—*Continued*
  with sulfisoxazole, in treatment of infectious diseases, 436*t*
  in treatment of
    infectious diseases, 437*t*
    neonatal chlamydial conjunctivitis, 518*t*
    pharyngitis, in pediatrics, 524*t*
    uvulitis, in pediatrics, 527*t*
Erythromycin-sulfisoxazole, 525*t*
Erythropoietin therapy, 500, 501
Escherichia coli
  as cause of neonatal conjunctivitis, 588
  enteropathic (traveler's diarrhea), diagnosis and treatment of, *324*, 327, 328
Esidrix (hydrochlorothiazide), 677
Esmolol
  FDA pregnancy safety classification of, 667*t*
  in treatment of
    arrhythmias, 213
    atrial fibrillation, 235
    atrial flutter, 235
    hyperthyroidism, 391
Esmolol hydrochloride, 239
Esophageal foreign bodies
  anatomical location of, 294
  causes of, 294
  diagnosis of, 294, 295
  emergency treatment for, 294–296
Esophagitis
  CMV, HIV related, diagnosis and treatment of, 497
  herpes, HIV related, diagnosis and treatment of, 497
  HIV related, diagnosis and treatment of, 497, 498
  idiopathic, HIV related, diagnosis and treatment of, 498
Esophagoscopy, 295
Estinyl (ethinyl estradiol), 677
Estrace (estradiol), 677
Estraderm (estradiol), 677
Estradiol (Estrace, Estraderm), 677
Estrogenic hormones, 677
Estrogens
  adverse drug interactions, with anticoagulants, 56*t*
  conjugated, in lactation, 677
  FDA pregnancy safety classification of, 669*t*
Ethacrynic acid
  adverse drug interactions, with anticoagulants, 56*t*
  FDA pregnancy safety classification of, 669*t*
Ethambutol
  FDA pregnancy safety classification of, 665*t*
  in lactation, 674
  recommendations and adverse reactions to, 427
  in treatment of
    HIV related
      Mycobacterium avium, 509
      tuberculosis, 507, 508
    septic arthritis, 641
Ethamide (ethoxzolamide), 600*t*
Ethanol
  abuse of, in psychiatric emergencies, 649, 653–655
  antidotal action of, 182*t*, 191, 192
  as cause of hyperthermia, 686, 689, 690*t*
  FDA pregnancy safety classification of, 670*t*
  in treatment of methanol ingestions, 364
Ethchlorvynol, 56*t*
Ether, 579
Ethinyl estradiol (Estinyl, Feminone), 677
Ethiodized oil (Ethiodol), 681
Ethiodol (ethiodized oil), 681

Ethosuximide
  FDA pregnancy safety classification of, 668*t*
  in lactation, 675
  in treatment of
    new onset seizures, 257*t*
    petit mal status epilepticus, 259
Ethoxzolamide (Ethamide), 600*t*
Ethylene glycol
  antidote for, 182*t*, 191, 192, 203
  ingestions of, diagnosis and treatment of, 364, 365
Etretinate
  FDA pregnancy safety classification of, 671*t*
  in lactation, 682
  in treatment of psoriasis vulgaris, 618
Eurax; *see* Crotamiton
Ex-Lax (phenolphthalein), 679
Expectorants, 677
Expectorants/antitussives 667*t*
Exposure keratopathy, 595*t*, 596
Extremity injuries
  diagnosis and treatment of, 562, 563
  pain control in, 565
Eyelid disorders, 584
  abscesses of, diagnosis and treatment of, 441
  diagnosis and treatment of
    blepharitis, 589
    chalazion, 589
    hordeolum, 589
  entropion/ectropion, diagnosis and treatment of, 596

F

Facial cellulitis, 438*t*, 439
Famotidine
  in lactation, 679
  in treatment of
    gastrointestinal bleeding, 300
    GERD, 298, 298*t*
Favism, 343*t*
Feen-a-Mint (phenolphthalein), 679
Felbamate, 257*t*
Felbatol (felbamate), 257*t*
Feldene (piroxicam), 672, 673
Feminone (ethinyl estradiol), 677
Fenoprofen
  in lactation, 672, 673
  in treatment of pain, 81*t*, 82, 83
Fenoterol, 667*t*
Fentanyl
  FDA pregnancy safety classification of, 665*t*
  oral narcotic equivalency table, 74*t*
  in parenteral treatment of pain, 99*t*
    alfentanil derivative of, 109
    in cardioversion, 122*t*
    contraindicated in pregnancy, 109
    lollipop form for children, 109
    parenteral/oral narcotic equivalency index, 101*t*
    recommendations and adverse reactions of, 97, 102, 103*t*, 109
    sufentanil derivative of, 109
  in parenteral treatment of painful procedures, 123*t*, 127, 128
  in treatment of tachycardias, *233*
Fetomaternal hemorrhages, 547, 548
FiberCon (polycarbophil), 679
Fibromyalgia, 95*t*
Fiorinal
  with codeine
    drug seekers feigning migraines for, 135*t*
    street price of, 133*t*

drug seekers of, 132
Fish poisonings, 343t, 344t
Flagyl (metronidazole), 674
Flecainide
  in lactation, 675
  in treatment of arrhythmias, 211
Fleet Phospho-soda (sodium phosphate/biphosphate), 679
Flexeril (cyclobenzaprine), 267t
Floctafenine
  as alternative for drug seekers
    with low back pain, 141, 142t
    with orthopedic injuries, 141, 142t
    with toothaches, 141, 142t
  in treatment of
    chest wall injuries, 95t
    dental pain, 95t
    dysmenorrhea, 95t
    fractures, 95t
    otitis externa, 569
    pain, 94t, 95t
    recommendations and adverse reactions of, 84, 85
    sprains, 96t
    strains, 96t
    trigeminal, 96t
Floxin; see Ofloxacin
Flubriprofen (Ansaid), 672
Flucinolide, 614t
Fluconazole
  adverse drug interactions, with anticoagulants, 56t
  recommendations and adverse reactions of, 425
  in treatment of
    candidal vaginitis, 446, 447t, 472t, 481
    HIV related candidiasis, 496
    HIV related esophagitis, 497
    moniliasis, 631, 632
Flucytosine, 490, 491
Flumazenil, 182t, 192, 193
Flumethasone, 569
Fluocinolone, 613t
Fluocinonide, 644
Fluorescein, 681
Fluorextine, 662
5-Fluorocytosine, 641
Fluoroquinolones
  in lactation, 674
  in treatment of conjunctivitis, 589
    contraindications to, 589
Fluoroquinones, , 665t, 666t
Fluoxetine, in treatment of
  pain, 88
  pain for fibromyalgia, 95t
Fluphenazine
  FDA pregnancy safety classification of, 671t
  precautions/contraindications for the elderly, 55t
  in treatment of pain, 89
Flurandrenolide, 613t
Flurazepam, 48t
Flurbiprofen, 81t, 82
Focal intracerebral lesions, HIV related
  diagnosis and treatment of, 491–494
  maintenance therapy, 494
  preventative medicine, 494
Foley catheters
  in emergency treatment
    for esophageal foreign bodies, 295
    for rectal foreign bodies, 310
  in treatment of
    gastrointestinal bleeding, 300

midgut volvulus and malrotation, 302
posterior epistaxis, 580
Folic acid
  antidotal action of, 182t, 193, 194
  FDA pregnancy safety classification of, 671t
  with pyrimethamine
    in treatment of
      HIV related encephalitis, 493
      HIV related focal intracerebral lesions, 493
      HIV related toxoplasmosis, 493
  in treatment of HIV related *Isospora belli,* 499
Folliculitis
  bacterial, HIV related
    antistaphylococcal agents in treatment of, 494
    diagnosis and treatment of, 494
    dicloxacillin in treatment of, 494
    eosinophilic pustular, HIV related, diagnosis and treatment of, 494
Food additives
  MSG, 332
  reactions to, 332, 333, 344t
  sulfite sensitivity, 332, 344t
  tartrazine (Yellow dye #5), 344t
Food poisoning
  B. cereus conditions, 328, 329
  botulism, 317–321
  campylobacter enteritis, *324,* 330
  cholera, 329, 330
  Clostridium perfringens conditions, 328
  diagnosis and treatment of, 316, 317, 343t, 344t
  Escherichia coli, enteropathic (traveler's diarrhea), *324,* 327, 328
  herbal remedies for, 338t, 339t, 340t, 341t
  listeriosis, 330
  miscellaneous, 342, 343t, 344t
  natural chemicals in food and plants, 333, 334, *335,* 336t, 337t, 338t, 339t, 340t, 341t
  salmonellosis, 322, 324t, 325, *326,* 327
  shellfish, 332
  shellfish-associated, 332, 344t
  shigellosis, 321, *322,* 323t
  staphylococcal, 330, 331
Forgeries of prescriptions by drug seekers, 138
Foscarnet, in treatment of HIV related
  CMV esophagitis, 497
  colorectal disease, 499, 500
  herpes esophagitis, 497
  herpes simplex virus, 495
  HSV proctitis, 500
  hyponatremia, 510
  retinitis, 503, 504
Fournier's Gangrene, 466
Fractures
  open, treatment of, 450
  treatment of, 95t, 565
Fungicides, 621
Fungizone; see Amphotericin B
Furazolidone, 404
Furoessemide, 13t
Furosemide
  as cause of orthostatic hypotension, 33t
  FDA pregnancy safety classification of, 669t
  in lactation, 677
  in treatment of
    acute renal failure, 399
    brain tumors, 271
    hypercalcemia, 383
    hyponatremia, 373
    intracranial hemorrhages, 263
    myxedema coma, 393

Furuncles, 439
Furunculosis
 definition of, 570
 diagnosis and treatment of, 438t, 439, 570
Fusobacterium, 578

G

G. lamblia; see Giardia lamblia
Gabapentin (Neurontin), 257t
Gadopentetate (Magnevist), 681
Gallstones; *see* Cholecystitis
Gamma globulin, 307
Ganciclovir
 precautions for use in pregnancy, 405
 in treatment of, HIV related
  CMV esophagitis, 497
  colorectal disease, 499, 500
  cutaneous CMV, 496
Gantrisin (sulfisoxazole), 586, 587t
Gastric disease, 498
Gastroenteritis, 520t, 521t
Gastroesophageal reflux disease (GERD), 297–299, 299t
 causes of, 298
 diagnosis of, 297
 differential diagnosis of, 297, 298, 298t
  with ischemic heart disease, 297
Gastrointestinal bleeding
 causes of, 299
 diagnosis and treatment of, 299, 300
Gastrointestinal drugs, 678, 679
Gastrointestinal emergencies
 treatment of, 294–312
  abdominal hernias, 311, 312
  acid and alkaline ingestions, 296, 297
  appendicitis, 308, 309
  cholecystitis, 305–307
  esophageal foreign bodies, 294–296
  gastroesophageal reflux disease, 297–299, 299t
  gastrointestinal bleeding, 299, 300
  hemorrhoids, 310, 311
  hepatitis, 307, 308
  hypertrophic pyloric stenosis, 301, 302
  intussusception, 300, 301
  pancreatitis, 303–305, 304t, 305t
  perirectal abscesses, 311
  rectal foreign bodies, 309, 310
  rectal prolapse, 310
  volvulus, 302, 303
Genital herpes, 448t, 449, 473t, 480
Genitourinary tract infections
 cystitis, 445, 446
 diagnosis and treatment of, 445, 446, 563
 epididymo-orchitis, 446
 prostatitis, 446
Gentamicin
 with ampicillin, in treatment of
  bacterial pneumonia, in pediatrics, 525t
  meningitis/sepsis, in pediatrics, 522t, 523t
  omphalitis, in pediatrics, 523t
  pyelonephritis, in pediatrics, 526t
 with ampicillin-sulbactam, in treatment of pneumonia in elderly, 530t
 with azithromycin, in treatment of pneumonia in elderly, 530t
 with clindamycin, in treatment of PID, 472t, 477
 FDA pregnancy safety classification of, 665t
 with metronidazole and nafcillin, in treatment of cellulitis in elderly, 532t

 with nafcillin, in treatment of acute bacterial endocarditis in elderly, 532t
 recommendations and adverse reactions of, 417
 with rifampin and vancomycin, in treatment of acute bacterial endocarditis in elderly, 532t
 in treatment of
  abdominal traumas, 566t
  bacterial conjunctivitis, 586, 587t
  conjunctivitis, 588
  corneal abrasions in uveitis, 592
  granuloma inguinale (donovanosis), 480
  necrotizing fasciitis, 466
  septic arthritis, 641
Gentian violet solutions, 570
Geocillin; *see* Indanyl carbenicillin
Geopen; *see* Carbenicillin
Germainin; *see* Suramin
Germicides, 673, 674
Giardia lamblia
 diagnosis and treatment of, *324,* 328, 450
 HIV related, diagnosis and treatment of, 499
Gingivitis, 578
Gingivostomatitis, 578, 579
Glancilovir, 503, 504
Glasgow coma scale, 554
 use in psychiatric emergencies of, 651
Glaucoma, 595t, 597, 598, 599t, 600t, 601
 angle-closure, diagnosis and treatment of, 595t, 598, 599t, 600t, 601, 601
 chronic open-angle
  definition of, 597
  diagnosis and treatment of, 585, 597, 598, 599t, 600t
 occlusive disease of retinal vessels, as symptom of, 594t
Glipizide, 44t
Glomerulopathies, 510–511
Glucagon
 adverse drug interactions, with anticoagulants, 56t
 antidotal action of, 182t, 190, 193
 in treatment of
  esophageal foreign bodies, 295, 296
  hypoglycemia, 390
Glucocorticoids
 deficiency of, diagnosis and treatment of, 393, 394
 prednisone, 636, 639, 644–646
 in treatment of
  hypercalcemia, 383
  osteoarthritis, 639
  pituitary hypofunction, 394
  rheumatoid arthritis, 636
Glucose, in treatment of
 hepatitis, 308
 hypoglycemia, 390
Glutethimide, 56t
Glyburide, 44t
Glycerol, in treatment of
 glaucoma, 599t, 601
  contraindications to, 599t
 thromboembolic strokes, 262
Glycopyrrolate, 667t
Glycosides, cardiac
 antidote for, 182t, 190, 191
 in lactation, 675, 676
Gold salts, in treatment of rheumatoid arthritis, 636
 pediatric, 638
Goldmann applanation tonometers, 584
Gonococcal conjunctivitis, 518t, 519t
Gonorrhea
 anorectal, treatment of, 477

antibiotic-resistant, treatment of, 476
cervical, treatment of, 471*t*
cervicitis, 476, 477
diagnosis and treatment of, 448*t*, 449, 476, 477
disseminated gonococcal infections, 478
rectal, treatment of, 471*t*
urethritis, 476, 477
Gout, 95*t*, 642, 643 *see also* Pseudogout
Grand mal status epilepticus
causes of, 258
diagnosis and treatment of, 258, 259
Granulocyte-macrophage colony stimulating factor, 501
Granulocytopenia, 500, 501
Granuloma inguinale (donovanosis), 480
Graves' disease, 594*t*
Griseofulvin
adverse drug interactions, with anticoagulants, 56*t*
contraindications of, in pregnancy, 404
FDA pregnancy safety classification of, 665*t*
recommendations and adverse reactions of, 425, 426
in treatment of tinea infections, 621
Guaifenesin, 667*t*
Guanethidine, 33*t*
Guanfacine (Tenex), 676
Guanidine, 33*t*
Guanidine hydrochloride, 321
Gunshot wounds, 559, 562
Gynecologic infections
cervicitis, 446
diagnosis and treatment of, 446, 447
PID, 447
salpingitis, 447
vaginitis, 446
Gyromitra esculenta, 182*t*

H

H₂ blockers, in treatment of
gastrointestinal bleeding, 300
GERD, 298, 298*t*
staphylococcal food poisoning, 331
Haemophilus influenzae
as cause of
bacterial conjunctivitis, 586
dacryocystitis, 590
epiglottitis, 582
meningitis/sepsis, 522*t*
neonatal conjunctivitis, 588
orbital cellulitis, 591
pediatric pneumonia, 525*t*
periorbital cellulitis, 590
sinusitis, 576
β-lactamase-producing
as cause of otitis media, 568*t*, 571, 572*t*
treatment of, 406
in pediatrics, 516*t*, 517*t*
Hairy leukoplakia, 495
Halcinonide, 613, 614*t*
Haldol (haloperidol), 680
Hallucinogens
acute psychosis and, 658
violent behavior in psychiatric emergencies and, 653
Haloperidol
FDA pregnancy safety classification of, 671*t*
in lactation, 680
in parenteral treatment of pain, 119, 120
in diagnostic imaging, 122*t*
precautions/contraindications for the elderly, 55*t*
in treatment of
acute agitation, 272
suicidal patients, 661
systemic lupus erythematosus, 644
violent behavior, 656, 657
Halothane
in lactation, 681
succinylcholine, as cause hyperthermia, 690*t*
HBIG (hepatitis B immune globulin), 307
Head injuries
diagnosis and treatment of, 555, 556, 565*t*
mild, treatment of, 259
severe, diagnosis and treatment of, 259, 260
Headaches
categories of, 266*t*
cluster
definition of, 265
diagnosis and treatment of, 95*t*, 123*t*, 127, 128, 265, 266, 267*t*, 269
ocular pain as symptom of, 597
diagnosis and treatment of, 265, 266, 267*t*, 269
differential diagnosis with subdural hematomas, 266
migraines
definition of, 265
diagnosis and treatment of, 95*t*, 98, 116, 117, 265, 266, 267*t*, 268
muscle contraction, diagnosis and treatment of, 265, 267*t*, 269
symptoms of, 265, 266
temporal arteritis, treatment of, 269
tension, diagnosis and treatment of, 123*t*, 127, 128
treatment of, 267*t*
vascular type, diagnosis and treatment of, 90
Heart disease, 594*t*
Heart failure; *see* Congestive heart failure (CHF)
Hemagglutination, 344*t*
Hematomas, 263, 264
Hematuria, 139
Hemodialysis, in treatment of
ethylene glycol ingestions, 365
methanol ingestions, 364
salicylates ingestions, 365
Hemodilution, 603
β-hemolytic streptococcus
as cause of dacryocystitis, 590
group A, as cause of peritonsillar abscesses, 580
Hemorrhages, 594*t*
Hemorrhagic strokes, 147*t*
Hemorrhoidal creams 311
Hemorrhoids, 310, 311
Henderson-Hasselbalch equation, 350, 351*t*
Heparin
antidote for, 201
FDA pregnancy safety classification of, 666*t*
in lactation, 674
in treatment of
myocardial infarction, 153
pulmonary embolism, 288, 289
thromboembolic strokes, 262
transient ischemic attacks (TIAs), 260
Hepatic encephalopathy, 308
Hepatitis, 307
Hepatitis A, 307, 308, 539, 540
Hepatitis B, 307, 308, 481, 540–542, 542*t*, 543
Hepatitis B immune globulin (HBIG), 307
Hepatitis B vaccines, 670*t*
Hepatitis C, 307, 308, 543
Hepatitis D, 307, 308

Hepatitis E, 307, 308
Hepatitis vaccines, 670*t*
Hepatobiliary disease, 498
Herbal remedies, 338*t*, 339*t*, 340*t*, 341*t*
Hernias, 311, 312
Herniation syndrome
  diagnosis and treatment of, 260
    with brain tumors, 271
    with intracranial hemorrhages, 363
    with thromboembolic strokes, 262
Heroin, 682
Herpes simplex keratitis
  necrotizing
    as cause of corneal ulcers, 596
    diagnosis and treatment of, 595*t*, 596
  treatment of, 588
Herpes simplex virus (HSV)
  as cause of
    meningitis/sepsis, 522*t*
    neonatal conjunctivitis, 518*t*, 519*t*
  as cause of herpetic gingivostomatitis, 578
  as cause of viral conjunctivitis, 588
  diagnosis and treatment of, 449, 480
  HIV related, diagnosis and treatment of, 495
  proctitis, treatment of, 473*t*, 480
Herpes varicella zoster (HVZ)
  HIV related, diagnosis and treatment of, 495
  ocular, HIV related, diagnosis and treatment of, 502
Herpes zoster
  diagnosis and treatment of, 91, 438*t*, 440
  vertigo with ear pain and herpetic vesicles, as symptoms of, 270
Herpes zoster ophthalmicus, 595*t*, 597
Herpes zoster oticus
  as cause of otitis externa, 567, 568*t*
  diagnosis and treatment of, 569, 570
  vertigo with ear pain and herpetic vesicles, as symptoms of, 270
Herpetic gingivostomatitis; *see* Gingivostomatitis, herpetic
Hetrazan; *see* Diethylcarbamazine
Hexamethonium, 33*t*
High blood pressure, nitroprusside, in treatment of
  with intracranial hemorrhages, 263
  with thromboembolic strokes, 262
Hiprex (methenamine hippurate), 673
Histamine receptor antagonists; *see* H$_2$ blockers
Histoplasmosis, 594*t*
HIV
  acute primary stage, diagnosis and treatment of, 483, 486
  advanced stage, diagnosis and treatment of, 487
  cardiac complications of, 489
    diagnosis and treatment of
      with congestive cardiomyopathy, 489
      with myocarditis, 489
  CDC classification system of, 484, 485*t*
  central nervous system disorders with, 489–494
  dermatologic manifestations of, 494–496
  diagnosis and treatment of, 483, 487–489
  early stage, diagnosis and treatment of, 486
  gastrointestinal complications of, 497–500
  hematologic complications of, 500, 501
  late stage, diagnosis and treatment of, 487
  middle stage, diagnosis and treatment of, 486, 487
  ocular infections with, 502–504
  pulmonary infections with, 504–506
  renal infections with, 510, 511
  syphilis with, diagnosis and treatment of, 448, 449

Homatropine
  FDA pregnancy safety classification of, 667*t*
  in treatment of uveitis, 591
Hordeolum
  definition of, 589
  diagnosis and treatment of, 589
  warm compresses in treatment of, 441
HPS; *see* Hypertrophic pyloric stenosis (HPS)
Human immunodeficiency syndrome; *see* HIV
Human papillamavirus (HVP), 495
Hunt-Hess Scale, 265, 265*t*
Hydralazine
  adverse side effects of, 31*t*
  as cause of orthostatic hypotension, 33*t*
  FDA pregnancy safety classification of, 668*t*
  in lactation, 676
Hydrazines, 182*t*, 201, 202
Hydrocephalus, 594*t*
Hydrochlorothiazide
  FDA pregnancy safety classification of, 669*t*
  in lactation, 677
Hydrochlorothiazide-triamterene, 575
Hydrocodone
  FDA pregnancy safety classification of, 665*t*
  in parenteral treatment of pain, 102
  recommendations and adverse reactions of, 76, 77
  in treatment of
    chest wall injuries, 95*t*
    fractures, 95*t*
    pain, 94*t*
    sprains, 96*t*
    strains, 96*t*
Hydrocortisone
  antidotal action of, 182*t*, 190
  in treatment of
    adrenocortical hypofunction (Addison's disease), 393
    botulism, 321
    dermatologic disorders, 613*t*
    glucocorticoid deficiency, 394
    myxedema coma, 392
    otitis externa, 568
Hydrocortisone valerate, 613*t*
HydroDIURIL (hydrochlorothiazide), 677
Hydrofluoric acid, 182*t*, 186
Hydrogen peroxide, 578
Hydrogen sulfide, 182*t*
Hydromorphone, 94*t*
  in cough syrups, street price of, 133*t*
  drug seekers of, 132
  oral narcotic equivalency table, 74*t*
  in parenteral treatment of pain, 99*t*
    restricted use of, 102
  parenteral/oral narcotic equivalency index, 101*t*
  plasma half lives of, 74*t*
  street price of, 133*t*
  in treatment of pain, 76, 77
Hydroxocobalamin, 182*t*, 189, 197, 198
Hydroxychloroquine
  in lactation, 673
  precautions for use, in pregnancy, 405
  in treatment of
    rheumatoid arthritis, 636
    pediatric, 638
    systemic lupus erythematosus, 644
Hydroxyzine
  FDA pregnancy safety classification of, 667*t*, 671*t*
  with meperidine, in treatment of migraines, 268
Hygroton (chlorthalidone), 677
Hypaque (diatrizoate), 681

Hypercalcemia, 382, 383
Hyperglycemia, 388, 389
Hyperkalemia, 378–380
Hypermagnesemia, 385
Hypernatremia
 diagnosis and treatment of, 374, 375
 medical causes of acute psychosis and, 658
Hyperosmotics, 599t, 601
Hyperphosphatemia, 384
Hypertension, 594t
Hypertensive retinopathy, 593, 594t
Hyperthermia
 causes of, 688–691
 differential diagnosis of, 691, 692
 treatment of, 692
Hyperthyroidism, 390–392
Hypertrophic pyloric stenosis (HPS), 301, 302
Hyperventilation, in emergency treatment
 of intracranial hemorrhages, 263
 of severe head injuries, 260
Hyperviscosity syndromes, 594t
Hypervitaminosis A, 315t
Hyphema, 593
Hypnotics
 FDA pregnancy safety classification of, 670t
 in lactation, 680
Hypocalcemia
 diagnosis and treatment of, 381, 382
 HIV related, diagnosis and treatment of, 510
Hypoglycemia
 diagnosis and treatment of, 389, 390
 medical causes of acute psychosis and, 658
 oral, FDA pregnancy safety classification of, 669t
Hypoglycemics, 182t, 190
Hypokalemia
 diagnosis and treatment of, 375–378
 HIV related, diagnosis and treatment of, 510
Hypomagnesemia, 384, 385
Hypomania, 651
Hyponatremia
 diagnosis and treatment of, 361t, 370–374
 HIV related, diagnosis and treatment of, 510
 medical causes of acute psychosis and, 658
Hypophosphatemia, 383, 384
Hypopyon keratitis, 596
Hypotension
 amaurosis fugax as symptom of, 594t
 orthostatic, drugs causing, 33t
 with thromboembolic strokes, 261
Hypothermia
 diagnosis of, 685–687
 medical causes of, 686, 687, 687t
 treatment of, 687, 688
Hypovitaminosis A, 315t

I

Ibuprofen
 FDA pregnancy safety classification of, 670t
 indicators of possible toxicity, 13t
 in lactation, 672
 in treatment of
  acute gout, 643
  dental pain, 95t
  dysmenorrhea, 95t
  osteoarthritis, 639
  pain, 80, 81t, 82, 83
Idoxuridine, in treatment of
 herpes simplex virus, 588
 necrotizing herpes simplex keratitis, 596
Imidazoles, cream
 in treatment of, HIV related seborrheic dermatitis, 496
 recommendations and adverse reactions to, 425
Imipenem
 recommendations and adverse reactions of, 413
 in treatment of
  clostridial anaerobic cellulitis, 465
  clostridial myonecrosis, 468
  Fournier's Gangrene, 466
  gram-negative synergistic necrotizing cellulitis, 465, 466
  pneumonia in immunocompromised adults, 463
  septicemia in immunocompromised adults, 461
Imipenem-cilastatin
 with aminoglycosides, in treatment of septicemia in nonimmunocompromised adults, 461
 with aztreonam, in treatment of septicemia in elderly, 461
 precautions for use, in pregnancy, 404
 in treatment of bacterial peritonitis in elderly, 531t
Imipramine
 FDA pregnancy safety classification of, 669t
 in lactation, 680
 in treatment of
  arrhythmias, 217
  panic disorders, 662
Imitrex (sumatriptan), 267t
Immune disorders, 689t
Immune globulins 670t
Immunization
 hepatitis A, 539, 540
 hepatitis B, 540–542, 542t, 543
 hepatitis C, 543
 for infectious diseases, by emergency department personnel, 452
 measles, 543, 544, 545t, 546
 rabies, 536, 537, 538, 539
 requirements in emergency medicine for, 533
 Rh isoimmunization, risks in pregnancy of, 547, 548
 schedule for adults, 534t
 schedule for infants and children, 533t
 tetanus, 534, 535, 536
  immunization schedule for, 534t–536t
 tetanus/diphtheria/and pertussis, immunization schedule for, 534t, 535t
 varicella, 546, 547
Immunosuppressives, 638
Imodium
 in lactation, 679
 in treatment of HIV related parasitic diarrhea, 499
Impacted cerumen, 570
Impetigo
 antimicrobial therapy for, in pediatrics, 521t
 diagnosis and treatment of, 438, 438t, 439
Inapsine (droperidol), 308
Indanyl carbenicillin, 408
Indapamide, 669t
Inderal (propranolol), 676
Indocin (indomethacin), 673
Indomethacin
 FDA pregnancy safety classification of, 670t
 in lactation, 673
 recommendations and adverse reactions of, 81t, 82, 83
 suppositories in treatment of renal colic, 96t
 in treatment of
  acute gout, 643
  pseudogout, 643

Indomethacin—*Continued*
  Reiter's syndrome, 640
  rheumatoid arthritis, 636
  systemic lupus erythematosus, 644
Infections
  caused by tumors, treatment of, 272
  conjunctivitis as symptom of, 594*t*
  viral, as cause of peripheral vertigo, 575
Infectious cutaneous disorders, 494–496
Infectious diseases; *see also* specific diseases, e.g., Bronchiolitis
  acute epiglottitis, 458, 459
  antimicrobial agents in treatment of, in pediatrics, 516t–527t
  conditions causing fever/hyperthermia, 689*t*
  diagnosis and treatment of, 436*t*, 437*t*
  diarrhea, 450
  emergency department personnel
    health care delivery practices, 452
    immunizations, 452
  genitourinary tract infections, 445, 446
  gynecologic infections, 446, 447
  meningitis, 451, 452
  ophthalmologic infections, 441
  pharyngitis, 456–458
  pneumonia, 461–464
  protection of emergency department personnel, 452
  respiratory tract infections
    lower, 443–445
    upper, 441–443
  septicemia, 459–461
  sexually transmitted diseases, 448, 449
  skin infections, 438–441
  soft tissue infections, 438–441
  vesiculoulcerative diseases, 449
Infestations, 441
Influenza vaccines, 670*t*
Inner ear infections; *see also* Ear infections
  as cause of vertigo, 270
Insect bites, 623, 624
Insecticides, 629
Insulin
  FDA pregnancy safety classification of, 669*t*
  in lactation, 678
  in treatment of
    hyperglycemia, 388
    hyperkalemia, 380
Interferon alpha, 307
Interferon-a-2b, 495
Intoxication, 139
Intracranial hemorrhages
  diagnosis and treatment of, 262–265, *264*
  extracerebral
    epidural hematomas, 264
    subarachnoid (SAH), 264, 265
    subdural hematomas, 263
  intracerebral
    cerebellar, 263
    definition of, 263, 263*t*
    parenchymal, 263
    treatment of, 263
    intracerebral vs. extracerebral, 263*t*
Intracranial infections, 256
Intraocular pressure (IOP)
  benign increased, papilledema as symptom of, 594*t*
  in diagnosis of, ophthalmologic disorders, 584, 585, *585*
  in uveitis, 591–593

Intravenous pyelograms, 140
Intussusception, 300, 301
Iodamide (Renovue), 681
Iodine, 674
Iodine compounds, 667*t*
Iododeoxyuridine, 519*t*
Iodoquinol
  recommendations and adverse reactions of, 428
  in treatment of HIV related symptomatic diarrhea, 499
Iohexol (Omnipaque), in lactation, 681
Iopanoic acid
  as cause of orthostatic hypotension, 33*t*
  in lactation, 681
Iridectomy 601
Iridocyclitis, 597
Iritis, 595*t*, 597
Iron, 182*t*, 188
Ischemic heart disease, 297
Isoethane, 277*t*, 280
Isoetharine, 667*t*
Isometheptene mucate, in treatment of
  migraine headaches, 95*t*
  vascular headaches, 90
Isoniazid
  FDA pregnancy safety classification of, 665*t*
  in lactation, 674
  recommendations and adverse reactions of, 426
  in treatment of
    HIV related tuberculosis, 507
    septic arthritis, 641
Isopropamide, 667*t*
Isopropyl alcohol, 570
Isoproterenol
  FDA pregnancy safety classification of, 667*t*
  in treatment of
    asthma, 280
    atrioventricular blocks, 241, *242, 243*
    cardiac arrest, 221
    sinus bradycardia, 241, *242, 243*
    torsades de pointes (TDP), 232
Isoptin (verapamil), 676
Isoptoatropine, 591
Isospora belli, 499
Isotonic fluids, 260
Isotretinoin
  FDA pregnancy safety classification of, 671*t*
  in lactation, 682
Itraconazole, in treatment of, HIV related
  candidiasis, 496
  corneal microsporidiosis, 502
Ivermectin, 432

J

Jaundice, 594*t*

K

Kanamycin, 665*t*
Kaolin, 678
Kaposi's Sarcoma
  diagnosis and treatment of, 494
  gastric, diagnosis and treatment of, 498
Keratitis, 441
  HIV related, diagnosis and treatment of, 502
Keratitis, herpetic; *see* Herpes simplex keratitis
Keratopathy, 595*t*, 596
Kerlone (betaxolol), 676
Kerorolac tromethamine (Toradol), 141, 142, 142*t*

Index 719

Ketamine
  in parenteral treatment of pain, 98, 104t, 114
  in parenteral treatment of pain in cardioversion, 122t
Ketoacidosis
  alcoholic (AKA), diagnosis and treatment of, 359t, 363, 364
  diabetic (DKA), diagnosis and treatment of, 385–387
  diagnosis and treatment of, 363, 364
  starvation, diagnosis and treatment of, 364
Ketoconazole
  recommendations and adverse reactions of, 425
  in treatment of
    candidal vaginitis, 481
    HIV related esophagitis, 497
    moniliasis, 631, 632
    oral candidiasis, 577
    tinea infections, 621
    tinea versicolor, 438t, 440, 441
Ketoprofen
  FDA pregnancy safety classification of, 670t
  recommendations and adverse reactions of, 81t, 82
Ketorolac
  analgesic dosage of, 81t
  FDA pregnancy safety classification of, 670t
  in lactation, 672, 673
  in parenteral treatment of pain
    in biliary colic, 125
    in costochondritis spasm, 126
    in migraine headaches, 123t, 127, 128
    in pericarditis, 126
    in rib fractures, 126
    in sickle crisis, 123t, 127, 128
  recommendations and adverse reactions of, 85
  in treatment of
    acute cholecystitis, 306
    biliary colic, 306
    chest wall injuries, 95t
    dental pain, 95t
    dysmenorrhea, 95t
    fractures, 95t
    otitis externa, 569
    pain, 94t
    renal colic, 96t
    sprains, 96t
    strains, 96t
Ketorolac tromethamine, 98, 104t, 112, 113
Killip classification, 146t
Klonopin (clonazepam)
  in lactation, 675
  in treatment of
    acute labyrinthitis, 270t
    positional vertigo, 269, 270t
Konsyl (psyllium), 679
Kwell; *see* Lindane

L

L. monocytogenes; *see* Listeria monocytogenes
Labetalol
  FDA pregnancy safety classification of, 667t
  in lactation, 676
  in treatment of pheochromocytoma, 395
Labyrinthitis, 269, 270t
Lacrimal disorders, 589, 590
β-lactam antibiotics, 461
Lactation
  breast feeding and
    categories of drugs in, 672
      analgesics, 672, 673
      antibiotics and antiinfectives, 673, 674
      anticoagulants, 674
      antiepileptics, 675
      antihypertensives and cardiovascular drugs, 675, 676
      antineoplastic, 676
      bronchodilators, 676, 677
      cold preparations, 677
      diuretics, 677
      endocrines, 677
      gastrointestinal, 678, 679
      miscellaneous, 681, 682
      nonmedical, 682
      psychotropic, 680
      sedatives and hypnotics, 680, 681
      vaccines, 681
      vitamins, 681
        uncategorized drugs in, 681, 682
      minimizing drug transfer to the infant, 682, 683
Lactic acidosis, 362t, 363
Lactulose enemas, 308
Lampit; *see* Nifurtimox
Lanoxin (digoxin), 675
Laparoscopy
  in diagnosis and treatment of appendicitis, 309
  in treatment of cholelithiasis, 306, 307
Larium; *see* Mefloquine
Laryngotracheobronchitis, viral; *see* Croup (viral laryngotracheobronchitis)
Lasix (furosemide), 677
Lathyrism, 344t
Laxative agents, 679
Lead, 182t, 188, 189
LES (lower esophageal sphincter), 294
Leucovorin; *see* Folinic acid (Leucovorin)
Leukemia, 594t
Leukocyte scans, radiolabeled autologous, 309
Levarterenol, 671t
Levodopa, 33t
Levonorgestrel implants, 677, 678
Levorphanol
  oral narcotic equivalency table, 74t
  in parenteral treatment of pain, 102
  parenteral/oral narcotic equivalency index, 101t
  plasma half lives of, 74t
  recommendations and adverse reactions of, 77, 78
Levothyroxine
  FDA pregnancy safety classification of, 669t
  in lactation, 678
  in treatment of myxedema coma, 392
LGV; *see* lymphogranuloma venereum
Lice, 438t, 441, 625–628
Lichen planus, 616, 617
Licorice poisoning, 344t
Lidocaine
  adverse drug interactions, with cimetidine, 61t
  as cause of orthostatic hypotension, 33t
  FDA pregnancy safety classification of, 668t
  in lactation, 675, 682
  in treatment of
    arrhythmias, 209, 210
    asystole, pediatric, 246, 247
    atrioventricular blocks, 241
    cluster headaches, 267t
    paroxysmal supraventricular tachycardia (PSVT), 239
    pulseless electrical activity (PEA), pediatric, 246, 247
    pulseless ventricular tachycardia (VT), 227

Index

Lidocaine—*Continued*
  pediatric, *246, 247*
  rapid sequence intubation, 292
  sinus bradycardia, 241
  tachycardias, *233*
  ventricular arrhythmias, 167
  ventricular ectopy, *230*
  ventricular fibrillation (VF), *227*
    pediatric, *246, 247*
  ventricular tachycardia, 237
  ventricular tachycardia with pulse, pediatric, *244*
Lidocaine gel, 91
Life-threatening arrhythmias; *see* Arrhythmias, life-threatening
Lindane
  contraindications of, in pregnancy, 404
  FDA pregnancy safety classification of, 666*t*
  in lactation, 674
  in treatment of
    lice, *438t, 441*, 626, 627
    scabies, *438t, 441*, 629, 630
      in pediatrics, 441
      precautions during pregnancy, 441
Lioresal (baclofen), 682
Liothyronine
  FDA pregnancy safety classification of, 669*t*
  in lactation, 678
Liquid cocaine, 123*t*, 127, 128
Lisinopril, 667*t*
Listeria, 522*t*
Listeria monocytogenes, 522*t*
Listeriosis, 330
Lithium
  as cause of hyperthermia, 690*t*
  FDA pregnancy safety classification of, 671*t*
  indicators of possible toxicity, 13*t*
  in lactation, 680
Liver cancer, 139
Liver disease, 139
Locacorten Vioform, 569
Lomefloxacin
  dosing frequencies for, 403*t*
  FDA pregnancy safety classification of, 666*t*
  recommendations and adverse reactions of, 416
Lomotil
  in lactation, 678
  in treatment of salmonellosis, *324,* 326
Loniten (minoxidil), 676
Loperamide
  drug seekers feigning colitis for, 135*t*
  FDA pregnancy safety classification of, 666*t*
  in lactation, 679
Lopressor (metoprolol), 676
Loracarbef
  dosing frequencies for, 403*t*
  recommendations and adverse reactions of, 410, 411
  in treatment of
    infectious diseases, 436*t*
    pharyngitis, group A β-hemolytic streptococcus, 458
Lorazepam
  anxiolytic effects on the elderly, 48*t*
  FDA pregnancy safety classification of, 670*t*
  in lactation, 680
  in treatment of
    acute psychosis, 659
    grand mal status epilepticus, 258
    suicidal patients, 661

violent behavior, 655–657
Lower esophageal sphincter (LES), 294
Loxapine, 671*t*
LSD; *see* Lysergic acid diethylamide
Ludiomil (maprotiline), 680
Lumbar punctures, 256
Lung abscesses, 444, 444*t,* 445
Lupus erythematosus, 644, 645
Lymphadenitis, 521*t*
Lymphogranuloma venereum, 448*t,* 449, 471*t,* 478, 479
Lymphoma
  non-Hodgkin's, diagnosis and treatment of, 498
  proptosis as symptom of, 594*t*
Lypressin, 669*t*
Lysergic acid diethylamide (LSD), 653

M

M. catarrhalis; see Branhamella catarrhalis
M. contagiosum; see Molluscum contagiosum
M. pneumoniae; see Mycoplasma pneumoniae
Maalox, 578
Macrobid (nitrofurantoin), 673
Macrodantin (nitrofurantoin), 673
Macrolides
  in treatment of
    abscesses, 438*t*
    carbuncles, 438*t,* 439
    cellulitis, 439
    community-acquired pneumonia, 443, 444, 444*t*
    erysipelas, 439
    furunculosis, 438*t*
    impetigo, 438*t*
    infectious diseases, 437*t*
    pharyngitis, 443
  with trimethoprim/sulfamethoxazole, in treatment of community-acquired pneumonia, 444*t*
Macular degeneration
  age and, 604
  diagnosis and treatment of, 605
  hereditary, 594*t*
  as symptom of
    cysts, 594*t*
    histoplasmosis, 594*t*
    senility, 594*t*
    trauma, 594*t*
Magnesium
  antidote for, 182*t,* 186
  disorders of
    hypermagnesemia, 385
    hypomagnesemia, 384, 385
  in treatment of
    hypomagnesemia, 385
    ventricular arrhythmias, 167
Magnesium citrate, 679
Magnesium hydroxide (milk of magnesia), 679
Magnesium sulfate
  antidotal action of, 182*t,* 186
  breast feeding and, 681
  FDA pregnancy safety classification of, 668*t*
  in lactation, 679, 681
  in treatment of
    asthma, 281
    torsades de pointes (TDP), 232
Magnevist (gadopentetate), 681
Malathion, 630
Malnutrition
  diagnosis and treatment of, 312*t,* 313, 315*t,* 316*t*
  protein-calorie, diagnosis and treatment of, 314*t*

Mandelamine (methenamine mandelate), 673
Mandol; *see* Cefamandole
Mannitol
   FDA pregnancy safety classification of, 669*t*
   in treatment of
      brain tumors, 271
      ethylene glycol ingestions, 365
      glaucoma, 599*t*, 601
         contraindications to, 599*t*
      intracranial hemorrhages, 263
      severe head injuries, 260
      thromboembolic strokes, 262
Maprotiline
   FDA pregnancy safety classification of, 669*t*
   in lactation, 680
Marcus Gunn pupils, 597
Marijuana, 682
Mastoiditis
   acute, antimicrobial therapy for, in pediatrics, 522*t*
   diagnosis and treatment of, 576
MAT; *see* Multifocal atrial tachycardia
Maxaquin; *see* Lomefloxacin
McMillan, Dr. Mary, 333
Measles, 543, 544, 545*t*, 546
Measles vaccines, 670*t*
Mebendazole
   in lactation, 673
   precautions for use, in pregnancy, 405
   recommendations and adverse reactions of, 431
Meclizine
   in emergency treatment of vertigo, 270*t*
   FDA pregnancy safety classification of, 666*t*
Meclizine hydrochloride (HCL), 575
Meclofenamate, 81*t*, 82, 84
Medihaler (ergotamine), 267*t*
Medrol (methylprednisolone), 678
Medroxyprogesterone (Provera), 677
Mefenamic acid
   adverse drug interactions, with anticoagulants, 56*t*
   in lactation, 673
Mefloquine
   precautions for use, in pregnancy, 405
   recommendations and adverse reactions of, 429
Mefoxin; *see* Cefoxitin
Melarsoprol, 430, 431
Meniere's disease, 574
Meningitis
   adult, diagnosis and treatment of, 451
   in alcoholic patients, diagnosis and treatment of, 451
   cryptococcal, HIV related
      diagnosis and treatment of, 489–491
      preventative medicine for, 489–491
   diagnosis and treatment of, 451, 452
   in elderly patients, diagnosis and treatment of, 451
   in neurosurgery/trauma patients, diagnosis and treatment of, 451
   in patients with CSF leak, diagnosis and treatment of, 451
   pediatric, diagnosis and treatment of, 451
   unprotected intimate contact, diagnosis and treatment of, 452
Meningitis/sepsis, 522*t*, 523*t*
Meningococcus vaccines, 670*t*
Meperidine
   drug seekers of, 132
   in emergency treatment of migraines, 267*t*
   FDA pregnancy safety classification of, 665*t*
   with hydroxyzine, in treatment of migraines, 268
   in lactation, 672

oral narcotic equivalency table, 74*t*
   in parenteral treatment of pain, 97, 99*t*, 102, 103*t*, 108
      precautions/contraindications
         for asthma, 108
         for the elderly, 108
      pain in biliary colic, 125
   parenteral/oral narcotic equivalency index, 101*t*
   plasma half lives of, 74*t*
   with promethazine, in treatment of migraines, 268
   recommendations and adverse reactions of, 78
   in treatment of tachycardias, *233*
Mephenytoin, 669*t*
Meprobamate, 670*t*
Mercury, 182*t*, 188, 189
Mesalamine, 679
Mesoridazine, 680
Mestinon (pyridostigmine), 682
Mestranol, 677
Metabolic acidosis
   anion gap, diagnosis and treatment of, 366*t*
   diagnosis and treatment of, 349*t*, 352*t*, 362*t*, 363–365, 366*t*, 367, 368
   ethylene glycol ingestions, 364, 365
   ketoacidosis, 363, 364
   lactic acidosis, 362*t*, 363
   methanol ingestions, 364
   nonanion gap, diagnosis and treatment of, 367, 368
   renal failure, 364
   salicylates ingestions, 365, 366
Metabolic alkalosis, 348, 349*t*, 368*t*, 369
Metabolic disorders
   case presentations of, 354–358
   caused by tumors, treatment of, 272
   diagnosis and treatment of, 346, 347*t*, 348, 349*t*, 350, 351*t*, 353–356, *357,* 358, 359*t*, 360, 361*t*
   diagnosis by
      anion gap, 350, 352*t*, 354, 355, 356, *357,* 358
      arterial blood gases, 348
      BUN/Cr ratio, 348
      emergency department battery (EDB), 347, 348
      Henderson-Hasselbalch equation, 350, 351*t*
      renal failure index (RIF), 348
      serum osmolality, 349
      urinary electrolytes, 348
      Winter's formula, 349
   types of, 347
Metabolic emergencies
   acid-base disorders and, 346–385
   diagnosis and treatment of, 346–400
   endocrine, 385–400
   seizures with, treatment of, 257
Metalazone, 669*t*
Metamucil (psyllium), 679
Metaproterenol
   FDA pregnancy safety classification of, 667*t*
   in treatment of asthma, 277*t*, 278*t*, 280
Metaraminol, 671*t*
Metastatic cancer, 135*t*
Metaxalone, 86
Methadone
   emergency use indications, 79
   in lactation, 673
   in parenteral treatment, restricted use of, 102
   plasma half lives of, 74*t*
   recommendations and adverse reactions of, 79
Methanol
   antidote for, 182*t*, 193, 194

Methanol—*Continued*
  ingestions of, diagnosis and treatment of, 364
  toxins of, optic neuritis as symptom of, 594*t*
Metharbital, 668*t*
Methazolamide
  in treatment of glaucoma, 600*t*
    adverse effects of, 607
    contraindications to, 600*t*
Methemoglobinemia, 182*t*, 194, 195
Methenamine hippurate, 673
Methenamine mandelate, 673
Methergine (methylergonovine), 682
Methicillin
  in treatment of
    parotitis, 576, 577
    omphalitis, in pediatrics, 523*t*
    septic arthritis, 641
Methimazole
  FDA pregnancy safety classification of, 669*t*
  in lactation, 678
  in treatment of hyperthyroidism, 391
Methixene, 667*t*
Methocarbamol
  in lactation, 682
  in parenteral treatment of pain, 105*t*, 115, 116
    in acute musculoskeletal injury, 124
    in tension headaches, 123*t*, 127, 128
  recommendations and adverse reactions of, 87*t*
Methotrexate
  antidote for, 182*t*
  in treatment of
    psoriasis vulgaris, 618
    Reiter's syndrome, 640
    rheumatoid arthritis, 636
      pediatric, 638
Methotrimeprazine, 33*t*
Methsuximide, 669*t*
4-Methyl pyrazole, 195
Methylcellulose (Citrucel), 679
Methyldopa
  adverse side effects of, 31*t*
  as cause of orthostatic hypotension, 33*t*
  FDA pregnancy safety classification of, 668*t*
  indicators of possible toxicity, 13*t*
  in lactation, 676
Methylene blue, 182*t*, 194, 195
Methylergonovine, 682
Methylphenidate
  drug seekers feigning attention deficit syndrome for, 135*t*
  drug seekers feigning narcolepsy for, 135*t*
  drug seekers of, 132
  street price of, 133*t*
Methylprednisolone
  in lactation, 678
  in treatment of
    acid and alkaline ingestions, 297
    asthma, 277*t*, 278*t*
    glucocorticoid deficiency, 394
    myasthenia gravis, 273
    systemic lupus erythematosus, 644
    temporal arteritis, 645
    vasculitis, 646
Methylprednisolone acetate, 613*t*
Methylxanthines, in treatment of
  asthma, 277*t*, 278*t*, 279–282
  COPD, 284
Methyprylon, 680
Methysergide, 33*t*
Metizan; *see* Ivermectin

Metoclopramide
  antidote for, 182*t*, 191
  as cause of dystonic reactions, 272
  FDA pregnancy safety classification of, 666*t*
  in lactation, 679
  in parenteral treatment of migraine, cluster, and tension headaches, 106*t*, 117
  in treatment of
    GERD, 298, 298*t*
    migraines, 267*t*, 268
      side effects of, 268
    vascular headaches, 90
Metoprolol
  FDA pregnancy safety classification of, 667*t*
  in lactation, 676
  in treatment of
    atrial fibrillation, 235
    atrial flutter, 235
    hyperthyroidism, 391
    myocardial infarction, 153
    Wolff-Parkinson-White syndrome (WPW), pediatric, 248
Metrizamide, 681
Metrizoate, 681
Metronidazole
  adverse drug interactions, with anticoagulants, 56*t*
  with aminoglycosides, in treatment of penetrating abdominal traumas, 450, 451
  with ampicillin and aminoglycosides, in treatment of
    Fournier's Gangrene, 466
    gram-negative synergistic necrotizing cellulitis, 466
  with ampicillin-sulbactam, in treatment of pneumonia in high risk aspiration adults, 464
  with ceftriaxone and tobramycin, in treatment of nonimmunocompromised elderly patients, 532*t*
  with ciprofloxacin, in treatment of diverticulitis in elderly, 531*t*
  contraindications of, in pregnancy, 404
  dosing frequencies for, 403*t*
  FDA pregnancy safety classification of, 666*t*
  in lactation, 674
  with mezlocillin, in treatment of bacterial cholangitis/biliary sepsis in elderly, 531*t*
  with nafcillin and gentamicin, in treatment of cellulitis in elderly, 532*t*
  with ofloxacin, in treatment of
    PID, 447, 447*t*, 471*t*
    salpingitis, 447, 447*t*
  with penicillin, in treatment of
    aspiration pneumonia, 444, 445
    dental abscesses, 443
    lung abscesses, 444, 445
    orofacial infections, 443
  with penicillin V, in treatment of
    aspiration pneumonia, 444*t*
    lung abscesses, 444*t*
    odontogenic infections, 443
  precautions for use, in pregnancy, 404
  recommendations and adverse reactions of, 422, 423, 428
  with ticarcillin/clavulanate, in treatment of pneumonia in high risk aspiration adults, 464
  in treatment of
    antibiotic-associated diarrhea, 450
    bacterial vaginitis, 446, 447*t*, 472*t*, 481
    clostridial anaerobic cellulitis, 465
    clostridial myonecrosis, 468

giardia, 450
gram-negative synergistic necrotizing cellulitis, 465
HIV related
giardia, 499
symptomatic diarrhea, 499
infectious diseases, 437t
necrotizing fasciitis, 466
shigellosis, 322
trichomoniasis vaginitis, 446, 447t, 472t, 480
Mexiletine
in lactation, 675
in treatment of arrhythmias, 210
Mexitil (mexiletine), 675
Mezlocillin
with metronidazole, in treatment of bacterial cholangitis/biliary sepsis in elderly, 531t
recommendations and adverse reactions of, 408
with tobramycin and vancomycin, in treatment of neutropenic elderly patients, 532t
in treatment of cholecystitis in elderly, 531t
MgSO$_4$, 227
Miconazole
FDA pregnancy safety classification of, 665t
in treatment of
candidal vaginitis, 446, 447t, 472t
moniliasis, 631, 632
tinea corporis, 438t, 440, 441
tinea cruris, 440, 441
tinea pedis, 440, 441
vaginal tablets, in treatment of HIV related candidiasis, 496
Midazolam
in lactation, 680
in parenteral treatment of pain, 104t, 118, 119
in cardioversion, 122t
in diagnostic imaging, 122t
in parenteral treatment of painful procedures, 123t, 127, 128
in treatment of
atrial fibrillation, 235
pediatric, 251
atrial flutter, 235
pediatric, 251
paroxysmal supraventricular tachycardia (PSVT), 238
supraventricular tachycardia (SVT), pediatric, 249
ventricular tachycardia, 237
ventricular tachycardia with pulse, pediatric, 244
Wolff-Parkinson-White syndrome (WPW), pediatric, 248
Middle ear disease; see also Ear infections
papilledema as symptom of, 594t
Midgut volvulus, 302, 303
Migraines
as cause of central vertigo, 575
chlorpromazine as, alternative for drug seekers with, 142, 142t
definition of, 265
diagnosis and treatment of, 265, 267t, 268
differential diagnosis with subarachnoid hemorrhages (SAH), 266
drug seekers feigning, for codeine with fiorinal, 135t
NSAIDs, as alternative for drug seekers, 141, 142t
ocular pain as symptom of, 597
prochlorperazine, as alternative for drug seekers with, 142, 142t
symptoms of, 265

Miliaria, 624, 625
Milk of magnesia (magnesium hydroxide), 679
Mineral oil
adverse drug interactions, with anticoagulants, 56t
in lactation, 679
Minocycline, in treatment of HIV related
encephalitis, 493
focal intracerebral lesions, 493
toxoplasmosis, 493
Minoxidil
as cause of orthostatic hypotension, 33t
in lactation, 676
Mintezol; see Thiabendazole
Miotics, in treatment of
glaucoma, 598, 599t, 601
adverse effects of, 606
Miradon (anisindione), 674
Mithramycin, 316t
Mitral regurgitation, 146t
Molluscum contagiosum, 495, 496
Moniliasis, 630–632
Monoamine oxidase inhibitors, 690t
Monocid; see Cefonicid
Monoctanoin, 306, 307
Monosodium glutamate; see MSG
Moricizine, 209
Morphine
drug seekers feigning metastatic cancer for, 135t
FDA pregnancy safety classification of, 665t
in lactation, 672
oral narcotic equivalency table, 74t
in parenteral treatment of pain, 97, 99t, 102, 103t, 107, 108
in acute musculoskeletal injury, 124
in biliary colic, 125
in cluster headaches, 123t, 127, 128
in migraine headaches, 123t, 127, 128
in myocardial infarction, 125
in pericarditis, 126
precautions/contraindications for asthma, 107
in renal colic, 128
in rib fractures, 126
in sickle crisis, 123t, 127, 128
in thoracic aortic aneurysm, 126
in parenteral treatment of painful procedures, 123t, 127, 128
parenteral/oral narcotic equivalency index, 101t
plasma half lives of, 74t
recommendations and adverse reactions of, 78, 79
in treatment of
cardiac arrest, 220, 221
tachycardias, 233
Morphine sulfate, 94t
Motility agents, in lactation, 679
Motrin (ibuprofen), in lactation, 672
MSG
as cause of vertigo, 270
reactions to, 332
Multifocal atrial tachycardia (MAT), 231, 232
Multiple sclerosis
as cause of central vertigo, 575
oculomotor paralysis as symptom of, 594t
optic neuritis as symptom of, 594t
vertigo as symptom of, 271
Mumps, 576
Mumps vaccines, 670t
Mupirocin, 521t
Mupirocin ointment, 438, 438t, 439
Muscle relaxants
in lactation, 682

724 Index

Muscle relaxants—*Continued*
  in pain control treatment of trauma, 565
  in parenteral treatment of pain, 114, 115
  skeletal, FDA pregnancy safety classification of, 671*t*
Musculoskeletal injuries, 122*t*, 124
Mushroom poisoning
  antidote for, 182*t*, 185, 186, 198, 199
  diagnosis and treatment of, 334, 335
Myambutol; *see* Ethambutol
Myasthenia gravis
  diagnosis and treatment of, 273, 274
  diagnosis of, 273
  differential diagnosis of, 274*t*
  as symptom of diplopia, 594*t*
  vs. cholinergic crisis, 274
Mycobacterial disease, 506–508
Mycobacterium avium, 508–510
Mycoplasma infections
  antimicrobial therapy for, in pediatrics, 517*t*
  pneumonia, with pharyngitis, treatment of, 458
Mycoplasma pneumoniae, 525*t*
Mycostatin, 631, 632
Mydriacyl (tropicamide), 606
Myocardial infarction
  acute, 144
  angiotensin-converting enzyme inhibitors in treatment of, 162, 163
  β-blockers in, 162
  cardiac enzyme indicators of, 148
  complications of, 164
  diagnosis by
    chest x-rays, 149
    echocardiography, 149
    electrocardiography, 146, 147, 147*t*
    serum indicators, 149
  diagnosis of, 145, 146
  drug precautions with, 163
  history of, 145, 146
  initial stabilization of, 150–152, 151*t*
  overview of, 155*t*, 156*t*
  parenteral treatment of, 122*t*, 125
  thrombolytic therapy of, 161
    patient selection in, 157, 158, 158*t*, 159, 160
  treatment of, 152–154, 162
Myocarditis, 489
Myopia, 594*t*
Myringotomy, 576
Mysoline (primidone)
  in lactation, 675
  in treatment of
    new onset seizures, 257*t*
    recurrent seizures, 258*t*
Myxedema comas, 392, 393

N

N-acetylcysteine (NAC,Mucomyst), 182*t*, 195, 196
NaCo$_3$, 229
Nadolol
  FDA pregnancy safety classification of, 667*t*
  in lactation, 676
Nafcillin
  with aminoglycoside, in treatment of suppurative arthritis, in pediatrics, 516*t*
  with cefotaxime, in treatment of suppurative arthritis, in pediatrics, 516*t*
  with chloramphenicol, in treatment of orbital cellulitis, 591
  with gentamicin, in treatment of acute bacterial endocarditis in elderly, 532*t*
  with gentamicin and metronidazole, in treatment of cellulitis in elderly, 532*t*
  recommendations and adverse reactions of, 409
  in treatment of
    acute mastoiditis, in pediatrics, 522*t*
    dacryocystitis, 590
    orbital cellulitis, 591
      in pediatrics, 517*t*
    osteomyelitis, in pediatrics, 523*t*
    periorbital cellulitis, 590
    preseptal/buccal cellulitis, in pediatrics, 517*t*
    septic arthritis, 641
    suppurative arthritis, in pediatrics, 516*t*
NaHCO$_3$; *see* Sodium bicarbonate
Nalbuphine
  oral narcotic equivalency table, 74*t*
  in parenteral treatment of pain, 98, 99*t*, 103*t*, 110, 111
    in abdomen, 122*t*
    in cluster headaches, 123*t*, 127, 128
    in migraine headaches, 123*t*, 127, 128
    in myocardial infarction, 125
    in rib fractures, 126
    in sickle crisis, 123*t*, 127, 128
    in tension headaches, 123*t*, 127, 128
    in thoracic aortic aneurysm, 126
  in parenteral treatment of painful procedures, 123*t*, 127, 128
  parenteral/oral narcotic equivalency index, 101*t*
  plasma half lives of, 74*t*
Nalfon (fenoprofen), 672, 673
Nalidixic acid
  adverse drug interactions, with anticoagulants, 56*t*
  in lactation, 674
Naloxone
  antidotal action of, 182*t*, 196, 197
  FDA pregnancy safety classification of, 670*t*
  in parenteral treatment of pain, 99*t*, 112
Naltrexone, 99*t*
Naphazoline hydrochloride, 585
Naproxen
  FDA pregnancy safety classification of, 670*t*
  in lactation, 672, 673
  recommendations and adverse reactions of, 81*t*, 83
  in treatment of
    acute gout, 643
    chest wall injuries, 95*t*
    dysmenorrhea, 95*t*
    fractures, 95*t*
    migraines, 268
    osteoarthritis, 639
    otitis externa, 569
    pseudogout, 643
    Reiter's syndrome, 640
    rheumatoid arthritis, 636
      pediatric, 637
    sprains, 96*t*
    strains, 96*t*
Narcolepsy, 135*t*
Narcotic agonists-antagonists
  in diagnosis of drug seekers, 141
  in parenteral treatment of pain, 97, 103*t*, 110–112
Narcotic analgesics, 73, 74*t*, 75*t*, 75–79, 79*t*
  drug seekers feigning
    orthopedic injuries for, 135*t*
    sickle crisis for, 135*t*
    tic douloureux for, 135*t*
    toothaches for, 135*t*
  equivalency index of, 74*t*
  opioid, 75*t*, 76–79, 79*t*

in parenteral treatment of pain, 100, 101t, 102
precautions/contraindications for the elderly, 73
recommendations and adverse reactions of, 73, 74t, 75, 75t, 96t
in treatment of
  migraines, 268
  pericarditis, 96t
  renal colic, 96t
  sickle crisis, 96t
Narcotic antagonists, 670t
Narcotics
  drug seekers feigning
    colitis for, 135t
    metastatic cancer for, 135t
    pain for, 135t
    renal colic for, 135t
  drug seekers of, 132
  FDA pregnancy safety classification of, 665t
  in lactation, 672
  in treatment of
    abdominal hernias, 312
    hemorrhoids, 311
    otitis media, 573
    perirectal abscesses, 311
    rectal foreign bodies, 310
Nardil (phenelzine), 680
Nasal balloons, 579, 580
Nasal decongestant sprays, 677
Nasal oxygen; see also Oxygen
  in treatment of
    cluster headaches, 95t
    vascular headaches, 90
Nasopharyngitis, purulent/sinusitis; see Sinusitis/purulent nasopharyngitis
Naturetin (bendroflumethiazide), 677
NBIN, 630
Neck traumas, 565t
Necrotizing fasciitis
  diagnosis and treatment of, 465–468
  Fournier's Gangrene, 466
  gram-negative synergistic necrotizing cellulitis, 466, 467
NegGram (nalidixic acid), 674
Neisseria gonorrhoeae
  as cause of
    bacterial conjunctivitis, 587
    neonatal conjunctivitis, 518t, 519t, 588
  treatment of, 406
Nembutal (pentobarbital), 680
Neomycin
  FDA pregnancy safety classification of, 665t
  ophthalmologic uses of, precautions with, 606
  with polymyxin B, in treatment of otitis externa, 568
  in treatment of
    conjunctivitis, 441
    seborrheic dermatitis, 616
Neonatal chlamydial conjunctivitis, 518t, 519t
Neonatal conjunctivitis; see Conjunctivitis, neonatal
Neoplasms, 594, 594t, 595
Neoplastic diseases, 689t
Neostigmine
  FDA pregnancy safety classification of, 669t
  in lactation, 682
  in treatment of
    myasthenia gravis, 273
    supraventricular tachycardia (SVT), pediatric, 249
Neptazane (methazolamide), in treatment of glaucoma, 600t

adverse effects of, 607
contraindications to, 600t
Nerve blocks, 141, 142t
Netilmicin, 417
Neuralgias, 96t
Neuroleptics
  extrapyramidal symptoms, antidote for, 182t, 191
  FDA pregnancy safety classification of, 671t
  in treatment of
    acute psychosis, 659
    violent behavior, 656, 657
Neurologic therapeutics, emergency, 255-274
  for acute agitation, 272, 273t
  for cerebrovascular disease, 260-265
  for dystonic drug reactions, 272, 273
  for head injuries, 259, 260
  for headaches, 265-269
  for myasthenia gravis, 273, 274
  for oncologic disorders, 271, 272
  for seizures, 255-259
  for vertigo, 269-271
Neurontin (gabapentin), 257t
Neuropathic disorders, 95t
Neuropathy, 597
Niacin, 314t
Niclosamide, 432, 433
Nicotine (smoking), 683
Nifedipine
  as cause of orthostatic hypotension, 33t
  FDA pregnancy safety classification of, 667t
  in lactation, 676
  in treatment of
    esophageal foreign bodies, 296
    pain in diffuse esophageal, 126
Nifurtimox, 431
Night cramps, 96t
Nimodipine
  FDA pregnancy safety classification of, 668t
  in treatment of subarachnoid hemorrhages (SAH), 265
Nitrate sticks, 579
Nitrates, 125
Nitrofurantoin
  contraindications of, in pregnancy, 404
  FDA pregnancy safety classification of, 666t
  in lactation, 673
  precautions for use, in pregnancy, 404
Nitrogen mustard, 575
Nitroglycerin
  in parenteral treatment of pain in myocardial infarction, 125
  in treatment of esophageal foreign bodies, 296
  in treatment of pain, in diffuse esophageal disorders, 126
Nitroprusside, in treatment of
  congestive heart failure/cardiogenic shock, precautions for, 165, 166
  high blood pressure
    with intracranial hemorrhages, 263
    with thromboembolic strokes, 262
  lactic acidosis, 363
  pheochromocytoma, 395
Nitrous oxide
  in parenteral treatment of pain, 105t, 115
    in cardioversion, 122t
    in rib fractures, 126
  in treatment of perirectal abscesses, 311
Nix, 627
Nizatidine
  in lactation, 679

726 Index

Nizatidine—*Continued*
  in treatment of GERD, 298, 298*t*
Noludar (methyprylon), 680
Nongonococcal urethritis, 478
Noninfectious pulmonary diseases; *see* Pulmonary diseases, noninfectious
Nonmedical drugs, 682, 683
Nonnarcotic analgesics, 96*t*
Nonsteroidal antiinflammatory drugs (NSAIDs)
  adverse drug interactions, with anticoagulants, 56*t*
  as alternative for drug seekers, 141, 142*t*
  current list of, 41*t*
  drug seekers of, 133
  FDA pregnancy safety classification of, 670*t*
  ibuprofen, 636, 638, 643
  indomethacin, 636, 638, 640, 643, 644
  naproxen, 636, 637, 639, 640, 643
  in parenteral treatment of pain, 98, 104*t*, 112, 113
  phenylbutazone, 639, 643
  piroxicam, 636, 639
  recommendations and adverse reactions of, 72, 80, 81*t*, 82–84
  salicylates, 636, 637
    aspirin, 636, 637, 639, 640, 644
  salsalate, 639
  sulindac, 636, 639, 643
  tolmetin sodium, 638
  in treatment of
    acute cholecystitis, 306
    biliary colic, 306
    migraines, 268
    muscle contraction headaches, 267*t*
    pericarditis, 96*t*
    rheumatoid arthritis, 636
    systemic lupus erythematosus, 644
Nonulcerative (seborrheic) blepharitis, 589
Norepinephrine, 363
Norethindrone, 677
Norethynodrel, 677
Norfloxacin
  contraindications of, in pregnancy, 404
  dosing frequencies for, 403*t*
  FDA pregnancy safety classification of, 665*t*
  in lactation, 674
  recommendations and adverse reactions of, 416
  in treatment of
    conjunctivitis, 441
    gonococcal cervicitis, 476, 477
    gonococcal urethritis, 476, 477
    gonorrhea, 448*t*, 449
    infectious diseases, 437*t*
Normal sinus rhythm, *223*
Normeperidine, 75*t*
Normodyne (labetalol), 676
Noroxin; *see* Norfloxacin
Norpace (disopyramide), 675
Norpramin (desipramine), 680
Nortriptyline
  adverse drug interactions, with anticoagulants, 56*t*
  FDA pregnancy safety classification of, 669*t*
  in lactation, 680
Nose bleeds; *see* Epistaxis
Nystatin
  FDA pregnancy safety classification of, 665*t*
  in treatment of
    HIV related candidiasis, 496
    oral candidiasis, 577

O

Obesity, 135*t*

Octreotide, 499
Ocular infections, 502
Ocular pain, 595*t*, 596, 597
Ocular tumors, 594*t*
Oculomotor palsies
  diplopia as symptom of, 594*t*
  with ocular pain, as symptom of carotid aneurysms, 597
Oculomotor paralysis, 594*t*
Odontogenic infections, 443
Ofloxacin
  with clindamycin, in treatment of
    PID, 447, 447*t*, 471*t*
    salpingitis, 447, 447*t*
  contraindications of, in pregnancy, 404
  dosing frequencies for, 403*t*
  FDA pregnancy safety classification of, 665*t*
  in lactation, 674
  with metronidazole, in treatment of
    PID, 447, 447*t*, 471*t*
    salpingitis, 447, 447*t*
  recommendations and adverse reactions of, 415, 416
  in treatment of
    cervical gonorrhea, 471*t*
    Chlamydia trachomatis, 448*t*, 449
    chronic bronchitis, 443, 444*t*
    epididymo-orchitis, 445*t*, 446
    gonococcal cervicitis, 471*t*, 476, 477
    gonococcal urethritis, 471*t*, 476, 477
    gonorrhea, 448*t*, 449
    infectious diseases, 437*t*
    rectal gonorrhea, 471*t*
Olsalazine (Dipentum), 679
Omeprazole, 298, 298*t*
Omnipaque (iohexol), 681
Omphalitis, 523*t*
Oncologic emergencies, 271
Ondansetron, 666*t*
Ontioconazole, 446
Ophthalmologic disorders
  acute vascular occlusions, 602, 603
  cataracts, 601, 602
  diagnosis of, 583–585
    intraocular pressure in, 584, 585
    lids and adnexa in, 584
    patient history in, 583
    peripheral vision in, 584
    visual acuity testing in, 583, 584
  glaucoma, 595*t*, 597, 598, 599*t*, 600*t*, 601
  macular degeneration, 604, 605
  ocular pain as symptom of, 595–597
  red eye, 585–593
  retinal detachments, 604
  as symptoms of systemic disease, 593–595, 594*t*
  temporal arteritis, 603, 604
Ophthalmologic drugs, 605–607
  adverse effects of
    antibiotics, 606
    β-blockers, 607
    carbonic anhydrase inhibitors, 607
    corticosteroids, 605
    cycloplegics, 606
    epinephrine, 606
    parasympathomimetic drugs, 606, 607
    phenylephrine, 606
  systemic reactions to, 605
  use with elderly, 605, 606*t*
Ophthalmologic infections, 441
Ophthalmoscopy

in diagnosis of temporal arteritis, 603, 604
for measurement of intraocular pressure (IOP), 584, 585
contraindications to, 584
Opiates, 98, 99t, 100t
Opioids, 76–79, 79T
antidote for, 182t, 196, 197
for mild pain, 76
codeine, 76
pentazocine, 76
propoxyphene, 76
for moderate pain, 76, 77
hydrocodone, 76, 77
oxycodone, 76, 77
plasma half-life of, 75T
for severe pain, 77, 78
hydromorphone, 77
levorphanol, 77, 78
meperidine, 78
methadone, 79
morphine, 78, 79
Opium powder (Paregoric), 678
Optic atrophy, 594t
Optic neuritis
ocular pain with Marcus Gunn pupils, as symptom of, 597
as symptom of
diabetes mellitus, 594t
Graves' disease, 594t
methanol toxins, 594t
multiple sclerosis, 594t
temporal arteritis, 594t
Optic neuropathy, 597
Oral candidiasis, 577
Oral contraceptives (OCs)
adverse drug interactions, with anticoagulants, 56t
in lactation, 677, 678
levonorgestrel implants, 677, 678
progestin-only, 677, 678
Oral pain management, 72–96
Orbital cellulitis
antimicrobial therapy for, in pediatrics, 517t
causes of, 591
diagnosis and treatment of, 590, 591
proptosis as symptom of, 594t
Orinase (tolbutamide), 678
Orofacial infections, 443
Oropharyngeal burns, 296
Orphenadrine
in parenteral treatment of pain, 105t, 115
in tension headaches, 128
recommendations and adverse reactions of, 86, 87t
Orthopedic injuries
drug seekers feigning, 136, 136t
diagnosis of, 139
for narcotic analgesics, 135t
radiographs for, 140
floctafenine for, as alternative for drug seekers, 141, 142t
NSAIDs, as alternative for drug seekers, 141, 142t
treatment of, 565t
Osteoarthritis (OA), 638, 639
Osteogenesis imperfecta, 594t
Osteomyelitis, 440
antimicrobial therapy for, in pediatrics, 523t
OTC drugs; *see* Over-the-counter drugs
Otitis externa
definition of, 567
diagnosis and treatment of, 441, 442, 567–569
differential diagnosis of, with otitis media, 568

ear drops in treatment of, 441, 442, 442t
malignant, diagnosis and treatment of, 567–569
Otitis malignant externa, 442
Otitis media
antimicrobial therapy for, in pediatrics, 524t
causes of, 571, 572, 572t
COME, treatment of, 573
definition of, 571
diagnosis and treatment of, 442, 442t, 571–573
pain management in, 573
recurrences of, 571
treatment for, 573
Otomycosis, 570
Over-the-counter drugs, 6, 7
Ovide lotion, 630
Oxacillin, 409
Oxamniquine, 404
Oxazepam
anxiolytic effects on the elderly, 48t
FDA pregnancy safety classification of, 670t
in lactation, 680
as preferred substance of drug seekers, 132
Oxycodone
with acetaminophen, in treatment of
dental pain, 95t
migraine headaches, 95t
drug seekers feigning renal colic for, 135t
drug seekers of, 132
FDA pregnancy safety classification of, 665t
in lactation, 672
oral narcotic equivalency table, 74t
parenteral/oral narcotic equivalency index, 101t
recommendations and adverse reactions of, 76, 77
street price of, 133t
in treatment of
chest wall injuries, 95t
fractures, 95t
otitis externa, 569
sprains, 96t
strains, 96t
Oxygen; *see also* Nasal oxygen
antidotal action of, 182t, 189, 197, 198
in treatment of
asthma, 279, 280
bacterial pneumonia, in pediatrics, 525t
bronchiolitis, in pediatrics, 517t
cardiac arrest, 218, 219
cluster headaches, 267t, 269
COPD, 283, 284
croup, in pediatrics, 519t
cyanide poisoning, 343t
midgut volvulus and malrotation, 303
trauma, 554
vascular headaches, 90
ventricular tachycardia, 236
Oxyphenbutazone
FDA pregnancy safety classification of, 670t
in treatment of acute gout, 643
Oxytocics, 682

P

Paget's disease, 594t
Pain
acute, Ketorolac tromethamine (Toradol), as alternative for drug seekers with, 141, 142, 142t
drug seekers feigning, for narcotics, 135t
physiology of, 98, 99t, 100t
Pain management
oral, 72–96
parenteral, 97–130

Palsies, 594t
Pamelor (nortriptyline), 680
Pancreatitis
  causes of, 303, 304t
  diagnosis and treatment of, 303, 304, 304t, 305t
    with CT scans, 304
    with serum lipase measurement, 303
    with ultrasound, 304
  drug seekers feigning, laboratory tests for, 139
  mortality with, 305t
Panic disorders, 661–663
Papaverine, 343t
Papilledema
  as symptom of
    benign increased IOP, 594t
    blood dyscrasias, 594t
    endocrine abnormalities, 594t
    hydrocephalus, 594t
    middle ear disease, 594t
    trauma, 594t
    tumors, 594t
Papulosquamous eruptions, 609
Paramethadione, 668t
Parapsoriasis, 618
Parasympathomimetic drugs, 606, 607
Parasympathomimetic/cholinergic agents, 682
Paregoric (opium powder), 678
Parent and child scams of prescription drug seekers in emergency rooms, 137
Parenteral pain management
  disease specific type of, 121, 122t, 123t, 124–130
  principles of, 120, 121
Parlodel (bromocriptine), 682
Paromomycin, 499
  symptomatic diarrhea, 499
Parotitis, 576, 577
Paroxysmal supraventricular tachycardia (PSVT), 236, 238, 239
Patient history in diagnosis of drug seekers, 138, 138t, 139, 140
PCP; see Phencyclidine (PCP)
PEA; see Pulseless electrical activity
Pectin, 678
Pediatric cardiac arrhythmias; see Arrhythmias, pediatric
Pediazole; see Sulfisoxazole
Pediculicides
  A-200 pyrinate shampoo, 626
  Kwell, 626, 627
  Nix, 627
  RID, 626
  Triple X, 626
PEEP; see Positive end-expiratory pressure (PEEP)
Pelvic inflammatory disease (PID), 471t, 472t, 477, 478
Pelvic injuries, 563, 564
Penetrating injuries, 556
Penetrex; see Enoxacin
Penicillamine, 636
Penicillin G
  antidotal action of, 182t, 198, 199
  in treatment of
    neonatal gonococcal conjunctivitis, 519t
    pharyngitis, in pediatrics, 524t
    retropharyngeal and peritonsillar abscesses, in pediatrics, 516t
    septic arthritis, 641
    uvulitis, 527t
Penicillin V
  with metronidazole, in treatment of
    aspiration pneumonia, 444t
    lung abscesses, 444t
    odontogenic infections, 443
  in treatment of
    acute necrotizing ulcerative gingivitis, 578
    infectious diseases, 436t
    peritonsillar abscesses, 580
    pharyngitis, 443, 581
Penicillin VK, in treatment of
  pharyngitis, in pediatrics, 524t
  uvulitis, in pediatrics, 527t
Penicillins
  with aminoglycosides, in treatment of
    clostridial anaerobic cellulitis, 465
    gram-negative synergistic necrotizing cellulitis, 465
    pneumonia in infants, 463
  aminopenicillins, 407, 408
    recommendations and adverse reactions of, 406, 407
  with amoxicillin/clavulanate, in treatment of
    dental abscesses, 443
    orofacial infections, 443
  bacterial resistance to, 406
  with clindamycin, in treatment of
    dental abscesses, 443
    orofacial infections, 443
  dosing frequencies for, 403t
  FDA pregnancy safety classification of, 666t
  β-lactamase-resistant
    recommendations and adverse reactions of, 408, 409
  in lactation, 673
  with metronidazole, in treatment of
    aspiration pneumonia, 444, 445
    dental abscesses, 443
    lung abscesses, 444, 445
    orofacial infections, 443
  natural, recommendations and adverse reactions of, 406, 407
  oxacillin, 409
  recommendations and adverse reactions of, 405–408
  tipseudomonal with aminoglycosides, in treatment of pneumonia in immunocompromised adults, 463
  in treatment of
    abscesses, 438t
    aerobic gram-negative bacilli, 406
    bacterial conjunctivitis, 587
    Bacteroides fragilis, 406
    botulism, 321
    carbuncles, 438t
    cellulitis, 438t, 439
    erysipelas, 439
    eyelid abscesses, 441
    furunculosis, 438t
    Haemophilus influenzae, 406
    herpes zoster, 438t, 440
    impetigo, 438, 438t, 439
    infectious diseases, 436t
    meningitis
      in adults, 451
      in alcoholic patients, 451
      in elderly, 451
      in patients with CSF leak, 451
      in pediatrics, 451
    mushroom poisoning, 335
    Neisseria gonorrhoeae, 406
    otitis externa, 569

Index

periorbital cellulitis, 590
pharyngitis, group A β-hemolytic streptococcus, 457
septic arthritis, 641
Staphylococcus aureus, 406
syphilis, 448, 619
Pentamidine, 426
Pentamidine isethionate, 505
Pentazocine, 94*t*
  drug seekers of, 132
  oral narcotic equivalency table, 74*t*
  in parenteral treatment of pain, 99*t*, 111, 112
  plasma half lives of, 74*t*
  precautions/contraindications for the elderly, 76
  recommendations and adverse reactions of, 76
  in treatment of sickle crisis, 96*t*
Pentobarbital (Nembutal), 680
Pentolinium, 33*t*
Pentostam; *see* Stibogluconate sodium
Pentothal (thiopental), 681
Pepcid (famotidine), 679
Pepto-Bismol (bismuth subsalicylate), 679
Pericardial disease, 489
Pericarditis
  ECG evaluation in, 147*t*
  myocardial infarction and, 146*t*
  parenteral treatment of, 122*t*, 125, 126
  treatment of, 96*t*
Perineal wounds, 564
Periorbital cellulitis
  antimicrobial therapy for, in pediatrics, 517*t*
  causes of, 590
  diagnosis and treatment of, 590
Peripheral nerve blocks, 565
Peripheral vascular injuries, 562, 563
Peripheral vision, 584
Perirectal abscesses, 311
Peritonitis, 301
Peritonsillar abscesses
  antimicrobials in treatment of, in pediatrics, 516*t*
  causes of, 580
  differential diagnosis of, 580
  treatment of, 580, 581
Permethrin
  FDA pregnancy safety classification of, 666*t*
  in treatment of
    lice, 438*t*, 441
    scabies, 438*t*, 441
Pernicious anemias; *see also* Anemias
  optic atrophy as symptom of, 594*t*
Perphenazine, 671*t*
Personnel, emergency department, 452
Pertussis, 534*t*, 535*t*
Petit mal status epilepticus, 259
Petrolatum, 627
Petroleum jelly iodoform gauze, 579
Pharyngitis
  antimicrobial therapy for, in pediatrics, 524*t*
  causes of, 581
  diagnosis and treatment of, 443, 456–458, 581, 582
  gonococcal, treatment of, 477
  group A β-hemolytic streptococcus
    treatment of, 457, 458
  secondary to *c. pneumonia,* treatment of, 458
  secondary to mycoplasma pneumonia, treatment of, 458
  viral, treatment of, 457
Pharyngodynia, 296
Phenacetin, 668*t*

Phencyclidine (PCP)
  as cause of hyperthermia, 690, 690*t*
  in lactation, 682
  violent behavior in psychiatric emergencies and, 653
Phenelzine, 680
Phenergan (promethazine)
  with meperidine, in treatment of migraines, 268
  in treatment of
    hepatitis, 308
    migraines, 268
    vertigo, 269, 270*t*
Phenmetrazine
  drug seekers feigning obesity for, 135*t*
  drug seekers of, 132
Phenobarbital
  FDA pregnancy safety classification of, 669*t*, 670*t*
  in lactation, 675, 680
  in treatment of
    grand mal status epilepticus, 259
    new onset seizures, 256, 257, 257*t*
      side effects of, 257
    recurrent seizures, 258*t*
    systemic lupus erythematosus, 644
Phenobarbital comas, 259
Phenolphthalein, 679
Phenothiazines
  antidote for, 182*t*, 191
  as cause of orthostatic hypotension, 33*t*
  as cause of dystonic reactions, 272
  as cause of hyperthermia, 689, 690*t*
  as cause of hypothermia, 686
  tranquilizers of, indicators of possible toxicity with, 13*t*
Phenoxybenzamine
  as cause of orthostatic hypotension, 33*t*
  in treatment of pheochromocytoma, 395
Phentermine, 671*t*
Phentolamine, 395
Phenylbutazone
  adverse drug interactions, with anticoagulants, 56*t*
  FDA pregnancy safety classification of, 670*t*
  in lactation, 673
  recommendations and adverse reactions of, 84
  in treatment of
    acute gout, 643
    osteoarthritis, 639
    pseudogout, 643
Phenylephrine
  ophthalmologic uses of, adverse effects of, 606
  in ophthalmoscopy, 584
  in treatment of supraventricular tachycardia (SVT), pediatric, *249*
  with xylocaine spray, in treatment of epistaxis, 579
Phenylpropanolamine
  FDA pregnancy safety classification of, 671*t*
  in treatment of sinusitis, 576
Phenytoin
  adverse drug interactions
    with anticoagulants, 56*t*
    with cimetidine, 61*t*
  FDA pregnancy safety classification of, 669*t*
  in lactation, 675
  in treatment of
    arrhythmias, 210, 211
    grand mal status epilepticus, 258, 259
    new onset seizures, 256, 257*t*
      side effects of, 256
    petit mal status epilepticus, 259
    recurrent seizures, 258*t*

730 Index

Phenytoin—*Continued*
  seizures with brain tumors, 271
  subarachnoid hemorrhages (SAH), 264, 265
  systemic lupus erythematosus, 644
  torsades de pointes (TDP), 232
  trigeminal, 96*t*
  ventricular tachycardia with pulse, pediatric, 244
Pheochromocytoma, 394, 395
Philadelphia collar, 260
Phosphorous, disorders of
  diagnosis and treatment of, 383, 384
  hyperphosphatemia, 384
  hypophosphatemia, 383, 384
Phosphorus, 388
Photocoagulation, 605
Phototherapy, 494
Physical examination, 139
Physiologic solutions, 592
Physostigmine
  antidotal action of, 182*t*, 199
  FDA pregnancy safety classification of, 669*t*
Phytonadione, 182*t*, 200, 201
Pilocarpine, in treatment of chronic open-angle glaucoma, 598, 599*t*
  adverse effects of, 606
  contraindications to, 599*t*
Pindolol, 667*t*
Piperacetazine, 671*t*
Piperacillin
  recommendations and adverse reactions of, 408
  with tobramycin and vancomycin, in treatment of neutropenic elderly patients, 532*t*
  in treatment of cholecystitis in elderly, 531*t*
Piperacillin/tazobactam, 414
Pirmenol, 216
Piroxicam
  in lactation, 672, 673
  recommendations and adverse reactions of, 81*t*, 82, 84
  in treatment of
    osteoarthritis, 639
    rheumatoid arthritis, 636
Pituitary hormones, 669*t*
Pituitary hypofunction, 394
Pityriasis rosea, 621, 622
Plant poisonings, 334, 335*t*, 336*t*, 337*t*
Plaquenil (hydroxychloroquine), 673
Plasma, in treatment of
  acute renal failure, 399
  clotting disorders with intracranial hemorrhages, 263
Plasmapheresis, in treatment of
  HIV related thrombotic thrombocytopenic purpura, 501
  myasthenia gravis, 274
Pneumococcal vaccines, 670*t*
Pneumococcus, 596
Pneumocystis carinii, 525*t*
Pneumocystis pneumonia, 504–506
Pneumonia
  in adults
    high risk aspiration, treatment of, 464
    immunocompromised, treatment of, 463
    treatment of, 463
  antibiotics for the elderly patient for, 528, 529
  aspiration, diagnosis and treatment of, 444, 444*t*, 445
  bacterial, antimicrobial therapy for, in pediatrics, 525*t*
  community-acquired, diagnosis and treatment of, 443, 444, 444*t*
  diagnosis and treatment of, 461–464
  pediatric
    treatment of, 463
    Ureaplasma urealyticum as cause of, 525*t*
  pneumocystic, HIV related, diagnosis and treatment of, 504–506
  during pregnancy, treatment of, 464
  treatment of, 464
Podophyllin, 481
Poison antidotes
  initial treatment of, 179, 180, 182*t*
  principles of antidotal action, 180, 181, 182*t*
Polio vaccines
  FDA pregnancy safety classification of, 670*t*
  in lactation, 681
Polyarteritis nodosa, 594*t*
Polycarbophil, 679
Polycythemia, 594*t*
Polymyxin, 441
Polymyxin B
  with colistin, in treatment of otitis externa, 568
  FDA pregnancy safety classification of, 666*t*
  with neomycin, in treatment of otitis externa, 568
Ponstel (mefenamic acid), 673
Positive end-expiratory pressure (PEEP)
  asthma and, 292
  pulmonary embolism and, 290
Potassium, 388
Potassium chloride, in treatment of
  hypokalemia, 377–378
  metabolic alkalosis, 369
Potassium iodide, 392
Potassium phosphate, 384
Pralidoxime
  antidotal action of, 182*t*, 199, 200
  antidote for, 199, 200
Prazepam, 680
Praziquantel, 432
Prazosin
  adverse side effects of, 31*t*
  as cause of orthostatic hypotension, 33*t*
  in treatment of pheochromocytoma, 395
Pred Forte, 591, 592
Prednisolone
  FDA pregnancy safety classification of, 669*t*
  in lactation, 678
Prednisolone acetate, 591, 592
Prednisone
  FDA pregnancy safety classification of, 669*t*
  in lactation, 678
  in treatment of
    asthma, 277*t*
    bacterial pneumonia, in pediatrics, 525*t*
    bronchiolitis, in pediatrics, 517*t*
    cluster headaches, 95*t*
    HIV related
      pneumocystis pneumonia, 505
      thrombocytopenia, 501
    myasthenia gravis, 273
    osteoarthritis, 639
    rheumatoid arthritis, 636
      pediatric, 638
    systemic lupus erythematosus, 644
    temporal arteritis, 645
    vascular headaches, 90
    vasculitis, 646
  with trimethoprim/sulfamethoxazole, in treatment of COME, 573

Pregnancy
  contraindications of
    amantadine, 404
    antibiotics in, 404
    antimicrobial agents in, 404, 405
    ciprofloxacin in, 404
    dehydroemetine/emetine in, 404
    erythromycin estolate in, 404
    fentanyl in, 109
    furazolidone in, 404
    griseofulvin in, 404
    lindane in, 404
    metronidazole in, 404
    nitrofurantoin in, 404
    norfloxacin in, 404
    ofloxacin in, 404
    oxamniquine in, 404
    primaquine in, 404
    quinolones in, 404
    ribavirin in, 404
    streptomycin in, 404
    sulfonamides in, 404
    tetracycline in, 404
  doxycycline in treatment of pneumonia in, 464
  fetomaternal hemorrhage and Rh isoimmunization, 547, 548
  over-the-counter and commonly prescribed medication in, 665t–671t
  precautions for
    acyclovir in, 405
    aminoglycosides in, 404
    antibiotics in, 405
    antihelminthics in, 405
    antimalarials in, 405
    antimicrobial agents in, 404, 405
    antituberculous medications in, 404, 405
    antiviral drugs in, 405
    chloramphenicol in, 404
    chloroquine in, 405
    clindamycin in, 404
    ganciclovir in, 405
    hydroxychloroquine in, 405
    Imipenem-cilastatin in, 404
    mebendazoles in, 405
    mefloquine in, 405
    metronidazole in, 404
    nitrofurantoin in, 404
    sulfonamides in, 404
    thiabendazole in, 405
    trimethoprim in, 404
    vidarabine in, 405
    zidovudine in, 405
  risk to fetus of medication in, 664
  salpingitis during, erythromycin in treatment of, 447, 447t
  syphilis during, benzathine penicillin G in treatment of, 448
  vaginitis during
    clotrimazole in treatment of, 446, 447t
    saline douches in treatment of, 446, 447t
Premarin, 677
Prerenal azotemia, 395, 396
Prescription drugs
  controlled
    drug seekers of, 131, 132
    street price of, 132, 133t
  drug seekers of
    diagnosis of, 138–141
      through laboratory tests, 139, 140
      through patient history, 138, 138t, 139, 140
      through physical examination, 139
    diseases feigned by, çt, 135, 136, 136t
      with flawed objective tests, 136, 136t
    drug addiction confession of, in emergency rooms, 138
    emergency room policies for, 141–143
    parent and child scams of, in emergency rooms, 137
    prescription forgeries of, 138
    psychologic tactics of, in emergency rooms, 136, 137
  noncontrolled, drug seekers of
    β-blockers, 132
    clonidine, 133
    NSAIDs, 133
Preseptal/buccal cellulitis, 517t
Preventative medicine
  HIV related
    cryptococcal meningitis, 489–491
    encephalitis, 494
    focal intracerebral lesions, 494
    Mycobacterium avium, 509–510
    pneumocystis pneumonia, 505–506
    toxoplasmosis, 494
    tuberculosis, 505, 506
  sexually transmitted diseases and, 474, 475
Prickly heat; *see* Miliaria
Primaquine
  contraindications of, in pregnancy, 404
  FDA pregnancy safety classification of, 666t
  in treatment of HIV related pneumocystis pneumonia, 505
Primaquine phosphate, 430
Primaxin; *see* Imipenem
Primidone
  FDA pregnancy safety classification of, 669t
  in lactation, 675
  in treatment of
    new onset seizures, 257t
    recurrent seizures, 258t
Probenecid
  with amoxicillin, in treatment of
    gonococcal cervicitis, 476, 477
    gonococcal urethritis, 476, 477
  with ampicillin, in treatment of
    gonococcal cervicitis, 476, 477
    gonococcal urethritis, 476, 477
  with cefoxitin and azithromycin, in treatment of PID, 471t
  with ceftriaxone, in treatment of gonococcal pharyngitis, 477
  with procaine penicillin, in treatment of
    gonococcal cervicitis, 476, 477
    gonococcal pharyngitis, 477
    gonococcal urethritis, 476, 477
  in treatment of septic arthritis, 641
Procainamide
  FDA pregnancy safety classification of, 668t
  indicators of possible toxicity from, 13t
  in lactation, 675
  in treatment of
    arrhythmias, 208
    asystole, pediatric, *247*
    atrial fibrillation, 235
      pediatric, *251*
    atrial flutter, 235
      pediatric, *251*
    paroxysmal supraventricular tachycardia (PSVT), *239*
    pulseless electrical activity (PEA)

Procainamide—*Continued*
  pediatric, *247*
  pulseless ventricular tachycardia (VT), *227*
    pediatric, *247*
  tachycardias, *233*
  ventricular arrhythmias, 167
  ventricular ectopy, *230*
  ventricular fibrillation (VF), *227*
    pediatric, *247*
  ventricular tachycardia, 237
  ventricular tachycardia with pulse, pediatric, *244*
  Wolff-Parkinson-White syndrome (WPW), *225*
    pediatric, *248*
Procaine penicillin
  with probenecid, in treatment of
    gonococcal cervicitis, 476, 477
    gonococcal pharyngitis, 477
    gonococcal urethritis, 476, 477
  recommendations and adverse reactions of, 407
  in treatment of septic arthritis, 641
Procan (procainamide), 675
Procarbazine, 33*t*
Procardia (nifedipine), 676
Prochlorperazine
  as alternative for drug seekers with migraines, 142, 142*t*
  as cause of dystonic reactions, 272
  FDA pregnancy safety classification of, 666*t*, 671*t*
  in parenteral treatment of pain, 106*t*, 117
    in migraine headaches, 123*t*, 127, 128
  in treatment of
    acute labyrinthitis, 269, 270*t*
    hepatitis, 308
Proctitis, 500
Professional patients, 133, 134, 134*t*
Progesterone, 677
Progestogenic hormones, 677
Progestogens, 669*t*
Promethazine
  in emergency treatment of vertigo, 269, 270*t*
  FDA pregnancy safety classification of, 667*t*
  with meperidine, in treatment of migraines, 268
  in treatment of
    hepatitis, 308
    migraines, 268
Promethazine HCL, 575
Pronestyl (procainamide), 675
Propafenone, in treatment of
  arrhythmias, 212
  atrial fibrillation, 235
    pediatric, *251*
  atrial flutter, 235
    pediatric, *251*
  Wolff-Parkinson-White syndrome (WPW), *225*
    pediatric, *248*
Propantheline bromide, 331
Propine (dipivefrin HCl), 600*t*
Propoxyphene
  drug seekers of, 132
  FDA pregnancy safety classification of, 668*t*
  in lactation, 672
  precautions in emergency medicine with, 76
  recommendations and adverse reactions of, 76
Propranolol
  adverse side effects of, 31*t*
  FDA pregnancy safety classification of, 667*t*
  in lactation, 676

  in treatment of
    arrhythmias, 212, 213
    atrial fibrillation, 235
      pediatric, *251*
    atrial flutter, 235
      pediatric, *251*
    hyperthyroidism, 391
    paroxysmal supraventricular tachycardia (PSVT), *239*
    ventricular tachycardia with pulse, pediatric, *244*
    Wolff-Parkinson-White syndrome (WPW), *225*
      pediatric, *248*
Proptosis, as symptom of
  aneurysms, 594*t*
  carotid-cavernous sinus fistula, 594*t*
  Graves' disease, 594*t*
  hemorrhages, 594*t*
  leukemia, 594*t*
  lymphoma, 594*t*
  ocular tumors, 594*t*
  orbital cellulitis, 594*t*
Propylthiouracil
  FDA pregnancy safety classification of, 669*t*
  in lactation, 678
  in treatment of hyperthyroidism, 391
Prostatitis, 446
Prostigmin (neostigmine), 682
Protamine, 666*t*
Provera (medroxyprogesterone), 677
Proxetil, 458
Pseudoephedrine
  FDA pregnancy safety classification of, 671*t*
  in treatment of barotitis, 571
Pseudogout, 643
Pseudomembranous candidiasis; *see* Oral candidiasis
Pseudomonas
  as cause of corneal ulcers, 596
  as pathogen in osteomyelitis, 523*t*
Pseudomonas aeruginosa, as cause of
  otitis externa, 567, 568*t*
  otitis media, 573
Pseudoxanthoma elasticum, 594*t*
Psoriasis vulgaris
  diagnosis and treatment of, 617, 618
  HIV related diagnosis and treatment of, 496
Psychiatric disorders, 135*t*
Psychiatric emergencies
  acute psychosis in, 658, 659
  causes of delirium in the elderly in, 650*t*, 651
  initial assessments in, 649, 650, 650*t*, 651, 652
  legal issues and, 652, 653
  referral and disposition in, 652
  responsibilities of the emergency physician and, 649–663
  the suicidal patient in, 659–661
  the violent patient in, 653–658
Psychologic tactics of prescription drug seekers in emergency rooms, 136, 137
Psychosis, acute
  amphetamines, cocaine, PCP, hallucinogens and, 658, 659
  diagnosis and treatment of, 658, 659
  medical causes of, 658
Psychotropic drugs, 680
Psyllium (Metamucil, Konsyl), 679
Ptosis, 594*t*
PTU (propylthiouracil), 678

Pulmonary diseases, noninfectious
  acute respiratory failure/rapid sequence intubation, 290, 291, 291*t*, 292
  asthma (acute), 276, 277, 277*t*, 278*t*, 278–285, 279*t*
  chronic obstructive, 283–285
  pulmonary embolism, 285–288, 289*t*
  requirements in emergency medicine of, 276
  respiratory distress syndrome, 289, 290
Pulmonary embolism, 285–288, 289*t*
Pulseless electrical activity (PEA)
  diagnosis and treatment of, *223, 224, 228, 229*
  treatment of, 167
Pulseless ventricular tachycardia (VT), diagnosis and treatment of, *223, 224, 226, 227*
Punctures
  diagnosis and treatment of, 440
  tetanus prophylaxis in treatment of, 438*t*, 440
Purulent nasopharyngitis/sinusitis; *see* Sinusitis/purulent nasopharyngitis
PUVA, 618
Pyelograms, 140
Pyelonephritis
  antimicrobial therapy for, in pediatrics, 526*t*
  diagnosis and treatment of, 445, 445*t*, 446
Pyloromyotomy, 302
Pyoderma, 521*t*
Pyogenic granuloma, 494
Pyrazinamide
  FDA pregnancy safety classification of, 665*t*
  recommendations and adverse reactions of, 427
  in treatment of HIV related tuberculosis, 507
Pyridostigmine
  in lactation, 682
  in treatment of myasthenia gravis, 273
Pyridoxine (vitamin B6), 182*t*, 201, 202
Pyrimethamine
  FDA pregnancy safety classification of, 666*t*
  in lactation, 673
  with leucovorin, in treatment of HIV related encephalitis, 493
    focal intracerebral lesions, 493
    toxoplasmosis, 493
  recommendations and adverse reactions of, 430
  in treatment of HIV related *Isospora belli*, 499
Pyrimethamine/sulfadoxine (fansidar), 493
PZA, 508

Q

Quazepam, 680
Quinacrine
  FDA pregnancy safety classification of, 666*t*
  in treatment of
    giardia, 450
    HIV related giardia, 499
Quinacrine HCl, 428
Quinalone, 281
Quinidine
  adverse drug interactions, with anticoagulants, 56*t*
  FDA pregnancy safety classification of, 668*t*
  in lactation, 675
  recommendations and adverse reactions of, 429, 430
  in treatment of
    atrial fibrillation, pediatric, *251*
    atrial flutter, pediatric, *251*
Quinidine gluconate, in treatment of
  atrial fibrillation, 235
  atrial flutter, 235
  Wolff-Parkinson-White syndrome (WPW), 225
Quinidine sulphate, in treatment of
  arrhythmias, 206, 208
  atrial fibrillation, 235
  atrial flutter, 235
  Wolff-Parkinson-White syndrome (WPW), 225
Quinine
  FDA pregnancy safety classification of, 666*t*
  in lactation, 673
  recommendations and adverse reactions of, 429, 430
Quinine sulfate
  recommendations and adverse reactions of, 90, 91
  in treatment of night cramps, 96*t*
Quinolines, 445, 445*t*, 446
Quinolones
  contraindications of, in pregnancy, 404
  with erythromycin, in treatment of
    diarrhea, 450
    dysentery, 450
  recommendations and adverse reactions, 414–416
  in treatment of
    diarrhea, 450
    dysentery, 450
    gonococcal cervicitis, 476, 477
    gonococcal urethritis, 476, 477
    infectious diseases, 437*t*

R

Rabies vaccines, 670*t*
Radiographic contrast enemas, 309
Radiographs
  in diagnosis of
    drug seekers, 140
    rectal foreign bodies, 309
  spine, in treatment of severe head injuries, 260
Radiopharmaceutical agents, 682
Ramapril, 667*t*
Ramsay Hunt syndrome; *see* Herpes zoster oticus
Ranitidine
  FDA pregnancy safety classification of, 666*t*
  in lactation, 679
  in treatment of
    gastrointestinal bleeding, 300
    GERD, 298, 298*t*
    staphylococcal food poisoning, 331
Rapid sequence intubation, 290, 291, 291*t*, 292
RDS; *see* Respiratory distress syndrome
Recombivax, 481
Rectal foreign bodies (RFB), 309, 310
Rectal prolapse, 310
Rectal traverse wounds, 564
Red Book, 404
Red eye
  causes of, 586*t*
  conjunctivitis, diagnosis and treatment of
    allergic, 585
    bacterial, 586, 587
    neonatal, 588
    viral, 587, 588
  diagnosis and treatment of, 585–592
  eyelid disorders, diagnosis and treatment of
    blepharitis, 589
    chalazion, 589
    hordeolum, 589
  lacrimal disorders, diagnosis and treatment of
    dacryoadenitis, 589, 590

Red eye—*Continued*
  dacryocystitis, 590
  orbital cellulitis, diagnosis and treatment of, 590, 591
  periorbital cellulitis, diagnosis and treatment of, 590
  uveitis
    from chemical injuries, 592, 593
    circumcorneal flush in, 591
    corneal abrasions in, 592
    diagnosis and treatment of, 591–593
    intraocular pressure in, 591–593
    traumatic hyphema in, 593
Red-free lights for measurement of intraocular pressure (IOP), 585
Reglan (metoclopramide)
  in lactation, 679
  in treatment of migraines, 267t
Rehydration, 520t
Reiter's syndrome, 639, 640
Renal colic
  diagnosis and treatment of, 96t
  drug seekers feigning, 136, 136t
    intravenous pyelograms for, 140
    for narcotics, 135t
  parenteral treatment of, 128
Renal disease, 396–398, 400
Renal failure
  acute
    causes of, 395
    diagnosis and treatment of, 398–400
    HIV related, diagnosis and treatment of, 510
  diagnosis and treatment of, 364
Renal failure index (RFI), 348
Renal injuries, 563
Renovue (iodamide), 681
Reserpine
  as cause of orthostatic hypotension, 33t
  as cause of hyperthermia, 686
  FDA pregnancy safety classification of, 668t
  in lactation, 676
Respiratory acidosis, 370
Respiratory alkalosis, 369t, 370
Respiratory distress syndrome, 289, 290
Respiratory failure, 290, 291, 291t, 292
Respiratory syncytial virus (RSV), 517t
Respiratory tract infections
  lower
    aspiration pneumonia, 443, 444
    chronic bronchitis, 443
    community-acquired pneumonia, 443, 444
    diagnosis and treatment of, 443–445
    lung abscesses, 443, 444
  upper
    diagnosis and treatment of, 441–443
    odontogenic infections, 443
    otitis externa, 441, 442
    otitis media, 442
    pharyngitis, 443
    sinusitis, 442, 443
Retin-A (tretinoin), 682
Retinal detachments
  cataracts as symptom of, 594t
  definition of, 604
  diagnosis and treatment of, 604
Retinal hemorrhages, 594t
Retinal vein occlusions
  central
    ocular pain as symptom of, 597

    as symptom of
      collagen vascular disease, 594t
      diabetes mellitus, 594t
      hypertension, 594t
      hyperviscosity syndromes, 594t
    diagnosis and treatment of, 603
    as symptom of
      abnormal blood viscosity syndromes, 594t
      atheromatous disease, 594t
      glaucoma, 594t
      hypertension, 594t
      temporal arteritis, 594t
Retinitis, 502–504
Retinoic acid, 495, 496
Retinoids, 681, 682
Retinopathy, 593
Retovir; *see* Zidovudine
Retropharyngeal abscess, 516t
Rh isoimmunization, 547, 548
Rheumatoid arthritis (RA)
  diagnosis and treatment of, 635, 636
  juvenile (JRA), diagnosis and treatment of, 636–638
  uveitis as symptom of, 594t
Rheumatoid emergencies
  acute gout, 642, 643
  diagnosis and treatment of, 635–648
  osteoarthritis, 638, 639
  pseudogout, 643
  Reiter's syndrome, 639, 640
  septic arthritis, 645
  systemic lupus erythematosus, 644, 645
  temporal arteritis, 640, 641
  vasculitis, 645, 646
Rib fractures, 122t, 126, 127
Ribavirin
  contraindications of, in pregnancy, 404
  FDA pregnancy safety classification of, 665t
  in treatment of
    pneumonia, in pediatrics, 463
    respiratory syncytial virus (RSV), in pediatrics, 517t
RID, 626
Rifabutin, in treatment of HIV related
  Mycobacterium avium, 509
  tuberculosis, 508
Rifampin
  adverse drug interactions, with anticoagulants, 56t
  FDA pregnancy safety classification of, 665t
  in lactation, 674
  in prevention of epiglottitis, 520t
  recommendations and adverse reactions of, 424, 427
  in treatment of
    angiokeratoma, 494
    HIV related
      dermal bacillary angiomatosis, 494
      Mycobacterium avium, 509
      tuberculosis, 507
    Kaposi's Sarcoma, 494
    meningitis in unprotected intimate contact, 452
    pyogenic granuloma, 494
    simple angioma, 494
  with vancomycin and gentamicin, in treatment of acute bacterial endocarditis in elderly, 532t
Rimantadine, 463
Ringworm; *see* Tinea corporis
Ritalin (methylphenidate), 132
Robaxin (methocarbamol), 682

Roentgenograms, 259, 260
Rowasa (mesalamine), 679
Roxcephin; *see* Ceftriaxone
RSI; *see* Rapid sequence intubation
RSV (respiratory syncytial virus), 517*t*
Rubella vaccines
    FDA pregnancy safety classification of, 670*t*
    in lactation, 681

S

S. aureus; see Staphylococcus aureus
S. epidermidis; see Staphylococcus epidermidis
S. pneumoniae; see Staphylococcus pneumoniae
Salicylates
    adverse drug interactions, with anticoagulants, 56*t*
    as cause of hyperthermia, 690*t*
    contraindications for, in treatment of chickenpox, in pediatrics, 518*t*
    ingestions of, diagnosis and treatment of, 365
    in lactation, 673
    in treatment of
        osteoarthritis, 639
        rheumatoid arthritis, 636
            pediatric, 638
Saline douches, 446, 447*t*
Saline nasal sprays, 576
Saline solutions
    with dextrose, in treatment of
        adrenocortical hypofunction (Addison's disease), 393
        migraines, 268
    isotonic, in treatment of myxedema coma, 392
    in treatment of
        acute renal failure, 399
        hypercalcemia, 382
        hyperglycemia, 388
        hypernatremia, 375
        hyponatremia, 372–374
Salmeterol, 280
Salmon, Dr., 322
Salmonella
    as cause of
        acute gastroenteritis, 520*t*
        osteomyelitis, 523*t*
    diagnosis and treatment of, 322, 324*t*, 325, *326*, 327
Salpingitis, 447, 447*t*
Salsalate, 639
Sarcoids, 594*t*
Scabicides, 666*t*
Scabies, 438*t*, 441, 628–630
Schiotz tonometers, 584
Schizophrenia
    acute psychosis and, 658
    diagnosis and treatment of, 651
Scintigraphy, 306
Scleral discoloration
    blue, as symptom of osteogenesis imperfecta, 594*t*
    brown, as symptom of alkaptonuria, 594*t*
    as symptom of jaundice, 594*t*
    yellow, as symptom of atabrine, 594*t*
Scopolamine
    FDA pregnancy safety classification of, 667*t*
    in treatment of acute labyrinthitis, 269, 270*t*
Seborrheic dermatitis
    diagnosis and treatment of, 615, 616
    HIV related, diagnosis and treatment of, 496
Seborrheic (nonulcerative) blepharitis, 589
Secobarbital (Seconal), 680

Seconal (secobarbital), 680
Sectral (acebutolol), 676
Sedatives
    as cause of vertigo, 270
    FDA pregnancy safety classification of, 670*t*
    in lactation, 680
Seizures
    causes of, 256*t*
    treatment of
        alcohol withdrawal seizures, with status epilepticus, 257
        with metabolic disturbances, 257
        new onset
            anticonvulsants for, 256, 257*t*
            with brain tumors, 256
            with intracranial infections, 256
            laboratory tests for, 255–257
            in pediatrics, 257
            with stroke, 256
        recurrent, 257, 258, 258*t*
            blood level measurement in, 257, 258, 258*t*
        in status epilepticus, 258, 259
Selenium sulfide, 440, 441
Sellick maneuver, 292
Senility, 594*t*
Senna (Senokot), 679
Senokot (senna), 679
Septic abortions, 447
Septicemia
    diagnosis and treatment of, 459–461
    in elderly, causes of, 529
    in immunocompromised adults, diagnosis and treatment of, 461
    in neonates, diagnosis and treatment of, 461
    in nonimmunocompromised adults, diagnosis and treatment of, 461
    in nonimmunocompromised children, diagnosis and treatment of, 461
Serax (oxazepam), 680
Serentil (mesoridazine), 680
Seromycin (cycloserine), 674
Serum lipase measurement, 303
Serum osmolality, 349
Serums, 670*t*
Sexually transmitted diseases
    chancroid, 479, 480
    diagnosis and treatment of, 448, 449, 469–474, 475, 476
    gonorrhea, 476–478
    granuloma inguinale (donovanosis), 480
    Hepatitis B, 481
    herpes simplex virus, 480
    lymphogranuloma venereum, 478, 479
    mucopurulent cervicitis, 449
    PID, 477, 478
    preventative medicine for, 474, 475
    syphilis, 448, 449, 479
    urethritis, 449
    vaginitis, 480, 481
    venereal warts, 481
    vesiculoulcerative diseases, 449
Shellfish, 332
Shigellosis, 321, 322, 323*t*
Shock
    contraindications in pain control, 565
    with intussusception, treatment of, 301
Sickle cell disease
    angioid streaks as symptom of, 594*t*
    drug seekers feigning, 136, 136*t*

736 Index

Sickle cell disease—*Continued*
  laboratory tests for, 139
   for narcotic analgesics, 135*t*
  parenteral treatment of, 123*t*, 127–129
  treatment of, 96*t*
Sigmoid volvulus, 302
Sigmoidoscope, 302
Sigmoidoscopy, 309
Silver nitrate, 634
Simethicone, 666*t*
Sinequan (doxepin), 680
Sinus bradycardia, *237, 240,* 241
Sinus rhythm, *223*
Sinus tachycardia, *231*
Sinusitis
  acute, diagnosis and treatment of, 442*t,* 443
  causes of, 576
  chronic, diagnosis and treatment of, 443
  diagnosis and treatment of, 442, 443, 575, 576
  uveitis as symptom of, 594*t*
Sinusitis/purulent nasopharyngitis, 527*t*
Sitz baths, 310, 311
Sjögren's syndrome, 594*t*
Skeletal muscle relaxants
  FDA pregnancy safety classification of, 671*t*
  recommendations and adverse reactions of, 72, 85, 86, 87*t*
Skin infections
  abscesses, 439
  bites, 439
  cellulitis, 439
  dermatophytoses, 440, 441
  diagnosis and treatment of, 438–441
  herpes zoster, 440
  impetigo, 438, 439
  infestations, 441
  punctures, 439
  tetanus prophylaxis, 440
Slit lamp examinations, 584, 585
Small bowel disease, 498
Smallpox vaccines, 670*t*
Smoking, 683
Snellen visual acuity test, 583, 584
Sodium bicarbonate
  antidotal action of, 182*t,* 202, 203
  in treatment of
    cardiac arrest, 220
    hyperkalemia, 380
    nonanion gap metabolic acidosis, 367–368
    pulseless electrical activity (PEA), *229*
    pulseless ventricular tachycardia (VT), *227*
    salicylates ingestions, 365
    ventricular fibrillation (VF), *227*
Sodium chloride solution, 369
Sodium iodide, 392
Sodium nitrite, 182*t,* 189, 197, 198
Sodium nitroprusside, 668*t*
Sodium pentobarbital, 122*t*
Sodium phosphate, 384
Sodium phosphate/biphosphatei, 679
Sodium sulamyd, 606
Sodium sulamyd ophthalmologic solution (sulfacetamide), 586, 587*t*
Sodium sulfacetamide, 588
Sodium thiosulfate, 182*t,* 189, 197, 198
Soft tissue infections
  abscesses, 439
  bites, 439
  cellulitis, 439
  clostridial anaerobic cellulitis, 464, 465
  dermatophytoses, 440, 441
  diagnosis and treatment of, 438–441
  Fournier's Gangrene, 466
  gram-negative synergistic necrotizing cellulitis, 465–467
  herpes zoster, 440
  HIV related, diagnosis and treatment of, 494
  impetigo, 438, 439
  infestations, 441
  necrotizing fasciitis, 465, 466
  punctures, 439
  requiring surgery, diagnosis and treatment of, 464–468
  tetanus prophylaxis, 440
  vibrio infections, 467
Somatostatin, 669*t*
Sotalol
  in lactation, 676
  in treatment of
    arrhythmias, 215
    atrial fibrillation, 235
      pediatric, 251
    atrial flutter, 235
      pediatric, 251
Spectinomycin, in treatment of
  cervical gonorrhea, 471*t*
  rectal gonorrhea, 471*t*
  septic arthritis, 641
Spermicides, 671*t*
Spinal cord compression, 271, 272
Spinal cord injuries, 555, 556
Spironolactone
  adverse side effects of, 31*t*
  FDA pregnancy safety classification of, 669*t*
  in lactation, 677
Sprains, 96*t*
Stadol (butorphanol), 672
Staphylococcal food poisoning, 330, 331
Staphylococcal (ulcerative) blepharitis, 589
Staphylococcus, 523*t*
Staphylococcus aureus
  as cause of
    acute lymphadenitis, 521*t*
    bacterial conjunctivitis, 586
    corneal ulcers, 596
    dacryocystitis, 586
    furunculosis, 570
    neonatal conjunctivitis, 588
    orbital cellulitis, 591
    osteomyelitis, 523*t*
    otitis externa, 567, 568*t*
    otitis media, 568*t,* 573
    parotitis, 576
    pediatric pneumonia, 525*t*
  treatment of, 406
Staphylococcus epidermidis, 568*t*
Staphylococcus pneumoniae, 525*t*
State regulations on narcotic prescriptions for emergency room physicians, 143
Status epilepticus
  with alcohol withdrawal seizures, treatment of, 257
  grand mal
    causes of, 258
    treatment of, 258, 259
  petit mal, treatment of, 259
STDs; *see* Sexually transmitted diseases
Steroids
  as cause of cataracts, 594*t*
  oral, in treatment of asthma, 282
  topical, in treatment of uveitis, 591, 592

in treatment of
  HIV related eosinophilic pustular folliculitis, 494
  HIV related psoriasis, 496
  HIV related thrombocytopenia, 501
  retinal vein occlusions, 603
  temporal arteritis, 604
Steven-Johnson syndrome, 632
Stibogluconate sodium, 431
Stool softeners, 310, 311
Strains, 96t
Streptococcus
  as cause of meningitis/sepsis, 522t
  group A β-hemolytic
    as cause of peritonsillar abscesses, 580
    as cause of pharyngitis, 581
Streptococcus pneumoniae, as cause of
  bacterial conjunctivitis, 586
  orbital cellulitis, 591
  otitis media, 568t, 571, 572t
  periorbital cellulitis, 590
  sinusitis, 576
Streptococcus pyogenes, as cause of
  orbital cellulitis, 591
  otitis externa, 567, 568t
  otitis media, 568t, 571
Streptokinase
  FDA pregnancy safety classification of, 671t
  in treatment of myocardial infarction, 153
Streptomycin
  as cause of vertigo, 270
  contraindications of, in pregnancy, 404
  FDA pregnancy safety classification of, 665t
  in lactation, 674
  recommendations and adverse reactions of, 427
Strokes
  diagnosis and treatment of, 262
  with new onset seizures, treatment of, 256
  thromboembolic
    with cardiac arrhythmias, 261
    with congestive heart failure, 261
    definition of, 261
    diagnosis and treatment of, 261, 262, 262t
    with hypertension, 261, 262
    with hypotension, 261
Subarachnoid hemorrhages (SAH)
  diagnosis and treatment of, 264, 265
  differential diagnosis with migraines, 266
  Hunt-Hess Scale of, 265, 265t
Subdural hematomas
  differential diagnosis with headaches, 266
  violent behavior in elderly patients with, 649
Succinylcholine, 291t, 292
Sucralfate
  in lactation, 679
  in treatment of
    GERD, 298, 298t
    HIV related idiopathic esophagitis, 498
Suicidal behavior, psychiatric emergencies and, 649, 651, 659–661
Sulfacetamide, in treatment of
  bacterial conjunctivitis, 586, 587t
  conjunctivitis, 441
  corneal abrasions in uveitis, 592
  ulcerative blepharitis, 589
  viral conjunctivitis, 588
Sulfadiazine, in treatment of HIV related
  encephalitis, 493
  focal intracerebral lesions, 493
  toxoplasmosis, 493

Sulfamethoxazole, 335
Sulfasalazine
  in lactation, 679
  in treatment of
    Reiter's syndrome, 640
    rheumatoid arthritis, pediatric, 638
Sulfinpyrazone, 56t
Sulfisoxazole
  with erythromycin, in treatment of otitis media, 572
  with erythromycin ethyl succinate, in treatment of infectious diseases, 436t
  with erythromycin ethylsuccinate, in treatment of
    otitis media, in pediatrics, 524t
    sinusitis/purulent nasopharyngitis, in pediatrics, 527t
  recommendations and adverse reactions of, 420, 421
  in treatment of
    bacterial conjunctivitis, 586, 587t
    lymphogranuloma venereum, 448t, 449
    recurrences of otitis media, 573
Sulfites, 332, 344t
Sulfonamides
  adverse drug interactions, with anticoagulants, 56t
  contraindications of, in pregnancy, 404
  with erythromycin, in treatment of otitis media, 442, 442t
  in lactation, 674
  precautions for use, in pregnancy, 404
  recommendations and adverse reactions of, 417, 418
Sulfonylureas, 56t
Sulfuric acid, 592
Sulindac
  analgesic dosage of, 81t
  in treatment of
    acute gout, 643
    osteoarthritis, 639
    pseudogout, 643
    rheumatoid arthritis, 636
Sulphur petrolatum, 630
Sumatriptan
  in parenteral treatment of acute migraine headaches, 98
  in treatment of
    cluster headaches, 269
    migraines, 267t, 268
    side effects of, 268
Suprax; *see* Cefixime
Suprofen, 81t, 82, 84
Suramin, 430
Surgical debridement, in treatment of
  clostridial myonecrosis, 468
  Fournier's Gangrene, 466
  gram-negative synergistic necrotizing cellulitis, 466
  HIV related corneal microsporidiosis, 502
Swan-Ganz catheterization, 692
Swimmer's ear; *see* Otitis externa
Symmetrel; *see* Amantadine
Sympatholytic agents, 36t
Sympathomimetics, 671t
Synchronized cardioversion, in treatment of
  atrial fibrillation, pediatric, *251*
  atrial flutter, pediatric, *251*
  supraventricular tachycardia (SVT), pediatric, *249*
  ventricular tachycardia with pulse, pediatric, *244*
  Wolff-Parkinson-White syndrome (WPW), pediatric, *248*
Synthroid (levothyroxine), 678

Syphilis
  cardiovascular, benzathine penicillin g in treatment of, 448
  diagnosis and treatment of, 448, 448t, 473t, 449, 479, 618, 619
  HIV patients, diagnosis and treatment of, 448, 449
  latent
    treatment of, 448
    penicillin in treatment of, 448
  during pregnancy, treatment of, 448
  tertiary, optic atrophy as symptom of, 594t
  tetracycline, in treatment of, 448t
Systemic lupus erythematosus (SLE), 644, 645

T

Tachycardias, 169, 170, 232
Tagamet (cimetidine), 679
Tambocor (flecainide), 675
Tapazole (methimazole), 678
Tar, 496
Taractan (chlorprothixene), 680
Tartrazine (Yellow dye #5), 344t
Tavist (clemastine), 677
TDP; *see* Torsades de pointes
Tegison (etretinate), 682
Tegretol (carbamazepine)
  in lactation, 675
  in treatment of new onset seizures, 257t
Telepaque (iopanoic acid), 681
Temazepam, 48t
Temporal arteritis
  diagnosis and treatment of, 269, 645
  occlusive disease of retinal vessels, as symptom of, 594t
TEN; *see* Toxic epidermal necrolysis
Tenex (guanfacine), 676
Tenormin (atenolol), 676
Terazosin, 395
Terbutaline
  FDA pregnancy safety classification of, 667t
  in lactation, 676
  in treatment of asthma, 277t, 278t
Terconazole
  cream, in treatment of candidal vaginitis, 481
  in treatment of candidal vaginitis, 446, 472t
Tetanus
  diagnosis and treatment of, 534, 535, 536
  diphtheria, pertussis, and, immunization schedule for, 534t, 535t
  immunization schedule for, 534t–536t
  prophylaxis
    in pain control treatment of
      fractures, 565
      trauma, 565
    in treatment of punctures, 438t, 440
  toxoid, 440
  vaccines, FDA pregnancy safety classification of, 670t
Tetanus immune globulin, 440
Tetracyclines
  with clindamycin, in treatment of
    animal bites, 438t, 439, 440
    human bites, 439, 440
  contraindications of, in pregnancy, 404
  dosing frequencies for, 403t
  FDA pregnancy safety classification of, 666t
  in lactation, 673
  recommendations and adverse reactions of, 422
  in treatment of
    acute necrotizing ulcerative gingivitis, 578
    acute nongonococcal urethritis, 478
    animal bites, 439, 440
    aphthous stomatitis, 578
    cholera, 324, 329, 330
    chronic prostatitis, 446
    community-acquired pneumonia, 443, 444, 444t
    gonococcal cervicitis, 476, 477
    gonococcal urethritis, 476, 477
    granuloma inguinale (donovanosis), 480
    human bites, 438t
    infectious diseases, 437t
    lymphogranuloma venereum, 478, 479
    nongonococcal urethritis, 478
    pharyngitis
      secondary to *c. pneumonia,* 458
      secondary to mycoplasma pneumonia, 458
    seborrheic dermatitis, 616
    syphilis, 448t
Tetrahydrozoline hydrochloride, 585
Theophylline
  adverse drug interactions, with cimetidine, 61t
  FDA pregnancy safety classification of, 667t
  indicators of possible toxicity with, 13t
  in lactation, 676, 677
  in treatment of asthma, 277t, 281
Thermoregulatory disorders
  hyperthermia, 688–692
  hypothermia, 685–688
Thiabendazole
  precautions for use, in pregnancy, 405
  recommendations and adverse reactions of, 431
Thiamine
  antidotal action of, 182t, 203
  deficiency of
    diagnosis and treatment of, 314t
    medical causes of acute psychosis and, 658
  FDA pregnancy safety classification of, 671t
  in treatment of
    grand mal status epilepticus, 258
    hypoglycemia, 390
Thiamine IV, 308
Thiazides, 31t
Thioctic acid, 335
Thiopental
  in lactation, 681
  in treatment of rapid sequence intubation, 291t, 292
Thioridazine
  FDA pregnancy safety classification of, 671t
  precautions/contraindications for the elderly, 55t
Thiothixene
  as cause of orthostatic hypotension, 33t
  FDA pregnancy safety classification of, 671t
  precautions/contraindications for the elderly, 55t
Thioxanthenes
  antidote for, 182t, 191
  as cause of dystonic reactions, 272
Thompson, Dr. S. C., 333
Thoracic aortic aneurysms, 122t, 126
Thorazine, 680
Thrombi, 602, 603
Thrombocytopenia, 501
Thrombolysis
  complications of, 160, 161
  heparin in treatment of myocardial infarction, 161
  in treatment of myocardial infarction, 152, 154
Thrombolytics, 671t
Thrombotic thrombocytopenic purpura, 501

Thyroid drugs
   adverse drug interactions, with anticoagulants, 56t
   in lactation, 678
Thyroid hormones
   as cause of hyperthermia, 689, 690t
   FDA pregnancy safety classification of, 669t
Thyrotropin, 669t
Tic douloureux, 135t
Ticarcillin
   with aminoglycosides, in treatment of malignant otitis externa, 569
   recommendations and adverse reactions of, 408
Ticarcillin/clavulanate
   with aminoglycosides, in treatment of septicemia in nonimmunocompromised adults, 461
   with aztreonam, in treatment of septicemia in elderly, 461
   with metronidazole, in treatment of pneumonia in high risk aspiration adults, 464
   in treatment of
      clostridial anaerobic cellulitis, 465
      gram-negative synergistic necrotizing cellulitis, 465
      pneumonia in adults, 463
Ticarcillin/clavulanic acid
   recommendations and adverse reactions of, 414
   with tobramycin, in treatment of bacterial peritonitis in elderly, 531t
   in treatment of
      cholecystitis in elderly, 531t
      septicemia in nonimmunocompromised children, 461
Tietze syndrome; see Costochondritis
Tigan (trimethobenzamide), 308
Timentin; see Ticarcillin/clavulanic acid
Timolol
   FDA pregnancy safety classification of, 667t
   in lactation, 676
   in treatment of glaucoma, 598, 600t
      adverse reactions of, 607
      contraindications to, 600t
Timoptic (timolol)
   in treatment of glaucoma, 598, 600t
      adverse reactions of, 607
      contraindications to, 600t
Tincture of opium, 499
Tinea corporis, 438t, 440, 441, 620, 621
Tinea cruris, 440, 441
Tinea infections, 620, 621
Tinea pedis, 440, 441
Tinea versicolor, 438t, 440, 441
Tipseudomonal penicillin, 463
TMP/SMX
   with azithromycin, in treatment of pneumonia in adults, 463
   with clarithromycin, in treatment of pneumonia in adults, 463
   with erythromycin, in treatment of pneumonia in adults, 463
   in treatment of HIV related
      bacterial diarrhea, 499
      Isospora belli, 499
      pneumocystis pneumonia, 504–506
TNS; see Transcutaneous nerve stimulation (TNS)
Tobramycin
   with ampicillin-sulbactam, in treatment of bacterial cholangitis/biliary sepsis in elderly, 531t
   bacterial peritonitis, in elderly, 531t
   cellulitis, in elderly, 532t
   diverticulitis, in elderly, 531t
   pyelonephritis, in elderly, 530t
   urinary tract infections, in elderly, 531t
   with ceftriaxone, in treatment of pneumonia, in elderly, 530t
   with clindamycin, in treatment of diverticulitis, in elderly, 531t
   FDA pregnancy safety classification of, 665t
   with metronidazole and ceftriaxone, in treatment of nonimmunocompromised elderly patients, 532t
   recommendations and adverse reactions of, 417
   with ticarcillin/clavulanate, in treatment of bacterial peritonitis, in elderly, 531t
   in treatment of
      conjunctivitis, 588
      corneal abrasions in uveitis, 592
      septic arthritis, 641
   with vancomycin and azlocillin, in treatment of neutropenic elderly patients, 532t
   with vancomycin and mezlocillin, in treatment of neutropenic elderly patients, 532t
   with vancomycin and piperacillin, in treatment of neutropenic elderly patients, 532t
Tocainide
   in lactation, 675
   in treatment of arrhythmias, 211
Tofranil (imipramine), 680
Tolazamide, 44t
Tolbutamide
   dosage, duration, and effects of, 44t
   in lactation, 678
Tolmetin
   FDA pregnancy safety classification of, 670t
   in lactation, 672, 673
   recommendations and adverse reactions of, 81t, 82, 84
Tolmetin sodium, 637
Tolmetin (Tolectin), 672, 673
Tolnaftate solutions 570
Tonocard (tocainide), 675
Tonometers, 584
Toothaches
   drug seekers feigning
      bupivacaine hydrochloride for, 141, 142t
      for narcotic analgesics, 135t
   floctafenine, as alternative for drug seekers with, 141, 142t
Toradol (ketorolac), 672, 673
Torsades de pointes (TDP), *232*
Toxic epidermal necrolysis (TEN), 633, 634
Toxins, 594t
Toxoids, 670t
Toxoplasmosis, 491–494
t-PA, 671t
Trabeculoplasty, 598
Tracheitis, 527t
Trandate (labetalol), 676
Tranquilizers
   as cause of dry eye syndrome, 594t
   FDA pregnancy safety classification of, 671t
   in treatment of
      acute agitation, 272
      eczema, 611
      lichen planus, 616, 617
Transcutaneous nerve stimulation (TNS), 72
Transcutaneous pacing, 168
Transderm Scop (scopolamine), 269, 270t
Transient ischemic attacks (TIAs)
   definition of, 260
   diagnosis and treatment of, 260, 261t

Transient ischemic attacks (TIAs)—*Continued*
differential diagnosis of, 261*t*
Trauma
blunt vs. penetrating, 552
cataracts as symptom of, 594*t*
as cause of peripheral vertigo, 575
comas in, 554
definitive emergency treatment of, 553, 554, 554*t*, 555
abdominal injuries, 560*t*, 560–562, 565*t*
chest injury, 557, 558, 558*t*, 559, 565*t*
extremity injuries, 562, 563
head injuries, 555, 556, 565*t*
pelvic injuries, 563, 564
penetrating wounds, 556
renal and genitourinary injuries, 563
spinal cord injuries, 555, 556
initial emergency treatment, 552
airway patency, 552
breathing ability, 553
circulation status, 553
disability assessment, 553
exposure and complete examination, 553
macular degeneration as symptom of, 594*t*
medical, conditions causing fever/hyperthermia, 689*t*
papilledema as symptom of, 594*t*
principles of care for, in emergency medicine, 551
resuscitation in, 553, 554, 554*t*, 555
Traveler's diarrhea; *see Escherichia coli,* enteropathic
Trazodone, 680
Trench mouth; *see* Gingivitis, acute necrotizing ulcerative
Treponema vincentii, 578
Tretinoin, 682
Triamcinolone, 644
Triamcinolone acetonide
dental paste, in treatment of aphthous stomatitis, 578
in treatment of dermatologic disorders, 613, 614*t*
Triamterene, 669*t*
Triazolam, 48*t*
Triazoles, 425
Trichiasis, 596
Trichinosis, 332
Tricyclic antidepressants, 13*t*
Trifluoperazine, 671*t*
Trifluridine, 519*t*
Trigeminal, 96*t*
Trigger point therapy, 91, 92
Trimethadione, 669*t*
Trimethaphan, 668*t*
Trimethobenzamide
FDA pregnancy safety classification of, 666*t*
in treatment of hepatitis, 308
Trimethoprim
FDA pregnancy safety classification of, 666*t*
precautions for use, in pregnancy, 404
recommendations and adverse reactions of, 418
Trimethoprim-sulfamethoxazole
dosing frequencies for, 403*t*
recommendations and adverse reactions of, 418, 419
in treatment of
acute gastroenteritis, in pediatrics, 520*t*
COPD, 285
Trimethoprim/sulfamethoxazole
with erythromycin, in treatment of
diarrhea, 450
dysentery, 450
with macrolides, in treatment of community-acquired pneumonia, 444*t*
with prednisone, in treatment of COME, 573
in treatment of
acute prostatitis, 446
acute sinusitis, 442*t*, 443
chronic bronchitis, 443, 444*t*
chronic prostatitis, 446
community-acquired pneumonia, 443, 444
cystitis, 445, 445*t*, 446
diarrhea, 450
epididymo-orchitis, 445*t*, 446
Escherichia coli, enteropathic (traveler's diarrhea), *324*, 328
lower urinary tract infections, in elderly, 530*t*
meningitis
in adults, 451
in pediatrics, 451
otitis media, 442, 442*t*, 572
pyelonephritis, 445, 445*t*, 446
recurrences of otitis media, 573
salmonellosis, 324, 327
shigellosis, 322, 324*t*
sinusitis, 576
in treatment of dysentery, 450
Trimethoprom/sulfamethoxazole, 437*t*
Triple X, 626
Tropicamide, 606
Tuberculosis, HIV related
diagnosis and treatment of, 506–508
preventative medicine, 505, 506
Tularemia vaccines, 670*t*
Tumors; *see also* Brain tumors
cerebellopontine-angle, as cause of central vertigo, 575
ocular, proptosis as symptom of, 594*t*
papilledema as symptom of, 594*t*
Typhoid vaccines, 670t

U

Ulcerative (staphylococcal) blepharitis, 589
Ultrasound, in diagnosis of
acute cholecystitis, 306
appendicitis, 309
cholelithiasis, 306
hypertrophic pyloric stenosis (HPS), 301, 302
pancreatitis, 304
Unasym; *see* Ampicillin-sulbactam
Upper GI, 302
Ureaplasma urealyticum, 525*t*
Urecholine (bethanechol), 682
Ureidopenicillins, 408
Urethritis
gonococcal, diagnosis and treatment of, 476, 477
nongonococcal, acute, diagnosis and treatment of, 478
Urex (methenamine hippurate), 673
Urinary electrolytes, 348
Urinary germicides, 673, 674
Urokinase, 671*t*
UroqidAcid (methenamine mandelate), 673
Ursodiol, 306
Uveal disease, 594*t*
Uveitis
circumcorneal flush in, 591
definition of, 591

Index

diagnosis and treatment of, 591–593
  chemical injuries in, 592, 593
  corneal abrasions in, 592
  traumatic hyphema in, 593
intraocular pressure in, 591–593
as symptom of
  Behcet's disease, 594t
  dental disease, 594t
  rheumatoid arthritis, 594t
  sarcoids, 594t
  sinusitis, 594t
  toxoplasmosis, 594t
Uvulitis, 527t

V

Vaccines
  breast feeding and, 681
  FDA pregnancy safety classification of, 670t
  in lactation, 681
  recombinant DNA, in treatment of hepatitis B, 307
  tularemia, FDA pregnancy safety classification of, 670t
  Typhoid, FDA pregnancy safety classification of, 670t
Vaginitis
  bacterial, treatment of, 446, 447t, 472t, 481
  butoconazole in, treatment of, 446
  candidal, treatment of, 446, 447t, 472t, 481
  diagnosis and treatment of, 446, 480, 481
  during pregnancy
    saline douches in treatment of, 446, 447t
    treatment of, 446, 447t
  treatment of, 446
  trichomoniasis
    clotrimazole vaginal suppositories in treatment of, 480
  treatment of, 446, 447t, 480
Valium (diazepam)
  in lactation, 680
  for treatment of, positional vertigo, 269, 270t
  in treatment of
    acute labyrinthitis, 270t
    grand mal status epilepticus, 258, 259
    side effects of, 258
    muscle contraction headaches, 267t, 268
    petit mal status epilepticus, 259
Valproic acid
  in emergency treatment, of new onset seizures, 257t
  FDA pregnancy safety classification of, 669t
  in lactation, 675
  in treatment of
    petit mal status epilepticus, 259
    of recurrent seizures, 258t
Vancomycin
  with azlocillin and tobramycin, in treatment of neutropenic elderly patients, 532t
  with cephalosporins, in treatment of pneumonia in immunocompromised adults, 463
  FDA pregnancy safety classification of, 666t
  in lactation, 674
  with mezlocillin and tobramycin, in treatment of neutropenic elderly patients, 532t
  with piperacillin and tobramycin, in treatment of neutropenic elderly patients, 532t
  recommendations and adverse reactions of, 423, 424
  with rifampin and gentamicin, in treatment of acute bacterial endocarditis, in elderly, 532t
  in treatment of parotitis, 577
  in treatment of
    antibiotic-associated diarrhea, 450
    meningitis
      in adults, 451
      in children, 451
      in neurosurgery/trauma patients, 451
    omphalitis, in pediatrics, 523t
    orbital cellulitis, 591
      in pediatrics, 517t
    orthopedic trauma, 566t
    osteomyelitis, in pediatrics, 523t
    septicemia in immunocompromised adults, 461
Vantin; see Cefpodoxime
Varicella zoster immune globulin (VZIG), 518t
Vascular accidents
  as cause of central vertigo, 575
  conditions causing fever/hyperthermia, 689t
Vascular disease, 594t
Vascular headaches, 89, 90
Vascular occlusions, 602, 603
Vasculitis, 645, 646
Vasocon-A, 585
Vasodilators, 603
Vasopressin, 669t
Vasotec (enalapril), 676
Venereal warts, 481
Ventricular aneurysms, 147t
Ventricular arrhythmias
  diagnosis and treatment of, 167
  fibrillation/pulseless ventricular tachycardia (VF/VT), diagnosis and treatment of, 167
Ventricular ectopy, *225, 230*, 231
Ventricular fibrillation (VF), *223, 224, 226, 227*
Ventricular tachycardia, 236, 237
Verapamil
  FDA pregnancy safety classification of, 667t
  in lactation, 676
  in treatment of
    arrhythmias, 215, 216
    atrial fibrillation, 235
    atrial flutter, 235
    paroxysmal supraventricular tachycardia (PSVT), *239*
    Wolff-Parkinson-White syndrome (WPW), pediatric, *248*
Vercuronium, 291t, 292
Vermox; see Mebendazole
Versed (midazolam), 680
Vertebral injuries, 556, 557
Vertigo
  acute labyrinthitis, diagnosis and treatment of, 269, 270t
  causes of, 270t
    alcohol, 270
    cerebellar hemorrhages, 270
    inner ear infections, 270
    monosodium glutamate, 270
    sedatives, 270
    streptomycin, 270
  central
    causes of, 575
    diagnosis and treatment of, 575
    vs. peripheral, 574t
  definition of, 269, 573
  diagnosis of, 574

Vertigo—*Continued*
  with ear pain and herpetic vesicles
    as symptom of Ramsay Hunt syndrome, 270
    as symptoms of herpes zoster, 270
  Meniere's disease, treatment of, 269, 270*t*
  peripheral
    diagnosis of, 574, 574*t*
    from drugs, diagnosis and treatment of, 575
    from Meniere's disease, diagnosis and treatment of, 574
    paroxysmal positional vertigo, diagnosis and treatment of, 575
    from trauma, diagnosis and treatment of, 575
    from viral infections, diagnosis and treatment of, 575
    vs. central, 574*t*
  positional, treatment of, 269, 270*t*
  as symptom of multiple sclerosis, 271
  vertebrobasilar insufficiency, emergency of, 269, 270
Vesiculoulcerative diseases, 449
Vestibular sedatives, 270*t*
VF; *see* Ventricular fibrillation
Vibrio infections, 467
Vidarabine
  FDA pregnancy safety classification of, 665*t*
  ointment, in treatment of necrotizing herpes simplex keratitis, 596
  ophthalmic ointment, in treatment of herpetic gingivostomatitis, 579
  precautions for use, in pregnancy, 405
  in treatment of neonatal gonococcal conjunctivitis, 519*t*
Vincent's angina; *see* Gingivitis, acute necrotizing ulcerative
Vinegar, 570
Violent behavior
  chemical restraints in treatment of, 655, 656
  in the elderly with subdural hematoma, 649
  ethanol intoxication, patients requiring restraint and, 649, 653–655
  LSD in psychiatric emergencies, 653–655
  psychiatric disorders associated with, 653
  psychiatric emergencies and, 649, 653–658
Viral infections, 575
Viral laryngotracheobronchitis; *see* Croup (viral laryngotracheobronchitis)
Visine AC, 585
Visual acuity testing, 583, 584
Vitamin A, 315*t*
Vitamin B$_6$; *see* Pyridoxine
Vitamin D, 315*t*, 316*t*
Vitamin E, 316*t*
Vitamin K
  adverse drug interactions, with anticoagulants, 56*t*
  antidotal action of, 182*t*, 200, 201
Vitamins
  A,B,D,D,E,K, in lactation, 681
  breast feeding and, 681
  FDA pregnancy safety classification of, 671*t*
  in lactation, 681
Volume expanders, 363
Volvulus, 302, 303
VoSol HC Otic Suspension, 568
VT; *see* Pulseless ventricular tachycardia

W

Warfarin
  adverse drug interactions, with cimetidine, 61*t*
  FDA pregnancy safety classification of, 666*t*
  in lactation, 674
Wernicke's encephalopathy; *see also* Encephalopathy
  oculomotor paralysis as symptom of, 594*t*
Winter's formula, 349
Wolff-Parkinson-White syndrome (WPW), 225
Wycillin; *see* Procaine penicillin

X

Xanax (alprazolam), 680
Xylocaine
  in lactation, 675
  spray
    with phenylephrine, in treatment of epistaxis, 579
    in treatment of peritonsillar abscesses, 580
  in treatment of
    aphthous stomatitis, 578
    cluster headaches, 267*t*

Y

Yeast infections, 630–632
Yellow fever vaccines, 670*t*
Yodoxin; *see* Iodoquinol

Z

Zantac (ranitidine), 679
Zarontin (ethosuximide)
  in lactation, 675
  in treatment of
    new onset seizures, 257*t*
    petit mal status epilepticus, 259
Zefazone; *see* Cefmetazole
Zentel; *see* Albendazole
Zidovudine
  precautions for use, in pregnancy, 405
  recommendations and adverse reactions of, 428
  in treatment of
    HIV, 487, 488
    HIV related thrombocytopenia, 501
Zinacef; *see* Cefuroxime
Zinc, 182*t*
Zinc sulfate, 585
Zithromax; *see* Azithromycin
Zosyn; *see* Piperacillin/tazobactam
Zovirax; *see* Amantadine